MW00711808

Critical Care Obstetrics

Critical Care Obstetrics

Fourth Edition

Editor-in-Chief

Gary A. Dildy III, MD
Professor, Department of Obstetrics and Gynecology
Louisiana State University Health Sciences Center, New Orleans, Louisiana

Editors

Michael A. Belfort, MBBCH, MD, PhD
Professor, Department of Obstetrics and Gynecology
University of Utah Health Services Center, Salt Lake City, Utah
Director, Department of Maternal Fetal Medicine
Utah Valley Regional Medical Center, Provo, Utah

George R. Saade, MD
Professor, Department of Obstetrics and Gynecology
Divisions of Maternal-Fetal Medicine and Reproductive Sciences
Director, Maternal-Fetal Medicine Fellowship
The University of Texas Medical Branch, Galveston, Texas

Jeffrey P. Phelan, MD, JD
Vice Chairman and Director of Quality Assurance, Department of Obstetrics and Gynecology
Citrus Valley Medical Center, West Covina, California
President and Director Clinical Research
Childbirth Injury Prevention Foundation, Pasadena, California

Gary D. V. Hankins, MD
Professor and Vice Chairman, Department of Obstetrics and Gynecology
Chief, Division of Maternal Fetal Medicine
The University of Texas Medical Branch, Galveston, Texas

Steven L. Clark, MD
Professor, Department of Obstetrics and Gynecology
University of Utah Health Services Center
LDS Hospital, Salt Lake City, Utah

WILEY

Published by John Wiley & Sons, Hoboken, NJ

For general information on our other products and services, please contact our Customer Care Department within the United States at 800-762-2974, outside the United States at 317-572-3993 or fax 317-572-4002.

For more information about Wiley products, visit our website at www.wiley.com.

ISBN: 0-632-04632-5

Library of Congress Cataloging-in-Publication Data

Critical care obstetrics.—4th ed. / edited by Gary A. Dildy III . . . [et al.].
p. ; cm.
Includes bibliographical references and index.
ISBN 0-632-04632-5
1. Pregnancy—Complications. 2. Obstetrical emergencies.
[DNLM: 1. Pregnancy Complications—therapy. 2. Critical Care—Pregnancy.
WQ 240 C9339 2003] I. Dildy, Gary A.

RG571.C68 2003
618.3'028—dc22

Contents

V. Special considerations

Preface

The 4th edition of *Critical Care Obstetrics* embodies the continuing accumulation of a rapidly expanding mass of knowledge, designed to assist clinicians caring for seriously ill gravidas. Around the time that the 1st edition of this book was published, obstetric critical care units were being established around the country. Countless patient admissions to the "OB/GYN Intensive Care Unit" at the University of Southern California Los Angeles County Woman's Hospital Medical Center, the "Yellow Room" at Baylor's Jefferson Davis Hospital, and to similar facilities provided the clinical experience for maternal–fetal medicine subspecialists interested in critical care to primarily manage pregnant patients of the highest acuity. With medical technology advancing at a meteoric pace, the era of one physician "doing it all" has long passed and is indeed an antiquated concept. The current American medical system is not structured to support a dedicated obstetric critical care unit in most hospitals, even in tertiary referral centers. This evolution in medicine does not portend the demise of the discipline of critical care obstetrics, but rather, further necessitates specialists in obstetrics who can provide complementary knowledge to the nonobstetrician. Thus, the purpose of this book is to assist OB/GYN and MFM clinicians in working integrally with intensivists, pulmonologists, cardiologists, and other members of the multidisciplinary team caring for the critically ill obstetric patient.

Chapters from the 3rd edition have been extensively revised for the 4th edition and new chapters have been added to cover topics concerning maternal morbidity trends, the organization of an obstetric critical care unit, neonatal resuscitation, noninvasive monitoring techniques, pulmonary edema, the acute abdomen, anesthesia considerations, the organ transplant patient, and ethical considerations of the critically ill pregnant woman. The 1st edition, published in 1987, contained 28 chapters; since then, this textbook has evolved into the current edition containing 46 chapters.

Certainly, the greatest strength of this book is its diverse group of authors; we sincerely thank everyone who contributed their time and expertise. We gratefully acknowledge Natalie George for meticulously reviewing the references. Finally, we are grateful to the staff at Blackwell Publishing, especially Julia Casson and Laura DeYoung, for their ongoing support of this book.

GAD, MAB, GRS, JPP, GDVH, SLC
May 2003

Dedications

To my parents, Gary and Barbara Dildy, who have provided ceaseless support and encouragement

Gary A. Dildy III

To my wife, Dr Joanne Belfort, and my children Sarah and Ben

Michael A. Belfort

To my wife, Yomna Tarek Monla, and daughters Lynnie and Mia

George R. Saade

To all the trench physicians and nurses throughout the United States and the world and, especially, at Citrus Valley Medical Center, Pomona Valley Hospital Medical Center, San Antonio Community Hospital, Beverly Hospital, Garfield Medical Center, and Arcadia Methodist Hospital for their untiring dedication to the health and safety of pregnant women and their unborn children and for sharing their insights into the science and art of medicine

Jeffrey P. Phelan

To my wife, Barbara Lynn Hankins

Gary D. V. Hankins

To my parents, Dave and Louise Clark

Steven L. Clark

Contributors

Audrey S. Alleyne, MD
Assistant Professor
Department of Anesthesiology
University of Rochester School of Medicine and Dentistry
and Attending Anesthesiologist
Strong Memorial Hospital
Rochester, New York, USA

Cande V. Ananth, PhD, MPH
Associate Professor of Obstetrics and Gynecology
Director, Section of Epidemiology and Biostatistics
Department of Obstetrics, Gynecology, and Reproductive Sciences
University of Medicine and Dentistry of New Jersey
Robert Wood Johnson Medical School
New Brunswick, New Jersey, USA

John Anthony, MB, ChB, FCOG (SA)
Associate Professor,
Department of Obstetrics and Gynecology
Groote Schuur Hospital,
University of Cape Town
Cape Town, South Africa

Peter L. Bailey, MD
Professor, Anesthesiology
and Director, Cardiac Anesthesia
University of Rochester
Strong Memorial Hospital
Rochester, New York, USA

William H. Barth, Col, USAF, MC, FS
Chairman, Department of Obstetrics and Gynecology
Wilford Hall Medical Center, Lackland AFB, Texas, USA
and Associate Professor of Obstetrics and Gynecology
Uniformed Services University of the Health Sciences
Military Consultant to the Surgeon General
for Maternal Fetal Medicine

Michael A. Belfort, MBBCH, MD, PhD
Professor
Department of Obstetrics and Gynecology
University of Utah Health Services Center,
Salt Lake City
and Director
Department of Maternal Fetal Medicine
Utah Valley Regional Medical Center
Provo, Utah, USA

Ron Bloom, MD
Professor, Department of Pediatrics
University of Utah
Salt Lake City, Utah, USA

Renee A. Bobrowski, MD
Assistant Professor
Department of Obstetrics and Gynecology
University of Connecticut
Farmington, Connecticut
and Attending Perinatologist
Hartford Hospital
Hartford, Connecticut, USA

D. Ware Branch, MD
Chairman of Obstetrics and Gynecology
LDS Hospital and Urban Central Region
and Professor and Vice-Chairman
Department of Obstetrics and Gynecology
University of Utah Health Sciences Center
Salt Lake City, Utah, USA

Rosie Burton, PhD, MRCOG
Perinatal Fellow
Department of Obstetrics and Gynecology
University of Cape Town
Observatory, South Africa

Steven L. Clark, MD
Professor
Department of Obstetrics and Gynecology
University of Utah Health Services Center
LDS Hospital
Salt Lake City, Utah, USA

Tawnya Constantino, MD
Assistant Professor of Neurology
and Director, Comprehensive Epilepsy Program
University of Utah, Department of Neurology
Salt Lake City, Utah, USA

Lowell E. Davis, MD
Professor
Department of Obstetrics and Gynecology
Oregon Health and Science University
Portland, Oregon, USA

Shad H. Deering, MD
Instructor, Department of Obstetrics/Gynecology
and Fellow, Maternal–Fetal Medicine
Georgetown University Hospital
Washington, DC, USA

Gary A. Dildy III, MD
Professor
Department of Obstetrics and Gynecology
Louisiana State University Health Sciences Center
New Orleans, Louisiana, USA

Donna Dizon-Townson, MD
Assistant Professor
Department of Obstetrics and Gynecology
Salt Lake City, Utah
and Co-Director, Maternal–Fetal Medicine
Utah Valley Regional Medical Center
Provo, Utah, USA

Michael R. Foley, MD
Clinical Professor
Department of Obstetrics and Gynecology
University of Arizona School of Medicine
Tucson, Arizona
and Medical Director
Phoenix Perinatal Associates/Obstetrics Medical Group of Phoenix
Phoenix, Arizona, USA

Alfredo F. Gei, MD
Assistant Professor
Division of Maternal–Fetal Medicine
Department of Obstetrics and Gynecology
University of Texas Medical Branch
Galveston, Texas, USA

Bernard Gonik, MD
Professor and Fann Srere Chair of Perinatal
Medicine–Feta;
and Director, Critical Care Obstetrics
Maternal–Fetal Medicine
Department of Obstetrics and Gynecology
Wayne State University School of Medicine
Sinai-Grace Hospital
Detroit, Michigan, USA

Cornelia R. Graves, MD
Associate Professor, Maternal–Fetal Medicine
and Director, Critical Care Obstetrics
Department of Obstetrics and Gynecology
Division of Maternal–Fetal Medicine
Nashville, Tennessee, USA

Nancy A. Hueppchen, MD, MS
Assistant Professor and Clerkship Director
Division of Maternal–Fetal Medicine
Department of Gynecology and Obstetrics
The Johns Hopkins University School of Medicine
Baltimore, Maryland, USA

Aristides Koutrouvelis, MD, FCCP
Assistant Professor of Anesthesiology
University of Texas Medical Branch
Galveston, Texas, USA

Cortney Kirkendall
Childbirth Injury Prevention Foundation
Pasadena, California, USA

Michael R. Leonardi, MD
Clinical Assistant Professor of Obstetrics and Gynecology
University of Illinois at Chicago
College of Medicine at Peoria, Peoria
and Attending Perinatologist
OSF/St. Francis Medical Center
Peoria, Illinois, USA

William C. Mabie, MD
Professor of Clinical Obstetrics and Gynecology
University of South Carolina—Greenville
Greenville, South Carolina, USA

Fergal D. Malone, MD
Director, Division of Maternal–Fetal Medicine
Columbia Presbyterian Medical Center
Columbia University College of Physicians and Surgeons
New York, USA

James N. Martin, Jr, MD
Professor, Department of Obstetrics and Gynecology
University of Mississippi Medical School
and Director, Division of Maternal–Fetal Medicine
University Hospitals, Wiser Hospital for Women and Infants
Jackson, Mississippi, USA

Brian A. Mason, MD
Associate Professor, Department of Obstetrics and Gynecology
Wayne State University
St. John Hospital and Medical Center
Detroit, Michigan, USA

Lisa E. Moore, MD
Associate Professor of Maternal Medicine
Department of Obstetrics and Gynecology
University of New Mexico Health Sciences Center
Albuquerque, New Mexico, USA

Errol R. Norwitz, MD, PhD
Division of Maternal–Fetal Medicine
Department of Obstetrics, Gynecology, and Reproductive Biology
Brigham and Women's Hospital
Harvard Medical School
Boston, Massachusetts, USA

Gayle Olson, MD
Associate Professor, Ob-Gyn, Maternal–Fetal Medicine
University of Texas Medical Branch
Galveston, Texas, USA

Luis Diego Pacheco, MD
Fellow, Maternal Fetal Medicine
Department of Obstetrics and Gynecology
University of Texas Medical Branch
Galveston, Texas, USA

Jeffrey P. Phelan, MD, JD
Vice Chairman and Director of Quality Assurance
Department of Obstetrics and Gynecology
Citrus Valley Medical Center
West Covina, California
and President and Director Clinical Research
Childbirth Injury Prevention Foundation
Pasadena, California, USA

T. Flint Porter, MD, MPH
Director, Maternal–Fetal Medicine
LDS Hospital
Urban Central Region, Intermountain Health Care
and Assistant Professor
Department of Obstetrics and Gynecology
University of Utah Health Sciences Center
Salt Lake City, Utah, USA

Fidelma B. Rigby, MD
Assistant Professor of Clinical Obstetrics and Gynecology
Assistant Program Director
Division of Maternal Fetal Medicine
Louisiana State University
New Orleans, Louisiana, USA

Scott Roberts, MD, MS
Associate Professor
Department of Obstetrics and Gynecology
University of Kansas School of Medicine, Kansas
and Attending Physician
Wesley Medical Center
Wichita, Kansas, USA

Julian N. Robinson, MD
Division of Maternal–Fetal Medicine
Department of Obstetrics and Gynecology
Columbia Presbyterian Medical Center
Columbia University, College of Physicians and Surgeons
New York, USA

Sheryl Rodts-Palenik, MD, FACOG
Fellow, Division of Maternal–Fetal Medicine
University of Mississippi Medical Center
Jackson, Mississippi, USA

David A. Sacks, MD
Clinical Professor
Department of Obstetrics and Gynecology
University of Southern California Keck School of Medicine
Los Angeles, California
and Director, Maternal–Fetal Medicine
Kaiser Foundation Hospital
Bellflower, California, USA

Andrew J. Satin, MD
Professor, Chair and Program Director
Department of Obstetrics and Gynecology
Uniformed Services University
Bethesda, Maryland, USA

Anthony Scardella, MD
Associate Professor of Medicine
University of Medicine and Dentistry of New Jersey
Robert Wood Johnson Medical School
New Brunswick
and Chief, Pulmonary Section
Saint Peter's University Hospital
New Brunswick, New Jersey, USA

William E. Scorza, MD, FACOG
Associate Professor
Department of Obstetrics, Gynecology, and Reproductive Sciences
University of Medicine and Dentistry of New Jersey
Robert Wood Johnson Medical School
New Brunswick
and Medical Director of Obstetric Services
Department of Obstetrics and Gynecology
Saint Peter's University Hospital
New Brunswick, New Jersey, USA

James R. Scott, MD
Professor, Department of Obstetrics and Gynecology
University of Utah Medical Center
Salt Lake City, Utah, USA

Gail L. Seiken, MD
Assistant Professor, Internal Medicine
Uniformed Services University
Washington Nephrology Association
Bethesda, Maryland, USA

Shailen S. Shah, MD
Clinical Associate Professor and
Associate Residency Director
Department of Obstetrics and Gynecology
and Co-Director Critical Care Obstetrics and
Director Student Medical Education
Division of Maternal–Fetal Medicine
Thomas Jefferson University Hospital
Philadelphia, Pennsylvania, USA

Howard T. Sharp, MD
Associate Professor
Department of Obstetrics and Gynecology
University of Utah School of Medicine
Salt Lake City, Utah, USA

John C. Smulian, MD, MPH
Associate Professor of Obstetrics and Gynecology
Director (acting), Division of Maternal–Fetal Medicine
Department of Obstetrics, Gynecology and Reproductive Sciences
University of Medicine and Dentistry of New Jersey
Robert Wood Johnson Medical School
Robert Wood Johnson University Hospital
New Brunswick, New Jersey, USA

Theresa L. Stewart, MD
Assistant Professor of Obstetrics and Gynecology
Uniformed Services University of the Health Sciences
Wilford Hall Medical Center
Lackland Air Force Base, Texas, USA

Victor R. Suárez, MD
Fellow, Division of Maternal–Fetal Medicine
Department of Obstetrics and Gynecology
University of Texas Medical Branch
Galveston, Texas, USA

Christopher A. Sullivan, MD
Director, Maternal/Fetal Medicine
Stamford Hosptial
Stamford, Connecticut, USA *and*
Assistant Professor, Obstetrics and Gynecology
New York Medical College,
Valhalla, New York, USA

Mark W. Tomlinson, MD
Clinical Assistant Professor
Department of Obstetrics and Gynecology
Oregon Health Sciences University
Portland, Oregon, USA

Rakesh B. Vadhera, MD, FRCA, FFARCS
Associate Professor
Department of Anesthesiology
University of Texas Medical Branch
Galveston, Texas, USA

James W. Van Hook, MD
Associate Professor
Division of Maternal–Fetal Medicine
Department of Obstetrics and Gynecology
University of Texas Medical Branch
Galveston, Texas, USA

Michael W. Varner, MD
Professor, Department of Obstetrics and Gynecology
University of Utah Health Sciences Center
Salt Lake City, Utah, USA

Janice E. Whitty, MD
Associate Professor, Obstetrics and Gynecology
and Director, Maternal Special Care Unit
Department of Obstetrics and Gynecology
Division of Maternal–Fetal Medicine
Wayne State University/Hutzel Hospital
Detroit, Michigan, USA

Carey L. Winkler, MD
Department of Obstetrics and Gynecology
Oregon Health and Science University
Portland, Oregon, USA

Jerome Yankowitz, MD
Director and Professor, Division of Maternal Fetal Medicine
and Fetal Diagnosis and Treatment Unit
Department of Obstetrics and Gynecology
University of Iowa Roy L and Lucille A Carver College of Medicine
Iowa City, Iowa, USA

Christian Con Yost, MD
Instructor, Department of Neonatology
Division of Neonatology
University of Utah
Salt Lake City, Utah, USA

Karen A. Zempolich, MD
Assistant Professor
Department of Obstetrics and Gynecology
Division of Gynecologic Oncology
University of Utah School of Medicine
Salt Lake City, Utah, USA

I Introduction to critical care obstetrics

1 Epidemiology of critical illness and outcomes in pregnancy

Cande V. Ananth
John C. Smulian

The successful epidemiologic evaluation of any particular disease or condition has several prerequisites. Two of the most important prerequisites are that the condition should be accurately defined and that there should be measurable outcomes of interest. Another requirement is that there must be some systematic way of data collection or surveillance that will allow the measurement of the outcomes of interest and associated risk factors. The epidemiologic evaluation of critical illness associated with pregnancy has met with mixed success on all of these counts.

Historically, surveillance of pregnancy-related critical illness has focused on the well-defined outcome of maternal mortality in order to identify illnesses or conditions that might have led to maternal death. Identification of various conditions associated with maternal mortality initially came from observations by astute clinicians. One of the best examples is the link described by Semmelweiss between hand-washing habits and puerperal fever. In most industrial and many developing countries, there are now population-based surveillance mechanisms in place to track maternal mortality. These often are mandated by law. In fact, the World Health Organization uses maternal mortality as one of the measures of the health of a population (World Health Organization, 1991).

Fortunately, in most industrialized nations the maternal mortality rates have fallen to very low levels. Recent statistics for the United States suggest that overall maternal mortality is 11.5 maternal deaths per 100,000 live births during 1991–97 (Morbidity and Mortality Weekly Report, 2001). Despite this impressively low rate of maternal mortality, tracking maternal deaths may not be the best way to assess pregnancy-related critical illnesses since the majority of such illnesses do not result in maternal death. As stated by Harmer (1997), "death represents the tip of the morbidity iceberg, the size of which is unknown." Unlike mortality, which is an unequivocal endpoint, critical illness in pregnancy as a morbidity outcome is difficult to define and, therefore, difficult to measure and study precisely.

There are many common conditions in pregnancy such as the hypertensive diseases, intrapartum hemorrhage, diabetes, thyroid disease, asthma, seizure disorders, and infection that occur frequently and require special medical care, but do not actually become critical illnesses. Most women with these complications have relatively uneventful pregnancies that result in good outcomes for both mother and infant. Nevertheless, each of these conditions can be associated with significant complications that have the potential for serious morbidity, disability and mortality. The stage where any condition becomes severe enough to be classified as a critical illness has not been clearly defined. However, it may be helpful to consider critical illness as impending, developing, or established significant organ dysfunction, which may lead to long-term morbidity or death. This allows some flexibility in the characterization of disease severity since it recognizes conditions that can deteriorate rather quickly in pregnancy.

Maternal mortality data collection is well established in many places, but specific surveillance systems that track severe complications of pregnancy not associated with maternal mortality are rare. It has been suggested that most women suffering a critical illness in pregnancy are likely to spend some time in an intensive care unit (Marmer, 1997; Mahutte et al., 1999; Hazelgrove et al., 2001). These cases have been described by some as "near-miss" mortality cases (Baskett & Sternadel, 1998; Mantel et al., 1998). Therefore, examination of cases admitted to intensive care units can provide insight into the nature of pregnancy-related critical illnesses and can compliment maternal mortality surveillance. However, it should be noted that nearly two-thirds of maternal deaths might occur in women who never reach an intensive care unit (Hazelgrove et al., 2001).

The following sections review much of what is currently known about the epidemiology of critical illness in pregnancy. Some of the information is based on published studies; however, much of the data are derived from publicly available data that are collected as part of nationwide surveillance systems in the United States.

Pregnancy-related hospitalizations

Pregnancy complications contribute significantly to maternal, fetal, and infant morbidity, as well as mortality (Scott et al., 1997). Many women with complicating conditions are hospitalized without being delivered. Although maternal complications of pregnancy are the fifth leading cause of infant mortality in the United States, little is known about the epidemiology of maternal complications associated with hospitalizations. Examination of complicating conditions associated with maternal hospitalizations can provide information on the types of conditions requiring hospitalized care. In the United States during the years 1991–92, it was estimated that 18.0% of pregnancies (per 100 births) were associated with nondelivery hospitalization with disproportionate rates between Black (28.1%) and White (17.2%) women (Bennett et al., 1998). This 18.0% hospitalization rate comprised 12.3% for obstetric conditions (18.3% among Blacks and 11.9% among Whites), 4.4% for pregnancy losses (8.1% among Blacks and 3.9% among Whites), and 1.3% for nonobstetric (medical or surgical) conditions (1.5% among Blacks and 1.3% among Whites). The likelihood of pregnancy-associated hospitalizations in the United States declined between 1986–87 and 1991–92 (Franks et al., 1992; Bennett et al., 1998).

More recent information about pregnancy-related hospitalization diagnoses could be found in the aggregated National Hospital Discharge Summary (NHDS) data for 1998–99. These data are assembled by the National Center for Health Statistics (NCHS) of the Centers for Disease Control and Prevention. The NHDS data is a survey of medical records from short-stay, nonfederal hospitals in the United States, conducted annually since 1965. A detailed description of the survey and the database can be found elsewhere (National Center for Health Statistics, 2000). Briefly, for each hospital admission, the NHDS data include a primary and up to six secondary diagnoses, as well as up to four procedures performed for each hospitalization. These diagnoses and procedures are all coded based on the International Classification of Diseases, ninth revision, clinical modification. We examined the rates (per 100 hospitalizations) of hospitalizations by indications (discharge diagnoses) during 1998–99 in the United States, separately for delivery (n = 7,965,173) and nondelivery (n = 960, 023) hospitalizations. We also examined the mean hospital lengths of stay (with 95% confidence intervals). Antepartum and postpartum hospitalizations were grouped as nondelivery hospitalizations.

During 1998–99, nearly 7.4% of all hospitalizations were for hypertensive diseases with delivery, and 6.6% were for hypertensive diseases not delivered (Table 1.1). Mean hospital length of stay (LOS) is an indirect measure of acuity for some illnesses. LOS was higher for delivery-related than nondelivery-related hospitalizations for hypertensive diseases. Hemorrhage, as the underlying reason for hospitalization (either as primary or secondary diagnosis), occurred much more frequently for delivery- than nondelivery-related hospitalizations. Nondelivery hospitalizations for genitourinary infections occurred three times more frequently (10.45%) than for delivery-related hospitalizations (3.19%), although the average LOS was shorter for nondelivery hospitalizations.

Hospitalizations for preterm labor occurred twice as frequently for nondelivery hospitalizations (21.21%) than delivery related (10.28%). This is expected since many preterm labor patients are successfully treated and some of these hospitalizations are for "false labor." Liver disorders were uncommonly associated with hospitalization. However, the mean hospital LOS for liver disorders that occurred with nondelivery hospitalizations was over 31 days, compared with a mean LOS of 3 days if the liver condition was delivery related. Coagulation-related defects required 14.9 days of hospitalization if not related to delivery compared with a mean LOS of 4.9 days if the condition was delivery related. Hospitalizations for embolism-related complications were infrequent, but generally required extended hospital stays.

The top 10 causes of hospital admissions, separately for delivery- and nondelivery-related events, are presented in Fig. 1.1. The chief cause for hospitalization (either delivery or nondelivery related) was for preterm labor. The second most frequent condition was hypertensive diseases (7.37% for delivery related and 6.61% for nondelivery related) followed by anemia (7.13% vs. 5.05%). Hospitalizations for infection-related conditions occurred twice more frequently for nondelivery periods (11.65%) than during delivery (5.75%). In contrast, hospitalization for hemorrhage was more frequent during delivery (4.43%) than nondelivery (3.26%). These data provide important insights into the most common complications and conditions associated with pregnancy hospitalization. The LOS data also give some indication of resource allocation needs. While this is important in understanding the epidemiology of illness in pregnancy, it does not allow a detailed examination of illness severity.

Maternal mortality

The National Health Promotion and Disease Prevention objectives of the *Healthy People 2010* indicators specifies a goal of no more than 3.3 maternal deaths per 100,000 live births in the United States (National Center for Health Statistics, 1993). The goal for maternal deaths among Black women was set at no more than 5.0 per 100,000 live births. As of 1997 (the latest available statistics on maternal deaths in the US) this objective remains elusive. The pregnancy-related maternal mortality ratio (PRMR) per 100,000 live births for the United States was 11.5 for 1991–97 (Morbidity and Mortality Weekly Report, 2001), with the ratio over threefold greater among Black compared with White women (Morbidity and Mortality Weekly Report, 1998). Several studies that have examined trends in

Table 1.1 Rate (per 100 hospitalizations) of delivery and nondelivery hospitalizations, and associated hospital lengths of stay (LOS) by diagnoses: United States, 1998–99

	Delivery hospitalization (*n* = 7,965,173)		Nondelivery hospitalization (*n* = 960,023)	
Hospital admission diagnosis*	**Rate (%)**	**Mean LOS (95% CI)**	**Rate (%)**	**Mean LOS (95% CI)**
Hypertensive diseases				
Chronic hypertension	3.05	3.0 (2.9, 3.2)	3.08	2.3 (1.9, 2.7)
Preeclampsia/eclampsia	4.08	3.7 (3.6, 3.9)	3.23	2.7 (1.8, 3.6)
Chronic hypertension + preeclampsia	0.24	6.3 (4.7, 7.8)	0.30	2.4 (1.8, 2.9)
Hemorrhage				
Placental abruption	1.02	3.9 (3.5, 4.3)	0.72	3.4 (2.2, 4.7)
Placenta previa	0.44	5.5 (4.6, 6.5)	0.13	3.2 (2.0, 4.4)
Hemorrhage (unassigned etiology)	0.24	4.0 (3.2, 4.9)	1.58	1.7 (1.3, 2.2)
Vasa previa	0.17	2.6 (2.0, 3.2)	—	—
Postpartum hemorrhage	2.56	2.6 (2.5, 2.7)	0.83	2.3 (1.3, 2.9)
Infection-related				
Viral infections (not malaria/rubella)	0.93	2.8 (2.6, 3.1)	1.04	2.6 (2.0, 3.2)
Genitourinary infections	3.19	3.4 (2.8, 3.9)	10.45	3.2 (2.5, 3.8)
Infection of the amniotic cavity	1.63	4.2 (3.7, 4.6)	0.16	4.2 (1.7, 6.7)
Anesthesia-related complications	0.02	4.7 (3.5, 5.9)	<0.01	—
Diabetes				
Preexisting diabetes	0.60	4.6 (3.7, 5.4)	2.40	3.2 (2.7, 3.7)
Gestational diabetes	3.15	2.9 (2.8, 3.1)	2.50	3.5 (3.0, 4.1)
Preterm labor	10.28	3.4 (3.3, 3.6)	21.21	2.5 (2.3, 2.7)
Maternal anemia	7.13	2.9 (2.8, 3.0)	5.05	3.9 (3.2, 4.5)
Drug dependency	0.19	3.0 (2.3, 3.7)	0.53	3.6 (2.3, 4.8)
Renal disorders	0.13	3.4 (2.6, 4.3)	0.86	2.7 (2.1, 3.2)
Liver disorders	0.06	3.0 (2.2, 3.8)	0.08	31.2 (2.7, 59.6)
Congenital cardiovascular disease	0.94	3.0 (2.7, 3.4)	0.98	3.1 (2.3, 3.8)
Thyroid disorders	0.17	2.3 (1.6, 3.0)	0.53	3.0 (1.7, 4.4)
Uterine tumors	0.54	3.8 (3.4, 4.2)	0.63	2.6 (1.5, 3.6)
Uterine rupture	0.11	4.8 (3.3, 6.2)	—	—
Postpartum coagulation defects	0.11	4.9 (3.7, 6.1)	0.07	14.9 (0.2, 47.8)
Shock/hypotension	0.09	3.3 (2.6, 4.0)	0.15	2.2 (0.4, 4.1)
Acute renal failure	0.02	6.9 (4.1, 9.7)	0.02	—
Embolism-related				
Amniotic fluid embolism	0.02	6.8 (1.8, 11.7)	—	—
Blood-clot embolism	<0.01	11.1 (2.7, 19.3)	0.19	5.2 (3.2, 7.5)
Other pulmonary embolism	<0.01	—	—	—

* The diagnoses associated with hospital admissions include both primary and secondary reasons for hospitalizations. Each admission may have had up to six associated diagnoses.

maternal mortality statistics have concluded that a majority of pregnancy-related deaths (including those resulting from ectopic pregnancies, and some cases of infection and hemorrhage) are preventable (Sachs et al., 1987; Syverson et al., 1991; World Health Organization, 1991). However, maternal deaths due to other complications such as pregnancy-induced hypertension, placenta previa, retained placenta, and thromboembolism, are considered by some as difficult to prevent (Mertz et al., 1992; Berg et al., 1996).

From the 1960s to the mid-1980s, the maternal mortality ratio in the United States declined from approximately 27 per 100,000 live births to about 7 per 100,000 live births (Fig. 1.2). Subsequently, the mortality ratio increased between 1987 (7.2 per 100,000 live births) and 1990 (10.0 per 100,000 live births).

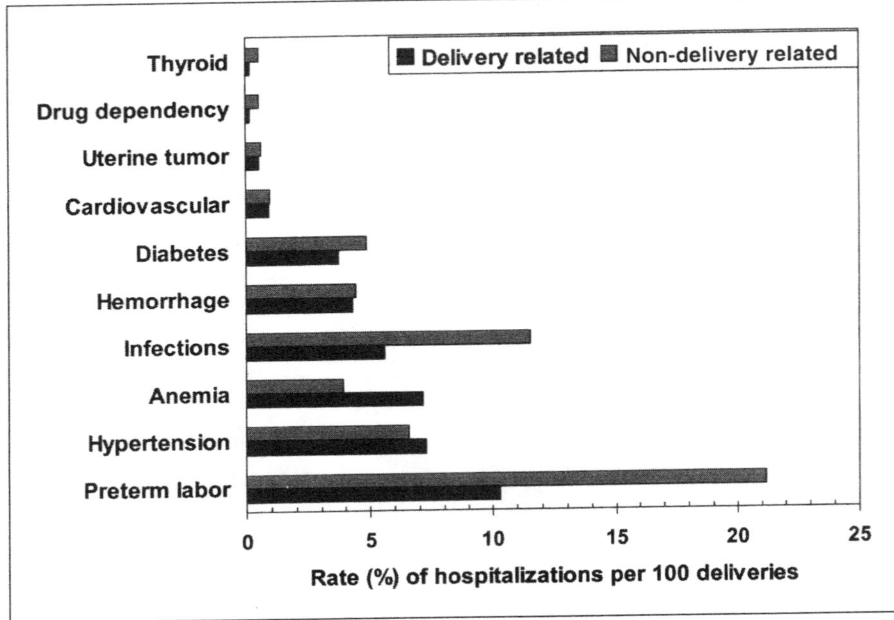

Fig. 1.1 Ten leading causes of delivery- and nondelivery-related maternal hospitalizations in the United States, 1998–99.

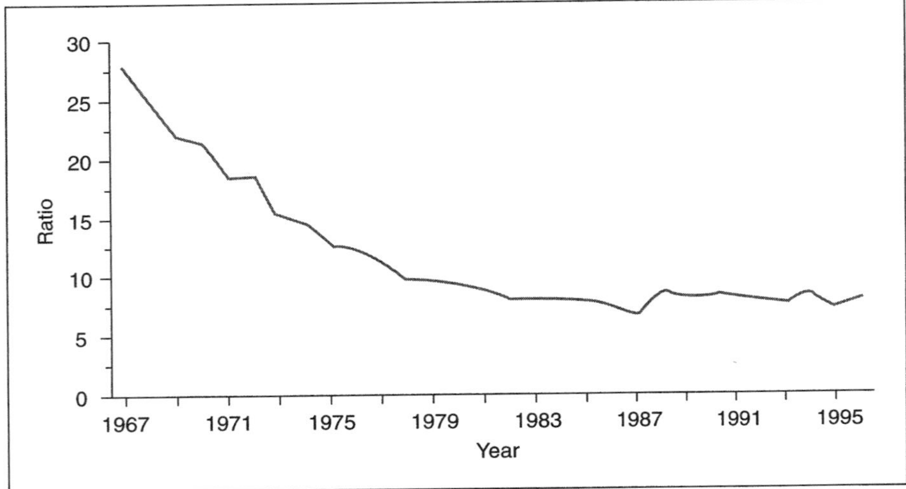

Fig. 1.2 Trends in maternal mortality ratio (number of maternal deaths per 100,000 live births) in the United States, 1967–96. The term "ratio" is used instead of rate because the numerator includes some maternal deaths that were not related to live births and thus were not included in the denominator.

During the period 1991 to 1997, the mortality ratio further increased to 11.5 per 100,000 live births—an overall relative increase of 60% between 1987 and 1997. The reasons for the recent increases are not clear.

Several maternal risk factors have been examined in relation to maternal deaths. Women aged 35–39 years carry a 2.6-fold (95% confidence interval 2.2, 3.1) increased risk of maternal death and those ≥40 years are at a 5.9-fold (95% confidence interval 4.6, 7.7) increased risk. Black maternal race confers a relative risk of 3.7 (95% confidence interval 3.3, 4.1) for maternal death compared with White women. Similarly, women without any prenatal care during pregnancy were almost twofold at increased risk of a maternal death relative to those who received prenatal care (Atrash et al., 1992).

The chief cause for a pregnancy-related maternal death depends on whether the pregnancy results in a live born, stillbirth, ectopic pregnancy, abortion, or molar gestation (Table 1.2). For the period 1987–90, hemorrhage was recorded in 28.8% of all deaths, leading to an overall pregnancy-related mortality ratio (PRMR) for hemorrhage of 2.6 per 100,000 live births, followed by embolism-related deaths (PRMR 1.8), and hypertensive diseases (PRMR 1.6). Among all live births, hypertensive diseases (23.8%) were the most frequent cause of death. Among stillbirths (27.2%) and ectopic (94.9%) pregnancies, the chief cause of death was hemorrhage, while infections (49.4%) were the leading cause of abortion-related maternal deaths.

Understanding the epidemiology of pregnancy-related deaths is essential in order to target specific interventions.

Table 1.2 Pregnancy-related maternal deaths by underlying cause: United States, 1987–90

	All outcomes		Outcome of pregnancy (% distribution)						
Cause of death	**%**	**PRMR***	**Live birth**	**Stillbirth**	**Ectopic**	**Abortions†**	**Molar**	**Undelivered**	**Unknown**
Hemorrhage	28.8	2.6	21.1	27.2	94.9	18.5	16.7	15.7	20.1
Embolism	19.9	1.8	23.4	10.7	1.3	11.1	0.0	35.2	21.1
Hypertension	17.6	1.6	23.8	26.2	0.0	1.2	0.0	4.6	16.3
Infection	13.1	1.2	12.1	19.4	1.3	49.4	0.0	13.0	9.0
Cardiomyopathy	5.7	0.5	6.1	2.9	0.0	0.0	0.0	2.8	13.9
Anesthesia	2.5	0.2	2.7	0.0	1.9	8.6	0.0	1.8	1.0
Others/unknown	12.8	1.2	11.1	13.6	0.6	11.1	83.3	27.5	19.3
Total	100.0	—	100.0	100.0	100.0	100.0	100.0	100.0	100.0

* Pregnancy-related mortality ratio per 100,000 live births.
† Includes both spontaneous and induced abortions.
(From Koonin et al. Pregnancy-related mortality surveillance—United States, 1987–1990. MMWR 1997;56:17–36.)

Table 1.3 Perinatal mortality rates among singleton and multiple gestations by gestational age and high-risk conditions: United States, 1995–98

	20–27 weeks		28–32 weeks		33–36 weeks		≥37 weeks	
High-risk conditions	**PMR**	**Relative risk (95% CI)**	**PMR**	**Relative risk (95% CI)**	**PMR**	**Relative risk (95% CI)**	**PMR**	**Relative risk (95% CI)**
Singletons								
Number of births	*N*=103,755		*N*=352,291		*N*=1,072,784		*N*=13,440,671	
Hypertension	200.4	0.6 (0.5, 0.7)	53.1	0.6 (0.5, 0.6)	13.5	0.6 (0.5, 0.7)	3.6	1.3 (0.5, 0.7)
Hemorrhage	308.9	1.1 (1.0, 1.2)	73.1	1.4 (1.3, 1.5)	19.9	1.6 (1.5, 1.7)	3.6	1.6 (1.5, 1.7)
Diabetes	287.0	1.0 (0.9, 1.1)	60.8	1.2 (1.1, 1.3)	19.5	1.8 (1.7, 1.9)	5.0	2.3 (2.1, 2.4)
SGA	467.4	2.3 (2.1, 2.5)	196.3	6.2 (6.0, 6.4)	56.3	7.8 (7.5, 8.1)	9.1	5.5 (5.4, 5.7)
No complications	297.6	1.0 (Referent)	38.8	1.0 (Referent)	7.0	1.0 (Referent)	1.5	1.0 (Referent)
Multiples								
Number of births	*N*=23,055		*N*=76,329		*N*=147,627		*N*=187,109	
Hypertension	183.5	0.7 (0.6, 0.8)	21.4	0.5 (0.4, 0.6)	5.3	0.6 (0.5, 0.7)	4.9	0.8 (0.6, 1.1)
Hemorrhage	251.6	1.0 (0.9, 1.1)	36.6	1.1 (1.0, 1.3)	9.6	1.2 (1.0, 1.4)	6.7	1.3 (1.1, 1.5)
Diabetes	214.9	0.8 (0.7, 1.1)	28.7	0.9 (0.7, 1.2)	9.7	1.3 (1.0, 1.7)	5.9	1.2 (0.9, 1.7)
SGA	394.5	2.0 (1.6, 2.4)	133.4	6.8 (6.3, 7.4)	36.8	7.5 (6.6, 8.4)	24.9	8.6 (7.6, 9.7)
No complications	251.1	1.0 (Referent)	23.4	1.0 (Referent)	5.2	1.0 (Referent)	2.8	1.0 (Referent)

CI, confidence interval; PMR, perinatal mortality rate per 1,000 births; SGA, small-for-gestational-age births.
Hypertension includes chronic hypertension, pregnancy-induced hypertension, and eclampsia.
Hemorrhage includes placental abruption, placenta previa, uterine bleeding of undermined etiology.
No complications include those that did not have any complications listed in the table.
Relative risk for each high-risk condition was adjusted for all other high-risk conditions shown in the table.

Improved population-based surveillance through targeted reviews of all pregnancy-related deaths, as well as additional research to understand the causes of maternal deaths by indication will help in achieving the *Healthy People 2010* goals.

Perinatal mortality

Perinatal mortality, defined by the World Health Organization as fetal deaths plus live born deaths within the first 28 days, is an important indicator of population health. Examination of the maternal conditions related to perinatal mortality can provide further information on the association and impact of these conditions on pregnancy outcomes. Table 1.3 shows the results of our examination of perinatal mortality rates among singleton and multiple births (twins, triplets and quadruplets) by gestational age and high-risk conditions. The study population comprises all births in the United States that occurred in

1995–98. Data were derived from the national linked birth/infant death files, assembled by the National Center for Health Statistics of the Centers for Disease Control and Prevention (MacDorman & Atkinson, 1998). Gestational age was predominantly based on the date of last menstrual period (Taffel et al., 1982), and was grouped as 20–27, 28–32, 33–36, and ≥37 weeks. Perinatal mortality rates were assessed for hypertension (chronic hypertension, pregnancy-induced hypertension, and eclampsia), hemorrhage (placental abruption, placenta previa, and uterine bleeding of undetermined etiology), diabetes (preexisting and gestational diabetes), and small for gestational age (SGA) births (defined as birth weight <10th centile for gestational age). We derived norms for the 10th centile birth weight for singleton and multiple births from the corresponding singleton and multiple births that occurred in 1995–98 in the United States. Finally, relative risks (with 95% confidence intervals) for perinatal death by each high-risk condition were derived from multivariable logistic regression models after adjusting for all other high-risk conditions.

Perinatal mortality rates progressively decline, among both singleton and multiple births, for each high-risk condition with increasing gestational age (Table 1.3). Among singleton and multiple gestations, with the exception of SGA births, mortality rates were generally higher for each high-risk condition, relative to the no complications group. Infants delivered small for their gestational age carried the highest risk of dying during the perinatal period compared with those born to mothers without complications. Among singleton births, the relative risks for perinatal death for SGA infants were 2.3, 6.2, 7.8, and 5.5 for those delivered at 20–27 weeks, 28–32, 33–36, and at term, respectively. Among multiple births, these relative risks were similar at 2.0, 6.8, 7.5, and 8.6, respectively, for each of the four gestational age categories.

Pregnancy-related intensive care unit admissions

Evaluation of obstetric admissions to intensive care units (ICU) may be one of the best ways to approach surveillance of critical illnesses in pregnancy. Unfortunately, there are no publicly available population-based databases for obstetric admissions to ICU that provide sufficiently detailed information to allow in-depth study of these conditions. Therefore, it is reasonable to examine descriptive case series to provide information on these conditions. We reviewed 22 studies involving 1,550,723 deliveries (DeMello & Restall, 1990; Mabie & Sibai, 1990; Stephens, 1991; Kilpatrick & Matthay, 1992; Ng et al., 1992; Collop & Sahn, 1993; Monoco et al., 1993; Lewinsohn et al., 1994; Bouvier-Colle et al., 1996; El-Sohl & Grant, 1996; Lapinsky et al., 1997; Platteau et al., 1997; Tang et al., 1997; Baskett & Sternadel, 1998; Mahutte et al., 1999; Cohen et al., 2000; Gilbert et al., 2000; Hogg et al., 2000; Panchal et al., 2000; Ryan et al., 2000; Afessa et al., 2001; Hazelgrove et al., 2001) and found an overall obstetric-related admission rate to ICU of 0.07–0.88% (Table 1.4). Some of the variation in the rates may be explained by the nature of the populations studied. Hospitals that are tertiary referral centers for large catchment areas typically receive a more concentrated high-risk population. These facilities would be expected to have higher rates of obstetric admissions to an ICU. Community-oriented facilities are probably less likely to care for critically ill obstetric patients unless the illnesses develop so acutely that they would preclude transport to a higher level facility. The largest study of pregnancy-related ICU admissions involved 37 maternity hospitals in Maryland and included hospitals at all care levels (Panchal et al., 2000). This study found a nearly 30% lower admission rate to ICUs for obstetric patients from community hospitals compared with major teaching hospitals. Another source of variation is the different criteria for admission to the ICU used at different institutions. Finally, there are major differences in the inclusion criteria used for these studies that further contributes to the variability in reported ICU utilization rates.

Reported maternal mortality for critically ill obstetric patients admitted to an ICU is approximately 5.0% (Table 1.4). This reflects the true seriousness of the illnesses of these women. The wide range of mortality from 0 to 21.3% is due to many factors. Most of the studies were small and just a few deaths may affect rates significantly. The populations studied also differ in underlying health status. The time period of the study can have an impact. In general, earlier studies had higher maternal mortality rates. These earlier studies represent the early stages of development of care mechanisms for critically ill obstetric patients. They probably reflect part of the "learning curve" of critical care obstetrics, as well as differences in available technology (Knaus et al., 1986). Regardless, the mortality rate from these ICU admissions is several orders of magnitude higher than the population maternal mortality rate of 11.5 per 100,000 live births. Therefore, these cases are a good representation of an obstetric population with critical illnesses.

Illnesses responsible for obstetric intensive care unit admissions

Examination of obstetric ICU admissions provides some insight into the nature of obstetric illnesses requiring critical care. Data were pooled from 18 published studies that provided sufficient details about the primary indication for the ICU admission (Mabie & Sibai, 1990; Stephens, 1991; Kilpatrick & Matthay, 1992; Ng et al., 1992; Collop & Sahn, 1993; Monoco et al., 1993; Lewinsohn et al., 1994; El-Sohl & Grant, 1996; Lapinsky et al., 1997; Platteau et al., 1997; Tang et al., 1997; Baskett & Sternadel, 1998; Mahutte et al., 1999; Cohen et al., 2000; Ryan et al., 2000; Afessa et al., 2001; Hazelgrove et al., 2001) (Table 1.5). It is no surprise that hypertensive diseases and obstetric hemorrhage were responsible for over 50% of the

Table 1.4 Obstetric admission rates to an intensive care unit (ICU) and corresponding maternal mortality rates from 22 studies

Reference	Year(s)	Location	Inclusion criteria	Total deliveries	Obstetric ICU admissions (rate)	Obstetric ICU deaths (rate)	Fetal/neonatal deaths (rate)
Mabie & Sibai, 1990	1986–89	United States	—	22,651	200 (0.88%)	7 (3.5%)	—
Kilpatrick & Matthay, 1992	1985–90	United States	Up to 6 weeks PP	8,000*	32 (0.4%)	4 (12.0%)	6 (18.8%)
Collop & Sahn, 1993	1988–91	United States	<42 weeks	—	20 (—)	4 (20.0%)	7 (35.0%)
El-Solh & Grant, 1996	1989–95	United States	Up to 10d PP	—	96 (—)	10/93 (10.8%)	10 (10.8%)
Monoco et al., 1993	1983–90	United States	16 weeks to 2 weeks PP	15,323	38 (0.25%)	7 (18.4%)	4 (10.5%)
Panchal et al., 2000	1984–97	United States	Delivering admission	822,591	1,023 (0.12%)	34 (3.3%)	—
Afessa et al., 2001	1991–98	United States	—	—	78 (—)	2 (2.7%)	13 (16.7%)
Gilbert et al., 2000	1991–98	United States	Up to 6 weeks PP	49,349	233 (0.47%)	8 (3.4%)	—
Hogg et al., 2000	1989–97	United States	15 weeks to 6 weeks PP	30,405	172 (0.57%)	23 (13.4%)	2 (1.2%)
Mahutte et al., 1999	1991–97	Canada	14 weeks to 6 weeks PP	44,340	131 (0.30%)	3 (2.3%)	—
Lapinsky et al., 1997	1997	Canada	—	25,000*	65 (0.26%)	0	7 (10.8%)
Baskett & Sternadel, 1998	1980–93	Canada	>20 weeks and PP	76,119	55 (0.07%)	2 (3.6%)	—
Hazelgrove et al., 2001	1994–96	England	Up to 6 weeks PP	122,850	210 (0.17%)	7 (3.3%)	40/200 (20.0%)
DeMello & Restall, 1990	1985–89	England	20–42 weeks	9,425	13 (0.14%)	0	—
Ryan et al., 2000	1996–98	Ireland	—	26,164	17 (0.07%)	0	—
Stephens, 1991	1979–89	Australia	Up to 4 weeks PP	61,435	126 (0.21%)	1 (0.8%)	—
Bouvier-Colle et al., 1996	1991	France	Up to 6 wkees PP	140,000*	435 (0.31%)	22 (5.1%)	58 (13.3%)
Cohen et al., 2000	1994–98	Israel	20 weeks to 2 weeks PP	19,474	46 (0.24%)	1 (2.3%)	10 (22.6%)
Lewinsohn et al., 1994	8 yrs	Israel	—	—	58 (—)	4 (6.9%)	—
Tang et al., 1997	1988–95	China	Up to 6 weeks PP	39,350	49 (0.12%)	2 (4.1%)	4 (8.2%)
Ng et al., 1992	1985–90	China	Delivery related	16,264	37 (0.22%)	2 (5.4%)	—
Platteau et al., 1997	1992	South Africa	—	—	80 (—)	17 (21.3%)	39 (48.6%)
Summary (pooled data)				1,550,723	2,905 (0.19%)	162/3,234 (5.0%)	200/1,308 (15.3%)
Summary (adjusted for study size)					(0.17%)		

PP, postpartum; —, data not provided or unable to be calculated (these values excluded from summaries of columns).
* Estimate calculated based on data in paper.

primary admitting diagnoses. Specific organ system dysfunction was responsible for the majority of the remaining admissions. Of those, pulmonary, cardiac, and infectious complications had the greatest frequency. From these reports, it is apparent that both obstetric and medical complications of pregnancy are responsible for the ICU admissions in similar proportions. There were eight studies that provided information on 531 patients as to whether the primary admitting diagnosis was related to an obstetric complication or a medical complication (Mabie & Sibai, 1990; Kilpatrick & Matthay, 1992; Ng et al., 1992; Monoco et al., 1993; El-Sohl & Grant, 1996; Tang et al., 1997; Mahutte et al., 1999; Ryan et al., 2000). The pooled data indicate that 54.2% ($n = 288$) were classified as obstetric-related and 45.8% ($n = 243$) were due to medical complications. These data clearly highlight the complex nature of obstetric critical care illnesses and provide support for a multidisciplinary approach to management since these patients are quite ill with a variety of diseases.

Causes of mortality in obstetric intensive care unit admissions

When specific causes of mortality for the obstetric ICU admissions were reviewed, 16 studies gave sufficient data to assign a primary etiology for the maternal death (Mabie & Sibai, 1990; Stephens, 1991; Kilpatrick & Matthay, 1992; Ng et al., 1992; Collop & Sahn, 1993; Monoco et al., 1993; Bouvier-Colle et al., 1996; El-Sohl & Grant, 1996; Lapinsky et al., 1997; Platteau et al., 1997; Tang et al., 1997; Baskett & Sternadel, 1998; Mahutte et al., 1999; Cohen et al., 2000; Afessa et al., 2001; Hazelgrove et al., 2001) (Table 1.6). Of a total of 93 maternal deaths, over 50% were related to complications of hypertensive diseases, pulmonary illnesses, and cardiac diseases. Other deaths were commonly related to complications of hemorrhage, bleeding into the central nervous system, malignancy, and infection. More importantly, despite an identified

Table 1.5 Complications primarily responsible for admission to the intensive care unit for obstetric patients: data summarized from 18 published studies (Mabie & Sibai, 1990; Stephens, 1991; Kilpatrick & Matthay, 1992; Ng et al., 1992; Collop & Sahn, 1993; Monoco et al., 1993; Lewinsohn et al., 1994; El-Sohl & Grant, 1996; Lapinsky et al., 1997; Platteau et al., 1997; Tang et al., 1997; Baskett & Sternadel, 1998; Mahutte et al., 1999; Cohen et al., 2000; Ryan et al., 2000; Afessa et al., 2001; Hazelgrove et al., 2001)

Category	Category examples	N	Percentage
Hypertensive diseases	Eclampsia, preeclampsia, HELLP syndrome, hypertensive crisis	417	30.8
Hemorrhage	Shock, abruption, previa, postpartum hemorrhage	275	20.3
Pulmonary	Pulmonary edema, pneumonia, adult respiratory distress syndrome, asthma, thromboembolic diseases, amniotic fluid embolus,	176	13.0
Cardiac	Valvular disease, arrhythmia, cardiomyopathy, infarction	95	7.0
Sepsis/infection	Chorioamnionitis, pyelonephritis	90	6.7
Central nervous system	Intracranial hemorrhage, seizure (noneclamptic), arteriovenous malformation	44	3.2
Anesthesia complication	Allergic reaction, failed intubation, high spinal	43	3.2
Gastrointestinal	Pancreatitis, acute fatty liver of pregnancy, inflammatory bowel disease, gallbladder disease	28	2.1
Renal	Renal failure	23	1.7
Hematologic	Thrombotic thrombocytopenic purpura, sickle cell disease, disseminated intravascular coagulation, aspiration	17	1.3
Endocrine	Diabetic ketoacidosis, thyroid storm	15	1.1
Malignancy	Various	7	0.5
Other	Insufficient information to assign to specific organ system	123	9.1
Total		1,354	100%

primary etiology for the maternal deaths, nearly all cases were associated with multiorgan dysfunction, which again emphasizes the complex nature of these critically ill women.

As noted earlier, obstetric and medical complications of pregnancy are equally represented in all admissions to the ICU (Table 1.5). However, 30% of all maternal deaths in the ICU were directly related to obstetric conditions (hypertensive diseases and hemorrhage) with the remaining 70% of deaths due to medical conditions (Table 1.6).

Comparison of population-based with intensive care unit etiologies for mortality and morbidity

When considering the implications of critical illness for obstetric patients, the focus is usually on the mother. However, it is important to reemphasize that many of these conditions also may have a significant impact on fetal and neonatal outcomes. There is surprisingly little detailed information available on these outcomes in pregnancies complicated by critical illnesses. However, there are data on perinatal outcomes based on specific disease conditions. Maternal high-risk conditions associated with perinatal mortality in the United States are presented in Table 1.3. However, these data do not separate outcomes by severity of maternal illness. We were able to identify 12 studies that provided information on fetal or neonatal mortality rates for obstetric admissions to the ICU (Table 1.4). Fetal and/or neonatal deaths were identified in 200 of the pooled 1,308 cases, resulting in an overall mortality rate of 15.3% (Kilpatrick & Matthay, 1992; Collop & Sahn, 1993; Monoco et al., 1993; Bouvier-Colle et al., 1996; El-Sohl & Grant, 1996; Platteau et al., 1997; Tang et al., 1997; Mahutte et al., 1999; Cohen et al., 2000; Hogg et al., 2000; Afessa et al., 2001; Hazelgrove et al., 2001). This proportion may not reflect a true perinatal mortality rate since some of these losses may have occurred prior to 20 weeks gestation. In addition, the denominator includes a number of postpartum admissions for conditions not expected to impact fetal or neonatal mortality. Nevertheless, the high loss rate highlights the importance of considering the fetus when managing critical illnesses in pregnancy.

Summary

In summary, understanding the nature of critical illness in pregnancy is an important and evolving process. We have clearly grown beyond simple mortality reviews for assessment of pregnancy-related critical illness. However, our currently available tools and databases for examining these patients still need improvement. Reports of critically ill women admitted to the ICU have further refined our understanding of these diseases. However, targeted surveillance of obstetric ICU admissions is needed to identify variations in care and disease that may affect management. As our understanding of these conditions continues to mature, we will hopefully gain greater insight into the specific nature of these

Table 1.6 Identified primary causes of mortality in obstetric admissions to intensive care units reported in 16 studies (Mabie & Sibai, 1990; Stephens, 1991; Kilpatrick & Matthay, 1992; Ng et al., 1992; Collop & Sahn, 1993; Monoco et al., 1993; Bouvier-Colle et al., 1996; El-Sohl & Grant, 1996; Lapinsky et al., 1997; Platteau et al., 1997; Tang et al., 1997; Baskett & Sternadel, 1998; Mahutte et al., 1999; Cohen et al., 2000; Afessa et al., 2001; Hazelgrove et al., 2001)

Identified etiology	Number	Percentage
Hypertensive diseases Hypertensive crisis with renal failure, HELLP syndrome, complications, eclampsia complications, other hypertensive disease complications	20	21.5
Pulmonary Pneumonia complications, amniotic fluid embolus, adult respiratory distress syndrome, pulmonary embolus	20	21.5
Cardiac Eisenmenger's complex, myocardial infarction, arrhythmia cardiomyopathy, unspecified	11	11.8
Hemorrhage	8	8.6
Central nervous system hemorrhage Arteriovenous malformation, brain stem hemorrhage, intracranial hemorrhage	8	8.6
Infection Sepsis, tuberculosis meningitis	6	6.4
Malignancy	6	6.4
Hematologic Thrombotic thrombocytopenic purpura	2	2.2
Gastrointestinal Acute fatty liver of pregnancy	1	1.1
Poisoning	1	1.1
Anesthesia complication	1	1.1
Unspecified	9	9.7
Total	93	100%

conditions that will lead to improved prevention strategies and better therapies for the diseases when they occur. In our view, these data will improve our ability to plan and allocate the necessary resources to adequately care for these often complex and severe illnesses.

Acknowledgments

We would like to express our sincere appreciation to Anthony Vintzileos, MD, from the Division of Maternal-fetal Medicine, University of Medicine and Dentistry of New Jersey, for critically reviewing the manuscript and offering several comments that improved its contents. We also appreciate the efficient and excellent assistance of Susan Fosbre during the preparation of this manuscript and thank Laura Smulian for critically proof-reading the chapter.

References

Afessa B, Green B, Delke I, Koch K. Systemic inflammatory response syndrome, organ failure, and outcome in critically ill obstetric patients treated in an ICU. Chest 2001;120:1271–1277.

Atrash HK, Rowley D, Hogue CJ. Maternal and perinatal mortality. Curr Opin Obstet Gynecol 1992;4:61–71.

Baskett TF, Sternadel J. Maternal intensive care and near-miss mortality in obstetrics. Br J Obstet Gynaecol 1998;105:981–984.

Bennett TA, Kotelchuck M, Cox CE, Tucker MJ, Nadeau DA. Pregnancy-associated hospitalizations in the United States in 1991 and 1992: A comprehensive review of maternal morbidity. Am J Obstet Gynecol 1998;178:346–354.

Berg CJ, Atrash HK, Koonin LM, Tucker M. Pregnancy-related mortality in the United States, 1987–1990. Obstet Gynecol 1996;88:161–167.

Bouvier-Colle MH, Salanave B, Ancel PY, et al. Obstetric patients treated in intensive care units and maternal mortality. Regional teams for the survey. Eur J Obstet Gynecol Reprod Biol 1996;65: 121–125.

Cohen J, Singer P, Kogan A, Hod M, Bar J. Course and outcome of obstetric patients in a general intensive care unit. Acta Obstet Gynecol Scand 2000;79:846–850.

Collop NA, Sahn SA. Critical illness in pregnancy. An analysis of 20 patients admitted to a medical intensive care unit. Chest 1993;103:1548–1552.

DeMello WF, Restall J. The requirement of intensive care support for the pregnant population. Anesthesia 1990;45:888.

El-Solh AA, Grant BJ. A comparison of severity of illness scoring systems for critically ill obstetrics patients. Chest 1996;110:1299–1304.

Franks AL, Kendrick JS, Olson DR, Atrash HK, Saftlas AF, Moien M. Hospitalization for pregnancy complications, United States, 1986 and 1987. Am J Obstet Gynecol 1992;166:1339–1344.

Gilbert TT, Hardie R, Martin A, et al. (Abstract). Obstetric admissions to the intensive care unit: demographic and severity of illness analysis. Am J Respir Crit Care Med 2000;161:A236.

Harmer M. Maternal mortality—is it still relevant? Anaesthesia 1997;52:99–100.

Hazelgrove JF, Price C, Pappachan GD. Multicenter study of obstetric admissions to 14 intensive care units in southern England. Crit Care Med 2001;29:770–775.

Hogg B, Hauth JC, Kimberlin D, Brumfield C, Cliver S. Intensive care unit utilization during pregnancy. Obstet Gynecol 2000;95 (Suppl):62S.

Kilpatrick SJ, Matthay MA. Obstetric patients requiring critical care. A five-year review. Chest 1992;101:1407–1412.

Knaus WA, Draper EA, Wagner DP, Zimmerman JE. An evaluation of outcome from intensive care in major medical centers. Ann Intern Med 1986;104:410–418.

Koonin LM, MacKay AP, Berg CJ, Atrash HK, Smith JC. Pregnancy-related mortality surveillance—United States, 1987–1990. MMWR, Morbidity and Mortality Weekly Report 1997;46:17–36.

Lapinsky SE, Kruczynski K, Seaward GR, Farine D, Grossman RF. Critical care management of the obstetric patient. Can J Anaesth 1997;44:325–329.

Lewinsohn G, Herman A, Lenov Y, Klinowski E. Critically ill obstetrical patients: Outcome and predictability. Crit Care Med 1994;22: 1412–1414.

Mabie WC, Sibai BM. Treatment in an obstetric intensive care unit. Am J Obstet Gynecol 1990;162:1–4.

MacDorman MF, Atkinson JO. Infant mortality statistics from the linked birth/infant death data set—1995 period data. Mon Vital Stat Rep 1998 Feb 26;46(6 Suppl 2):1–22.

Mahutte NG, Murphy-Kaulbeck L, Le Q, Solomon J, Benjamin A, Boyd ME. Obstetrics admissions to the intensive care unit. Obstet Gynecol 1999;94:263–266.

Mantel GD, Buchmann E, Rees H, Pattinson RC. Severe acute maternal morbidity: A pilot study of a definition for a near-miss. Br J Obstet Gynaecol 1998;105:985–990.

Mertz KJ, Parker AL, Halpin GJ. Pregnancy-related mortality in New Jersey, 1975–1989. Am J Public Health 1992;82:1085–1088.

Monoco TJ, Spielman FJ, Katz VL. Pregnant patients in the intensive care unit: a descriptive analysis. South Med J 1993;86:414–417.

Morbidity and Mortality Weekly Report—MMWR. Maternal mortality—United States, 1982–1996. US Department of Health and Human Services 1998;47:705–707.

Morbidity and Mortality Weekly Report—MMWR. Pregnancy-related deaths among Hispanic, Asian/Pacific Islander, and American Indian/Alaska Native women—United States, 1991–1997. US Department of Health and Human Services 2001;50: 361–364.

National Center for Health Statistics. Healthy people 2000 review, 1992. Hyattsville, MD: US Department of Health and Human Services, Public Health Service, CDC, 1993.

National Center for Health Statistics. Design and operation of the National Hospital Discharge Survey: 1988 redesign. Series I. Programs and collection procedures. US Department of Health and Human Services, CDC 2000; DHHS Publication 2001-1315 (number 39).

Ng Tl, Lim E, Tweed WA, Arulkumaran S. Obstetric admissions to the intensive care unit—a retrospective review. Ann Acad Med Singapore 1992;21:804–806.

Panchal S, Arria AM, Harris AP. Intensive care utilization during hospital admission for delivery: Prevalence, risk factors, and outcomes in a statewide population. Anesthesiology 2000;92:1537–1544.

Platteau P, Engelhardt T, Moodley J, Muckart DJ. Obstetric and gynaecological patients in an intensive care unit: A 1 year review. Trop Doctor 1997; 27:202–206.

Ryan M, Hamilton V, Bowen M, McKenna P. The role of a high-dependency unit in a regional obstetric hospital. Anaesthesia 2000;55:1155–1158.

Sachs BP, Brown DA, Driscoll SG, et al. Maternal mortality in Massachusetts: trends and prevention. N Engl J Med 1987;316: 667–672.

Scott CL, Chavez GF, Atrash HK, Taylor DJ, Shah RS, Rowley D. Hospitalizations for severe complications of pregnancy, 1987–1992. Obstet Gynecol 1997;90:225–229.

Stephens ID. ICU admissions from an obstetrical hospital. Can J Anaesth 1991;38:677–681.

Syverson CJ, Chavkin W, Atrash HK, Rochat RW, Sharp ES, King GE. Pregnancy-related mortality in New York City, 1980 to1984: Causes of death and associated factors. Am J Obstet Gynecol 1991;164: 603–608.

Taffel S, Johnson D, Heuser R. A method of imputing length of gestation on birth certificates. Vital Health Stat 2, 1982 May;93:1–11.

Tang LC, Kwok AC, Wong AY, Lee YY, Sun KO, So AP. Critical care in obstetrical patients: An eight-year review. Chinese Med J (English) 1997;110:936–941.

World Health Organization. Maternal mortality: A global factbook. Geneva: World Health Organization, 1991.

2 Organizing a critical care obstetric unit

Cornelia R. Graves

The discipline of *intensive care* dates from the 1952 Copenhagen polio epidemic. During this time doctors were able to reduce patient morbidity and mortality by caring for patients in a specific area of the hospital instead of across different wards (Bennett & Bion, 1999). The discipline of *critical care* arose from the need to observe patients more closely in the postoperative period. In 1863, Florence Nightingale established small areas near the operating room for patients recovering from surgery (Mabie & Sibai, 1990). It was noted that having an attendant at the bedside improved quality of care.

Since the first critical care unit was established in the United States in 1958, there has been a proliferation of critical care units in this country and around the world. It is now estimated that there are over 800 units in the United States alone. Critical care units have expanded such that each unit meets a certain patient population and need. For example, data show that children cared for in an adult intensive care unit fare less well than those cared for in a dedicated pediatric facility (Pollack et al., 1991). The benefits of units established to address the unique needs of patients with neurological injury, complex medical diseases, and/or surgical complications are clearly established.

The evolution of critical care for the obstetric patient began in the late 1970s. van Geldren reported a 10-month experience of managing patients in a maternal intensive care unit (ICU) in South Africa (van Gelderen, 1978). In the same year, Young and colleagues reported their 3-year experience, citing a reduction in perinatal mortality. Their experience led to the conclusion that the obstetric-ICU system provided the ideal mechanism for optimizing maternal and fetal outcomes (Young, 1978). Since that time, there has been increasing knowledge regarding the complex interactions between pregnancy-induced physiologic changes, fetal response, and the effects of critical illness. In addition, maternal–fetal medicine fellowship programs have begun to emphasize the need for specialists to be able to attend to the unique requirements of the critically ill mother and her fetus. It is against this backdrop that many labor and delivery (L&D) units have attempted to establish facilities to address another unique population of critically ill patients.

Evaluating your patient population

In 1992, indications for the use of invasive central hemodynamic monitoring (Swan–Ganz catheter) were outline by the American College of Obstetricians and Gynecologists (1992). Conditions for which invasive monitoring may be of assistance in the obstetric population include sepsis, preeclampsia with persistent oliguria or pulmonary edema, cardiovascular decompensation, massive blood loss, certain cardiac diseases, adult respiratory distress syndrome, and shock.

Academic referral centers may provide care for up to 100 patients per year who would qualify for obstetric intensive care services. Smaller units may rarely deal with this patient population. In considering the need for critical care facilities, it is important to keep in mind the following factors. A small patient base may not provide sufficient clinical experience to maintain a fully trained staff of critical care providers. While a large patient population may allow the staff to maintain their skills, patients requiring long-term critical care services on a busy L&D unit may stress the staff and lead to a decrease in the quality of care for the general L&D patient population. In addition, the continuing debate regarding health care quality versus cost remains an issue unanswered. It has been estimated that 1% of the obstetric population would require specialized obstetric intensive care services in order for the unit to be economically feasible (Mabie & Sibai, 1990).

Staffing

Once the need for an intensive care unit has been established, staffing becomes the next priority. The staff should consist of a multidisciplinary team which includes nurses, physicians, respiratory therapists, pharmacists, and ancillary health care members. Each member of the team should understand the issues of providing critical care to the obstetric patient and her family.

Nursing

The critical care obstetric nurse is an integral part of the team. Critical care nursing traditionally includes but is not limited to the roles of the staff nurse, nurse manager, clinical nurse specialist, and acute care nurse practitioner (Brilli et al., 2001). Critical care nurses perform the majority of patient assessment, evaluation, and care in the intensive care unit. In obstetrics, the patient-to-nurse ratio is usually 1 : 1, as the obstetric critical care nurse must not only monitor the mother but also the fetus. If the patient is in labor, we have found in our experience, that a ratio of 1 : 2 may provide optimal care to the patient and her fetus.

The bedside nurse should partner with the physician to provide care and oversee and communicate the plan of care. The maternal–fetal nurse has a unique understanding of the issues that are involved in taking care of the critically ill obstetric patient.

Organization of the nursing staff requires evaluating the unit needs and determining which obstetric nurses may be interested in long-term critical care. Some units are staffed by a separate set of nurses who control their own schedules to insure availability on a 24-hour basis (Mabie & Sibai, 1990). Other units have designated nursing staff that function in the regular rotation, insuring that a critical care obstetric nurse is available at all times. Because few units have a large volume of critically ill obstetric patients, all nursing staff are required to have some basic knowledge of obstetric physiology, hemodynamic monitoring, and electronic fetal monitoring. The staff should have at least a year of experience in a labor and delivery unit. Formal instruction in obstetric intensive care is recommended. All nurses are encouraged to become certified in advanced life support techniques. In addition, continuing medical education is strongly suggested to keep the staff abreast of the latest technology.

Nursing responsibilities in the care of the critically ill obstetric patient are expanded dramatically. Besides assisting in the medical needs of the critically ill obstetric patient, the nurse should be able to guide the patient's family members through the waves of anxiety that accompany severe illness. As only a minority of childbearing women experience complications that require intensive care during pregnancy, and because having a baby is usually not perceived by patients and their families as life-threatening in current times, the psychosocial needs are unique. Because obstetric patients tend to be young, many patients and their families have not given thought to end-of-life issues. If delivery of a healthy infant has occurred, thought must be given to the long-term care plans of the infant if the mother has a lengthy illness and remains hospitalized after discharge of the neonate. Special care should be taken to educate the patient and her family on the illness, the treatment that may be necessary, and the outcome that can be expected for both the mother and the fetus (May & Salyer, 1992).

Physician staffing

In order for the critical care obstetric unit to function to its fullest, there must be a maternal–fetal medicine specialist or specialists that have experience and interest in taking care of the critically ill obstetric patient. They should have a full understanding of obstetric physiology, hemodynamic monitoring, and the impact of pregnancy on disease states. The physician should be able to communicate well with the staff and take an interest in the function of the unit. While one specialist can, with the assistance of the nursing staff, take care of all the patients in the unit, the availability of a group of perinatalogists ensures that physician "burn-out" does not become an issue if long-term care is foreseen.

Most units have a medical director, who is responsible for running the unit. The director should also assist in obtaining continuing medical education for all of the staff in the unit. We have found that monthly meetings allow the staff to address issues and to debrief others about patient care concerns. The medical director should have considerable critical care experience in addition to specialized training in maternal–fetal medicine.

Other staffing

Designated anesthesia staff are a necessity for the proper functioning of the unit. In addition to providing pain management services, the anesthesiologist can offer valuable advice regarding airway and ventilator management. A dedicated respiratory therapist is also needed to assist in ventilator changes and management. Because of the needs of immediate access to pressors and other medications, a satellite pharmacy is recommended. The neonatalogist should be continually updated regarding fetal issues including maternal medications that may affect fetal resuscitation.

In addition to the staff mentioned above, access to a nutritionist, pulmonologist and cardiologist who have experience with the critically ill obstetric patient is required. Staff that are frequently overlooked but that are integral in caring for the patient include a social worker and a chaplin to aid in addressing long-term care needs and end-of-life issues.

Designing the unit

Few hospitals have critical care units designed for the critically ill obstetric patient. In fact, a review of the literature published to date has failed to identify any reports on the efforts required to set up an obstetric ICU. While the patient population which may benefit from an obstetric ICU has been targeted, the challenges of setting up and designing a unit remain uncharted.

As the care of two patients is involved, the unit should be organized so that both sets of needs can be met. The phrase, "form follows function", should be the basis for the design of any unit. As each state has different regulations regarding the actual structure of the unit (windows, etc.), the purpose of this section will be to give general guidelines for design.

There are three aspects that should be addressed when taking care of the critically ill obstetric patient. The first is the need for invasive maternal monitoring. Numerous studies have supported the use of invasive monitoring in the treatment of the critically ill obstetric patient (Gilbert et al., 2000). Pulmonary artery catherization has been proved to be a safe and effective way of monitoring this population. Arterial catherization can also be utilized to assist in gathering data to stabilize the patient. Therefore, bedspace is of paramount importance in allowing adequate care to be delivered. In the nonobstetric literature, 200–250 square feet have been recommended for private room design. In addition, the room should be organized so that the nurses, physicians, therapists, and others can have easy access to the patient. Central monitoring, while not a necessity, reduces the need for 1 : 1 nursing for critical care patients who have been stabilized and do not require continued nursing support.

The second aspect that should be addressed is the need for specialized treatments. Mechanical ventilation is the most common treatment that is required in the critically ill obstetric population. Gases and appropriate connections should be available and easily accessible in order to facilitate rapid changes in patient management. On occasion, space is needed for other equipment, such as dialysis or neurological monitoring. In some situations, consideration should be given to portable anesthesia equipment to be used if an emergency delivery needs to be performed.

The third aspect is the ability to monitor and intervene on behalf of the fetus. The need to manage two patients and to rapidly assess the risk : benefit of the mother or the fetus, makes the discipline of critical care obstetrics unique. Central fetal monitoring is preferable as this allows others to monitor the fetal status in addition to the assigned nurse. The ability to deliver the patient, whether she is having a vaginal delivery or a cesarean section, without having to transfer her to another room is also desirable.

The unit should be designed so that immediate assistance for the primary nurse is available. The unit should have a feel of community. The number of beds needed should be determined by the patient population. Rapid lab and radiographic access are essential in order to provide assistance in treating the patient's ever-changing status.

In some centers, a recovery room can be transformed into a critical care area by moving mobile monitors for critical care services.

The Task Force on Critical Care has provided specific guidelines for the development of an ICU. These guidelines should be reviewed prior to meeting with the design team. A multidisciplinary approach involving physicians, nursing, and ancillary staff will allow for each area to address their concerns and to provide valuable input (Task Force on Guidelines, 1988).

Maintaining the unit

As the number of critically ill obstetric patients is relatively small, maintaining the facility and staff competency may be the greatest challenge. Panchal et al. (2000) noted that the ICU admission rate for obstetric patients who were delivered in Maryland was 0.12%. At Vanderbilt Hospital, approximately 1–3% of our patient population requires critical care obstetric services. However, only 0.5% of these patients will require long-term care. Frequently, patients present in clusters so that the staff may go long periods of time without managing such a patient. Competencies can be maintained through continuing medical education. Several courses that specifically address critical care issues, offered throughout the USA and Europe, facilitate obtaining and maintaining nursing competency. Pairing with another unit, such as a surgical intensive care unit, can allow nurses to exchange information and to maintain technical skills.

Staff burn-out can be minimized in a number of ways. One way is to have a large number of qualified staff available in order to facilitate shift rotation and relief. This is a difficult task because of the small number of patients as previously mentioned. Another solution is to have different levels of skilled care available, so that the staff qualified and trained to take care of the sickest of patients will not need to take care of every patient that needs invasive monitoring. Therefore, all staff might be trained in arterial line monitoring in a large territory care unit, freeing up other staff to assist with central hemodynamic monitoring.

Taking care of critically ill obstetric patients in other units

The utilization of ICU resources for the critically ill obstetric patient may vary among patient populations. Therefore, it may not be efficacious for every hospital to have a separate intensive care facility for the critically ill obstetric patient. Critical care interventions are expensive and have a narrow margin of safety (Hanson et al., 1999). In addition, outcome data are particularly difficult to assess, given current techniques that are standard of care.

In the era of cost-effectiveness, not all hospitals will have the desire to allocate resources to a separate or designated area for critically ill obstetric patients. Therefore, these patients may need to be transferred to surgical or medical intensive care units within the facility, or out to another hospital. Because of limited space in many L&D areas, critically ill obstetric patients that have been delivered are often transferred to other units for long-term care.

Preeclampsia, eclampsia, and massive hemorrhage are common conditions requiring intensive care admission (Gilbert et al., 2000). These complications and the normal physiological changes in pregnancy are unique to our patient population. Lastly, it should be remembered that delivery does not immediately reverse pregnancy physiology which may persist up to 4 weeks after delivery.

When it is necessary to transfer these patients for care in other units, continued involvement of those who are knowledgeable in obstetric pathophysiology and complications is essential in order to provide optimal care. Ideally, a multidisciplinary approach involving obstetric and critical care personel will be required to address needs as they arise. If the patient remains undelivered, then special attention should be given to fetal monitoring and bedside delivery capabilities in case of an obstetric emergency.

The bottom line

While there are little formal data regarding the establishment of a critical care obstetric unit, there are a number of units or designated areas in existence. Each of these units has a different set of issues to address. However, the goal of every unit should be to offer optimal care to its patients. Due to the relatively small numbers in this population and numerous other limitations, it has been difficult to assess whether patients in an obstetric ICU have any different outcome that those treated in standard units.

The theoretical advantages of maintaining critically ill patients in an obstetric setting have been noted in the literature (Mabie & Sibai, 1990). Perinatalogists, anesthesiologists, and others who are involved in the care of these patients recognize that many issues in this population are more easily addressed in facilities that are prepared to specifically respond to the complications that are unique to pregnancy and the puerperium. A better understanding of maternal physiology and applicable pharmacology results in prompt treatment. Closer nursing supervision and organization of the unit may assist in early recognition of complications. Continuity of care can be maintained before and after delivery. The importance of bonding, breastfeeding, and family involvement are more easily addressed in an environment familiar with these issues. The unit also allows for focused training of perinatal fellows and obstetric residents in complex complications of pregnancy.

As the maternal population ages and general medical care improves, the need for critical care obstetric services will continue to increase. It is through our understanding of this complex patient population that an impact will possibly be made toward reducing perinatal morbidity and mortality.

References

American College of Obstetricians and Gynaecologists. *Hemodynamic Monitoring in Pregnancy*. Technical Bulletin No. 175. American College of Obstetricians and Gynecologist, Washington DC, 1992.

Bennett D, Bion J. ABC of intensive care: Organisation of intensive care. BMJ 1999;318(1796):1468–1470.

Brilli RJ, Spevetz A, Branson RD, et al. Critical care delivery in the intensive care unit: Defining clinical roles and the best practice model. Crit Care Med 2001;29(10):2007–2019.

van Gelderen CJ. Maternal intensive care. S Afr Med J 1978;53(21):838–841.

Gilbert W, Towner DR, Field NT, Anthony JMB. The safety and utility of pulmonary artery catherization in severe preeclampsia and eclampsia. Am J Obstet Gynecol 2000;182(6):1397–1403.

Hanson CW, Deutschman CS, Anderson HL, et al. Effects of an organized critical care service on outcomes and resource utilization: A cohort study. Crit Care Med 1999;27(2):270–274.

Mabie WC, Sibai BM. Treatment in an obstetrical intensive care unit. Am J Obstet Gynecol 1990;162(1):1–4.

May KA, Salyer S. Psychosocial implications of high-risk intrapartum care. In: Mandeville LK, Troiano NH, eds. High Risk and Critical Care Nursing. JB Lippincott, 1992:51–64.

Panchal S, Arria AM, Harris AP. Intensive care utilization during hospital admission for delivery: Prevalence, risks factors and outcomes in a statewide population. Anesthesiology 2000;92(6):1537–1544.

Pollack MM, Alexander SR, Clarke N, et al. Improved outcomes from a tertiary center pediatric intensive care: A statewide comparison of tertiary and nontertiary care facilities. Crit Care Med 1991;19: 150–159.

Task Force on Guidelines, Society of Critical Medicine. Recommendations for critical care unit design. Crit Care Med 1988;16:796–806.

Young RK, Weinstein HN, Katz M. Intrapartum maternal and fetal monitoring: the obstetrical intensive care unit. Int J Gynaecol Obsetet 1978;15(6):526–529.

II Pregnancy physiology

3 Pregnancy-induced physiologic alterations

Errol R. Norwitz
Julian N. Robinson
Fergal D. Malone

Physiologic adaptations occur in the mother in response to the demands of pregnancy. These demands include support of the fetus (volume support, nutritional and oxygen supply, and clearance of fetal waste), protection of the fetus (from starvation, drugs, toxins), preparation of the uterus for labor, and protection of the mother from potential cardiovascular injury at delivery. Variables such as maternal age, multiple gestation, ethnicity, and genetic factors affect the ability of the mother to adapt to the demands of pregnancy. All maternal systems are required to adapt; however, the quality, degree, and timing of the adaptation varies from one individual to another and from one organ system to another. This chapter serves to review in detail the normal physiologic adaptations that occur within each of the major maternal organ systems. A detailed discussion of fetal physiology is beyond the scope of this review. A better understanding of the normal physiologic adaptations of pregnancy will improve the ability of clinicians to anticipate the effects of pregnancy on underlying medical conditions and to manage pregnancy-associated complications.

Cardiovascular system

Critical illnesses that compromise the cardiovascular system are among the most challenging problems affecting pregnant women. When evaluating patients for cardiovascular compromise, it is important to be aware of the pregnancy-associated changes and how these changes influence the various maternal hemodynamic variables, including blood volume, blood pressure (BP), heart rate, stroke volume, cardiac output, and systemic vascular resistance (SVR). Factors such as maternal age, multiple pregnancy, gestational age, body habitus, positioning, labor, and blood loss may further complicate the management of such patients. This section reviews in detail the effects of pregnancy on the maternal cardiovascular system, and the relevance of this information in the management of the critically ill obstetric patient.

Blood volume

Maternal plasma volume increases by 10% as early as the 7th week of pregnancy. As summarized in Fig. 3.1, this increase reaches a plateau of around 45–50% at 32 weeks, remaining stable thereafter until delivery (McLennon & Thouin, 1948; Caton et al., 1951; Hytten & Paintin, 1963; Lund & Donovan, 1967; Scott, 1972; Clapp et al., 1988). Although the magnitude of the hypervolemia varies considerably between women, there is a tendency for the same plasma volume expansion pattern to be repeated during successive pregnancies in the same woman (Pritchard, 1965a; Lund & Donovan, 1967). Moreover, the magnitude of the hypervolemia varies with the number of fetuses (Pritchard, 1965a; Rovinsky & Jaffin, 1965). In a longitudinal study comparing blood volume estimations during term pregnancy with that in the same patient after pregnancy, Pritchard (1965a) demonstrated that blood volume in a singleton pregnancy increased by an average of 1,570 mL (+48%) as compared with 1,960 mL in a twin pregnancy (Table 3.1). There is a similar but less pronounced increase in red cell mass during pregnancy (Fig. 3.1), likely due to the stimulatory effect of placental hormones (chorionic somatomammotropin, progesterone, and possibly prolactin) on maternal erythropoiesis (Jepson, 1968; Letsky, 1995). These changes account for the maternal dilutional anemia that develops in pregnancy despite seemingly adequate iron stores (Cavill, 1995). Hemodilution is maximal at around 30–32 weeks of gestation.

The physiologic advantage of maternal hemodilution of pregnancy remains unclear. It may have a beneficial effect on the uteroplacental circulation by decreasing blood viscosity, thereby improving uteroplacental perfusion and possibly preventing stasis and resultant placental thrombosis (Koller, 1982). Blood volume changes are closely related to maternal morbidity, and hypervolemia likely serves as a protective mechanism against excessive blood loss at delivery. Preeclamptic women, for example, are less tolerant of peripartum blood loss, because they have a markedly reduced intravascular volume as compared with normotensive parturients, due primarily to an increase in capillary permeability

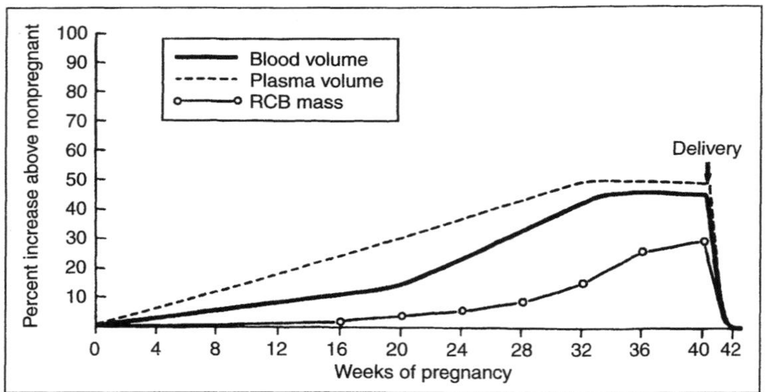

Fig. 3.1 Blood volume changes during pregnancy. (Reproduced by permission from Scott DE. Anemia during pregnancy. Obstet Gynecol Annu 1972;1:219.)

Table 3.1 Blood and red-cell volumes in normal women late in pregnancy and again when not pregnant

	Late pregnancy	Nonpregnant	Increase (mL)	Increase (%)
Single fetus (n = *50*)				
Blood volume	4,820	3,250	1,570	48
RBC volume	1,790	1,355	430	32
Hematocrit	37.0	41.7	—	—
Twins (n = *30*)				
Blood volume	5,820	3,865	1,960	51
RBC volume	2,065	1,580	485	31
Hematocrit	35.5	41.0	—	—

(Reproduced by permission from Pritchard JA. Changes in the blood volume during pregnancy and delivery. Anesthesiology 1965;26:393.)

(Table 3.2) (Pritchard et al., 1984). Normal maternal blood volume expansion also appears to be important for fetal growth. Salas et al. (1993) compared maternal plasma volume as measured by Evans blue dye dilution in term pregnancies with normal and growth-restricted fetuses. Pregnancies complicated by fetal intrauterine growth restriction (IUGR) had significantly lower mean maternal plasma volumes as compared with pregnancies with well grown fetuses (2,976 ± 76 mL vs 3,594 ± 103 mL, respectively).

The physiologic mechanisms responsible for these pregnancy-associated changes in blood volume are not fully understood. Pregnancy may best be regarded as a state of volume overload resulting primarily from renal sodium and water retention, with a shift of fluid from the intravascular to the extravascular space. Indeed, in addition to fetal growth, a substantial part of maternal weight gain during pregnancy results from fluid accumulation. Unlike other arterial vasodilatory states, pregnancy is associated with an increase in renal glomerular filtration and filtered sodium load (Schrier & Briner, 1991), leading to an increase in urinary sodium and water excretion (Oparil et al., 1975). To prevent excessive fluid loss and resultant compromise to uteroplacental perfusion, mineralocorticoid activity increases to promote sodium and water retention by the distal renal tubules. The increased mineralocorticoid activity results primarily from extra-adrenal conversion of progesterone to deoxycorticosterone (Winkel et al., 1980). It is also possible that another as yet unidentified vasodilator(s) may be responsible for the volume expansion, since studies in pregnant baboons have demonstrated that systemic vasodilation precedes the measured increase in maternal blood volume (Phippard et al., 1986). The net result of these two opposing mechanisms is an accumulation during

Table 3.2 Blood volume changes in five women

	Nonpregnant	Normal pregnancy	Eclampsia
Blood volume (mL)	3,035	4,425	3,530
Change (%)*	—	+47	+16
Hematocrit (%)	38.2	34.7	40.5

Blood volume estimation (chromium 51) during antepartum eclampsia, again when non-pregnant, and finally at a comparable time in a second pregnancy uncomplicated by hypertension.
* Change in blood volume (%) as compared with non-pregnant women.
(Adapted by permission from Pritchard JA, Cunningham FG, Pritchard SA. The Parkland Memorial Hospital protocol for treatment of eclampsia: evaluation of 245 cases. Am J Obstet Gynecol 1984;148:951.)

pregnancy of approximately 500–900 mEq of sodium and 6–8 L of total body water (Seitchik, 1967; Lindheimer & Katz, 1973).

There is also evidence to suggest that the fetus may contribute to the increase in maternal plasma volume. Placental estrogens are known to promote aldosterone production by directly activating the renin–angiotensin system, and the capacity of the placenta to synthesize estrogens is dependent in large part on the availability of estrogen precursor (dehydroepiandrosterone) from the fetal adrenal. As such, the fetus may regulate maternal plasma volume through its effect on the placental renin–angiotensin system (Longo & Hardesty, 1984). In support of this mechanism, pregnancies complicated by IUGR have lower circulating levels of aldosterone and other vasodilator substances (prostacyclin, kallikrein) as compared with pregnancies with well-grown fetuses (Salas et al., 1993). However, the fetus is not essential for the development of gestational hypervolemia, because it develops also in complete molar pregnancies (Pritchard, 1965b).

Blood pressure

Blood pressure (BP) is the product of cardiac output and SVR, and reflects the ability of the cardiovascular system to maintain perfusion to the various organ systems, including the fetoplacental unit. Maternal BP is influenced by several factors, including gestational age, measurement technique, and positioning.

Gestational age is an important factor when evaluating BP in pregnancy. For example, a maternal sitting BP of 130/84 mmHg would be considered normal at term, but concerningly high at 20 weeks of gestation. A sustained elevation in BP of ≥140/90 should be regarded as abnormal at any stage of pregnancy. Earlier reports suggested that an increase in BP of ≥30 mmHg systolic or ≥15 mmHg diastolic over first or early second trimester BP should be used to define hypertension; however, this concept is no longer valid since many women exhibit such changes in normal pregnancy (Villar & Sibai, 1989; ACOG, 1996).

BP normally decreases approximately 10% by the 7th week of pregnancy (Clapp et al., 1988). This is likely due to systemic vasodilatation resulting from hormonal (progesterone) changes in early pregnancy. Indeed, studies in baboons have shown that the fall in arterial BP that occurs very early in pregnancy is due entirely to the decrease in SVR (Phippard et al., 1986). The resultant increase in cardiac output does not fully compensate for the diminished afterload, thereby providing a reasonable explanation for a lower mean arterial BP during the first trimester.

Systolic and diastolic BP continue to decrease until mid-pregnancy, and then gradually recover to nonpregnant values by term. A longitudinal study of 69 women during normal pregnancy demonstrated that the lowest arterial BP occur at around 28 weeks of gestation (Fig. 3.2) (Wilson et al., 1980). BP measurements can be affected by maternal positioning. In this same series, BP was lowest when measured with the patient in the left lateral decubitus position, and increased by approximately 14 mmHg when patients were rotated into the supine position (Wilson et al., 1980) (Fig. 3.3). Despite the difference in absolute measurements, the pattern of BP change throughout pregnancy was unaffected (Fig. 3.3) For the sake of consistency and standardization, all BP measurements in pregnancy should be taken with the patient in the sitting position.

BP measurements are also subject to change depending on the technique used to attain the measurements. In a series of 70 pregnant women, Ginsberg and Duncan (1969) demonstrated

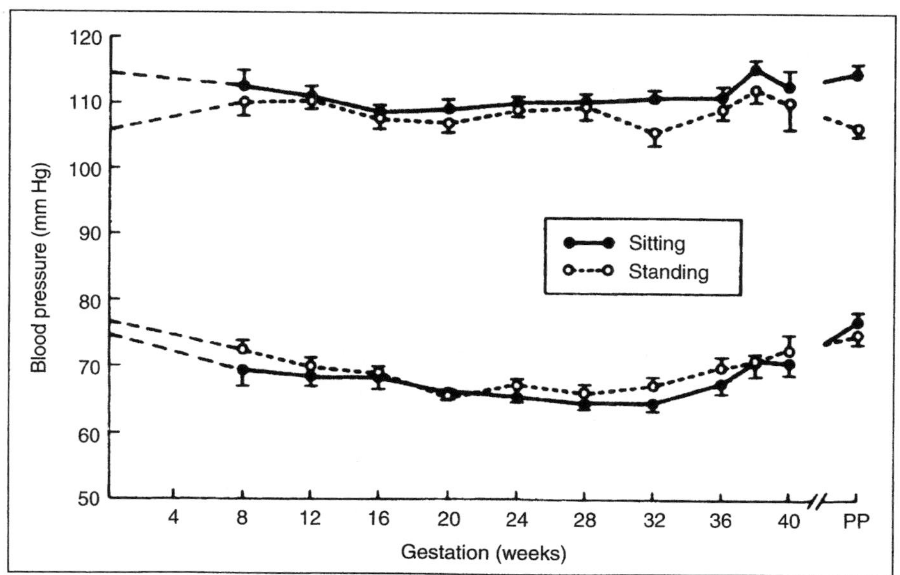

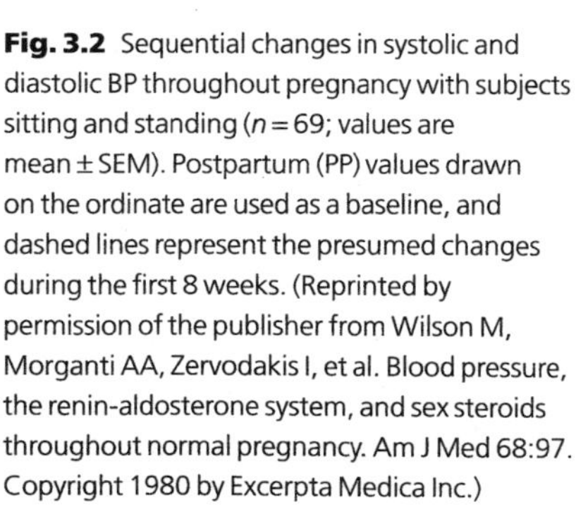
Fig. 3.2 Sequential changes in systolic and diastolic BP throughout pregnancy with subjects sitting and standing ($n = 69$; values are mean ± SEM). Postpartum (PP) values drawn on the ordinate are used as a baseline, and dashed lines represent the presumed changes during the first 8 weeks. (Reprinted by permission of the publisher from Wilson M, Morganti AA, Zervodakis I, et al. Blood pressure, the renin-aldosterone system, and sex steroids throughout normal pregnancy. Am J Med 68:97. Copyright 1980 by Excerpta Medica Inc.)

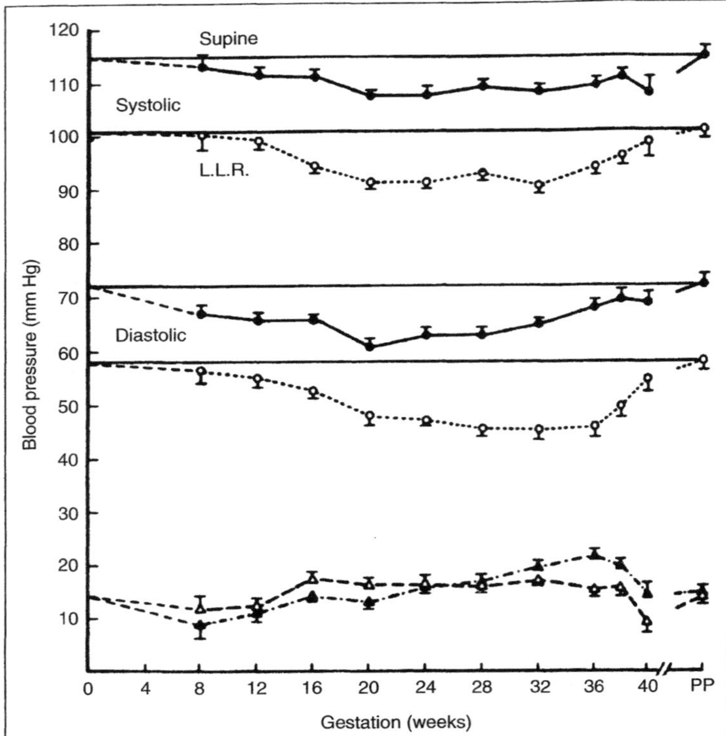

Fig. 3.3 Sequential changes in BP throughout pregnancy with subjects in the supine and left lateral decubitus positions ($n = 69$; values are mean ± SEM). The calculated change in systolic (open triangles) and diastolic (closed triangles) BP produced by repositioning from the left lateral decubitus to the supine position is illustrated. LLR, left lateral recumbent; PP, postpartum. (Reprinted by permission of the publisher from Wilson M, Morganti AA, Zervodakis I, et al. Blood pressure, the renin-aldosterone system, and sex steroids throughout normal pregnancy. Am J Med 68:97. Copyright 1980 by Excerpta Medica Inc.)

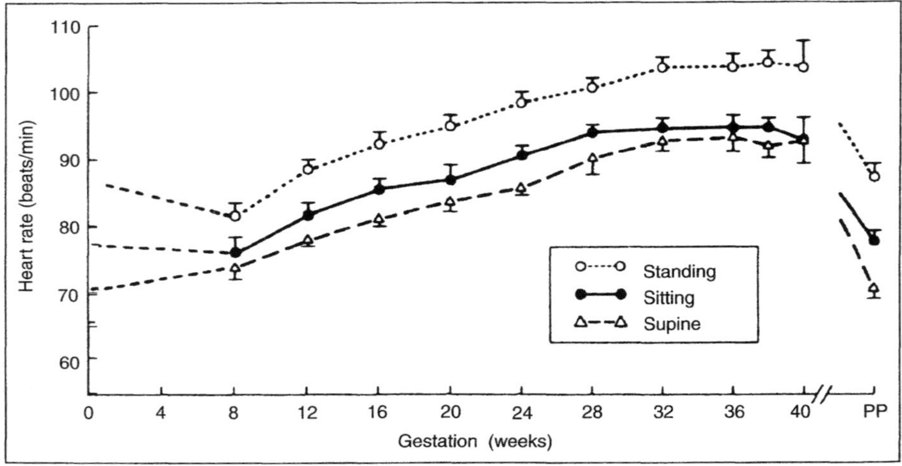

Fig. 3.4 Sequential changes in mean heart rate in three positions throughout pregnancy ($n = 69$; values are mean ± SEM). PP, postpartum. (Reprinted by permission of the publisher from Wilson M, Morganti AA, Zervodakis I, et al. Blood pressure, the renin-aldosterone system, and sex steroids throughout normal pregnancy. Am J Med 68:97. Copyright 1980 by Excerpta Medica Inc.)

that mean systolic and diastolic BP were lower (by −6 mmHg and −15 mmHg, respectively) when measurements were taken directly using a radial intra-arterial line as compared with indirect measurements using a standard sphygmomanometer. Conversely, Kirshon and colleagues (1987) found a significantly lower systolic (but not diastolic) BP when using an automated sphygmomanometer as compared with direct radial intra-arterial measurements in a series of 12 postpartum patients.

Heart rate

Maternal heart rate increases as early as the 7th week of pregnancy and by late pregnancy is increased approximately 20% as compared with postpartum values (Wilson et al., 1980) (Fig. 3.4). It is likely that the increase in heart rate is a secondary (compensatory) effect resulting from the decline in SVR during pregnancy (Duvekot et al., 1993). However, a direct effect of hormonal factors cannot be entirely excluded. Although human chorionic gonadotropin (hCG) is an unlikely candidate (Glinoer et al., 1990), free thyroxine levels increase by 10 weeks and remain elevated throughout pregnancy (Harada et al., 1979; Glinoer et al., 1990). The possibility that thyroid hormones may be responsible for the maternal tachycardia warrants further investigation.

In addition to pregnancy-associated changes, maternal tachycardia can also result from other causes (such as fever, pain, blood loss, hyperthyroidism, respiratory insufficiency, and cardiac disease) which may have important clinical implications for critically ill parturients. For example, women with severe mitral stenosis must rely on diastolic ventricular filling to achieve satisfactory cardiac output. Because left ventricular diastolic filling is heart rate dependent, maternal tachycardia can severely limit the capacity of such women to maintain an adequate BP, and can lead to cardiovascular shock and fetal distress. As such, the management of patients with severe mitral stenosis should include, among other parameters, careful control of maternal heart rate and cardiac preload.

Cardiac output and stroke volume

Cardiac output is the product of heart rate and stroke volume, and reflects the overall capacity of the left ventricle to maintain systemic BP and thereby organ perfusion. Cardiac index is calculated by dividing cardiac output by body surface area (Table 3.3). Although useful in nonpregnant women, cardiac index is less useful in pregnant women, because the normal correlation between cardiac output and body surface area is lost in pregnancy (van Oppen et al., 1995). This may be explained, in part, by the observation that the Du Bois and Du Bois (1916) body surface area nomogram widely used to calculate cardiac index is based on nine nongravid subjects and, as such, may not apply to pregnant women.

Linhard (1915) was the first to report a 50% increase in cardiac output during pregnancy using the indirect Fick method. Others have studied maternal cardiac output by invasive catheterization (Hamilton, 1949; Palmer & Walker, 1949; Bader et al., 1955; Clark et al., 1989), dye dilution (Walters et al., 1966; Lees et al., 1967; Ueland et al., 1969a,b,c), impedance cardiography (Atkins et al., 1981a,b), and echocardiography or Doppler ultrasound (Katz et al., 1978; Laird-Meeter et al., 1979; Mashini et al., 1987; Easterling et al., 1990; van Oppen et al., 1996). Despite controversy about the relative contributions of stroke volume and heart rate, maternal cardiac output increases as early as 10 weeks' gestation and peaks at 30–50% over nonpregnant values by the latter part of the second trimester. This rise, from 4.5 to 6.0 L/min, is sustained for the remainder of the pregnancy. Nulliparous women have a higher mean cardiac output than multiparous women (van Oppen et al., 1996).

Table 3.3 Cardiovascular parameters

Parameter	Units	Comment/derivation
	Measured directly using minimally invasive techniques	
Systolic blood pressure (SBP)	mmHg	
Diastolic blood pressure (DBP)	mmHg	
Heart rate	beats/min (bpm)	
	Measured directly using invasive techniques	
Central venous pressure (CVP)	mmHg	Reflects right ventricular preload
Pulmonary artery SBP	mmHg	
Pulmonary artery DBP	mmHg	
Pulmonary capillary wedge pressure (PCWP)	mmHg	Reflects left ventricular preload
	Derived from measured values	
Pulse pressure	mmHg	= SBP – DBP
Mean arterial pressure (MAP)	mmHg	= DBP + (pulse pressure/3)
Systemic vascular resistance (SVR)	dynes/sec/cm^{-5}	= (MAP – CVP) (80)/CO
Peripheral vascular resistance (PVR)	dynes/sec/cm^{-5}	= (MPAP – PCWP) (80)/CO
Cardiac output (CO)	L/min	= MAP/SVR = HR (beats/min) × SV (mL/beat)
Stroke volume (SV)	mL/beat	= CO (L/min)/HR (beats/min)
Cardiac index (CI)	L/min/m^2	= CO (L/min)/body surface area (m^2)
Stroke volume index (SVI)	mL/beat/m^2	= SV (mL/beat)/body surface area (m^2)

Beginning in the late 1940s, right heart catheterization provided a more refined, although invasive, method for studying cardiac output. Hamilton (1949) measured cardiac output in 24 nongravid and 68 normal pregnant women by this technique. Cardiac output averaged 4.51 ± 0.38 L/min in nonpregnant women. In pregnancy, cardiac output began to increase at approximately 10–13 weeks' gestation, reached a maximum of 5.73 L/min at 26–29 weeks, and returned to nonpregnant levels by term. These observations have been confirmed by subsequent cross-sectional right heart catheterization studies in pregnant women (Palmer & Walker, 1949; Bader et al., 1955).

Longitudinal studies using Doppler and M-mode echocardiography to interrogate maternal cardiac output throughout pregnancy report conflicting results about the relative contributions of heart rate and stroke volume. Katz and colleagues (1978) attributed the elevation in cardiac output (+59% by the third trimester; $n = 19$) to increases in both heart rate and stroke volume, whereas the study by Mashini et al. (1987) showed that the increase (+32% in the third trimester; $n = 16$) was due almost exclusively to maternal tachycardia. Laird-Meeter et al. (1979) have suggested that the initial increase in cardiac output prior to 20 weeks' gestation is due to maternal tachycardia, whereas that observed after 20 weeks results from an increase in stroke volume due primarily to reversible myocardial hypertrophy. Mabie and colleagues (1994), on the other hand, attributed the increase in cardiac output (from 6.7 ± 0.9 L/min at 8–11 weeks to 8.7 ± 1.4 L/min at 36–39 weeks; $n = 18$) to augmentation of both heart rate (+29%) and stroke volume (+18%) (Fig. 3.5). The conflicting nature of these studies can be attributed, in part, to the positioning of the patient during examination (lateral recumbent versus supine position). It must also be emphasized that, although M-mode echocardiographic estimation of stroke volume correlates well with angiographic studies in nongravid subjects, similar validation studies have not been carried out during pregnancy (Pombo et al., 1971; Murray et al., 1972). For this reason, ultrasound measurements of maternal volume flow in pregnancy have been validated only against similar measurements attained by thermodilution techniques (Easterling et al., 1987; Robson et al., 1987a,b,c; Lee et al., 1988).

One criticism of the above studies is that the maternal hemodynamic measurements in pregnancy are usually compared with those from postpartum control subjects. This comparison may not be valid, however, because cardiac output remains elevated for many weeks after delivery (Robson et al., 1987c; Capeless & Clapp, 1991). To address this issue, Robson et al. (1989a) measured cardiac output by Doppler echocardiography in 13 women before conception and again at monthly intervals throughout pregnancy. Maternal heart rate was significantly elevated by 5 weeks' gestation, and continued to increase thereafter, reaching a plateau at around 32 weeks (+17% above midpregnancy values). Stroke volume was increased by 8 weeks, with maximal values (+32% over midpregnancy levels) attained at 16–20 weeks. Overall, maternal cardiac output increased from 4.88 L/min at 5 weeks to 7.21 L/min (+48%) at 32 weeks.

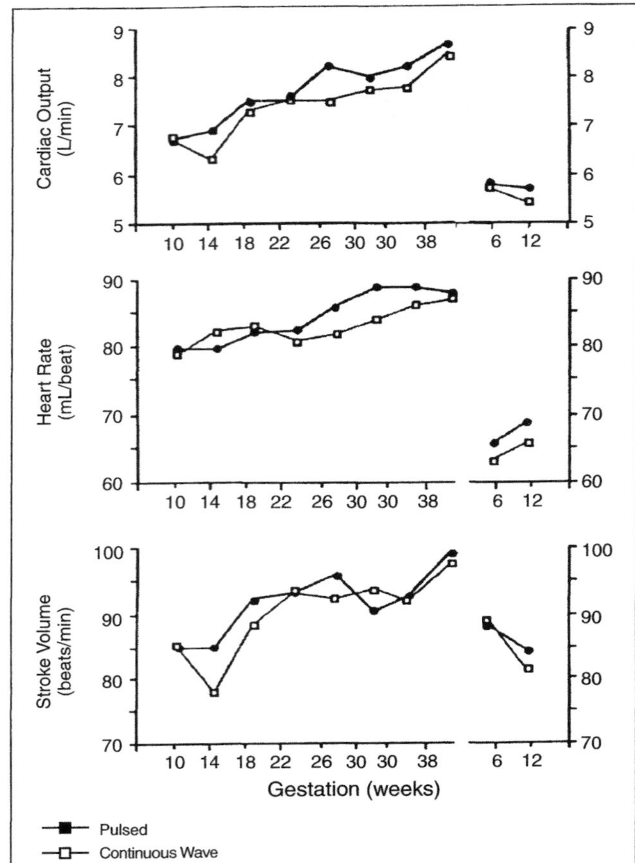

Fig. 3.5 Hemodynamic changes during pregnancy and postpartum. (Reproduced by permission from Mabie W, DiSessa TG, Crocker LG, et al. A longitudinal study of cardiac output in normal human pregnancy. Am J Obstet Gynecol 1994;170:849.)

The mechanisms responsible for the increase in maternal cardiac output during pregnancy remain unclear. An increase in circulating blood volume is unlikely to contribute significantly to this effect, because hemodynamic studies in pregnant baboons have shown that the increase in cardiac output develops much earlier than does the gestational hypervolemia (Phippard et al., 1986). Burwell et al. (1938) noted that the increase in plasma volume, cardiac output, and heart rate during pregnancy was similar to that seen in patients with arteriovenous shunting, and proposed that these hemodynamic changes are the result of the low-pressure, high-volume arteriovenous shunting that characterizes the uteroplacental circulation. A third hypothesis is that hormonal factors (possibly steroid hormones) may act directly on the cardiac musculature to increase stroke volume and hence cardiac output, analogous to the mechanisms responsible for the decrease in venous tone seen in normal pregnancy (McCalden, 1975) or after oral contraceptive administration (Wook & Goodrich, 1964). In support of this hypothesis, high-dose estrogen administration has been shown to increase stroke volume and cardiac output in male transsexuals (Slater et al., 1986). To further investigate this hypothesis, Duvekot and colleagues (1993) studied serial echocardiographic, hormonal, and renal electrolyte measurements in 10 pregnant women. The authors propose that the inciting event may be the fall in SVR that leads, in turn, to a compensatory tachycardia with activation of volume-restoring mechanisms. In this manner, the increased stroke volume may be a direct result of "normalized" vascular filling in the setting of systemic afterload reduction. These data support the conclusion of Morton and co-workers (1984) that early stroke volume increases are caused by a "shift to the right" of the left ventricular pressure–volume curve (Frank–Starling mechanism).

Systemic vascular resistance

Systemic vascular resistance (SVR) is a measure of the impedance to the ejection of blood into the maternal circulation (i.e. afterload). Bader et al. (1995) used cardiac catheterization to investigate the effect of pregnancy on SVR. They demonstrated that SVR decreases in early pregnancy, reaching a nadir at around 980 dynes/sec/cm^{-5} at 14–24 weeks. Thereafter, SVR rises progressively for the remainder of pregnancy, approaching a prepregnancy value of around 1,240 dynes/sec/cm^{-5} at term. These findings are consistent with subsequent studies (Clark et al., 1989), which found a mean SVR of 1210 ± 266 dynes/sec/cm^{-5} during late pregnancy.

When describing the physiologic relationship between pressure and flow, it is customary to report vascular impedance as a ratio of pressure to flow (Table 3.3). The observed decrease in SVR during pregnancy results primarily from a decrease in mean arterial pressure coupled with an increase in cardiac output. It is important to recognize the inverse relationship between cardiac output and SVR.

Peripheral arterial vasodilation with relative underfilling of the arterial circulation is likely the primary event responsible for the decrease in SVR seen in early pregnancy (Schrier, 1988; 1990). The factors responsible for this vasodilatation are not clear, but likely include hormonal factors (progesterone) and peripheral vasodilators such as nitric oxide (Seligman et al., 1996). The existence of a pregnancy-specific vasodilatory substance has been postulated, but has yet to be characterized. Cardiac afterload is further reduced by the progressive development of the low-resistance uteroplacental circulation. The decrease in SVR in early pregnancy leads to activation of compensatory homeostatic mechanisms designed to maintain arterial blood volume by increasing cardiac output and promoting sodium and water retention (summarized in Fig. 3.6). This is accomplished through activation of arterial baroreceptors, upregulation of vasopressin, stimulation of the sympathetic nervous system, and increased mineralocorticoid activity.

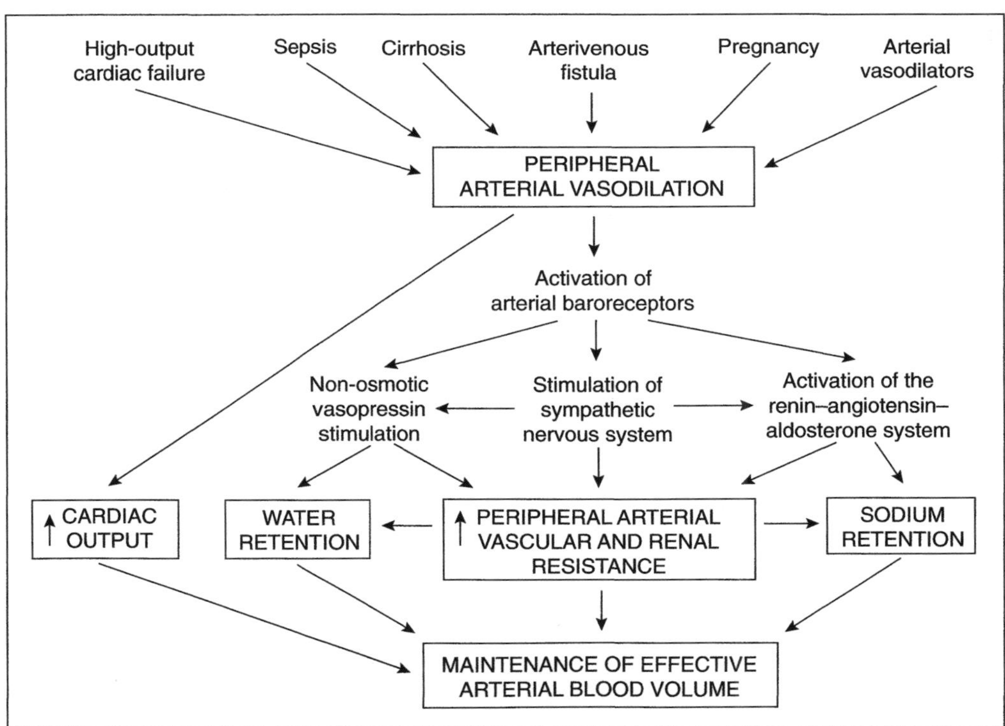

Fig. 3.6 Unifying hypothesis of renal sodium and water retention initiated by peripheral arterial vasodilation. (Reprinted by permission from the American College of Obstetricians and Gynecologists [Obstetrics and Gynecology, 1991;77:632].)

Whether atrial natriuretic peptide (ANP) has a role to play in the regulation of SVR in pregnancy is still unclear. ANP is a peptide hormone produced by atrial cardiocytes, which promotes renal sodium excretion and diuresis in nonpregnant subjects (Brenner et al., 1990). In vitro, ANP has been shown to promote vasodilatation in vascular smooth muscle pretreated with angiotensin II. Circulating ANP levels increase in pregnancy, suggesting that ANP may have a role to play in decreasing maternal SVR (Cusson et al., 1985; Thomsen et al., 1988). Earlier cross-sectional studies did not correlate ANP levels with blood volume and hemodynamic measurements. In a prospective longitudinal study, Thomsen et al. (1993) demonstrated that plasma ANP levels were positively correlated with Doppler ultrasound estimates of peripheral vascular resistance. Although their results substantiate the physiologic importance of ANP in the regulation of blood volume, the authors conclude that ANP does not function as a significant vasodilator during pregnancy.

Regional blood flow

Significant regional blood flow changes have been documented during pregnancy. For example, renal blood flow increases by 30% over nonpregnant values by midpregnancy, and remains elevated for the remainder of pregnancy (Chesley, 1960; Gabert & Miller, 1985). As a result, glomerular filtration rate increases 30–50% (Schrier, 1988). Similarly, skin perfusion increases slowly to 18–20 weeks' gestation, but rises rapidly thereafter reaching a plateau at 20–30 weeks that persists until approximately 1 week postpartum (Katz & Sokal, 1980). This is likely due to vasodilation of dermal capillaries (Burt, 1949; Herbert et al., 1958), and may serve as a mechanism by which the excess heat of fetal metabolism is allowed to dissipate the maternal circulation. Pulmonary blood flow increases during pregnancy from 4.88 L/min in early pregnancy to 7.19 L/min at 38 weeks, an increase of around 32% (Kitabatake et al., 1983; Robson et al., 1991). A small decrease in pulmonary vascular resistance was noted at 8 weeks without any subsequent significant change thereafter. However, both noninvasive (Kitabatake et al., 1983) and invasive studies (Werko, 1954; Bader et al., 1955; Clark et al., 1989) have shown that mean pulmonary artery pressure remains stable at around 14 mmHg, which is not significantly different from the nongravid state.

The most dramatic change in regional blood flow in pregnancy occurs in the uterus. Uterine blood flow increases from approximately 50 mL/min at 10 weeks to 500 mL/min at term (Metcalfe et al., 1955; Assali et al., 1960). At term, therefore, uterine blood flow accounts for over 10% of maternal cardiac output. This increase in blood flow is likely related to hormonal factors, because animal studies have shown a significant decrease in uterine vascular resistance in response to exogenous administration of estrogen and progesterone (Ueland & Parer, 1966; Caton et al., 1974).

Effect of posture on maternal hemodynamics

Prior to the 1960s, clinical investigators did not fully appreciate the effects of postural change on maternal hemodynamics and patients were often studied in the supine position. The unique angiographic studies of Bieniarz et al. (1966, 1968) demonstrate that the gravid uterus can significantly impair vena caval blood flow in >90% of women studied in the supine position, thereby predisposing pregnant women to dependent edema and varicosities of the lower extremities. Moreover, impairment of central venous return in the supine position can result in decreased cardiac output, a sudden drop in BP, bradycardia, and syncope (Kerr, 1968). These clinical features were initially described by Howard et al. (1953), and are now commonly referred to as the "supine hypotensive syndrome." Symptomatic supine hypotension occurs in 8% (Holmes, 1960) to 14% (Calvin et al., 1988) of women during late pregnancy. It is likely that women with poor collateral circulation through the paravertebral vessels may be predisposed to symptomatic supine hypotension, because these vessels usually serve as an alternate route for venous return from the pelvic organs and lower extremities (Kinsella & Lohmann, 1994). In addition to impairing venous return, compression by the gravid uterus in the supine position can also result in partial obstruction of blood flow through the aorta and its ancillary branches leading, for example, to diminished renal blood flow (Chesley, 1960; Lindheimer & Katz, 1972).

The clinical significance of supine hypotension is not clear. Vorys et al. (1961) demonstrated an immediate 16% reduction in cardiac output when women in the latter half of pregnancy were moved from the supine to the dorsal lithotomy position, likely due to the compressive effect of the gravid uterus on the vena cava (Table 3.4). To investigate the effect of gestational age on the maternal cardiovascular response to posture, Ueland et al. (1969) measured changes in resting heart rate, stroke volume, and cardiac output for 11 normal gravid women in various positions (sitting, supine, and left lateral decubitus) throughout their pregnancies (Fig. 3.7). Maternal heart rate was maximal (range, +13% to +20% compared with

Table 3.4 Changes in cardiac output with maternal position

Late-trimester women ($n = 31$)	Change from supine (%)
Horizontal left side	+14
Trendelenberg left side	+13
Lithotomy	−16
Supine Trendelenberg	−18

(Reproduced by permission from Vorys N, Ullery JC, Hanusek GE. The cardiac output changes in various positions in pregnancy. Am J Obstet Gynecol 1961;82:1312.)

postpartum values) at 28–32 weeks of pregnancy, and was further elevated in the sitting position. Stroke volume increased early in pregnancy, with maximal values by 20–24 weeks (range, +21% to +33%), followed by a progressive decline towards term that was most striking in the supine position. Indeed, measurements of stroke volume and cardiac output in the supine position at term were even lower than the corresponding values in the postpartum period (Fig. 3.7). On an optimistic note, Calvin and associates (1988) were able to demonstrate that supine hypotension does not normally result in significant oxygen desaturation.

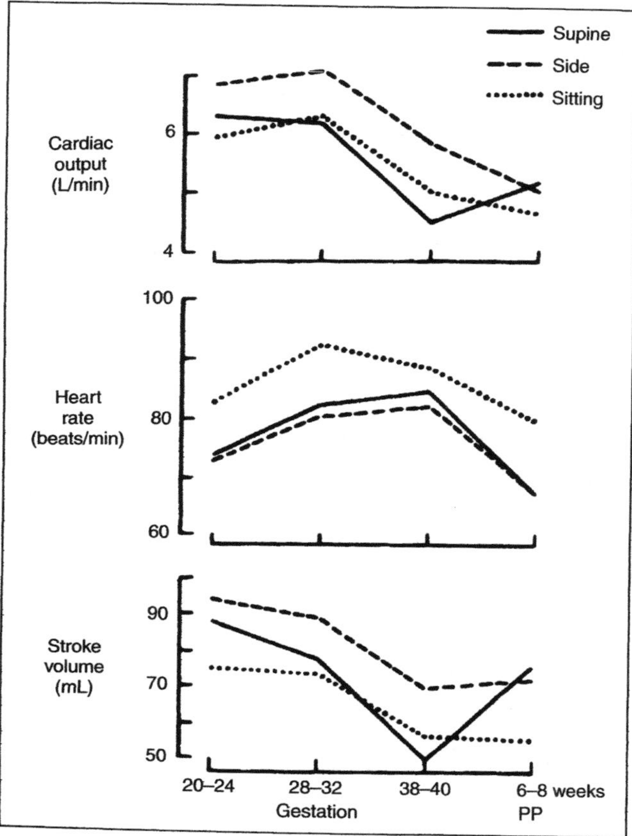

Fig. 3.7 Effect of posture on maternal hemodynamics. PP, postpartum. (Reproduced by permission from Ueland K, Metcalfe J. Circulatory changes in pregnancy. Clin Obstet Gynecol 1975;18:41; modified from Ueland K, Novy MJ, Peterson EN, et al. Maternal cardiovascular dynamics. IV. The influence of gestational age on the maternal cardiovascular response to posture and exercise. Am J Obstet Gynecol 1969;104:856.)

To investigate the effect of standing on the maternal hemodynamic profile, Easterling et al. (1988) measured cardiac output and SVR in the recumbent, sitting, and standing positions in women during early (11.1 ± 1.4 weeks) and late (36.7 ± 1.6 weeks) pregnancy. A change from the recumbent to standing position resulted in a decrease in cardiac output of around 1.7 L/min at any stage of gestation with a compensatory SVR augmentation (Table 3.5). Of note, the compensatory increase in SVR was significantly blunted in late pregnancy as compared with nonpregnant subjects, which may be related to the altered response to norepinephrine observed during pregnancy (Barron et al., 1986; Nisell et al., 1988). In addition to confirming these findings, Clark et al. (1991) were able to demonstrate that maternal BP was essentially unaffected by standing in the third trimester of pregnancy, despite varying effects on cardiac output (Table 3.6). The observed decrease in left ventricular stroke work index on standing (−22%) was attributed to the subject's inability to compensate for the decrease in stroke volume by heart rate alone as a result of Starling forces. Intrapulmonary shunting is not affected by maternal position (Hankins et al., 1996). Whether such postural changes have any clinical significance in terms of placental perfusion, birthweight, and/or preterm delivery is unclear at this time (Naeye & Peters, 1982; Henriksen et al., 1995).

Central hemodynamic changes associated with pregnancy

To establish normal values for central hemodynamics, Clark and colleagues (1989) interrogated the maternal circulation by invasive hemodynamic monitoring. Ten primiparous women underwent right heart catheterization during late pregnancy

Table 3.5 Net change in hemodynamic parameters from recumbent to standing positions

	Nonpregnant	Early pregnancy	Late pregnancy	P*
MAP (mmHg)	78 ± 8.3	3.7 ± 7.7	5.0 ± 11.3	NS
Heart rate (bpm)	15.5 ± 9.2	25.7 ± 11.8	16.7 ± 11.2	NS
CO (L/min)	−1.8 ± 0.84	−1.8 ± 0.79	−1.7 ± 1.2	NS
Stroke volume (mL/beat)	−41.1 ± 15.8	−38.7 ± 13.5	−30.8 ± 17.5	NS
SVR (dynes/sec/cm^{-5})	732 ± 363	588 ± 246	379 ± 214	0.005

Data are presented as mean ± SD.
* Determined by analysis of variance.
CO, cardiac output; MAP, mean arterial pressure; NS, not significant; SVR, systemic vascular resistance.
(Reproduced by permission from the American College of Obstetricians and Gynecologists (Obstetrics and Gynecology 1988;72:550).)

Table 3.6 Hemodynamic alterations in response to position change late in third trimester of pregnancy

Hemodynamic parameter	Position			
	Left lateral	Supine	Sitting	Standing
MAP (mmHg)	90 ± 6	90 ± 8	90 ± 8	91 ± 14
CO (L/min)	6.6 ± 1.4	6.0 ± 1.4*	6.2 ± 2.0	5.4 ± 2.0*
Heart rate (bpm)	82 ± 10	84 ± 10	91 ± 11	107 ± 17*
SVR (dynes/sec/cm^{-5})	1,210 ± 266	1,437 ± 338	1,217 ± 254	1,319 ± 394
PVR (dynes/sec/cm^{-5})	76 ± 16	101 ± 45	102 ± 35	117 ± 35*
PCWP (mmHg)	8 ± 2	6 ± 3	4 ± 4	4 ± 2
CVP (mmHg)	4 ± 3	3 ± 2	1 ± 1	1 ± 2
LVSWI (g/min/m^{-2})	43 ± 9	40 ± 9	44 ± 5	34 ± 7*

* $P < 0.05$, compared with left lateral position.

CO, cardiac output; CVP, central venous pressure; LVSWI, left ventricular stroke work index; MAP, mean arterial pressure; PCWP, pulmonary capillary wedge pressure; PVR, pulmonary vascular resistance; SVR, systemic vascular resistance.

(Reproduced by permission from Clark SL, Cotton DB, Pivarnik JM, et al. Position change and central hemodynamic profile during normal third-trimester pregnancy and postpartum. Am J Obstet Gynecol 1991;164:883.)

Table 3.7 Central hemodynamic changes associated with late pregnancy

	Nonpregnant	Pregnant	Change (%)
MAP (mmHg)	86 ± 8	90 ± 6	NS
PCWP (mmHg)	6 ± 2	8 ± 2	NS
CVP (mmHg)	4 ± 3	4 ± 3	NS
Heart rate (bpm)	71 ± 10	83 ± 10	+17
CO (L/min)	4.3 ± 0.9	6.2 ± 1.0	+43
SVR (dynes/sec/cm^{-5})	1,530 ± 520	1,210 ± 266	−21
PVR (dynes/sec/cm^{-5})	119 ± 47	78 ± 22	−34
Serum COP (mmHg)	20.8 ± 1.0	18.0 ± 1.5	−14
COP–PCWP gradient (mmHg)	14.5 ± 2.5	10.5 ± 2.7	−28
LVSWI (g/min/m^{-2})	41 ± 8	48 ± 6	NS

Measurements from the left lateral decubitus position are expressed as mean ± SD ($n = 10$). Significant changes are noted at the $P < 0.05$ level, paired two-tailed *t*-test.

CO, cardiac output; COP, colloid osmotic pressure; CVP, central venous pressure; LVSWI, left ventricular stroke index; MAP, mean arterial pressure; NS, non-significant; PCWP, pulmonary capillary wedge pressure; PVR, pulmonary vascular resistance; SVR, systemic vascular resistance.

(Adapted by permission from Clark SL, Cotton DB, Lee W, et al. Central hemodynamic assessment of normal term pregnancy. Am J Obstet Gynecol 1989;161:1439.)

(35–38 weeks) and again 11–13 weeks postpartum (Table 3.7). When compared with postpartum values, late pregnancy was associated with a significant increase in heart rate (+17%), stroke volume (+23%), and cardiac output (+43%) as measured in the left lateral recumbent position. Significant decreases were noted in SVR (−21%), pulmonary vascular resistance (−34%), serum colloid osmotic pressure (−14%), and the colloid osmotic pressure to pulmonary capillary wedge pressure gradient (−28%). No significant changes were found in the pulmonary capillary wedge or central venous pressures which confirmed prior studies (Bader et al., 1955).

Hemodynamic changes during labor

Repetitive and forceful uterine contractions (but not Braxton-Hicks contractions) have a significant effect on the cardiovascular system during labor. Each uterine contraction in labor expresses 300–500 mL of blood back into the systemic circulation (Adams & Alexander, 1958; Hendricks & Quilligan, 1958). Moreover, angiographic studies have shown that the change in shape of the uterus during contractions leads to improved blood flow from the pelvic organs and lower extremities back to the heart. The resultant increase in venous return during uterine contractions leads to a transient maternal bradycardia followed by an increase in cardiac output and compensatory bradycardia. Indeed, using a modified pulse pressure method for estimating cardiac output, Hendricks and Quilligan (1958) showed a 31% increase in cardiac output with contractions as compared with the resting state.

Other factors that may be responsible for the observed increase in maternal cardiac output during labor included pain, anxiety, valsalva, and maternal positioning (Winner & Romney, 1966; Ueland et al., 1969a,b; 1976). Using the dye-dilution technique to measure hemodynamic parameters in 23 pregnant women in early labor with central catheters inserted into their brachial artery and superior vena cava, Ueland and co-workers (1969a,b) demonstrated that change in position from the supine to the lateral decubitus position was associated with an increase in both cardiac output (+21.7%) and stroke volume (+26.5%), and a decrease in heart rate (−5.6%). Figure 3.8 summarizes the effect of postural changes and uterine contractions on maternal hemodynamics during the first stage of labor. Under these conditions, uterine contrac-

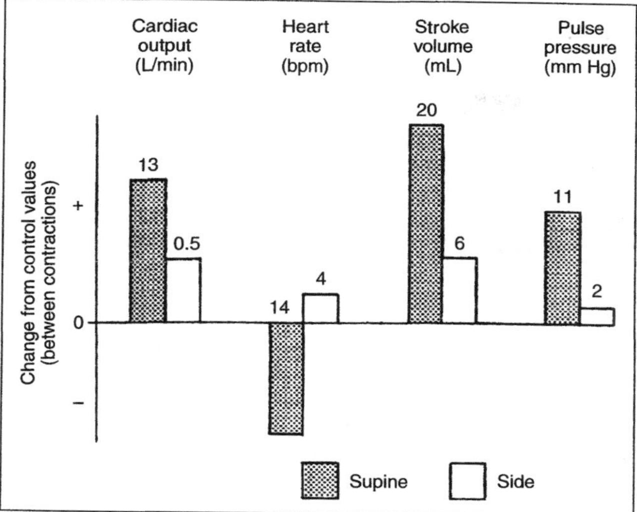

Fig. 3.8 Effect of posture on the maternal hemodynamic response to uterine contractions in early labor. (Reproduced by permission from Ueland K, Metcalfe J. Circulatory changes in pregnancy. Clin Obstet Gynecol 1975;18:41; modified from Ueland K, Hansen JM. Maternal cardiovascular dynamics. II. Posture and uterine contractions. Am J Obstet Gynecol 1969;103:8.)

tions resulted in a 15.3% rise in cardiac output, a 7.6% heart rate decrease, and a 21.5% increase in stroke volume. These hemodynamic changes were of less magnitude in the lateral decubitus position, although cardiac output measurements between contractions were actually higher when patients were on their side.

The first stage of labor is associated with a progressive increase in cardiac output. Kjeldsen (1979) found that cardiac output increased by 1.10 L/min in the latent phase, 2.46 L/min in the accelerating phase, and 2.17 L/min in the decelerating phase as compared with antepartum values. Ueland and Hansen (1969b) described a similar increase in cardiac output between early and late first stages of labor. In a more detailed analysis, Robson and colleagues (1987a) used Doppler ultrasound to measure cardiac output serially throughout labor in 15 women in the left lateral position under meperidine labor analgesia. Cardiac output measured between contractions increased from 6.99 L/min to 7.88 L/min (+13%) by 8-cm cervical dilation, primarily as a result of increased stroke volume. A further increase in cardiac output was evident during contractions, due to augmentation of both heart rate and stroke volume. Of interest, the magnitude of the contraction-associated augmentation in cardiac output increased as labor progressed: ≤3 cm (+17%), 4–7 cm (+23%), and ≥8 cm (+34%). Similar results were reported by Lee et al. (1989b) using Doppler and M-mode echocardiography to study the effects of contractions on cardiac output in women with epidural analgesia. Under epidural analgesia, however, the effect of contractions on heart rate was minimal. Although a detailed discussion of the effect of labor analgesia on maternal hemodynamics is beyond the scope of this chapter and is dealt with in detail elsewhere in this book, the increase in cardiac output during the labor was not as pronounced in women with regional anesthesia as compared with women receiving local anesthesia (paracervical or pudendal). These data suggest that the relative lack of pain and anxiety in women with regional analgesia may limit the absolute increase in cardiac output encountered at delivery. Alternatively, the fluid bolus required for regional anesthesia may itself affect cardiac output. Indeed, Robson and co-workers (1989b) found that in fusion of 800 mL of Ringer's lactate prior to epidural anesthesia resulted in a 12% increase in stroke volume and an overall augmentation of cardiac output from 7.01 to 7.70 L/min. It is likely that this change is responsible, at least in part, for the altered response of the maternal cardiovascular system to labor in the setting of regional anesthesia.

Hemodynamic changes during the postpartum period

The postpartum period is associated with significant hemodynamic fluctuations, due largely to the effect of blood loss at delivery. Using chromium-labeled erythrocytes to quantify blood loss, Pritchard and colleagues (1962) found that the average blood loss associated with cesarean delivery was 1,028 mL, approximately twice that of vaginal delivery (505 mL). They also demonstrated that healthy pregnant women can lose up to 30% of their antepartum blood volume at delivery with little or no change in their postpartum hematocrit. These findings were similar to those of other investigators (Wilcox et al., 1959; Newton et al., 1961).

Ueland (1976) compared blood volume and hematocrit changes in women delivered vaginally ($n = 6$) with those delivered by elective cesarean ($n = 34$) (Fig. 3.9). The average blood loss at vaginal delivery was 610 mL, compared with 1,030 mL at cesarean. In women delivered vaginally, blood volume decreased steadily for the first 3 days postpartum. In women delivered by cesarean, however, blood volume dropped off precipitously within the first hour of delivery, but remained fairly stable thereafter. As a result, both groups had a similar drop off in blood volume (–16.2%) at the third postpartum day (Fig. 3.9). The differences in postpartum hematocrit between women delivered vaginally (+5.2% on day 3) and those delivered by cesarean (–5.8% on day 5) suggests that most of the volume loss following vaginal delivery was due to postpartum diuresis. This diuresis normally occurs between day 2 and day 5 postpartum, and allows for loss of the excess extracellular fluid accumulated during pregnancy (Cunningham, 1993a) with a resultant 3 kg weight loss (Chesley et al., 1959). Failure to adequately diurese in the first postpartum week may lead to excessive accumulation of intravascular fluid, elevated pulmonary capillary wedge pressure, and pulmonary edema (Hankins et al., 1984).

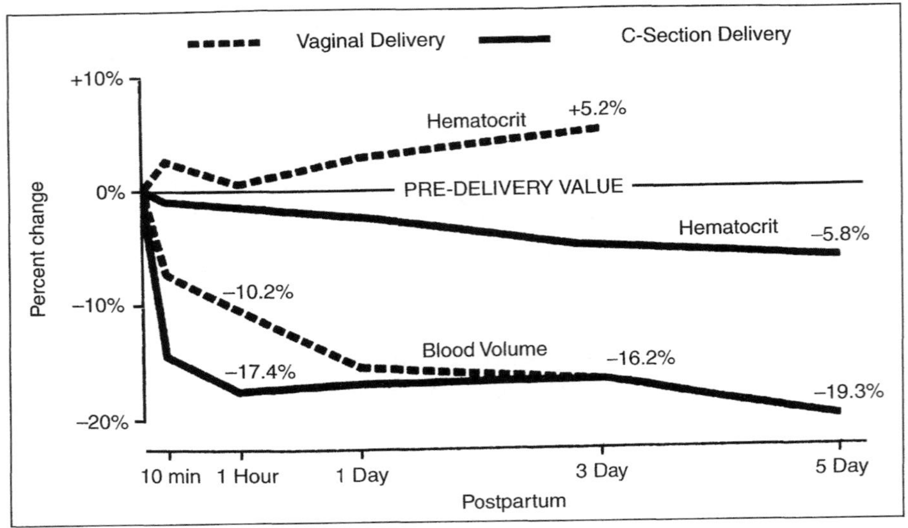

Fig. 3.9 Percentage change in blood volume and venous hematocrit following vaginal or cesarean delivery. (Reproduced by permission from Metcalfe J, Ueland K. Heart disease and pregnancy. In: Fowler NO, ed. Cardiac Diagnosis and Treatment, 3rd edn. Hagerstown, MD: Harper and Row, 1980:1153–1170.)

Significant changes in cardiac output, stroke volume, and heart rate also occur after delivery (Kjeldsen, 1979). Ueland and Hansen (1969b) demonstrated a dramatic increase in cardiac output (+59%) and stroke volume (+71%) within the first 10 minutes after delivery in 13 women who delivered vaginally under regional anesthesia. At 1 hour, cardiac output (+49%) and stroke volume (+67%) in these women were still elevated, with a 15% decrease in heart rate and no significant change in BP. The increase in cardiac output following delivery likely results from increased cardiac preload due to the autotransfusion of blood from the uterus back into the intravascular space, the release of vena caval compression from the gravid uterus, and the mobilization of extravascular fluid into the intravascular compartment.

These changes in maternal cardiovascular physiology resolve slowly after delivery. Using M-mode and Doppler echocardiography, Robson et al. (1987c) measured cardiac output and stroke volume in 15 healthy parturients at 38 weeks (not in labor) and then again at 2, 6, 12, and 24 weeks postpartum. Their results show a decrease in cardiac output from 7.42 L/min at 38 weeks to 4.96 L/min at 24 weeks postpartum, which was attributed to a reduction in both heart rate (–20%) and stroke volume (–18%). By 2 weeks postpartum, there was a substantial decrease in left ventricular size and contractility as compared with term pregnancy. By 24 weeks postpartum, however, echocardiographic studies demonstrated mild left ventricular hypertrophy that correlated with a slight diminution in left ventricular contractility as compared with age-matched nongravid control. Because the echocardiographic parameters in the control subjects were similar to that in previously published reports, it is likely that this small diminution in myocardial function 6 months after delivery is a real observation. This is an interesting finding, because patients with peripartum cardiomyopathy usually develop their disease within 5–6 months of delivery (Lee & Cotton, 1989).

Respiratory system

There are numerous changes in the maternal respiratory system during pregnancy. These changes result initially from the endocrine changes of pregnancy and, later, from the physical and mechanical changes brought about by the enlarging uterus. The net physiologic result of these changes is a lowering of the maternal $P\text{CO}_2$ to less than that of the fetus, thereby facilitating effective exchange of CO_2 from the fetus to the mother.

Changes in the upper airways

The elevated estrogen levels and increases in blood volume associated with pregnancy may contribute to mucosal edema and hypervascularity in the upper airways of the respiratory system. Although a recent study failed to demonstrate an increased prevalence or severity of upper airway symptomatology in pregnancy, this study was of modest numbers (33 pregnant patients) and confined only to the first trimester (Sobol et al., 2001). The weight of evidence in the literature suggests that such changes do lead to an increased prevalence of nasal stuffiness, rhinitis, and epistaxis during pregnancy. Epistaxis can be severe and recurrent. Indeed, there are several case reports of epistaxis severe enough to cause "fetal distress" (Braithwaite & Economides, 1995) and to be life threatening to the mother (Howard, 1985). The peculiar condition of "rhinitis of pregnancy" was recognized as far back as 1898 (MacKenzie, 1898). It has been reported to complicate up to 30% of pregnancies (Mabry, 1986), although—since, in some cases, the condition likely predated the pregnancy—the incidence of rhinitis attributable to pregnancy is somewhat lower at around 18% (Mabry, 1986). Symptoms of eustachian tube dysfunction are also frequently reported in pregnancy (Schatz & Zieger, 1988).

The factors responsible for the changes in the upper airways are not clearly understood. Animal studies have reported nasal mucosa swelling and edema in response to exogenous estrogen administration (Mortimer et al., 1936; Taylor, 1961) and in pregnancy (Taylor, 1961). Increased cholinergic activity has been demonstrated in the nasal mucosa of pregnant women (Toppozada et al., 1982) and following estrogen administration to animals (Reynolds & Foster, 1940). Although an estrogen-mediated cholinergic effect may explain the maternal rhinitis seen in pregnancy, other factors such as allergy, infection, stress, and/or medications may also be responsible (Mabry, 1986). As such, the occurrence of rhinitis in pregnancy should not be attributed simply to a normal physiological process until other pathological mechanisms have been excluded.

Changes in the mechanics of respiration

The mechanics of respiration change throughout pregnancy. In early pregnancy, these changes result primarily from hormonally-mediated relaxation of the ligamentous attachments of the chest. In later pregnancy, the enlarging uterus leads to changes in the shape of the chest. The lower ribs flare outwards resulting in a 50% increase in the subcostal angle from around 70 degrees in early pregnancy (Contreras et al., 1991). Although this angle decreases after delivery, it is still significantly greater (by approximately 20%) at 24 weeks postpartum than that measured at the beginning of pregnancy (Contreras et al., 1991). The thoracic circumference increases by around 8% during pregnancy and returns to normal shortly after delivery (Contreras et al., 1991). Both the antero-posterior and transverse diameters of the chest increase by around 2 cm in pregnancy (Weinberger et al., 1980; Elkus & Popovich, 1992). The end result of these anatomic changes is elevation of the diaphragm by approximately 5 cm (Elkus & Popovich, 1992) and increase in excursion (Gilroy et al., 1988). On the other hand, both respiratory muscle function and rib cage compliance are unaffected by pregnancy (Contreras et al., 1991). The relative contribution of the diaphragm and intercostal muscles to tidal volume is also similar in late pregnancy and after delivery (Macklem et al., 1978). As such, there is no significant difference in maximum respiratory pressures before and after delivery (Gilroy et al., 1988; Contreras et al., 1991).

In later pregnancy, abdominal distention and loss of abdominal muscle tone may necessitate greater use of the accessory muscles of respiration during exertion. The perception of increased inspiratory muscle effort may contribute to a subjective experience of dyspnea (Nava et al., 1992). Indeed, 15% of pregnant women report an increase in dyspnea in the first trimester as compared with almost 50% by 19 weeks and 76% by 31 weeks' gestation (Milne et al., 1978). Labor is a condition requiring considerable physical exertion with extensive use of the accessory muscles. Acute diaphragmatic fatigue has been reported in labor (Nava et al., 1992).

Physiologic changes in pregnancy

Static lung volumes change significantly throughout pregnancy (Table 3.8; Fig. 3.10). There is a modest reduction in the total lung capacity (TLC) (Elkus & Popovich, 1992). The functional reserve capacity (FRC) also decreases because of a progressive reduction in expiratory reserve volume (ERV) and residual volume (RV) (Thomson & Cohen, 1938; Cugell et al., 1953; Rubin et al., 1956; Gee et al., 1967; Baldwin et al., 1977; Contreras et al., 1991; Elkus & Popovich, 1992). The inspiratory capacity (IC) increases as the FRC decreases. It is important to note that these changes are relatively small and vary considerably between individual parturients as well as between reported studies. In one report, for example, the only parameter that consistently changed in all women studied was the FRC (Cugell et al., 1953). Data from a recent review (Crapo, 1996) of three large studies comparing static lung volumes is pregnant and nonpregnant women (Cugell et al., 1953; Alaily & Carrol, 1978; Norregard et al., 1989) is summarized in Table 3.8.

It is commonly accepted that the decrease in ERV and FRC results primarily from the upward displacement of the diaphragm in pregnancy. It has also been suggested that this displacement further reduces the negative pleural pressure leading to earlier closure of the small airways, an effect that is especially pronounced at the lung bases (Baldwin et al., 1977). The modest change in TLC and lack of change in vital capacity (VC) suggests that this upward displacement of the diaphragm in pregnancy is compensated for by such factors as the increase in transverse thoracic diameter, thoracic circumference, and subcostal angle (Contreras et al., 1991).

Respiratory rate and mean inspiratory flow are unchanged in pregnancy (Contreras et al., 1991). On the other hand, ventilatory drive (measured as mouth occlusion pressure) is increased during pregnancy, leading to a state of hyperventilation as evidenced by an increase in minute ventilation, alveolar ventilation, and tidal volume (Contreras et al., 1991; Crapo, 1996). Moreover, these changes are evident very early in pregnancy. Minute ventilation, for example, is already increased by around 30% in the first trimester of pregnancy as compared with postpartum values (Pernoll et al., 1975; Alaily & Carrol,

Table 3.8 Changes in static lung volumes in pregnant women at term

Static lung volumes	Change from nonpregnant state
Total lung capacity (TLC)	↓ 200–400 mL (–4%)
Functional residual capacity (FRC)	↓ 300–500 mL (–17% to –20%)
Expiratory reserve volume (ERV)	↓ 100–300 mL (–5% to –15%)
Reserve volume (RV)	↓ 200–300 mL (–20% to –25%)
Inspiratory capacity (IC)	↑ 100–300 mL (+5% to +10%)
Vital capacity (VC)	Unchanged

(Data from Baldwin GR, Moorthi DS, Whelton JA, MacDonnell KH. New lung functions in pregnancy. Am J Obstet Gynecol 1977;127:235.)

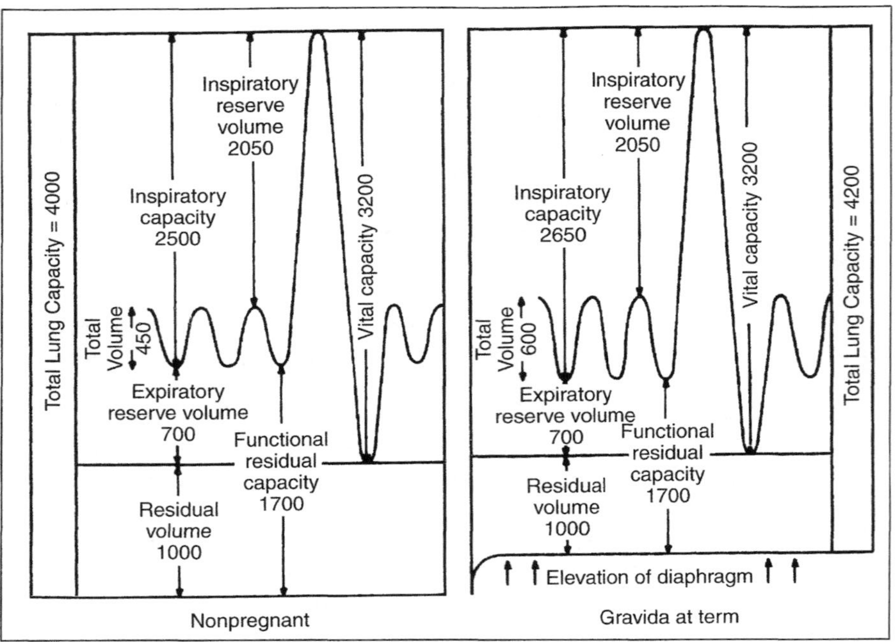

Fig. 3.10 Respiratory changes during pregnancy. (Reproduced by permission from Bonica JJ. Principles and Practice of Obstetrical Analgesia and Anesthesia. Philadelphia: FA Davis, 1962.)

1978; Milne, 1979; Contreras et al., 1991). Overall, pregnancy is associated with a 30–50% (approximately 3 L/min) increase in minute ventilation, a 50–70% increase in alveolar ventilation, and a 30–50% increase in tidal volume (Crapo, 1996). Although ventilatory dead space may increase by approximately 50% in pregnancy, the net effect on ventilation may be so small (approximately 60 mL) that it may not even be detectable (Crapo, 1996). Another reported change in ventilation during pregnancy is a decrease in airway resistance (Rubin et al., 1956), while pulmonary compliance is thought to remain unchanged (Gee et al., 1967; Contreras et al., 1991). The hyperventilation of pregnancy has been attributed primarily to a progesterone effect. Indeed, minute ventilation had been shown to increase in men following exogenous progesterone administration (Zwillich et al., 1978). However, other factors—such as the increased metabolic rate associated with pregnancy—may also have a role to play (Bayliss & Millhorn, 1992).

Changes in maternal acid–base status

Pregnancy represents a state of compensated respiratory alkalosis. CO_2 diffuses across membranes far faster than oxygen. As such, it is rapidly removed from the maternal circulation by the increased alveolar ventilation, with a concomitant reduction in the P_aCO_2 from a normal level of 35–45 mmHg to a lower level of 27–34 mmHg (Elkus & Popovich, 1992; Crapo, 1996). This leads in turn to increased bicarbonate excretion by the maternal kidneys, which serves to maintain the arterial blood pH between 7.40 and 7.45 (as compared with 7.35–7.45 in the nonpregnant state) (Weinberger et al., 1980; Elkus & Popovich, 1992; Crapo, 1996). As a result, serum bicarbonate levels decrease to 18–21 mEq/L in pregnancy (Elkus & Popovich, 1992; Crapo, 1996). The increased minute ventilation in pregnancy leads to an increase in P_aO_2 to 101–104 mmHg as compared with 80–100 mmHg in the nonpregnant state (Weinberger et al., 1980; Elkus & Popovich, 1992; Crapo, 1996) and a small increase in the mean alveolar–arterial (A–a) O_2 gradient to 14.3 mmHg (Awe et al., 1979). It should be noted, however, that a change from the sitting to supine position in pregnant women can decrease the capillary PO_2 by 13 mmHg (Ang et al., 1969) and increase the mean (A–a) O_2 gradient to 20 mmHg (Awe et al., 1979).

Genitourinary system

Alterations in renal tract anatomy

Because of the increased blood volume, the kidneys increase in length by approximately 1 cm during pregnancy (Cietak & Newton, 1985). The urinary collecting system also undergoes marked changes during pregnancy, with dilation of the renal calyces, renal pelvices, and ureters (Shulman & Herlinger, 1975). This dilation is likely secondary to the smooth muscle relaxant effects of progesterone, which may explain how it is that dilation of the collecting system can be visualized as early as the first trimester. However, an obstructive component to the dilation of the collecting system is also possible, due to the enlarging uterus compressing the ureters at the level of the pelvic brim (Dure-Smith, 1970). Indeed, the right-sided collecting system tends to undergo more marked dilation than the left side, likely due to dextrorotation of the uterus

(Hertzberg et al., 1993). These anatomic alterations may persist for up to 4 months postpartum (Fried et al., 1983).

The end result of these anatomic changes is physiologic obstruction and urinary stasis during pregnancy, leading to an increased risk of pyelonephritis in the setting of asymptomatic bacteriuria. Moreover, interpretation of renal tract imaging studies needs to take into account the fact the mile hydronephrosis and bilateral hydroureter are normal feature of pregnancy, and do not necessarily imply pathologic obstruction.

Alterations in renal physiology

The glomerular filtration rate (GFR), as measured by creatinine clearance, increases by approximately 50% by the end of the first trimester to a peak of around 180 mL/min (Davison & Hytten, 1975). Effective renal plasma flow also increases by around 50% during early pregnancy, and remains at this level until the final weeks of pregnancy at which time it declines by 15–25% (Lindheimer & Barron, 1998). These physiologic changes result in a decrease in serum blood urea nitrogen (BUN) and creatinine levels during pregnancy, such that a serum creatinine value of greater than 0.8 mg/dL may be an indicator of abnormal renal function. An additional effect of the increased GFR is an increase in urinary protein excretion. Indeed, urinary protein loss of up to 260 mg/day can be considered normal during pregnancy (Higby et al., 1994).

Renal tubular function is also significantly changed during pregnancy. The filtered load of sodium increases significantly due to the increased GFR and to the action of progesterone as a competitive inhibitor of aldosterone. Despite this increased filtered load of sodium, the increase in tubular reabsorption of sodium results in a net retention of up to 1 g of sodium per day. The increase in tubular reabsorption of sodium is likely a result of increased circulating levels of aldosterone and deoxycorticosterone (Barron & Lindheimer, 1984). Renin production increases early in pregnancy in response to rising estrogen levels, resulting in increased conversion of angiotensinogen to angiotensin I and II and culminating in increased levels of aldosterone. Aldosterone acts directly to promote renal tubular sodium retention.

Loss of glucose in the urine (glycosuria) is a normal finding during pregnancy, resulting from increased glomerular filtration and decreased distal tubular reabsorption (Davison & Hytten, 1975). This observation makes urinalysis an unreliable screening tool for gestational diabetes mellitus. Moreover, glycosuria may be a further predisposing factor to urinary tract infection during pregnancy.

Pregnancy is a period of marked water retention. During pregnancy, intravascular volume expands by around 1–2 L and extravascular volume by approximately 4–7 L (Lindheimer & Barron, 1998). This water retention results in a decrease in plasma sodium concentration from 140 to 136 mmol/L (Davison et al., 1981) and in plasma osmolality from 290 to 280 mosmol/kg (Davison et al., 1981). Plasma osmolality is maintained at this level throughout pregnancy due to a re-setting of the central osmoregulatory system.

Gastrointestinal system

Alterations in gastrointestinal anatomy

Gingival hyperemia and swelling are common in pregnancy, and the resultant pregnancy gingivitis often presents as an increased tendency for bleeding gums during pregnancy. The principal anatomic alterations of the gastrointestinal tract result from displacement or pressure from the enlarging uterus. Intragastric pressure rises in pregnancy, likely contributing to heartburn and to an increased incidence of hiatal hernia in pregnancy. The appendix is displaced progressively superiorly and laterally as pregnancy advances, such that the pain associated with appendicitis is localized to the right upper quadrant and term (Baer et al., 1932). Another anatomic alteration commonly seen in pregnancy is an increased incidence of hemorrhoids, which likely results both from the progesterone-mediated relaxation of the hemorrhoidal vasculature and from the increased constipation associated with pregnancy.

Alterations in gastrointestinal physiology

Many of the physiologic changes affecting gastrointestinal physiology during pregnancy are the result of a progesterone-mediated smooth muscle relaxant effect. Lower esophageal sphincter tone is decreased, resulting in increased gastroesophageal reflux and symptomatic heartburn (Van Thiel et al., 1977). Gastric and small bowel motility may also be decreased, leading to delayed gastric emptying and prolonged intestinal transit times (Parry et al., 1970). Such effects may contributed to pregnancy-related constipation by facilitating increased large intestine water reabsorption, and may explain, at least in part, the increased risk of regurgitation and aspiration with induction of general anesthesia in pregnancy. Of interest, more recent studies have suggested that delayed gastric emptying is only significant around the time of delivery and, rather than a pregnancy-related phenomenon, may result primarily from anesthetic medications given during labor (Radberg et al., 1989).

Early studies suggested that the progesterone dominant milieu of pregnancy resulted in a decrease in gastric acid secretion and an increase in gastric mucin production (Vasicka et al, 1957), and that these changes accounted for the apparent rarity of symptomatic peptic ulcer disease during pregnancy. However, more recent studies have shown no significant change in gastric acid production during pregnancy (Waldum et al., 1980). It is possible that the apparent protective effect of pregnancy on peptic ulcer disease may be a result of underreporting, since dyspeptic symptoms may be attributed to pregnancy-related heartburn without a complete evaluation.

Hepatobiliary changes in pregnancy

Although the liver does not change in size during pregnancy, its position is shifted upwards and posteriorly, especially during the third trimester. Other physical signs commonly attributed to liver disease in nonpregnant women (such as spider nevi and palmar erythema) can be normal features of pregnancy, and are likely due to increased circulating estrogen levels. Pregnancy is associated with dilation of the gallbladder and biliary duct system, which most likely represents a progesterone-mediated smooth muscle relaxant effect (Braverman et al., 1980).

Liver function tests change during pregnancy. Circulating levels of transaminases, including aspartate transaminase (AST) and alanine transaminase (ALT), as well as γ-glutamyl transferase (γGT) and bilirubin are normal or slightly diminished in pregnancy (Girling et la., 1997). Knowledge of the normal range for liver function tests in pregnancy as compared with nonpregnant patients is important, for example, when evaluating patients with preeclampsia. Prothrombin time (PT) and lactic acid dehydrogenase (LDH) levels are unchanged in pregnancy. Serum albumin and protein levels are decreased in pregnancy, most likely as a result of hemodilution from the increased plasma volume. Serum alkaline phosphatase (ALP) levels are markedly increased, especially during the third trimester of pregnancy, and this is almost exclusively as a result of the placental isoenzyme fraction.

Gallbladder function is considerably altered during pregnancy. This is due primarily to progesterone-mediated inhibition of cholecystokinin, which results in decreased gallbladder motility and stasis of bile within the gallbladder (Braverman et al., 1980). In addition, pregnancy is associated with an increase in biliary cholesterol concentration and a decrease in the concentration of select bile acids (especially chenodeoxycholic acid), both of which contribute to the increased lithogenicity of bile. Such changes serve to explain why cholelithiasis is more common during pregnancy.

Hematologic system

The functions of the hematologic system include supplying tissues and organ systems with oxygen and nutrients, removal of CO_2 and other metabolic waste products, regulation of temperature, protection against infection, and humoral communication. In pregnancy, the developing fetus and placenta impose further demands and the maternal hematologic system must adapt in order to meet these demands. Such adaptations included changes in plasma volume as well as the numbers of constituent cells and coagulation factors. All of these changes are designed to benefit the mother and/or fetus. However, some changes may also bring with them potential risks. It is important for the obstetric care provider to have a comprehensive understanding of both the positive and negative effects of the pregnancy-associated changes to the maternal hematologic system.

Changes in red blood cell mass

Red blood cell mass increase throughout pregnancy. In a landmark study using chromium (^{51}Cr)-labeled red blood cells, Pritchard (1965a) reported an average increase in red blood cell mass of around 30% (450 mL) in both singleton and twin pregnancies. Of note, the increase in red blood cell mass lags significantly behind the change in plasma volume and, as such, occurs later in pregnancy and continues until delivery (Lund & Donovan, 1967; Pirani et al., 1973; Peck & Arias, 1979). The difference in timing between the increase in red blood cell mass and plasma volume expansion results in a physiologic fall of the hematocrit in the first trimester (so-called physiologic anemia of pregnancy), which persists until the end of the second trimester. Erythropoiesis is stimulated by erythropoietin (which increases in pregnancy) as well as by human placental lactogen, a hormone produced by the placenta which is more abundant in later pregnancy (Jepson & Lowenstein, 1968). There are different opinions as to what ought to be regarded as the definition of anemia in pregnancy, but an historical and widely accepted value is that of a hemoglobin concentration <10.0 g/dL (Pritchard, 1965a). The increase in red blood cell mass serves to optimize oxygen transport to the fetus, while the decrease in blood viscosity resulting from the physiological anemia of pregnancy will improve placental perfusion and offer the mother some protection from obstetric hemorrhage.

Iron stores in healthy reproductive-age women are marginal, with two-thirds of such women having suboptimal iron stores (Scott & Pritchard, 1967). The major reason for low iron stores is thought to be menstrual blood loss. The total iron requirement for pregnancy has been estimated at around 980 mg. This amount of iron is not provided by a normal diet. As such, iron supplementation is recommended for all reproductive-age and pregnant women.

Changes in white blood cell count

Serum white blood cell count increases in pregnancy due to a selective bone marrow granulopoiesis (Peck & Arias, 1979). This results in a "left shift" of the white cell count, with a granulocytosis and increased numbers of immature white blood cells. The white blood cell count is increased in pregnancy, and peaks at around 30 weeks' gestation (Pitkin & Witte, 1979; Peck & Arias, 1979; Table 3.9). Although a white blood cell count of 5,000–12,000/mm^3 is considered normal in pregnancy, only around 20% of women will have a white blood cell count of

Table 3.9 White blood cell count in pregnancy

	White blood cell count (cells/mm³)	
	Mean	Normal range
First trimester	8,000	5,110–9,900
Second trimester	8,500	5,600–12,200
Third trimester	8,500	5,600–12,200
Labor	25,000	20,000–30,000

(Data from Pitkin R, Witte D. Platelet and leukocyte counts in pregnancy. JAMA 1979;242:2696.)

greater than 10,000/mm^3 in the third trimester (Peck & Arias, 1979).

Changes in platelet count

Most studies suggest that platelet counts decrease in pregnancy (Sejeny et al., 1975; O'Brien, 1976), although some studies show no change (Fenton et al., 1977). Since pregnancy does not appear to change the lifespan of platelets (Wallenburg & van Kessel, 1978), it is likely that the decrease in platelet count with pregnancy is primarily a dilutional effect. Whether there is increased consumption of platelets in pregnancy is controversial. Fay et al. (1985) reported a decrease in platelet count due to both hemodilution and increased consumption that reached a nadir at around 30 weeks' gestation. This study, along with the observation that the mean platelet volume increase in pregnancy indicative of a younger platelet population (Rakoczi et al., 1979), suggests that there may indeed be some increased platelet consumption in pregnancy.

The lower limit of normal for platelet counts in pregnancy is commonly accepted as the same as that for nonpregnant women (i.e. 150,000/mm^3). A maternal platelet count less than 150,000/mm^3 should be regarded as abnormal, although the majority of cases of mild thrombocytopenia (i.e. 100,000–150,000/mm^3)will have no identifiable cause. Such cases are thought to result primarily from hemodilution. This condition has been termed "gestational thrombocytopenia." It is evident in around 8% of pregnancies (Burrows & Kelton, 1990) and poses no apparent risk to either mother or fetus.

Changes in coagulation factors

Pregnancy is associated with changes in the coagulation and fibrinolytic cascades that favor thrombus formation. These changes include an increase in circulating levels of factors XII, X, IX, VII, VIII, von Willebrand factor, and fibrinogen (Hellgren, 1996). Factor XIII, high molecular weight kininogen, prekallikrein, and fibrinopeptide A (FPA) levels are also increased, although reports are conflicting (Hellgren, 1996). Factor XI decreases, and levels of prothrombin and factor V are unchanged (Hellgren, 1996). In contrast, antithrombin III and protein C levels are either unchanged or increased, and protein S levels are generally seen to decreases in pregnancy (Hellgren, 1996). The observed decrease in fibrinolytic activity in pregnancy is likely due to the marked increase in the plasminogen activator inhibitors, PAI-I and PAI-2 (Davis, 2000). The net result of these changes is an increased predisposition to thrombosis during pregnancy and the puerperium. Genetic risk factors for coagulopathy may also be present. Such factors include, among others, deletions or mutations of genes encoding for protein C, protein S, antithrombin III, heparin co-factor II (HC-II), factor V Leiden, prothrombin 20210A, and methylenetetrahydrofolate reductase (a condition leading to hyperhomocysteinemia).

The hypercoagulable state of pregnancy helps to minimize blood loss at delivery. However, these same physiological changes also put the mother at increased risk of thromboembolic events, both in pregnancy and in the puerperium. In a recent large epidemiologic study, the incidence of pregnancy-related thromboembolic complications was 1.3 per 1,000 deliveries (Lindqvist et al., 1999).

Endocrine system

The pituitary gland

The pituitary gland enlarges by as much as 135% during normal pregnancy (Gonzalez et al., 1988). This enlargement is generally not sufficient to cause visual disturbance from compression of the optic chiasma, and pregnancy is not associated with an increased incidence of pituitary adenoma.

Pituitary hormone function can vary considerably during normal pregnancy. Plasma growth hormone levels begin to increase at around 10 weeks' gestation, plateau at around 28 weeks, and can remain elevated until several months postpartum (Kletzky et al., 1985). Prolactin levels increase progressively throughout pregnancy, reaching a peak at term. The role of prolactin in pregnancy is not clear, but appears to be important in preparing breast tissue for lactation by stimulating glandular epithelial cell mitosis and increasing production of lactose, lipids, and certain proteins (Anderson, 1982).

The thyroid gland

A relative deficiency of iodide is common during pregnancy, due often to a relative dietary deficiency and increased urinary excretion of iodide. There are also increased demands on the thyroid gland to increase its uptake of available iodide from the circulation during pregnancy, leading to glandular hypertrophy. The thyroid gland also enlarges as a result of increased vascularity and cellular hyperplasia (Glinoer et al., 1990). However, evidence of frank goiter is not a feature of normal pregnancy, and its presence always warrants appropriate investigation.

Thyroid-binding globulin increases significantly during pregnancy under the influence of estrogen, and this leads to an increase in the total and bound fraction of thyroxine (T_4) and triiodothyronine (T_3). This increase begins as early as 6 weeks' gestation and reaches a plateau at around 18 weeks (Glinoer et al., 1990). However, the free fraction of T_4 and T_3 remain relatively stable throughout pregnancy and are similar to non-pregnant values. Thyroid-stimulating hormone (TSH) levels fall slightly in early pregnancy as a result of the high circulating hCG levels, which have a mild thyrotropic effect (Ballabio et al., 1991). TSH levels generally return to normal later in pregnancy. These physiologic changes in thyroid hormone levels have important clinical implications when selecting appropriate laboratory tests for evaluating thyroid status during pregnancy. As a general rule, total T_4 and T_3 levels are unhelpful in pregnancy. The most appropriate test to detect thyroid dysfunction is the high-sensitivity TSH assay. If this is abnormal, free T_4 and free T_3 levels should be measured.

The adrenal glands

Although the adrenal glands do not change in size during pregnancy, there are significant changes in adrenal hormone levels. Serum cortisol levels increase significantly in pregnancy, although the vast majority of this cortisol is bound to cortisol-binding globulin, which increases in the circulation in response to estrogen stimulation. However, free cortisol levels also increase in pregnancy by around 30% (Nolten & Rueckert, 1981).

Serum aldosterone levels increase throughout pregnancy, reaching a peak during the third trimester (Watanabe et al., 1963). This increase likely reflects an increase in renin substrate production, which results in increased levels of angiotensin II that, in turn, stimulates the adrenal glands to secrete aldosterone. Aldosterone functions to retain sodium at the level of the renal tubules, and likely acts to balance the natriuretic effects of progesterone.

Circulating levels of adrenal androgens are also increased in pregnancy. This is due in part to increased levels of sex-hormone binding globulin, which serves to retard their clearance from the maternal circulation. The conversion of adrenal androgens (primarily androstenedione and testosterone) to estradiol-17β by the placenta effectively protects the fetus from androgenic side effects.

The endocrine pancreas

β-cells in the islets of Langerhans within the pancreas are responsible for insulin production. β-cells undergo hyperplasia during pregnancy, resulting in increased insulin secretion. This insulin hypersecretion is likely responsible for the fasting hypoglycemia seen in early pregnancy. Peripheral resistance to circulating insulin increases as pregnancy progresses, due primarily to the increased production of insulin antagonists such as human placental lactogen. Such placental insulin antagonists result in the normal postprandial hyperglycemia seen in pregnancy (Phelps et al., 1981).

Immune system

One of the more interesting issues is not why some pregnancies fail, but how is it that any pregnancies succeed? Immunologists would argue that the fetus acquires its genetic information equally from both parents and, as such, represents a foreign tissue graft (hemi-allograft). It should therefore be identified as "foreign" by the maternal immune system and destroyed. This is the basis of transplant rejection. Successful pregnancy, on the other hand, is dependent on maternal tolerance (immunononreactivity) to paternal antigen. How is it that the hemi-allogeneic fetus is able to evade the maternal immune system? In 1953, Medawar proposed that mammalian viviparous reproduction represents a unique example of successful transplantation (known colloquially as *nature's transplant*). Several hypotheses have been put forward to explain this apparent discordance, which include the following:

1 The conceptus is not immunogenic and, as such, does not evoke an immunologic response.
2 Pregnancy alters the systemic maternal immune response to prevent immune rejection.
3 The uterus is an immunologically privileged site.
4 The placenta is an effective immunological barrier between mother and fetus.

The answer to this intriguing question likely incorporates a little of each of these hypotheses (Norwitz et al., 2001). Pregnancy is not a state of non-specific systemic immunosuppression. In experimental animals, for example, mismatched tissue allografts (including paternal skin grafts and ectopic fetal tissue grafts) are not more likely to be accepted in pregnant as compared with nonpregnant animals. However, there is evidence to suggest that the intrauterine environment is a site of partial immunologic privilege. For example, foreign tissue allograft placed within the uterus will ultimately be rejected, even in hormonally primed animals, but this rejection is often slower and more protracted than tissue grafts at other sites (Wilder, 1998).

Trophoblast (placental) cells are presumed to be essential to this phenomenon of immune tolerance, because they lie at the maternal–fetal interface where they are in direct contact with cells of the maternal immune system. It has been established that chorionic villous trophoblasts do not express classical major histocompatibility complex (MHC) class II molecules (Redman, 1983). Surprisingly, cytotrophoblasts upregulate a MHC class Ib molecule, HLA-G, as they invade the uterus (Kovats et al., 1990). This observation, and the fact that HLA-G exhibits limited polymorphism (Bainbridge et al., 1999), suggests functional importance. The exact mechanisms involved are not known, but may include upregulation of the inhibitory immunoglobulin-like transcript 4, an HLA-G receptor that is expressed on macrophages and a subset of natural killer (NK) lymphocytes (Allan et al., 1999). Cytotrophoblasts that express HLA-G come in direct contact with maternal lymphocytes that are abundant in the uterus during early pregnancy. Although estimates vary, a minimum of 10–15% of all cells found in the decidua are leukocytes (Starkey et al., 1988; King et al., 1998). Like invasive cytotrophoblasts, these maternal lymphocytes have unusual properties. Most are CD56+ NK cells. However, compared with peripheral blood lymphocytes, decidual leukocytes have low cytotoxic activity (Deniz et al., 1994). Trophoblast cells likely help to recruit these unusual maternal immune cells through the release of specific chemokines (Drake et al., 2001).

Cytotoxicity against trophoblast cells must be selectively inhibited to prevent immune rejection and pregnancy loss. The factors responsible for this localized immunosuppression are unclear, but likely include cytotrophoblast-derived interleukin-10, a cytokine that inhibits alloresponses in mixed lymphocyte reactions (Roth et al., 1996). Steroid hormones, including progesterone, have similar effects (Pavia et al., 1979). The complement system may also be involved, since deletion of the complement regulator, Crry, in mice leads to fetal loss secondary to placental inflammation (Xu et al., 2000). Finally, pharmacological data, also from studies in mice, suggest that trophoblasts express an enzyme, indoleamine 2,3-dioxygenase, that rapidly degrades tryptophan, which is essential for T-cell activation (Munn et al., 1998). Whether this mechanism occurs in humans is not known, although human syncytiotrophoblasts express indoleamine 2,3-dioxygenase (Kamimura et al., 1991) and maternal serum tryptophan concentrations fall during pregnancy (Schrocksnadel et al., 1996).

Although pregnancy does not represent a state of generalized maternal immunosuppression, there is evidence of altered immune function (Wilder, 1998). The major change in the maternal immune system during pregnancy is a move away from cell-mediated immune responses toward humoral or antibody-mediated immunity. Absolute numbers and activity of T-helper 1 cells and NK cells decline, whereas that of T-helper 2 cells increase. Clinically, the decrease in cellular immunity during pregnancy leads to an increased susceptibility to intracellular pathogens (including cytomegalovirus, varicella, and malaria). The decrease in cellular immunity may also explain why cell-mediated immunopathologic diseases (such as rheumatoid arthritis) frequently improve during pregnancy (Wilder, 1998). Although pregnancy is characterized by enhanced antibody-mediated immunity, the levels of immunoglobulins A (IgA), IgG, and IgM all decrease in pregnancy. This decrease in titers is due primarily to the hemodilutional effect of pregnancy and has little, if any, clinical implications (Baboonian & Griffiths, 1983). The peripheral white blood cell (leukocyte) count rises progressively during pregnancy (Pitkin & Witte, 1979; Table 3.9), primarily because of increased numbers of circulating segmented neutrophils and granulocytes. The reason for this leukocytosis is not clear, but is likely secondary to elevated estrogen and cortisol levels. It probably represents the reappearance in the circulation of leukocytes previously shunted out of the circulation.

Although maternal IgM and IgA are effectively excluded from the fetus, maternal IgG does cross the placenta (Gitlin et al., 1972; Cunningham et al., 1993b). Fc receptors are present on trophoblast cells, and the transport of IgG across the placenta is accomplished by way of these receptors through a process known as endocytosis. IgG transport from mother to fetus begins at around 16 weeks' gestation and increases as gestation proceeds. However, the vast majority of IgG acquired by the fetus from the mother occurs during the last 4 weeks of pregnancy (Gitlin et al., 1971; 1972). The human fetus begins to produce IgG shortly after birth, but adult values are not attained until approximately 3 years of age (Cunningham et al., 1993b).

Conclusions

Physiologic adaptations occur in all maternal organ systems during pregnancy; however, the quality, degree, and timing of the adaptation vary from one organ system to another and from one individual to another. Moreover, maternal adaptations to pregnancy occur before they appear to be necessary. Such physiologic modifications may be prerequisite for implantation and normal placental and fetal growth. It is important that obstetric care providers have a clear understanding of such physiologic adaptations, and how preexisting variables (such as maternal age, multiple gestation, ethnicity, and genetic factors) and pregnancy-associated factors (including gestational age, labor, and intrapartum blood loss) interact to affect the ability of the mother to adapt to the demands of pregnancy. A better understanding of the normal physiologic adaptations of pregnancy will improve the ability of clinicians to anticipate the effects of pregnancy on underlying medical conditions and to better manage pregnancy-associated complications, such as preeclampsia, pulmonary edema, and pulmonary embolism.

References

Adams JQ, Alexander AM. Alterations in cardiovascular physiology during labor. Obstet Gynecol 1958;12:542.

Alaily AB, Carrol KB. Pulmonary ventilation in pregnancy. Br J Obstet Gynaecol 1978;85:518–524.

Allan DS, Colonna M, Lanier LL, et al. Tetrameric complexes of human histocompatibility leukocyte antigen (HLA)-G bind to peripheral blood myelomonocytic cells. J Exp Med 1999;189:1149–1156.

American College of Obstetricians and Gynecologists. Hypertension in pregnancy. ACOG Technical Bulletin Number 219. Washington, DC: ACOG, 1996.

Anderson JR. Prolactin in amniotic fluid and maternal serum during uncomplicated human pregnancy. Dan Med Bull 1982;29:266.

Ang CK, Tan TH, Walters WA, et al. Postural influence on maternal capillary oxygen and carbon dioxide tension. Br Med J 1969;4:201–203.

Assali NS, Rauramo L, Peltonen T. Measurement of uterine blood flow and uterine metabolism. VIII. Uterine and fetal blood flow and oxygen consumption in early human pregnancy. Am J Obstet Gynecol 1960;79:86–98.

Atkins AF, Watt JM, Milan P. A longitudinal study of cardiovascular dynamic changes throughout pregnancy. Eur J Obstet Reprod Biol 1981a;12(4):215–224.

Atkins AFJ, Watt JM, Milan P, et al. The influence of posture upon cardiovascular dynamics throughout pregnancy. Eur J Obstet Gynecol Reprod Biol 1981b;12(6):357–372.

Awe RJ, Nicotra MB, Newsom TD, et al. Arterial oxygenation and alveolar–arterial gradients in term pregnancy. Obstet Gynecol 1979;53:182–186.

Baboonian C, Griffiths P. Is pregnancy immunosuppressive? Humoral immunity against viruses. Br J Obstet Gynaecol 1983;90:1168–1175.

Bader RA, Bader MG, Rose DJ, et al. Hemodynamics at rest and during exercise in normal pregnancy as studied by cardiac catheterization. J Clin Invest 1955;34:1524.

Baer JL, Reis RA, Artens RA. Appendicitis in pregnancy with changes in position and axis of the normal appendix in pregnancy. JAMA 1932;98:1359.

Bainbridge DR, Ellis SA, Sargent IL. Little evidence of HLA-G mRNA polymorphism in Caucasian or Afro-Caribbean populations. J Immunol 1999;163:2023–2027.

Baldwin GR, Moorthi DS, Whelton JA, MacDonnell KF. New lung functions in pregnancy. Am J Obstet Gynecol 1977;127:235–239.

Ballabio M, Poshyachinda M, Ekins RP. Pregnancy-induced changes in thyroid function: role of human chorionic gonadotropin as putative regulator of maternal thyroid. J Clin Endocrinol Metab 1991;73:824–831.

Barron WM, Lindheimer MD. Renal sodium and water handling in pregnancy. Obstet Gynecol Annu 1984;13:35–69.

Barron WM, Mujais SK, Zinaman M, et al. Plasma catecholamine responses to physiologic stimuli in normal human pregnancy. Am J Obstet Gynecol 1986;154:80–84.

Bayliss DA, Millhorn DE. Central neural mechanisms of progesterone action: application to the respiratory system. J Appl Physiol 1992;73:393–404.

Bieniarz J, Maqueda E, Caldeyro-Barcia R. Compression of aorta by the uterus in late human pregnancy. I. Variations between femoral and brachial artery pressure with changes from hypertension to hypotension. Am J Obstet Gynecol 1966;95:795–808.

Bieniarz J, Crottogini JJ, Curuchet E, et al. Aortocaval compression by the uterus in late human pregnancy. II. An arteriographic study. Am J Obstet Gynecol 1968;100:203.

Braithwaite JM, Economides DL. Severe recurrent epistaxis causing antepartum fetal distress. Int J Gynaecol Obstet 1995;50:197–198.

Braverman DZ, Johnson ML, Kern F. Effects of pregnancy and contraceptive steroids on gallbladder function. N Engl J Med 1980;302:262–264.

Brenner BM, Ballermann BJ, Gunning ME, Zeidel ML. Diverse biological actions of atrial natriuretic peptide. Physiol Rev 1990;70:665–669.

Burrows RF, Kelton JG. Thrombocytopenia at delivery: a prospective survey of 6,715 deliveries. Am J Obstet Gynecol 1990;162:731–734.

Burt CC. Peripheral skin temperature in normal pregnancy. Lancet 1949;2;787.

Burwell CS, Strayhorn WD, Flickinger D, et al. Circulation during pregnancy. Arch Intern Med 1938;62:979.

Calvin S, Jones OW, Knieriem K, Weinstein L. Oxygen saturation in the supine hypotensive syndrome. Obstet Gynecol 1988;71:872–877.

Capeless EL, Clapp JF. When do cardiovascular parameters return to their preconception values? Am J Obstet Gynecol 1991;165:883–886.

Caton WL, Roby CC, Reid DE, et al. The circulating red cell volume and body hematocrit in normal pregnancy and the puerperium. Am J Obstet Gynecol 1951;61:1207.

Caton D, Abrams RM, Clapp JF, et al. The effect of exogenous progesterone on the rate of blood flow of the uterus of ovariectomized sheep. Q J Exp Physiol Cogn Med Sci 1974;59:225–231.

Cavill I. Iron and erythropoiesis in normal subjects and in pregnancy. J Perinat Med 1995;23:47–50.

Chesley LC. Renal functional changes in normal pregnancy. Clin Obstet Gynecol 1960;3:349.

Chesley LC, Valenti C, Uichano L. Alterations in body fluid compartments and exchangeable sodium in early puerperium. Am J Obstet Gynecol 1959;77:1054.

Cietak KA, Newton JR. Serial quantitative maternal nephrosonography in pregnancy. Br J Radiol 1985;58:405–413.

Clapp JF, Seaward BL, Sleamaker RH, et al. Maternal physiologic adaptations to early human pregnancy. Am J Obstet Gynecol 1988;159:1456–1460.

Clark SL, Cotton DB, Lee W, et al. Central hemodynamic assessment of normal term pregnancy. Am J Obstet Gynecol 1989;161:1439–1442.

Clark SL, Cotton DB, Pivarnik JM, et al. Position change and central hemodynamic profile during normal third-trimester pregnancy and postpartum. Am J Obstet Gynecol 1991;164:883–887.

Contreras G, Guitierrez M, Beroiza T, et al. Ventilatory drive and respiratory muscle function in pregnancy. Am Rev Respir Dis 1991;144:837–841.

Crapo RO. Normal cardiopulmonary physiology during pregnancy. Clin Obstet Gynecol 1996;39:3–16.

Cugell DW, Frank NR, Gaensler EA, Badger TL. Pulmonary function in pregnancy. I. Serial observations in normal women. Am Rev Tuberc 1953;67:598.

Cunningham FG, MacDonald PC, Gant NF, Leveno KJ, Gilstrap LC III. The Puerperium. In: Cunningham FG, MacDonald PC, Gant NF, Leveno KJ, Gilstrap LC III, eds. Williams Obstetrics, 19th edn. Norwalk, CT: Appleton & Lange, 1993a:467.

Cunningham FG, MacDonald PC, Gant NF, Leveno KJ, Gilstrap LC III. The Morphological and Functional Development of the Fetus. In: Cunningham FG, MacDonald PC, Gant NF, Leveno KJ, Gilstrap LC III, eds. Williams Obstetrics, 19th edn. Norwalk, CT: Appleton & Lange, 1993b:165–207.

Cusson JR, Gutkowska, J, Rey E, et al. Plasma concentration of atrial natriuretic factor in normal pregnancy. N Engl J Med 1985;313:1230–1231.

Davis GL. Hemostatic changes associated with normal and abnormal pregnancies. Clin Lab Sci 2000;13:223–228.

Davison JM, Hytten FE. The effect of pregnancy on the renal handling of glucose. Br J Obstet Gynaecol 1975;82:374–381.

Davison JM, Vallotton MB, Lindheimer MD. Plasma osmolality and urinary concentration and dilution during and after pregnancy. Br J Obstet Gynaecol 1981;88:472–479.

Deniz G, Christmas SE, Brew R, Johnson PM. Phenotypic and functional cellular differences between human CD3-decidual and peripheral blood leukocytes. J Immunol 1994;152:4255–4261.

Drake PM, Gunn MD, Charo IF, et al. Human placental cytotrophoblasts attract monocytes and CD56 (bright) natural killer cells via the actions of monocyte inflammatory protein 1-alpha. J Exp Med 2001;193:1199–1212.

Du Bois D, Du Bois EF. A formula to estimate the approximate area if height and weight be known. Arch Intern Med 1916;17:863.

Dure-Smith P. Pregnancy dilatation of the urinary tract: the iliac sign and its significance. Radiology 1970;96:545–550.

Duvekot JJ, Cheriex EC, Pieters FA, et al. Early pregnancy changes in hemodynamics and volume homeostasis are consecutive adjustments triggered by a primary fall in systemic vascular tone. Am J Obstet Gynecol 1993;169:1382–1392.

Easterling TR, Watts DH, Schmucker BC, Benedetti TJ. Measurement of cardiac output during pregnancy: validation of Doppler technique and clinical observations in preeclampsia. Obstet Gynecol 1987;69:845–850.

Easterling TR, Schmucker BC, Benedetti TJ. The hemodynamic effects of orthostatic stress during pregnancy. Obstet Gynecol 1988;72:550–552.

Easterling TR, Benedetti TJ, Schmucker BC, Millard SP. Maternal hemodynamics in normal and preeclamptic pregnancies: a longitudinal study. Obstet Gynecol 1990;76:1061–1069.

Elkus R, Popovich J. Respiratory physiology in pregnancy. Clin Chest Med 1992;13:555–565.

Fay RA, Bromham DR, Brooks JA, et al. Platelets and uric acid in the prediction of pre-eclampsia. Am J Obstet Gynecol 1985;152: 1038–1039.

Fenton V, Saunders K, Cavill I. The platelet count in pregnancy. J Clin Pathol 1977;30:68–69.

Fried A, Woodring JH, Thompson TJ. Hydronephrosis of pregnancy. J Ultrasound Med 1983;2:255–259.

Gabert HA, Miller JM. Renal disease during pregnancy. Obstet Gynecol Surv 1985;40:449–461.

Gee JB, Packer BS, Millen JE, Robin ED. Pulmonary mechanics during pregnancy. J Clin Invest 1967;46:945–952.

Gilroy RJ, Mangura BT, Lavietes MH. Rib cage and abdominal volume displacements during breathing in pregnancy. Am Rev Respir Dis 1988;137:668–672.

Ginsberg J, Duncan SL. Direct and indirect blood pressure measurement in pregnancy. J Obstet Gynaecol Br Commonw 1969;76:705.

Girling JC, Dow E, Smith JH. Liver function tests in preeclampsia: importance of comparison with a reference range derived for normal pregnancy. Br J Obstet Gynaecol 1997;104:246–250.

Gitlin D. Development and metabolism of the immune globulins. In: Kagan BM, Stiehm ER, eds. Immunologic Incompetence. Chicago, IL: Year Book Inc., 1971.

Gitlin D, Kumate J, Morales C, Noriega C, Arevalo N. The turnover of amniotic fluid protein in the human conceptus. Am J Obstet Gynecol 1972;113:632–645.

Glinoer D, De Nayer P, Bourdoux P, et al. Regulation of maternal thyroid during pregnancy. J Clin Endocrinol Metab 1990;71:276–287.

Gonzalez JG, Elizondo G, Saldivar D, Nanez H, Todd LE, Villarreal JZ. Pituitary gland growth during normal pregnancy: an in vivo study using magnetic resonance imaging. Am J Med 1988;85:217–220.

Hamilton HGH. The cardiac output in normal pregnancy as determined by the Cournard right heart catheterization technique. J Obstet Gynaecol Br Emp 1949;56:548.

Hankins GD, Wendel GD, Cunningham FG, et al. Longitudinal evaluation of hemodynamic changes in eclampsia. Am J Obstet Gynecol 1984;150:506–512.

Hankins GDV, Harvey CJ, Clark SL, et al. The effects of maternal position and cardiac output on intrapulmonary shunt in normal third-trimester pregnancy. Obstet Gynecol 1996;88:327–330.

Harada A, Hershman JM, Reed AW, et al. Comparison of thyroid stimulators and thyroid hormone concentrations in the sera of pregnant women. J Clin Endocrinol Metab 1979;48:793–797.

Hellgren M. Hemostasis during pregnancy and puerperium. Hemostasis 1996;26(Suppl 4):244–247.

Hendricks ECH, Quilligan EJ. Cardiac output during labor. Am J Obstet Gynecol 1958;76:969.

Henriksen TB, Hedegaard M, Secher NJ, Wilcox AJ. Standing at work and preterm delivery. Br J Obstet Gynaecol 1995;102:198–206.

Herbert CM, Banner EA, Wakim KG. Variations in the peripheral circulation during pregnancy. Am J Obstet Gynecol 1958;76:742.

Hertzberg BS, Carroll BA, Bowie JD, et al. Doppler US assessment of maternal kidneys: analysis of intrarenal resistivity indexes in normal pregnancy and physiologic pelvicaliectasis. Radiology 1993;186:689–692.

Higby K, Suiter CR, Phelps JY, Siler-Khodr T, Langer O. Normal values of urinary albumin and fetal protein excretions during pregnancy. Am J Obstet Gynecol 1994;171:984–989.

Holmes F. Incidence of the supine hypotensive syndrome in late pregnancy. J Obstet Gynaecol Br Emp 1960;67:254.

Howard BK, Goodson JH, Mengert WF. Supine hypotensive syndrome in late pregnancy. Obstet Gynecol 1953;1:371.

Howard DJ. Life-threatening epistaxis in pregnancy. J Laryngol Otol 1985;99:95–96.

Hytten FE, Paintin DB. Increase in plasma volume during normal pregnancy. J Obstet Gynaecol Br Commonw 1963;70:402.

Jepson JH. Endocrine control of maternal and fetal erythropoiesis. Can Med Assoc J 1968;98:844–847.

Jepson JH, Lowenstein L. Role of erythropoietin and placental lactogen in the control of erythropoiesis during pregnancy. Can J Physiol Pharmacol 1968;46:573–576.

Kamimura S, Eguchi K, Yonezawa M, Sekiba K. Localization and developmental change of indoleamine 2,3-dioxygenase activity in the human placenta. Acta Med Okayama 1991;45:135–139.

Katz M, Sokal MM. Skin perfusion in pregnancy. Am J Obstet Gynecol 1980;137:30–33.

Katz R, Karliner JS, Resnik R. Effects of a natural volume overload state (pregnancy) on left ventricular performance in normal human subjects. Circulation 1978;58:434–441.

Kerr MG. Cardiovascular dynamics in pregnancy and labour. Br Med Bull 1968;24:19.

King A, Burrows T, Verma S, Hiby S, Loke YW. Human uterine lymphocytes. Hum Reprod Update 1998;4:480–485.

Kinsella SM, Lohmann G. Supine hypotensive syndrome. Obstet Gynecol 1994:774–788.

Kirshon B, Lee W, Cotton DB, Giebel R. Indirect blood pressure monitoring in the postpartum patient. Obstet Gynecol 1987;70:799–801.

Kitabatake A, Inoue M, Asao M, et al. Noninvasive evaluation of pulmonary hypertension by a pulsed Doppler technique. Circulation 1983;68:302–309.

Kjeldsen J. Hemodynamic investigations during labor and delivery. Acta Obstet Gynecol Scand 1979;89(Suppl):1–252.

Kletzky OA, Rossman F, Bertolli SI, Platt LD, Mischel DR Jr. Dynamics of human chorionic gonadotropin, prolactin, and growth hormone in serum and amniotic fluid throughout normal human pregnancy. Am J Obstet Gynecol 1985;151:878–884.

Koller O. The clinical significance of hemodilution during pregnancy. Obstet Gynecol Surv 1982;37:649–652.

Kovats S, Main EK, Librach C, Stubblebine M, Fisher SJ, DeMars R. A class I antigen, HLA-G, expressed in human trophoblasts. Science 1990;248:220–223.

Laird-Meeter K, van de Ley G, Bom TH, et al. Cardiocirculatory adjustments during pregnancy—an echocardiographic study. Clin Cardiol 1979;2:328–332.

Lee W, Cotton DB. Peripartum cardiomyopathy: current concepts and clinical management. Clin Obstet Gynecol 1989;32:54–67.

Lee W, Rokey R, Cotton DB. Noninvasive maternal stroke volume and cardiac output determinations by pulsed Doppler echocardiography. Am J Obstet Gynecol 1988;158:505–510.

Lee W, Rokey R, Cotton DB, Miller JF. Maternal hemodynamic effects of uterine contractions by M-mode and pulsed-Doppler echocardiography. Am J Obstet Gynecol 1989;161:974–977.

Lees MM, Taylor SH, Scott DB, et al. A study of cardiac output at rest throughout pregnancy. J Obstet Gynaecol Br Commonw 1967;74:319–328.

Letsky EA. Erythropoiesis in pregnancy. J Perinat Med 1995;23:39–45.

Lindheimer MD, Barron WM. Renal function and volume homeostasis. In: Gleicher N, Buttino L, Elkayam U, Evans MI, Galbraith RM, Gall SA, Sibai BM, eds. Principles and Practice of Medical Therapy in Pregnancy, 3rd edn. Stanford, CT. Appleton & Lange, 1998: 1043–52.

Lindheimer MD, Katz AI. Renal function in pregnancy. Obstet Gynecol Annu 1972;1:139–176.

Lindheimer MD, Katz AI. Sodium and diuretics in pregnancy. N Engl J Med 1973;288:891–894.

Lindqvist P, Dahlback B, Marsal K. Thrombotic risk during pregnancy: a population study. Obstet Gynecol 1999;94:595–599.

Linhard J. Uber das minutevolumens des herzens bei ruhe und bei muskelarbeit. Pflugers Arch 1915;1612:233.

Longo LD, Hardesty JS. Maternal blood volume: measurement, hypothesis of control, and clinical considerations. Rev Perinatal Med 1984;5:35.

Lund CJ, Donovan JC. Blood volume during pregnancy. Significance of plasma and red cell volumes. Am J Obstet Gynecol 1967; 98:394–403.

Mabie WC, DiSessa TG, Crocker LG, et al. A longitudinal study of cardiac output in normal human pregnancy. Am J Obstet Gynecol 1994;170:849–856.

Mabry RL. Rhinitis of pregnancy. South Med J 1986;79:965.

McCalden RA. The inhibitory action of oestradiol-17β and progesterone on venous smooth muscle. Br J Pharmacol 1975;53: 183–192.

MacKenzie JN. The physiological and pathological relations between the nose and the sexual apparatus of man. Alienist & Neurol 1898;19:219.

Macklem PT, Gross D, Grassino GA, Roussos C. Partitioning of inspiratory pressure swings between diaphragm and intercostals/accessory muscles. J Applied Physiol 1978;44:200–208.

McLennon CE, Thouin LG. Blood volume in pregnancy. Am J Obstet Gynecol 1948;55:1189.

Mashini IS, Albazzaz SJ, Fadel HE, et al. Serial noninvasive evaluation of cardiovascular hemodynamics during pregnancy. Am J Obstet Gynecol 1987;156:1208–1213.

Medawar PB. Some immunological and endocrinological problems raised by the evolution of viviparity in vertebrates. Symposium of the Society of Experimental Biology 1953;7:320.

Metcalfe J, Romney SL, Ramsy LH, et al. Estimation of uterine blood flow in normal human pregnancy at term. J Clin Invest 1955;34:1632.

Milne JA. The respiratory response to pregnancy. Postgrad Med J 1979;55:318–324.

Milne JA, Howie AD, Pack AI. Dyspnoea during normal pregnancy. Br J Obstet Gynaecol 1978;85:260–263.

Mortimer H, Wright RP, Collip JB. The effect of the administration of oestrogenic hormones on the nasal mucosa of the monkey (Macata mulatta). Can Med Assoc J 1936;35:503.

Morton M, Tsang H, Hohimer R, et al. Left ventricular size, output, and structure during guinea pig pregnancy. Am J Physiol 1984;246:R40–48.

Munn DH, Zhou M, Attwood JT, et al. Prevention of allogeneic fetal rejection by tryptophan catabolism. Science 1998;281:1191–1193.

Murray JA, Johnston W, Reid JM. Echocardiographic determination of left ventricular dimensions, volumes, and performance. Am J Cardiol 1972;30:252–257.

Naeye RL, Peters EC. Working during pregnancy: effects on the fetus. Pediatrics 1982;69:724–727.

Nava S, Zanotti E, Ambrosino N, Fracchia C, Scarabelli C, Rampulla C. Evidence of acute diaphragmatic fatigue in a "natural" condition. The diaphragm during labor. Am Rev Respir Dis 1992;146:1226–1230.

Newton M, Mosey LM, Egli GE, et al. Blood loss during and immediately after delivery. Obstet Gynecol 1961;17:9.

Nisell H, Lunell N, Linde B. Maternal hemodynamics and impaired fetal growth in pregnancy-induced hypertension. Obstet Gynecol 1988;71:163–166.

Nolten WE, Rueckert PA. Elevated free cortisol index in pregnancy: possible regulatory mechanisms. Am J Obstet Gynecol 1981;139:492–498.

Norregard O, Shultz P, Ostergaard A, Dahl R. Lung function and postural changes during pregnancy. Respir Med 1989;83:467.

Norwitz ER, Schust DJ, Fisher SJ. Implantation and the survival of early pregnancy. N Engl J Med 2001;345:1400–1408.

O'Brien JR. Platelet counts in normal pregnancy. J Clin Pathol 1976;29:174.

Oparil S, Ehrlich EN, Lindheimer MD. Effect of progesterone on renal sodium handling in man: relation to aldosterone excretion and plasma renin activity. Clin Sci Mol Med 1975;49:139–147.

van Oppen AC, van der Tweel I, Duvekot JJ, Bruinse HW. Use of cardiac output in pregnancy: is it justified? Am J Obstet Gynecol 1995;173:923–928.

van Oppen ACC, van der Tweel I, Alsbach GPJ, et al. A longitudinal study of maternal hemodynamics during normal pregnancy. Obstet Gynecol 1996;88:40–46.

Palmer AJ, Walker AHC. The maternal circulation in normal pregnancy. J Obstet Gynaecol Br Emp 1949;56:537.

Parry E, Shields R, Turnbull AC. Transit time in the small intestine in pregnancy. J Obstet Gynaecol Br Commonw 1970;77:900–901.

Pavia C, Siiteri PK, Perlman JD, Stites DP. Suppression of murine allogeneic cell interactions by sex hormones. J Reprod Immunol 1979;1:33–38.

Peck TM, Arias F. Hematologic changes associated with pregnancy. Clin Obstet Gynecol 1979;22:785–798.

Pernoll ML, Metcalfe J, Kovach PA, Wachtel R, Dunham MJ. Ventilation during rest and exercise in pregnancy and postpartum. Respir Physiol 1975;25:295–310.

Phelps RL, Metzger BE, Freinkel N. Carbohydrate metabolism in pregnancy. XVII. Diurnal profiles of plasma glucose, insulin, free fatty acids, triglycerides, cholesterol, and individual amino acids in late normal pregnancy. Am J Obstet Gynecol 1981;140:730–736.

Phippard AF, Horvath JS, Glynn EM. Circulatory adaptation to pregnancy—serial studies of hemodynamics, blood volume, renin and aldosterone in the baboon (*Papio hamadryas*). J Hypertens 1986;4:773–779.

Pirani BBK, Campbell DM, MacGillivray I. Plasma volume in normal first pregnancy. J Obstet Gynaecol Br Commonw 1973;80:884–887.

Pitkin R, Witte D. Platelet and leukocyte counts in pregnancy. JAMA 1979;242:2696–2698.

Pombo JF, Troy BL, Russell RO. Left ventricular volumes and ejection fraction by echocardiography. Circulation 1971;43:480–490.

Pritchard JA. Changes in the blood volume during pregnancy and delivery. Anesthesiology 1965a;26:393.

Pritchard JA. Blood volume changes in pregnancy and the puerperium. IV. Anemia associated with hydatidiform mole. Am J Obstet Gynecol 1965b;91:621.

Pritchard JA, Baldwin RM, Dickey JC, Wiggins KM. Blood volume changes in pregnancy and the puerperium. II. Red blood cell loss and changes in apparent blood volume during and following vaginal delivery, cesarean section, and cesarean section plus total hysterectomy. Am J Obstet Gynecol 1962;84:1271.

Pritchard JA, Cunningham FG, Pritchard SA. The Parkland Memorial Hospital protocol for treatment of eclampsia: evaluation of 245 cases. Am J Obstet Gynecol 1984;148:951.

Radberg G, Asztely M, Cantor P, Rehfeld JF, Jarnfeldt-Samsioe A, Svanvik J. Gastric and gall bladder emptying in relation to the secretion of cholecystokinin after a meal in late pregnancy. Digestion 1989;42:174–180.

Rakoczi I, Tallian F, Bagdany S, Gati I. Platelet lifespan in normal pregnancy and pre-eclampsia as determined by a non-radioisotope technique. Thromb Res 1979;15:553–556.

Redman CW. HLA-DR antigen on human trophoblast: a review. Am J Reprod Immunol 1983;3:175–177.

Reynolds SRM, Foster FI. Acetylcholine—equivalent content of the nasal mucosa in rabbits and cats, before and after administration of estrogen. Am J Physiol 1940;131:422.

Robson SC, Dunlop W, Boys RJ, Hunter S. Cardiac output during labor. Br Med J 1987a;295:1169–1172.

Robson SC, Dunlop W, Moore M, Hunter S. Combined Doppler and echocardiographic measurement of cardiac output: theory and application in pregnancy. Br J Obstet Gynaecol 1987b;94:1014–1027.

Robson SC, Hunter S, Moore M, Dunlop W. Haemodynamic changes during the puerperium: a Doppler and M-mode echocardiographic study. Br J Obstet Gynaecol 1987c;94:1028–1039.

Robson SC, Hunter S, Boys RJ, Dunlop W. Serial study of factors influencing changes in cardiac output during human pregnancy. Am J Physiol 1989a;256:H1060–1065.

Robson SC, Hunter R, Boys W, et al. Changes in cardiac output during epidural anaesthesia for caesarean section. Anaesthesia 1989b;44:475–479.

Robson SC, Hunter S, Boys J, Dunlop W. Serial changes in pulmonary haemodynamics during human pregnancy: a non-invasive study using Doppler echocardiography. Clin Sci 1991;80:113–117.

Roth I, Corry DB, Locksley RM, Abrams JS, Litton MJ, Fisher SJ. Human placental cytotrophoblasts produce the immunosuppressive cytokine interleukin 10. J Exp Med 1996;184:539–548.

Rovinsky JJ, Jaffin H. Cardiovascular hemodynamics in pregnancy. I. Blood and plasma volumes in multiple pregnancy. Am J Obstet Gynecol 1965;93:1.

Rubin A, Russo N, Goucher D. The effect of pregnancy upon pulmonary function in normal women. Am J Obstet Gynecol 1956;72:963.

Salas SP, Rosso P, Espinoza R, et al. Maternal plasma volume expansion and hormonal changes in women with idiopathic fetal growth retardation. Obstet Gynecol 1993;81:1029–1033.

Schatz M, Zieger RS. Diagnosis and management of rhinitis during pregnancy. Allergy Proc 1988;9:545–554.

Schrier RW. Pathogenesis of sodium and water retention in high-output and low-output cardiac failure, nephrotic syndrome, cirrhosis, and pregnancy. N Engl J Med 1988;319:1127–1134.

Schrier RW. Body fluid volume regulation in health and disease: a unifying hypothesis. Ann Intern Med 1990;113:155–159.

Schrier RW, Briner VA. Peripheral arterial vasodilation hypothesis of sodium and water retention in pregnancy: implications for pathogenesis of preeclampsia-eclampsia. Obstet Gynecol 1991;77:632–639.

Schrocksnadel H, Baier-Bitterlich G, Dapunt O, Wachter H, Fuchs D. Decreased plasma tryptophan in pregnancy. Obstet Gynecol 1996;88:47–50.

Scott DE. Anemia during pregnancy. Obstet Gynecol Annu 1972;1:219–244.

Scott DE, Pritchard JA. Iron deficiency in healthy young college women. JAMA 1967;199:897–900.

Seitchik J. Total body water and total body density of pregnant women. Obstet Gynecol 1967;29:155–166.

Sejeny SA, Eastham RD, Baker SR. Platelet counts during normal pregnancy. J Clin Pathol 1975;28:812–813.

Seligman SP, Kadner SS, Finlay TH. Relationship between preeclampsia, hypoxia, and production of nitric oxide by the placenta. Am J Obstet Gynecol 1996;174:abstract.

Shulman A, Herlinger H. Urinary tract dilatation in pregnancy. Br J Radiol 1975;48:638–645.

Slater AJ, Gude N, Clarke IJ, Walters WA. Haemodynamic changes and left ventricular performance during high-dose oestrogen administration to male transsexuals. Br J Obstet Gynaecol 1986; 93:532-538.

Sobol SE, Frenkiel S, Nachtigal D, Wiener D, Teblum C. Clinical manifestations of sinonasal pathology during pregnancy. J Otolaryngol 2001;30:24–28.

Starkey PM, Sargent IL, Redman CW. Cell populations in human early pregnancy decidua: characterization and isolation of large granular lymphocytes by flow cytometry. Immunology 1988;65: 129–134.

Taylor M. An experimental study of the influence of the endocrine system on the nasal respiratory mucosa. J Laryngol Otol 1961;75:972.

Thomsen JK, Storm TL, Thamsborg G, et al. Increased concentration of circulating atrial natriuretic peptide during normal pregnancy. Eur J Obstet Gynecol Reprod Biol 1988;27:197–201.

Thomsen JK, Fogh-Anderson N, Jaszczak P, Giese J. Atrial natriuretic peptide (ANP) decrease during normal pregnancy as related to hemodynamic changes and volume regulation. Acta Obstet Gynecol Scand 1993;72:103–110.

Thomson JK, Cohen ME. Studies on the circulation in pregnancy. II. Vital capacity observations in normal pregnant women. Surg Gynecol Obstet 1938;66:591.

Toppozada H, Michaels L, Toppozada M, et al. The human respiratory mucosa in pregnancy. J Laryngol Otol 1982;96:613–626.

Ueland K. Maternal cardiovascular dynamics. VII. Intrapartum blood volume changes. Am J Obstet Gynecol 1976;126:671–677.

Ueland K, Hansen JM. Maternal cardiovascular dynamics. II. Posture and uterine contractions. Am J Obstet Gynecol 1969a; 103:1–7.

Ueland K, Hansen JM. Maternal cardiovascular hemodynamics. III. Labor and delivery under local and caudal anesthesia. Am J Obstet Gynecol 1969b;103:8–18.

Ueland K, Metcalfe J. Circulatory changes in pregnancy. Clin Obstet Gynecol 1975;18:41–50.

Ueland K, Parer JT. Effects of estrogens on the cardiovascular system of the ewe. Am J Obstet Gynecol 1966;96:400–406.

Ueland K, Novy MJ, Peterson EN, et al. Maternal cardiovascular dynamics. IV. The influence of gestational age on the maternal cardiovascular response to posture and exercise. Am J Obstet Gynecol 1969;104:856–864.

Van Thiel DH, Gavaler JS, Joshi SN, Sara RK, Stremple J. Heartburn of pregnancy. Gastroenterology 1977;72:666–668.

Vasicka A, Lin TJ, Bright RH. Peptic ulcer and pregnancy: review of hormonal relationships and a report of one case of massive hemorrhage. Obstet Gynecol Surv 1957;12:1.

Villar MA, Sibai BM. Clinical significance of elevated mean arterial pressure in second trimester and threshold increase in systolic and diastolic blood pressure during third trimester. Am J Obstet Gynecol 1989;160:419–423.

Vorys N, Ullery JC, Hanusek GE. The cardiac output changes in various positions in pregnancy. Am J Obstet Gynecol 1961;82:1312.

Waldum HL, Straume BK, Lundgren R. Serum group I pepsinogens during pregnancy. Scand J Gastroenterol 1980;15:61–63.

Wallenburg HC, van Kessel PH. Platelet lifespan in normal pregnancy as determined by a nonradioisotopic technique. Br J Obstet Gynaecol 1978;85:33–36.

Walters WAW, MacGregor WG, Hills M. Cardiac output at rest during pregnancy and the puerperium. Clin Sci 1966;30:1–11.

Watanabe M, Meeker CI, Gray MJ, Sims EA, Solomon S. Secretion rate of aldosterone in normal pregnancy. J Clin Invest 1963;42:1619.

Weinberger SE, Weiss ST, Cohen WR, Weiss JW, Johnson TS. Pregnancy and the lung: state of the art. Am Rev Respir Dis 1980;121:559–581.

Werko L. Pregnancy and heart disease. Acta Obstet Gynecol Scand 1954;33:162.

Wilcox CF, Hunt AR, Owen FA. The measurement of blood lost during cesarean section. Am J Obstet Gynecol 1959;77:772.

Wilder R. Hormones, pregnancy, and autoimmune diseases. Ann N Y Acad Sci 1998;840:45–50.

Wilson M, Morganti AA, Zervodakis I, et al. Blood pressure, the renin-aldosterone system, and sex steroids throughout normal pregnancy. Am J Med 1980;68:97–107.

Winkel CA, Milewich L, Parker CR Jr, et al. Conversion of plasma progesterone to desoxycorticosterone in men, nonpregnant, and pregnant women, and adrenalectomized subjects. J Clin Invest 1980;66:803–812.

Winner W, Romney SL. Cardiovascular responses to labor and delivery. Am J Obstet Gynecol 1966;96:1004.

Wook JE, Goodrich SM. Dilation of the veins with pregnancy or with oral contraceptive therapy. Trans Am Clin Climatol Assoc 1964; 76:174.

Xu C, Mao D, Holers VM, Palanca B, Cheng AM, Molina H. A critical role for murine complement regulator crry in fetomaternal tolerance. Science 2000;287:498–501.

Zwillich CW, Natalino MR, Sutton FD, Weil JV. Effects of progesterone on chemosensitivity in normal men. J Lab Clin Med 1978; 92:262–269.

4 Maternal–fetal blood gas physiology

Renee A. Bobrowski

Abnormalities in acid–base and respiratory homeostasis are common among patients requiring intensive medical support, but many clinicians find the physiology cumbersome. As a result of both their illness and our therapeutic interventions, critically ill patients frequently require assessment of metabolic and respiratory status. An understanding and clinical application of basic physiologic principles is therefore essential to the care of these patients. It is also important that clinicians involved in the care of critically ill gravidas be familiar with the metabolic and respiratory changes of pregnancy as well as their effect on arterial blood gas interpretation.

The arterial blood gas provides information regarding acid–base balance, oxygenation, and ventilation. A blood gas should be considered when a patient has significant respiratory symptoms, experiences oxygen desaturation, or as a baseline in the evaluation of preexisting cardiopulmonary disease. In this chapter we focus on fundamental physiology, analytical considerations, effective interpretation of an arterial blood gas, and acid–base disturbances.

Essential physiology

Acid–base homeostasis

Normal acid–base balance depends on production, buffering, and excretion of acid. The delicate balance that is crucial for survival is maintained by buffer systems, the lungs and kidneys. Each day, approximately 15,000 mEq of volatile acids (e.g. carbonic acid) are produced by the metabolism of carbohydrates and fats. These acids are transported to and removed via the lungs as carbon dioxide (CO_2) gas. Breakdown of proteins and other substances results in 1–1.5 mEq/kg/day of nonvolatile or fixed acids (predominantly phosphoric and sulfuric acids) that are removed by the kidney.

Buffers are substances that can absorb or donate protons and thereby resist or reduce changes in H^+ ion concentration. Acids produced by cellular metabolism move out of cells and into the extracellular space where buffers absorb the protons. These protons are then transported to the kidney and excreted in urine. The intra- and extracellular buffer systems that maintain homeostasis in the human include the carbonic acid–bicarbonate system, plasma proteins, hemoglobin, and bone.

The carbonic acid–bicarbonate system is the principal extracellular buffer. Its effectiveness is predominantly due to the ability of the lungs to excrete carbon dioxide. In this system, bicarbonate, carbonic acid, and carbon dioxide are related by the equation:

$$\underset{\substack{\text{Gaseous}\\\text{phase}\\\downarrow\\\textit{Lung}}}{CO_2} \leftrightarrow \underset{\text{Dissolved}}{H_2O + CO_2} \leftrightarrow \underset{\substack{\text{Carbonic}\\\text{acid}}}{H_2CO_3} \underset{\substack{\textit{Carbonic}\\\textit{anhydrase}}}{\leftrightarrow} \underset{\substack{\text{Bicarbonate}\\\downarrow\\\textit{Kidney}}}{H^+ + HCO_3^-}$$

Carbon dioxide is produced as an end product of aerobic metabolism and physically dissolves in body fluids. A portion of dissolved CO_2 reacts with water to form carbonic acid, which dissociates into bicarbonate and hydrogen ions. The concentration of carbonic acid is normally very low relative to that of dissolved CO_2 and HCO_3^-. If the H^+ ion concentration increases, however, the acid load is buffered by bicarbonate, and additional carbonic acid is formed. The equilibrium of the equation is then driven to the left, and excess acid can be excreted as carbon dioxide gas.

The Henderson–Hasselbalch equation expresses the relationship between the reactants of the carbonic acid–bicarbonate system under conditions of equilibrium:

$$\mathrm{pH} = \mathrm{pK} + \log\frac{[HCO_3^-]}{(s)P\text{CO}_2} = \frac{\text{metabolic}}{\text{respiratory}}$$

As the equation demonstrates, the ratio of $[HCO_3^-]/P\text{CO}_2$ determines pH (H^+ ion concentration) and not individual or absolute concentrations. This ratio is influenced to a large extent by the function of the kidneys (HCO_3^-) and lungs ($P\text{CO}_2$). The constant s represents the solubility coefficient of CO_2 gas in plasma and relates $P\text{CO}_2$ to the concentration of dissolved CO_2 and HCO_3^-. The value of s is 0.03 mmol/L/mmHg at 37°C. The dissociation constant (pK) of blood carbonic acid is equivalent to 6.1 at 37°C.

The lungs are the second component of acid–base regulation. Alveolar ventilation controls $P\text{CO}_2$ independent of bicarbonate excretion. When the bicarbonate concentration is altered, respiratory changes attempt to return the ratio of $[HCO_3^-]/P\text{CO}_2$ toward the normal 20:1. Thus, in the presence of metabolic acidosis (decreased HCO_3^-), ventilation increases, $P\text{CO}_2$ is lowered, and the ratio normalizes. In metabolic alkalosis, the opposite occurs as $P\text{CO}_2$ rises in response to the primary increase in HCO_3^-.

The kidney is the final element of acid–base regulation. The main functions of the renal system are excretion of fixed acids and regulation of plasma bicarbonate levels. Carbonic acid that has been transported to the kidney dissociates into H^+ and HCO_3^- in renal tubular cells. Each H^+ ion secreted into the tubular lumen is exchanged for sodium, and HCO_3^- is passively reabsorbed into the blood. Essentially all bicarbonate must be reabsorbed by the kidney before acid can be excreted, because the loss of one HCO_3^- is equivalent to the addition of one H^+ ion. Mono- and diphasic phosphates and ammonia are urinary buffers that combine with H^+ ions in the renal tubules and are excreted. Under normal conditions, the amount of H^+ excreted approximates the amount of nonvolatile acids produced.

The buffer systems, the lungs and kidneys interact to maintain very tight control of the body's acid–base balance. The sequence of responses to a H^+ ion load and the time required for each may be summarized:

Extracellular buffering by HCO_3^- (immediate)	→	Respiratory buffering $P\text{CO}_2\downarrow$ (minutes to hours)	→	Renal exretion of $H^+\uparrow$ (hours to days)

In contrast, when $P\text{CO}_2$ changes:

Intracellular buffering (minutes)	→	Renal excretion of $H^+\uparrow$ (hours to days)

Unlike the response to an acid load, no extracellular buffering occurs with a change in $P\text{CO}_2$. Since HCO_3^- is not an effective buffer against H_2CO_3, the only protection against respiratory acidosis or alkalosis is intracellular buffering (i.e. by hemoglobin) and renal H^+ ion excretion.

Acid–base disturbances

Disturbances in acid–base balance are classified according to whether the underlying process results in an abnormal rise or fall in arterial pH. The suffix *-osis* refers to a pathologic process that causes a gain or loss of acid or base. Thus, *acidosis* describes any condition that leads to a fall in blood pH if the process continues uncorrected. Conversely, *alkalosis* characterizes any process that will cause a rise in pH if unopposed. The terms acidosis and alkalemia do not require the pH to be abnormal. The suffix *-emia* refers to the state of the blood, and *acidemia* and *alkalemia* are appropriately used when blood pH is abnormally low (<7.36) or high (>7.44), respectively (Kruse, 1993).

In addition, alterations in acid–base homeostasis are classified based upon whether the underlying mechanism is metabolic or respiratory. If the primary abnormality is a net gain or loss of CO_2, this is respiratory acidosis or alkalosis, respectively. Alternatively, a net gain or loss of bicarbonate results in metabolic alkalosis or acidosis, respectively. If only one primary process is present, then the acid–base disturbance is simple, and bicarbonate and $P\text{CO}_2$ always deviate in the same direction. A mixed disturbance develops when two or more primary processes are present, and the changes in HCO_3^- and $P\text{CO}_2$ are in opposite directions.

The compensatory response attempts to normalize the $[HCO_3^-]/P\text{CO}_2$ ratio and maintain pH. Renal and pulmonary function must be adequate for these responses to be effective and adequate time must be allowed for the complete response. The compensatory response for a primary respiratory abnormality is via the bicarbonate system or acid excretion by the kidney and requires several days for a complete response. Compensation for a metabolic aberration is through ventilation changes and occurs quite rapidly.

Compensatory responses cannot, however, completely return the pH to normal, with the exception of chronic respiratory alkalosis. The more severe the primary disorder, the more difficult it is for the pH to return to normal. When the pH is normal but $P\text{CO}_2$ and HCO_3^- are abnormal or the expected compensatory responses do not occur, then a second primary disorder exists. The four types of acid–base abnormalities and the compensatory response associated with each are listed in Table 4.1.

Respiratory and acid–base changes during pregnancy

A variety of physiologic changes occur during pregnancy, affecting maternal respiratory function and gas exchange. As a result, an arterial blood gas obtained during pregnancy must be interpreted with an understanding of these alterations. Since these changes begin early in gestation and persist into the puerpurium, they must be taken into consideration regardless of the stage of pregnancy (MacRae & Palavradji, 1967). In addition, the altitude at which a patient lives will affect arterial blood gas values, and normative data for each individual population should be established (Hankins et al., 1996a).

Minute ventilation increases by 30–50% during pregnancy (Artal et al., 1986; Cruikshank & Hays, 1991) and alveolar and arterial $P\text{CO}_2$ decrease. Normal maternal arterial $P\text{CO}_2$ levels range from 26 to 32 mmHg (Andersen et al., 1969; Dayal et al., 1972; Liberatore et al., 1984). Since the fetus depends upon the

Table 4.1 Summary of acid–base disorders: the primary disturbance, compensatory response, and expected degree of compensation

	Primary disturbance	Compensatory response	Expected degree of compensation
Metabolic acidosis	Decreased HCO_3^-	Decreased $P\text{CO}_2$	$P_a\text{CO}_2 = [1.5 \times (\text{serum bicarbonate})] + 8$ $P_a\text{CO}_2$ = last two digits of pH
Metabolic alkalosis	Increased HCO_3^-	Increased $P\text{CO}_2$	$P_a\text{CO}_2 = [0.7 \times (\text{serum bicarbonate})] + 20$
Respiratory acidosis	Increased $P\text{CO}_2$	Increased HCO_3^-	Acute: pH $\Delta = 0.08 \times (\text{measured } P_a\text{CO}_2 - 40)/10$ Chronic: pH $\Delta = 0.03 \times (\text{measured } P_a\text{CO}_2 - 40)/10$
Respiratory alkalosis	Decreased $P\text{CO}_2$	Decreased HCO_3^-	Acute: pH $\Delta = 0.08 \times (40 - \text{measured } P_a\text{CO}_2)/10$ Chronic: pH $\Delta = 0.03 \times (40 - \text{measured } P_a\text{CO}_2)/10$

maternal respiratory system for carbon dioxide excretion, the decreased maternal $P\text{CO}_2$ creates a gradient that allows the fetus to offload carbon dioxide. Nevertheless, fetal $P\text{CO}_2$ is approximately 10 mmHg higher than the maternal level when uteroplacental perfusion is normal.

Maternal alveolar oxygen tension increases as alveolar carbon dioxide tension decreases, and arterial $P\text{CO}_2$ levels rise as high as 106 mmHg during the first trimester (Anderson et al., 1969; Templeton & Kelman, 1976). Airway closing pressures increase with advancing gestation, causing a slight fall in arterial $P\text{CO}_2$ in the third trimester (101–104 mmHg) (Anderson et al., 1969; Pernoll et al., 1975; Templeton & Kelman, 1976). The arterial $P\text{CO}_2$ level, however, is dependent upon the altitude at which the patient resides. The mean arterial $P\text{CO}_2$ for gravidas at sea level ranges from 95 to 102 mmHg (Templeton & Kelman, 1976; Awe et al., 1979), while the average values reported for those living at 1,388 m are 87 mmHg (Hankins, 1996b) and 61 mmHg at 4,200 m (Sobrevilla et al., 1971). As with carbon dioxide transfer, the fetus depends upon the oxygen gradient for continued diffusion across the placenta. Maternal arterial oxygen content, uterine artery perfusion, and maternal hematocrit contribute to fetal oxygenation and compromise of any of these factors can cause fetal hypoxemia and eventually acidemia (Novy & Edwards, 1967).

Despite the increased ventilation, maternal arterial pH remains essentially unchanged during pregnancy (Anderson et al., 1969; Weinberger et al., 1980). A slightly higher pH value has been noted in women living at a moderate altitude, with a reported mean of 7.46 at 1,388 m above sea level (Hankins, 1996a). Bicarbonate excretion by the kidney is increased during normal pregnancy to compensate for the lowered $P\text{CO}_2$, and serum bicarbonate levels are normally 18–21 mEq/L (MacRae & Palavradji, 1967; Andersen et al., 1969; Lucius et al., 1970; Dayal et al., 1972). Thus, the metabolic state of pregnancy is a chronic respiratory alkalosis with a compensatory metabolic acidosis (Table 4.2).

Table 4.2 Arterial blood gas values during pregnancy at mild to moderate altitude. Normative data should be established for individual populations residing at high altitude

Parameter	Normal range
pH	7.40–7.46
$P\text{CO}_2$	26–32 mmHg
$P\text{O}_2$	75–106 mmHg
HCO_3^-	18–21 mEq/L

Oxygen delivery and consumption

All tissues require oxygen for the combustion of organic compounds to fuel cellular metabolism. The cardiopulmonary system serves to deliver a continuous supply of oxygen and other essential substrates to tissues. Oxygen delivery is dependent on oxygenation of blood in the lungs, oxygen carrying capacity of the blood and cardiac output. Under normal conditions, oxygen delivery ($D\text{O}_2$) exceeds oxygen consumption ($V\text{O}_2$) by about 75% (Cain, 1983). The amount of oxygen delivered is determined by the cardiac output (CO L/min) times the arterial oxygen content ($C_a\text{O}_2$ mL/O_2/dL):

$$D\text{O}_2 = \text{CO} \times C_a\text{O}_2 \times 10\,\text{dL/L}$$

Arterial oxygen content ($C_a\text{O}_2$) is determined by the amount of oxygen that is bound to hemoglobin ($S_a\text{O}_2$) and by the amount of oxygen that is dissolved in plasma ($P_a\text{O}_2 \times 0.003$):

$$C_a\text{O}_2 = (1.39 \times \text{Hb} \times S_a\text{O}_2) + (P_a\text{O}_2 \times 0.003)$$

It is clear from this formula that the amount of oxygen dissolved in plasma is negligible and, therefore, that arterial oxygen is dependent largely on hemoglobin concentration and arterial oxygen saturation. Oxygen delivery can be impaired by conditions that affect either cardiac output (flow), arterial oxygen content, or both (Table 4.3). Anemia leads to low arterial oxygen content because of a lack of hemoglobin binding sites for oxygen (Stock et al., 1986). The patient with hypoxemic respiratory failure will not have sufficient oxygen available to saturate the hemoglobin molecule. Furthermore, it has been demonstrated that desaturated hemoglobin is altered structurally in such a fashion as to have a diminished affinity for oxygen (Bryan-Brown et al., 1973). It must be kept in mind that the amount of oxygen actually available to tissues also is

Table 4.3 Commonly used formulas for assessment of oxygenation

	Formula	Normal value
Est. alveolar oxygen tension	$P_{A}O_2 = 145 - P_{a}CO_2$	
Pulmonary capillary oxygen content	$C_{c}O_2 = [Hb](1.39) + (P_{A}O_2)(0.003)$	
Arterial oxygen content	$C_{a}O_2 = (1.39 \times Hb \times S_{a}O_2) + (P_{a}O_2 \times 0.003)$	18–21 mL/dL
Mixed venous oxygen content	$C\bar{v}O_2 = (1.39 \times Hb \times S\bar{v}O_2) + (P\bar{v}O_2)(0.003)$	
Oxygen delivery	$DO_2 = CaO_2 \times Q_T \times 10$	640–1,200 mL O_2/min
Oxygen consumption	$VO_2 = Q_T(C_{a}O_2 - C_{v}O_2) = 13.8\,(Hb)\,(Q_T)\,(S_{a}O_2 - S_{v}O_2)/100$	180–280 mL O_2/min
Shunt equation	$\dfrac{Q_{sp}}{Q_t} = \dfrac{Cc'O_2 - C_{a}O_2}{Cc'O_2 - C\bar{v}O_2}$	3–8%
Estimated shunt	$\text{Est. } Q_{sp}/Q_t = \dfrac{Cc'O_2 - C_{a}O_2}{[Cc'O_2 - C_{a}O_2] + [C_{a}O_2 - C\bar{v}O_2]}$	

$P_{a}CO_2$, partial pressure of arterial carbon dioxide; $P_{a}O_2$, partial pressure of arterial oxygen; $P\bar{v}O_2$, partial pressure of venous oxygen; Hb, hemoglobin; $S_{a}O_2$, arterial oxygen saturation; $S\bar{v}O_2$, venous oxygen saturation; Q_T, cardiac output.

affected by the affinity of the hemoglobin molecule for oxygen. Thus, the oxyhemoglobin dissociation curve (Fig. 4.1) and those conditions that influence the binding of oxygen either negatively or positively must be considered when attempts are made to maximize oxygen delivery (Perutz, 1978). An increase in the plasma pH level, or a decrease in temperature or 2,3-diphosphoglycerate (2,3-DPG) will increase hemoglobin affinity for oxygen, shifting the curve to the left and resulting in diminished tissue oxygenation. If the plasma pH level falls, or temperature or 2,3-DPG increases, hemoglobin affinity for oxygen will decrease and more oxygen will be available to tissues (Perutz, 1978).

In certain clinical conditions, such as septic shock and adult respiratory distress syndrome (ARDS), there is maldistribution of flow relative to oxygen demand, leading to diminished delivery and loss of vascular autoregulation, producing regional and microcirculatory imbalances in blood flow (Rakow, 1991). This mismatching of blood flow with metabolic demand causes excessive blood flow to some areas, with relative hypoperfusion of other areas, limiting optimal systemic utilization of oxygen (Rackow & Astiz, 1991).

The patient with diminished cardiac output secondary to hypovolemia or pump failure is unable to distribute oxygenated blood to tissues. Therapy directed at increasing volume with normal saline, or with blood if the hemoglobin level is less than 10 g/dL, increases oxygen delivery in the hypovolemic patient. The patient with pump failure may benefit from inotropic support and afterload reduction in addition to supplementation of intravascular volume.

Relationship of oxygen delivery to consumption

Oxygen consumption (VO_2) is the product of the arteriovenous oxygen content difference ($C_{(a-v)}O_2$) and cardiac output. Under

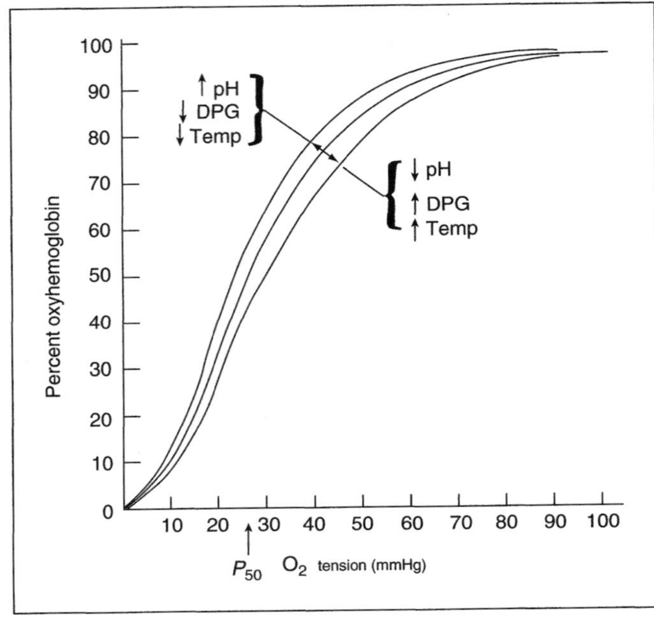

Fig. 4.1 The oxygen binding curve for human hemoglobin A under physiologic conditions (middle curve). The affinity is shifted by changes in pH, diphosphoglycerate (DPG) concentration, and temperature, as indicated. P_{50} represents the oxygen tension at half saturation. (Reproduced by permission from Bunn HF, Forget BG. Hemoglobin: molecular, genetic, and clinical aspects. Philadelphia: WB Saunders, 1986.)

normal conditions, oxygen consumption is a direct function of the metabolic rate (Shoemaker et al., 1989).

$$VO_2 = C_{(a-v)}O_2 \times CO \times 10\,dL/L$$

The oxygen extraction ratio (OER) is the fraction of delivered oxygen that is actually consumed:

$$OER = VO_2/DO_2$$

The normal OER is about 0.25. A rise in the OER is a compensatory mechanism employed when oxygen delivery is inadequate for the level of metabolic activity. An OER less than 0.25 suggests flow maldistribution, peripheral diffusion defects, or fractional shunting (Shoemaker et al., 1989). As the supply of oxygen is reduced, the fraction extracted from blood increases and oxygen consumption is maintained. If a severe reduction in oxygen delivery occurs, the limits of oxygen extraction are reached, tissues are unable to sustain aerobic energy production, and consumption decreases. The level of oxygen delivery at which oxygen consumption begins to decrease has been termed the "critical $D\text{o}_2$" (Shibutani et al., 1983). At the critical $D\text{o}_2$, tissues begin to use anaerobic glycolysis, with resultant lactate production and metabolic acidosis (Shibutani et al., 1983). If this oxygen deprivation continues, irreversible tissue damage and death ensue.

Oxygen delivery and consumption in pregnancy

The physiologic anemia of pregnancy results in a reduction in the hemoglobin concentration and arterial oxygen content. Oxygen delivery is maintained at or above normal despite this because cardiac output increases 50%. It is important to remember, therefore, that the pregnant woman is more dependent on cardiac output for maintenance of oxygen delivery than the nonpregnant patient (Barron & Lindheimer, 1991). Oxygen consumption increases steadily throughout pregnancy and is greatest at term, reaching an average of 331 mL/min at rest and 1,167 mL/min with exercise (Pernoll et al., 1975). During labor, oxygen consumption increases by 40–60%, and cardiac output increases by about 22% (Gemzell et al., 1957; Ueland & Hansen, 1969). Because oxygen delivery normally far exceeds consumption, the normal pregnant patient usually is able to maintain adequate delivery of oxygen to herself and her fetus, even during labor. When a pregnant patient's oxygen delivery decreases, however, she very quickly can reach the critical $D\text{o}_2$, especially during labor, compromising both herself and her fetus. The obstetrician, therefore, must make every effort to optimize oxygen delivery before allowing labor to begin in the compromised patient.

Blood gas analysis

The accuracy of a blood gas determination relies upon many factors, including blood collection techniques, specimen transport, and laboratory equipment. Up to 16% of specimens may be improperly handled, diminishing diagnostic utility in a number of cases (Walton et al., 1981). Factors that can influence blood gas results include excessive heparin in the collection syringe, catheter dead space, air bubbles in the blood sample, time delays to laboratory analysis as well as other less common causes. This section highlights considerations for obtaining a blood sample and potential sources of error, and briefly describes laboratory methods.

Sample collection

The collection syringe typically contains heparin to prevent clotting of the specimen. Excessive heparin in the syringe prior to blood collection, however, can significantly decrease the $P\text{co}_2$ and bicarbonate of the sample. The spurious $P\text{co}_2$ level results in a falsely lowered bicarbonate concentration when calculated using the Henderson–Hasselbalch equation. Although sodium heparin is an acid, pH is minimally affected because whole blood is an adequate buffer. Expelling all heparin except that in the dead space of the syringe and needle and ensuring adequate dilution by obtaining a minimum of 3 mL of blood will help avoid anticoagulant-related errors (Bloom et al., 1985).

In the intensive care setting, an arterial catheter is often placed when frequent blood sampling is anticipated. Dilutional errors occur when a blood sample is contaminated with fluids in the catheter (Ng et al., 1984). An adequate volume of maintenance fluid or flush solution must be withdrawn from the catheter and discarded prior to obtaining the sample for analysis, but estimating the appropriate amount can be difficult. Although a 2.5 mL discard volume has been suggested, it has also been recommended that each intensive care unit establish its own policy based upon individual catheter and connection systems (Al-Ameri et al., 1986; Bhaskaran & Lawler, 1988; Kruse, 1993).

Air bubbles in the collection syringe cause time-dependent changes in the arterial blood gas. Air trapped as froth accelerates these changes because of their increased surface area (Biswas et al., 1982). The degree of change in $P\text{o}_2$ depends upon the initial $P\text{o}_2$ of the sample. Since an air bubble has a $P\text{o}_2$ of 150 mmHg (room air), the bubble will cause a falsely elevated $P\text{o}_2$ if the sample $P\text{o}_2$ is <150 mmHg. The opposite occurs if the sample has an initial $P\text{o}_2$ >150 mmHg (Mueller & Lang, 1982; Kruse, 1993). Oxygen saturation is most significantly affected when the sample $P\text{o}_2$ is <60 mmHg since saturation changes rapidly with changes in $P\text{o}_2$, as predicted by the oxyhemoglobin dissociation curve. $P\text{co}_2$ in the sample decreases within several minutes of exposure to ambient air (Biswas et al., 1982; Harsten et al., 1988).

When a blood sample remains at room temperature following collection, $P\text{o}_2$ and pH may decrease while $P\text{co}_2$ increases. Specimens analyzed within 10–20 min of collection give accurate results even when transported at room temperature (Madiedo et al., 1980; Nanji & Whitlow, 1984). In most clinical settings, however, the time between sampling and laboratory analysis of the specimen exceeds this limit. Therefore, the syringe should be placed into an ice bath immediately after sample collection. The combination of ice and water provides better cooling of the syringe than ice alone, and a sample may be stored for up to 1 hour without adversely affecting blood gas results (Harsten et al., 1988).

Several additional factors can influence blood gas results (Urbina & Kruse, 1993). Insufficient time between an adjustment in fractional inspired oxygen or mechanical ventilator settings and blood gas analysis may not accurately reflect the change. Equilibration is quite rapid, however, and has been reported to occur as soon as 10 min after changing ventilator settings of postoperative cardiac patients (Schuch & Price, 1986). General anesthesia with halothane will falsely elevate Po_2 determination as it mimics oxygen during sample analysis (Dent & Netter, 1976; Douglas et al., 1978; McHugh et al., 1979; Maekawa et al., 1980). Finally, severe leukocytosis causes a false lowering of Po_2 due to consumption by the cells in the collection syringe (Hess et al., 1979). The effect of the white blood cells may be minimized, but not necessarily eliminated, by cooling the sample immediately after it is obtained.

The blood gas analyzer

The blood gas analyzer is designed to simultaneously measure the pH, Po_2, and Pco_2 of blood. An aliquot of heparinized blood is injected into a chamber containing one reference and three measuring electrodes. Each measuring electrode is connected to the reference electrode by a Ag/AgCl wire. The electrodes and injected sample are kept at a constant 37°C by a warm water bath or heat exchanger. The accuracy of the measurements depends upon routine calibration of equipment, proper sample collection, and constant electrode temperature.

Blood pH and Pco_2 are potentiometric determinations, with the potential difference between each electrode and the reference electrode quantitated. The pH electrode detects hydrogen ions, and the electrical potential developed by the electrode varies with the H^+ ion activity of the sample. The potential difference between the pH and reference electrode is measured by a voltmeter and converted to the pH. The Pco_2 electrode is actually a modified pH electrode. A glass electrode is surrounded with a weak bicarbonate solution and enclosed in a silicone membrane. Carbon dioxide in the sample diffuses through this membrane that is permeable to CO_2 but not water and H^+ ions. As CO_2 diffuses through the membrane, the pH of the bicarbonate solution changes. Thus, the pH measured by the electrode is related to CO_2 tension.

The measurement of Po_2 is amperometric, as the current generated between an anode and cathode estimates the partial pressure of oxygen. The Po_2 electrode surrounds a membrane permeable to oxygen but not other blood constituents. The electrode consists of an anode and a cathode, and constant voltage is maintained between them. An electrolytic process that occurs in the presence of oxygen produces current, and the magnitude of the current is proportional to the partial pressure of oxygen in the sample. As oxygen tension increases, the electrical current generated between the anode and cathode increases.

Bicarbonate concentration as reported on a blood gas result is not directly measured in the blood gas laboratory. Once pH and Pco_2 are determined, bicarbonate concentration is calculated using the Henderson–Hasselbalch equation or determined from a nomogram. In contrast, the total serum CO_2 (tCO_2) content is measured by automated methods and reported with routine serum electrolyte measurements.

Oxygen saturation (So_2) is the ratio of oxygenated hemoglobin to total hemoglobin. It can be plotted graphically once Po_2 is determined, calculated using an equation that estimates the oxyhemoglobin dissociation curve, or determined spectrophotometrically by a co-oximeter. The latter is the most accurate method since saturation is determined by a direct reading.

Pulse oximetry

The oximetry system determines arterial oxygen saturation by measuring the absorption of selected wavelengths of light in pulsatile blood flow (New, 1985). Oxyhemoglobin absorbs much less red and slightly more infrared light than reduced hemoglobin. Oxygen saturation is therefore the ratio of red to infrared absorption.

Red and infrared light from light-emitting diodes are projected across a pulsatile tissue bed and analyzed by a photodetector. The absorption of each wavelength of light varies cyclically with pulse. The patient's heart rate, therefore, is also determined. When assessing the accuracy of the arterial saturation measured by the pulse oximeter, correlation of the oximeter-determined heart rate and the patient's actual pulse rate indicates proper electrode placement. The oximetry probe is usually placed on a nail bed or ear lobe. Under ideal circumstances, most oximeters measure saturation (S_po_2) to within 2% of S_ao_2 (New, 1985).

Pulse oximetry is ideal for noninvasive arterial oxygen saturation monitoring near the steep portion of the oxyhemoglobin dissociation curve, namely at a P_ao_2 less than or equal to 70 mmHg (Demling & Knox, 1993). P_ao_2 levels greater than or equal to 80 mmHg result in very small changes in oxygen saturation, namely 97–99%. Large changes in the P_ao_2 from 90 mmHg to 60 mmHg can occur without significant change in arterial oxygen saturation. This technique, therefore is useful as a continuous monitor of the adequacy of blood oxygenation and not as a method to quantitate the level of impaired gas exchange (Huch et al., 1988).

Poor tissue perfusion, hyperbilirubinemia, and severe anemia may cause inaccurate oximetry readings (Demling & Knox, 1993). Carbon monoxide poisoning leads to an overestimation of the P_ao_2. When methemoglobin levels exceed 5%, the pulse oximeter cannot reliably predict oxygen saturation. Methylene blue, the treatment for methemoglobinemia, will also lead to inaccurate oximetry readings. Normal values for maternal pulse oximetry readings (S_po_2) are dependent upon gestational age, position, and altitude of residence (Dildy et al., 1998, 1999; Richlin et al., 1998).

Mixed venous oxygenation

The mixed venous oxygen tension (P_vO_2) and mixed venous oxygen saturation (S_vO_2) are parameters of tissue oxygenation (Shoemaker et al., 1989). P_vO_2 is 40 mmHg with a saturation of 73%. Saturations less than 60% are abnormally low. These parameters can be measured directly by obtaining a blood sample from the distal port of the pulmonary artery catheter. The S_vO_2 also can be measured continuously with a fiberoptic pulmonary artery catheter. Mixed venous oxygenation is a reliable parameter in the patient with hypoxemia or low cardiac output, but findings must be interpreted with caution. When the S_vO_2 is low, oxygen delivery can be assumed to be low. However, normal or high does not guarantee that tissues are well oxygenated. In conditions such as septic shock and ARDS, the maldistribution of systemic flow may lead to abnormally high S_vO_2 in the face of severe tissue hypoxia (Rackow & Astiz, 1991). The oxyhemoglobin dissociation curve must be considered when interpreting the S_vO_2 as an indicator of tissue oxygenation (Bryan-Brown et al., 1973). Conditions that result in a left shift of the curve cause the venous oxygen saturation to be normal or high, even when the mixed venous oxygen content is low. The S_vO_2 is useful for monitoring trends in a particular patient, because a significant decrease will occur when oxygen delivery has decreased secondary to hypoxemia or a fall in cardiac output.

Blood gas interpretation

The processes leading to acid–base disturbances are well described, and blood gas analysis may facilitate identification of the cause of a serious illness. Since many critically ill patients have metabolic and respiratory derangements, correct interpretation of a blood gas is fundamental to their care. Misinterpretation, however, can result in treatment delays and inappropriate therapy. Several methods of acid–base interpretation have been devised, including graphic nomograms and step-by-step analysis. Each method is detailed in this section to aid in rapid and correct diagnosis of disturbances in acid–base balance.

Blood gas results are not a substitute for clinical evaluation of a patient, and laboratory values do not necessarily correlate with the degree of clinical compromise. A typical example is the patient with an acute exacerbation of asthma who experiences severe dyspnea and respiratory compromise prior to developing hypercapnea and hypoxemia. Thus, a blood gas is an adjunct to clinical judgment, and decision making should not be based on a single test.

Graphic nomogram

Nomograms are a graphic display of an equation and have been designed to facilitate identification of simple acid–base disturbances (Arbus, 1973; Goldberg et al., 1973; Davenport, 1974; Cogan, 1986). Figure 4.2 is an example of a nomogram with arterial blood pH represented on the x-axis, HCO_3^- concentration on the y-axis, and arterial PCO_2 on the regression lines. Nomograms are accurate for simple acid–base disturbances, and a single disorder can be identified by plotting measured blood gas values. When blood gas values fall between labeled areas, a mixed disorder is present and the nomogram does not apply. These complex disorders must then be characterized by quantitative assessment of the expected compensatory changes (Table 4.1).

A systematic approach to an acid–base abnormality

Several different approaches for blood gas interpretation have been devised (Haber, 1991; Tremper & Barker, 1992). A six-step approach modified from Narins and Emmett provides a simple and reliable method to analyze a blood gas, particularly when a complicated mixed disorder is present (Narins & Emmett, 1980; Morganroth, 1990a, b). This method, adjusted for pregnancy, is as follows (Fig. 4.3):

1 *Is the patient acidemic or alkalemic?* If the arterial blood pH is <7.36, the patient is acidemic, while a pH >7.44 defines alkalemia.
2 *Is the primary disturbance respiratory or metabolic?* The primary alteration associated with each of the four primary disorders is shown in Table 4.1.
3 *If a* respiratory *disturbance is present, is it acute or chronic?* The equations listed in Table 4.1 are used to determine the acuteness of the disturbance. The expected change in the pH is calculated and the measured pH is compared to the pH that would be expected based on the patient's PCO_2.
4 *If a* metabolic acidosis *is present, is the anion gap increased?* Metabolic acidosis is classified according to the presence or absence of an anion gap.
5 *If a* metabolic *disturbance is present, is the respiratory compensation adequate?* The expected PCO_2 for a given degree of metabolic acidosis can be predicted by Winter's formula (Table 4.1), since the relationship between PCO_2 and HCO_3^- is linear. Predicting respiratory compensation for metabolic alkalosis, however, is not nearly as consistent as with acidosis.
6 *If the patient has an anion gap metabolic acidosis, are additional metabolic disturbances present?* The excess anion gap represents bicarbonate concentration before the anion gap acidosis developed. By calculating the excess gap, an otherwise undetected nonanion gap acidosis or metabolic alkalosis may be detected.

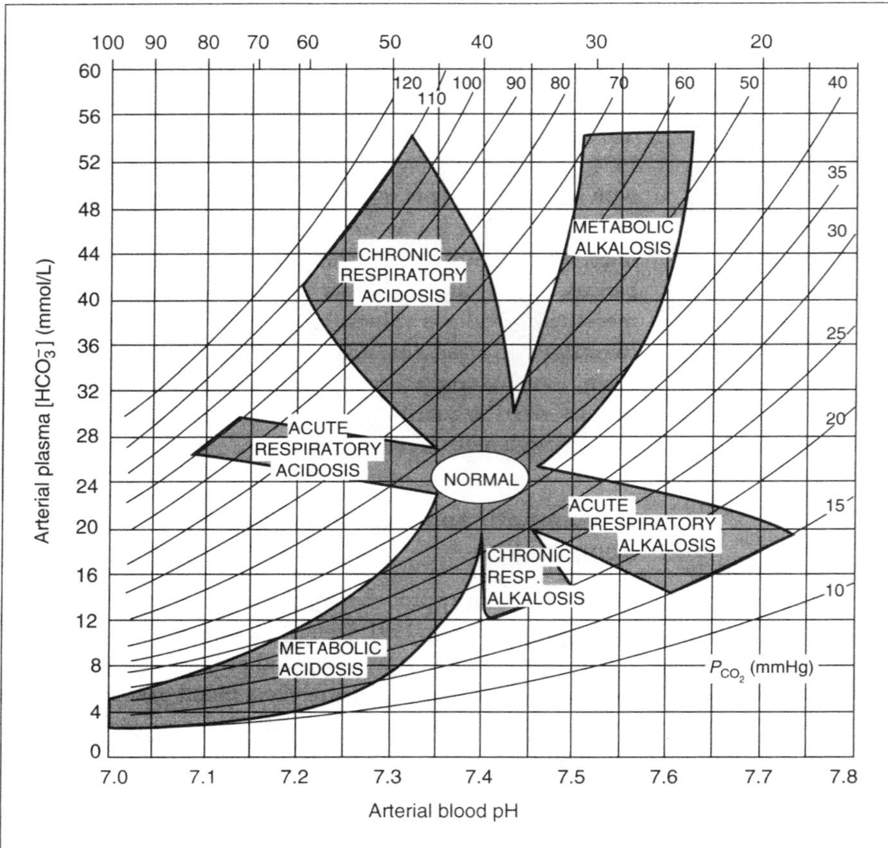

Fig. 4.2 Nomogram for interpretation of simple acid–base disorders. (Reproduced by permission from Cogan MJ. In: Brenner BM, Rector FC Jr, eds. The Kidney. Philadelphia: WB Saunders, 1986:473.)

Respiratory components of the arterial blood gas

Partial pressure of arterial oxygen (P_ao_2)

The P_ao_2 reflects the lung's ability to provide adequate arterial oxygen. Normal arterial oxygen tension during pregnancy ranges from 87 to 106 mmHg, depending upon the altitude at which a patient lives. Although P_ao_2 has been reported to decrease by 25% when samples are obtained from gravidas in the supine position (Awe et al., 1979), arterial blood gas values were recently shown to be unaffected by a change in maternal position (Hankins et al., 1996a). Abnormal gas exchange, inadequate ventilation or both can lead to a fall in P_ao_2. Hypoxemia is defined as a P_ao_2 below 60 mmHg or a saturation less than 90%. At this level, the oxygen content of blood is near its maximum for a given hemoglobin concentration and any additional increase in arterial oxygen tension will increase oxygen content only a small amount.

The amount of oxygen combined with hemoglobin is related to the P_ao_2 by the oxyhemoglobin dissociation curve and influenced by a variety of factors (Fig. 4.4). The shape of the oxyhemoglobin dissociation curve allows P_ao_2 to decrease faster than oxygen saturation until the P_ao_2 is approximately 60 mmHg. A left shift of the curve increases hemoglobin's affinity for oxygen and oxygen content, but decreases release of O_2 in peripheral tissues. The fetal or neonatal oxyhemoglobin dissociation curve is shifted to the left as a result of fetal hemoglobin and lower levels of 2,3-DPG (Fig. 4.4). The increased affinity of hemoglobin for oxygen allows the fetus to extract maximal oxygen from maternal blood. A shift to the right has the opposite effect, with decreased oxygen affinity and content but increased release in the periphery.

Assessment of lung function

Impairment of lung function can be estimated using an oxygen tension- or oxygen content-based index. Oxygen tension-based indices include: (i) expected P_ao_2 for a given fraction of inspired oxygen (F_io_2); (ii) P_ao_2/F_io_2 ratio; and (iii) alveolar–arterial oxygen gradient ($P_{(A-a)}o_2$). These methods are quick and easy to use but have limitations in the critically ill patient (Cane et al., 1988). The shunt calculation (Q_{sp}/Q_t) is an oxygen content-based index and is the most reliable method of determining the extent to which pulmonary disease is contributing to arterial hypoxemia. The need for a pulmonary artery blood sample is a disadvantage, however, as not all patients require invasive monitoring. The estimated shunt calculation (est. Q_{sp}/Q_t) is derived from the shunt equation and is the optimal

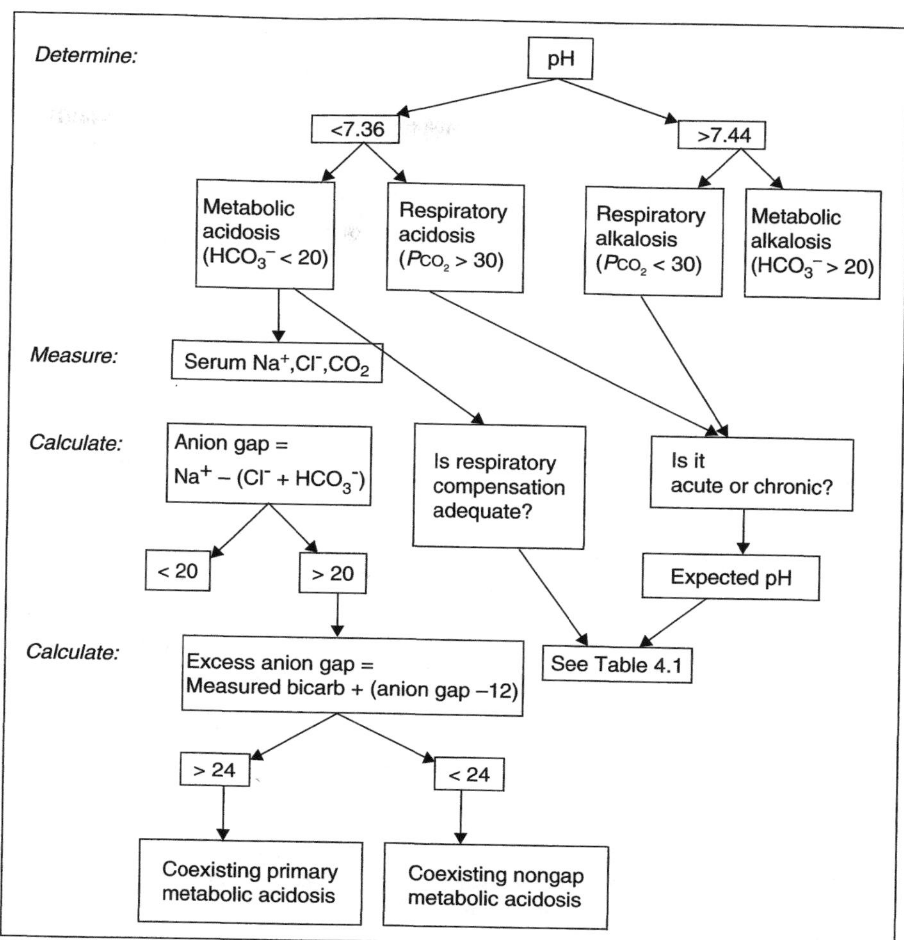

Fig. 4.3 A systematic approach to the interpretation of an arterial blood gas during pregnancy.

method to estimate lung compromise when a pulmonary artery catheter is not in place.

The expected P_aO_2 is an oxygen tension-based calculation and can be quickly estimated by multiplying the actual percentage of inspired oxygen by 6 (Wilson, 1992a). Thus, a patient receiving 50% oxygen has an expected PO_2 of (50 × 6) or 300 mmHg. Alternatively, the F_iO_2 (e.g. 0.50 in a patient receiving 50% oxygen) may be multiplied by 500 to estimate the minimum PO_2 (Shapiro & Peruzzi, 1992). The P_aO_2/F_iO_2 ratio has been used to estimate the amount of shunt. The normal ratio is 500–600 and correlates with a shunt of 3–5% while a shunt of 20% or more is present when the ratio is less than 200.

Calculation of the alveolar–arterial oxygen gradient is also an oxygen tension calculation. The A–a gradient is most reliable when breathing room air and is normally less than 20. An increased gradient indicates pulmonary dysfunction. A–a gradient values, however, can change unpredictably with changes in F_iO_2 and vary with alterations in oxygen saturation and consumption. Thus, the utility of this measurement in critically ill patients has been questioned since these patients often require a high F_iO_2 and have unstable oxygenation (Nearman & Sampliner, 1982). Additionally, the A–a gradient appears to be unreliable in the assessment of lung impairment during pregnancy (Awe et al., 1979).

Oxygen content-based indices include the shunt equation and estimated shunt as derived from the shunt equation (Table 4.3) The estimated shunt has been shown to be superior to the oxygen tension-based indices described above (Cane et al., 1988). The patient is given 100% oxygen for at least 20 min prior to determining arterial and venous blood gases and hemoglobin. Since the estimated shunt equation does not require a pulmonary artery blood sample, the $C_{(a-v)}O_2$ difference is assumed to be 3.5 mL/dL. A normal shunt in nonpregnant patients is less than 10%, while a 20–29% shunt may be life-threatening in a patient with compromised cardiovascular or neurologic function, and a shunt of 30% and greater usually requires significant cardiopulmonary support.

Intrapulmonary shunt values during normal pregnancy, however, have been reported to be nearly three times above the mean for nonpregnant individuals (Hankins, 1996b). The mean Q_s/Q_t in normotensive primiparous women at 36–38 weeks' gestation ranges from 10% in the knee–chest position to 13% in the standing position and 15% in the lateral position. The increased Q_s/Q_t can be explained by the physiologic

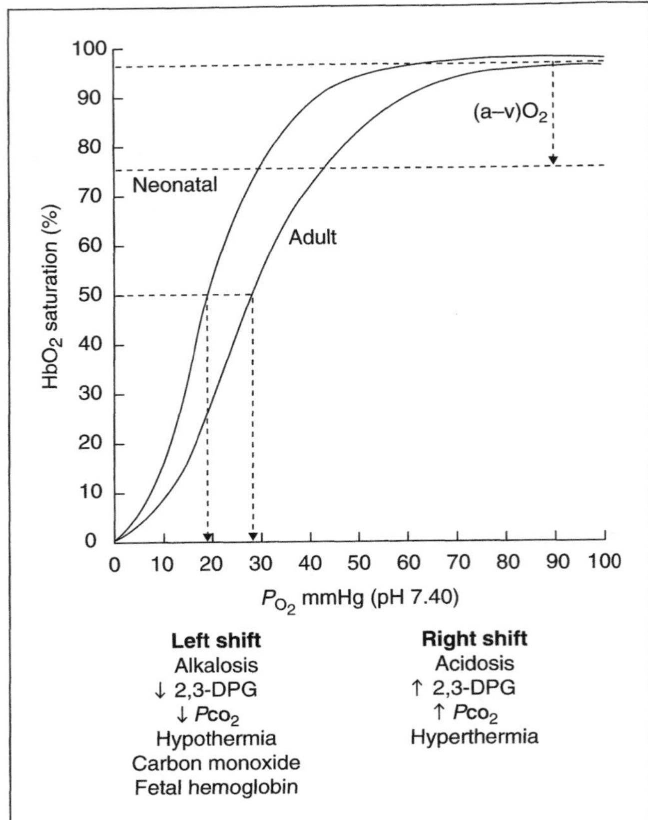

Fig. 4.4 Maternal and fetal oxyhemoglobin dissociation curves. 2,3-DPG, 2,3-diphosphoglycerate. (Reproduced by permission from Semin Perinatol. WB Saunders, 1984;8:168.)

changes of pregnancy as follows. Lung volumes decrease during gestation and the amount of shunt increases. In addition, pulmonary blood flow increases secondary to increased cardiac output. The combined effect of decreased lung volumes and increased pulmonary flow results in a higher intrapulmonary shunt during pregnancy.

Oxygenation of peripheral tissues

An adequate P_ao_2 is only the initial step in oxygen transport, however, and it does not guarantee well-oxygenated tissues. The degree of intrapulmonary shunt, oxygen delivery, and oxygen consumption all contribute to adequate tissue oxygenation. Accurate assessment of peripheral oxygenation requires measurement of arterial and venous partial pressures of oxygen, arterial and venous oxygen saturation, hemoglobin, and cardiac output (Table 4.3).

The amount of O_2 (mL) contained in 100 mL of blood defines oxygen content. Oxygen delivery (Do_2) is the volume of O_2 brought to peripheral tissues in 1 min and consumption (Vo_2) is the volume used by the tissues in 1 min. Under normal conditions, delivery of oxygen is 3–4 times greater than consumption. Oxygen extraction measures the amount of O_2 transferred to tissues from 100 mL of blood and can be thought of as $C_ao_2 - C\bar{v}o_2$. Thus, an O_2 extraction of 3–4 mL/dL suggests adequate cardiac reserve to supply additional oxygen if demand increases. Inadequate cardiac reserve is indicated by an O_2 extraction of 5 mL/dL or greater, and tissue extraction must be increased to meet changing metabolic needs (Shapiro & Peruzzi, 1995).

Mixed venous oxygen tension (P_vo_2) and saturation (S_vo_2) are measured from pulmonary artery blood. These measurements are better indicators of tissue oxygenation than arterial values since venous blood reflects peripheral tissue extraction. Normal arterial oxygen saturation is 100% and venous saturation is 75%, yielding a normal arteriovenous difference ($S_ao_2 - S_vo_2$) of 25%. An increased S_vo_2 (>80%) can occur when oxygen delivery increases, oxygen consumption decreases (or some combination of the two), cardiac output increases, or the pulmonary artery catheter tip is in a pulmonary capillary instead of the artery. A decrease in S_vo_2 (<50–60%) may be due to increased oxygen consumption, decreased cardiac output or compromised pulmonary function. The venous oxygen saturation may not change at all, however, even with significant cardiovascular changes.

Partial pressure of arterial carbon dioxide (P_aco_2)

The metabolic rate determines the amount of carbon dioxide that enters the blood. Carbon dioxide is then transported to the lung as dissolved CO_2, bicarbonate, and carbamates. It diffuses from blood into alveoli and is removed from the body by ventilation, or the movement of gas into and out of the pulmonary system. Measurement of the arterial pressure of carbon dioxide allows assessment of alveolar ventilation in relation to the metabolic rate.

Ventilation (V_E) is the amount of gas exhaled in 1 minute and is the sum of alveolar and dead space ventilation ($V_E = V_A + V_{DS}$). Alveolar ventilation (V_A) is that portion of the lung that removes CO_2 and transfers O_2 to the blood while dead space (V_{DS}) has no respiratory function. As dead space increases, ventilation must increase to maintain adequate alveolar ventilation. Dead space increases with a high ventilation–perfusion ratio (V/Q) (i.e. an acute decrease in cardiac output, acute pulmonary embolism, acute pulmonary hypertension, or ARDS) and positive pressure ventilation.

Because P_aco_2 reflects the balance between production and alveolar excretion of carbon dioxide, accumulation of CO_2 indicates failure of the respiratory system to excrete the products of metabolism. The primary disease process may be respiratory or a process outside the lungs. Extrapulmonary processes that increase metabolism and CO_2 production include fever, shivering, seizures, sepsis, or physiologic stress. Parenteral nutrition with glucose providing more than 50% of nonprotein calories can also contribute to high CO_2 production.

Recognizing respiratory acid–base imbalance is important because of the need to assist in CO_2 elimination. As V_E increases, the work of breathing can cause fatigue and respiratory failure. It is important to recognize that the P_aco_2 may initially be normal, but rises as the work of breathing exceeds a patient's functional reserve. Ventilatory failure occurs when the pulmonary system can no longer provide adequate excretion of CO_2. Clinically, this is recognized as tachypnea, tachycardia, intercostal muscle retraction, accessory muscle use, diaphoresis and paradoxical breathing.

The metabolic component of the arterial blood gas: bicarbonate

Measurement of bicarbonate reflects a patient's acid–base status. The bicarbonate concentration reported with a blood gas is calculated using the Henderson–Hasselbalch equation and represents a single ionic species. tCO_2 content is measured with serum electrolytes and is the sum of the various forms of CO_2 in serum. Bicarbonate is the major contributor to tCO_2, and additional forms include dissolved CO_2, carbamates, carbonate, and carbonic acid. The calculated bicarbonate concentration does not include carbonic acid, carbonate, and carbamates.

Frequently, arterial and venous blood samples are obtained simultaneously, making arterial blood gas bicarbonate and venous serum tCO_2 measurements available. Venous serum tCO_2 content is 2.5–3 mEq/L higher than arterial blood gas bicarbonate, since CO_2 content is higher in venous than arterial blood and all species of carbon dioxide are included in the determination of tCO_2. If the blood sample is arterial, the tCO_2 content reported on the electrolyte panel should be 1.5–2 mEq/L higher than the calculated bicarbonate. the tCO_2 measured directly with serum electrolytes will be higher because it includes the different forms of CO_2. Since both blood gas bicarbonate and electrolyte tCO_2 determinations are usually available, the clinical utility of one compared with the other has been a subject of controversy (Kruse et al., 1989). A recent review, however, concludes that calculated and measured bicarbonate values are close enough in most cases that either is acceptable for clinical use (Kruse, 1995).

Disorders of acid–base balance

Metabolic acidosis

Metabolic acidosis is diagnosed on the basis of a decreased serum bicarbonate and arterial pH. The baseline bicarbonate concentration during pregnancy should, of course, be kept in mind when interpreting bicarbonate concentration. Metabolic acidosis develops when fixed acids accumulate or bicarbonate is lost. Accumulation of fixed acid occurs with overproduction as in diabetic ketoacidosis or lactic acidosis, or with decreased acid excretion as in renal failure. Diarrhea, a small bowel fistula, and renal tubular acidosis can all result in loss of extracellular bicarbonate.

Although the clinical signs associated with metabolic acidosis are not specific, multiple organ systems may be affected. Tachycardia develops with the initial fall in pH, but bradycardia usually predominates as the pH drops below 7.10. Acidosis causes venous constriction and impairs cardiac contractility, increasing venous return while cardiac output decreases. Arteriolar dilation occurs at pH < 7.20. Respiratory rate and tidal volume increase in an attempt to compensate for the acidosis. Maternal acidosis can result in fetal acidosis as H^+ ions equilibrate across the placenta, and fetal pH is generally 0.1 pH units less than the maternal pH.

The compensatory response to metabolic acidosis is an increase in ventilation that is stimulated by the fall in the pH. Hyperventilation lowers Pco_2 as the body attempts to return the $[HCO_3^-] / Pco_2$ ratio toward normal. The respiratory response is proportional to the degree of acidosis and allows calculation of the expected Pco_2 for a given bicarbonate level (Table 4.1). When the measured Pco_2 is higher or lower than expected for the measured serum bicarbonate, a mixed acid–base disorder must be present. This formula is ideally applied once the patient has reached a steady state, when Pco_2 nadirs 12–24 hours after the onset of acidosis (Narins & Emmett, 1980).

The classification of metabolic acidosis as nonanion gap or anion gap acidosis helps determine the pathologic process. Once a metabolic acidosis is detected, serum electrolytes should be obtained to calculate the anion gap. Frequently the clinical history and a few additional diagnostic studies can identify the underlying abnormality (Fig. 4.5) (Battle et al., 1998).

Electroneutrality in the body is maintained because the sum of all anions equals the sum of all cations. Na^+, K^+, Cl^-, and HCO^-_3 are the routinely measured serum ions while Mg^+, Ca^{++}, proteins (particularly albumin), lactate, HPO^-_4, and SO^-_4 are the unmeasured ions. Na^+ and K^+ account for 95% of cations while HCO^-_3 and Cl^- represent 85% of anions (Preuss, 1993). Thus, unmeasured anions are greater than unmeasured cations. The anion gap is the difference between measured plasma cations (Na^+) minus measured anions (Cl^-, HCO^-_3) and is derived:

$$\text{Total anions} = \text{Total cations}$$

$$\textbf{Measured anions} + \text{Unmeasured anions} = \textbf{Measured cations} + \text{Unmeasured cations}$$

$$([\mathbf{Cl^-}] + [\mathbf{tCO_2^-}]) + \text{Unmeasured anions} = [\mathbf{Na^+}] + \text{Unmeasured cations}$$

$$\text{Unmeasured anions} - \text{Unmeasured cations} = [\mathbf{Na^+}] - ([\mathbf{Cl^-}] + [\mathbf{tCO_2^-}])$$

$$\textit{Anion gap} = [Na^+] - ([Cl^-] + [tCO_2^-])$$

A normal anion gap is 8–16 mEq/L. Potassium may be included as a measured cation, although it contributes little to the accuracy or utility of the gap. If K^+ is included in the calcu-

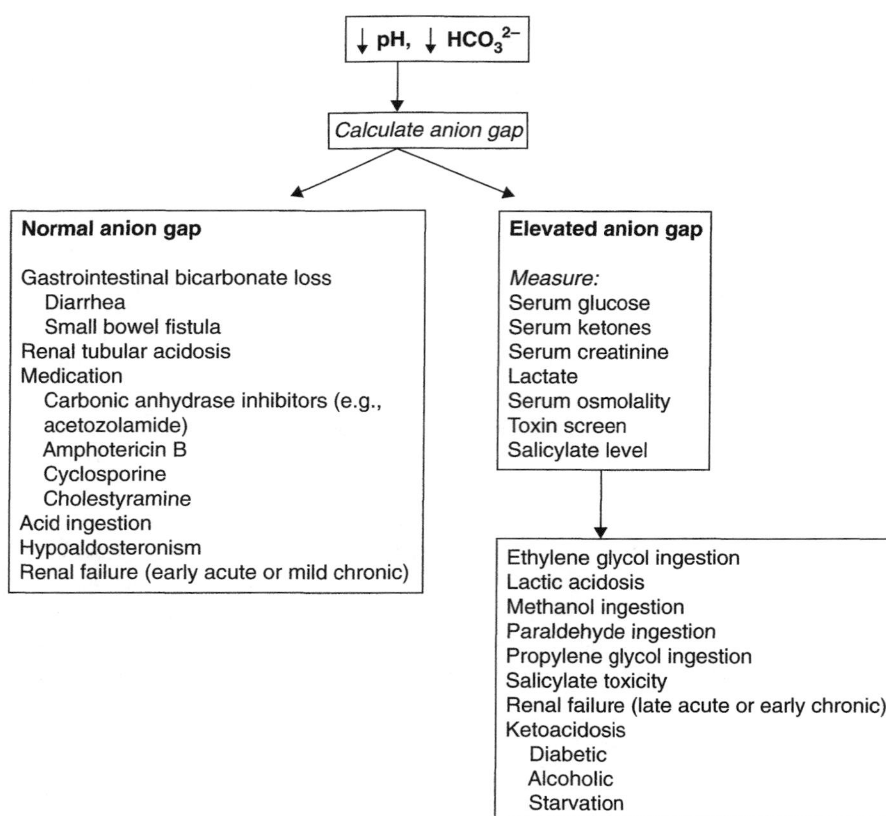

Fig. 4.5 Etiology and evaluation of metabolic acidosis.

lation, however, the normal range becomes 12–20 mEq/L (Kruse, 1994).

A change in the gap involves a change in unmeasured cations or anions. An elevated gap is most commonly due to an accumulation of unmeasured anions that include organic acids (i.e. ketoacids or lactic acid), or inorganic acids (i.e. sulfate and phosphate) (Oh & Carroll, 1977). A decrease in cations, i.e. magnesium and calcium, will also increase the gap, but the serum level is usually life-threatening.

The following example demonstrates use of the anion gap in a patient who had been experiencing dysuria, polyuria, and polydypsia of several days duration. Initial evaluation of this 19-year-old gravida at 24 weeks gestation was notable for a serum glucose level of 460 mg/dL and 4+ urinary ketones. Further investigation revealed: arterial pH of 7.30 and HCO^-_3 of 14 mEq/L, serum Na^+ of 133 mEq/L, K^+ of 4.1 mEq/L, tCO_2 of 15 mEq/L, and Cl^- of 95 mEq/L. The anion gap was determined:

$$\begin{aligned} \textit{Anion gap} &= [Na^+] - [Cl^-] + [tCO_2^-] \\ &= 133\,mEq/L - (95\,mEq/L + 15\,mEq/L) \\ &= 133\,mEq/L - 110\,mEq/L \\ \text{Anion gap} &= 23\,mEq/L \end{aligned}$$

The elevated anion gap is the result of unmeasured organic anions or ketoacids that have accumulated and decreased serum bicarbonate. As this patient with type I diabetes mellitus receives insulin therapy, the anion gap will normalize, reflecting disappearance of the ketoacids from serum.

The limitations of the anion gap, however, should be recognized. Various factors can lower the anion gap, but its importance is not so much in the etiology of the decrease as in its ability to mask an elevated gap. Since albumin accounts for the majority of unmeasured anions, the gap decreases as albumin levels fall. For each 1 g decrease in albumin, the gap may be lowered by 2.5–3 mEq/L. The most common cause of a lowered gap is decreased serum albumin. Other less common causes include markedly elevated levels of unmeasured cations (K^+, Mg^+, and Ca^{++}), hyperlipidemia, lithium carbonate intoxication, multiple myeloma, and bromide or iodide intoxication.

Although an elevated anion gap is traditionally associated with metabolic acidosis, it may also occur in the presence of severe metabolic alkalosis. The ionic activity of albumin changes with increasing pH and protons are released. The net negative charge on each molecule increases, thereby increasing unmeasured anions. Volume contraction leads to hyperproteinemia and augments the anion gap.

If an anion gap acidosis is present, the ratio of the change in the anion gap (the delta gap) to the change in HCO^-_3 can be helpful in determining the type of disturbances present:

$$\frac{\Delta\ \text{gap}}{\Delta\ HCO_3^-} = \frac{\text{Anion gap} - 12}{24 - [HCO_3^-]}$$

In simple anion gap metabolic acidosis, the ratio approximates 1.0, since the decrease in bicarbonate equals the increase in anions. The delta gap for the patient with diabetes and ketoacidosis previously described is calculated as follows:

$$\frac{\Delta\ \text{gap}}{\Delta\ HCO_3^-} = \frac{\text{Anion gap} - 12}{24 - [HCO_3^-]} = \frac{23-12}{24-14} = \frac{11}{10} = 1.1$$

The delta gap is 0 when the acidosis is a pure nonanion gap acidosis. A delta gap of 0.3–0.7 is associated with one of two mixed metabolic disorders: (i) a high anion gap acidosis and respiratory alkalosis; or (ii) high anion gap with a preexisting normal or low anion gap. A ratio greater than 1.2 implies a metabolic alkalosis superimposed on a high anion gap acidosis or a mixed high anion gap acidosis and chronic respiratory acidosis. The use of the delta gap is, however, limited by the wide range of normal values for the anion gap and bicarbonate, and its accuracy has been questioned (Salem & Mujais, 1992).

When a normal anion gap metabolic acidosis is present, the urinary anion gap may be helpful in distinguishing the cause of the acidosis:

$$\text{Urinary anion gap} = [\text{Urine } Na^+] + [\text{Urine } K^+] - [\text{Urine } Cl^-]$$

The urinary anion gap is a clinically useful method to estimate urinary ammonium (NH^+_4) excretion. Since the amount of NH^+_4 excreted in the urine cannot be directly measured, the urinary anion gap helps determine whether the kidney is responding appropriately to a metabolic acidosis (Halperin, 1988). Normally, the urine anion gap is positive or close to zero. A negative gap ($Cl^- > Na^+$ and K^+) occurs with gastrointestinal bicarbonate loss and NH^+_4 excretion by the kidney increases appropriately. In contrast, a positive gap ($Cl^- < Na^+$ and K^+) in a patient with acidosis suggests impaired distal urinary acidification with inappropriately low NH^+_4 excretion.

A variety of processes can lead to metabolic acidosis and therapy will depend on the underlying condition. Adequate oxygenation should be ensured and mechanical ventilation instituted for impending respiratory failure. The use of bicarbonate solutions to correct acidosis has been suggested when arterial pH is less than 7.10 or bicarbonate is lower than 5 mEq/L. Bicarbonate solutions must be administered with caution since an "overshoot" alkalosis can lower seizure threshold, impair oxygen availability to peripheral tissues, and stimulate additional lactate production.

Metabolic alkalosis

Metabolic alkalosis is characterized by a rise in serum bicarbonate concentration and an elevated arterial pH. The most impressive clinical effects of metabolic alkalosis are neurologic and include confusion, obtundation, and tetany. Cardiac arrhythmias, hypotension, hypoventilation, and various metabolic aberrations may accompany these neurologic changes.

Metabolic alkalosis results from a loss of acid or the addition of alkali. The development of metabolic alkalosis occurs in two phases, with the initial addition or generation of HCO^-_3 followed by the inability of the kidney to excrete the excess HCO^-_3. The two most common causes of metabolic alkalosis are excessive loss of gastric secretions and diuretic administration. Once established, volume contraction, hypercapnea, hypokalemia, glucose loading, and acute hypercalcemia promote HCO^-_3 reabsorption by the kidney and sustain the alkalosis.

The degree of respiratory compensation for metabolic alkalosis is more variable than with metabolic acidosis, and formulas to estimate the expected P_aco_2 have not proven useful (Narins & Emmett, 1980). Alkalosis tends to cause hypoventilation but P_aco_2 rarely exceeds 55 mmHg (Narins & Emmett, 1980; Wilson, 1992b). Tissue and red blood cells attempt to lower HCO^-_3 by exchanging intracellular H^+ ions for extracellular Na^+ and K^+.

Once metabolic alkalosis is diagnosed, determination of urinary chloride concentration can be helpful in determining the etiology (Fig. 4.6). Urinary chloride is a more reliable indicator of volume status than urinary sodium concentration in this group of patients. Sodium is excreted in the urine with bicarbonate to maintain electroneutrality and occurs independently of volume status. Therefore low urinary chloride in patients with volume contraction accurately reflects sodium chloride retention by the kidney.

A urinary chloride concentration <10 mEq/L that improves with sodium chloride administration is a chloride-responsive metabolic alkalosis. In contrast, a urine chloride >20 mEq/L indicates the alkalosis will not improve with saline administration and is a chloride-resistant alkalosis. Urine chloride levels must be interpreted with caution since levels are falsely elevated when obtained within several hours of diuretic administration.

Treatment of metabolic alkalosis is aimed at eliminating excess bicarbonate and reversing factors responsible for maintaining the alkalosis. If the urinary chloride level indicates a responsive disorder, infusion of sodium chloride will correct the abnormality. Conversely, saline administration will not correct a chloride-resistant disorder and can be harmful. Treatment of the primary disease will concurrently correct the alkalosis. Although mind alkalemia is generally well tolerated, critically ill surgical patients with a pH ≥ 7.55 have increased mortality (Rimmer & Gennari, 1987; Wilson et al., 1992b).

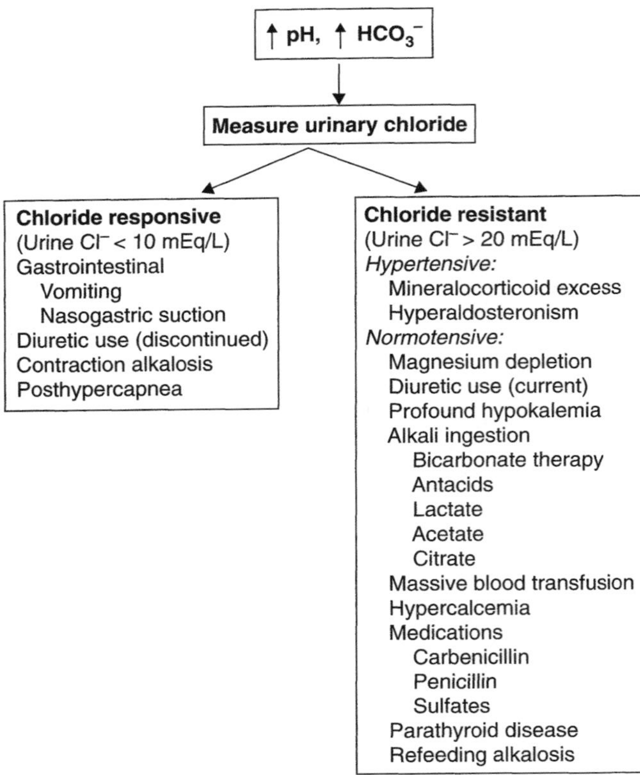

Fig. 4.6 Etiology and evaluation of metabolic alkalosis.

Table 4.4 Causes of respiratory acidosis

Airway obstruction
Aspiration
Laryngospasm
Severe bronchospasm
Impaired ventilation
Pneumothorax
Hemothorax
Severe pneumonia
Pulmonary edema
Adult respiratory distress syndrome
Circulatory collapse
Massive pulmonary embolism
Cardiac arrest
CNS depression
Medication
Sedatives
Narcotics
Cerebral infarct, trauma or encephalopathy
Obesity–hypoventilation syndrome
Neuromuscular disease
Myasthenic crisis
Severe hypokalemia
Guillain–Barré
Medication

Respiratory acidosis

Respiratory acidosis is characterized by hypercapnea (a rise in $P\text{co}_2$) and a decreased arterial pH. The development of respiratory acidosis indicates the failure of carbon dioxide excretion to match CO_2 production. A variety of disorders can contribute to this acid–base abnormality (Table 4.4). It is important to remember that the normal $P\text{co}_2$ in pregnancy is 30 mmHg, and normative data for nonpregnant patients do not apply to the gravida.

The clinical manifestations of acute respiratory acidosis are particularly evident in the central nervous system. Since carbon dioxide readily penetrates the blood–brain barrier and cerebrospinal fluid buffering capacity is not as great as blood, $P\text{co}_2$ elevations quickly decrease the pH of the brain. Thus, neurologic compromise may be more significant with respiratory acidosis than metabolic acidosis (Wilson, 1992b). Acute hypercapnia also decreases cerebral vascular resistance, leading to increased cerebral blood flow and intracranial pressure.

The compensatory response depends on the duration of the respiratory acidosis. In acute respiratory acidosis, the respiratory center is stimulated to increase ventilation. Carbon dioxide is neutralized in erythrocytes by hemoglobin and other buffers, and bicarbonate is generated. An acute disturbance implies that renal compensation is not yet complete. Sustained respiratory acidosis (longer than 6–12 hours) stimulates the kidney to increase acid excretion, but this mechanism usually requires 3–5 days for full compensation (Narins, 1994).

The primary goal in the management of respiratory acidosis is to improve alveolar ventilation and decrease arterial $P\text{co}_2$. Assessment and support of pulmonary function are paramount when a patient has respiratory acidosis. Carbon dioxide accumulates rapidly, and $P\text{co}_2$ rises 2–3 mmHg/min in a patient with apnea. The underlying condition should be rapidly corrected and may include relief of an airway obstruction or pneumothorax, administration of bronchodilator therapy, narcotic reversal, or a diuretic.

Adequate oxygenation is crucial because hypoxemia is more life-threatening than hypercapnia. In the pregnant patient, hypoxemia also compromises the fetus. Uterine perfusion should be optimized and maternal oxygenation ensured since the combination of maternal hypoxemia and uterine artery hypoperfusion profoundly affects the fetus. When a patient cannot maintain adequate ventilation despite aggressive support, endotracheal intubation and mechanical ventilation should be performed without delay.

Respiratory alkalosis

Respiratory alkalosis is characterized by hypocapnea (decreased $P\text{CO}_2$) and an increased arterial pH. Acute hypocapnea frequently is accompanied by striking clinical symptoms, including paresthesias, circumoral numbness, and confusion. Tachycardia, chest tightness, and decreased cerebral blood flow are some of the prominent cardiovascular effects. Chronic respiratory alkalosis, however, is usually asymptomatic.

Respiratory alkalosis is the result of increased alveolar ventilation (Table 4.5). Hyperventilation can develop from stimulation of brainstem or peripheral chemoreceptors and nociceptive lung receptors. Higher brain centers can override chemoreceptors and this occurs with involuntary hyperventilation. Respiratory alkalosis is commonly encountered in critically ill patients in response to hypoxemia or acidosis, or secondary to central nervous system dysfunction.

The compensatory response is divided into acute and chronic phases. In acute alkalosis, there is an instantaneous decrease in H^+ ion concentration due to tissue and red blood cell buffer release of H^+ ions. If the duration of hypocapnea is greater than a few hours, renal excretion of bicarbonate is increased and acid excretion is decreased. This response requires at least several days to reach a steady state. Chronic respiratory alkalosis is the only acid–base disorder in which the compensatory response can return the pH to normal.

Table 4.5 Causes of respiratory alkalosis

Pulmonary disease
Pneumonia
Pulmonary embolism
Pulmonary congestion
Asthma
Drugs
Salicylates
Xanthines
Nicotine
CNS disorders
Voluntary hyperventilation
Anxiety
Neurologic disease
Infection
Trauma
Cerebrovascular accident
Tumor
Other causes
Pregnancy
Pain
Sepsis
Hepatic failure
Iatrogenic mechanical hyperventilation

Respiratory alkalosis may be diagnostic of an underlying condition and is usually corrected with treatment of the primary problem. Hypocapnea itself is not life-threatening but the disease causing the alkalosis may be. The presence of respiratory alkalosis should always raise suspicion for hypoxemia, pulmonary embolism, or sepsis. These conditions, however, can be overlooked if the only concern is correction of the alkalosis. Mechanical ventilation may lead to iatrogenic respiratory alkalosis and the $P\text{CO}_2$ can usually be corrected by lowering the machine-set respiratory rate.

References

Al-Ameri MW, Kruse JA, Carlson RW. Blood sampling from arterial catheters: minimum discard volume to achieve accurate laboratory results. Crit Care Med 1986;14:399.

Andersen GJ, James GB, Mathers NP, et al. The maternal oxygen tension and acid-base status during pregnancy. J Obstet Gynaecol Br Commonw 1969;76:16–19.

Arbus GS. An in vivo acid-base nomogram for clinical use. Can Med Assoc J 1973;109:291–293.

Artal R, Wiswell R, Romem Y, Dorey F. Pulmonary responses to exercise in pregnancy. Am J Obstet Gynecol 1986;154:378–383.

Awe RJ, Nicotra MB, Newsom TD, Viles R. Arterial oxygenation and alveolar-arterial gradients in term pregnancy. Obstet Gynecol 1979;53:182–186.

Barron WM, Lindheimer MD. Medical disorders during pregnancy, 1st edn. St. Louis: Mosby-Year Book, 1991:234.

Battle DC, Hizon M, Cohen E, et al. The use of the urinary anion gap in the diagnosis of hyperchloremic metabolic acidosis. N Engl J Med 1988;318:594.

Bhaskaran NC, Lawler PG. How much blood for a blood gas? Anesthesiology 1988;43:811–812.

Biswas CK, Ramos JM, Agroyannis B, Kerr DN. Blood gas analysis: effect of air bubbles in syringe and delay in estimation. Br Med J 1982;284:923–927.

Bloom SA, Canzanello VJ, Strom JA, Madias NE. Spurious assessment of acid-base status due to dilutional effect of heparin. Am J Med 1985;79:528–530.

Bryan-Brown CW, Baek SM, Makabali G, et al. Consumable oxygen: availability of oxygen in relation to oxyhemoglobin dissociation. Crit Care Med 1973;1:17–21.

Cain SM. Peripheral oxygen uptake and delivery in health and disease. Clin Chest Med 1983;4:139–148.

Cane RD, Shapiro BA, Templin R, Walther K. Unreliability of oxygen tension-based indices in reflecting intrapulmonary shunting in critically ill patients. Crit Care Med 1988;16:1243–1245.

Cogan MJ. In: Brenner BM, Rector FC Jr, eds. The Kidney, 3rd edn. Philadelphia: WB Saunders, 1986:473.

Cruikshank DP, Hays PM. Maternal physiology in pregnancy. In: Gabbe S, Niebyl J, Simpson JL, eds. Obstetrics: normal and problem pregnancies, 2nd edn. New York: Churchill Livingstone, 1991:129.

Davenport HW. Normal acid-base paths. In: The ABC of acid-base chemistry, 6th edn. Chicago: University of Chicago Press, 1974:69.

Dayal P, Murata Y, Takamura H. Antepartum and postpartum acid-base changes in maternal blood in normal and complicated pregnancies. J Obstet Gynaecol Br Cwlth 1972;79:612–624.

Demling BK, Knox JB. Basic concepts of lung function and dysfunction: oxygenation, ventilation and mechanics. New Horiz 1993;1:362–370.

Dent JG, Netter KJ. Errors in oxygen tension measurements caused by halothane. Br J Anaesth 1976;48:195–197.

Dildy GA, Loucks CA, Porter TF, Sullivan CA, Belfort MA, Clark SL. Many normal pregnant women residing at moderate altitude have lower arterial oxygen saturations than expected. Society for Gynecologic Investigation, Atlanta, GA, March 1998.

Dildy GA, Sullivan CA, Moore LG, Richlin ST, Loucks CA, Belfort MA, Clark SL. Altitude reduces and pregnancy increases maternal arterial oxygen saturation. Society for Maternal-Fetal Medicine, San Francisco, CA, January 1999.

Douglas IH, McKenzie PJ, Ledingham I, Smith G. Effect of halothane on PO_2 electrode. Lancet 1978;2:1370–1371.

Gemzell CA, Robbe H, Strom G, et al. Observation on circulatory changes and muscular work in normal labor. Acta Obstet Gynecol Scand 1957;36:75.

Goldberg M, Green SB, Moss ML, et al. Computer-based instruction and diagnosis of acid-base disorders. JAMA 1973;223:269.

Haber RJ. A practical approach to acid-base disorders. West J Med 1991;155:146–151.

Halperin ML, Richardson RM, Bear RA, et al. Urine ammonium: the key to the diagnosis of distal renal tubular acidosis. Nephron 1988;50:1–4.

Hankins GD, Harvey CJ, Clark SL, Uckan EM, Van Hook JW. The effects of maternal position and cardiac output on intrapulmonary shunt in normal third-trimester pregnancy. Obstet Gynecol 1996a;88:327–330.

Hankins GD, Clark SL, Uckan EM, et al. Third trimester arterial blood gas and acid-base values in normal pregnancy at moderate altitude. Obstet Gynecol 1996b;88:347–350.

Harsten A, Berg B, Inerot S, Muth L. Importance of correct handling of samples for the results of blood gas analysis. Acta Anesthesiol Scand 1988;32:365–368.

Hess CE, Nichols AB, Hunt WB, Suratt PM. Pseudohypoxemia secondary to leukemia and thrombocytopenia. N Engl J Med 1979;301:361–363.

Huch A, Huch R, Konig V, et al. Limitations of pulse oximetry. Lancet 1988;1:357–358.

Kruse JA. Acid-base interpretations. Crit Care 1993;14:275.

Kruse JA. Use of the anion gap in intensive care and emergency medicine. In: Vincent MJ, ed. Yearbook of intensive care and emergency medicine. New York: Springer, 1994:685–696.

Kruse JA. Calculation of plasma bicarbonate concentration versus measurement of serum CO_2 content. pK revisited. Clin Int Care 1995;6:15.

Kruse JA, Hukku P, Carlson RW. Relationship between the apparent dissociation constant of blood carbonic acid and severity of illness. J Lab Clin Med 1989;114:568–574.

Liberatore SM, Pistelli R, Patalano F, et al. Respiratory function during pregnancy. Respiration 1984;46:145–150.

Lucius H, Gahlenbeck H, Kleine HO, et al. Respiratory functions, buffer system, and electrolyte concentrations of blood during human pregnancy. Respir Physiol 1970;9:311–317.

McHugh RD, Epstein RM, Longnecker DE. Halothane mimics oxygen in oxygen microelectrodes. Anesthesiology 1979;50:47–49.

MacRae DJ, Palavradji D. Maternal acid-base changes in pregnancy. J Obstet Gynaecol Br Cwlth 1967;74:11–16.

Madiedo G, Sciacca R, Hause L. Air bubbles and temperature effect on blood gas analysis. J Clin Pathol 1980;33:864–867.

Maekawa T, Okuda Y, McDowall DG. Effect of low concentrations of halothane on the oxygen electrode. Br J Anaesth 1980;52:585–587.

Morganroth ML. An analytic approach to diagnosing acid-base disorders. J Crit Ill 1990a;5:138.

Morganroth ML. Six steps to acid-base analysis: clinical applications. J Crit Ill 1990b;5:460.

Mueller RG, Lang GE. Blood gas analysis: effect of air bubbles in syringe and delay in estimation. Br Med J 1982;285:1659–1660.

Nanji AA, Whitlow KJ. Is it necessary to transport arterial blood samples on ice for pH and gas analysis? Can Anaesth Soc J 1984;31:568–571.

Narins RG. Acid-base disorders: definitions and introductory concepts. In: Narins RG, ed. Clinical disorders of fluid and electrolyte metabolism, 5th edn. New York: McGraw-Hill, 1994:755–767.

Narins RG, Emmett M. Simple and mixed acid-base disorders: a practical approach. Medicine 1980;59:161–187.

Nearman HS, Sampliner JE. Respiratory monitoring. In: Berk JL, Sampliner JE, eds. Handbook of critical care, 3rd edn. Boston: Little Brown, 1982;125–143.

New W. Pulse oximetry. J Clin Monit 1985;1:126–129.

Ng RH, Dennis RC, Yeston N, et al. Factitious cause of unexpected arterial blood-gas results. N Engl J Med 1984;310:1189–1190.

Novy MJ, Edwards MJ. Respiratory problems in pregnancy. Am J Obstet Gynecol 1967;99:1024–1045.

Oh MS, Carroll HJ. The anion gap. N Engl J Med 1977;297:814–817.

Pernoll ML, Metcalfe J, Kovach PA, et al. Ventilation during rest and exercise in pregnancy and postpartum. Respir Physiol 1975;25:295–310.

Perutz MF. Hemoglobin structure and respiratory transport. Sci Ann 1978;239:92–125.

Preuss HG. Fundamentals of clinical acid-base evaluation. Clin Lab Med 1993;13:103–116.

Rackow EC, Astiz M. Pathophysiology and treatment of septic shock. JAMA 1991;266:548–554.

Richlin S, Cusick W, Sullivan C, Dildy GA, Belfort MA. Normative oxygen saturation values for pregnant women at sea level. The American College of Obstetricians and Gynecologists, New Orleans, LA, May 1998.

Rimmer JM, Gennari FJ. Metabolic alkalosis. J Intens Care Med 1987;2:137.

Salem MM, Mujais SK. Gaps in the anion gap. Arch Intern Med 1992;152:1625–1629.

Schuch CS, Price JG. Determination of time required for blood gas homeostasis in the intubated, post-open-heart surgery adult following a ventilator change. NTI Res Abs 1986;15:314.

Shapiro BA, Peruzzi WT. Blood gas analysis. In: Civetta J, Taylor R, Kirby J, eds. Critical care, 2nd edn. Philadelphia: Lippincott, 1992:325–342.

Shapiro BA, Peruzzi WT. Interpretation of blood gases. In: Ayres SM, Grenvik A, Holbrook PR, Shoemaker WC, eds. Textbook of critical care, 3rd edn. Philadelphia: WB Saunders, 1995:278–294.

Shibutani K, Komatsu T, Kubal K, et al. Critical levels of oxygen delivery in anesthetized man. Crit Care Med 1983;11:640–643.

Shoemaker WC, Ayres S, Grenvik A, et al. Textbook of Critical Care, 2nd edn. Philadelphia: WB Saunders, 1989.

Sobrevilla LA, Cassinelli MT, Carcelen A, et al. Human fetal and maternal oxygen tension and acid-base status during delivery at high altitude. Am J Obstet Gynecol 1971;111:1111–1118.

Stock MC, Shapiro BA, Cane RD. Reliability of $S_v O_2$ in predicting A-VDO_2 and the effect of anemia. Crit Care Med 1986;14:402.

Templeton A, Kelman GR. Maternal blood-gases, $P_AO_2 - PaO_2$ physiological shunt and VD/VT in normal pregnancy. Br J Anaesth 1976;48:1001–1004.

Tremper KK, Barker SJ. Blood-gas analysis. In: Hall JB, Schmidt GA, Wook LDH, eds. Principles of critical care. New York: McGraw-Hill, 1992:181–196.

Ueland K, Hansen JM. Maternal cardiovascular hemodynamics: II. Posture and uterine contractions. Am J Obstet Gynecol 1969;103:1–7.

Urbina LR, Kruse JA. Blood gas analysis and related techniques. In: Carlson RW, Geheb MA, eds. Principles and practice of medical intensive care. Philadelphia: WB Saunders, 1993:235–250.

Walton JR, Shapiro BA, Wine C. Pre-analytic error in arterial blood gas measurement. Respir Care 1981;26:1136.

Weinberger SE, Weiss ST, Cohen WR, et al. Pregnancy and the lung. Am Rev Respir Dis 1980;121:559–581.

Wilson RF. Acid-base problems. In: Critical Care Manual: Applied Physiology and principles of therapy, 2nd edn. Philadelphia: FA Davis, 1992a:715–756.

Wilson RF. Blood gases: pathophysiology and interpretation. In: Critical care manual: applied physiology and principles of therapy, 2nd edn. Philadelphia: FA Davis, 1992b:389–421.

Wilson RF, Gibson D, Percinel AK, et al. Severe alkalosis in critically ill surgical patients. Arch Surg 1972;105:197–203.

5 Fluid and electrolyte balance

William E. Scorza
Anthony Scardella

The physiologic effects of pregnancy on normal fluid dynamics and renal function

The infusion of fluid remains a cornerstone of therapy when treating critically ill pregnant women with hypovolemia. An understanding of the distribution and pharmacokinetics of plasma expanders, as well as knowledge of normal renal function and fluid dynamics during pregnancy, is needed to allow for prompt resuscitation of patients in various forms of shock, as well as to provide maintenance therapy for other critically ill patients.

The total body water (TBW) ranges from 45% to 65% of total body weight in the human adult. TBW is distributed between two major compartments, the intracellular fluid (ICF) space and the extracellular fluid (ECF) space. Two-thirds of the TBW resides in the ICF space and one-third in the ECF space. The ECF is further subdivided into the interstitial and intravascular spaces in a ratio of 3:1. Regulation of the ICF is mostly achieved by changes in water balance, whereas the changes in plasma volume are related to the regulation of sodium balance. Because water can freely cross most cell membranes, the osmolalities within each compartment are the same. When water is added into one compartment, it distributes evenly throughout the TBW, and the amount of volume added to any given compartment is proportional to its fractional representation of the TBW. Infusions of fluids that are isotonic with plasma are distributed initially within the ECF; however, only one-fourth of the infused volume remains in the intravascular space after 30 minutes. Because most fluids are a combination of free water and isotonic fluids, one can predict the space of distribution and thus the volume transfused into each compartment.

During pregnancy, the ECF accumulates 6–8 L of extra fluid, with the plasma volume increasing by 50% (Gallery & Brown, 1987). Both plasma and red cell volumes increase during pregnancy. The plasma volume increases slowly but to a greater extent than the increase in total blood volume during the first 30 weeks of pregnancy and is then maintained at that level until term (Wittaker & Lind, 1993). The plasma volume to ECF ratio is also increased in pregnancy (Brown et al., 1992). Plasma volume is increased by a greater fraction in multiple pregnancies (MacGillivray et al., 1971; Thomsen et al., 1993), with the increase being proportional to the number of fetuses (Fullerton et al., 1965). Reduced plasma volume expansion has been shown to occur in pregnancies complicated by fetal growth restriction (Hytten & Paintin, 1973; Salas et al., 1993), hypertensive disorders (Arias, 1965; MacGillivray et al., 1971; Gallery et al., 1979; Goodlin et al., 1981; Sibai et al., 1983; Brown et al., 1992), prematurity (Raiha, 1964; Goodlin et al., 1981), oligohydramnios (Goodlin et al., 1981; 1983), and maternal smoking (Pirani & MacGillivray, 1978). In pregnancy-induced hypertension the total ECF is unchanged (Brown et al., 1989; 1992), supporting an altered distribution of ECF between the two compartments, possibly secondary to the rise in capillary permeability. A similar mechanism may occur in other conditions in which the plasma volume is reduced; the clinician needs to be cognizant of this when choosing fluids for resuscitation. Blood volume decreases over the first 24 hours postpartum (Ueland, 1976), with nonpregnant levels reached at 6–9 weeks postpartum (Lund & Donovan, 1967). With intrapartum hemorrhage, ICF can be mobilized to restore the plasma volume (Ueland, 1976).

Red cell mass is increased by 24% during the course of pregnancy (Thomsen et al., 1993), resulting in physiologic hemodilution and relative anemia. The decrease in the hematocrit is characterized by a gradual fall until week 30, followed by a gradual rise afterward (Peeters & Buchan, 1989). This is also associated with a decrease in whole blood viscosity, which may be beneficial for intervillous perfusion (Peeters et al., 1987). With hemorrhagic shock and mobilization of fluid from the ICF, the hematocrit, and thus oxygen-carrying capacity, would be further reduced, requiring replacement with appropriate fluids.

The glomerular filtration rate (GFR) increases during pregnancy, and peaks approximately 50% above nonpregnant levels by 9–11 weeks' gestation. This level is sustained until the 36th week (Dafinis & Sabatini, 1992). The cause of this increase in GFR is unknown. Postulated mechanisms include an increased plasma and ECF volume, a fall in intrarenal oncotic pressure due to decreased albumin and an increased level of a number of hormones including prolactin (Chesley, 1978a; Baylis, 1980; Walker & Garland, 1985).

Several aspects of tubular function are affected during pregnancy. Sodium retention occurs throughout pregnancy. The total amount of sodium retained during the course of pregnancy is approximately 950 mEq. A number of factors may contribute to the enhanced sodium reabsorption seen in pregnant patients. Increased levels of aldosterone, deoxycortisone, progesterone, and plactental lactogen as well as decreased plasma albumin have all been implicated (Dafinis & Sabatini, 1992). The tendency to retain sodium is offset in part by factors that favor sodium excretion in pregnancy, among which the most important is a higher GFR. Heightened levels of progesterone favor sodium excretion by competitive inhibition of aldosterone (Oparil et al., 1975). Increased calcium absorption from the small intestine occurs in order to meet the increased needs of the pregnant woman for calcium. Calcium excretion does increase during pregnancy, serum calcium and albumin are both decreased, but total ionized calcium remains unchanged. During the first and second trimester plasma uric acid levels decrease but gradually reach prepregnancy values in the third trimester.

The effects of pregnancy on acid–base balance are well known. There is a partially compensated respiratory alkalosis that begins early in pregnancy and is sustained throughout. The expected reduction in arterial $P\text{CO}_2$ is to about 30 mmHg with a concomitant rise in the arterial pH to approximately 7.44 (Elkus & Popovich, 1992). The pH is maintained in this range by increased bicarbonate excretion that keeps serum bicarbonate levels between 18 and 21 mEq/L (Elkus & Popovich, 1992). The chronic hyperventilation seen in pregnancy is thought to be secondary to increased levels of circulating progesterone, which may act directly on brainstem respiratory neurons (Skatrud et al., 1978).

Fluid resuscitation

Controversy exists as to the appropriate intravenous (IV) solutions to use in the management of hypovolemic shock. As long as physiologic endpoints are used to guide therapy and adjustments are made based on the individual's needs, side effects associated with inadequate or overaggressive resuscitation can be avoided. In most types of critical illness, intravascular volume is decreased. Hemorrhagic shock has been shown to deplete the ECF compartment with an increase in intracellular water secondary to cell membrane and sodium–potassium pump dysfunction (Skillman et al., 1967, 1975, 1976; Carrico et al., 1976). After trauma, surgical patients are found to have an expanded ECF, while the intravascular volume is depleted (Shoemaker et al., 1973). Most available studies of fluid balance have been conducted in patients in the nonpregnant state; very little data exist documenting these changes in pregnant women. Whatever the underlying pathology, intravascular volume is decreased in many types of critical illness. Successful resuscitation thus remains dependent on the prompt restoration of intravascular volume.

Crystalloid solutions

The most commonly employed crystalloid products for fluid resuscitation are 0.9% saline and lactated Ringer's solutions. The contents of normal saline and Ringer's lactate solutions are shown in Table 5.1. These are isotonic solutions that distribute evenly throughout the extracellular space but will not promote ICF shifts.

Isotonic crystalloids

Isotonic crystalloid solutions are generally readily available, easily stored, nontoxic, and reaction-free. They are an inexpensive form of volume resuscitation. The infusion of large volumes of 0.9% saline and Ringer's lactate is not a problem clinically; when administered in large volumes to patients with traumatic shock, acidosis does not occur (Lowery et al., 1971). The excess circulating chloride ion resulting from saline infusion is excreted readily by the kidney. In a similar manner, the lactate load in Ringer's solution does not potentiate the lactacidemia associated with shock (Trudnowski et al., 1967), nor has it been shown to effect the reliability of blood lactate measurements (Lowery et al., 1971).

Using the Starling–Landis–Staverman equation for fluid flux across a microvascular wall, one can predict that crystal-

Table 5.1 Characteristics of various volume-expanding agents

Agent	Na^+ (mEq/L)	Cl^- (mEq/L)	Lactate (mEq/L)	Osmolarity (mosmol/L)	Oncotic pressure (mmHg)
Ringer's lactate	130	109	28	275	0
Normal saline	154	154	0	310	0
Albumin (5%)	130–160	130–160	0	310	20
Hetastarch (6%)	154	154	0	310	30

loids will distribute rapidly between the ICF and ECF. Equilibration within the extracellular space occurs within 20–30 minutes after infusion. In healthy nonpregnant adults, approximately 25% of the volume infused remains in the intravascular space after 1 hour. In the critically ill or injured patient, however, only 20% or less of the infusion remains in the circulation after 1–2 hours (Carey et al., 1970; Hauser et al., 1980). The volemic effects of various crystalloid solutions compared with albumin and whole blood are shown in Table 5.2. At equivalent volumes, crystalloids are less effective than colloids for expansion of the intravascular volume. Two to 12 times the volume of crystalloids are necessary to achieve similar hemodynamic and volemic endpoints (Hanshiro & Weil, 1967; Skillman et al., 1976; Hauser et al., 1980; Dawidson et al., 1981; Moss et al., 1981; Dawidson & Eriksson, 1982). The rapid equilibration between the ICF and ECF seen with crystalloid infusion reduces the incidence of pulmonary edema (Virgilio, 1979; Virgilio et al., 1979a), whereas exogenous colloid administration promotes the accumulation of interstitial fluid (Siegel et al., 1970; Lucas et al., 1988).

Indications

Shock

Crystalloids—either normal saline or Ringer's lactate—are used to replenish plasma volume deficits and replace fluid and electrolyte losses from the interstitium (Takaori & Safer, 1967; Moss et al., 1971; 1981; Shoemaker et al., 1973; Lowe et al., 1977; Virgilio et al., 1979b). Patients in shock from any cause should receive immediate volume replacement with crystalloid solution during the initial clinical evaluation. Aggressive administration of crystalloid may promptly restore BP and peripheral perfusion. Given in a quantity of 3–4 times the amount of blood lost, they can adequately replace an acute loss of up to 20% of the blood volume, although 3–5 L of crystalloid may be required to replace a 1-L blood loss (Baue et al., 1967; Siegel et al., 1970; Virgilio et al., 1979b; Waxman et al., 1989; Singh et al., 1992). After the initial resuscitation with crystalloid, the selection of fluids becomes controversial, especially if microvascular integrity is not preserved (as in sepsis, burns, trauma, and anaphylaxis). Further fluid resuscitation should be guided by continuous bedside observation of urine output, mental status, heart rate, pulse pressure, respiratory rate, BP, and temperature monitoring, together with serial measurements of hematocrit, serum albumin, platelet count, prothrombin, and partial thromboplastin times. More aggressive monitoring is required in patients who remain in shock or fail to respond to the initial resuscitatory efforts and in patients with poor physiologic reserve who are unlikely to tolerate imprecisions in resuscitation efforts.

Table 5.2 Typical volemic effects of various resuscitative fluids after 1 L infusion

Fluid*	ICV (mL)	ECV (mL)	IV (mL)	PV (mL)
0.5% Dextrose/water	660	340	255	85
Normal saline or lactated Ringer's	−100	1,100	825	275
Albumin	0	1,000	500	500
Whole blood	0	1,000	0	1,000

* Based on infusion of 1 L volumes.

ECV, extracellular volume; IV, interstitial volume; IVC, intracellular volume; PV, plasma volume.

(From Carlson RW, Rattan S, Haupt M. Fluid resuscitation in conditions of increased permeability. Anesth Rev 1990;17(suppl 3):14.)

Diagnosis of oliguria

In critically ill patients, it is often extremely difficult to distinguish volume depletion from congestive heart failure (CHF). Because prerenal hypoperfusion resulting in a urine output of less than 0.5 mL/kg/hr can result in renal failure, it is extremely important to separate the two conditions and treat accordingly. An adequate fluid challenge consists of at least 500 mL of Ringer's lactate or normal saline administered over 5–10 minutes. Increasing the patient's IV infusion rate to 200 mL/hr or giving the bolus over 30 minutes or longer will not expand the intravascular volume sufficiently to help differentiate the etiology or treat the volume depletion. If there is no response from the initial fluid challenge, one may repeat it. If no increase in urine output occurs, one is probably not dealing with intravascular depletion, and further fluid management should be guided by invasive monitoring with a pulmonary artery catheter or repetitive echocardiograms. Patients with CHF do not experience a prolonged increase in vascular volume because crystalloid fluids distribute out of the intravascular space rapidly with only a transient increase in intravascular volume.

Side effects

Crystalloid solutions are generally nontoxic and free of side effects. However, fluid overload may result in pulmonary, cerebral, myocardial, mesenteric, and skin edema; hypoproteinemia; and altered tissue oxygen tension.

Pulmonary edema

Isotonic crystalloid resuscitation lowers the colloid oncotic pressure (COP) (Lewis, 1980; Haupt & Rackow, 1982), although it is uncertain whether such alterations in COP actually worsen lung function (Skillman et al., 1967; Virgilio 1979; Virgilio et al., 1979a; Hauser et al., 1980). The lung has a variety of mechanisms that act to prevent the development of pulmonary edema. These include increased lymphatic flow, diminished pulmonary interstitial oncotic pressure, and increased interstitial hydrostatic pressure. Together they limit the effect of the lowered COP (Lewis, 1980). In patients with intact microvascular integrity, studies have failed to demonstrate an increase in extravascular lung water after appropriate crystalloid loading (Miller et al., 1971). Irrespective of the amount of fluid administered, strict attention to physiologic endpoints and oxygenation is essential in order to prevent pulmonary edema.

Peripheral edema

Peripheral edema is a frequent side effect of fluid resuscitation but can be limited by appropriate monitoring of the resuscitatory effort. Excess peripheral edema may result in decreased oxygen tension in the soft tissue, promoting complications such as poor wound healing, skin breakdown, and infection (Myers et al., 1967; Hohn et al., 1976; Kaufman et al., 1984). Despite this, burn patients have shown improvement in survival after massive crystalloid resuscitation (Barone & Snyder, 1991).

Bowel edema

Edema of the gastrointestinal system seen with aggressive crystalloid resuscitation may result in ileus and diarrhea, probably secondary to hypoalbuminemia (Granger et al., 1984). This may be limited by monitoring of the COP and correction of hypo-oncotic states.

Central nervous system

Under normal circumstances, the brain is protected from volume-related injury by the blood–brain barrier and cerebral autoregulation. However, a patient in shock may have a primary or coincidental CNS injury, which may damage either or both of these protective mechanisms. In this situation, the COP and osmotic gradients should be monitored closely to prevent edema.

Colloid solutions

Colloids are large-molecular-weight substances to which cell membranes are relatively impermeable. They increase COP resulting in the movement of fluid from the interstitial compartment to the intravascular compartment. Their ability to remain in the intravascular space prolongs their duration of action. The net result is a lower volume of infusate necessary to expand the intravascular space when compared with crystalloid solutions.

Albumin

Albumin is the colloidal agent against which all others are judged (Tullis, 1977). Albumin is produced in the liver and represents 50% of hepatic protein production (Rothschild et al., 1972). It contributes to 70–80% of the serum COP (Thompson, 1975; Lewis, 1980). A 50% reduction in the serum albumin concentration will lower the COP to one-third of normal (Thompson, 1975).

Albumin is a highly water-soluble polypeptide with a molecular weight ranging from 66,300 to 69,000 daltons (Thompson, 1975) and is distributed unevenly between the intravascular (40%) and interstitial (60%) compartments (Thompson, 1975). The normal serum albumin concentration is maintained between 3.5 and 5 g/dL and is affected by albumin secretion, volume of distribution, rate of loss from the intravascular space, and degradation. The albumin level also is well correlated with nutritional status (Grant et al., 1981). Hypoalbuminemia secondary to diminished production (starvation) or excess loss (hemorrhage) results in a decrease in its degradation and a compensatory increase in its distribution in the interstitial space (Rothschild et al., 1972; Rosenoer et al., 1980). In acute injury or stress with depletion of the intravascular compartment, interstitial albumin is mobilized and transported to the intravascular department by lymphatic channels or transcapillary refill (Moss et al., 1966). Albumin synthesis is stimulated by thyroid hormone (Rothschild et al., 1958) and cortisol (Rothschild et al., 1957) and decreased by an elevated COP (Liljedahl & Rieger, 1968).

The capacity of albumin to bind water is related to the amount of albumin given as well as to the plasma volume deficit (Rothschild et al., 1957; Lamke & Liljedahl, 1976a). One gram of albumin increases the plasma volume by approximately 18 mL (Molcroft & Trunkey, 1974; Granger et al., 1978; Lewis, 1980). Albumin is available as a 5% or 25% solution in isotonic saline. Thus, 100 mL of 25% albumin solution increases the intravascular volume by approximately 450 mL over 30–60 minutes (Hauser et al., 1980). With depletion of the ECF, this equilibration is not sufficiently brisk or complete unless supplementation with isotonic fluids is provided as part of the resuscitation regimen (Lewis, 1980). A 500-mL solution of 5% albumin containing 25 g of albumin will increase the intravascular space by 450 mL. In this instance, however, the albumin is administered in conjunction with the fluid to be retained.

Infused albumin has an initial plasma half-life of 16 hours, with 90% of the albumin dose remaining in the plasma 2 hours after administration (Berson & Yalow, 1957; Lewis, 1980). The albumin equilibrates between the intravascular and interstitial compartments over a 7–10-day period (Sterling, 1951), with 75% of the albumin being absent from the plasma in 2 days. In patients with shock, the administration of plasma albumin has been shown to significantly increase the COP for at least 2 days after resuscitation (Haupt & Rackow, 1982).

Indications

Albumin is used primarily for the resuscitation of patients

with hypovolemic shock. In the United States, 26% of all albumin administered to patients is given to treat acute hypovolemia (surgical blood loss, trauma, hemorrhage) while an additional 12% is given to treat hypovolemia due to other causes, such as infection (Boldt, 2000). A major goal in the resuscitation of a patient in acute shock is to replace the intravascular volume in order to restore tissue perfusion. In patients with acute blood loss of greater than 30% of blood volume, it probably should be used early in conjunction with a crystalloid infusion to maintain peripheral perfusion. Treatment goals are to maintain a serum albumin of greater than 2.5 g/dL in the acute period of resuscitation. With nonedematous patients, 5% albumin and crystalloid can be used, but with edematous patients, 25% albumin may assist the patient in mobilizing her own interstitial volume. In patients with suspected loss of capillary wall integrity (especially in the lung in patients at risk for the subsequent development of acute respiratory distress syndrome), the use of albumin should be limited, because it crosses the capillary wall and exerts an oncotic influence in the interstitial space, worsening pulmonary edema. Albumin may be used in patients with burns (Rothschild et al., 1972) once capillary integrity is restored, approximately 24 hours after the initial event.

The use of albumin in patients with volume depletion regardless of the cause is not without controversy. In one meta-analysis of 30 relatively small randomized clinical trials comparing the use of albumin or plasma protein fraction with no administration or the administration of crystalloids in critically ill patients with hypovolemia or burns, the authors found no evidence that albumin decreased mortality (Cochrane Injuries Group, 1998). A later meta-analysis of randomized clinical trials of albumin use found that in many trials included for analysis, problems with randomization were present. In addition there was significant heterogeneity among the various studies (Ferguson et al., 1999). The authors of this study concluded that there was no hard evidence that albumin was beneficial. They surmised that albumin and large volume crystalloid infusions were equivalent in terms of mortality in critically ill patients. Finally, given the lack of data supporting a beneficial effect of albumin on mortality in critically ill patients, the cost of this therapy also becomes a factor. One study projected that compared to albumin, the use of the least expensive, fully approved colloid would save nearly $300 million per year in the United States (Boldt, 2000).

Side effects

A number of potential adverse effects of albumin have been reported. This agent may accentuate respiratory failure and contribute to the development of pulmonary edema. However, the presence or absence of infection, together with the method of resuscitation and volumes used, affect respiratory function far more than the type of fluid infused (Vito et al., 1974; Virgilio et al., 1979a,c; Shoemaker et al., 1981; Poole et al., 1982). Albumin may lower the serum ionized calcium concentration, resulting in a negative inotropic effect on the myocardium (Weaver et al., 1978; Lucas et al., 1980; Kovalik et al., 1981; Lucas et al., 1988), and it may impair immune responsiveness. Infusion of albumin results in moderate to transient abnormalities in prothrombin time, partial thromboplastin time, and platelet counts (Cogbill et al., 1981). However, the clinical implications of these defects, if any, are unknown. Albumin-induced anaphylaxis is reported in 0.47–1.53% of recipients (Rothschild et al., 1972). These reactions are short lived and include urticaria, chills, fever and rarely, hypertension. Although albumin is derived from pooled human plasma, there is no known risk of hepatitis or acquired immune deficiency syndrome. This is because it is heated and sterilized by ultrafiltration.

Hetastarch

Hetastarch is a synthetic colloid molecule that closely resembles glycogen. It is prepared by incorporating hydroxyethyl ether into the glucose residues of amylopectin (Solanke et al., 1971). Hetastarch is available clinically as a 6% solution in normal saline. The molecular weight of the particles is 480,000 daltons, with 80% of the molecules in the range of 30,000–2,400,000 daltons. Hetastarch is metabolized rapidly in the blood by alpha-amylase (Farrow et al., 1970; Yacobi et al., 1982; Ferber et al., 1985), with the rate of degradation dependent on the dose and the degree of glucose hydroxyethylation or substitution (Thompson et al., 1962; Mishler et al., 1980; Ferber et al., 1985).

There is an almost immediate appearance of smaller-molecular-weight particles (molecular weight, 50,000 daltons or less) in the urine after IV infusion of hetastarch (Mishler et al., 1977). Forty percent of this compound is excreted in the urine after 24 hours, with 46% excreted by 2 days and 64% by 8 days (Puri et al., 1981; Yacobi et al., 1982). Bilirubin excretion accounts for less than 1% of total elimination in humans (Ring & Messmer, 1977). The larger particles are metabolized by the reticuloendothelial system (Bogan et al., 1969; Metcalf et al., 1970; Thompson et al., 1970) and remain in the body for an extended period (Mishler et al., 1979, 1980). Blood alpha-amylase also degrades larger particles to smaller starch polymers and free glucose. The smaller particles eventually are cleared through the urine and bowel. The amount of glucose thus produced does not cause significant hyperglycemia in a diabetic animal model (Hofer & Lanier, 1992). The half-life of hetastarch represents a composite of the half-lives of the various-sized particles. Ninety percent of a single infusion of hetastarch is removed from the circulation within 42 days, with a terminal half-life of 17 days (Yacobi et al., 1982).

Indications

Hetastarch is an effective long-acting plasma volume-expanding agent that can be used in patients suffering from shock secondary to hemorrhage, trauma, sepsis, and burns. It initially expands plasma volume by an amount equal to or greater than the volume infused (Ballinger, 1966; Kilian et al., 1975; Lamke & Liljedahl, 1976a). The volume expansion seen after the infusion of hetastarch is equal to or greater than that produced by dextran 70 (Lee et al., 1968; Metcalf et al., 1970; Khosropour et al., 1980) or 5% albumin. The plasma volume remains 70% expanded for 3 hours after the infusion and 40% expanded for 12 hours after the infusion (Metcalf et al., 1970). At 24 hours after infusion, the plasma volume expansion is approximately 28%, with 38% of the drug actually remaining intravascular (Laks et al., 1974a). The increase in intravascular volume has been associated with improvement in hemodynamic parameters in critically ill patients (Puri et al., 1981; Diehl et al., 1982; Shatney et al., 1983; Kirklin et al., 1984). Hetastarch also has been shown to increase the COP to the same degree as albumin (Haupt & Rackow, 1982; Kirklin et al., 1984). The maximum recommended daily dose for adults is 1,500 mL/70 kg of body weight.

Side effects

Starch infusions increase serum amylase levels two- to threefold. Peak levels occur 12–24 hours after infusion, with elevated levels present for 3 days or longer (Boon et al., 1976; Kohler et al., 1977; Mishler et al., 1977; Korttila et al., 1984). No alterations in normal pancreatic function have been noted (Kohler et al., 1977). Liver dysfunction with ascites secondary to intrahepatic obstruction after hetastarch infusions has been reported (Lucas et al., 1988).

Hetastarch does not seem to promote histamine release (Lorenz et al., 1975) or to be immunogenic (Maurer & Berardinelli, 1968; Ring et al., 1976). Anaphylactic reactions occur in less than 0.1% of the population, with shock or cardiopulmonary arrest occurring in 0.01% (Ring & Messmer, 1977). When given in doses below 1,500 mL/day, hetastarch has not been associated with clinical bleeding, but minor alterations in laboratory measurements may be seen (Lee et al., 1968; Muller et al., 1977). There is a transient decrease in the platelet count, prolonged prothrombin and partial thromboplastin times, acceleration of fibrinolysis, reduced levels of factor VIII, a decrease in the tensile clot strength and platelet adhesion, and an increased bleeding time (Solanke, 1968; Weatherbee et al., 1974; Strauss et al., 1985; Mattox et al., 1991). Hetastarch-induced disseminated intravascular coagulation (Chang et al., 1980) and intracranial bleeding in patients with subarachnoid hemorrhage have been documented (Cully et al., 1987; Damon et al., 1987).

Electrolyte disorders

Although almost any metabolic disorder can occur coincidentally with pregnancy, there are a few electrolyte disturbances of special importance that can specifically complicate pregnancy such as:

- water intoxication (hyponatremia)
- hyperemesis gravidarum
- hypokalemia associated with betamimetic tocolysis
- hypocalcemia with magnesium sulfate treatment for preeclampsia
- hypermagnesemia in treatment for preeclampsia.

Physiologic control of volume and osmolarity

Under normal physiologic conditions sodium and water are major molecules responsible for determining volume and tonicity of the ECF. These are in turn controlled by the influence of the renin–angiotensin aldosterone system and the action of antidiuretic hormone (ADH) otherwise known as vasopressin.

A decrease in ECF volume for any reason causes the juxtaglomerular complex in the kidney to sense a decrease in pressure resulting in an outpouring of renin, which through angiotensin I and angiotensin II, stimulates the adrenal cortex to secrete aldosterone. This results in an increase in sodium reabsorption in the renal collecting tubule. Water follows the sodium, restoring the extracellular volume to normal.

When the osmolarity of the ECF increases above a predetermined set point (usually 280–300 mosmol/L), the posterior pituitary is stimulated via the hypothalamus to release ADH which acts at the level of the collecting tubule to maximally stimulate the reabsorption of water into the circulation. The reabsorbed water dilutes the plasma solute, restoring normal tonicity. When osmolarity of the ECF decreases, ADH secretion is shut down and water reabsorption is inhibited. Therefore, normal tonicity is once again restored. Although this is the main regulatory mechanism for the control of osmolarity, there are other physiologic stimuli for controlling the secretion of ADH. Decreased blood pressure and decreased blood volume are problems commonly encountered in obstetric hemorrhage. These stimuli result in an increase in ADH. In addition, vomiting is also a potent stimulus for the release of ADH (Guyton & Hall, 1996). Pregnancy is associated with a decrease in tonicity and plasma osmolarity beginning in early gestation resulting in a new steady state. It appears that the osmotic threshold for release of ADH and thirst (which stimulates drinking and is another way of increasing ECF water) are decreased. In general, this leads to a decrease of about 10 mosmol/L below nonpregnant levels (Lindheimer & Davison, 1995). The serum osmolarity can be measured in the laboratory but it can also be estimated for clinical purposes. Sodium and the ions associated with it account for almost 95% of the solute in ECF. To estimate the plasma osmolarity the following formula can be used (Guyton & Hall, 1996):

$$P_{osm} = 2.1 \times \text{plasma sodium concentration}$$

Disturbances in sodium metabolism

Hyponatremia

Hyponatremia is defined as plasma sodium concentration of less than 135 mEq/L. Lowering the plasma osmolarity results in water movement into cells, leading to cellular over hydration, which is responsible for most of the symptoms associated with this disorder. Hyponatremia occurs when there is the addition of free water to the body or an increased loss of sodium. After ingestion of the water load there is a fall in plasma osmolarity (P_{osm}) resulting in decreased secretion and synthesis of ADH. This leads to decreased water reabsorption in the collecting tubule, the production of dilute urine and rapid excretion of excess water. When the plasma sodium is less than 135 mEq/L and/or the P_{osm} is below 275 mosmol/kg, ADH secretion generally ceases. A defect in renal water excretion will thus lead to hyponatremia. A reduction in free water excretion is caused by either decreased generation of free water in the loop of Henle and distal tubule or enhanced water permeability of the collecting tubules due to the presence of ADH (see Table 5.3). Hyponatremia may occur with normal renal water excretion in primary polydipsia and in conditions where there is a resetting of the plasma osmostat, such as in psychosis and malnutrition (Anderson et al., 1985). Levels of atrial natriuretic peptide (ANP) and aldosterone lead to significant alteration in serum sodium excretion in twins as opposed to singleton pregnancy (Thomsen et al., 1994). True hyponatremia may be accompanied by a normal plasma osmolality because of hyperglycemia, azotemia or after the administration of hypertonic mannitol (Weisberg, 1989).

Table 5.3 Common causes of decreased renal water excretion

Effective circulation volume depletion
Gastrointestinal losses (vomiting, diarrhea)
Renal losses (diuretics, hypoaldosteronism)
Skin losses (burns)
Edematous states (heart failure, nephrotic syndrome, cirrhosis)
Renal failure
Administration of diuretics
Syndrome of inappropriate ADH secretion
Drugs (e.g. indomethacin, chlorpropanamide, barbiturates)
Tumors
CNS diseases
Pulmonary diseases
Physical and emotional distress
Glucocorticoid deficiency
Adrenal insufficiency
Hypothyroidism

Etiology

Oxytocin is a polypeptide hormone secreted by the posterior pituitary. It differs from the other posterior pituitary polypeptide hormone, ADH, by only two amino acids. Although oxytocin serves an entirely different physiologic function, there is some ADH effect exerted by oxytocin. When oxytocin is infused at a rate of about 45 mU/min the antidiuretic effect is maximal and equal to the maximal effect of ADH. At a rate of 20 mU/min, the antidiuretic effect is about half the maximal effect of ADH (Abdul-Karim & Assali, 1961; Chesley, 1978b). When oxytocin is infused in high concentrations or for prolonged periods of time in dextrose 5% water or hypotonic solutions, oxytocin-induced water intoxication can occur. This provides a classic example of the clinical presentation of hyponatremia. The use of a balanced salt solution such as 0.9% normal saline as the vehicle for administration of oxytocin virtually eliminates the problem. Oxytocin infusion for the treatment of stillbirth, and prolonged induction of labor still results in this problem (Josey et al., 1969; Morgan et al., 1977; Wang et al., 2000).

Hyperemesis is another example of a disorder unique to pregnancy that can lead to severe electrolyte disturbance. Hyperemesis gravidarum complicates between 0.3% and 2% of all pregnancies. It can result in depletion of sodium, potassium, chloride, and other electrolytes. Hyponatremia can occur in severe cases causing lethargy, seizures, and rarely Wernicke's encephalopathy. Wernicke's encephalopathy, secondary to thiamin deficiency, is characterized by confusion, ataxia, and abnormal eye movement. Over aggressive treatment of hyponatremia in these patients can lead to central pontine myelinolysis (Theunissen & Parer, 1994).

Clinical presentation

Patients initially complain of headache, nausea, and vomiting, progressing to disorientation and obtundation, followed by seizure and coma. Hyponatremia may result in cerebral edema, permanent neurologic deficits, and death. The severity of the symptoms correlates with the degree of cerebral over hydration together with the speed at which this occurs, as well as the degree in reduction in the plasma sodium concentration (Pollock & Arieff, 1980; Arieff, 1986). (See Table 5.4.)

The diagnosis of hyponatremia is established through a good history and physical examination and appropriate laboratory tests. The history should focus on fluid volume losses

Table 5.4 Neurologic symptoms associated with an acute reduction in plasma sodium

Plasma sodium level (mEq/L)	Symptoms
120–125	Nausea, malaise
115–120	Headache, lethargy, obtundation
<115	Seizures, coma

such as vomiting and diarrhea and whether replacement fluids were hypotonic or isotonic. Symptoms of renal failure should be sought as well as diuretic use or other medications including nicotine, tricyclic antidepressants, antipsychotic agents, antineoplastic drugs, narcotics, nonsteroidal anti-inflammatory medications, methylxanthines, chlorpropamide, and barbiturates. Psychiatric history and an assessment of physical and emotional status is also important because compulsive water drinking may also cause hyponatremia. Laboratory evaluation should include serum electrolytes, BUN, creatinine, urinalysis with urine electrolytes, and an estimation of the serum osmolarity as described previously. The presence of a low plasma sodium and normal osmolarity suggests pseudohyponatremia but does not confirm it. The cause of pseudohyponatremia is investigated by examining the serum, which may have a milky appearance in patients with hyperlipidemia, and measurement of the serum lipid profile, plasma proteins, plasma sodium, osmolarity, and glucose. A urine osmolarity below 100 mosmol/kg (specific gravity <1.003) is seen with primary polydipsia or a reset osmostat. A urine osmolarity of greater than 100 mosmol/kg is seen in patients with a syndrome of inappropriate ADH secretion (SIADH). When evaluating hyponatremia associated with hypo-osmolarity, one needs to distinguish between SIADH, effective circulating volume depletion, adrenal insufficiency, and hypothyroidism. Urinary sodium excretion is less than 25 mEq/L in hypovolemic states and greater than 40 mEq/L in SIADH, reset osmostat, renal disease, and adrenal insufficiency. A BUN <10 mg/dL (Decaux et al., 1980), a serum creatinine <1 mg/dL and a serum urate <4.0 mg/dL (Beck, 1979) are all suggestive of normal circulating volume.

In the treatment of hyponatremia the plasma sodium concentration should be raised at a safe rate while treating the underlying cause. Treatment involves the administration of sodium to volume-depleted patients and restriction of water intake in normal volemic and edematous patients. Water is removed in hyponatremic states with normal or increased body sodium content. Vigorous therapy with hypertonic saline is required with acute hyponatremia (developing over 1–3 days) when symptoms are present or the sodium concentration is <110 mEq/L.

Overly rapid correction of hyponatremia can be harmful, leading to central demyelinating lesions (central pontine myelinolysis). This is characterized by paraparesis or quadraparesis, dysarthria, dysphagia, coma, and less commonly seizures. It is best diagnosed by magnetic resonance imaging, but it may not be detected radiologically for 4 weeks (Sterns, 1990). The risk of central pontine myelinolysis is lower in patients with acute hyponatremia who have cerebral edema. To minimize this complication chronic hyponatremia should be corrected at a speed of less than 0.5 mEq/L per hour (Sterns, 1990). The degree of correction over the first day (<12 mEq/L), however, seems to be more important than the rate at which it is corrected (Soupart et al., 1992). Rapid correction at a rate of 1.5–2 mEq/L per hour for 3–4 hours should be restricted to only those patients with acute symptomatic hyponatremia. With concomitant hypokalemia, replacement potassium may raise the plasma sodium at close to the maximum rate (Kamel & Bear, 1993); therefore, the appropriate treatment is 0.45% sodium chloride containing 40 mEq of potassium in each liter. For rapid replacement of sodium depletion in patients with symptomatic hypo-osmolality, the IV administration of sodium as hypertonic saline will effectively correct the hypo-osmolality. The sodium needed to raise the sodium concentration to a chosen level is approximated to 0.5 × lean body weight (kg) × (Na) where Na is the desired serum sodium minus the actual serum sodium. Sodium may be administered as a 3% or 5% sodium chloride solution. With hyponatremia secondary to the excessive water accumulation, the water may be removed rapidly by administration of IV furosemide together with hypertonic saline. Furosemide results in the loss of water and sodium but the latter is given back as hypertonic saline with the net result being the loss of water only (Hantman et al., 1973). In extreme cases peritoneal dialysis or hemodialysis may be required. The usual adult starting dose of furosemide for this purpose is 40 mg, IV. The same dose can be repeated at 2–4 hour intervals while hypertonic saline is being given. Potassium supplements are usually needed with this therapy. Chronic hyponatremia may be treated by water restriction or by an increase in renal water excretion. Water restriction may be difficult to achieve in patients with heart failure. In these and similar patients, administration of a loop diuretic such as furosemide in conjunction with an angiotensin-converting enzyme inhibitor (Packer et al., 1984) is effective. Recently, mannitol has been administered with furosemide as a proposed alternative to 3% hypertonic saline for the treatment of acute hyponatremia (<48 hours duration). This therapy may be considered in the acute setting when hypertonic saline is not available and significant neurologic symptoms or seizures are present with acute hyponatremia (Berl, 2000; Porzio et al., 2000).

Hypernatremia

Etiology

Hypernatremia is defined as an increased sodium concentration in plasma water. This is characterized by a serum sodium of >145 mosmol/L and represents a hyperosmolar state. The increased P_{osm} results in water moving extracellularly with cellular dehydration occurring. However, the extracellular volume in hypernatremia may be normal, decreased, or increased (Oh et al., 1992). Hypernatremia represents water loss, sodium retention, or a combination of both (see Table 5.5). Loss of water is due to either increased loss or reduced intake and gain of sodium is due to either increased intake or reduced renal excretion. As shown in Table 5.5, there are numerous disorders responsible for hypernatremia. However, there are two important conditions specific to pregnancy that can result in hypernatremia. The first is iatrogenic and caused by hypertonic saline used for second trimester induced abortion. Twenty percent hypertonic saline, which is infused into the amniotic sac as an abortifacient, can gain access to the maternal vascular compartment resulting in acute, profound hypernatremia, hyperosmolar crisis, and disseminated intravascular coagulopathy. Fortunately, this method has mostly been abandoned in the United States, but it is still performed in other countries.

Transient diabetes insipidus of pregnancy (TDIP) has become a well recognized, although unusual condition. It is characterized by polyuria, polydipsia, and normal or increased serum sodium. Most importantly, a majority of these patients develop preeclampsia or liver abnormalities such as acute fatty liver of pregnancy.

As noted previously, pregnancy is associated with a lower threshold for thirst and a lower osmolarity threshold for ADH release. In addition, the placenta produces vasopressinase, which is a cysteine-aminopeptidase that breaks down the bond between 1-cysteine and 2-tyrosine of vasopressin (ADH), effectively neutralizing the antidiuretic effect of the hormone (Sjoholm & Ymam, 1967; Krege et al., 1989). The liver is believed to be the major site for degradation of vasopressinase and active liver disease can decrease the clearance of vasopressinase.

Table 5.5 Causes of hypernatremia

Water loss
Insensible loss: burns, respiratory infection, exercise
Gastrointestinal loss: gastroenteritis, malabsoption syndromes, osmotic diarrhea
Renal loss: central diabetes insipidus (transient diabetes insipidus of pregnancy, Sheehan's syndrome, cardiopulmonary arrest), nephrogenic diabetes insipidus (X-linked recessive, sickle-cell disease, renal failure, drugs—lithium, diuresis with mannitol, or glucose)
Decreased water intake
Hypothalamic disorders
Loss of consciousness
Limited access to water or inability to drink
Sodium retention
Increased intake of sodium or administration of hypertonic solutions
Saline-induced abortion

Women who are symptomatic or mildly symptomatic prior to pregnancy develop progressively increasing polyuria and polydipsia as the ability of endogenous ADH to effect reabsorption of water in the kidney is overwhelmed. There are probably at least two subsets of women who develop TDIP. In the first group women are minimally symptomatic prior to pregnancy and have subclinical cranial diabetes insipidus (DI). The inability to produce enough ADH, combined with increased vasopressinase activity, leads to clinically evident DI. In this group preeclampsia and liver abnormalities do not seem to develop. In the second subset, abnormal liver function leading to decreased metabolism of vasopressinase causes increased inactivation of ADH in clinical manifestations of DI (Williams et al., 1993). It is in the second group that the incidence of preeclampsia and abnormal liver function seems to be increased. Interestingly, it appears that there is a higher preponderance of male infants in mothers who develop TDIP. In one report, which reviewed 17 pregnancies with TDIP, 16 had abnormal liver function tests, 12 had diastolic blood pressures ≥90 mmHg and six had significant proteinuria (Krege et al., 1989).

This form of TDIP tends not to recur in subsequent pregnancies (Tur-Kasm et al., 1998). Patients who present with polyuria and polydipsia must be evaluated for previously unrecognized diabetes mellitus, preeclampsia, and liver disease. If these are excluded, serum electrolytes, creatinine, liver enzymes, bilirubin, uric acid, complete blood count with differential and peripheral smear, urinalysis for electrolytes, specific gravity, osmolality, protein and 24-hour urine collection for total protein, and creatinine clearance should be ordered. The diagnosis of diabetes insipidus can be made by a water deprivation test. Water is withheld and hourly serum sodium and osmolality are determined as well as urine osmolality and specific gravity. Normally, when water is withheld, sodium and therefore osmolality, should rise as the urine becomes more concentrated, urine osmolality increases and urine volume decreases. In DI the urine osmolality fails to rise and dilute urine continues to be produced. After exogenous ADH is administered (DDAVP should be used in pregnancy), patients with TDIP should respond by concentrating the urine. Failure to concentrate the urine suggests a rarer form of nephrogenic diabetes insipidus. In nephrogenic diabetes insipidus the collecting tubule of the kidney is unable to respond to ADH. Caution is advised if a water deprivation test is performed in pregnancy because as plasma volume decreases, uterine hypoperfusion could be of consequence, especially in a patient who may have surreptitious preeclampsia. Electronic fetal monitoring should be performed during the test. Because osmolarity is reduced in pregnancy, lower serum osmolarity criteria for the diagnosis of DI in pregnancy are recommended. Administration of DDAVP will help differentiate nephrogenic DI from cranial DI.

DDAVP (1-desamino-8-D-argenine-vasopressin) is a synthetic analog of ADH and is not subject to breakdown by vasopressinase. Therefore, this is an ideal drug for the treatment of TDIP. It can be administered by a nasal spray (10–20 μg) or subcutaneously (1–4 μg). DDAVP has negligible pressor or oxytoxic effects. Failure to respond to DDAVP suggests nephrogenic DI.

Clinical presentation

The symptoms are primarily neurologic. The earliest findings are lethargy, weakness, and irritability. These may progress to seizures, coma, and death (Ross & Christie, 1969; Arieff & Guisado, 1976). It is often difficult to discern whether the symptoms are secondary to neurologic disease or hypernatremia. Patients may also exhibit signs of volume expansion or volume depletion. With DI the patient may complain of nocturia, polyuria, and polydipsia.

Diagnosis

Hypernatremia usually causes altered mental status; therefore, obtaining a good history is difficult. Physical examination should help to evaluate the volume status of the patient as well as demonstrate any focal neurologic abnormalities. A urine specific gravity of less than 1.010 usually indicates diabetes insipidus. Administration of ADH in this situation will differentiate central diabetes insipidus (ADH response is an increase in specific gravity with a decrease in urine volume) from nephrogenic diabetes insipidus (no change) (Miller et al., 1970). A specific gravity greater than 1.023 is often seen with excessive insensible or gastrointestinal water losses, primary hypodipsia, and excessive administration of hypertonic fluids. Urine volume should be recorded, because volumes in excess of 5 L/day are seen with lithium toxicity, primary polydipsia, hypercalcemia, central diabetes insipidus, and congenital nephrogenic diabetes insipidus. A water restriction test may be the only way to differentiate the etiologies of CDI and NDI.

Management

Hypernatremia is treated by either the addition of water or removal of sodium, the choice of which depends on the status of the body's sodium and water content. If water depletion is the cause of hypernatremia, water is added. If sodium excess is the cause, sodium needs to be removed. Rapid correction of hypernatremia can cause cerebral edema, seizures, permanent neurologic damage, and death (Pollock & Arieff, 1980). The plasma sodium content should be lowered slowly to normal unless the patient has symptomatic hypernatremia. Hypernatremia of TDIP is generally mild because the thirst mechanism is uninhibited. Hypernatremia secondary to other causes tends to be more severe. When hypernatremia is secondary to water loss calculation of the water deficit is essential. The water deficit can be estimated by the following equation:

$$\text{Water deficit} = \text{body weight (kg)} \times 0.55 \times \text{Na}/\text{Na}_b$$

Where Na_b is the desired sodium level and Na is the difference between the desired and observed serum sodium. This relationship allows calculation of the volume of fluid replacement necessary to reduce the sodium to the desired level. In acute, symptomatic, hypernatremia sodium may be reduced by 6–8 mEq/L in the first 4 hours. But thereafter, the rate of decline should not exceed 0.5 mEq/L/hr. As with hyponatremia, chronic hypernatremia usually does not cause CNS symptoms and therefore does not require rapid correction. As with hyponatremia, a safe rate of correction is 0.7 mEq/L/hr or 12 mEq/L/day (Blum et al., 1986). The type of fluid administered to correct losses depends on the patient's clinical state. Dextrose in water, either orally or IV, can be given to patients with pure water loss. If sodium depletion is also present, such as in vomiting or diarrhea, 0.25 mol/L saline is recommended. In hypotensive patients, normal saline should be used until tissue perfusion has been corrected. Thereafter, a more dilute saline solution should be used.

In patients with excess sodium, the restoration of normal volume usually initiates natriuresis, but if natriuresis does not occur promptly, sodium may be removed with diuretics. Furosemide with a dextrose 5% solution can be used in this situation, but care must be taken not to allow serum sodium concentration to decline too rapidly. Furosemide can be administered at doses of up to 60 mg, IV every 2–4 hours. Patients with renal failure can be treated with dialysis.

Nephrogenic diabetes, which does not respond to ADH or DDAVP, requires treatment with a thiazide diuretic combined with a low sodium, low protein diet. Subjects with primary hypodipsia should be educated to drink on schedule. Stimulation of the thirst center with chlorpropamide has met with some success in these patients (Bode et al., 1971).

Potassium metabolism

Total body potassium (K^+) averages approximately 50 mEq/kg body weight, or about 3,500 mEq in a 70 kg nonpregnant individual, but only 2% of it is extracellular (Lindeheimer et al., 1987). During pregnancy there is an accumulation of 300–320 mEq of potassium (Godfrey & Wadsworth, 1970; Lindeheimer et al., 1987). Approximately 200 mEq of it is in the products of conception. Serum plasma levels change little from the nonpregnant state, with an average decrease in serum potassium (K^+) of approximately 0.2–0.3 mEq/L. The serum K^+ level is determined by three factors: K^+ consumption, whether taken in by diet or administered by parenteral solutions; K^+ loss through the kidney and GI tract; and the shifting between extracellular and intracellular compartments. Renal excretion of potassium is determined by the reabsorption of potassium and most importantly by the secretion of potassium in the distal and collecting tubule of the kidney. Aldosterone enhances the secretion of potassium in the distal tubules and collecting ducts and also increases the permeability of the luminal cellular membranes of the tubules, further facilitating K^+ excretion (Guyton & Hall, 1996). Acute acidosis decreases the kidneys' ability to secrete K^+, while alkalosis enhances the secretion of potassium into the distal tubules. The shifting of K^+ between the extracellular space and the intracellular space is controlled by the sodium potassium ATP-ase pump (Na^+–K^+ ATPase pump), which actively transports sodium (Na^+) out of the cell and in turn moves K^+ into the cell. Acid–base balance plays a critical role in the function of the Na^+–K^+ ATPase pump. In simple terms, acidosis inhibits the function of the Na^+–K^+ ATPase pump and alkalosis enhances it. Thus, acidosis will result in flux of K^+ out of the cell and decreased secretion of K^+ into the distal renal tubules and collecting ducts, leading to hyperkalemia. Alkalosis has the opposite effect, resulting in hypokalemia.

Hypokalemia

Etiology

The causes of hypokalemia are listed in Table 5.6. One particular cause of hypokalemia of special interest in obstetrics is the administration of intravenous β_2-adrenergic agonists for the treatment of preterm labor. β_2-receptor stimulation by agents such as terbutaline, ritodrine, and fenoterol has widespread metabolic effects. Stimulation of the β_2-receptors in the liver results in glycogenolysis, gluconeogenesis, and causes an elevation in serum glucose. The increase in glucose as well as direct stimulation of β_2-receptors in the pancreatic eyelet cells causes secretion of insulin. Most importantly the Na^+–K^+ ATPase pump is directly stimulated by these agents. A significant decrease in serum potassium occurs within minutes of intravenous administration of β_2-agonists, even before glucose and insulin levels increase. As glucose levels rise and insulin secretion increases, K^+ levels fall even further as K^+ is shifted into the cell (Braden et al., 1997). Although an intracellular shift of K^+ caused by insulin-induced glucose uptake may contribute to the hypokalemia, it seems that the most important cause is the direct β_2-adrenergic stimulation (Cano et al., 1985). Renal excretion does not seem to be a factor in β_2-agonist-induced hypokalemia (Braden et al., 1997).

The severity of the hypokalemia is dependent upon the pretreatment concentration of serum K^+. The effect is more pronounced when the pretreatment K^+ concentration is high and the effect is reduced in patients with preexisting hypokalemia. Nevertheless, patients with preexisting hypokalemia may be at greater risk of developing the complications of hypokalemia (Hildebrandt et al., 1997). Since the hypokalemia associated with intravenous administration of β_2-agonists represents an intracellular shift with unchanged total body K^+ and side effects are uncommon, serum K^+ of 2.5 mmol/L generally does not require K^+ replacement. At levels <2.5 mmol/L serious cardiac arrhythmias have been reported with β_2-agonist tocolysis and replacement of K^+ is recommended (Braden et al., 1997).

Bartter's syndrome is an autosomal recessive disorder characterized by hypokalemia, hyperaldosteronism, sodium wasting, normal blood pressure, hypochloremic alkalosis, and hyperplasia of the juxtaglomerular apparatus (O'Sullivan et al., 1997). Increasing numbers of cases are being reported in the literature (Johnson et al., 2000; Nohira et al., 2001). Hypokalemia is responsible for most of the symptoms of Bartter's syndrome and therapy is directed toward increasing the K^+ concentration with supplements and K^+ sparing diuretics. Over one-third of patients with Bartter's syndrome also suffer magnesium wasting and increased magnesium supplementation may also be required for treatment.

Table 5.6 Causes of hypokalemia

Redistribution within the body
β_2-agonists
Glucose and insulin therapy
Acute alkalosis or correction of acute acidosis
Familial periodic paralysis
Barium poisoning
Reduced intake
Chronic starvation
Increased loss
Gastrointestinal loss
Prolonged vomiting or nasogastric suction
Diarrhea or intestinal fistula
Villous adenoma
Renal loss
Primary hypoaldosteronism
Secondary hypoaldosteronism (renal artery stenosis, diuretic therapy, malignant hypertension)
Cushing's syndrome and steroid therapy
Bartter's syndrome
Carbenoxolone
Licorice-containing substances
Renal tubular acidosis
Acute myelocytic and monocytic leukemia
Magnesium deficiency

Clinical presentation

Muscle weakness, hypotonia and mental status changes may occur when the serum K^+ is below 2.5 mmol/L. ECG changes occur in 50% of patients with hypokalemia (Flakeb et al., 1986) and involve a decrease in T-wave amplitude in addition to the development of prominent U-waves. Hypokalemia can potentiate arrhythmias due to digitalis toxicity (Flakeb et al., 1986).

Diagnosis

After obtaining a history and physical examination, serum and urine electrolytes plus serum calcium and magnesium should be obtained. The urine potassium will help differentiate renal from extrarenal losses. A urine potassium below 30 mEq/L signifies extrarenal losses, seen commonly in patients with diarrhea or redistribution within the body (see Table 5.6). A urine potassium of greater than 30 mEq/L is seen with renal losses. In this situation, a serum bicarbonate will help separate renal tubular acidosis (<24 mEq/L) from other causes. A urine chloride less than 10 mEq/L is seen with vomiting, nasogastric suctioning, and overventilation. A level greater than 10 mEq/L is seen with diuretic and steroid therapy.

Management

Hypokalemia is treated either by the administration of potassium or by preventing the renal loss of potassium. Once the potassium falls below 3.5 mEq/L, there is already a 200 mEq deficit in potassium; therefore, any additional decrease in potassium is significant regardless of the magnitude (Marino, 1991c).

If the serum potassium level is below 2.5 mEq/L, clinical symptoms or ECG changes are generally present, and one should initiate IV therapy. While it is theoretically useful to estimate the potassium deficit prior to initiating therapy, such calculations are of limited value because they can vary considerably secondary to transcellular shifts. As a rough estimate, a serum potassium of 3.0 mEq/L is associated with a potassium deficit of 350 mEq, and a potassium level of 2.0 mEq/L with a deficit of 700 mEq. The recommended IV replacement dose is 0.7 mEq/kg lean body weight over 1–2 hours (Smith et al., 1985). In obese patients, 30 mEq/m^2 body surface area is administered. The dose should not increase the serum potassium by more than 1.0–1.5 mEq/L unless an acidosis is present. In life-threatening situations, a rate in excess of 100 mEq/hr may be used (Smith et al., 1985). If aggressive replacement therapy does not correct the serum potassium, magnesium depletion should be considered and the magnesium then replaced.

With an underlying metabolic alkalosis, one should use potassium chloride for replacement of hypokalemia. The chloride salt is necessary to correct the alkalosis, which otherwise would result in the administered potassium being lost in the urine. When rapidly replacing potassium chloride, glucose-containing solutions should not be used because they will stimulate release of insulin, which will drive potassium into the cells. Potassium at concentrations exceeding 40 mEq/L may produce pain at the infusion site and may lead to sclerosis of smaller vessels; thus, it is advisable to split the dosage and administer each portion via a separate peripheral vein. One should avoid central venous infusion of potassium at high concentrations because this can produce life-threatening cardiotoxicity.

Renal loss of potassium is prevented either by treating its cause or by the administration of potassium-sparing diuretics. Spironolactone (25–150 mg twice a day), triamterine (50–100 mg twice a day), or amiloride (5–20 mg/day) is effective in reducing potassium loss. Amiloride should be administered with food to avoid gastric irritation. Mild potassium loss can be replaced orally in the form of potassium chloride or KPO_4.

Hyperkalemia

Hyperkalemia is defined as a serum potassium greater than 5.5 mEq/L. Because of its potential for producing dysrhythmias, hyperkalemia should be managed far more aggressively than hypokalemia. Pseudohyperkalemia is defined as an increase in potassium concentration only in the local blood vessel or in vitro and has no physiologic consequences. Hemolysis during venepuncture, thrombocytosis (greater than 1 million/μL), and severe leukocytosis (over 50,000) cause psuedohyperkalemia. Pseudohyperkalemia should always be investigated immediately, with careful attention paid to avoiding cell trauma during blood collection. Both thrombocytosis and leukocytosis release potassium from the platelets and WBC during blood clotting (Hartman et al., 1958; Robertson, 1984). Suspected pseudohyperkalemia should be investigated by obtaining simultaneous serum potassium specimens from clotted and unclotted specimens. The potassium in the clotted sample should be 0.3 mEq/L higher than in the unclotted specimen.

Etiology

The causes of hyperkalemia can be classified according to three basic mechanisms: redistribution within the body, increased potassium intake, or reduced renal potassium excretion (Table 5.7). Severe tissue injury leads to direct release of potassium due to disruption of cell membranes. Rhabdomyolysis and hemolysis cause hyperkalemia only when causing renal failure. Metabolic acidosis results in increased potassium shift across membranes, with reduced renal excretion of potassium. This can increase the serum potassium by up to 1 mEq/L (Smith et al., 1985). Hyperkalemia is less predictable with organic causes of acidosis, such as diabetic and lactic acidosis, when compared with the inorganic causes of acidosis (Oster et al., 1978). Respiratory acidosis does not often produce hyperkalemia. Digitalis toxicity leads to disruption of the membrane sodium–potassium pump, which normally keeps potassium intracellular (Bismuth et al., 1973).

Diminished renal potassium excretion is due to renal failure, reduced aldosterone or aldosterone responsiveness, or reduced distal delivery of sodium. Renal failure usually does not cause hyperkalemia until the GFR is below 10 mL/min or urine output is less than 1 liter (Williams & Rosa, 1988). Deficiency of aldosterone may be due to an absence of hormone, such as occurs in Addison's disease, or may be part of a selective process, such as occurs in hyporeninemic hypoaldosteronism, which is the most common cause of chronic hyperkalemia (Phelps et al., 1980). Heparin in a small dose can reversibly inhibit aldosterone synthesis causing hypokalemia. Angiotensin-converting enzyme inhibitors, potassium-sparing diuretics, and nonsteroidal anti-inflammatory agents limit the supply of renin or angiotensin II, resulting in decreased aldosterone and hyperkalemia. Severe dehydration may result in the delivery of sodium to the distal nephron being markedly reduced with the development of hyperkalemia (Oh, 1982). Life-threatening arrhythmias and cardiac arrest have been reported in patients treated for preterm labor with prolonged bed rest intravenous magnesium sulfate infusion combined with β_2-adrenergic agonists who underwent induction of general anesthesia for cesarean section with succinylcholine. Sudden increases in serum potassium concentrations ranging from 5.7 to 7.2 occurred in patients shortly after induction of anesthesia with the muscle blocking agent succinylcholine. The administration of succinylcholine in immobilized patients may cause a hazardous hyperkalemic response. In addition, patients with burns, infections, or neuromuscular disease are at risk for massive hyperkalemia after succinylcholine injection. It is speculated that extrajunctional acetylcholine receptors develop in these patients so that potassium is released from the entire muscle instead of the neuromuscular junction alone. This increase of potassium release is referred to as upregulation of acetylcholine receptors (Sato et al., 2000). Severe hyperkalemia has also been reported in intravenous drug abusers treated with prolonged parenteral magnesium sulfate in the absence of an obvious cause (Spital & Greenwell, 1991).

Table 5.7 Causes of hyperkalemia

Redistribution within the body
Severe tissue damage (e.g. myonecrosis)
Insulin deficiency
Metabolic acidosis
Digitalis toxicity
Severe acute starvation
Hypoxia
Increased potassium intake
Overly aggressive potassium therapy
Failure to stop therapy when depletion corrected
Reduced renal excretion of potassium
Adrenal insufficiency
Drugs
Angiotensin-converting enzyme inhibitors
Potassium-sparing diuretics
Nonsteroidal anti-inflammatory agents
Heparin
Succinylcholine
Renal glomerular failure
Magnesium sulfate

Clinical presentation

Skeletal muscle and cardiac conduction abnormalities are the dominant features of clinical hyperkalemia. Neuromuscular weakness may occur, with severe flaccid quadriplegia being common (Villabona et al., 1987). ECG changes begin when the serum potassium reaches 6.0 mEq/L and are always abnormal when a serum level of 8.0 mEq/L is reached (Williams & Rosa, 1988). The earliest changes are tall, narrow T-waves in precordial leads V2–4. The T-wave in hyperkalemia has a narrow base, which helps to separate it from other causes of tall T-waves. As the serum potassium level increases, the P-wave amplitude decreases with lengthening of the P–R interval until the P-waves disappear. The Q–R–S complex may be prolonged, resulting in ventricular asystole. Occasionally, gastrointestinal symptoms occur.

Diagnosis

After obtaining a history and physical examination, serum and urine electrolytes plus serum calcium and magnesium should be obtained. The urine potassium will help differentiate renal from extrarenal losses. A urine potassium above 30 mEq/L suggests a transcellular potassium shift; below this level, reduced renal excretion is suggested.

Management

Therapy always should be initiated when the serum potassium exceeds 6.0 mEq/L, irrespective of ECG finding, because ventricular tachycardia can appear without premonitory ECG signs (Smith et al., 1985). Therapy should be monitored by frequent serum potassium level sampling and ECG. The plan is to acutely manage the hyperkalemia and then achieve and maintain a normal serum level (Table 5.8).

Table 5.8 Management of hyperkalemia

Acute management
Calcium gluconate
10 mL (10% solution) IV over 3 min; repeat in 5 min if no response
Insulin-glucose infusion
10 units regular insulin in 500 mL of 20% dextrose and infuse over 1 hour
Sodium bicarbonate
1–2 ampules (44–88 mEq) over 5–10 min
Furosemide
40 mm IV
Dialysis
Chronic management
Kayexalate
Oral: 30 g in 50 mL of 20% sorbitol
Rectal: 50 g in 200 mL of 20% sorbitol retention enema

The mainstay of therapy for patients with acute and severe hyperkalemia is administration of calcium. This may be a life-saving medication in an emergency. Calcium directly antagonizes the action of potassium and decreases excitation potential at the membrane. Calcium gluconate is the preferred agent because inadvertent extravasation of calcium chloride into soft tissues can cause a severe inflammation and tissue necrosis. Ten milliliters of a 10% solution of calcium gluconate (approximately 1 g) can be infused over 2–3 minutes. The effect is rapid, occurring over a few minutes, but is short lived, lasting only about 30 minutes. If no effect is noted, characterized by changes in the ECG, the dose can be repeated once. Measures must be taken to achieve a more prolonged effect to lower potassium levels. Another time-honored, proven therapy is to effect a shift of potassium into the cells by infusing glucose and insulin. Ten units of regular insulin can be mixed in 500 ml of 20% dextrose in water (D20%W) and infused over 1 hour. Diluting standard D50%W can make 20% glucose. Alternatively 10–20 units of regular insulin can be infused more rapidly in D50%W. The onset of action should occur over 15–30 minutes and the duration of action is hours. The serum glucose should fall by 1 mEq/L within about an hour. Sodium bicarbonate has been recommended as a tertiary agent to lower the serum potassium; however its efficacy for treatment of patients with renal failure has been called into doubt (Allon & Shanklin, 1996; Greenberg, 1998). It may be more efficacious in patients suffering with concomitant metabolic acidosis. In theory raising the pH of blood will increase uptake of potassium by the cells. One to three ampules of $NaHCO_3$, 44–132 mEq, can be mixed with D5% water and infused over 1 hour or 1–2 ampules can be administered over 10 minutes. β_2-adrenergic agents such as salbutamol and albuterol administered parenterally or by nebulizer have been shown to be efficacious in the treatment of hyperkalemia. The mechanism of action has been described previously. β_2-adrenergic agents are familiar to most obstetricians and can be considered in the less acute management of patients with hyperkalemia. A paradoxical initial rise in serum potassium has been reported and caution is advised if considering this in initial treatment (Mandelberg et al., 1999). Dialysis may be necessary in patients with acute or chronic renal failure if these measures fail to return potassium to safe levels.

In less acute situations any offending agents contributing to hyperkalemia should be stopped, potassium intake adjusted, and therapy instituted. Removal of potassium may be accomplished by several routes including through the gastrointestinal tract, through the kidneys, or by hemodialysis or peritoneal dialysis. A potassium exchange resin, sodium polystyrene sulfonate (Kayexalate), may be administered either orally or by enema. It is more effective when given with sorbitol or mannitol, which cause osmotic diarrhea. One tablespoon of Kayexalate mixed with 100 mL of 10% sorbitol or mannitol can be given by mouth 2–4 times a day. Loop diuretics, mineralocorticoids or increased salt intake enhance the urinary excretion of potassium. Finally, in cases of severe refractory or life-threatening hyperkalemia, either hemodialysis or peritoneal dialysis may be necessary.

Abnormalities in calcium metabolism

Calcium circulates in the blood in one of three forms. 40–50% of calcium is bound to serum protein, mostly albumin, and is nondiffusible. Approximately 10% is bound to other anions such as citrate or phosphate and is diffusible. The remainder is unbound ionized calcium, which is diffusible and the most physiologically active form. The normal serum range for the ionized fraction is between 1.1 and 1.3 mmol/L (Marino, 1991a). The total serum calcium levels may not accurately reflect the ionized calcium level. Alteration of the patient's serum albumin concentration can influence the protein bound fraction, leading to an incorrect assessment of the ionized calcium level. It is the ionized calcium that determines the normalcy of the physiologic state. Therefore, measurement of the ionized calcium is preferred for clinical decision making. If the ionized calcium cannot be measured by the laboratory the total calcium and serum albumin should be measured simultaneously and a correction factor used to estimate whether hypocalcemia is present. The normal range of serum calcium is 9–10.5 mg/dL and the normal range for serum albumin is 3.5–5.5 g/dL. One simply adds 0.8 mg/dL for every 1 g/dL albumin concentration below 4 g/dL. For example, if the total serum calcium is 7.8 mg/dL and the serum albumin is 3.0 g/dL, using the correction factor $1 \times 0.8 + 7.8 = 8.6$. Therefore, this patient would not be in the hypocalcemic range. In pregnancy, serum albumin concentration drops with a compensatory increase in ionized calcium activity. In a condition such as preeclampsia albumin levels may drop even further. Calcium levels are also influenced by blood pH. Acidosis leads to decreased binding of calcium to serum proteins and an increase in the ionized calcium level. Alkalosis has the opposite effect. Free fatty acids increase calcium binding to albumin. Serum levels of free fatty acids are often increased during critical illness as a result of illness-induced elevations of plasma concentrations of epinephrine, glucagon, growth hormone, and corticotropin as well as decreases in serum insulin concentrations.

Serum calcium levels are normally maintained within a very narrow range. Calciferol, obtained either in the diet or formed in the skin, is converted to 1α, 25-dihydroxycalciferol by reactions in the liver and kidney and is commonly referred to as 1,25-dihydroxyvitamin D. This substance enhances calcium absorption in the gut. Parathyroid hormone (PTH) is secreted in accordance to a feedback relationship with calcium. As calcium levels drift lower, PTH is secreted and as calcium levels increase, PTH secretion is inhibited. Calcitonin stimulates calcium entry into bone due to the action of osteoblasts and its effect is less important in calcium control than PTH.

PTH stimulates osteoclastic absorption of bone leading to release of calcium into the extracellular fluid. In addition, PTH stimulates calcium reabsorption in the distal tubules of the kidney.

Calcium imbalances

Hypocalcemia

The most commonly encountered derangement in calcium homeostasis in pregnancy is hypocalcemia associated with magnesium sulfate ($MgSO_4{\cdot}7H_2O$) therapy used to treat preeclampsia, eclampsia, and preterm labor. Magnesium sulfate is usually administered as a 3–6 g bolus over 15–30 minutes, followed by a 1–3 g/hr continuous infusion (ACOG Technical Bulletin, 1996). Within 1 hour of initiation of intravenous magnesium sulfate infusion, both total and ionized calcium levels decline rapidly. Serum ionized and total calcium concentrations have been shown to decline 11% and 22% respectively during infusion for the treatment of preeclampsia. These levels are 4–6 standard deviations below the mean normal serum calcium concentration (Cruikshank et al., 1979, 1993). Serum albumin is often significantly decreased in preeclampsia and can contribute to the lower serum calcium levels; however, other mechanisms are probably responsible for this effect. Urinary calcium excretion increases 4.5-fold during magnesium sulfate infusions at a rate three times greater than observed in normal controls (Cruikshank et al., 1981). Some have noted decreased PTH levels in response to magnesium sulfate administration, an effect that would cause decreased calcium reabsorption in the kidney and decreased serum calcium levels (Cholst et al., 1984). Cruikshank demonstrated not only increased levels of PTH, but also increased levels of 1,25-dihydroxyvitamin D, during magnesium sulfate infusions. It is hypothesized that magnesium ions compete with calcium ions for common reabsorptive sites or mechanisms in the nephron. The increased delivery of magnesium to the distal tubule and collecting duct results in increased magnesium reabsorption and less availability for resorptive sites for calcium, leading to increased urinary calcium loss (Carney et al., 1980; Cruikshank et al., 1981).

Etiology

Common nonobstetric causes of hypocalcemia include both metabolic and respiratory alkalosis, sepsis, magnesium depletion, and renal failure (Table 5.9). Magnesium deficiency is common in critically ill patients and also may cause hypocalcemia (Anast et al., 1976; Zaloga et al., 1987). One cannot correct a calcium deficiency until the magnesium deficit has been corrected.

Sepsis can lead to hypocalcemia, presumably as a result of calcium efflux across a disrupted microcirculation (Zaloga & Chernow, 1987). This effect may be linked to an underlying respiratory alkalosis; this combination confers a poor prognosis. Hypocalcemia commonly is seen in patients with acute pancreatitis and also is associated with a poor prognosis (Zaloga & Chernow, 1985b). Renal failure leads to phosphorus retention, which may cause hypocalcemia as a result of calcium precipitation, inhibition of bone resorption, and suppression of renal 1-hyroxylation of vitamin D (Chernow et al., 1981; Zaloga, 1990). Thus, the treatment of hypocalcemia in this setting is to lower the serum PO_4 level. Citrated blood (massive blood transfusion), albumin, and radiocontrast dyes are the most common chelators that cause hypocalcemia in critically ill patients. Primary hypoparathyroidism is seen rarely, whereas secondary hypoparathyroidism after neck surgery is a common cause of hypocalcemia (Nagant De Deuxchaisnes & Krane, 1978).

Table 5.9 Causes of hypocalcemia

Magnesium sulfate infusion
Massive blood transfusion
Acid–base disorders
Respiratory and metabolic alkalosis
Shock
Renal failure
Malabsorption syndrome
Magnesium depletion
Hypoparathyroidism
Surgically produced
Idiopathic
Pancreatitis
Fat embolism syndrome
Drugs
Heparin, aminogylcosides, cis-platinum, phenytoin, phenobarbital, and loop diuretics

Clinical presentation

Hypocalcemia may present with a variety of clinical signs and symptoms. The most common manifestations are caused by increased neuronal irritability and decreased cardiac contractility (Zaloga & Chernow, 1985b). Neuronal symptoms include seizures, weakness, muscle spasm, paresthesias, tetany, and Chvostek's and Trousseau's signs. Neither Chvostek's nor Trousseau's signs are sensitive or specific (Zaloga & Chernow, 1985a). Cardiovascular manifestations include hypotension, cardiac insufficiency, bradycardia, arrhythmias, left ventricular failure, and cardiac arrest. ECG findings include Q–T and S–T interval prolongation and T-wave inversion. Other clinical findings include anxiety, irritability, confusion, brittle nails, dry scaly skin, and brittle hair.

Serum calcium levels may drop to very low levels during continuous intravenous administration of magnesium. Although hypocalcemic tetany has been reported during treat-

Table 5.10 Calcium preparations

Parenteral	*Rate*
Calcium gluconate	1.0 mL/min
Calcium chloride	0.5 mL/min
Oral	*Contents*
Calcium carbonate	500 mg calcium
Calcium gluconate	500 mg calcium

ment for preeclampsia, it is so rare that compensatory protective mechanisms must be acting (Monif & Savory, 1972).

Parathyroid hormone levels have been shown to rise 30–50% after infusion of magnesium sulfate and its associated hypocalcemia. 1,25-dihydroxyvitamin D rises by more than 50% and the placenta is a significant source of this vitamin. Such a response leads to increased calcium released from bone and increased gastrointestinal absorption, perhaps limiting the progressive decline in calcium concentration. It is not necessary to replace depleted calcium in preeclamptic patients with magnesium-induced hypocalcemia, unless the ionized calcium levels fall dangerously low and obvious clinical signs of hypocalcemia ensue. In the authors' and editors' collective experience it has not been necessary to replace calcium in severely preeclamptic or eclamptic patients. The administration of calcium could interfere with the therapeutic effect of magnesium sulfate.

Treatment

All patients with an ionized calcium concentration below 0.8 mmol/L should receive treatment. Life-threatening arrhythmias can develop when the ionized calcium level approaches 0.5–0.65 mmol/L. Acute symptomatic hypocalcemia is a medical emergency that necessitates IV calcium therapy (Table 5.10). With acute symptoms, a calcium bolus can be given at an initial dose of 100–200 mg IV over 10 minutes, followed by a continuous infusion of 1–2 mg/kg/h. This will raise the serum total calcium by 1 mg/dL, with levels returning to baseline by 30 minutes after injection. Intravenous calcium preparations are irritating to veins and should be diluted (10 mL vial in 100 mL of D5W and warmed to body temperature). If IV access is not available, calcium gluceptate may be given intramuscularly (IM) (Haynes & Murad, 1985).

Anticonvulsant drugs, sedation, and paralysis may help eliminate signs of neuronal irritability. Once the serum calcium is in the low normal range, oral replacement with enteral calcium is recommended.

Hypercalcemia

Etiology

The finding of hypercalcemia is a relatively rare occurrence in women of the reproductive age group. The most common cause of hypercalcemia in the general population is hyperparathyroidism secondary to a benign adenoma. Approximately 80% are single, benign adenomas, while multiple adenomas or hyperplasia of the four parathyroid glands also may cause hyperparathyroidism. In patients treated in the intensive care unit hypercalcemia is more likely to be related to malignancy. Ten to 20% of patients with malignancy develop hypercalcemia because of direct tumor osteolysis of bone and secretion of humoral substances that stimulate bone resorption (Benabe & Martinez-Maldonado, 1987; Mundy, 1989). Other causes of hypercalcemia are listed in Table 5.11. There are rare reports cases of parathyroid carcinoma in pregnancy accounting for a minority of cases (Montoro et al., 2000).

Table 5.11 Causes of hypercalcemia

Malignancy
Hyperparathyroidism
Chronic renal failure
Recovery from acute renal failure
Immobilization
Calcium administration
Hypocalciuric hypercalcemia
Granulomatous disease
Sarcoidosis
Tuberculosis
Hyperthryroidism
AIDS
Drug-induced
Lithium, theophylline, thiazides, and vitamin D or A

Clinical presentation

Although women are twice as common as men to develop hyperparathyroidism, the peak incidence is in women over the age of 45 years. In nonpregnant individuals the disorder is generally asymptomatic and detected on screening metabolic profiles. This is not the case in pregnancy, where approximately 70% of individuals exhibit symptoms of hypercalcemia (Mestamen, 1998). Constipation, anorexia, nausea, and vomiting are common. Severe hypertension and arrhythmias have been reported in patients with hypercalcemia during pregnancy. Other symptoms include fatigue, weakness, depression, cognitive dysfunction, and hyporeflexia. ECG changes include Q–T segment shortening. Nephrolithiasis may occur in a third of these patients and pancreatitis in 13%. This is in contrast to nonpregnant individuals with hyperparathyroidism who have an incidence of 1.5% of pancreatitis (Mestamen, 1998).

Diagnosis

Calcium derangements in neonates and infants may indicate

disorders of maternal calcium metabolism. Hypocalcemic tetany and seizures in infants have been reported in mothers diagnosed with hypercalcemia. Therefore, serum calcium levels should be measured in mothers whose infants are born with metabolic bone disease or abnormal serum calcium levels (Thomas et al., 1999). After a complete history and physical examination is obtained, serum electrolytes, total and ionized calcium, magnesium, PO_4, and albumin should be obtained. Serum PTH, thyroid-stimulating hormone (TSH), T_3 and T_4 should be obtained and an ECG performed. Renal function should be assessed with a 24-hour urine collection for calcium, creatinine, creatinine clearance, and total volume to help distinguish hypocalciuric from hypercalciuric syndromes.

Treatment

Surgical removal of the abnormal parathyroid gland is the only long-term effective treatment for primary hyperparathyroidism. Surgery is optimally performed in the first and second trimester on symptomatic patients with serum calcium over 11 mg/dL. The major complication from surgical treatment is hypocalcemia, which can be treated with a calcium gluconate infusion. Calcium gluconate can be diluted in 5% dextrose and infused at a rate of 1 mg/kg body weight per hour (Mestamen, 1998). Medical therapy (Table 5.12) needs to be initiated when the serum calcium reaches 13 mg/dL or patients are symptomatic at levels greater than 11. Patients with hypercalcemia are usually dehydrated. Hyperuricemia resulting from hypercalcemia compounds the volume deficit and further elevates the serum calcium level. The first step in management of hypercalcemia is restoration of intravascular volume. Volume expansion will not only dilute the serum calcium, but volume expansion with isotonic saline inhibits sodium reabsorption and increases calcium excretion. After the intravascular volume is restored, furosemide or ethacrynic acid, the loop diuretics, may be administered. Their major effect is in preventing volume overload in patients predisposed to CHF. Although they may increase sodium and calcium excretion, the additional benefit is questionable and their administration necessitates vigilant monitoring and replacement of potassium and magnesium. Thiazide diuretics inhibit renal calcium excretion and are contraindicated in the treatment of hypercalcemia. Bisphosphonates are medications that inhibit osteoclast-mediated bone reabsorption. Pamidronate is most commonly used and should be administered early in the therapy of hypercalcemia after volume restoration with normal saline has been accomplished. A single dose of 30–60 mg, diluted 500 mL of 0.9% saline or 5% dextrose in water can be infused over 4 hours. However, for severe hypercalcemia 90 mg can be infused over 24 hours. The maximal hypocalcemic effect is observed in 1–2 days and its effect generally lasts for weeks. Pamidronate has been used in pregnancy for the treatment of malignant hypercalcemia with no ill effect reported on the fetus (Illidge et al., 1996). Animal studies have failed to demonstrate a teratogenic effect of the medication (Graepel et al., 1992). However, it does bind to fetal bone and limited experience with its use in pregnancy warrants caution. Calcitonin inhibits bone resorption and increases urinary calcium excretion. Its effect is rapid and can lower serum calcium 1–2 mg/dL within several hours. It can be administered subcutaneously or intramuscularly in doses of 4–8 IU/kg every 6–12 hours. Unfortunately, tachyphylaxis develops over days and its effectiveness is decreased. Nevertheless, it is safe, relatively free of side effects and compatible with use in renal failure. Glucocorticoids may be beneficial in hypercalcemia secondary to sarcoidosis, multiple myeloma and vitamin D intoxication. They are generally considered a secondary or tertiary agent and require doses of 50–100 mg of prednisone in divided doses per day. Oral phosphate, which has been a mainstay of therapy in the past, has fallen out of common usage because of more effective medications noted above. It can have a modest effect in decreasing calcium levels by inhibiting calcium absorption and promoting calcium deposition in bone. Mithramycin is another agent whose use has been supplanted by pamidronate. It is associated with serious side effects such as thrombocytopenia, coagulopathy, and renal failure.

Hemodialysis can be highly effective in the treatment of severe hypercalcemia or hypercalcemia refractory to other methods of treatment. It is generally reserved as a last line of therapy.

Table 5.12 Acute management of hypercalcemia

Agent	Dose	Comments
0.9% Saline	300–500 mL/hr	Adjust infusion to maintain urine output at ≥200 mL/hr. Add furosemide if volume overload or CHF
Pamidronate	30–60 mg in 500 mL of 0.9% saline or D5%W over 4 hr	Maximal effect in 2 days; lasts for weeks
Calcitonin	4 IU/kg IM or subcutaneously q 12 hr	Tachyphylaxis develops
Steroids	Prednisone 20–50 mg b.i.d.	Multiple myeloma, sarcoidosis, vitamin D toxicity
Phosphates	0.5–1 g p.o. t.i.d.	Requires normal renal function
Hemodialysis		Severe hypercalcemia, renal failure, CHF

Magnesium imbalances

Hypomagnesemia

Magnesium (Mg^{2+}) is the second most abundant intracellular cation in the body. It is a cofactor for all enzyme reactions involved in the splitting of high-energy adenosine triphosphate (ATP) bonds required for the activity of phosphatases. Such enzymes are essential and provide energy for the sodium–potassium ATPase pump, proton pump, calcium ATPase pump, neurochemical transmission, muscle contraction, glucose–fat–protein metabolism, oxidative phosphorylation, and DNA synthesis (Quamme & Dirks, 1987; Zaloga & Roberts, 1990; Salem et al., 1991). Magnesium is also required for the activity of adenylate cyclase.

Magnesium is not distributed uniformly within the body. Less than 1% of total body magnesium is found in the serum, with 50–60% found in the skeleton and 20% in muscle (Quamm & Dirks, 1987). Serum levels, thus, may not reflect true intracellular stores accurately and may be normal in the face of magnesium depletion or excess (Reinhart, 1988; Zaloga & Roberts, 1990). In the blood, there are three fractions: an ionized fraction (55%), which is physiologically active and homeostatically regulated; a protein-bound fraction (30%); and a chelated fraction (15%).

Magnesium can be viewed as a calcium-channel blocker. Intracellular calcium levels rise as magnesium becomes depleted. Many calcium channels have been shown to be magnesium dependent and higher concentrations of magnesium inhibit the flux of calcium through both intracellular, extracellular channels and from the sarcoplasmatic reticulum. Hypomagnesemia enhances the vasoconstrictive effect of catecholemines and angiotensin II in smooth muscle (Dacey, 2001).

It is estimated that at least 65% of critically ill patients develop hypomagnesemia. The normal magnesium concentration is between 1.7 and 2.4 mg/dL (1.4–2.0 mEq/L); however, a normal reading should not deter one from considering hypomagnesemia in the presence of a suggestive clinical presentation (Marino, 1991b).

Etiology

Hypomagnesemia results from at least one of three causes. These are: decreased intake, increased losses from the gastrointestinal tract or kidney, and cellular redistribution. Hypomagnesemia is common in patients receiving TPN and increased supplementation may be required to assure adequate magnesium intake. Increase renal losses secondary to the use of diuretics and amnioglycosides constitute the most common cause of magnesium loss in a hospital setting (Table 5.13). Diuretics such as furosemide and ethacrynic acid and amnioglycosides inhibit magnesium reabsorption in the loop of Henle and also block absorption at this site, leading to increased urinary losses (Ryan, 1987). Up to 30–40% of patients receiving aminoglycosides will develop hypomagnesemia (Zaloga et al., 1984; Elin, 1988).

Hypomagnesemia can result from internal redistribution of magnesium. Following the administration of glucose or amino acids, magnesium shifts into cells (Berkelhammer & Bear, 1985; Brauthbar & Massry, 1987). A similar effect is seen with increased catecholemine levels, correction of acidosis, and hungry bone syndromes. Lower gastrointestinal tract secretions are rich in magnesium; thus, severe diarrhea leads to hypomagnesemia.

Table 5.13 Causes of hypomagnesemia

Drug-induced
Diuretics (furosemide, thiazides, mannitol)
Aminoglycosides
Neoplastic agents (cis-platinum, carbenicillin, cyclosporine)
Amphotericin B
Digoxin
Thyroid hormone
Insulin
Malabsorption, laxative abuse, fistulas
Malnutrition
Hyperalimentation and prolonged IV therapy
Renal losses
Glomerulonephritis, interstitial nephritis
Tubular disorders
Hyperthyroidsm
Diabetic ketoacidosis
Pregnancy and lactation
Sepsis
Hypothermia
Burns
Blood transfusion (citrate)

Clinical presentation

The signs and symptoms of hypomagnesemia are very similar to those of hypocalcemia and hypokalemia, and it is not entirely clear whether hypomagnesemia alone is responsible for these symptoms (Kingston et al., 1986; Zaloga, 1989). Most symptomatic patients have levels below 1.0 mg/dL. Cardiovascular symptoms include hypertension, heart failure, arrhythmias, increased risk for digitalis toxicity, and decreased pressor response (Iseri et al., 1975; Burch & Giles, 1977; Berkelhammer & Bear, 1985; Rasmussen et al., 1986; Abraham et al., 1987; Brauthbar & Massry, 1987). The ECG may demonstrate a prolonged P–R and Q–T interval with S–T depression. Tall, peaked T-waves occur early and slowly broaden with decreased amplitude together with the development of a widened Q–R–S interval as the magnesium level falls. As with hypocalcemia, there is increased neuronal irritability with weakness, muscle spasms, tremors, seizures, tetany, confusion, psychosis, and coma. Patients also complain of anorexia, nausea, and abdominal cramps.

Diagnosis

Following a complete history, physical examination, and ECG, serum electrolyte, calcium, magnesium, and PO_4 levels should be obtained. A 24-hour urine magnesium measurement is helpful in separating renal from nonrenal causes. An increased urinary magnesium level suggests increased renal loss of magnesium as the etiology of hypomagnesemia.

Treatment

Patients with life-threatening arrhythmias, acute symptomatic hypomagnesemia, or severe hypomagnesemia are best treated with IV magnesium sulfate (Flink, 1969; Mordes & Wacker, 1977; Heath, 1980; Rude & Singer, 1981; Cronin & Knochel, 1983; Whang et al., 1985). A 2 g bolus of magnesium sulfate is administered IV over 1–2 minutes, followed by a continuous infusion at a rate of 2 g/hr. After a few hours, this can be reduced to a 0.5–1.0 g/hr maintenance infusion. Magnesium chloride is used in patients with concurrent hypocalcemia, because sulfate can bind calcium and worsen hypocalcemia. During magnesium replacement, one should monitor the serum levels of magnesium, calcium, potassium, and creatinine. Blood pressure, respiratory status, and neurologic status (mental alertness, deep tendon reflexes) should be assessed periodically. As magnesium sulfate is renally excreted, its dose should be reduced in patients with renal insufficiency.

With moderate magnesium deficiency, 50–100 mEq magnesium sulfate per day (600–1,200 mg elemental magnesium) can be administered in patients without renal insufficiency. Mild asymptomatic magnesium deficiency can also be replaced with diet alone. It can take up to 3–5 days to replace intracellular stores.

Magnesium is important for the maintenance of normal potassium metabolism (Whang et al., 1985; Zaloga & Roberts, 1990). Magnesium deficiency can lead to renal potassium wasting, resulting in a cellular potassium deficiency. Magnesium levels must, therefore, be adequate prior to successful correction of potassium deficiency.

Hypermagnesemia

Hypermagnesemia, like hypomagnesemia, is difficult to detect because of the unreliability of serum levels in predicting clinical symptoms. New technology has been developed to more accurately measure ionized magnesium levels and this is gaining wider acceptance in practice. However, the clinical utility of measuring serum ionized magnesium levels has not been substantiated. Hypermagnesemia (serum magnesium >3 mg/dL or 2.4 mEq/L or 1.2 mmol/L) occurs in up to 10% of hospitalized patients (Iseri et al., 1975), most commonly secondary to iatrogenic causes (Mordes & Wacker, 1977; Stewart et al., 1980; Rude & Singer, 1981; Zaloga & Roberts, 1990).

Etiology

The most common cause of hypermagnesemia in the critically ill obstetric population is treatment for preeclampsia/eclampsia and preterm labor with magnesium sulfate infusion. Magnesium sulfate remains the mainstay for the treatment of preeclampsia and has been shown to be a better agent for the prevention of eclampsia than phenytoin. The most common medical illness associated with hypermagnesemia is renal failure usually in combination with excess magnesium ingestion. The usual sources of excess magnesium ingestion are magnesium-containing antacids and cathartics. Other causes include diabetic ketoacidosis, pheochromocytoma, hypothyroidism, Addison's disease, and lithium intoxication.

Clinical presentation

Hypermagnesemia can lead to neuromuscular blockade and depressed skeletal muscle function. Conduction through the cardiac conducting system is slowed, with ECG changes noted at a serum concentration as low as 5 mEq/L and heart block seen at 7.5 mEq/L (Reinhart, 1988). In patients not suffering from preeclampsia, hypotension may be seen at levels between 3.0 and 5.0 mEq/L (Reinhart, 1988). Loss of deep tendon reflexes occurs at a serum concentration of 10 mEq/L (12 mg/dL), with respiratory paralysis occurring at a serum concentration of 15 mEq/L (18 mg/dL). Cardiac arrest occurs at a serum concentration of greater than 25 mEq/L (30 mg/dL).

Diagnosis

A complete history and physical examination should be performed. Special attention should be directed at soliciting a history of concomitant calcium-channel blocker use with magnesium sulfate for treatment of preterm labor. Neuromuscular blockade, profound hypotension, and myocardial depression have been associated with this practice (Waisman et al., 1988; Snyder & Cardwill, 1989; Kurtzman et al., 1993). ECG, serum electrolyte, calcium, magnesium, and PO_4 levels should be obtained.

Treatment

Intravenous calcium gluconate (10 mL of 10% solution over 3 minutes) is effective in reversing the physiologic effects of hypermagnesemia (Fassler et al., 1985). Calcium gluconate should not be administered to patients being treated for preeclampsia/eclampsia with magnesium levels in the therapeutic range of 4–8 mg/dL because this may counteract the therapeutic effect of magnesium in the prevention of seizures. In patients with other disorders hemodialysis is the recommended therapy. In patients who can tolerate fluid therapy, aggressive infusion of IV saline with furosemide may be effective in increasing renal magnesium losses. All agents containing magnesium should be discontinued.

References

Abdul-Karim R, Assali NS. Renal function in human pregnancy, V Effects of oxytocin on renal hemodynamics and water electrolyte excretion. J Lab Clin Med 1961;57:522–532.

Abraham AS, Rosenmann D, Kramer M, et al. Magnesium in the prevention of lethal arrhythmias in acute myocardial infarction. Arch Intern Med 1987;147:753–755.

ACOG Technical Bulletin No. 219, January 1996:518.

Allon M, Shanklin N. Effect of bicarbonate administration on plasma potassium in dialysis patients: interactions with insulin and albuterol. Am J Kidney Dis 1996;28(4):508–514.

Anast CS, Winnacker JL, Forte LR, Burns TW. Impaired release of parathyroid hormone in magnesium deficiency. J Clin Endocrinol Metab 1976;42:707–717.

Anderson RJ, Chung H-M, Kluge R, Schrier RW. Hyponatremia: a prospective analysis of its epidemiology and pathogenetic role of vasopressin. Ann Intern Med 1985;102:164–168.

Arias F. Expansion of intravascular volume and fetal outcome in patients with chronic hypertension and pregnancy. Am J Obstet Gynecol 1965;123:610.

Arieff AI. Hyponatremia, convulsions, respiratory arrest, and permanent brain damage after elective surgery in healthy women. N Engl J Med 1986;314:1529–1535.

Arieff AI, Guisado R. Effects on the central nervous system of hypernatremic and hyponatremic states. Kidney Int 1976;10:104–116.

Ballinger WF. Preliminary report on the use of hydroxyethyl starch solution in man. J Surg Res 1966;6:180–183.

Barone JE, Snyder AB. Treatment strategies in shock: use of oxygen transport measurements. Heart Lung 1991;20:81–85.

Baue AE, Tragus ET, Wolfson SK. Hemodynamic and metabolic effects of Ringer's lactate solution in hemorrhagic shock. Ann Surg 1967;166:29–38.

Baylis C. The mechanism of the increase in glomerular filtration rate in the twelve-day pregnant rat. J Physiol 1980;305:405–414.

Beck LH. Hypouricemia in the syndrome of inappropriate secretion of antidiuretic hormone. N Engl J Med 1979;301:528–530.

Benabe JE, Martinez-Maldonado R. Disorders of calcium metabolism. In: Maxwell MH, Kleeman CR, Narins RG, eds. Clinical disorders of fluid and electrolyte metabolism, 4th edn. New York: McGraw-Hill, 1987:758.

Berkelhammer C, Bear RA. A clinical approach to common electrolyte problems: hypomagnesemia. Can Med Assoc J 1985;132:360–368.

Berl T. Mannitol a therapeutic alternative in the treatment of acute hyponatremia. Crit Care Med 2000;28(6):2152–2153.

Berson SA, Yalow RS. Distribution and metabolism of I^{131} labeled proteins in man. Fed Proc 1957;16:13S–18S.

Bismuth C, Gaultier M, Conso F, et al. Hyperkalemia in acute digitalis poisoning: prognostic significance and therapeutic implications. Clin Toxicol 1973;6:153–162.

Blum D, Brasseur D, Kahn A, Brachet E. Safe oral rehydration of hypertonic dehydration. J Pediatr Gastroenterol Nutr 1986;5: 232–235.

Bode HH, Harley BM, Crawford JD. Restoration of normal drinking behavior by chlorpropamide in patients with hypodipsia and diabetes insipidus. Am J Med 1971;51:304–313.

Bogan RK, Gale GR, Walton RP. Fate of 14C-label hydroxyethyl starch in animals. Toxicol Appl Pharmacol 1969;15:206–211.

Boldt J. The good, the bad and the ugly: Should we completely banish human albumin from our intensive care units? Anesth Analg 2000;91:887–895.

Boon JC, Jesch F, Ring J, et al. Intravascular persistence of hydroxyethyl starch in man. Eur Surg Res 1976;8:497–503.

Braden GL, von Oeyen PT, Germain MJ. Ritodrine and terbutaline-induced hypokalemia in preterm labor: Mechanisms and consequences. Kidney Int 1997;51:1867–1875.

Brauthbar N, Massry SG. Hypomagnesemia and hypermagnesemia. In: Maxwell MH, Kleeman CR, Narins RG, eds. Clinical disorders of fluid and electrolyte metabolism, 4th edn. New York: McGraw-Hill, 1987:831.

Brown MA, Zammit VC, Lowe SA. Capillary permeability and extracellular fluid volumes in pregnancy-induced hypertension. Clin Sci (Lond) 1989;77:599–604.

Brown MA, Zammitt VC, Mitar DM. Extracellular fluid volumes in pregnancy-induced hypertension. J Hypertens 1992;10:61–68.

Burch GE, Giles TD. The importance of magnesium deficiency in cardiovascular disease. Am Heart J 1977;94:649–651.

Cano A, Tovar I, Parrilla JJ, et al. Metabolic disturbances during intravenous use of ritodrine: Increased insulin levels and hypokalemia. Obstet Gynecol 1985;65:356–360.

Carey JS, Scharschmidt BF, Culliford AT et al. Hemodynamic effectiveness of colloid and electrolyte solutions for replacement of simulated operative blood loss. Surg Gynecol Obstet 1970;131:679–686.

Carney SL, Wong NL, Quamme GA, et al. Effect of magnesium deficiency on renal magnesium and calcium transport in the rat. J Clin Invest 1980;65:180–188.

Carrico CJ, Canizaro PC, Shires GT. Fluid resuscitation following injury; rational for the use of balanced salt solutions. Crit Care Med 1976;4:46–54.

Chang JC, Gross HM, Jang NS. Disseminated intravascular coagulation due to intravenous administration of hetastarch. Am J Med Sci 1990;300:301–303.

Chernow B, Rainey TG, Georges LP, O'Brian JT. Iatrogenic hyperphosphatemia: a metabolic consideration in critical care medicine. Crit Care Med 1981;9:772–774.

Chesley LC. The kidney. In: Chesley LC, ed. Hypertensive disorders in pregnancy. New York: Appleton-Century-Crofts 1978a: 154–197.

Chesley LC. Management of preeclampsia and eclampsia. In: Chesley LC, ed. Hypertensive disorders in pregnancy. New York: Appleton-Century-Crofts, 1978b:345.

Cholst IN, Steinberg SF, Tropper PJ, et al. The influence of hypermagnesemia on serum calcium and parathyroid hormone levels in human subjects. N Engl J Med 1984;310:1221–1225.

Cochrane Injuries Group. Human albumin administration in critically ill patients: systematic review of randomised controlled trials. BMJ 1998;317:235–240.

Cogbill TH, Moore EE, Dunn EI, et al. Coagulation changes after albumin resuscitation. Crit Care Med 1981;9:22–26.

Cronin RE, Knochel JP. Magnesium deficiency. Adv Intern Med 1983;28:509–533.

Cruikshank DP, Pitkin RM, Reynolds WA, et al. Effects of magnesium sulfate treatment on perinatal calcium metabolism. I—Maternal and fetal responses. Am J Obstet Gynecol 1979;134:243–249.

Cruikshank DP, Pitkin RM, Donnelly E, et al. Urinary magnesium, calcium and phosphate excretion during magnesium sulfate infusion. Obstet Gynecol 1981;58:430–434.

Cruikshank DP, Chan GM, Doerrfeld D. Alterations in vitamin D and calcium metabolism with magnesium sulfate treatment of preeclampsia. Am J Obstet Gynecol 1993;168:1170–1177.

Cully MD, Larson CP, Silverberg GD. Hetastarch coagulopathy in a neurosurgical patient. Anesthesiology 1987;66:706–707.

Dacey MJ. Hypomagnesemic disorders. Crit Care Clin 2001;17(1): 155–173.

Dafinis E, Sabatini, S. The effect of pregnancy on renal function: physiology and pathophysiology. Am J Med Sci 1992;303:184–205.

Damon L, Adams M, Striker RB, et al. Intracranial bleeding during treatment with hydroxyethyl starch. N Engl J Med 1987;317:964–965.

Dawidson I, Eriksson B. Statistical evaluations of plasma substitutes based on 10 variables. Crit Care Med 1982;10:653–657.

Dawidson I, Gelin LE, Hedman L, et al. Hemodilution and recovery from experimental intestinal shock in rats: a comparison of the efficacy of three colloids and one electrolyte solution. Crit Care Med 1981;9:42–46.

Decaux G, Genette F, Mockel J. Hypouremia in the syndrome of inappropriate secretion of antidiuretic hormone. Ann Intern Med 1980;93:716–717.

Diehl JT, Lester JL 3rd, Cosgrove DM. Clinical comparison of hetastarch and albumin in postoperative cardiac patients. Ann Thorac Surg 1982;34:674–679.

Elin RJ. Magnesium metabolism in health and disease. Dis Mon 1988;34:161–218.

Elkus R, Popovich J Jr. Respiratory physiology in pregnancy. Clin Chest Med 1992;13:555–565.

Farrow SP, Hall M, Ricketts CR. Changes in the molecular composition of circulating hydroxyethyl starch. Br J Pharmacol 1970;38:725–730.

Fassler CA, Rodriguez RM, Badesch DB, et al. Magnesium toxicity as a cause of hypotension and hypoventilation. Arch Intern Med 1985;14:1604–1606.

Ferber HP, Nitsch E, Forster H. Studies on hydroxyethyl starch. Part II: changes of the molecular weight distribution for hydroxyethyl starch types 450/0.7, 450/0.3, 300/0.4, 200/0.7, 200/0.5, 200/0.3, 200/0.1 after infusion in serum and urine of volunteers. Arzneimittelforschung 1985;35:615–622.

Ferguson N, Stewart T, Etchells. Human albumin administration in critically ill patients. Intensive Care Med 1999;25:323–325.

Flakeb G, Villarread D, Chapman D. Is hypokalemia a cause of ventricular arrhythmias? J Crit Illness 1986;1:66.

Flink EB. Therapy of magnesium deficiency. Ann NY Acad Sci 1969;162:901–905.

Fullerton WT, Hytten FE, Klopper AL, et al. A case of quadruplet pregnancy. J Obstet Gynaecol Br Cmwlth 1965;72:791–796.

Gallery EDM, Brown MA. Volume homeostasis in normal and hypertensive human pregnancy. Baillieres Clin Obstet Gynecol 1987;1:835–851.

Gallery ED, Hunyor SN, Gyory AZ. Plasma volume contraction: a significant factor in both pregnancy-associated hypertension (preeclampsia) and chronic hypertension in pregnancy. Q J Med 1979;48:593–602.

Godfrey BE, Wadsworth GR. Total body potassium in pregnant women. J Obstet Gynaecol Br Cmwlth 1970;77:244–246.

Goodlin RC, Quaife MA, Dirksen JW. The significance, diagnosis, and treatment of maternal hypovolemia as associated with fetal/maternal illness. Semin Perinatol 1981;5:163–174.

Goodlin RC, Anderson JC, Gallagher TF. Relationship between amniotic fluid volume and maternal plasma volume expansion. Am J Obstet Gynecol 1983;146:505–511.

Graepel P, Bentley P, Fritz H, et al. Reproductive studies with pamidronate. Arzneimittelforschung 1992;42(5);654–667.

Granger DN, Gabel JC, Drahe RE, et al. Physiologic basis for the clinical use of albumin solutions. Surg Gynecol Obstet 1978;146:97–104.

Granger DW, Udrich M, Parks DA, et al. Transcapillary exchange during intestinal fluid absorption. In: Sheppard AP, Granger DW, eds. Physiology of the intestinal circulation. New York: Raven, 1984:107.

Grant JP, Custer PB, Thurlow J. Current techniques of nutritional assessment. Surg Clin North Am 1981;61:437–463.

Greenberg A. Hyperkalemia treatment options. Semin Nephrol 1998;18(1):46–57.

Guyton AC, Hall JE. Regulation of extracellular fluid, osmolarity and sodium concentration. In: Guiton AC, Hall JE, eds. Textbook of medical physiology, 9th edn. Philadelphia, Pennsylvania: WB Saunders Company, 1996:349–365.

Hanshiro PK, Weil MH. Anaphylactic shock in man. Arch Intern Med 1967;119:129–140.

Hantman D, Rossier B, Zohlman R, et al. Rapid correction of hyponatremia in the syndrome of appropriate secretion of antidiuretic hormone. Ann Intern Med 1973;78:870–875.

Hartman RC, Auditore JC, Jackson DP. Studies in thrombocytosis. I. Hyperkalemia due to release of potassium from platelets during coagulation. J Clin Invest 1958;37:699.

Hauser CJ, Shoemaker WC, Turpin I, et al. Oxygen transport responses to colloids and crystalloids in critically ill surgical patients. Surg Gynecol Obstet 1980;150:811–816.

Haupt MT, Rackow EC. Colloid osmotic pressure and fluid resuscitation with hetastarch, albumin and saline solutions. Crit Care Med 1982;10:159–162.

Haynes RC, Murad F. Agents affecting calcification: calcium, parathyroid hormone, calcitonin, vitamin D, and other compounds. In: Gilman AG, Goodman LS, Rall TW, Murad F, eds. Goodman and Gilman's The pharmacological basis of therapeutics. New York: Macmillan, 1985:1517.

Heath DA. The emergency management of disorders of calcium and magnesium. Clin Endocrinol Metab 1980;9:487–502.

Hildebrandt R, Weitzel HK, Gundert-Remy U. Hypokalemia in pregnant women treated with β_2 mimetic drug fenoterol—A concentration and time dependent effect. J Perinat Med 1997;25(2): 173–179.

Hofer RE, Lanier WL. Effect of hydroxyethyl starch solutions on blood glucose concentrations in diabetic and nondiabetic rats. Crit Care Med 1992;20:211–215.

Hohn DC, Makay RD, Holliday B, et al. Effect of oxygen tension on microbicidal function of leukocytes in wounds and in vitro. Surg Forum 1976;27:18–20.

Holcroft JW, Trunkey DD. Extravascular lung water following hemorrhagic shock in the baboon: comparison between resuscitation with Ringer's lactate and plasmanate. Ann Surg 1974;180:408–417.

Hytten FE, Paintin DB. Increase in plasma volume during normal pregnancy. J Obstet Gynaecol Br Cmwlth 1973;70:402.

Illidge TM, Hussey M, Godden CW. Malignant hypercalcaemia in pregnancy and antenatal administration of intravenous pamidronate. Clin Oncol (R Coll Radiol) 1996;8(4):257–258.

Iseri LT, Freed J, Bures AR. Magnesium deficiency and cardiac disorders. Am J Med 1975;58:837–846.

Johnson JR, Miller RS, Samuels P. Bartter syndrome in pregnancy. Obstet Gynecol 2000;95(6 Part 2):1035.

Josey WE, Pinto AP, Plante RF. Oxytocin induced water intoxication. Am J Obstet Gynecol 1969;104:926.

Kamel KS, Bear RA. Treatment of hyponatremia: a quantitative analysis. Am J Kidney Dis 1993;21:439–443.

Kaufman BS, Rackow EC, Falk JL. The relationship between oxygen delivery and consumption during fluid resuscitation of hypovolemic and septic shock. Chest 1984;85:336–340.

Khosropour R, Lackner F, Steinbereithner K, et al. Comparison of the effect of pre- and intraoperative administration of medium molecular weight hydroxyethyl starch (HES 200/0.5) and dextran 40 (60) in vascular surgery. Anaesthesist 1980;29:616–622. (In German.)

Kilian J, Spilker D, Borst R. Effect of 6% hydroxyethyl starch, 45% dextran 60 and 5.5% oxypolygelatine on blood volume and circulation in human volunteers. Anaesthesist 1975;24:193–197. (In German.)

Kingston ME, Al-Siba'i MB, Skooge WC. Clinical manifestations of hypomagnesemia. Crit Care Med 1986;14:950–954.

Kirklin JK, Lell WA, Kouchoukos NT. Hydroxyethyl starch vs. albumin for colloid infusion following cardiopulmonary bypass in patients undergoing myocardial revascularization. Ann Thorac Surg 1984;37:40–46.

Kohler H, Kirch W, Horstmann HJ. Hydroxyethyl starch-induced macroamylasemia. Int J Clin Pharmacol Biopharm 1977;15:428–431.

Korttila K, Grohn P, Gordin A, et al. Effect of hydroxyethyl starch and dextran on plasma volume and blood hemostasis and coagulation. J Clin Pharmacol 1984;24:273–282.

Kovalik SG, Ledgerwood AM, Lucas CE, et al. The cardiac effect of altered calcium homeostasis after albumin resuscitation. J Trauma 1981;21:275–279.

Krege J, Katz VL, Bowes WA Jr. Transient diabetes insipidus of pregnancy. Obstet Gynecol Surv 1989;44(11):789–795.

Kurtzman JL, Thorp JM Jr, Spielman FJ, Mueller RC, Cerfalo RC. Do nifedipine and verapamil potentiate the cardiac toxicity of magnesium sulfate? Am J Perinatol 1993;10(6):450–452.

Laks H, Pilon RN, Anderson W, et al. Acute normovolemic hemodilution with crystalloid vs colloid replacement. Surg Forum 1974a;25:21–22.

Lamke LO, Liljedahl SO. Plasma volume changes after infusion of various plasma expanders. Resuscitation 1976a;5:93–102.

Lamke LO, Liljedahl SO. Plasma volume expansion after infusion of 5%, 20%, and 25% albumin solutions in patients. Resuscitation 1976b;5:85–92.

Lee WH, Cooper N, Weidner MG. Clinical evaluation of a new plasma expander: hydroxyethyl starch. J Trauma 1968;8:381–393.

Lewis RT. Albumin: role and discriminative use in surgery. Can J Surg 1980;23:322–328.

Liljedahl SO, Rieger A. Blood volume and plasma protein. IV. Importance of thoracic-duct lymph in restitution of plasma volume and plasma proteins after bleeding and immediate substitution in the splenectomized dog. Acta Chir Scand 1968;379(suppl):39–51.

Lindheimer MD, Davison JM. Osmo regulation, the secretion of arginine vasopressin and its metabolism during pregnancy. Eur J Endocrinol 1995;132(2):133–143.

Lindeheimer MD, Richardson DA, Ehrlich EN. Potassium homeostasis in pregnancy. J Repro Med 1987;32(7):517–532.

Lorenz W, Doenicke A, Freund M, et al. Plasma histamine levels in man following infusion of hydroxyethyl starch: a contribution to the question of allergic or anaphylactoid reactions following administration of a new plasma substitute. Anaesthesist 1975: 24:228–230.

Lowe RJ, Moss GS, Jilek J, et al. Crystalloid vs. colloid in the etiology of pulmonary failure after trauma: a randomized trial in man. Surgery 1977;81:676–683.

Lowery BD, Cloutier CT, Carey LC. Electrolyte solutions in resuscitation in human hemorrhagic shock. Surg Gynecol Obstet 1971;133:273–284.

Lucas CE, Ledgerwood AM, Higgins RF, et al. Impaired pulmonary function after albumin resuscitation from shock. J Trauma 1980;20: 446–451.

Lucas CE, Denis R, Ledgerwood AM, et al. The effects of hespan on serum and lymphatic albumin, globulin and coagulant protein. Ann Surg 1988;207:416–420.

Lund CJ, Donovan JC. Blood volume during pregnancy. Significance of plasma and red cell volumes. Am J Obstet Gynaecol 1967;98:394–403.

MacGillivray I, Campbell D, Duffus GM. Maternal metabolic response to twin pregnancy in primigravidae. J Obstet Gynaecol Br Cmwlth 1971;78:530–534.

Mandelberg A, Krupnik Z, Houri S, et al. Salbutamol metered-dose inhaler with spacer for hyperkalemia: how fast? How safe? Chest 1999;115(3):617–622.

Marino P. Calcium and phosphorous. In: Marino P, ed. The ICU book. Philadelphia: Lea & Febiger, 1991a:499.

Marino P. Magnesium: the hidden ion. In: Marino P, ed. The ICU book. Philadelphia: Lea & Febiger, 1991b:489.

Marino P. Potassium. In: Marino P, ed. The ICU book. Philadelphia: Lea & Febiger, 1991c:478.

Mattox KL, Maningas PA, Moore EE, et al. Prehospital hypertonic saline/dextran infusion for post-traumatic hypotension. Ann Surg 1991;213:482–491.

Maurer PH, Berardinelli B. Immunologic studies with hydroxyethyl starch (HES): a proposed plasma expander. Transfusion 1968;8:265–268.

Mestamen JH. Parathyroid disorders of pregnancy. Semin Perinatal 1998;22(6):485–496.

Metcalf W, Papadopoulos A, Tufaro R, et al. A clinical physiologic study of hydroxyethyl starch. Surg Gynecol Obstet 1970;131:255–267.

Miller M, Dalakos T, Moses AM, et al. Recognition of partial defects in antidiuretic hormone secretion. Ann Intern Med 1970;73:721–729.

Miller RD, Robbins TO, Tong MJ, et al. Coagulation defects associated with massive blood transfusions. Ann Surg 1971;174:794–801.

Mishler JM, Borberg H, Emerson PM. Hydroxyethyl starch, an agent for hypovolemic shock treatment. II. Urinary excretion in normal volunteers following three consecutive daily infusions. Br J Pharmacol 1977;4:591–595.

Mishler JM, Ricketts CR, Parkhouse EJ. Changes in molecular composition of circulating hydroxyethyl starch following consecutive daily infusions in man. Br J Clin Pharmacol 1979;7:505–509.

Mishler JM, Ricketts CR, Parkhouse EJ. Post transfusion survival of hydroxyethyl starch 450/0.7 in man: a long term study. J Clin Pathol 1980;33:155–159.

Monif GR, Savory J. Iatrogenic maternal hypocalcemia following magnesium sulfate therapy. JAMA 1972;219(11):1469–1470.

Montoro MN, Paler RJ, Goodwin TM, et al. Parathyroid carcinoma during pregnancy. Obstet Gynecol 2000;96(5 Part 2):841.

Mordes JP, Wacker WE. Excess magnesium. Pharmacol Rev 1977;29:273–300.

Morgan DB, Kirwan NA, Hancock KW, et al. Water intoxication and oxytocin infusion. Br J Obstet Gynaecol 1977;84:6–12.

Moss GS, Proctor JH, Homer LD. A comparison of asanguineous fluids and whole blood in the treatment of hemorrhagic shock. Surg Gynecol Obstet 1966;129:1247–1257.

Moss GS, Siegel DC, Cochin A, et al. Effects of saline and colloid solutions on pulmonary function in hemorrhagic shock. Surg Gynecol Obstet 1971;133:53–58.

Moss GS, Lower RJ, Jilek J, et al. Colloid or crystalloid in the resuscitation of hemorrhagic shock. A controlled clinical trial. Surgery 1981;89:434–438.

Muller N, Popov-Cenic S, Kladetzky RG, et al. The effect of hydroxyethyl starch on the intra- and postoperative behavior of haemostasis. Bibl Anat 1977;16:460–462.

Mundy GR. Calcium homeostasis: hypercalcemia and hypocalcemia. London: Martin Dunitz 1989:1.

Myers MB, Cherry G, Heimburger S, et al. Effect of edema and external pressure on wound healing. Arch Surg 1967;94:218–222.

Nagant De Deuxchaisnes C, Krane SM. Hypoparathyroidism. In: Avioli LV, Krane SM, eds. Metabolic bone disease, vol 2. Orlando, FL: Academic, 1978:217.

Nohira T, Nakada T, Akutagawa O, et al. Pregnancy complicated with Bartter's syndrome: A case report. J Obstet Gynaecol Res 2001; 27(5):267–274.

Oh MS. Selective hypoaldosteronism. Resident Staff Phys 1982;28:46S.

Oh MS, Carroll HJ. Hypernatremia. In: Hurst JW, ed. Medicine for the practicing physician, 3rd edn. Boston: Butterworth-Heinemann, 1992:1293.

Oparil S, Ehrlich EN, Lindheimer MD. Effect of progesterone on renal sodium handling in man: Relation to aldosterone excretion and plasma renin activity. Clin Sci Mol Med 1975;44:139–147.

O'Sullivan E, Monga M, Graves W. Bartter's syndrome in pregnancy—a case report and review. Am J Perinatol 1997;14(1):55–57.

Oster JR, Perez GO, Vaamonde CA. Relationship between blood pH and phosphorus during acute metabolic acidosis. Am J Physiol 1978;235:F345–351.

Packer M, Medina N, Yushnak M. Correction of dilutional hyponatremia in severe chronic heart failure by converting-enzyme inhibition. Ann Intern Med 1984;100:782–789.

Peeters LL, Buchan PC. Blood viscosity in perinatology. Rev Perinatol Med 1989;6:53.

Peeters LL, Verkeste CM, Saxena PR, et al. Relationship between maternal hemodynamics and hematocrit and hemodynamic effects of isovolemic hemodilution and hemoconcentration. I. The awake late-pregnancy guinea pig. Pediatr Res 1987;21:584–589.

Pirani BBK, MacGillivray I. Smoking during pregnancy. Its effect on maternal metabolism and fetoplacental function. Obstet Gynecol 1978;52:257–263.

Phelps KR, Lieberman RL, Oh MS, et al. Pathophysiology of the syndrome of hyporeninemic hypoaldosteronism. Metabolism 1980;29: 186–199.

Pollock AS, Arieff AL. Abnormalities of cell volume regulation and their functional consequences. Am J Physiol 1980;239:F195–205.

Poole GV, Meredith JW, Pernell T, et al. Comparison of colloids and crystalloids in resuscitation from hemorrhagic shock. Surg Gynecol Obstet 1982;154:577–586.

Porzio P, Halberthal M, Bohn D, et al. Treatment of acute hyponatremia: Ensuring the excretion of a predictable amount of electrolyte-free water. Crit Care Med 2000;28(6):1905–1910.

Puri VK, Paidipaty B, White L. Hydroxyethyl starch for resuscitation of patients with hypovolemia in shock. Crit Care Med 1981;9:833–837.

Quamme GA, Dirks KJ. Magnesium metabolism. In: Maxwell MH, Kleeman CR, Narins RG, eds. Clinical disorders of fluid and electrolyte metabolism, 4th edn. New York: McGraw-Hill 1987:297.

Raiha CE. Prematurity, perinatal mortality, and maternal heart volume. Guy's Hosp Rep 1964;113:96.

Rasmussen HS, McNair P, Norregard P, et al. Intravenous magnesium in acute myocardial infarction. Lancet 1986;1:234–236.

Reinhart RA. Magnesium metabolism. A review with special reference to the relationship between intracellular content and serum levels. Arch Intern Med 1988;148:2415–2420.

Ring J, Messmer K. Incidence and severity of anaphylactoid reactions to colloid volume substitutes. Lancet 1977;1:466–469.

Ring J, Seifert B, Messmer K, et al. Anaphylactoid reactions due to hydroxyethyl starch infusion. Eur Surg Res 1976;8:389–399.

Robertson GL. Abnormalities of thirst regulation. Kidney Int 1984;25:460–469.

Rosenoer VM, Skillman JJ, Hastings PR, et al. Albumin synthesis and nitrogen balance in postoperative patients. Surgery 1980;87:305–312.

Ross EJ, Christie SB. Hypernatremia. Medicine 1969;48:441–473.

Rothschild MA, Bauman A, Yalow RS, et al. The effect of large doses of desiccated thyroid on the distribution and metabolism of albumin-I^{131} in euthyroid subjects. J Clin Invest 1957;36:422–428.

Rothschild MA, Schreiber SS, Oratz M, et al. The effects of adrenocortical hormones on albumin metabolism studies with albumin-I^{131}. J Clin Invest 1958;37:1229–1235.

Rothschild MA, Oratz M, Schreiber SS. Albumin synthesis. N Engl J Med 1972;286:748–756, 816–820.

Rude RK, Singer FR. Magnesium deficiency and excess. Annu Rev Med 1981;32:245–259.

Ryan MP. Diuretics and potassium/magnesium depletion. Direction Am J Med 1987;82:38A.

Salas SP, Rosso P, Espinoza R, et al. Maternal plasma volume expansion and hormonal changes in women with idiopathic fetal growth retardation. Obstet Gynecol 1993;81:1029–1033.

Salem M, Munoz R, Chernow B. Hypomagnesemia in critical illness. A common and clinically important problem. Crit Care Clin 1991;7:225–252.

Sato K, Nishiwaki K, Kuno N, et al. Unexpected hyperkalemia following succinylcholine administration in prolonged immobilized parturients treated with magnesium and ritodrine. Anesthesiology 2000;93(6):1539–1541.

Shatney CH, Deapiha K, Militello PR, et al. Efficacy of hetastarch in the resuscitation of patients with multisystem trauma and shock. Arch Surg 1983;118:804–809.

Shoemaker WC, Bryan-Brown CW, Quigley L, et al. Body fluid shifts in depletion and post-stress states and their correction with adequate nutrition. Surg Gynecol Obstet 1973;136:371–374.

Shoemaker WC, Schluchter M, Hopkins JA, et al. Comparison of the relative effectiveness of colloids and crystalloids in emergency resuscitation. Am J Cardiol 1981;142:73–84.

Sibai BM, Anderson GD, Spinnato JA, et al. Plasma volume findings in patients with mild pregnancy-induced hypertension. Am J Obstet Gynecol 1983;147:16–19.

Siegel DC, Moss GS, Cochin A, et al. Pulmonary changes following treatment for hemorrhagic shock: saline vs. colloid infusion. Surg Forum 1970;921:17–19.

Singh G, Chaudry KI, Chaudry IH. Crystalloid is as effective as blood in resuscitation of hemorrhagic shock. Ann Surg 1992;215:377–382.

Sjoholm I, Ymam L. Degradation of oxytocin lysine—vasopressin, angiotensin II, angiotensin II-amide by oxytocinase. Acta Pharmacol Suecca 1967;4:65–76.

Skatrud J, Dempsey J, Kaiser DG. Ventilatory response to medroxyprogesterone acetate in normal subjects: Time course and mechanism. J Appl Physiol 1978;44:393–394.

Skillman JJ, Awwad HK, Moore FD. Plasma protein kinetics of the early transcapillary refill after hemorrhage in man. Surg Gynecol Obstet 1967;125:983–996.

Skillman JJ, Restall DS, Salzman EW. Randomized trial of albumin vs. electrolyte solutions during abdominal aortic operations. Surgery 1975;78:291–303.

Skillman JJ, Rosenoer VM, Smith PC. Improved albumin synthesis in postoperative patients by amino acid infusion. N Engl J Med 1976;295:1037–1040.

Smith JD, Bia MJ, DeFronzo RA. Clinical disorders of potassium metabolism. In: Arieff AI, DeFronzo RA, eds. Fluid, electrolyte and acid-base disorders. New York: Churchill Livingstone, 1985:413.

Snyder SW, Cardwill MS. Neuromuscular blockade with magnesium sulfate and nifedipine. Am J Obstet Gynecol 1989;161(1):35–36.

Solanke TF. Clinical trial of 6% hydroxyethyl starch (a new plasma expander). Br Med J 1968;3:783–785.

Solanke TF, Khwaja MS, Madojemu EI. Plasma volume studies with four different plasma volume expanders. J Surg Res 1971;11:140–143.

Soupart A, Penninckx R, Stenuit A, et al. Treatment of chronic hyponatremia in rats by intravenous saline: comparison of rate versus magnitude of correction. Kidney Int 1992;41:1662–1667.

Spital A, Greenwell R. Severe hyperkalemia during magnesium sulfate therapy in two pregnant drug abusers. South Med J 1991;84(7):919–921.

Sterling K. The turnover rate of serum albumin in man as measured by I-131 tagged albumin. J Clin Invest 1951;30:1228–1237.

Sterns RH. The treatment of hyponatremia: first, do no harm. Am J Med 1990;88:557–560.

Stewart AF, Horst R, Deftos LJ, et al. Biochemical evaluation of patients with cancer-associated hypercalcemia: evidence for humoral and nonhumoral groups. N Engl J Med 1980;303:1377–1383.

Strauss RG, Stump DC, Henriksen RA. Hydroxyethyl starch accentuates von Willebrand's disease. Transfusion 1985;25:235–237.

Takaori M, Safer P. Acute severe hemodilution with lactated Ringer's solution. Arch Surg 1967;94:67–73.

Theunissen IM, Parer JT. Fluids and electrolytes in pregnancy. Clin Obstet Gynecol 1994;34(1):3–15.

Thomas AK, McVie R, Levine SN. Disorders of maternal calcium metabolism implicated by abnormal calcium metabolism in the neonate. Am J Perinatol 1999;16(10):515–520.

Thompson WL. Rational use of albumin and plasma substitutes. Johns Hopkins Med J 1975;136:220–225.

Thompson WL, Britton JJ, Walton RP. Persistence of starch derivatives and dextran when infused after hemorrhage. Pharmacol Exp Ther 1962;136:125–132.

Thompson WL, Fukushima T, Rutherford RB, et al. Intravascular persistence, tissue storage, and excretion of hydroxyethyl starch. Surg Gynecol Obstet 1970;131:965–972.

Thomsen JK, Fogh-Andersen N, Jaszczak P, et al. Atrial natriuretic peptide decrease during normal pregnancy as related to hemodynamic changes and volume regulation. Acta Obstet Gynecol Scand 1993;72:103–110.

Thomsen JK, Fogh-Andersen N, Jaszczak P. Atrial natriuretic peptide, blood volume, aldosterone, and sodium excretion during twin pregnancy. Acta Obstet Gynecol Scand 1994;73:14–20.

Trudnowski RJ, Goel SB, Lam FT, et al. Effect of Ringer's lactate solution and sodium bicarbonate on surgical acidosis. Surg Gynecol Obstet 1967;125:807–814.

Tullis JL. Albumin. I. Background and use. JAMA 1977;237:355–360.

Tur-Kasm I, Paz I, Gleicher W. Disorders of the pituitary and hypothalamus. In: Gleicher N, Butino L, et al., eds. Principles and practice of medical therapy in pregnancy, 3rd edn. Stamford, Connecticut: Appleton & Lange, 1998:424–430.

Ueland K. Maternal cardiovascular dynamics. VII. Intrapartum blood volume changes. Am J Obstet Gynecol 1976;126:671–677.

Villabona C, Rodriguez P, Joven J. Potassium disturbances as a cause of metabolic neuromyopathy. Intensive Care Med 1987;13:208–210.

Vito L, Dennis RC, Weisel RD. Sepsis presenting as acute respiratory insufficiency. Surg Gynecol Obstet 1974;138:896–900.

Virgilio RW. Crystalloid vs. colloid resuscitation [reply to letter to editor]. Surgery 1979;86:515.

Virgilio RW, Rice CL, Smith DE. Crystalloid vs colloid resuscitation: is one better? A randomized clinical study. Surgery 1979a;85:129–139.

Virgilio RW, Smith DE, Zarins CK. Balanced electrolyte solutions: experimental and clinical studies. Crit Care Med 1979b;7:98–106.

Waisman GD, Mayorga LM, Camera MI, Vignolo CA, Martinotti A. Magnesium plus nifedipine: potentiation of hypotensive effect in preeclampsia? Am J Obstet Gynecol 1988;159(2):308–309.

Walker J, Garland HO. Single nephron function during prolactin-induced pseudopregnancy in the rat. J Endocrinol 1985;107:127–131.

Wang JY, Shih HL, Yuh FL, et al. An unforgotten cause of acute hyponatremia: water intoxication due to oxytocin administration in a pregnant woman. Nephron 2000;86:342–343.

Waxman K, Holness R, Tominaga G, et al. Hemodynamic and oxygen transport effects of pentastarch in burn resuscitation. Ann Surg 1989;209:341–345.

Weatherbee L, Spencer HH, Knopp CT, et al. Coagulation studies after the transfusion of hydroxyethyl starch protected frozen blood in primates. Transfusion 1974;14:109–115.

Weaver DW, Ledgerwood AM, Lucas CE, et al. Pulmonary effects of albumin resuscitation for severe hypovolemic shock. Arch Surg 1978;113:387–392.

Weisberg LS. Pseudohyponatremia: a reappraisal. Am J Med 1989;86:315–318.

Whang R, Flink EB, Dyckner T, et al. Magnesium depletion as a cause of refractory potassium repletion. Arch Intern Med 1985;145:1686–1689.

Williams DJ, Metcalf KA, Skingle AI. Pathophysiology of transient cranial diabetes insipidus during pregnancy. Clin Endocrinol (Oxf) 1993;38:595–600.

Williams ME, Rosa RM. Hyperkalemia: disorders of internal and external potassium balance. J Intensive Care Med 1988;3:52.

Wittaker PG, Lind T. The intravascular mass of albumin during human pregnancy: A serial study in normal and diabetic women. Br J Obstet Gynaecol 1993;100:587–592.

Yacobi A, Stoll RG, Sum CY, et al. Pharmacokinetics on hydroxyethyl starch in normal subjects. J Clin Pharmacol 1982;22:206–212.

Zaloga GP, Chernow B, Pock A, et al. Hypomagnesemia is a common complication of aminoglycoside therapy. Surg Gynecol Obstet 1984;158:561–565.

Zaloga GP. Interpretation of the serum magnesium level. Chest 1989;95:257–258.

Zaloga GP. Phosphate disorders. Probl Crit Care 1990;4:416.

Zaloga GP, Chernow B. Calcium metabolism. Clin Crit Care Med 1985a;5.

Zaloga GP, Chernow B. Stress-induced changes in calcium metabolism. Semin Respir Med 1985b;7:56.

Zaloga GP, Chernow B. The multifactorial basis for hypocalcemia during sepsis. Studies of the parathyroid hormone-vitamin D axis. Ann Intern Med 1987;107:36–41.

Zaloga GP, Roberts JE. Magnesium disorders. Probl Crit Care 1990;4:425.

Zaloga GP, Wilkens R, Tourville J, et al. A simple method for determining physiologically active calcium and magnesium concentrations in critically ill patients. Crit Care Med 1987;15:813–816.

III Procedures and interventions

6 Cardiopulmonary resuscitation

Nancy A. Hueppchen
Andrew J. Satin

Over 300,000 Americans suffer from cardiac arrest each year. Cardiopulmonary arrest occurs in 1 in 30,000 pregnancies, contributing to nearly 10% of all maternal deaths (Syverson et al., 1991; Dildy & Clark, 1995). Consequently, obstetricians in busy practices or tertiary referral centers will eventually encounter a "peripartum code" and should, therefore, have an understanding of current cardiopulmonary resuscitation (CPR) techniques. A century ago, most maternal deaths stemmed from chronic illnesses, not wholly unexpected as an arrest is usually the endpoint of other serious medical problems. More recently, the leading causes of maternal death include embolism, intrapartum cardiac arrest, complications of hypertensive disease, stroke, anesthetics, acute respiratory failure, sepsis, tocolysis, and hemorrhage. The advent of assisted reproduction and advanced pharmacologies have enabled more women with advanced age or chronic disease to conceive. Consequently, we may now have a larger population at risk for cardiopulmonary arrest during pregnancy.

Cardiopulmonary arrest is the abrupt cessation of spontaneous and effective ventilation and systemic perfusion. Cardiopulmonary resuscitation provides artificial ventilation and perfusion until advanced cardiac life support (ACLS) can be initiated and spontaneous cardiopulmonary function restored. Emergency cardiac care (ECC) in pregnancy includes basic life support (BLS), ACLS, and neonatal resuscitation. Preparation for successful CPR in the pregnant patient requires the availability of ACLS equipment, cesarean section instruments, and equipment for neonatal resuscitation. The American Heart Association and the National Academy of Sciences—National Research Council periodically review advances and research in ECC and publish texts in BLS, ACLS, and neonatal resuscitation (American Heart Association, 2000).

Since the publication of the third edition of this text, the International Guidelines 2000 conference on cardiopulmonary resuscitation made several important changes in managing CPR and ECC (Satin, 1997; Guidelines, 2000). The primary purpose of CPR in a pregnant woman who has arrested is the improved survival of both the mother and the neonate. This chapter includes a markedly revised bibliography, updated CPR recommendations, as well as a review of maternal and fetal physiology and their unique relationship, which require adjustment in both physical and pharmacologic aspects of ECC. The new ACLS recommendations for treatment of tachyarrhythmias and their effects on the fetus will be reviewed. The issue of perimortem cesarean section and survival data for mother and infant will also be addressed.

Physiology and techniques of cardiopulmonary resuscitation

The initial objective of ECC is to maintain adequate oxygenation and vital organ perfusion. CPR has been shown to restore hemodynamic stability in 40–60% of arrested patients; however, prolonged survival is lower with underlying illness and postresuscitation syndrome (Thel & O'Connor, 1999). Overall outcome, particularly full neurologic recovery, is improved by early initiation of CPR and defibrillation. There is usually enough oxygen in the lungs and bloodstream to support life for up to 6 minutes (American Heart Association, 1994). If breathing stops first, the heart often continues to pump blood for several minutes. When the heart stops, oxygen in the lungs and bloodstream cannot be circulated to vital organs. The patient whose heart and breathing have stopped for less than 4 minutes has an excellent chance for recovery if CPR is administered immediately and is followed by ACLS within 4 minutes (Eisenberg, 1979). By 4–6 minutes, brain damage may occur, and after 6 minutes, brain damage will almost always occur. The initial goals of CPR, therefore, are: (i) delivery of oxygen to the lungs; (ii) providing a means of circulation to the vital organs (via closed-chest compression), followed by (iii) ACLS, with restoration of the heart as the mechanism of circulation. Practically speaking these goals are achieved by remembering the "A–B–C–Ds" of the primary and secondary survey (Table 6.1).

The primary survey consists of airway management using noninvasive techniques, breathing with positive pressure

Table 6.1 The systematic survey approach to emergency cardiac care

		Primary	Secondary
A	**A**irway	Open	Intubate/Advanced airway devices
B	**B**reathing	PPV	Assess bilateral chest rise and ventilation/PPV
C	**C**irculation	Chest compressions/ Doppler FHT	IV access, pharmacologic interventions, assess rhythm
D	**D**efibrillate	Shock VF/pulseless VT	**D**ifferential diagnosis —treat reversible causes; consider **D**elivery

FHT, fetal heart tones; IV, intravenous; PPV, positive pressure ventilation; VF, ventricular fibrillation; VT, ventricular tachycardia.

Table 6.2 Potentially reversible causes of cardiac arrest

Hypovolemia
Hypoxia
Hydrogen ion—acidosis
Hyper-/hypokalemia, other metabolic
Hypothermia
Tablets (drug overdose, accidents)
Tamponade, cardiac
Tension pneumothorax
Thrombosis, coronary
Thrombosis, pulmonary

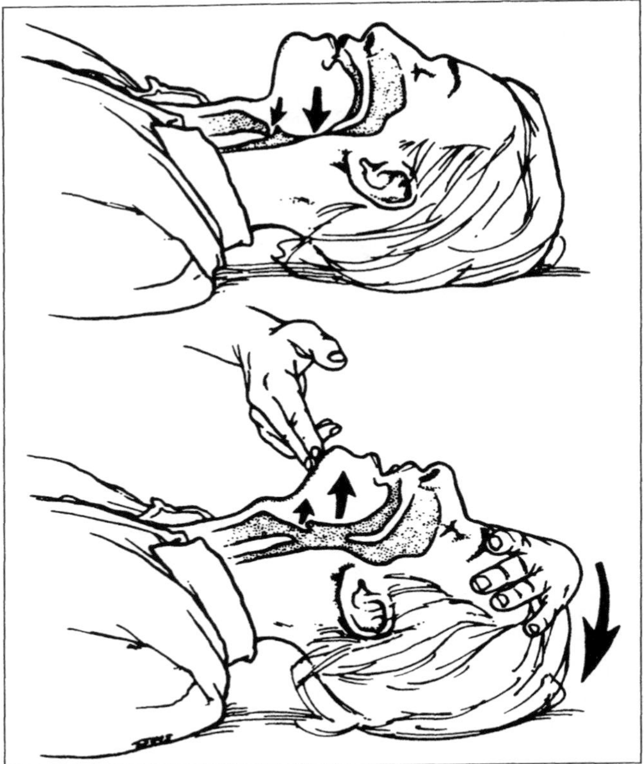

Fig. 6.1 Opening the airway. Airway obstruction produced by the tongue and epiglottis (top). Relief via head-tilt and chin-lift maneuvers (below). (Reproduced by permission from Textbook of Basic Life Support for Healthcare Providers, 1994. Copyright American Heart Association.)

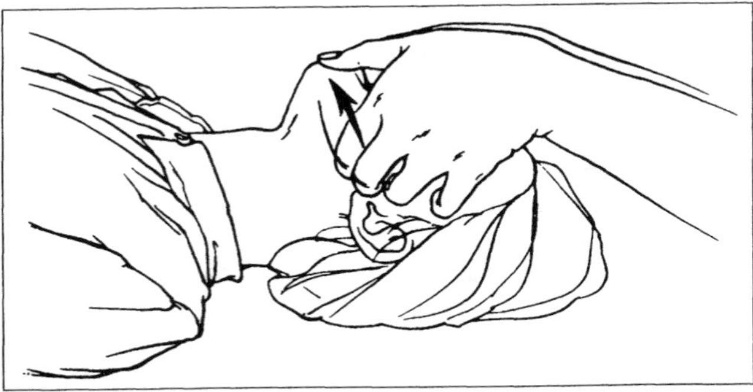

Fig. 6.2 Jaw-thrust maneuver. Rescuer grasps the angles of the patient's lower jaw and lifts with both hands, one on each side, displacing the mandible forward while tilting the head backward. (Reproduced by permission from Textbook of Basic Life Support for Healthcare Providers, 1994. Copyright American Heart Association.)

ventilations, and performing CPR until an automated external defibrillator (AED) arrives. Tools required include gloved hands, a barrier device for CPR, and an AED for defibrillation. The secondary survey requires the use of advanced, invasive techniques as the rescuer attempts to resuscitate, stabilize, and transfer the patient to a higher level of care (i.e. hospital or intensive care setting). Potentially reversible causes of cardiopulmonary arrest should also be considered and addressed at this stage (Table 6.2).

Delivery of oxygen is achieved by positioning the patient, opening the airway, and rescue breathing. In the absence of muscle tone, the tongue and epiglottis frequently obstruct the airway. The head-tilt with the chin-lift maneuver (Fig. 6.1) or the jaw-thrust maneuver (Fig. 6.2) may provide airway access. If foreign material appears in the mouth, it should be removed either manually or with active suction if available. If air does not enter the lungs with rescue breathing, reposition the head and repeat the attempt at rescue breathing. Persistent obstruction may require the Heimlich maneuver (subdiaphragmatic abdominal thrusts), chest thrusts, removal of foreign body if now visualized, and rescue breathing (Table 6.3). Importantly, the Heimlich maneuver cannot be used in the late stages of pregnancy or in the obese choking victim. Airway obstruction may occur in a choking victim as well as a patient experiencing a cardiopulmonary arrest. The conscious woman with only partial airway obstruction should be allowed to attempt to

Table 6.3 Management of a foreign-body obstruction

Conscious patient
1 Perform the Heimlich maneuver (chest thrusts if in latter half of gestation)
2 Repeat until the obstruction is relieved or the patient is unconscious

Unconscious patient
1 Activate emergency medical system (EMS)
2 Position the head, tongue–jaw lift
3 Perform a finger sweep, or use a Kelly clamp or Magill forceps if there is direct visualization of the foreign body
4 Attempt ventilation, reposition the head, and repeat ventilation
5 Repeat the sequence of up to five abdominal thrusts (chest thrusts in latter half of gestation), finger sweep, and attempt at ventilation until the obstruction is relieved

clear the obstruction herself, and finger sweeps by the rescuer are avoided. Finally, failure of nonsurgical procedures to relieve the airway obstruction is an indication for emergency cricothyroidotomy or jet-needle insufflation, if appropriate equipment is available.

Abdominal thrusts are accomplished by wrapping your hands around the victim's waist, making a fist with one hand and placing the thumb side of the fist against the victim's abdomen in the midline slightly above the navel and well below the top of the xiphoid process. The rescuer grasps the fist with the other hand and presses the fist into the victim's abdomen with quick, distinct, upward thrusts. The thrusts are continued until the object is expelled or the victim is unconscious. Abdominal thrusts may be impeded by the gravid uterus. The unconscious victim is placed supine, and the heel of one hand remains against the victim's abdomen, in the midline slightly above the navel but below the top of the xiphoid. The second hand lies directly on top of the first, and quick upward thrusts are administered.

The gravid uterus or obesity may necessitate the use of chest thrusts instead of abdominal thrusts. Chest thrusts in a conscious sitting or standing victim require placing the thumb side of the fist on the middle of the sternum, avoiding the xiphoid and the ribs. The rescuer then grabs her or his own fist with the other hand and performs chest thrusts until either the foreign object dislodges or the patient loses consciousness (Fig. 6.3). The unconscious patient is placed supine. The rescuer's hand closest to the patient's head is placed two finger breadths above the xiphoid. The long axis of the heel of the provider's hand rests in the long axis of the sternum (Fig. 6.4). The other hand lies over the first, with fingers either extended or interlaced. The elbows are extended, and the chest is compressed 1.5–2 inches. Up to five abdominal or chest thrusts are given, followed by repetition of the jaw-lift, foreign body visualization, and attempted ventilation. These steps are repeated until effective.

If the patient is unresponsive, but now breathing spontaneously, she is placed in the recovery position to keep the airway open (American Heart Association, 2000). The pregnant victim is placed on her left side. The left arm is placed at a right angle to the victim's torso, while the right arm is placed across her chest with the back of her hand under the lower cheek. The victim's right thigh is flexed at a right angle to the torso, across the left leg, with the right knee resting on the surface. The victim's head is tilted back to maintain the airway, using the right hand to maintain the head tilt. Breathing is monitored regularly, and if breathing stops, the emergency medical system is activated and the ABCDs of CPR are begun.

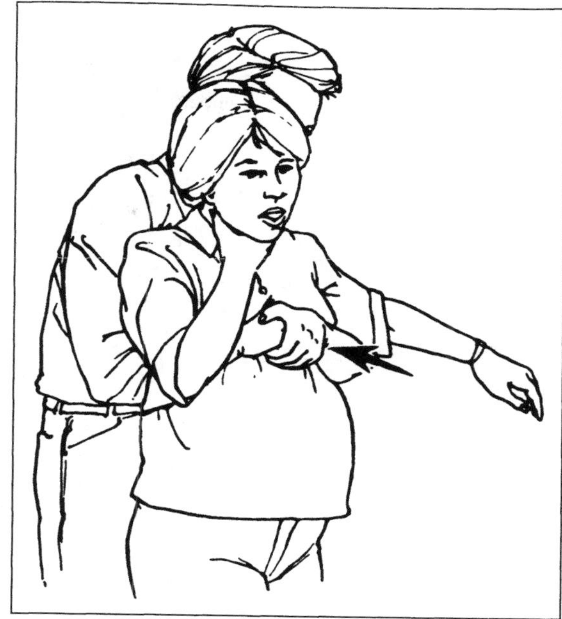

Fig. 6.3 Chest thrusts administered to a standing conscious patient. (Reproduced by permission from Textbook of Basic Life Support for Healthcare Providers, 1994. Copyright American Heart Association.)

Rescue breathing may be facilitated by mouth-to-mouth, mouth-to-nose, mouth-to-mask, or bag valve-to-mask resuscitation, or ultimately by endotracheal intubation. Endotracheal intubation by direct laryngoscopy is the preferred method for maintaining airway patency for the gravid arrest victim. Alternative techniques for airway management include endotracheal intubation by lighted stylet, esophageal tracheal combitube, laryngeal mash airway, and transtracheal ventilation. The reader is referred to the extensive review by Reed (1995). Tracheal intubation offers several advantages, including security and protection of the airway, as well as facilitation of oxygenation and ventilation, and it provides a route for administration of drugs during a cardiac arrest.

If the patient undergoes endotracheal intubation, new guidelines require immediate confirmation of the tracheal tube using nonphysical examination techniques, such as end-tidal carbon dioxide (ET CO_2) indicators (European Resuscitation Council, 2000). The presence of ET CO_2 is a reliable

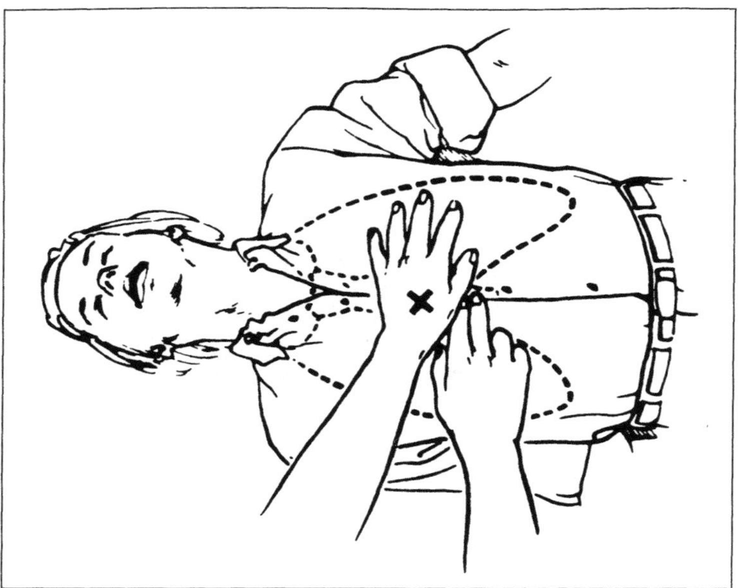

Fig. 6.4 The technique for chest thrusts for an unconscious supine patient of foreign body airway obstruction is identical to closed chest compressions for cardiac arrest. (Reproduced by permission from Textbook of Basic Life Support for Healthcare Providers, 1994. Copyright American Heart Association.)

measure of pulmonary perfusion and, therefore, can measure the efficacy of CPR. Esophageal detector devices may also be used to confirm tracheal tube position; however, a false negative result may be obtained in women late in gestation. False negatives are due to decreased functional residual capacity (FRC) and tracheal compression in late pregnancy. Consequently, the gold standard for confirmation in the pregnant woman is repeat direct visualization (Barnes et al., 2001).

In the absence of a spontaneous heartbeat, external chest compressions provide a means of circulation, as originally described by Kouwenhoven and colleagues in 1960. They believed that the chest compressions caused direct compression of the heart between the sternum and the spine, leading to a rise in ventricular pressure, a closure of the mitral and tricuspid valves, and a forcing of blood into the pulmonary artery and aorta. Subsequently, fluctuations in intrathoracic pressure and creation of an arteriovenous pressure gradient peripherally have been implicated as the mechanism of circulation with external chest compressions (Rudikoff et al., 1980). External chest compressions cause a rise in intrathoracic pressure, which is distributed to all intrathoracic structures. Competent venous valves prevent transmission of this pressure to extrathoracic veins, whereas the arteries transmit the increased pressure to extrathoracic arteries, creating an arterial venous pressure gradient and forward blood flow (Fig. 6.5). Werner et al. (1981), using echocardiography, showed that the mitral and tricuspid valves remain open during CPR, supporting the concept of the heart as a passive conduit rather than a pump during CPR.

BLS guidelines call for a ratio of two ventilations to 15 compressions in one or two person CPR, pausing for ventilation with an unprotected airway. A one to five ratio is used with a protected airway (American Heart Association, 2000). A chest compression rate of approximately 100 per minute is used in both airway circumstances. ACLS involves the addition of electrical and pharmacologic therapy, invasive monitoring, and therapeutic techniques to correct cardiac arrhythmias, metabolic imbalances, and other causes of cardiac arrest. A defibrillator can be used without significant complications for the fetus in a pregnant woman (Ogburn et al., 1992). The fetus has a relatively high fibrillation threshold and the current den-

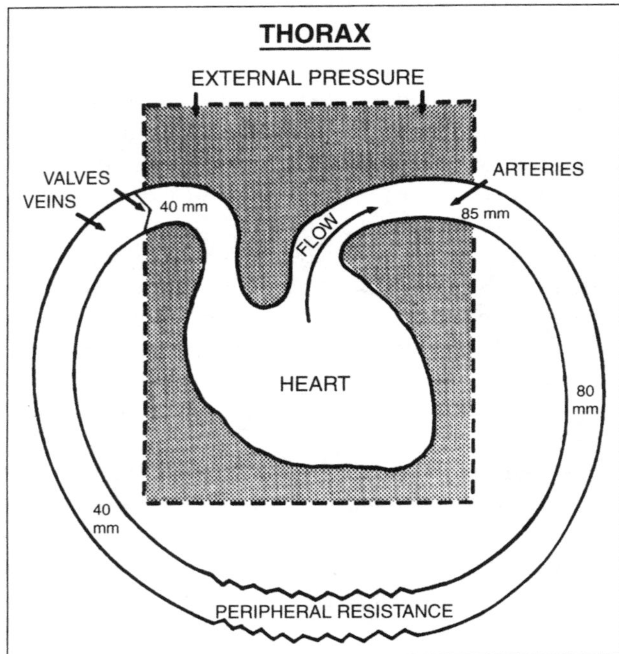

Fig. 6.5 Hypothesized mechanism for circulation prompted by external chest compressions.

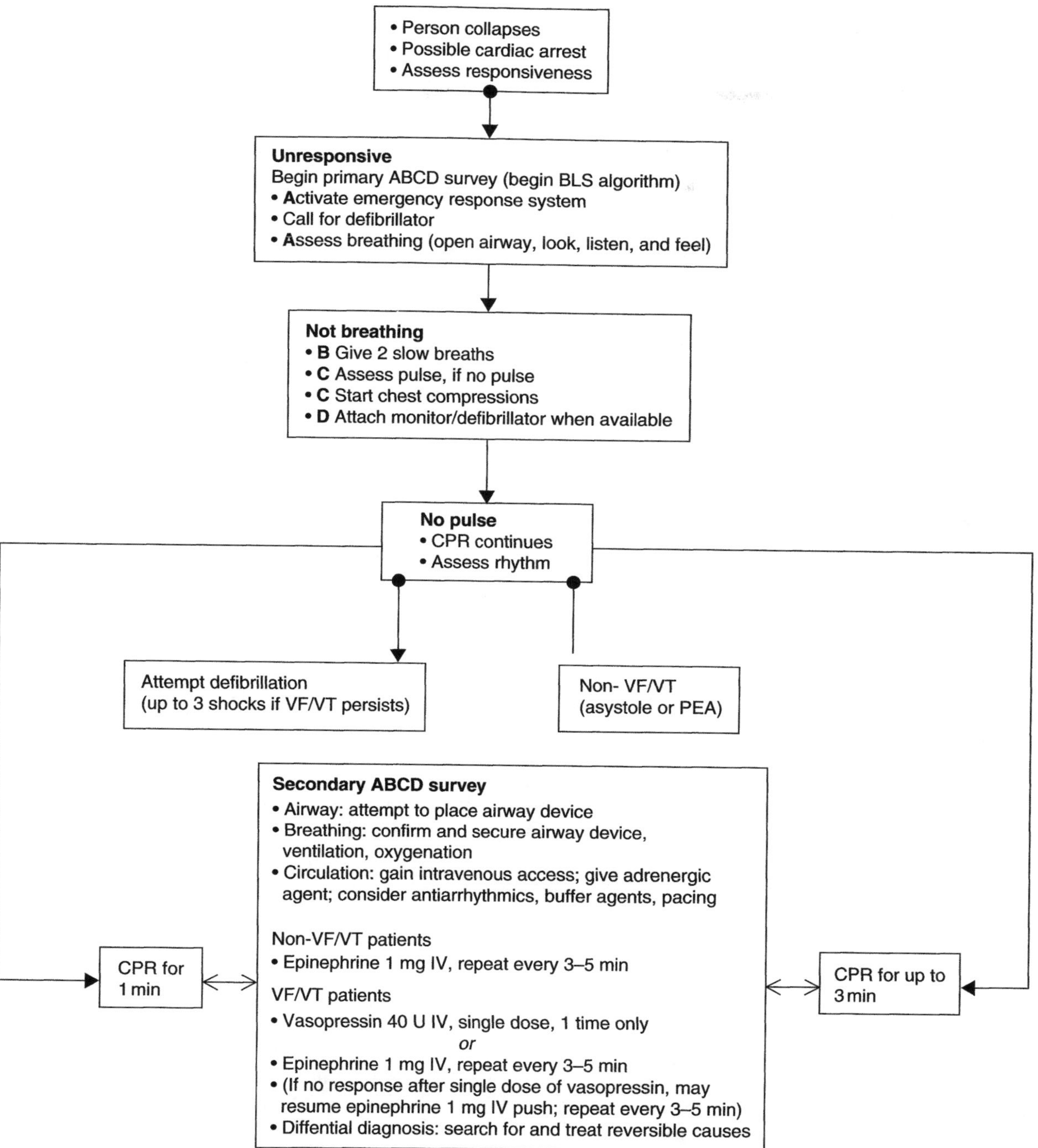

Fig. 6.6 Comprehensive ECC algorithm. BLS, basic life support; CPR, cardiopulmonary resuscitation; IV, intravenous; PEA, pulseless electrical activity; VF/VT, ventricular fibrillation/ventricular tachycardia. (Adapted from Guidelines 2000 for Cardiopulmonary Resuscitation and Emergency Cardiovascular Care. Circulation 2000;102 (Suppl 1).)

sity reaching the fetus is small. Standard algorithms recommended by the American Heart Association are reviewed in Figs 6.6–6.15. Major changes in ECC recommended by the international guidelines conference in 2000 are listed in Table 6.4.

Morris and colleagues (1996) evaluated neonatal survival following emergency cesarean section in trauma patients presenting to nine Level I trauma centers nationwide. They suggested adding Doppler fetal heart tone (FHT) assessment to the primary survey along with assessment of maternal circulation. If FHTs were not present, the pregnancy would otherwise be

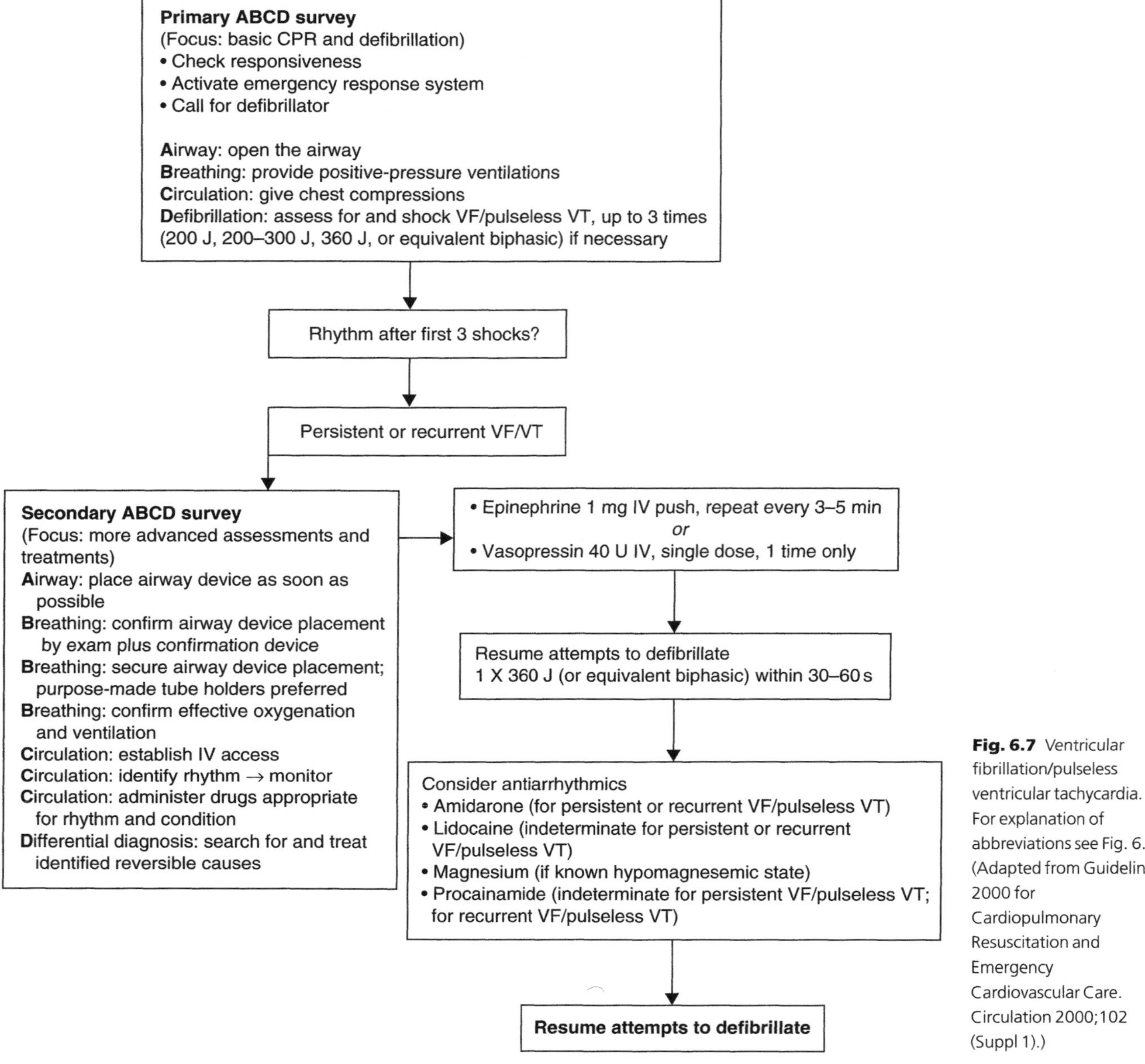

Fig. 6.7 Ventricular fibrillation/pulseless ventricular tachycardia. For explanation of abbreviations see Fig. 6.6. (Adapted from Guidelines 2000 for Cardiopulmonary Resuscitation and Emergency Cardiovascular Care. Circulation 2000;102 (Suppl 1).)

ignored and treatment directed toward maternal survival alone. Delivery of the fetus can be considered in the secondary survey if fetal distress is present, and more importantly, as a means of improving effectiveness of maternal CPR efforts.

The effect of pregnancy on cardiopulmonary resuscitation

Pregnancy produces physiologic changes that have a dramatic effect on cardiopulmonary resuscitation (Table 6.5). Pregnancy represents a high-flow, low-resistance state with a high cardiac output (CO) and low systemic vascular resistance (SVR). CO increases to 150% of nonpregnant norms. The uterus, with minimum resistance, receives up to 30% of CO, as compared with 2–3% in the nongravid patient. The increases in CO satisfy the increase in oxygen demands of the growing fetus, the placenta, and the mother.

Effective CPR in pregnancy is hindered by structural and physiologic changes that occur. Enlarging breast tissue which decreases chest wall compliance and increasing pharyngeal edema make ventilation more difficult. The enlarging uterus imposes changes on the respiratory system as well. Upward displacement of the diaphragm leads to a decrease in the FRC of the lungs. Maternal minute ventilation increases, probably due to a central effect of progesterone (DeSwiet, 1999). The decrease in FRC combines with the increase in oxygen demand to predispose the pregnant woman to a decrease in arterial and

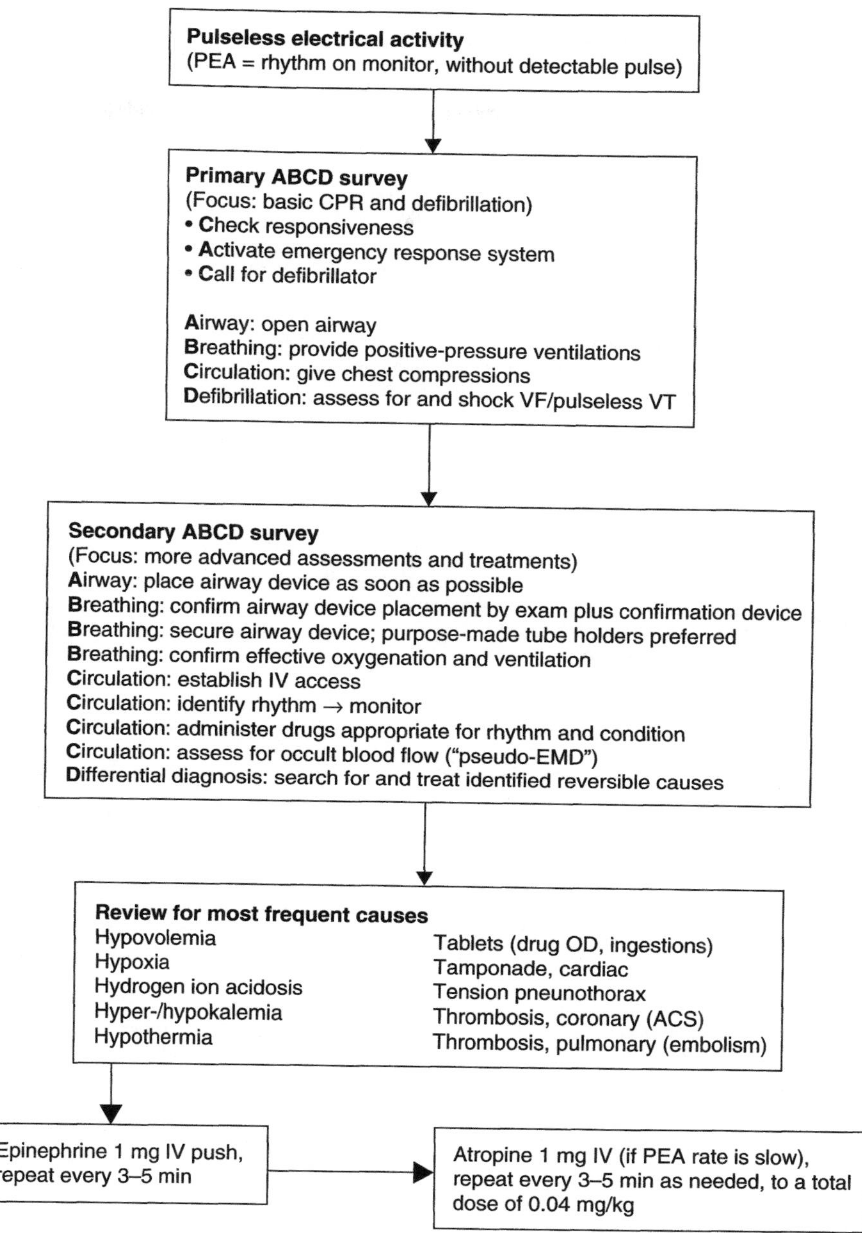

Fig. 6.8 Pulseless electric activity (PEA) algorithm. ACS, acute coronary syndrome; EMD, electromechanical dissociation; OD, overdose. For explanation of other abbreviations, see Fig. 6.6. (Adapted from Guidelines 2000 for Cardiopulmonary Resuscitation and Emergency Cardiovascular Care. Circulation 2000;102 (Suppl 1).)

venous oxygen tension during periods of decreased ventilation. Furthermore, the increase in ventilation in pregnancy leads to a decline in arterial carbon dioxide tension. The maternal kidney compensates for this respiratory alkalosis by reducing serum bicarbonate concentration. Maternal hypocapnia and respiratory alkalosis enhance renal excretion of carbon dioxide by the fetus. Hence, increases in maternal carbon dioxide may lead to fetal acidosis. The mother also compensates for hypoxia by decreasing uteroplacental blood flow. Therefore, during maternal cardiopulmonary arrest, the physiologic changes of pregnancy and tendency toward hypoxia in the presence of apnea make it more difficult to resuscitate the mother. Superimposed on an already compromised maternal circulation characterized by hypercarbia and hypoxia, normal physiologic compensatory mechanisms that decrease uteroplacental flow during the arrest lead to further fetal acidosis.

For the patient in the latter half of pregnancy, aortocaval compression by the gravid uterus renders resuscitation more difficult than in her nonpregnant counterpart. It does so by decreasing venous return, causing supine hypotension, and decreasing the effectiveness of thoracic compressions. The pregnant uterus exerts pressure on the inferior vena cava, iliac vessels, and abdominal aorta. In the supine position, such uterine compression may lead to sequestration of up to 30% of circulating blood volume (Lee, 1986). Furthermore, the en-

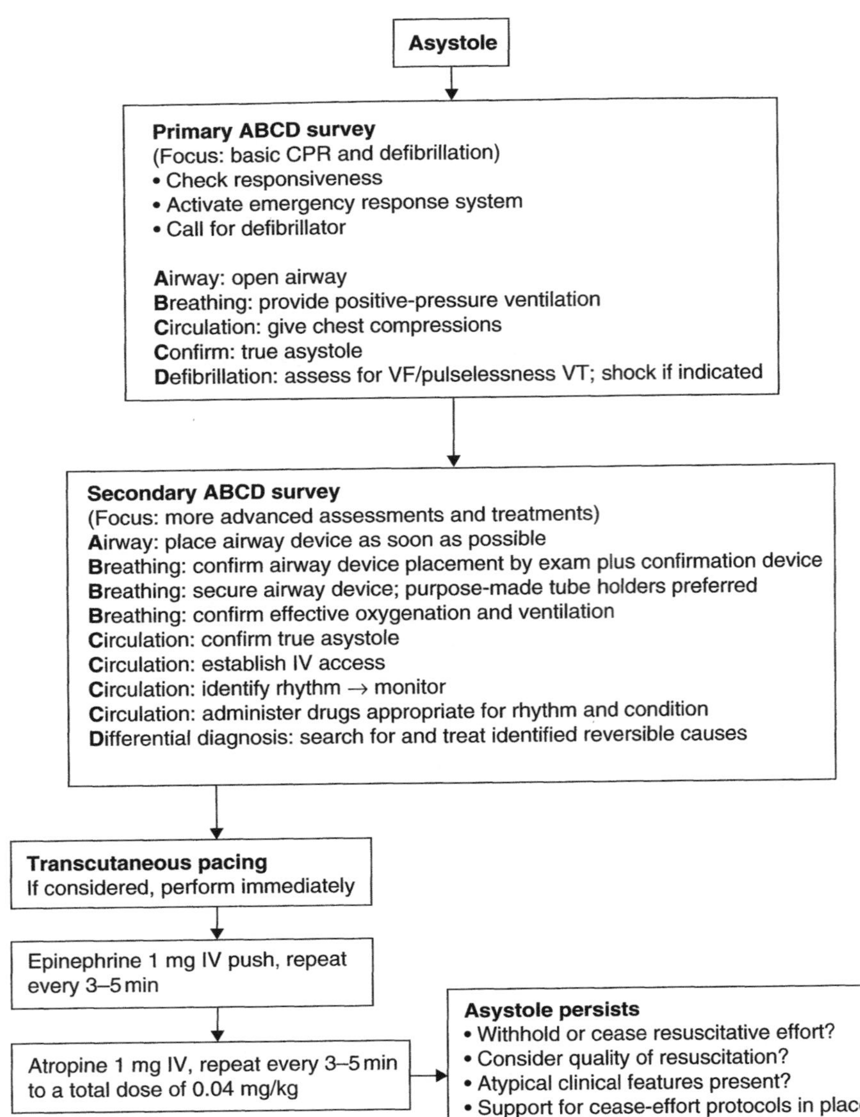

Fig. 6.9 Asystole algorithm. For explanation of abbreviations see Fig. 6.6. (Adapted from Guidelines 2000 for Cardiopulmonary Resuscitation and Emergency Cardiovascular Care. Circulation 2000;102 (Suppl 1).)

larged uterus poses an obstruction to forward blood flow, particularly when arterial pressure and volume are decreased, as in a cardiac arrest.

Changes in the gravid woman's response to drugs and alterations in the maternal gastrointestinal system also hinder effective resuscitation. Vasopressors used in ACLS, especially alpha-adrenergic or combined alpha and beta agents, are capable of producing uteroplacental vasoconstriction, leading to decreased fetal oxygenation and carbon dioxide exchange. Decreases in gastrointestinal motility and relaxation of the lower esophageal sphincter lead to an increased risk of aspiration prior to or during endotracheal intubation. Thus, physiologic and anatomic changes of pregnancy involving the cardiac, respiratory, and gastrointestinal systems; the enlarging uterus; and the patient's response to pressors all adversely affect resuscitation of the pregnant patient.

Modifications of basic life support and advanced cardiac life support in pregnancy

The anatomic and physiologic changes of pregnancy require several modifications in ECC (Table 6.6). Most important, to effect an increase in venous return and reduce supine hypotension, the uterus must be displaced to the left. Left lateral displacement can be achieved by: (i) manual displacement of the uterus by a member of the resuscitation team; (ii) positioning the patient on an operating room table that can be tilted laterally; (iii) positioning a wedge under the right hip; (iv) using a Cardiff resuscitation wedge (Rees & Willis, 1988); or (v) using a human wedge (Goodwin & Pearce, 1992). The human wedge kneels on the floor with the victim's back placed on the thighs of the human wedge. The wedge uses one arm to stablilize the

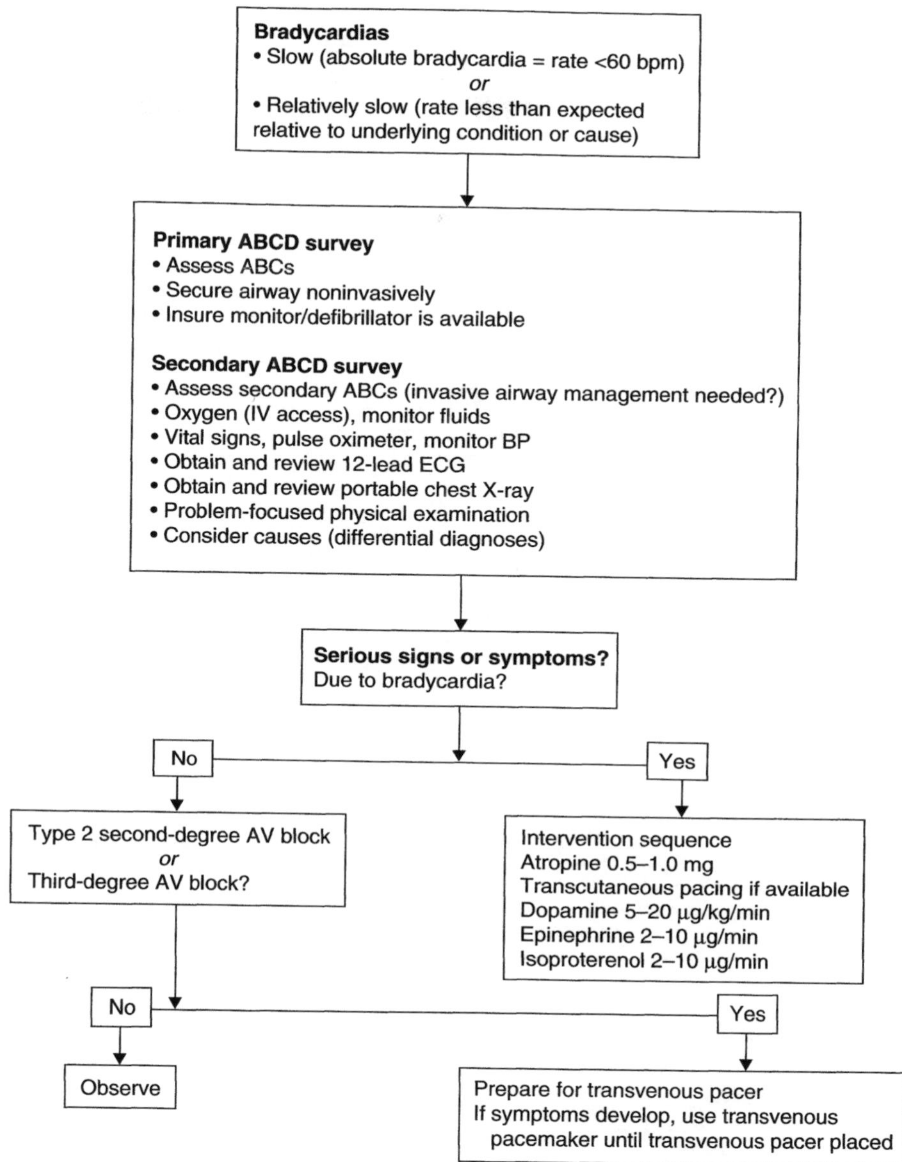

Fig. 6.10 Bradycardia algorithm for patient not in cardiac arrest. AV, arterioventricular; BP, blood pressure; ECG, electrocardiogram; IV, intravenous. (Adapted from Guidelines 2000 for Cardiopulmonary Resuscitation and Emergency Cardiovascular Care. Circulation 2000;102 (Suppl 1).)

victim's shoulder and the other arm to stabilize the pelvis. The human wedge maneuver has the advantage that it may be employed without equipment, utilizing an untrained person. Its obvious disadvantage is the wedge must be displaced when defibrillation is necessary.

While the maternal propensity for hypoxia and hypercapnia (which lead to decreases in uteroplacental perfusion) suggests that the pregnant woman may benefit from sodium bicarbonate in an arrest situation in order to keep maternal pH greater than 7.10, it must be kept in mind that sodium bicarbonate only very slowly crosses the placenta. Accordingly, with rapid correction of maternal metabolic acidosis, her respiratory compensation will cease with normalization of her $P\text{CO}_2$. If the maternal $P\text{CO}_2$ increases from 20 to 40 mmHg as a result of bicarbonate administration, the fetal $P\text{CO}_2$ will also increase. However, the fetus will not receive the benefit of the bicarbonate. If the fetal pH was 7.00 before maternal bicarbonate administration, the normalization of maternal pH will be achieved at the expense of increasing the fetal $P\text{CO}_2$ by 20 mmHg, with a resultant fall in fetal pH to approximately 6.84. Accordingly, the merits of such treatment must be questioned. Indeed, sodium bicarbonate is not indicated and is possibly harmful in patients with hypoxic lactic acidosis, such as occurs in nonintubated patients with prolonged cardiopulmonary arrest. Current understanding of the acid–base pathophysiology during cardiopulmonary arrest indicates that carbon dioxide generated in tissues is not well cleared by low blood flow (Adrogue et al., 1989). Adequate ventilation and

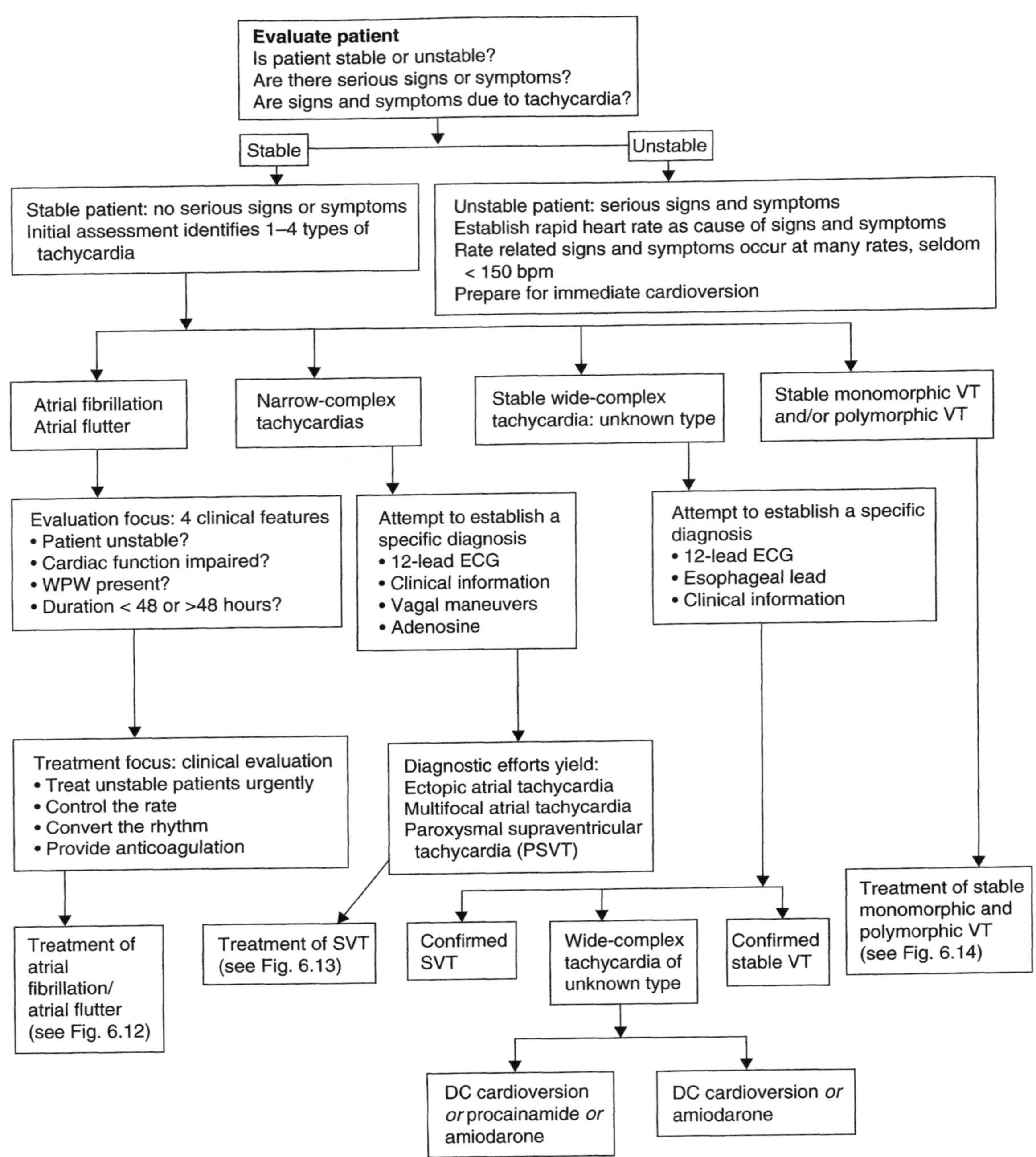

Fig. 6.11 Tachycardia algorithm. DC, direct current; ECG, electrocardiogram; SVT, supraventricular tachycardia; VT, ventricular tachycardia; WPW, Wolff–Parkinson–White syndrome. (Adapted from Guidelines 2000 for Cardiopulmonary Resuscitation and Emergency Cardiovascular Care. Circulation 2000;102 (Suppl 1).)

restoration of perfusion are the mainstays of control of acid–base balance during cardiac arrest. Buffering the blood with bicarbonate does not benefit the patient (Niemann, 1992; American Heart Association, 2000; European Resuscitation Council, 2000).

Both the increased oxygen utilization in pregnancy and the

Atrial fibrillation/ atrial flutter with: • Normal heart • Impaired heart • WPW	**1. Control rate** Heart function preserved	**1. Control rate** Impaired heart EF < 40% or CHF	**2. Convert rhythm** Duration < 48 h	**2. Convert rhythm** Duration > 48 h or unknown
Normal cardiac function	**Note**: If AF > 48 h duration, use agents with potential to convert rhythm with extreme caution in patients not receiving adequate anticoagulation because of possible embolic complications Use only one of the following agents (see note below): • Calcium-channel blockers (class 1) • Beta-blockers (class 1) • For additional drugs that are class 2b recommendations, see guidelines or ACLS text	Does not apply	**Consider** • DC cardioversion Use only one of the following agents (see note below): • Amiodarone (class 2b) • Flecainide (class 2a) • Propafenone (class 2a) • Procainamide (class 2a) • For additional drugs that are class 2b recommendations, see guidelines or ACLS text	• Avoid nonemergent cardioversion unless anticoagulation or clot precautions are taken (see below) • **Note**: Conversion of AF to NSR with drugs or shock may cause embolization of atrial thrombi unless patient has adequate anticoagulation • Use antiarrhthymic agents with extreme caution if AF > 48 h *or* **Delayed cardioversion anticoagulation × 3 weeks at proper levels** • Cardioversion, then • Anticoagulation × 4 weeks more *or* **Early cardioversion** • Begin IV heparin at once • TEE to exclude atrial clot *then* • Cardioversion within 24 h *then* Anticoagulation × 4 more weeks
Impaired heart (EF < 40% or CHF)	Does not apply	**Note**: If AF > 48 h duration, use agents with potential to convert rhythm with extreme caution in patients not receiving adequate anticoagulation because of possible embolic complications Use only one of the following agents • Digoxin (class 2b) • Dilitiazem (class 2b) • Amiodarone (class 2b)	**Consider** • DC cardioversion *or* • Amiodarone (class 2b)	• Avoid nonemergent cardioversion unless anticoagulation or clot precautions are taken (see above) • Anticoagulation as described above *followed by* • DC cardioversion
WPW	**Note**: If AF > 48 h duration, use agents with potential to convert rhythm with extreme caution in patients not receiving adequate anticoagulation because of possible embolic complications *or* • Primary antiarrhythmic agents (see note below) • Amiodarone (class 2b) • Flecainide (class 2b) • Procainamide (class 2b) • Propafenone (class 2b) Class 3 (can be harmful) • Adenosine • Beta-blockers • Calcium blockers • Digoxin	**Note**: If AF > 48 h duration, use agents with potential to convert rhythm with extreme caution in patients not receiving adequate anticoagulation because of possible embolic complications *or* • DC cardioversion *or* • Amiodarone (class 2b)	**Consider** • DC cardioversion Use only one of the following agents (see note below): • Amiodarone (class 2b) • Flecainide (class 2a) • Propafenone (class 2a) • Procainamide (class 2a) • For additional drugs that are class 2b recommendations, see guidelines or ACLS text	• Avoid nonemergent cardioversion unless anticoagulation or clot precautions are taken (see above) • Anticoagulation as described above *followed by* • DC cardioversion

Note: Occasionally two of the named antiarrhythmics may be used, but use of these agents in combination may have proarrhythmic potential. The classes listed represent the class of recommendation rather than the Vaughn–Williams classification of antiarrhythmics.

Fig. 6.12 Tachycardia treatment of atrial fibrillation (AF) and flutter. ACLS, advanced cardiac life support; CHF, congestive heart failure; DC, direct current; EF, ejection fraction; IV, intravenous; NSR, normal sinus rhythm; TEE, transesophageal echocardiogram; WPW, Wolff–Parkinson–White syndrome. (Adapted from Guidelines 2000 for Cardiopulmonary Resuscitation and Emergency Cardiovascular Care. Circulation 2000;102 (Suppl 1).)

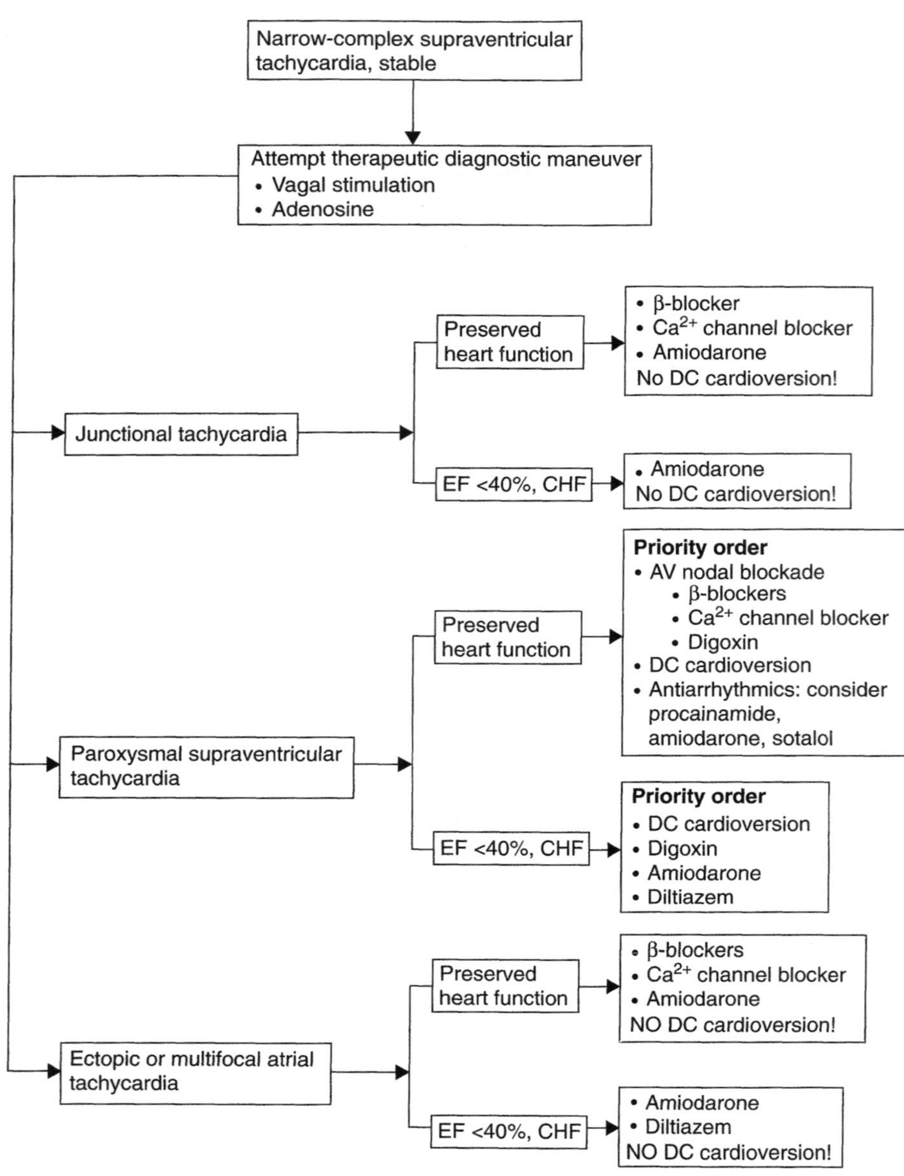

Fig. 6.13 Narrow complex tachycardia algorithm. AV, arterioventricular; CHF, congestive heart failure; DC, direct current; EF, ejection fraction. (Adapted from Guidelines 2000 for Cardiopulmonary Resuscitation and Emergency Cardiovascular Care. Circulation 2000;102 (Suppl 1).)

increased risk of aspiration suggest that the airway should be managed aggressively, and prompt endotracheal intubation should be performed in all pregnant women during arrest situations. With an obstructed airway, abdominal thrusts must be avoided in the latter half of pregnancy and chest compressions substituted.

Clinical experience with the pharmacologic agents used in ACLS is limited in pregnancy. Most of the data concerning fetal effects of these drugs comes from chronic use rather than limited dosing in the acute arrest setting. The use of certain antiarrhythmics represents a major area of change in the ACLS guidelines. Amiodarone is emerging as the drug of choice for treatment of wide-complex tachycardia, stable narrow-complex tachycardia, monomorphic and polymorphic VT, and potentially for shock-refractory VF/VT. Placental transfer occurs with amiodarone, a category D drug. With chronic use, fetal effects such as growth restriction, hypothyroid goiter, enlarged fontanelle, and transient bradycardia in the newborn have all been reported (Page, 1995; Briggs & Garite, 1997). Thus, use of amiodarone in pregnancy should be reserved for life-threatening conditions only. Adenosine, lidocaine, procainamide, and beta-blockers, also used in the treatment of tachyarrythmias, all appear to be safe in pregnancy (Rubin, 1981). Vasopressin, instead of epinephrine, appears to be a more effective pressor agent in cardiac arrest. In addition, vasopressin appears to have a lower adverse effect profile than

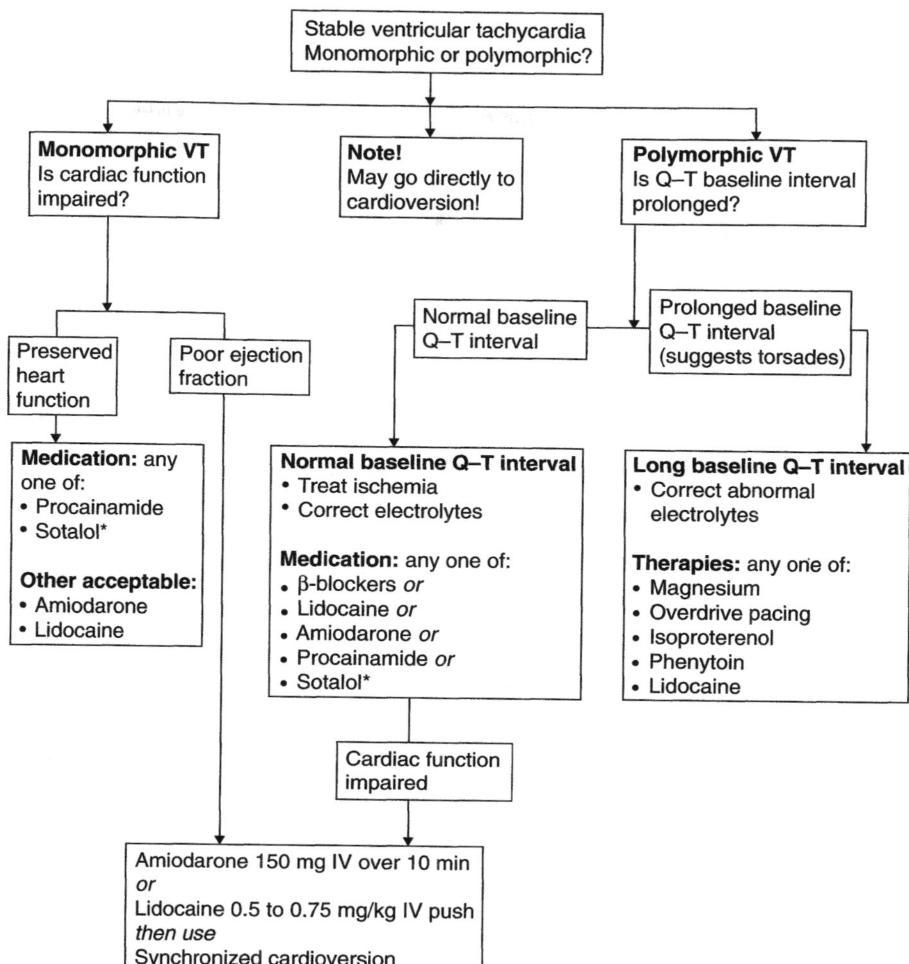

Fig. 6.14 Stable ventricular tachycardia algorithm, for monomorphic and polymorphic VT. *Not available in the United States. (Adapted from Guidelines 2000 for Cardiopulmonary Resuscitation and Emergency Cardiovascular Care. Circulation 2000;102 (Suppl 1).)

epinephrine. Cardiac arrest survivors who received high-dose epinephrine suffer from more postresuscitation complications (European Resuscitation Council, 2000).

Importantly, the volume of distribution and drug metabolism may vary from nonpregnant norms. Page (1995) eloquently described the multiple factors contributing to altered therapeutic blood levels of drugs in pregnancy: increased intravascular volume, reduced drug protein binding, increased clearance of renally excreted drugs, progesterone-activated increased hepatic metabolism, and altered gastrointestinal absorption due to changes in gastric secretion and gut motility. The agents used in ACLS are recommended in standard doses. However, if the victim does not respond to standard doses, higher doses should be considered to account for the expanded plasma volume of pregnancy.

Although volume administration, which can lead to decreased cerebral and coronary blood flow, is generally not recommended during treatment of cardiac arrest, it should be strongly considered in cardiopulmonary arrest related to postpartum hemorrhage or circulatory collapse as seen with amniotic fluid embolism. Finally, there are no data suggesting modifications in defibrillation guidelines should be made due to pregnancy. Early return of maternal circulation and ventilation is of primary importance to the mother and the fetus.

Complications of cardiopulmonary resuscitation during pregnancy

Cardiopulmonary resuscitation during pregnancy may impose complications on both mother and fetus. Maternal injuries may include: (i) fractures of ribs and sternum; (ii) hemothorax and hemopericardium; (iii) rupture of internal organs (especially the spleen and uterus); and (iv) lacerations of organs (most notably the liver). Damaging effects to the fetus consist of central nervous toxicity from medications, altered uterine activity, and reduced uteroplacental perfusion, with possible fetal hypoxemia and acidemia. Fetal monitoring may be used to assess ongoing fetal status; however, maternal resuscitation should be the primary goal.

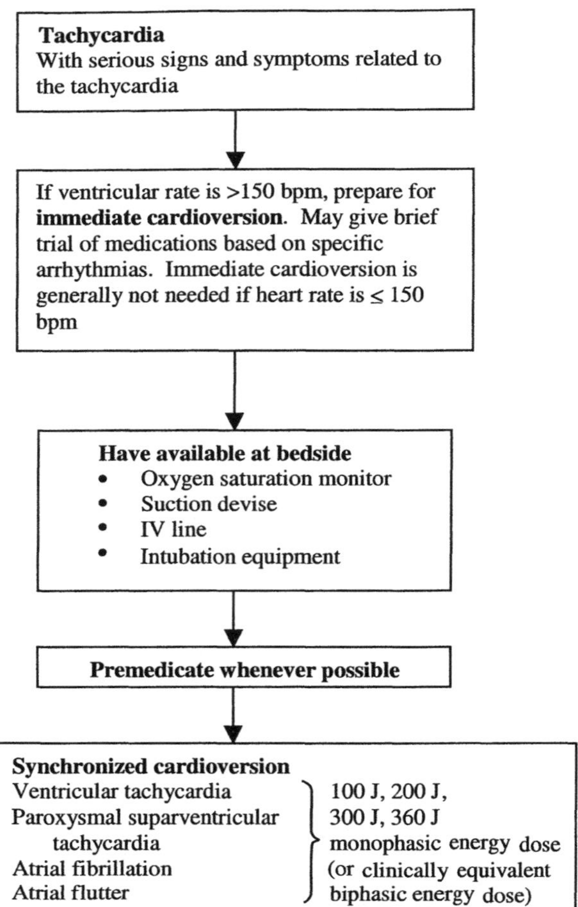

Notes:

1. Effective regimes have included a sedative (e.g. diazepam, midazolam, barbiturates, etomidate, ketamine, methohexital) with or without an analgesic agent (e.g. fentanyl, morphine, meperidrine). Many experts recommend anesthesia if service is readily available.
2. Both monophasic and biphasic waveforms are acceptable and documented as clinically equivalent to reports of monophasic success.
3. Note possible need to resynchronize after each cardioversion.
4. If delays in synchronization occur and clinical condition is critical, go immediately to unsynchronized shocks.
5. Treat polymorphic ventricular tachycardia (irregular form and rate) like ventricular fibrillation: see Fig.6.7.
6. Paroxysmal supraventricular tachycardia and trial flutter often respond to lower energy levels (start with 50 J)

Steps for synchronized cardioversion

1. Consider sedation.
2. Turn on defibrillator (monophasic or biphasic).
3. Attach monitor leads to the patient ("white to right, red to rib, what's left over to the left shoulder") and insure proper display of the patient's rhythm.
4. Engage the synchronization mode by pressing the "sync" control button.
5. Look for makers on R waves indicating sync mode.
6. If necessary, adjust monitor gain until sync markers occur with each R wave.
7. Select appropriate energy level.
8. Position conductor pads on patient (or apply gel to paddles).
9. Position paddle on patient (sternum–apex).
10. Announce to team members: **"Charging defibrillator – stand clear."**
11. Press "charge" button on apex paddle (right hand).
12. When the defibrillator is charged, begin the final clearing chant. State firmly in a forceful voice the following chant before shock:
    "I am going to shock on three. One, I'm clear." (Check to make sure you are clear of contact with the patient, the stretcher, and the equipment.)
    "Two, you are clear." (Make a visual check to insure that no one continues to touch the patient or stretcher. In particular, do not forget the person giving ventilations. That person's hands should not be touching the ventilatory adjuncts, including the tracheal tube!)
    "Three, everybody's clear." Check yourself one more time before pressing the "shock" buttons.
13. Apply 25 lb pressure on both paddles.
14. Press the "discharge" buttons simultaneously.
15. Check the monitor. If tachycardia persists, increase the joules according to the electrical cardioversion algorithm.
16. Reset the sync mode after each synchronized cardioversion because most defibrillators default back to unsynchronized mode. This default allows immediate shock if the cardioversion produces VF.

Fig. 6.15 Electrical cardioversion algorithm. (Adapted from Guidelines 2000 for Cardiopulmonary Resuscitation and Emergency Cardiovascular Care. Circulation 2000;102 (Suppl 1).)

Table 6.4 Recently recommended changes in basic life support and advanced cardiac life support*

Basic life support
Assessment of circulation includes observation for "signs of circulation", not necessarily a pulse check
Signs include breathing, coughing, or movement
Compression/ventilation ratio of 15 : 2 for one or two rescuers with an unprotected airway
Advanced cardiac life support
May use alternative airways in the absence of a bag-mask device or authorization to perform tracheal intubation
Must confirm tracheal tube position immediately using nonphysical examination techniques, such as ET CO_2 indicators
Mechanically ventilated patients should not be hyperventilated, unless there are signs of cerebral herniation after resuscitation
High dose epinephrine not recommended because of potential for harm
Vasopressin may be substituted for epinephrine
Amiodarone and procainamide recommended ahead of lidocaine and adenosine for stable wide-complex techycardia
Bretylium omitted from the VF/pulseless VT algorithm
rtPA administered within 3 hr of stroke onset in patients who meet fibrinolytic criteria
Following cardiac arrest, do not actively rewarm patients who are mildly hypothermic
Nitrates are first-line therapy together with benzodiazepines in cocaine-associated acute coronary syndromes
Induction of systemic alkalosis is treatment of choice for hypotension or arrhythmias related to tricyclic overdose
Acute respiratory failure due to opiate overdose should be reversed by mechanical ventilation prior to naloxone

* New, detailed protocols are outlined in subsequent tables.
ET, end-tidal; rtPA, recombinant tissue plasminogen activator; VF, ventricular fibrillation; VT, ventricular tachycardia.

Table 6.5 Maternal physiologic changes of pregnancy

Cardiovascular	
CO	Increases
Blood volume	Increases
HR	Increases
SVR	Decreases
COP	Decreases
PCWP	Decreases
Hematologic	
Clotting factors	Increases
Respiratory	
Pharyngeal edema	Increases
Minute ventilation	Increases
Oxygen consumption	Increases
FRC	Decreases
Arterial P_{CO_2}	Decreases
Serum bicarbonate	Decreases
Breast	
Chest wall compliance	Decreases
Gastrointestinal	
Motility	Decreases
Lower esophageal sphincter tone	Decreases
Renal	
Compensated respiratory alkalosis	Increases
Uteroplacental	
Blood flow	Increases
Aortocaval compression	Increases

CO, cardiac output; HR, heart rate; COP, colloid oncotic pressure; FRC, functional residual capacity; PCWP, pulmonary capillary wedge pressure; SVR, systemic vascular resistance.

Table 6.6 Modifications in emergency cardiac care for the pregnant patient

Heimlich maneuver—chest thrust in latter half of gestation
Left uterine displacement
Aggressive airway management
Cricoid pressure to avoid aspiration
Increase chest wall compression force
Delivery within 5 minutes if fetus is viable
Aggressive restoration of circulatory volume if appropriate

Successful resuscitation

In contrast to the image popularized in the media, CPR is rarely effective in restoring spontaneous circulation and permitting neurologically intact recovery to hospital discharge. Successful resuscitation is reported in 6–15% of patients suffering inhospital cardiac arrest (Karetzky et al., 1995; Diem et al., 1996). Survival in pregnancy is unusual given the physiologic changes outlined above any compounded by aortocaval compression.

Cesarean delivery and cardiopulmonary arrest

In ancient times, cesarean section was performed postmortem, not to save the child but to remove it from the mother prior to burial. Numa Pompilus, the king of Rome (715–673 BC) decreed that if a woman died while pregnant, the infant was to be immediately cut out of her abdomen (Ritter, 1961). This decree became part of the *Lex Regia* and subsequently part of the *Lex Caesare* (Emperor's law), hence, the origin of the "cesarean operation." By the first half of this century, the operation was performed in a desperate attempt to save the infant of a dying mother. By 1960, 120 successful postmortem cesarean sections were reported (Ritter, 1961). It was noted that fetal prognosis was better in cases of sudden maternal death than after chronic illnesses.

In the twenty-first edition of *Williams Obstetrics*, Cunningham and colleagues (2001) suggest that delivery within 5 minutes of cardiopulmonary arrest would not only benefit the infant but also may facilitate maternal resuscitation. This recommendation was based primarily on the report by Katz and colleagues (1986) who analyzed reports of successful results. They recognized that the gravid uterus may prevent proper CPR techniques from restoring adequate cardiac output. The low-resistance, high-volume uteroplacental unit sequesters blood, hindering effective CPR, In the nonpregnant state, external chest compressions produce a cardiac output approximately 30% of normal. The gravid uterus in the supine position obstructs venous return and CO. Left lateral tilt causes the torso to roll, and part of the compression force is lost. Therefore, optimal chest compressions in pregnancy will yield less than 30% of normal cardiac output. Because without adequate cerebral perfusion irreversible brain damage from anoxia occurs within 4–6 minutes, they argue for cesarean section within 4–5 minutes, especially when the woman is pulseless despite CPR. Pulselessness may persist until the uterus is evacuated (DePace et al., 1982; O'Connor & Sevarino, 1994). Delivery leads to a decrease in aortocaval obstruction, an increase in effectiveness of compressions, and an increase in maternal CO. Uterine evacuation will increase the CO up to 25%. Vasopressors used in ACLS cause uterine vasoconstriction (Prentice-Bjerkeseth, 1999). Delivery might actually assist CPR efforts, allow a viable fetus to survive, and decrease fetal exposure to ACLS drugs. Therefore, cesarean section should be considered part of CPR as it may improve outcome for both the mother and the fetus.

Clearly, the timing of the operation is critical for infant survival, which appears proportional to the time between the mother's cardiac arrest and her delivery (Table 6.7). If delivery is accomplished within 5 minutes of maternal cardiac arrest, intact neurologic neonatal survival is likely (Katz et al., 1986; Clark et al., 1995). Beyond 15 minutes, neonatal death or impaired survival is generally seen. Primate studies confirm brain damage in utero with as little as 6 minutes of complete asphyxia; severe cellular damage occurs by 8 minutes (Windle, 1968). Scattered reports describe infant survival at longer intervals following arrest, implying that cesarean delivery should be performed postarrest if signs of fetal life are present (Selden & Binke, 1988; Kaiser, 1994).

Table 6.7 Perimortem cesarean delivery with the outcome of surviving infants from the time of death until delivery

Time interval (min)	Surviving infants	Intact neurologic status of survivors
0–5	45	98%
6–15	18	83%
16–25	9	33%
26–35	4	25%
36+	1	0%

(Data from Katz VL, Dotters DJ, Droegemueller W. Perimortem cesarean delivery. Obstet Gynecol 1986; 68; 571 and Clark SI, Hankins GDV, Dudley DA, et al. Amniotic fluid embolism: Analysis of the national registry. Am J Obstet Gynecol 1995; 172: 1939.)

In light of the evolving definition of fetal viability, one group of authors attempted to develop an algorithm to assist clinicians in determining when and who would benefit from a perimortem cesarean section (Morris, 1996). The "potentially salvageable" infant was defined as an estimated gestational age of greater than or equal to 26 weeks with confirmation of fetal cardiac activity by Doppler ultrasound. In this group, 75% of the infants survived. The authors postulated that 60% of the infant deaths may have been avoided by earlier recognition of fetal distress and earlier cesarean section.

Women with chronic illness are less likely to have a normal surviving infant by perimortem cesarean section, as compared with those suffering an acute arrest. Because the latter is now relatively more common, a more compelling argument is made for a cesarean section within minutes of an arrest. Thus if a pregnant woman suffers a cardiopulmonary arrest beyond the stage of viability for a given institution, a cesarean section should be considered. The 4-minute limit to initiate delivery, as advocated by Katz and colleagues (1986, 1995), the American College of Obstetricians and Gynecologists, and several texts, is derived from theoretical physiologic advantages for resuscitating the mother, as well as from extrapolation of data on infant survival. While such data suggest an ideal arrest-to-delivery interval, in actual practice these goals can be achieved only rarely. Further, it must be emphasized that no data exist to document actual maternal benefits of perimortem cesarean section; maternal death clearly remains, by far, the most likely outcome regardless of arrest-to-delivery interval. In the setting of perimortem cesarean section performed for the likely salvageable fetus, the staff should be well versed in the techniques of neonatal resuscitation as these infants are likely to suffer from respiratory and circulatory depression at birth.

Conclusion

Since the publication of the last edition of this text, the most significant clinical change in CPR has been in the area of pharmacology, particularly treatment of tachyarrhythmias. The revised American Heart Association algorithms are outlined in Figs 6.6–6.15. Late pregnancy requires certain modifications to ECC, including aggressive airway management and left lateral uterine displacement. Physiologic alterations of pregnancy may require larger doses of pharmacologic agents than in the nonpregnant patient. Once cardiopulmonary arrest is confirmed, initiation of delivery within 4 minutes appears to offer the best chance for both maternal and neonatal survival. Fetal outcome appears to be directly related to the condition of the mother. It cannot be overemphasized that the resuscitation efforts of the mother take precedence over the fetus. Delivery of the infant may have maternal resuscitative benefit by improving cardiac return and hence cardiac output.

References

Adrogue HJ, Rashad MN, Gorin AB, et al. Assessing acid-base status in circulatory failure: differences between arterial and central venous blood flow. N Engl J Med 1989;320:1312–1316.

American Heart Association. Textbook of basic life support for healthcare providers. Dallas: American Heart Association, 1994.

American Heart Association. Handbook of emergency cardiovascular care. Dallas: American Heart Association, 2000.

Barnes TA, Macdonald D, Nolan J, et al. Cardiopulmonary resuscitation and emergency cardiovascular care. Airway devices. Ann Emerg Med 2001;37(4):S145–S151.

Briggs GG, Garite TJ. Effects on the fetus of drugs used in critical care. In: Clark SL, Cotton DB, Hankins GD, Phelan J, eds. Critical care obstetrics. Malden, Massachusetts: Blackwell Science, 1997:696.

Clark SL, Hankins GD, Dudley DS, et al. Amniotic fluid embolism: Analysis of the national registry. Am J Obstet Gynecol 1995;172 (4 Part 1):1158–1167; discussion 1167–1169.

Cunningham FG, Gant NF, Levino KJ, et al. Williams obstetrics, 21st edn. New York, NY: McGraw-Hill, 2001:1176–1177.

DePace NL, Betesh JS, Kotler MN. "Postmortem" cesarean section with recovery of both mother and offspring. JAMA 1982;248:971–973.

DeSwiet M. Pulmonary disorders. In: Creasy RK, Resnick R, eds. Maternal-fetal medicine: principles and practice. Philadelphia: WB Saunders, 1999:921–934.

Diem SJ, Lantos JD, Tulsky JA. Cardiopulmonary resuscitation on television. Miracles and misinformation. N Engl J Med 1996;334:1578–1582.

Dildy GA, Clark SL. Cardiac arrest during pregnancy. Obstet Gynecol Clin N Am 1995;22:303–314.

Eisenberg MS, Bergner I, Hallstrom A. Cardiac resuscitation in the community. Importance of rapid provision and implications for program planning. JAMA 1979;24:1905–1907.

European Resuscitation Council. Part 6: Advanced cardiovascular life support. Section 1: Introduction to ACLS 2000: Overview of recommended changes in ACLS from the guidelines 2000 conference. Resuscitation 2000;46:103–107.

Goodwin AP, Pearce AJ. The human wedge. A manoeuvre to relieve aortocaval compression during resuscitation in late pregnancy. Anesthesia 1992;47:433–434.

Guidelines 2000 for Cardiopulmonary Resuscitation and Emergency Cardiovascular Care. Circulation 2000;102(8):I1–I291.

Kaiser RT. Air embolism death of a pregnant woman secondary to orogenital sex. Acad Emerg Med 1994;1:555–558.

Karetzky M, Zubair M, Parikh J. Cardiopulmonary resuscitation in intensive care unit and non-intensive care unit patients: immediate and long term survival. Arch Intern Med 1995;155:1277–1280.

Katz VL, Dotters DJ, Droegemueller W. Perimortem cesarean delivery. Obstet Gynecol 1986;68:571–576.

Katz VL, Wells Sr, Kuller JA, et al. Cesarean delivery: a reconsideration of terminology. Obstet Gynecol 1995;86:152–153.

Kouwenhoven WB, Jude JR, Knickerbocker GG. Closed-chest cardiac massage. JAMA 1960;173:94.

Lee RV, Rogers BD, White LM, Harvey RC. Cardiopulmonary resuscitation of pregnant women. Am J Med 1986;81:311.

Morris JA, Rosenbower TJ, Jurkovich GJ, et al. Infant survival after cesarean section for trauma. Ann Surg 1996;223:481–488.

Niemann JT. Cardioplmonary resuscitation. N Engl J Med 1992;327: 1075–1080.

O'Connor RL, Sevarino FB. Cardiopulmonary arrest in a pregnant patient: a report of a successful resuscitation. J Clin Anesth 1994; 6:66–68.

Ogburn PL, Schmidt G, Linman J, Cefalo RC. Paroxysmal tachycardia and cardioversion during pregnancy. J Reprod Med 1992;27:359–366.

Page RL. Treatment of arrythmias during pregnancy. Am Heart J 1995;130:871–876.

Prentice-Bjerkeseth R. Perioperative anesthetic management of trauma in pregnancy. Anes Clin N Am 1999;17(1):277.

Reed AP. Current concepts in airway management for cardiopulmonary resuscitation. Mayo Clin Proc 1995;70:1172–1184.

Rees GA, Willis BA. Resuscitation in late pregnancy. Anesthesia 1988;43:347–349.

Ritter JW. Postmortem cesarean section. JAMA 1961;175:715.

Rubin PC. Current concepts: Beta blockers in pregnancy. N Engl J Med 1981;305:1323–1326.

Rudikoff MT, Maughan WI, Effon M, et al. Mechanisms of blood flow during cardiopulmonary resuscitation. Circulation 1980;61:345–352.

Satin AJ. Cardiopulmonary resuscitation in pregnancy. In: Clark SL, Cotton DB, Hankins GD, Phelan J, eds. Critical care obstetrics. Malden, Massachusetts: Blackwell Science, 1997:219.

Selden BS, Burke TJ. Complete maternal and fetal recovery after prolonged cardiac arrest. Ann Emerg Med 1988;17:346–349.

Syverson CJ, Chavkin W, Atrash HK, et al. Pregnancy related mortality in New York City, 1980 to 1984: causes of death and associated risk factors. Am J Obstet Gynecol 1991;164:603–608.

Thel MC, O'Connor CM. Cardiopulmonary resuscitation: Historical perspective to recent investigations. Am Heart J 1999;137:39–48.

Werner JA, Greene JL, Janko CL, Cobb LA. Visualization of cardiac valve motion in man during external chest compressions using two-dimensional echocardiography: Implications regarding the mechanism of blood flow. Circulation 1981;63:1417–1421.

Windle WF. Brain damage at birth. JAMA 1968;206:1967–1972.

7 Neonatal resuscitation

Christian Con Yost
Ron Bloom

Under normal circumstances, the transition from the womb to the world is a series of dramatic and rapid physiologic changes leading to the birth of an infant prepared to continue the processes of growth and development. The goal of delivering a healthy child ready to continue normal development is, unfortunately, not always technically feasible. Pregnancies and/or deliveries complicated by common and uncommon conditions discussed throughout this text, are, at times, not always successful in making the transition to extrauterine life. Modern diagnostic tools often, but not always, allow for anticipation of infants at risk of not making a successful transition, and, thus, permit the perinatal team to plan for neonatal resuscitation and/or medically necessary inventions. However, more acute and often unanticipated conditions such as a sudden prolapsed cord or abruption or a previously unrecognized congenital anomaly may preclude the availability of a neonatal resuscitation team.

At birth, neonatal resuscitation may be medically necessary. Thus, the ability to conduct effective resuscitation of the newborn infant is an integral part of the considerations and planning for delivery. Regardless of the level of care, a trained and experienced team capable of neonatal resuscitation is an integral part of perinatal care (International Guidelines for Neonatal Resuscitation, 2000).

Basic principles

Causes of asphyxia

While all deliveries involve a complex physiologic transition at birth, infants of those mothers cared for by the high-risk obstetric team, especially if premature, are at a greater risk of birth depression. Birth depression requiring resuscitation of a neonate cannot always be predicted, and the newborn infant may be depressed at birth through a variety of mechanisms, unrelated to asphyxia.

Maternal or placental conditions can result in birth depression. For example, diminished uterine blood flow may result from maternal hypotension, eclampsia, regional anesthesia, or uterine contractions. Placental abnormalities such as abruption, edema, or inflammatory changes may reduce placental gaseous exchange. Fetoplacental blood flow may also be compromised due to sustained and unrelieved cord compression from a nuchal or prolapsed umbilical cord.

Compromising conditions or events may also be primarily fetal in origin. These include drug-induced central nervous system (CNS) depression, CNS anomalies, spinal cord injury, mechanical airway obstruction, pulmonary immaturity, congenital anomalies, and infection. All of these events or conditions, maternal and fetal, may occur at the time of delivery or significantly prior to the events of parturition. It is important to note that intrauterine ischemic events, even those quite remote from the delivery of the infant, may extend into the newborn period by reducing the infant's ability to adapt to air breathing life.

Response to hypoxia

In the normal fetal circulation, blood returning to the heart from the body and placenta is primarily shunted through the foramen ovale to the left side of the heart facilitating the movement of oxygenated blood to the head and heart. Blood that reaches the right ventricle is shunted through the ductus arteriosus to the aorta, bypassing the lungs due to high pulmonary vascular resistance (Rudolf & Yuan, 1966). This serves the fetus well as the major organ of gas exchange is the placenta (Fig. 7.1).

However, if the fetus or neonate is subjected to "hypoxic" conditions, the physiologic response is to exacerbate or maintain an increase in pulmonary vascular resistance. For the neonate, maintenance of the fetal circulation serves only to shunt blood away from the lungs.

In the circumstances of progressive asphyxia, the fetus or newborn responds with an increase in systemic vascular resistance or vasoconstriction. This results in intrafetal or neonatal shunting by decreasing blood flow to the musculature and intestines, while attempting to increase blood flow to the head

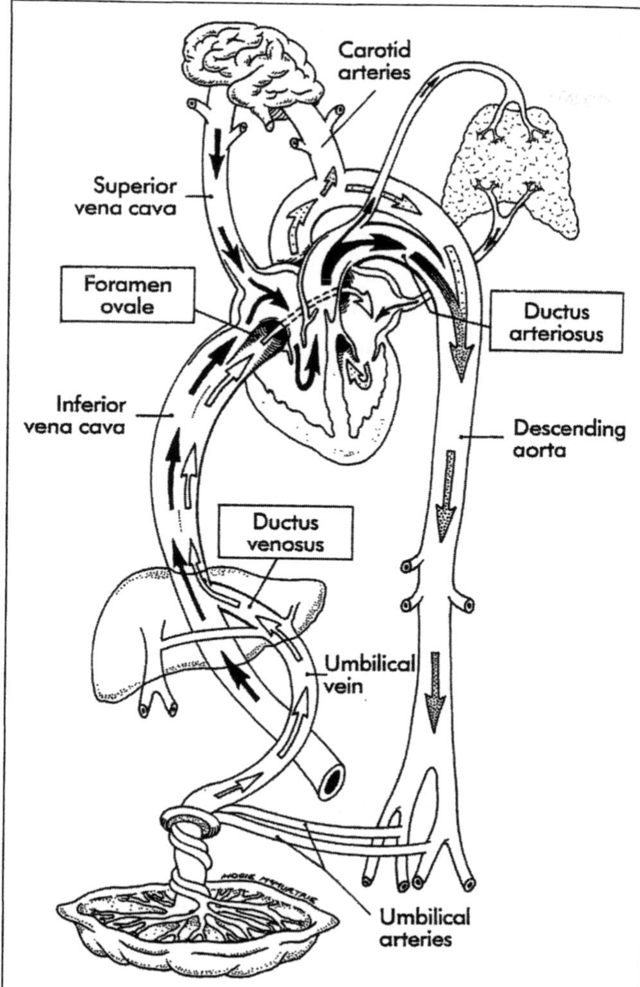

Fig. 7.1 Fetal circulation. (Reproduced by permission from Neonatal-Perinatal Medicine: Diseases of the Fetus and Newborn; 7th edn; Editors: Faranoff, AA and Martin, RJ; p. 417, St Louis, Mosby, 2002.)

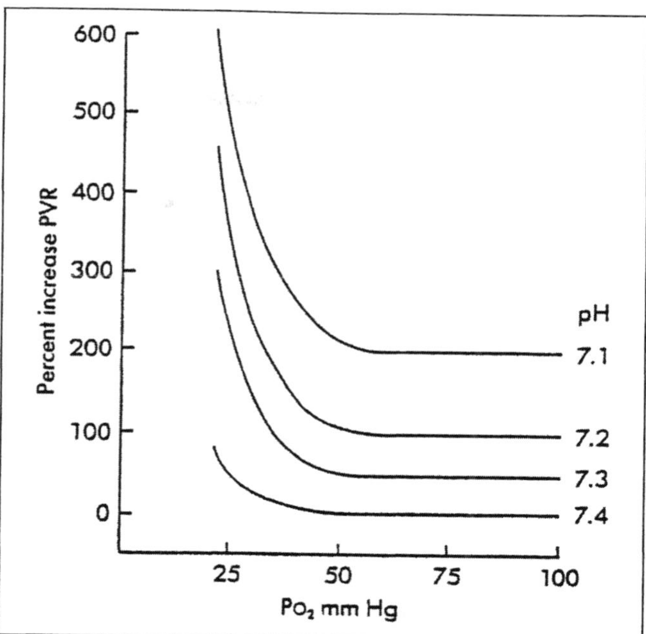

Fig. 7.2 Pulmonary vascular resistance (PVR) in the calf. (From Rudolph AM, Yuan S. Response of the pulmonary vasculature to hypoxia and H^+ ion concentration changes. J Clin Invest 1966;45:339.)

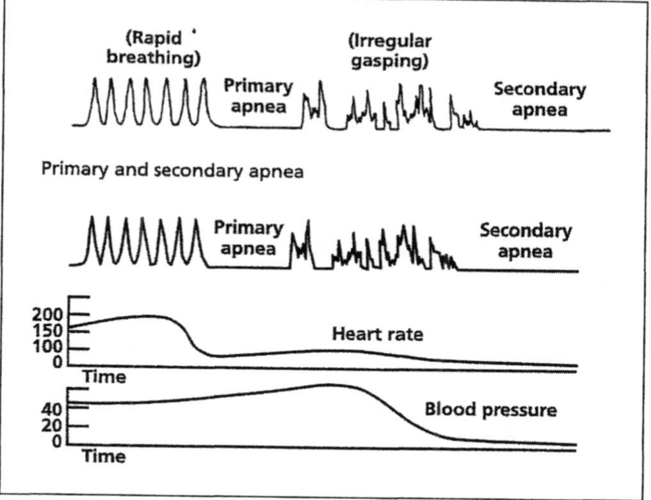

Fig. 7.3 Heart rate and blood pressure changes during apnea. (Reproduced by permission from Textbook of Neonatal Resuscitation, 4th edn, p. 1–7; Elk Grove, IL; American Academy of Pediatrics/American Heart Association, 2000.)

and heart. Thus, blood flow to the cardiac and cerebral vessels is maximized at the expense of "nonvital" organs. This pattern of blood flow, if prolonged, can through redistribution result in increasing acidosis (Rudolf, 1988; Morin & Weiss, 1992). The vasospastic process, if uncorrected, further increases the pulmonary vascular resistance (Fig. 7.2). For both fetus and newborn, cardiac output and blood pressure are maintained to the vital organs initially, but will ultimately fail with myocardial failure (Downing et al., 1966).

Primary and secondary apnea

Superimposed on these circulatory and hemodynamic changes is believed to be the respiratory response to asphyxia. The fetus or neonate will initiate gasping respiration (which may occur in utero) and, should the asphyxia persist, enter an apnea phase known as primary apnea. If the asphyxia continues, the primary apnea in the neonate will be followed by a period of irregular gasping respirations. Continued asphyxia will lead to a period of unremitting apnea known as secondary apnea. Figure 7.3 illustrates the respiratory and cardiovascular effects of asphyxia.

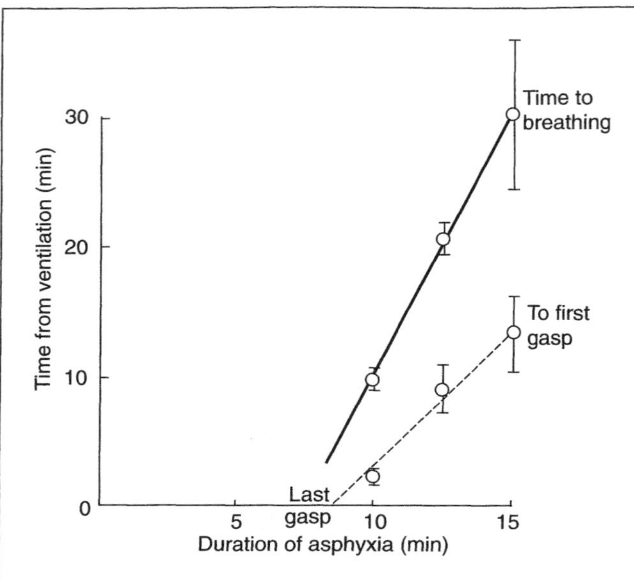

Fig. 7.4 Time from ventilation to first gasp and to rhythmic breathing in newborn monkeys asphyxiated for 10, 12.5, and 15 minutes at 30°C. (From Adamsons K, et al. Resuscitation by positive pressure ventilation and tris-hydroxymethyl-aminomethane of rhesus monkeys asphixiated at birth. J Pediatr 1964;65:807.)

If an infant is in primary apnea and exposed to oxygen when gasping respirations ensue, oxygen exposure is usually sufficient to reverse the process. However, once the infant reaches secondary apnea, positive pressure ventilation is required to initiate spontaneous ventilation. Furthermore, the longer the duration of secondary apnea, the longer it will take for spontaneous respiratory effort to return following the administration of positive pressure ventilation (Adamsons et al., 1964; Dawes, 1968) (Fig. 7.4).

Asphyxia may begin in utero such that the infant may undergo primary apnea in utero, and then be born in secondary apnea. Thus, it is extremely difficult to assess the degree of asphyxia at the time of birth. For this reason, the resuscitative efforts should begin immediately for infants born with any degree of depression and should reduce the need, in selected circumstances, of a potentially prolonged resuscitation with an increased risk of neonatal brain damage.

Importance of resuscitation

While the long-term effects of asphyxia are sometimes unavoidable, a prompt and effective resuscitation may, in most cases, restore spontaneous respiratory effort and reverse the underlying vasospastic process (Box 7.1). In the vast majority of resuscitations of depressed infants, the initiation of effective positive-pressure ventilation is sufficient to restore spontaneous respirations. In a large series, a very small percentage of neonates (0.12%) required chest compressions or medication. In those neonates with persistent neonatal depression, 75% were believed due to ineffective or improper ventilatory support (Perlman & Risser, 1995).

The Apgar score reflects the level of resuscitation required in a given neonate. For example, if an infant is born in secondary apnea, intervention should be initiated immediately rather than waiting 1 minute. Thus, the Apgar score is intended to provide a "snapshot" look at the neonatal condition for one moment in time and the level of resuscitation required in a neonate (Table 7.1).

Box 7.1 Consequences of asphyxia

Central nervous system
- Cerebral hemorrhage
- Cerebral edema
- Hypoxic-ischemic encephalopathy
- Seizures

Lung
- Delayed onset of respiration
- Respiratory distress syndrome
- Meconium aspiration syndrome

Cardiovascular system
- Myocardial failure
- Papillary muscle necrosis
- Persistent fetal circulation

Renal system
- Cortico/tubular/medullary necrosis

Gastrointestinal tract
- Necrotizing enterocolitis

Blood
- Disseminated intravascular coagulation

(From Neonatal-Perinatal Medicine: Diseases of the Fetus and Newborn; 7th edn; Editors: Faranoff, AA and Martin, RJ; p. 420, St Louis, Mosby, 2002.)

Elements of a resuscitation

Overview (Fig. 7.5)

The ability to provide for a prompt and effective resuscitation should be available for all infants regardless of the relative risk for resuscitation as estimated by prenatal complications, fetal heart tracings, or complications of labor. For infants at risk of being born depressed based on the clinical circumstances, the

Table 7.1 Apgar scoring

	Score		
Sign	**0**	**1**	**2**
Heart rate	Absent	Slow (<100 bpm)	≥100 bpm
Respirations	Absent	Slow, irregular	Good, crying
Muscle tone	Limp	Some flexion	Active motion
Reflex irritability (catheter in nares, tactile stimulation)	No response	Grimace	Cough, sneeze, cry
Color	Blue or pale	Pink body, blue extremities	Completely pink

(Reproduced by permission from International Guidelines for Neonatal Resuscitation: Pediatrics 2000; 106(3). URL: http://www.pediatrics.org/cgi/content/full/106/3/e29.)

need for resuscitation should be anticipated, when possible, and preparations made for the time of delivery.

With each delivery, a quick assessment permits effective triaging of the infant. If the infant is term, crying, vigorous, and pink, there is obviously no further need for resuscitation and the infant can be handed to an eager mother. The infant with a congenital anomaly, an early gestational age, meconium, or poor respiratory effort, tone, color, or general morphology may, but not always, require a longer assessment.

If the neonate is placed on a radiant warmer, the initial steps include, but are not limited to, warming and drying, correct airway positioning, suctioning of the mouth and nose, and assessment of respiratory effort, heart rate, and color. After the initial period of assessment, subsequent efforts are dictated by the clinical assessment of respiratory effort, heart rate, and color.

Gasping or absent respiration, or a neonatal heart rate below 100, should prompt initiation of positive-pressure ventilation. Most infants will respond to positive-pressure ventilation

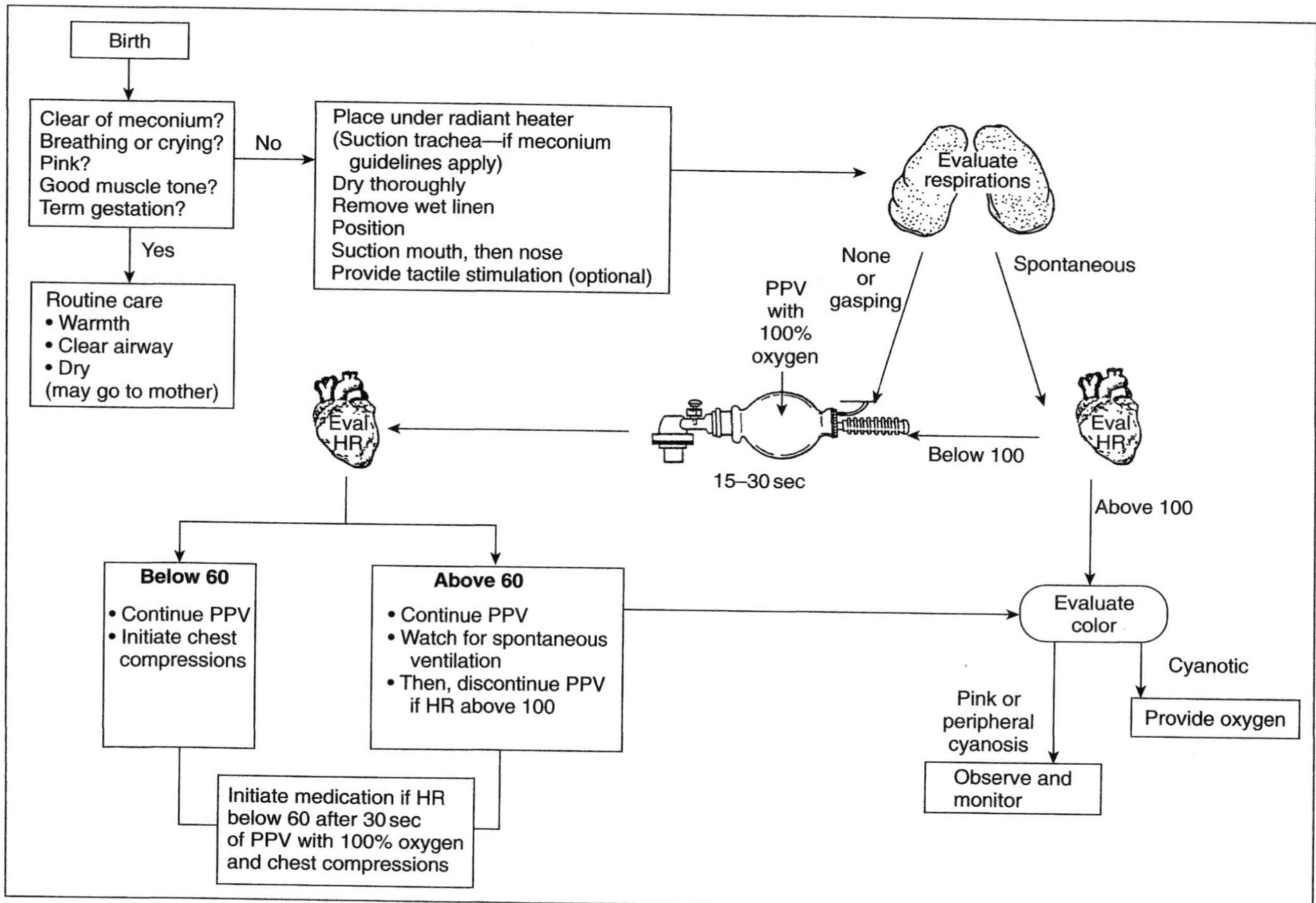

Fig. 7.5 Overview of resuscitation in the delivery room. (Modified from Textbook of Neonatal Resuscitation, 4th edn; Elk Grove, IL; American Academy of Pediatrics/American Heart Association, 2000. Originally published in Neonatal-Perinatal Medicine: Diseases of the Fetus and in Newborn; 7th edn; Editors: Faranoff, AA and Martin, RJ; p. 434, St Louis, Mosby, 2002.)

alone. If an infant has central cyanosis but adequate spontaneous respirations and a heart rate greater than 100 beats per minute (bpm), free-flow oxygen is usually sufficient until color improves.

Chest compressions are reserved for infants whose heart rate remains below 60 bpm for longer than 30 seconds after the initiation of assisted ventilation. If after an additional 30 seconds of positive-pressure ventilation and chest compression, the heart rate does not begin to rise medications may be indicated. Chest compressions should be continued until the infant's heart rate exceeds 60 bpm. Assisted ventilation is continued until the infant has spontaneous respiration which is adequate to sustain the neonatal heart rate above 100.

The resuscitative steps for infants with special circumstances such as thick meconium-stained amniotic fluid, pneumothorax, congenital diaphragmatic hernia or erythroblastosis/hydrops will be discussed later in this chapter.

Preparation for a resuscitation

Anticipation

The infant delivered of a mother requiring critical care to support and maintain a pregnancy may require complex resuscitation. Thus, preparation is the first step to assure neonatal resuscitation. A careful review of the antepartum and peripartum maternal history as well as an assessment of the infant's response to labor will frequently identify the potential for delivering a depressed infant (Box 7.2).

Traditionally, cesarean delivery of any type has been considered high risk. Enough information is now available to state that the uncomplicated repeat cesarean section carries no greater risk for the infant than a vaginal delivery (Press et al., 1985).

The need for neonatal resuscitation has been made easier by technologic advances allowing better prenatal assessment of the fetus. But, not all events compromising an infant's response to labor may be predicted. For this reason, equipment and personnel must be immediately available to intervene on behalf of the infant requiring an unanticipated resuscitation.

Box 7.2 Factors associated with neonatal depression and asphyxia

Antepartum risk factors
Maternal diabetes
Pregnancy-induced hypertension
Chronic hypertension
Chronic maternal illness
- Cardiovascular
- Thyroid
- Neurological
- Pulmonary
- Renal

Anemia or isoimmunization
Previous fetal or neonatal death
Bleeding in second or third trimester
Maternal infection
Polyhydramnios
Oligohydramnios
Premature rupture of membranes
Post-term gestation
Multiple gestation
Size–dates discrepancy
Drug therapy, e.g.
- Lithium carbonate
- Magnesium
- Adrenergic-blocking drugs

Maternal substance abuse
Fetal malformation
Diminished fetal activity
No prenatal care
Age <16 or >35 years

Intrapartum risk factors
Emergency cesarean section
Forceps or vacuum-assisted delivery
Breech or other abnormal presentation
Premature labor
Precipitous labor
Chorioamnionitis
Prolonged rupture of membranes (>18 hours before delivery)
Prolonged labor (>24 hours)
Prolonged second stage of labor (>2 hours)
Fetal bradycardia
Nonreassuring fetal heart rate patterns
Use of general anesthesia
Uterine tetany
Narcotics given to mother within 4 hours of delivery
Meconium-stained amniotic fluid
Prolapsed cord
Abruptio placentae
Placenta previa

(Modified from Textbook of Neonatal Resuscitation; 4th edn; Elk Grove, IL; American Academy of Pediatrics/American Heart Association, 2000. Originally published in Neonatal-Perinatal Medicine: Diseases of the Fetus and Newborn; 7th edn; Editors: Faranoff, AA and Martin, RJ; p. 420, St Louis, Mosby, 2002.)

Equipment

Appropriate equipment must be close at hand and in good working order (Box 7.3).

Adequate personnel

Individuals vested with the responsibility of resuscitating infants should be adequately trained, readily available, and capable of working together as a team. Adequate training involves not only satisfactory completion of a course such as the Neonatal Resuscitation Program of the American Heart Association/American Academy of Pediatrics but also sufficient experience. Those having completed a course, but still lacking the expertise gained through experience should be supervised and supported by experienced personnel. Ultimately, the ability to resuscitate neonates is based on the training, skill, and experience of the resuscitator.

Neonatal resuscitation is a team effort. If individuals are aware of and able to fulfill their respective responsibilities as well as anticipate the needs of other team members, difficult resuscitations are made easier. In those institutions where resuscitations are uncommon events, frequent mock code drills may help to maintain skills and develop coordination among various team members.

Initial steps and evaluation

To its mother or not?

The healthy vigorous term infant may be given directly to its mother, thereby facilitating maternal–neonatal bonding.

Whether to bypass resuscitative efforts should, however, be based on information obtained during the initial triage of the infant. The infant born at term without obvious deformity or the passage of meconium in utero, who immediately after birth is vigorous, breathing easily, and exhibits good tone and color may be able to bond with its mother in keeping with the wishes of the parents. A light blanket and some drying of the infant by the mother and delivery room staff will help to estab-

Box 7.3 Neonatal resuscitation supplies and equipment

Suction equipment
Bulb syringe
Mechanical suction
Suction catheter: Size 5 (or 6), 8, 10, or 12 Fr
Size 8 Fr feeding tube and 20 mL syringe
Meconium aspirator

Bag-and-mask equipment
Neonatal resuscitation bag with a pressure-release valve or pressure gauge; the bag must be capable of delivering 90–100% oxygen
Face masks—newborn and premature sizes (cushioned-rim masks preferred)
Oral airways—newborn (size 0) and premature sizes (size 00)
Oxygen source with intact flowmeter and tubing

Intubation equipment
Laryngoscope with straight blades—no. 0 (premature) and no. 1 (term newborn)
Extra bulbs and batteries for laryngoscope
Endotracheal tubes—sizes 2.0, 2.5, 3.0, 3.5, 4.0 mm ID
Stylet (optional)
Scissors
Gloves
Tape or securing device for endotracheal tube

Medications
Epinephrine 1 : 10,000 (0.1 mg/mL) 3 mL or 10 mL ampules
Naloxone hydrochloride, 0.4 mg/mL in 1 mL ampules or 1.0 mg/mL in 2 mL ampules
Isotonic crystalloid (normal saline or Ringer's lactate) for volume expansion—100 or 250 mL
Sodium bicarbonate 4.2% (5 mEq/10 mL) in 10 mL ampules
Dextrose 5% and 10%, 250 mL
Sterile water

Other equipment and supplies
Radiant warmer
Stethoscope
Blood pressure monitor with transducer (desirable)
Adhesive tape—½-inch or ¾-inch wide
Syringes—1, 3, 5, 10, 20, 50 mL
Needles—25, 21, 18 gauge
Alcohol sponges
Umbilical artery catheterization tray
Umbilical tape
Umbilical catheters size 3.5, 5 Fr
Three-way stopcocks
Size 5 Fr feeding tube
Cardiotachometer with electrocardiographic oscilloscope (desirable)
Pressure transducer and monitor (desirable)
Pulse oximeter

(Originally published in Neonatal-Perinatal Medicine: Diseases of the Fetus and Newborn; 7th edn; Editors: Faranoff, AA and Martin, RJ; p. 422, St Louis, Mosby, 2002.)

lish an appropriate thermal environment but should not hinder frequent and adequate assessments of the neonate's condition.

If, however, the infant is premature, has passed meconium in utero, or exhibits any degree of respiratory distress, cyanosis, pallor, hypotonia, or obvious malformations, the infant should be evaluated in the radiant warmer. There, a more thorough assessment can be performed and possible further resuscitative interventions begun.

Initial steps

Thermal management

Since temperatures in the delivery rooms are typically lower than the neonate's core temperature, the neonate needs to be dried quickly. If there is any concern regarding neonatal status, the neonate should be placed in a preheated radiant warmer. There simple measures can minimize the significant drop in infant core body temperature experienced immediately after birth (Miller & Oliver, 1966). These measures are particularly important for the infant with any degree of compromise. The infant's homeostatic response to cold stress is incompletely developed, and, as a result, a greater than normal drop in core body temperature may result (Bruck, 1961; Adamsons et al., 1965).

Clearing the airway

With delivery of the fetal head, the oropharynx is normally cleared with the use of a bulb syringe or suction catheter. Both devices are equally efficacious. The primary purpose is to clear secretions in the oropharynx and to potentially prevent their aspiration should deep breaths occur with nasal suctioning. Gentle suctioning of the oropharynx will frequently, but not always, avoid the reflex bradycardia associated with vigorous suctioning (Cordero & Hon, 1971). If a suction catheter is used, Kattwinkel recommends that the catheter be inserted no more than 5 cm from the lips and that the duration of suctioning be no more than 5 seconds (Kattwinkel et al., 1999).

Tactile stimulation

Drying and suctioning are generally sufficient to stimulate respirations in the newborn infant. Other methods such as flicking the feet or rubbing the back are also useful to stimulate a more vigorous respiratory response in a sluggish newborn. If, however, there is no immediate response to these supplemental methods, positive-pressure ventilation should be initiated. Positive-pressure ventilation is typically necessary in the infant who exhibits gasping respirations or respirations inadequate to sustain a heart rate ≥ 100 bpm.

Free flow oxygen

The infant breathing spontaneously with a heart rate >100 bpm but with persistent central cyanosis should receive 100% free flow oxygen until the oxygen saturation meets or exceeds 85% or the neonate fails to respond to 100% oxygen such as in neonates with cyanotic congenital heart disease.

Free flow oxygen in high concentrations can easily be administered by oxygen mask (with escape holes) or by cupping the hand around the end of the oxygen tubing and holding this close to the infant's nose and mouth (Fig. 7.6). A flow-inflating (anesthesia) bag and mask held lightly over the infant's nose and mouth may also deliver a high concentration of inspired oxygen. Caution should be used to avoid a tight seal so as to avoid providing positive pressure to the lung.

Cold, dry oxygen can be given in an emergency; however, a persistent need for free flow oxygen should prompt humidification and heating of the oxygen. An oxygen blender and oxygen saturation monitor are useful in determining the concentration of oxygen an individual infant requires.

Positive-pressure ventilation

The vast majority of infants requiring resuscitation will respond to timely positive-pressure ventilation. Under most circumstances, positive-pressure ventilation can be quickly and effectively provided with a bag and mask. Those with extensive experience in the placement of endotracheal tubes in newborn infants may choose this route for ventilation, but for most neonates, bag-mask ventilation is usually sufficient.

Resuscitation bags

Regardless of the type of bag used, the volume should be geared to the gestational age and size of the neonate (250–750 mL total volume), and capable of delivering high concentrations of oxygen. A flow-inflating or a self-inflating bag may be used to administer positive-pressure ventilation. While opinions differ as to the effectiveness of one bag over the other (Kanter, 1987), self-inflating bags are easier for the resuscitator to use.

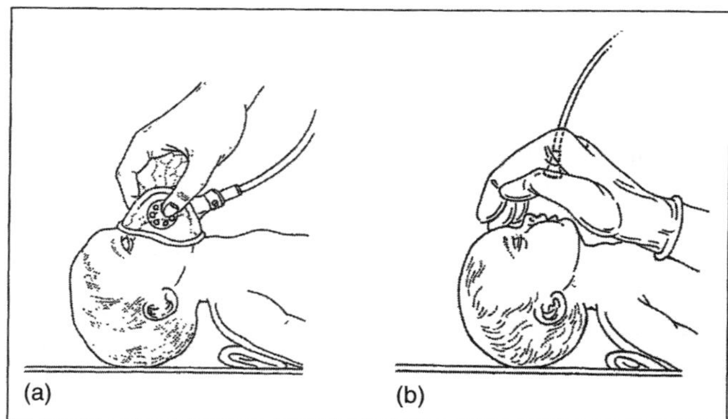

Fig. 7.6 (a) Oxygen mask held close to baby's face. (b) Oxygen delivered by tubing held in cupped hand. (Reproduced by permission from from Textbook of Neonatal Resuscitation; p. 2–32; Elk Grove, IL; American Academy of Pediatrics/American Heart Association, 1994, rev. 1996.)

To protect an infant's lungs from excessive pressures, resuscitation bags should be equipped with a pressure gauge, a pressure-relief valve (pop-off valve) or both. Pop-off valves vent pressures in excess of 30–40 cmH_2O, but there is considerable variability between individual bags (Finer et al., 1986). Should excessive pressures be required to establish adequate chest rise, a finger can easily be placed over the pop-off valve.

Prior to each potential resuscitation, the bag and mask apparatus should be checked. To check a bag for proper function, simply occlude the air outlet and squeeze the bag. A properly functioning bag should be able to generate pressures in excess of 30–40 cmH_2O.

Table 7.2 Endotracheal tube sizes

Tube size (mm ID)	Weight (g)	Gestational age (weeks)
2.0*	500–600 or less	25–26 or less
2.5	<1,000	<28
3.0	1,000–2,000	28–34
3.5	2,000–3,000	34–38
3.5–4.0	>3,000	>38

* May be needed if a size 2.5 Fr tube does not fit.
ID, internal diameter.
(Reproduced by permission from Neonatal-Perinatal Medicine: Diseases of the Fetus and Newborn; 7th edn; Editors: Faranoff, AA and Martin, RJ; p. 426, St Louis, Mosby, 2002.)

Bag/mask ventilation

An adequate seal for delivery of positive-pressure ventilation depends on using an appropriately sized and properly placed mask. A mask with a cushioned rim is preferred because these masks conform more fully to the contours of the infant face and usually require less pressure to maintain a good seal. Given the wide range of neonates that may require resuscitation, masks should be available for infants ranging in weight from 500 to 4,500 g.

When prolonged ventilation with a bag and mask is necessary, an 8 French feeding tube is helpful to vent air built up in the stomach and to remove gastric contents to reduce the risk of aspiration.

Whenever positive-pressure ventilation with bag and mask fails to establish adequate ventilation, an endotracheal tube or oral airway may need to be inserted. The need for these devices typically arises in infants with unusual facial contours, such as the Pierre-Robin Sequence infant, or in small or large infants without an appropriately sized mask.

Bag/endotracheal tube ventilation

Endotracheal intubation is more easily accomplished by two people. One person inserts the tube into the airway, while the other assists and then assesses for correct placement of the tube by listening for equal breath sounds on both sides of the chest. Uncuffed endotracheal tube sizes ranging from 2.0 to 4.0 are typically available in the delivery suite. A 2.5 endotracheal tube is usually sufficient for most infants with the exception of the extremely low-birth-weight infant (Table 7.2). If a soft, flexible wire stylet is used to assist with endotracheal tube placement, it should not extend past the tip of the endotracheal tube, ensuring that the stylet does not harm the tracheal wall or carina.

For endotracheal intubation, the neonatal neck should be in a position of slight extension to provide a direct line of sight for visualization of the glottis. The simplest approach is to use a modest shoulder roll coupled by gentle extension at the neck. If the neck is hyperextended, the glottis is displaced anteriorly, hindering visualization of the glottis and placement of the endotracheal tube through the vocal cords (Fig. 7.7).

With the neonate in the proper position for intubation, a correctly sized straight blade for the infant's size, usually either a 0 or 1 blade, should be used. Prior to its use, check for adequate lumination.

The ability to visualize the glottis and vocal cords depends upon landmark recognition and proper neonatal positioning. Figure 7.8 demonstrates both positioning and possible corrective actions based on the landmarks visualized. If necessary, visualization of the anteriorly set glottis can be improved with gentle, downward pressure at the infant's cricoid cartilage either by the operator or by the assistant.

During the insertion of the endotracheal tube, direct visualization of both the glottis and tip of the tube should be maintained at all times. Simultaneously, the intubator should gently insert the tube through the vocal cords until the vocal cord guide (black line near the tip of the endotracheal tube) is at the level of the vocal cords. A tip to lip distance in centimeters should be used to estimate depth of placement (Table 7.3). As a general guideline, adding 6 cm to the number representing the weight of the infant in kilograms will provide a safe initial depth in centimeters from lip to tip.

Insertion of the endotracheal tube should be done quickly, and each attempt should usually last less than 20 seconds. Prolonged attempts at endotracheal intubation should be avoided. If intubation is not achieved, bag mask ventilation should be used between attempts and, if possible, the heart rate brought to above 100 bpm. For severely asphyxiated infants who may need prolonged positive-pressure ventilation, placement of an endotracheal tube is desirable at some time during the resuscitation because it is easier to ventilate the neonate.

When the tube is placed in the airway, a bag should be attached to the endotracheal tube and a series of breaths initiated. Endotracheal tube placement should initially be checked by auscultation of equal breath sounds on both sides of the chest. Further evidence of a properly placed endotra-

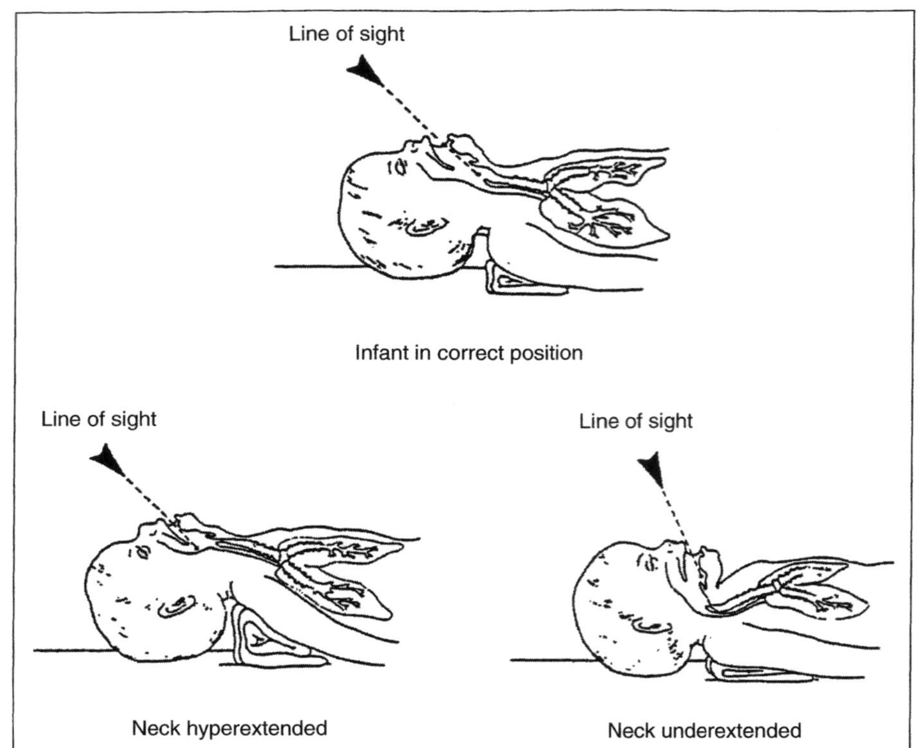

Fig. 7.7 Effects of flexion and hyperextension on ability to visualize the glottis. (Reproduced by permission from Textbook of Neonatal Resuscitation; p. 5–16; Elk Grove, IL; American Academy of Pediatrics/American Heart Association, 1994, rev. 1996.)

cheal tube is the presence of a gentle chest rise and the lack of significant auscultated gastric breath sounds or significant gastric distension.

Possible complications of endotracheal intubation include hypoxia, bradycardia, infection, and contusions or lacerations to the structures of the upper airway, including the vocal cords themselves. Rarely, the trachea or esophagus may become perforated. Of note, these complications can and do arise in the presence of an appropriately managed intubation.

Table 7.3 Endotracheal tube placement

Weight (kg)	Depth of insertion (cm from upper lip)
1	7*
2	8
3	9
4	10

* Infants weighing less than 750 g may require only 6 cm insertion. (Reproduced by permission from Textbook of Neonatal Resuscitation; 4th edn, p. 5–19; Elk Grove, IL; American Academy of Pediatrics/American Heart Association, 2000.)

Positive-pressure ventilation

Positive-pressure ventilation is used to establish the functional residual capacity (FRC), provide an adequate tidal volume and to halt any asphyxial process. Pressures ranging from 12 to 42 cmH_2O may be necessary depending on the health and maturity of the infant's lungs. Overexpansion of the lungs, when possible, should be avoided to potentially prevent volu- and barotrauma to the lungs (Hernandez et al., 1989; Carlton et al., 1990).

Although there is a split of opinion on how to accomplish this goal, current guidelines suggest that initial breaths be delivered with pressures of 30–40 cmH_2O which are sufficient to cause a gentle rise and fall of the chest. At times, however, the conventional recommendations for inspiratory pressures may not be sufficient. When this happens, a higher inspiratory pressure is medically necessary. After establishing an adequate FRC and tidal volume, inspiratory pressure requirements will drop (Upton & Milner, 1991). During positive-pressure ventilation, a rate of 40–60 breaths per minute is currently recommended.

With the initiation of positive-pressure ventilation, the assisting team member should monitor the quality and symmetry of breath sounds, chest expansion, and heart rate. To assist the clinician, Table 7.4 illustrates the common problems associated with inadequate chest expansion and potential corrective actions that can be easily performed in the delivery room.

Room air versus 100% oxygen

There is an emerging split of opinion whether to use room air or 100% oxygen during the resuscitation of asphyxiated

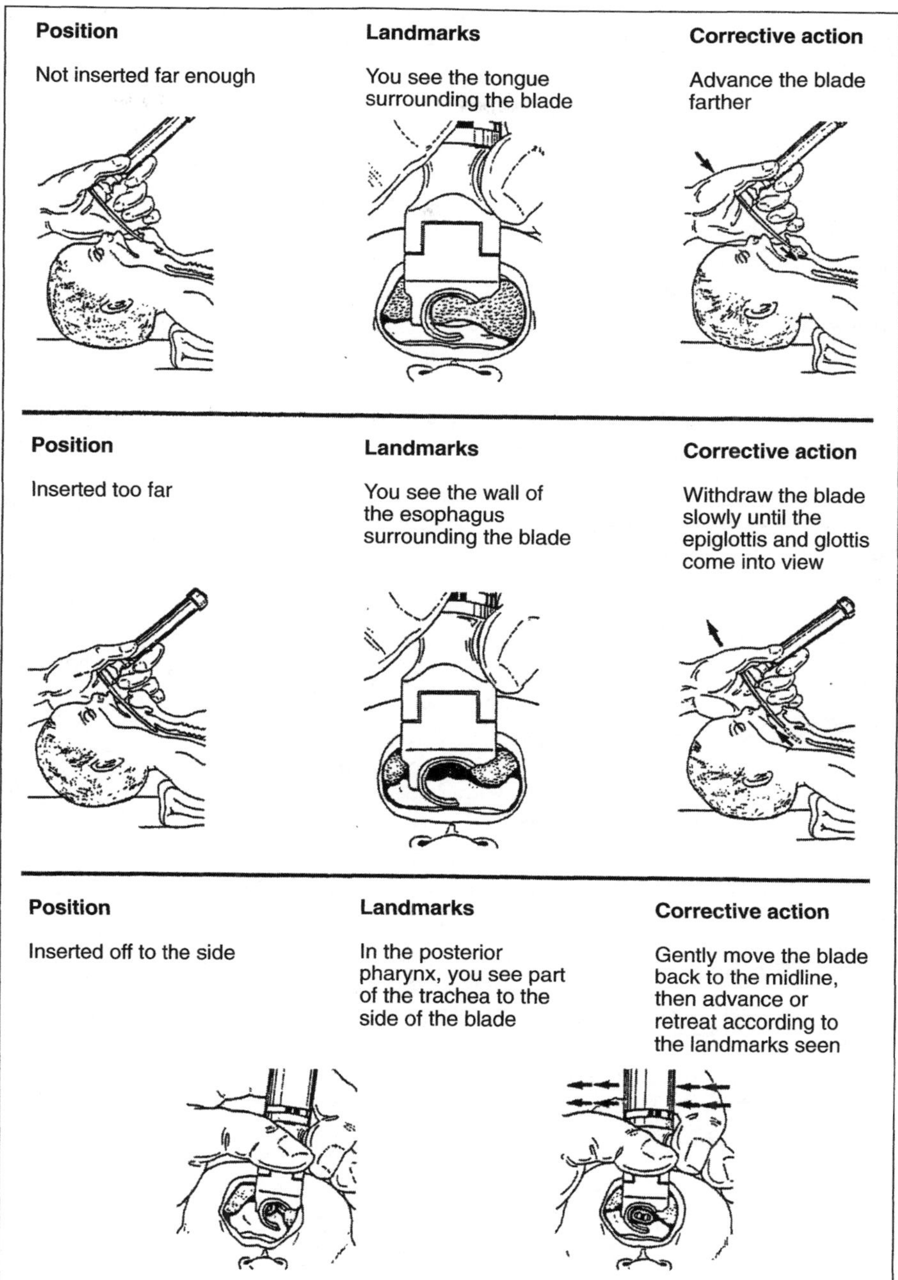

Fig. 7.8 Examples of incorrect positioning of laryngoscope and how to take corrective action. (Reproduced by permission from Textbook of Neonatal Resuscitation; p. 5–23; Elk Grove, IL; American Academy of Pediatrics/American Heart Association, 1994, rev. 1996.)

neonates. Resuscitation of the potentially asphyxiated infant with room air may provide potential benefits and may not be harmful. The concern is that oxygen administration may be harmful because the generation of oxygen free-radicals during the reperfusion phase of ischemic injury may be associated with increased damage (Rootwelt et al., 1980; Saugsta, 1990; Poulson et al., 1993). After a pilot study demonstrating no difference in neonatal outcomes with room air versus 100% oxygen (Ramji et al., 1993), a large multicenter controlled study of 609 infants found that the use of room air did not increase neonatal morbidity and mortality. Of note, there were no significant differences in mortality, incidence, and severity of hypoxic-ischemic encephalopathy, acid–base status, oxygen saturations, or arterial oxygen concentrations (Saugstad et al., 1998). At this time, both approaches appear to be equally efficacious.

Chest compressions

In the vast majority of compromised infants, positive-pressure ventilation alone is usually sufficient to overcome any bradycardia and lead to spontaneous respirations. If, however, after 30 seconds of ventilation with 100% oxygen, the newborn remains bradycardic, chest compressions will be needed to maintain systemic blood flow.

The American Heart Association/American Academy of Pediatrics currently recommends beginning chest compressions for a heart rate of less than 60 bpm. This can be accomplished with either the two finger or thumb methods (Fig. 7.9). With both methods, the lower third of the sternum is compressed. When performing the compressions, the resuscitator should be careful not to apply pressure to the xyphoid process. Thus, to find the lower third of the sternum, draw an imaginary line between the two nipples of the infant. This will demarcate the upper two-thirds from the lower third of the sternum. When conducting chest compressions with the thumb technique, the pressure is applied by encircling the chest with both hands and applying pressure with both thumbs over the lower third of the sternum. In contrast, two fingers are placed perpendicular to the chest and apply pressure over the lower third of the sternum (Todres & Rogers, 1975; David, 1988). During chest compressions, the goal is to generate a palpable pulse. Along with 90 compressions per minute, ventilation should be sufficient to produce 30 respirations per minute (American Heart Association/American Academy of Pediatrics, 2000).

Table 7.4 Problems associated with inadequate chest expansion

Problem	Correction
Inadequate face mask seal	Reapply mask to face Alter position of hand that holds mask
Blocked airway	Bag and mask: Check infant's position Suction mouth, oropharynx, and nose Insert oral airway if indicated (Pierre Robin, macroglossia) Bag and endotracheal tube: Suction the tube
Misplaced endotracheal tube	Remove endotracheal tube, ventilate with bag and mask, replace tube
Inadequate pressure	Increase pressure, taking care not to overexpand the chest; may require adjusting or overriding the pop-off valve

(Reproduced by permission from Neonatal-Perinatal Medicine: Diseases of the Fetus and Newborn; 7th edn; Editors: Faranoff, AA and Martin, RJ; p. 429, St Louis, Mosby, 2002.)

Simultaneous ventilation and compression (SVC/CPR) holds no advantage over interposing ventilations between compressions. But, there is the potential for compromise of neonatal tidal volumes and the need for higher ventilatory pressures. SVC/CPR increases the likelihood of inadequate gas exchange, increased gastric air accumulation and barotrauma (Rudikoff et al., 1980; Chandra et al., 1981; Swenson et al., 1988; Berkowitz et al., 1989; Krischer et al., 1989).

Intermittently, chest compressions should be stopped to check for a spontaneous heart rate. If the spontaneous heart rate is greater than 60 bpm, compressions may be stopped.

If well-coordinated chest compressions and ventilation do not raise the infant's heart rate above 60 bpm within 30 seconds, support of the cardiovascular system with medications is indicated.

Medications

Medications are indicated when, in the rare infant, positive-pressure ventilation and chest compressions fail to correct neonatal bradycardia. Depending upon the medication, it may be given via an umbilical venous catheter or endotracheal tube. Because of the potential for organ injury from infusion of medications, any concerns about the position of the umbilical catheter should prompt removal and reinsertion of the

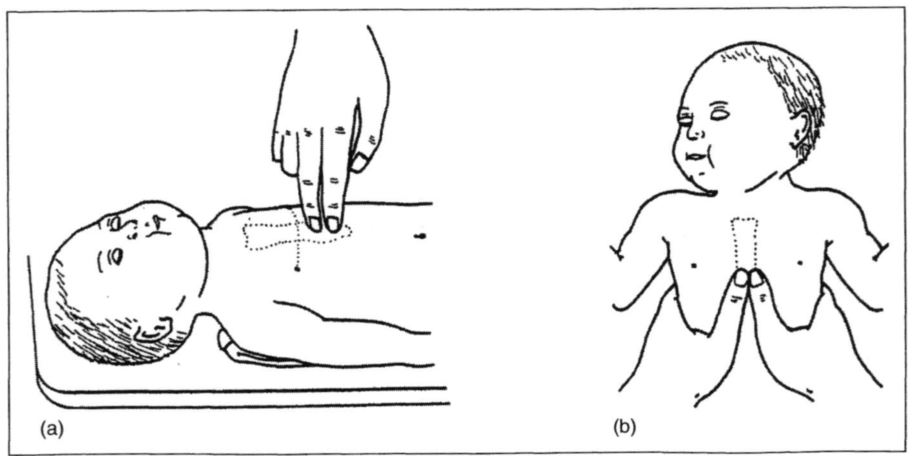

Fig. 7.9 Two methods of applying chest compression: (a) the two finger method; and (b) the thumb method (Reproduced by permission from Textbook of Neonatal Resuscitation; p. 4–12; Elk Grove, IL; American Academy of Pediatrics/American Heart Association, 1994, rev. 1996.)

catheter to the level of the skin. Table 7.5 presents an overview of the various resuscitative medications with their concentrations, dosages, routes of administration, and precautions.

Epinephrine

Epinephrine 1:10,000 (0.1–0.3 mL/kg) is the first-line agent for persistent bradycardia, and may be given via intravenous catheter or endotracheal tube. Epinephrine may be re-administered every 3–5 minutes as needed for any persistent bradycardia. Whether an increase in the standard intravenous (IV) epinephrine dosage should routinely be given when epinephrine is administered via the endotracheal tube (Quinton et al., 1987; Orlowski et al., 1990) remains uncertain. Thus, the current dosage recommendations for IV and endotracheal tube administration are the same. While higher doses of epinephrine have been used in pediatric (Goetting & Paradis, 1991) and adult (Paradis et al., 1991) resuscitations, there is concern about adverse outcomes among high-dose epinephrine recipients. Thus, routine use of higher epinephrine doses is not recommended.

Epinephrine has two effects on the cardiovascular system. First, via stimulation of the beta-1 adrenergic receptors, it has a direct effect on the heart. The second effect is to increase systemic vascular resistance via stimulation of alpha-1 adrenergic receptors. The increase in systemic vascular resistance increases blood flow to the coronary arteries, thus increasing myocardial oxygenation (Berkowitz et al., 1991). Animal models also suggest that metabolic acidosis significantly blunts the cardiac and peripheral vasculature response to epinephrine (Preziosi et al., 1993). Therefore, if epinephrine alone is ineffective, consideration should be given to the possibility of hypovolemic shock and/or significant metabolic acidosis.

Volume expanders

After administration of epinephrine, the infant with poor capillary refill, evidence or suspicion of acute blood loss, or other signs of hypovolemia should receive a volume expander. Infusion of volume expanders should consist of a volume of 10 mL/kg given over 5–10 minutes. If necessary, the infusion can be repeated. In the acute setting, isotonic normal saline is the volume expander of choice. A solution of 5% albumin does not appear to offer any advantage over normal saline and may make fluid retention more likely (Fleck et al., 1985; So et al., 1997).

The preferred volume expander, although rarely available, is whole O-negative blood cross-matched against the mother's blood. This provides volume, oxygen-carrying capacity, and colloid. In emergent circumstances, the blood from the freshly delivered placenta may be recovered and infused into the hypovolemic infant and is very rarely necessary. If this technique is used, sterile technique should be employed as soon as possible after the placenta is delivered. Withdrawing blood from the placenta requires a heparinized syringe attached to a filter to prevent microclots from entering the syringe. Before infusion of the blood back into the infant, the filter should be changed and the blood passed through a second filter to prevent the infusion of microclots into the infant.

Sodium bicarbonate

The use of sodium bicarbonate in the acute phase of a delivery room resuscitation should be discouraged. Since the initial acidosis may consist of both respiratory and metabolic components, the respiratory acidosis is more easily corrected with the establishment of adequate ventilation. Metabolic acidosis is best corrected by establishing adequate circulation and oxygenation and adequate fuel substrates. This physiologic approach will halt the production of additional anaerobic metabolites, lead to the breakdown of lactic acid and help clear the remaining metabolic acidosis.

Sodium bicarbonate is useful to correct persistent metabolic acidosis associated with prolonged resuscitation.

In the absence of adequate ventilation, the acute generation of carbon dioxide may be harmful because carbon dioxide permeates all biological membranes and will acutely lower the pH in all major organs, including the brain and heart (Bersin, 1992). If ventilation is inadequate, excess carbon dioxide will be generated. Thus, sodium bicarbonate is reserved, if at all, for neonates with adequate ventilation.

If sodium bicarbonate is required, the recommended dose is 2 mEq/kg. To avoid a sudden increase in osmolality, with its potential risk of intraventricular hemorrhage, the concentration of bicarbonate should be 0.5 mEq/mL, infused at a rate of no more than 1 mEq/kg/min. This would require approximately 2 minutes to infuse the dose. The rapid infusion of sodium bicarbonate is associated with an increased risk of intraventricular hemorrhage, especially in the preterm infant (Papile et al., 1978).

Dopamine

When the severely asphyxiated infant has poor cardiac output following initial resuscitative efforts, dopamine should be implemented at an intravenous infusion rate of 5 μg/kg/min, increasing, if necessary, to 20 μg/kg/min. If the dose of 20 μg/kg/min is reached without improvement, further increases in the infusion rate are unlikely to make a difference. By the time one has reached the point at which dopamine is needed, consultation with a neonatologist or pediatrician experienced in taking care of sick newborns would appear necessary.

The drug-depressed infant

Neonatal respiratory depression following inhalational

Table 7.5 Medications for neonatal resuscitation

Medication	Concentration to administer	Preparation	Dosage/route	Total dose/infant			Rate/precautions
				Weight		*Total dose*	
Epinephrine	1 : 10,000	1 mL	0.1–0.3 mL/kg IV or ET	1 kg		0.1–0.3 mL	Give rapidly
				2 kg		0.2–0.6 mL	May dilute with normal saline solution to 1–2 mL if giving ET
				3 kg		0.3–0.9 mL	
				4 kg		0.4–1.2 mL	
				Weight		*Total dose*	
Volume expanders	Normal saline solution Ringer's lactate solution Whole blood 5% albumin–saline solution	40 mL	10 mL/kg IV	1 kg		10 mL	Give over 5–10 min
				2 kg		20 mL	
				3 kg		30 mL	
				4 kg		40 mL	
				Weight	*Total dose*	*Total dose*	
Sodium bicarbonate	0.5 mEq/mL (4.2% solution)	20 mL or two 10 mL prefilled syringes	2 mEq/kg IV	1 kg	2 mEq	4 mL	Give *slowly*, over at least 2 min
				2 kg	4 mEq	8 mL	Give only if infant is being effectively ventilated
				3 kg	6 mEq	12 mL	
				4 kg	8 mEq	16 mL	
				Weight	*Total dose*	*Total dose*	
Naloxone hydrochloride	0.4 mg/mL	1 mL	0.1 mg/kg (0.25 mL/kg) IV, ET IM, SQ	1 kg	0.1 mg	0.25 mL	Give rapidly IV, ET preferred. IM, SQ acceptable
				2 kg	0.2 mg	0.50 mL	
				3 kg	0.3 mg	0.75 mL	
				4 kg	0.4 mg	1.00 mL	
	1.0 mg/mL	1 mL	0.1 mg/kg (0.1 mL/kg) IV, ET IM, SQ	1 kg	0.1 mg	0.1 mL	Do not give if mother is suspected of narcotic addiction or on methadone maintenance (may result in severe seizures)
				2 kg	0.2 mg	0.2 mL	
				3 kg	0.3 mg	0.3 mL	
				4 kg	0.4 mg	0.4 mL	
				Weight		*Total dose*	
Dopamine $\frac{6 \times \text{Weight (kg)} \times \text{Desired dose } (\mu g/kg/min)}{\text{Desired fluid (mL/hr)}}$ = mg of dopamine per 100 mL of solution			Begin at 5 μg/kg/min (may increase to 20 μg/kg/min if necessary) IV	1 kg		5–20 μg/min	Give as a continuous infusion, using an infusion pump
				2 kg		10–40 μg/min	Monitor heart rate and blood pressure closely
				3 kg		15–60 μg/min	Seek consultation
				4 kg		20–80 μg/min	

ET, endotracheal; IM, intramuscular; IV, intravenous; SQ, subcutaneous.
(Reproduced by permission from Textbook of Neonatal Resuscitation; p. 6–51; Elk Grove, IL; American Academy of Pediatrics/American Heart Association, 1994, rev. 1996.)

anesthetic during a cesarean or a narcotic analgesic less than 4 hours prior to birth is relatively uncommon. With inhalational anesthetics, adequate ventilation will effectively clear them from the infant. If a narcotic analgesic was administered less than 4 hours prior to delivery, naloxone (Narcan) can be useful in antagonizing the narcotic agent's respiratory depression. The standard dose is 0.1 mg/kg administered preferentially via umbilical venous catheter or endotracheal tube. Administration may also be intramuscularly or subcutaneously; but these routes may be associated with a lag between the time of the dose and its reversal effects. Repeated doses of Narcan may also be necessary because of its short duration of action. In infants of a mother addicted to narcotics, naloxone administration should be avoided because of the potential for acute withdrawal symptoms and seizures.

Immediate care after establishing adequate ventilation and circulation

Once an infant is stabilized after a resuscitation, the future course of ventilation is related to the degree of cardiorespiratory compromise. Many infants will quickly improve, developing good lung compliance, adequate pulmonary blood flow, and spontaneous respiratory drive. In these infants, assisted ventilation can be withdrawn in a matter of minutes. At the same time, some degree of inspired oxygen may be medically necessary to support the recovering term or preterm infant after an effective resuscitation.

Prolonged assisted ventilation

Prolonged ventilatory assistance is often linked to the time required to resume spontaneous respirations. Some asphyxiated infants, as well as premature infants, may also demonstrate some degree of lung disease and, hence, may require ventilatory assistance even after the resumption of spontaneous respirations. At times, infants with lung disease start out well on their own, but very shortly require ventilatory assistance, in the form of intermittent mechanical ventilation (IMV) or continuous positive airway pressure (CPAP), to maintain adequate ventilation and oxygenation. Whenever an infant requires prolonged ventilatory support, the infant should be in a center skilled at providing assisted ventilation to neonates.

Glucose

As soon as the neonatal resuscitation has been completed, a glucose infusion at a rate of 5 mg/kg/min may be necessary (approximately 80 ml/kg/day of 10% glucose) to help maintain neonatal glucose levels. Adjustments of the glucose infusion rate should be based on subsequent neonatal blood glucose measurements to avoid potential hypoglycemia.

Fluids

If a fetus undergoes "asphyxia", neonatal urine output should be carefully monitored. If oliguria is observed, fluids should be restricted until the neonate demonstrates adequate urine output. Under these circumstances and when glucose infusion is contemplated, the glucose infusion should be given in terms of milligrams per kilogram of body weight per minute, rather than in the amount of 10% glucose to be given. Thus, the concentration of glucose will depend on how much fluid can be given to the infant.

Feeding

During the asphyxial process, ischemia of the intestine may rarely occur as a result of vasoconstriction of the mesenteric blood vessels. Due to the association between gut ischemia and the development of necrotizing enterocolitis, enteral feeding of the asphyxiated infant may need to be withheld for a few days.

Other problems

Other complications of the postasphyxial infant include but are not limited to hypocalcemia, disseminated intravascular coagulation, seizures, cerebral edema, and intracerebral hemorrhage.

Special problems during resuscitation

Meconium aspiration

Meconium-stained amniotic fluid is the sign of the patent anus. Infants who pass meconium are at an increased risk of meconium aspiration syndrome. Aspiration of meconium into the lungs may create ball-valve obstructions throughout the lung, leading to possible air trapping and pneumothorax. Aspirated meconium may further create a reactive inflammation in the lungs that will hinder gas exchange and may be associated with persistent pulmonary hypertension. This perpetuates the fetal circulation pattern and further impairs ventilation and oxygenation of the infant.

Recommendations for neonatal management in cases of meconium-stained fluid have been changed to reflect the neonatal condition at birth and the need for tracheal suctioning (Wiswell et al., 2000). All infants born through thick or thin meconium-stained amniotic fluid should have their hypopharynx and nares suctioned on the perineum with delivery of the head. If the neonate is depressed direct tracheal suctioning should be done. Vigorous, term infants do not need to be handled in a special way.

To remove meconium from the trachea, an endotracheal tube is inserted into the trachea under direct visualization.

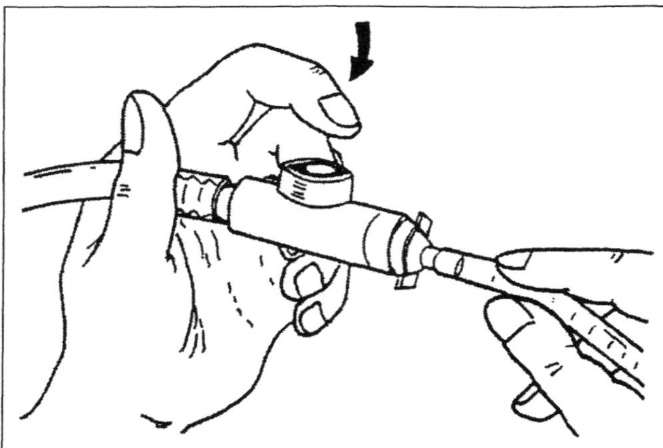

Fig. 7.10 Adapter to connect endotracheal tube to mechanical suction. (Reproduced by permission from Textbook of Neonatal Resuscitation; p. 5–68; Elk Grove, IL; American Academy of Pediatrics/American Heart Association, 1994, rev. 1996.)

An adapter attached to a regulated wall suction apparatus at approximately 100 mmHg is connected to the endotracheal tube as the tube is withdrawn (Fig. 7.10). The trachea can then be reintubated and suctioned again, if necessary. Because some infants with thick meconium-stained amniotic fluid may be severely asphyxiated, it may not be possible to clear the trachea completely before beginning positive-pressure ventilation. Clinical judgment will dictate the number of medically necessary reintubations.

Pneumothorax

Whenever positive-pressure ventilation is used, a pneumothorax, or popped lung, is a potential. A pneumothorax should be suspected in an improving infant that suddenly deteriorates. This complication may also present with unequal breath sounds and distant heart sounds or the heart sounds may be shifted to the other side of the chest. Clincially, the affected side may be slightly more distended and less mobile with ventilation than the unaffected side. Additional signs of pneumothorax include sudden oxygen desaturations and cyanosis. If the pleural air generates enough tension, cardiac venous return may be impaired. This may result in hypotension due to a significant drop in cardiac output.

Diaphragmatic hernia

Congenital diaphragmatic hernia undiagnosed prior to birth is an unusual but not an uncommon event in the contemporary practice of perinatal medicine. In any infant suspected of having a diaphragmatic hernia one should always use an endotracheal tube for ventilation to prevent gas from entering the intestines. An orogastric tube should be placed as soon as possible to remove as much air as possible from the intestines. Forcing air into the intestine with bag-and-mask positive-pressure ventilation increases the chances of inflating the intrathoracic bowel and further compromising pulmonary function.

Erythroblastosis/hydrops

The hydropic infant is likely to not only be severely anemic, but also to have marked ascites, pleural effusions, and pulmonary edema. These infants are also more likely to be asphyxiated in utero as well as to be born prematurely, adding respiratory distress syndrome to the list of complications. Thus, successful resuscitation of an infant with hydrops demands preparation and a coordinated team with preassigned responsibilities. The team should be prepared at delivery to perform a thoracentesis, paracentesis, and a complete resuscitation, in addition to a partial (or rarely, a complete) exchange transfusion, with O-negative blood cross-matched against the mother.

Establishment of adequate positive-pressure ventilation with immediate tracheal intubation is paramount. Poor lung compliance and marked pulmonary edema are the rule in this setting. High ventilatory pressures are commonly needed to recruit alveoli in the face of significant pulmonary edema. If adequate ventilation cannot be established and significant abdominal distension is noted, paracentesis with removal of significant ascites will often allow improved diaphragmatic excursion and improve ventilation and oxygenation. Consideration should be given to performing a thoracentesis for removal of significant pleural effusions if evidence for significant fluid accumulations exists. Information obtained from prenatal ultrasound examinations can help predict the amount of fluid present. Careful attention must be paid to the maintenance of intravascular volume and the prevention of shock, especially after the removal of large amounts of peritoneal or pleural fluid.

An hematocrit obtained in the delivery room will determine the need for an exchange transfusion (usually partial) in the delivery room. If the infant is extremely anemic and in need of immediate oxygen-carrying capacity, catheters should be inserted into both the umbilical artery and vein to permit a slow, isovolemic exchange with packed red cells. This should result in minimal impact on the hydropic infant's already tenuous hemodynamic status. These lines can also be transduced for central venous and central arterial pressures. Then, critical information for managing the hydropic infant's volume needs can be more easily accomplished. This information is even more essential if large fluid volumes are removed from either the chest or the abdomen.

Screening for congenital anomalies

Two to three percent of infants born will have a congenital anomaly that may require intervention soon after birth. Those that commonly require some form of immediate intervention include bilateral choanal atresia, congenital diaphragmatic hernia or aspiration pneumonia due to esophageal atresia or high intestinal obstruction. A rapid screen for congenital defects can easily be performed by the delivery room staff to help identify many of these defects which may require intervention.

External physical examination

A rapid external physical examination will identify obvious abnormalities such as abnormal facies and limbs, abdominal wall or spinal column defects. A scaphoid abdomen may indicate a diaphragmatic hernia, whereas a two-vessel umbilical cord would suggest the potential of latent congenital abnormalities.

Internal physical examination

Bilateral choanal atresia of the nares will present with respiratory distress and require a secure airway at birth. This defect can be quickly ruled in or out by assessing the infant's ability to breath with its mouth held closed. Some infants with unilateral choanal atresia will appear normal and only exhibit respiratory distress when the mouth is held closed and the patent nostril is occluded. The inability to insert a soft nasogastric tube with obstruction noted within 3–4 cm suggests possible choanal atresia.

Insertion of a nasogastric tube may help identify esophageal atresia or a high intestinal obstruction. If the tube does not reach the stomach, an esophageal atresia, commonly associated with a tracheoesophageal fistula, should be suspected. If the tube is in the correct position, a few milliliters of air forced through the tube into the stomach will be auscultated in the gastric area. Additionally, stomach contents may be aspirated. The presence of 15–20 mL of gastric contents on initial aspiration suggests a high intestinal obstruction. The same tube can then be removed and inserted into the anal opening. Easy passage of the tube for 3 cm into the anus makes anal atresia unlikely. A minute or so spent screening for congenital defects in this way may help avert many future problems.

References

Adamsons K, Behrman R, Dawes GS, James LS, Koford CO. Resuscitation by positive pressure ventilation and tris-hydroxymethylaminomethane of rhesus monkeys asphyxiated at birth. J Pediatr 1964;65:807.

Adamsons K, Gandy GM, James LS. The influence of thermal factors upon oxygen consumption of the newborn human infant. J Pediatr 1965;66:495.

American Heart Association / American Academy of Pediatrics. Textbook of Neonatal Resuscitation, 4th edn. Dallas: American Heart Association National Center, 2000.

Berkowitz ID, Chantarojanasiri T, Koehler RC, et al. Blood flow during cardiopulmonary resuscitation with simultaneous compression and ventilation in infant pigs. Pediatr Res 1989;26:558–564.

Berkowitz ID, Gervais H, Schleien CL, et al. Epinephrine dosage effects on cerebral and myocardial blood flow in an infant swine model of cardiopulmonary resuscitation. Anesthesiology 1991;75: 1041–1050.

Bersin RM. Effects of sodium bicarbonate on myocardial metabolism and circulatory function during hypoxia. In: Arieff AI, ed. Hypoxia, Metabolic Acidosis, and the Circulation. Oxford, UK: Oxford University Press, 1992.

Bruck K. Temperature regulation in the newborn infant. Biol Neonate 1961;3:65.

Carlton DP, Cummings JJ, Scheerer RG, et al. Lung overexpansion increases pulmonary microvascular protein permeability in lambs. J Appl Physiol 1990;69:577–583.

Chandra N, Weisfeldt ML, Tsitlik J, et al. Augmentation of carotid flow during cardiopulmonary resuscitation by ventilation at high airway pressure simultaneous with chest compression. Am J Cardiol 1981;48:1053–1063.

Cordero L Jr, Hon EH. Neonatal bradycardia following nasopharyngeal stimulation. J Pediatr 1971;78:441–447.

David R: Closed chest massage in the newborn infant. Pediatrics 1988;81:552–554.

Dawes GS. Birth asphyxia, resuscitation, brain damage. In: Foetal and Neonatal Physiology. Chicago: Year Book Medical, 1968:141.

Downing SE, Talner NS, Gardner TH. Influences of arterial oxygen tension and pH on cardiac function in the newborn lamb. Am J Physiol 1966;211:1203–1208.

Finer NN, Barrington KJ, Al-Fadley F, Peters KL. Limitations of self-inflating resuscitators. Pediatrics 1986;77:417–420.

Fleck A, Raines G, Hawker F, et al. Increased vascular permeability: A major cause of hypoalbuminemia in disease and injury. Lancet 1985;1:781–784.

Goetting MG, Paradis NA. High-dose epinephrine improves outcome from pediatric cardiac arrest. Ann Emerg Med 1991;20:22–26.

Hernandez LA, Peevy KJ, Moise AA, Parker JC. Chest wall restriction limits high airway pressure-induced lung injury in young rabbits. J Appl Physiol 1989;66:2364–2368.

International Guidelines for Neonatal Resuscitation: An excerpt from the Guidelines 2000 for cardiopulmonary resuscitation and emergency cardiovascular care: International Consensus on Science. Pediatrics 2000;106. Available at: http://www.pediatrics.org/cgi/content/full/106/3/e29.

Kanter RK. Evaluation of mask-bag-ventilation in resuscitation of infants. Am J Dis Child 1987;141:761–763.

Kattwinkel J, Niermeyer S, Nadkarni V, et al. ILCOR advisory statement: Resuscitation of the newly born infant. Pediatrics 1999;103(4):e56. Available at: http://www.pediatrics.org/cgi/content/full/103/4/e56.

Krischer JP, Fine EG, Weisfeldt ML, et al. Comparison of pre-hospital conventional and simultaneous compression-ventilation cardiopulmonary resuscitation. Crit Care Med 1989;17:1263.

Miller DL, Oliver TK Jr. Body temperature in the immediate neonatal period: The effect of reducing thermal losses. Am J Obstet Gynecol 1966;94:964–969.

Morin CM, Weiss KI. Response of the fetal circulation to stress. In: Polin RA, et al., eds. Fetal and Neonatal Physiology. Philadelphia: WB Saunders Co, 1992:620.

Orlowski JP, Gallagher JM, Porembka DT. Endotracheal epinephrine is unreliable. Resuscitation 1990;19:103–113.

Papile LA, Burstein J, Burstein R, et al. Relationship of intravenous sodium bicarbonate infusion and cerebral intraventricular hemorrhage. J Pediatr 1978;93:834–836.

Paradis NA, Martin GB, Rosenberg J, et al. The effect of standard- and high-dose epinephrine on coronary perfusion pressure during prolonged cardiopulmonary resuscitation. JAMA 1991;265:1139–1144.

Perlman JM, Risser R. Cardiopulmonary resuscitation in the delivery room: Associated clinical events. Arch Pediatr Adolesc Med 1995;149:20–25.

Poulson JP, Oyasaeter S, Saugstad OD. Hypoxanthine, xanthine, and uric acid in newborn pigs during hypoxemia followed by resuscitation with room air or 100% oxygen. Crit Care Med 1993;21:1058–1065.

Press S, Tellechea C, Pregen S. Cesarean delivery of full-term infants: Identification of those at high risk for requiring resuscitation. J Pediatr 1985;106:477–479.

Preziosi MP, Roig JC, Hargrove N, Burchfield DJ. Metabolic acidemia with hypoxia attenuates the hemodynamic responses to epinephrine during resuscitation in lambs. Crit Care Med 1993;21:1901–1907

Quinton DN, O'Byrne G, Aitkenhead AR. Comparison of endotracheal and peripheral intravenous adrenaline in cardiac arrest: Is the endotracheal route reliable? Lancet 1987;1:828–829.

Ramji S, Ahuja S, Thirupuram S, et al. Resuscitation of asphyxic newborn infants with room air or 100% oxygen. Pediatr Res 1993;34:809–812.

Rootwelt T, Loberg EM, Moen A, Oyasaeter S, Saugstad OD. Hypoxemia and reoxygenation with 21% or 100% oxygen in newborn pigs: Changes in blood pressure, base deficit, and hypoxanthine and brain morphology. Pediatr Res 1980;32:107–113.

Rudikoff MT, Maughan WL, Effron M, et al. Mechanisms of blood flow during cardiopulmonary resuscitation. Circulation 1980;61:345–352.

Rudolph AM, Yuan S. Response of the pulmonary vasculature to hypoxia and H+ ion concentration changes. J Clin Invest 1966;45:339–411.

Rudolph AM. Fetal cardiovascular response to stress. In: Wiknjosastro WH, et al., eds. Perinatology. New York: Elsevier Science, 1988.

Saugstad OD. Oxygen toxicity in the neonatal period. Acta Paediatr Scand 1990;79:881–892.

Saugstad OD, Rootwelt T, Aalen O. Resuscitation of asphyxiated newborn infants with room air or oxygen: An international controlled trial: The Resair 2 Study. Pediatrics 1998;102:e1. Available at: http://www.pediatrics.org/cgi/contnet./full/102/1/e1.

So KW, Fok TF, Ng PC, et al. Randomized controlled trial of colloid or crystalloid in hypotensive preterm infants. Arch Dis Child 1997;76:F43–46.

Swenson RD, Weaver WD, Niskanen RA, et al. Hemodynamics in humans during conventional and experimental methods of cardiopulmonary resuscitation. Circulation 1988;78:630–639.

Todres ID, Rogers MC. Methods of external cardiac massage in the newborn infant. J Pediatr 1975;86:781–782.

Upton CJ, Milner AD. Endotracheal resuscitation of neonates using a rebreathing bag. Arch Dis Child 1991;66:39–42.

Wiswell TC, Gannon CM, Jacob J, et al. Delivery room management of the apparently vigorous meconium-stained neonate: Results of the multicenter, international collaborative trial. Pediatrics 2000;105: 1–7.

8 Airway management in critical illness

Janice E. Whitty

Maternal mortality decreased from 15.3 to 7.8 per every 100,000 live births between 1975 and 1985. Currently, one of the most important remaining causes of maternal mortality is acute respiratory failure (Kaunitz et al., 1985; United States Public Health Service, 1988). Thromboembolism, amniotic fluid embolism, and venous air embolism together account for approximately 20% of maternal deaths. Other causes of respiratory failure probably account for a further 10–15% of maternal deaths (Kaunitz et al., 1985). Not only does maternal respiratory failure affect the mother but it also contributes to considerable fetal morbidity and mortality. The purpose of this chapter is to familiarize the reader with the general principles of airway management in the pregnant patient who has suffered acute respiratory failure, whatever the underlying etiology. To that end, we will present information to facilitate a timely recognition of respiratory compromise or failure. We will also discuss methods of respiratory support, including mechanical ventilation.

Respiratory failure

The respiratory system functions to ensure an adequate exchange of oxygen (O_2) and carbon dioxide (CO_2). When functioning adequately, this system both transfers enough oxygen to saturate the circulating hemoglobin, and eliminates adequate carbon dioxide to maintain a normal arterial pH. Respiratory failure results when either of these two endpoints of gas exchange is not met.

Hypoxemia results when the lungs fail to adequately exchange oxygen. Hypoxemia can be accompanied by either normocapnia or hypocapnia. Usually, if there is a failure of the ventilatory apparatus, this results in hypoventilation with accompanying hypercapnia and, to a lesser extent, hypoxemia. The most commonly encountered causes of acute respiratory failure in pregnancy are listed in Table 8.1. Hypoxemic respiratory failure is the most frequently seen of these. It should be remembered that respiratory failure in pregnancy results in decreased oxygen delivery not only to the mother, but also the fetus.

The normal respiratory changes that occur in pregnancy are presented in Table 8.2. The team caring for the pregnant patient with respiratory failure should keep these changes in mind when managing respiratory failure both during pregnancy, and in the postpartum period. These patients should be managed by a team that includes an obstetrician, an obstetric and/or medical intensivist, a neonatologist, and a skilled ICU nursing team. Additional consultation from other subspecialists should be obtained when appropriate, in order to optimize outcome for mother and fetus.

Ventilation/perfusion mismatch

Shunt (Q_S/Q_T)

A mismatch of ventilation to perfusion (V_A/Q) is a major cause of lung dysfunction (Demling & Knox, 1993). Oxygenation does not occur in an area of the lung without ventilation even in the face of normal perfusion. This perfused but nonventilated area of the lung is known as a shunt. The shunt fraction (Q_S/Q_T) is the total amount of pulmonary blood flow that perfuses nonventilated areas of the lung. In normal lungs, the value of the shunt fraction is 2–5% (Pontoppidan et al., 1972). A shunt of 10–15% is evidence of significant impairment in oxygenation. A shunt fraction ≥25%, in spite of therapy, suggests active adult respiratory distress syndrome (ARDS). Although, a true shunt does not respond to the administration of oxygen, most shunts are not the result of a total lack of ventilation, and therefore, some response to the administration of oxygen is usually seen (Demling & Knox, 1993). The causes of pulmonary shunting include alveolar consolidation or edema, alveolar collapse and atelectasis, and anatomic right to left shunt (e.g. thebesian veins, septal defects). The shunt fraction (Q_S/Q_T) can be calculated using the following formula:

$$Q_S/Q_T = C_cO_2 - C_aO_2/C_cO_2 - C_vO_2$$

C_cO_2 is the oxygen content of pulmonary capillary blood. C_aO_2 is the oxygen content of arterial blood and C_vO_2 is the oxygen content of mixed venous blood. The oxygen content of pulmonary capillary blood is approximated by the alveolar oxygen content. Therefore, administering an $F_{I}O_2$ of 1.0 (100%) simplifies the calculation of the shunt fraction (Demling & Knox, 1993).

Table 8.1 Causes of lung injury and acute respiratory failure in pregnancy

Hypoxic
Thromboembolism
Amniotic fluid embolism
Venous air embolism
Pulmonary edema
Aspiration of gastric contents
Pneumonia
Pneumothorax
Acute respiratory distress syndrome (ARDS)
Hypercapnic/hypoxic
Asthma
Drug overdose
Myasthenia gravis
Guillain–Barré syndrome

Dead space

When an area of the lung is ventilated but not perfused, it is referred to as dead space (Demling & Knox, 1993). The portion of tidal volume (V_t) that is dead space (V_d) is calculated as a ratio, V_d/V_t.

$$V_d/V_t = \frac{P_aCO_2 - PECO_2}{P_aCO_2} \quad (PECO_2 = \text{expired } CO_2)$$

Causes of increased dead space include shallow breathing, vascular obstruction, pulmonary hypertension, pulmonary emboli, low cardiac output, hypovolemia, ARDS, impaired perfusion, positive-pressure ventilation, and increased airway pressure. Acute increases in physiologic dead space significantly increase ventilatory requirements and may result in respiratory acidosis and ventilatory failure. Increased dead space may impose a higher minute ventilation and hence, work of breathing. A value of dead space to tidal volume ratio ≥0.6 usually requires mechanical ventilatory assistance (Demling & Knox, 1993).

Arterial oxygen tension (P_aO_2)

P_aO_2 is a measure of the amount of oxygen dissolved in plasma.

Table 8.2 Normal pulmonary values in pregnant and nonpregnant women

Term	Definition	Nonpregnant value	Pregnant value	Clinical significance in pregnancy
Tidal volume (V_T)	The amount of air moved in one normal respiratory cycle	450 mL	600 mL (increases up to 40%)	
Respiratory rate (RR)	Number of respirations per minute	16/min	Changes very little	
Minute ventilation	The volume of air moved per minute; product of RR and V_T	7.2 L	9.6 L (increases up to 40% because of the increase in V_T)	Increases oxygen available for the fetus
Forced expiratory volume in 1 second (FEV_1)		Approximately 80–85% of the vital capacity	Unchanged	Valuable to measure because there is no change due to pregnancy
Peak expiratory flow rate (PEFR)		30	Unchanged	Valuable to measure because there is no change due to pregnancy
Forced vital capacity (FVC)	The maximum amount of air that can be moved from maximum inspiration to maximum expiration	3.5 L	Unchanged	If over 1 L, pregnancy is usually well tolerated
Residual volume (RV)	The amount of air that remains in the lung at the end of maximal expiration	1,000 mL	Decreased by around 200 mL to around 800 mL	Improves gas transfer from alveoli to blood

(Reproduced by permission from ACOG Technical Bulletin: Pulmonary Disease in Pregnancy 1996;224:2.)

P_aO_2 determines the percent saturation of hemoglobin, which is the major factor in determining blood oxygen content. P_aO_2 changes with position and age, and is increased during pregnancy (Anderson et al., 1969; Templeton & Kelman, 1976). P_aO_2 is affected by pulmonary disorders that impair oxygen exchange. These include impaired diffusion, increased shunt, and ventilation perfusion mismatch. P_aO_2 is also affected by the degree of mixed venous oxygen saturation especially in the presence of an increased shunt (Demling & Knox, 1993). Hypercarbia also effects affects the P_aO_2 (especially when breathing room air), as CO_2 displaces oxygen.

Alveolar–arterial oxygen tension gradient

The alveolar–arterial oxygen tension gradient $[P_{(A-a)}O_2]$ is a sensitive measure of impairment of oxygen exchange from lung to blood (Demling & Knox, 1993). Alveolar–oxygen tension (P_AO_2) is estimated as:

$$P_AO_2 = (P_B - P_{H_2O}) \times F_IO_2 - P_aCO_2/RQ$$

P_B is barometric pressure, P_{H_2O} is water vapor pressure, and RQ is the respiratory quotient.

The alveolar–arterial oxygen tension gradient is equal to:

$$P_AO_2 - P_aO_2$$

Under the clinical circumstances where the P_AO_2 value is less than 60 mmHg, and especially when oxygen therapy is administered, it is acceptable to discount the respiratory quotient disparity and use the simplified version of the ideal alveolar gas equation:

$$P_AO_2 = [P_B - P_{H_2O}]F_IO_2 - P_aCO_2$$

This is best measured when the patient is breathing 100% oxygen (Demling & Knox, 1993). Under these circumstances, the alveolar–arterial oxygen tension gradient is a reflection of physiologic shunting in the lung. The normal alveolar–arterial oxygen tension gradient is less than 50 torr on when the F_IO_2 is 1.0 (less than 30 torr on room air).

Oxygen delivery and consumption

All tissues require oxygen for the combustion of organic compounds to fuel cellular metabolism. The cardiopulmonary system serves to deliver a continuous supply of oxygen and other essential substrates to tissues. Oxygen delivery is dependent upon oxygenation of blood in the lungs, the oxygen-carrying capacity of the blood, and the cardiac output (Barcroft, 1920). Under normal conditions, oxygen delivery (DO_2) exceeds oxygen consumption (VO_2) by about 75% (Cain, 1983).

$$DO_2 = CO \times C_aO_2 \times 10 \text{ (normal range} = 700\text{–}1{,}400\,\text{mL/min)}$$

Arterial oxygen content (C_aO_2) is determined by the amount of oxygen that is bound to hemoglobin (S_aO_2) and by the amount of oxygen that is dissolved in plasma ($P_aO_2 \times 0.0031$):

$$C_aO_2 = (\text{Hgb} \times 1.34 \times S_aO_2) + (P_aO_2 \times 0.0031)$$
$$\text{(normal range} = 16\text{–}22\text{ mL } O_2/\text{dL)}$$

It is clear from the above formula that the amount of oxygen dissolved in plasma is negligible (unless the patient is receiving hyperbaric oxygen therapy) and, therefore, the arterial oxygen content is largely dependent on the hemoglobin concentration and the arterial oxygen saturation. Oxygen delivery can be impaired by conditions that affect either cardiac output (flow), arterial oxygen content, or both (Table 8.3). Anemia leads to a low arterial oxygen content because of a lack of hemoglobin binding sites for oxygen. Carbon monoxide poisoning, likewise, will decrease oxyhemoglobin because of blockage of the oxygen binding sites. The patient with hypoxemic respiratory failure will not have sufficient oxygen available to saturate the hemoglobin molecule. Furthermore, it has been demonstrated that desaturated hemoglobin is altered structurally in such a fashion as to have a diminished affinity for oxygen (Bryan-Brown et al., 1973).

It must be kept in mind that the amount of oxygen actually available to the tissues is also affected by the affinity of the hemoglobin molecule for oxygen. Thus, the oxyhemoglobin dissociation curve (Fig. 8.1) and those conditions that influence the binding of oxygen either negatively or positively must be considered when attempts are made to maximize oxygen delivery (Perutz, 1978). An increase in the plasma pH level, or a decrease in temperature or 2,3-diphosphoglycerate (2,3-DPG) will increase hemoglobin affinity for oxygen, shifting the oxygen–hemoglobin dissociation curve to the left ("left shift") and resulting in diminished tissue oxygenation. If the plasma pH level falls or temperature rises, or if 2,3-DPG increases, he-

Table 8.3 Causes of impaired oxygen delivery

Low arterial oxygen content
Anemia
Hypoxemia
Carbon monoxide
Hypoperfusion
Shock
Hemorrhagic
Cardiogenic
Distributive
Septic
Anaphylactic
Neurogenic
Obstructive
Tamponade
Massive pulmonary emboli
Hypovolemia

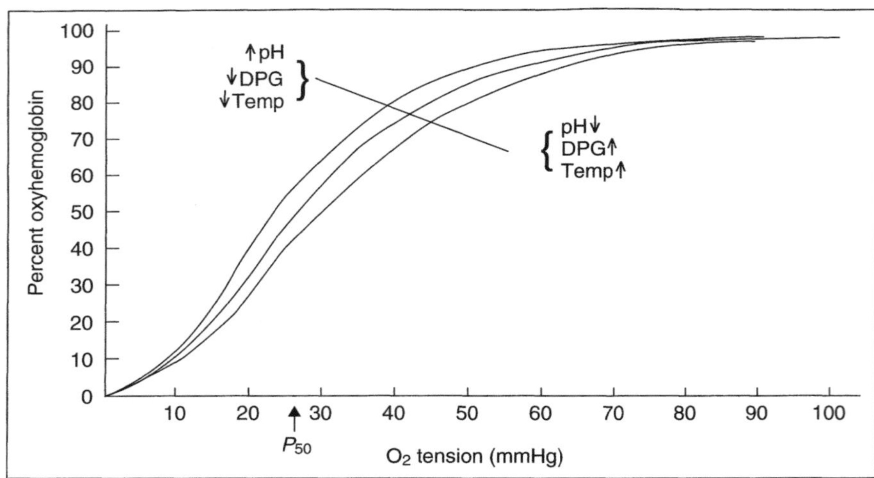

Fig. 8.1 The oxygen-binding curve for human hemoglobin A under physiologic conditions (middle curve). The affinity is shifted by changes in pH, diphosphoglycerate (DPG) concentration, and temperature, as indicated. P_{50} represents the oxygen tension at half saturation. (Reproduced by permission from Bunn HF, Forget BG: Hemoglobin: Molecular, Genetic, and Clinical Aspcets. Philadelphia, Saunders, 1986.)

moglobin affinity for oxygen will decrease ("right shift") and more oxygen will be available to tissues (Perutz, 1978).

In certain clinical conditions, such as septic shock and ARDS, there is maldistribution of blood flow relative to oxygen demand, leading to diminished delivery and consumption of oxygen. The release of vasoactive substances is hypothesized to result in the loss of normal mechanisms of vascular autoregulation, producing regional and microcirculatory imbalances in blood flow (Rackow & Astiz, 1991). This mismatching of blood flow with metabolic demand causes excessive blood flow to some areas, with relative hypoperfusion of other areas, limiting optimal systemic utilization of oxygen (Rackow & Astiz, 1991).

The patient with diminished cardiac output secondary to hypovolemia or pump failure is unable to distribute oxygenated blood to the tissues. Therapy directed at increasing volume with normal saline, or with blood if the hemoglobin level is less than 10 g/dL, increases oxygen delivery in the hypovolemic patient. The patient with pump failure may benefit from inotropic support and afterload reduction in addition to supplementation of intravascular volume. It is taken for granted that in such patients every effort is made to ensure adequate oxygen saturation of the hemoglobin by optimizing ventilatory parameters.

Relationship of oxygen delivery to consumption

Oxygen consumption (Vo_2) is the product of the arteriovenous oxygen content difference ($C_{a-v}o_2$) and cardiac output. Under normal conditions, oxygen consumption is a direct function of the metabolic rate (Shoemaker et al., 1989).

$$Vo_2 = C_{(a-v)}o_2 \times \text{CO} \times 10 \quad \text{(normal range} = 180\text{–}280\ \text{mL/min)}$$

The oxygen extraction ratio (OER) is the fraction of delivered oxygen that actually is consumed:

$$\text{OER} = Vo_2/Do_2$$

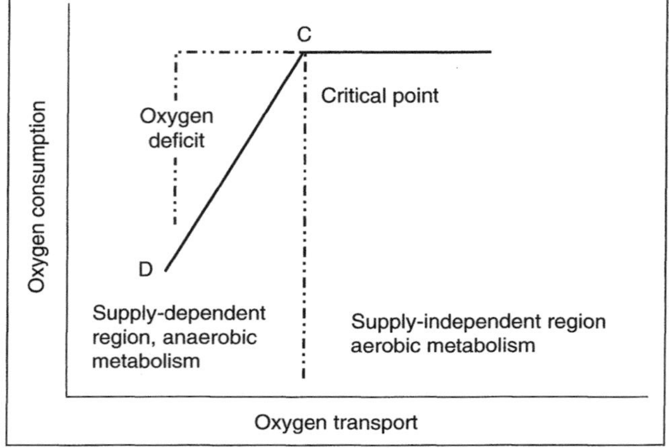

Fig. 8.2 The nonlinear relationship between oxygen transport and oxygen consumption is observed during carefully controlled animal experiments. (Reprinted by permission from Gutierrez G. Oxygen transport and consumption. Curr Pulmonol 1995;16:121–168.)

The normal oxygen extraction ratio is about 25%. A rise in OER is a compensatory mechanism employed when oxygen delivery is inadequate for the level of metabolic activity. A subnormal value suggests flow maldistribution, peripheral diffusion defects, or functional shunting (Shoemaker et al., 1989). As the supply of oxygen is reduced, the fraction extracted from the blood increases and oxygen consumption is maintained. If a severe reduction in oxygen delivery occurs, the limits of O_2 extraction are reached, tissues are unable to sustain aerobic energy production, and consumption decreases. The level of oxygen delivery at which oxygen consumption begins to decrease has been termed the "critical Do_2" (Shibutani et al., 1983; Gutierrez & Brown, 1995) (Fig. 8.2). At the critical Do_2, tissues begin to use anaerobic glycolysis, with resultant lactate production and metabolic acidosis (Shibutani et al., 1983). If this oxygen deprivation continues, irreversible tissue damage and death ensue.

Oxygen delivery and consumption in pregnancy

The physiologic anemia of pregnancy results in a reduction in the hemoglobin concentration and arterial oxygen content. Oxygen delivery is maintained at or above normal in spite of this because of the 50% increase that occurs in cardiac output. It is important to remember, therefore, that the pregnant woman is more dependent on cardiac output for maintenance of oxygen delivery than is the nonpregnant patient (Barron & Lindheimer, 1991). Oxygen consumption increases steadily throughout pregnancy and is greatest at term, reaching an average of 331 mL/min at rest and 1,167 mL/min with exercise (Pernoll et al., 1975). During labor, oxygen consumption increases by 40–60% and cardiac output increases by about 22% (Gemzell et al., 1957; Ueland & Hansen, 1969). Because oxygen delivery normally far exceeds consumption, the normal pregnant patient usually is able to maintain adequate delivery of oxygen to herself and her fetus even during labor. When a pregnant patient has a low oxygen delivery, however, she very quickly can reach the critical Do_2 during labor, compromising both herself and her fetus. Preeclampsia is known to significantly adversely affect oxygen delivery and consumption and this is believed to result from a tissue level disturbance that makes their oxygen consumption dependent on their oxygen delivery, i.e. there is loss of the normal reserve (Belfort et al., 1991, 1993).

The obstetrician, therefore, must make every effort to optimize oxygen delivery before allowing labor to begin in the compromised patient.

Assessing oxygenation

Arterial blood gases (ABG) are important for evaluating pH, arterial oxygen concentration, arterial carbon dioxide concentration, and oxygen saturation. Arterial blood gas values differ in pregnancy compared to nonpregnant values (ACOG, 1996) (Table 8.4). Interpreting the ABG is useful for identifying respiratory and metabolic derangements. Measured P_ao_2 is required for calculating $P_{(A-a)}o_2$. In addition, acid–base disturbances can be diagnosed (Shapiro et al., 1994). An indwelling arterial line is useful for obtaining arterial blood gas measurements and monitoring blood pressure when patients are receiving ventilatory support. However, arterial oxygen saturation can be assessed continuously and noninvasively by pulse oximetry. End tidal CO_2 can be measured noninvasively as well.

Table 8.4 Arterial blood gas values in the pregnant and nonpregnant woman

Status	pH	P_ao_2 (mmHg)	Pco_2 (mmHg)
Nonpregnant	7.4	93	35–40
Pregnant	7.4	100–105	30

Pulse oximetry

The oximetry system determines arterial oxygen saturation by measuring the absorption of selected wavelengths of light in pulsatile blood flow (New, 1985). Oxyhemoglobin absorbs much less red and slightly more infrared light than reduced hemoglobin. The degree of oxygen saturation of the hemoglobin thereby determines the ratio of red to infrared light absorption. Red and infrared light are detected from light-emitting diodes projected onto a photo detector across a pulsatile tissue bed with the absorption of each wavelength of the tissue bed varying cyclically with each pulse. The pulse rate is therefore also determined. When assessing the accuracy of the arterial saturation measured by the pulse oximeter, correlation of the pulse rate determined by the oximeter and the patient's heart rate is an indication of proper placement of the electrode. The sites usually used for measurement are the nail bed on the finger and the ear lobe. Most oximeters under ideal circumstances measure saturation (S_po_2) to within 2% of S_ao_2 (New, 1985).

Pulse oximetry is ideal for noninvasive monitoring of the arterial oxygen saturation near the steep portion of the oxygen hemoglobin dissociation curve, namely at a P_ao_2 of 70 torr (Demling & Knox, 1993). P_ao_2 levels >80 torr result in very small changes in oxygen saturation, namely 97–99%. Large changes in the P_ao_2 value in the range of 90 torr to a possible 600 torr can occur without significant change in arterial oxygen saturation (Fig. 8.1). This technique, therefore, is useful as a continuous monitor of the adequacy of blood oxygenation and not as a method to quantitate the level of impaired gas exchange.

Poor tissue perfusion, hyperbilirubinemia, and severe anemia may lead to oximetry inconsistencies (Demling & Knox, 1993). Carbon monoxide poisoning will lead to an overestimation of the P_ao_2. If methemoglobin levels reach greater than 5%, the pulse oximeter no longer accurately predicts oxygen saturation. The administration of methylene blue will also lead to oximetry inaccuracies.

Mixed venous oxygenation

The mixed venous oxygen tension (P_vo_2) and mixed venous oxygen saturation (S_vo_2) are parameters of tissue oxygenation (Shoemaker et al., 1989). Normally, the P_vo_2 is 40 mmHg with a saturation of 73%. Saturations less than 60% are abnormally low. These parameters can be measured directly by obtaining a blood sample from the distal port of the pulmonary artery catheter when the catheter tip is well positioned for a wedge pressure reading and the balloon is not inflated. The S_vo_2 also can be measured continuously with special pulmonary artery catheters equipped with fiberoptics.

Mixed venous oxygenation is a reliable parameter in the patient with hypoxemia or low cardiac output, but findings must be interpreted with caution. When the $S_{V}O_2$ is low, oxygen delivery can be assumed to be low. However, normal or high $S_{V}O_2$ does not guarantee that tissues are well oxygenated. In conditions such as septic shock and ARDS, the maldistribution of systemic flow may lead to abnormally high $S_{V}O_2$ in the face of severe tissue hypoxia (Rackow & Astiz, 1991). The oxygen dissociation curve must be considered when interpreting the $S_{V}O_2$ as an indicator of tissue oxygenation (Bryan-Brown et al., 1973) (Fig. 8.1). Conditions that result in a left shift of the curve cause the venous oxygen saturation to be normal or high, even when the mixed venous oxygen content is low. The $S_{V}O_2$ is useful for monitoring trends in a particular patient, as a significant decrease will occur when oxygen delivery has decreased secondary to hypoxemia or a fall in cardiac output.

Impairment of oxygenation

A decrease in arterial oxygen saturation ($P_{a}O_2$) below 90% is one definition of hypoxemia. However, the degree to which the alveolar–arterial oxygen tension gradient is increased is a more accurate measurement of the degree of impairment. A shunt of greater than 20% reflects respiratory failure. This degree of shunt will result in an alveolar–arterial oxygen tension gradient of greater than 400 torr (Demling & Knox, 1993). It is important to understand the interrelationship between shunt, the level of mixed venous oxygen saturation, and the arterial oxygen saturation. As more oxygen is extracted from the blood, the mixed venous oxygen saturation decreases resulting in a lower $P_{a}O_2$ (depending on the severity of the shunt). Therefore, a marked change in $P_{a}O_2$ can occur in the absence of any change in lung pathology (Demling & Knox, 1993).

Therapy

Hypoxemia is treated by increasing the fraction of inspired oxygen ($F_{I}O_2$) while at the same time attempting to correct the underlying problem. Processes causing increased shunt, such as atelectasis and bronchial pneumonia, can usually be treated effectively with pulmonary toilet, position change, and antibiotic therapy. Since a component of hypoxemia is often due to ventilation perfusion mismatching, an increase in $F_{I}O_2$ usually results in some improvement in oxygenation (Demling & Knox, 1993). Table 8.5 lists some available noninvasive oxygen delivery systems and approximate $F_{I}O_2$ obtained (Woodley & Whelan, 1993). When the shunt is large (>25%), $P_{a}O_2$ is not significantly improved by increasing $F_{I}O_2$. This clinical situation usually arises in processes such as ARDS or cardiogenic pulmonary edema. In this situation, mechanical ventilation is indicated.

Continuous positive airway pressure (CPAP)

Continuous positive airway pressure (CPAP) is the most widely used method of noninvasive positive pressure ventilatory support. This method consists of a continuous high flow

Table 8.5 Oxygen delivery systems

Type	$F_{I}O_2$ capability	Comments
Nasal cannula		
Standard	True $F_{I}O_2$ uncertain and highly dependent on inspiratory flow rate	Flow rates should be limited to <5 L/min
Reservoir type	True $F_{I}O_2$ uncertain and highly dependent on inspiratory flow rate	Severalfold less flow required than with standard cannula
Transtracheal cannula	$F_{I}O_2$ less dependent on inspiratory flow rate	Usual flow rates of 0.25–3.0 L/min
Ventimask	Available at 24, 28, 31, 35, 40, and 50%	Less comfortable, but provides a relatively controlled $F_{I}O_2$. Poorly humidified gas at maximum $F_{I}O_2$
High humidity mask	Variable from 28 to nearly 100%	Levels >60% may require additional oxygen bleed-in. Flow rates should be 2–3 times minute ventilation. Excellent humidification
Reservoir mask		
Nonrebreathing	Not specified, but about 90% if well fitted	Reservoir fills during expiration and provides an additional source of gas during inspiration to decrease entrainment of room air
Partial rebreathing	Not specified, but about 60–80%	
Face tent	Variable; same as high humidity mask	Mixing with room air makes actual O_2 concentration inspired unpredictable
T-tube	Variable; same as high humidity mask	For spontaneous breathing through endotracheal or tracheostomy tube. Flow rates should be 2–3 times minute ventilation

of gas and an expiratory resistance valve attached to a tight fitting mask. Airway pressure in CPAP is consistently higher than atmospheric pressure even though all of the patient's breaths are spontaneous. The best CPAP level is one in which oxygenation is adequate and there is no evidence of depressed cardiac function and carbon dioxide retention. CPAP prevents the development of alveolar collapse and increases the pressure in the small airways (including those in which the critical closing pressure has been elevated) thus increasing functional residual capacity. CPAP has the advantage of convenience, lower cost, and morbidity sparing potential when compared with standard invasive positive pressure ventilation. Unfortunately, CPAP also suffers from some disadvantages (i.e. a heightened risk of volu-trauma and hypotension). An additional problem is the potential for developing pressure sores from the tight fitting mask (Meyer & Hill, 1994).

Noninvasive positive pressure ventilation

Another type of noninvasive ventilation is called noninvasive positive pressure ventilation. It differs from CPAP, which does not provide ventilatory assistance, but instead applies a sustained positive pressure. Noninvasive positive pressure ventilation on the other hand delivers intermittent positive airway pressure through the upper airway and actively assists ventilation (Meyer & Hill, 1994).

Noninvasive positive pressure ventilation requires patient cooperation (Carrey et al., 1990). Patients must learn to coordinate their breathing efforts with the ventilator so that spontaneous breathing is assisted even during sleep. This type of ventilatory assistance is particularly efficacious in treating patients with chronic obstructive sleep apnea.

Noninvasive approaches have been most effective for managing episodes of acute respiratory failure in which rapid improvement is expected such as during episodes of cardiogenic pulmonary edema or acute exacerbations of chronic obstructive pulmonary disease (COPD). Selection guidelines for noninvasive positive pressure ventilation in acute respiratory failure are presented in Table 8.6.

Table 8.6 Selection guidelines for noninvasive positive pressure ventilation use in acute respiratory failure

Respiratory failure or insufficiency without need for immediate intubation with the following:
Acute respiratory acidosis
Respiratory distress
Use of accessory muscles or abdominal paradox
Cooperative patient
Hemodynamic stability
No active cardiac arrhythmias or ischemia
No active upper gastrointestinal bleeding
No excessive secretions
Intact upper airway function
No acute facial trauma
Proper mask fit achieved

(Reproduced by permission from Meyer TJ, Hill NS. Non-invasive positive pressure ventilation to treat respiratory failure. Ann Intern Med 1994;120:760.)

The pregnant patient suffering hypoxemia may respond positively to initial intervention with noninvasive means of increasing $F_{I}O_2$. However, clinical deterioration can be acute. Therefore, these gravida require intense surveillance with frequent evaluation of clinical status, S_pO_2 or S_aO_2. If viable (⩾24 weeks), the fetal status should be assessed frequently as well. This can be accomplished with continuous electronic fetal heart rate monitoring, or intermittent nonstress testing or biophysical profile scoring as appropriate.

Mechanical ventilatory support in pregnancy

Clinical recognition of the gravida who is experiencing respiratory failure and needs mechanical ventilation is extremely important, because maternal and fetal reserve is likely impaired in the gravida who has been hypoxic. This is particularly important for the laboring patient, who may rapidly reach the "critical DO_2" level, i.e. that point at which oxygen consumption becomes directly dependent on oxygen delivery.

In addition to the parameters noted in Table 8.7, the onset of changes in the fetal heart rate pattern consistent with hypoxemia may signal respiratory failure in the pregnant patient. These fetal heart rate patterns include persistent late decelerations, tachycardia, bradycardia, and absent beat-to-beat variability (Freeman et al., 1991). One should not intervene on behalf of the fetus unless the maternal condition is stabilized. Intervention, in an unstable hypoxemic gravida, may lead to increased morbidity or even mortality for the patient as well as her fetus. One should also recognize that stabilization of the gravida and the institution of mechanical ventilatory support will likely rescue the fetus as well. However, if maternal death appears iminent or cardiac arrest unresponsive to resuscitation occurs, the potentially viable fetus (⩾24 weeks) should be delivered abdominally within 5 minutes. In this situation, delivery may actually improve maternal survival (Katz et al., 1986).

Intubation

In general, indications for intubation and mechanical ventilation do not vary with pregnancy. However, because of the reduced PCO_2 seen in normal pregnancy, intubation may be indicated once the PCO_2 reaches 35–40 mmHg since this may signal impending respiratory failure (especially in a patient with asthma). In addition to the criteria in Table 8.7, one should

Table 8.7 Definition of acute respiratory failure

Parameter	Normal range	Indication for ventilatory assistance
Mechanics		
Respiratory rate (breaths/min)	12–20	>35
Vital capacity (mL/kg body weight)*	65–75	<15
Inspiratory force (cmH_2O)	–(75–100)	<–25
Compliance (mL/cmH_2O)	100	<25
FEV_1 (mL/kg body weight)*	50–60	<10
Oxygenation		
P_ao_2† (torr)	80–95	<70
(kPa)	10.7–12/7	<9.3
$P_{(A-a)}o_2$‡ (torr)	25–50	>450
(kPa)	3.3–6.7	>60
Q_S/Q_T (%)	5	>20
Ventilation		
P_aco_2 (torr)	35–45	55§
(kPa)	4.7–6.0	7.3
V_D/V_T	0.2–0.3	0.60

FEV_1, forced expiratory volume in 1 min; $P_{(A-a)}o_2$, alveolar–arterial oxygen tension gradient; Q_S/Q_T, shunt fraction; V_D/V_T, dead space to tidal volume ratio. * Use ideal body weight; † room air; ‡ $F_io_2 = 1.0$; § exception is chronic lung disease.

(Reproduced by permission from Van Hook JW: Ventilator therapy and airway management, Crit Care Obstet 1997, 8:143.)

include: apnea, upper airway obstruction, inability to protect the airway, respiratory muscle fatigue, mental status deterioration, and hemodynamic instability.

Intubation of the pregnant patient should be accomplished by skilled personnel. Intubation in pregnancy differs somewhat from that of nonpregnant patients. Pregnancy, particularly at term, has been associated with slow gastric emptying and increased residual gastric volume (Sutherland et al., 1986). This implies a slightly increased risk of aspiration of gastric contents during intubation of the gravid patient. The use of sodium bicarbonate preoperatively neutralizes gastric contents (Gibbs & Banner, 1984). This should be administered prior to intubation if possible. In addition, intubation should proceed using techniques that preserve airway reflexes (e.g. awake intubation). Alternatively, use of an "in rapid sequences," induction of general anesthesia and Sellick's maneuver (cricoid pressure) may be employed to prevent passive reflex of gastric contents into the pharynx (Sellick, 1961). Another difference is that hyperemia associated with pregnancy can narrow the upper airways sufficiently so that patients are at increased risk for upper airway trauma during intubation (Cheek & Gutsche, 1987). Relatively small endotracheal tubes may be required (6–7 mm). Nasal tracheal intubation should probably be avoided as well unless no other way to secure an airway is available.

Decreased functional residual capacity in pregnancy may lower oxygen reserve such that, at the time of intubation, a short period of apnea may be associated with a precipitous decrease in the Po_2 (Cheek & Gutsche, 1987). Therefore, 100% oxygen should be administered either by mask or by ambubag when the patient requires intubation. Over-enthusiastic hyperventilation should be avoided because the associated respiratory alkalosis may actually decrease uterine blood flow. In addition, if ambubreaths are given with too high a pressure, the stomach will fill with air and increase the risk of aspiration. In cases where intubation is not successful after 30 seconds, one should stop and resume ventilation with bag and mask prior to repeating the attempt in order to avoid prolonged hypoxemia (Deem & Bishop, 1995). Once the patient is intubated, the cuff should be inflated and the patient should be ventilated with the ambubag while auscultation over the chest and stomach is performed to ensure proper endotracheal tube placement. In addition, a chest X-ray should be ordered for confirmation of tube placement. Complications of endotracheal intubation are listed in Table 8.8.

The recommended initial ventilator settings are: F_Io_2: 0.9–1 and rate of 12–20 breaths per minute. Traditionally, a tidal volume (V_T) of 10–15 mL/kg was recommended. It has recently been recognized that these volumes result in abnormally high ariway pressures and volu-trauma. Therefore V_T should be instituted at 5–8 mL/kg to prevent excessive alveolar distention (Bidani et al., 1994; Baudouin, 2001; Brower et al., 2001).

Traditional ventilator modes

Controlled mechanical ventilation

When controlled mechanical ventilation (CMV) is instituted, the patient makes no effort and the ventilator assumes all respiratory work by delivering a preset volume of gas at a preset rate (Hinson & Marini, 1992). This mode of mechanical ventilation is typically used during general anesthesia, certain drug overdoses, in coma, and when paralytic agents and sedation are used.

Assist control

In assist control (A/C) mode (Fig. 8.3), every inspiratory effort by the patient triggers a ventilator delivered breath at the selected tidal volume (Hinson & Marini, 1992). Controlled ventilator initiated breaths are automatically delivered when the spontaneous rate falls below a selected back-up rate. All breaths are delivered by the ventilator, therefore the work of breathing is minimized in this mode. Because a full selected tidal volume is delivered with each inspiratory effort initiated by the patient, respiratory alkalosis may develop in patients with tachypnea. Patients with rapid shallow respiration may

Table 8.8 Complications of endotracheal intubation

During intubation: immediate
Failed intubations
Main stem bronchial or esophageal intubation
Laryngospasm
Trauma to naso/oropharynx or larynx
Perforation of trachea or esophagus
Cervical spine fracture
Aspiration
Bacteremia
Hypoxemia/hypercarbia
Arrhythmias
Hypertension
Increased intracranial/intraocular pressure
During intubation: later
Accidental extubation
Endobronchial intubation
Tube obstruction or kinking
Aspiration, sinusitis
Tracheoesophageal fistula
Vocal cord ulcers, granulomata
On extubation
Laryngospasm, laryngeal edema
Aspiration
Hoarseness, sore throat
Non-cardiogenic pulmonary edema
Laryngeal incompetence
Swallowing disorders
Soreness, dislocation of jaw
Delayed
Laryngeal stenosis
Tracheomalacia/tracheal stenosis

(Modified from Stehling LC. Management of the airway. In: Barash PG, Cullen BF, Stoelting RK, eds. Clinical Anesthesia, 2nd edn. Philadelphia: JB Lippincott, 1992: 685–708.)

generate very high intrathoracic pressure with consequent baro-trauma resulting from attempts to exhale during a ventilator-driven inflation cycle.

Intermittent mandatory ventilation

During intermittent mandatory ventilation (IMV), the patient can breathe at a spontaneous rate and tidal volume without triggering the ventilator (Hinson & Marini, 1992). In addition, the ventilator adds mechanical breaths at a preset rate and tidal volume. Potential advantages of IMV included less respiratory alkalosis, fewer adverse cardiovascular effects of mechanical ventilation because of lower intrathoracic pressures, less requirement for sedation or paralysis, maintenance of respiratory muscle function, and facilitation of weaning. However, there is little scientific support for these proposed advantages. Potential disadvantages of IMV include a lack of response to increased ventilatory demand, increased work of breathing, potential respiratory muscle fatigue, and inappropriately prolonged weaning. The amount of respiratory work varies inversely with the ventilator rate in IMV.

Synchronized intermittent mandatory ventilation

Synchronized intermittent mandatory ventilation (SIMV) (Fig. 8.3) incorporates a demand valve that must be patient activated with each spontaneous breath and that allows a mechanical breath to be delivered in concert with the patient's effort (Hinson & Marini, 1992). In most ventilators, the opening of the demand valve is triggered by a fall in pressure. Once the preset pressure of flow sensitivity is reached, the ventilator adds fresh gas into the circuit to meet the patient's ventilatory demand. Since machine and patient breaths are better synchronized, SIMV promotes greater patient comfort and tolerance and avoids high airway pressures. The SIMV system has a major drawback in that the work of breathing is increased. This increase in the work of breathing is due to the large airway pressure drop required to open the demand valve. Additional potential problems are the time delay between the initiation of a breath and the delivery of the fresh gas and insufficient fresh gas flows to meet the patient's ventilatory demands.

New ventilator modes

Because of limitations of the traditional forms of mechanical ventilation, alternative modes have been developed. Management of severe ARDS, which entails extremely noncompliant lungs with extensive shunting, has been particularly challenging (Kollef & Schuster, 1985).

Inverse ratio ventilation

Conventional mechanical ventilation devotes approximately one-third of the respiratory cycle to inspiration and two-thirds to expiration. In contrast, this ratio (I : E) is reversed in inverse ratio ventilation (IRV). The objective of IRV is to achieve better oxygenation as a result of higher mean alveolar, pressure and volume. In IRV, inspiration is set at equal or longer duration than expiration. This results in slower inspiratory flow for a given tidal volume and therefore lower peak airway pressures (Lain et al., 1989). This type of ventilation is desirable in patients with ARDS who are experiencing worsening compliance and refractory hypoxemia. Growing clinical experience with IRV suggests that it can be useful in improving gas exchange in patients with ARDS whose oxygenation cannot be maintained with more conventional approaches. In this type of ventilatory mode, oxygenation is improved as atelectatic areas are recruited and maintained as functional units, thereby lowering the dead space to tidal volume ration. Lower peak

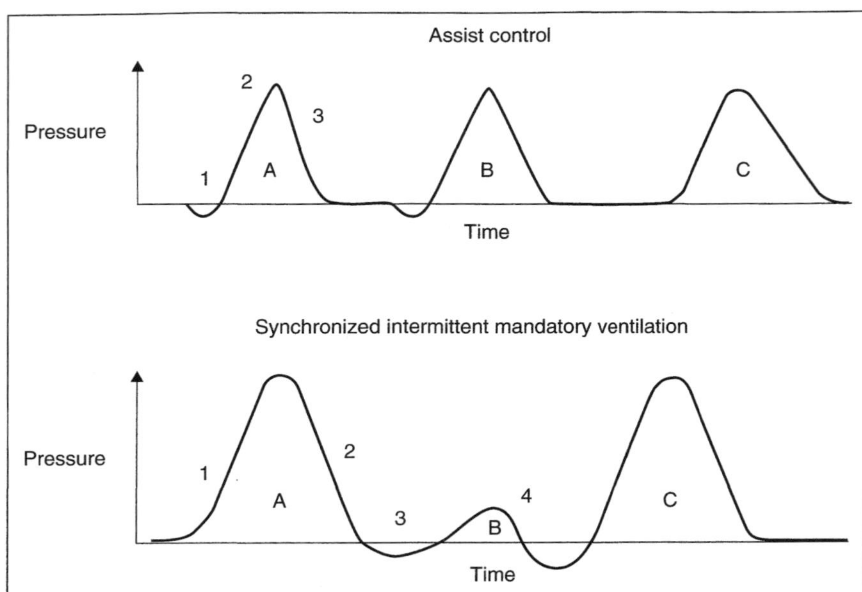

Fig. 8.3 Modes of ventilation. *Assist Control*: 1, patient initiation of breath; 2, inspiration; 3, expiration; A, B, patient-triggered breaths; C, machine-triggered breaths. *Synchronized intermittent mandatory ventilation*: 1, machine breath inspiration; 2, machine breath expiration; 3, spontaneous inspiration; 4, spontaneous expiration; A, B, patient-triggered breaths; C, synchronized machine breath.

airway pressures reduce the volu-trauma involved with increasing peak airway pressure.

There are a number of drawbacks associated with IRV (Tharratt et al., 1988). It is a very unpleasant mode of ventilation necessitating both sedation and paralysis when used in nonanesthetized patients. Neuromuscular blockade during the management of respiratory failure is occasionally associated with prolonged weakness and paralysis (Douglass et al., 1992; Segredo et al., 1992). Also, expiratory time is encroached upon and air trapping and hyperinflation may occur which may result in volu-trauma or hemodynamic compromise secondary to increased intrathoracic pressure (Biddle, 1993).

Airway pressure release ventilation

In airway pressure release ventilation (APRV), the patient receives continuous positive airway pressure ventilation that intermittently decreases pressure from the preset value to a lower value as the airway pressure release valve opens (Stock et al., 1987). Mean airway pressure is thereby lowered during an assisted breath. As in IRV, the I : E ratio is inverted in APRV. This mode of ventilation is most effective in a primary crisis of oxygenation, in which ventilatory requirements are not the overriding problem. The theoretical utility of this strategy is based upon its ability to augment alveolar ventilation as well as opening, recruiting, and stabilizing previously collapsed alveoli without risk of volu-trauma or detriment to the cardiac output (Stock et al., 1987). Limited human trials that have been performed have shown that peak airway pressures tend to be only 50% of those seen with conventional, mechanical ventilation, while oxygenation and CO_2 removal are highly satisfactory (Rasanen et al., 1991). Reported clinical experience with this mode for treatment in ARDS, however, is limited.

Pressure support ventilation

Pressure support ventilation (PSV) (Fig. 8.4) is used in awake patients who are assuming part of the work of breathing. In PSV, the ventilator provides a preset level of positive pressure in response to the patient's inspiratory effort (MacIntyre et al., 1990). Thus, PSV augments the patient's inspiratory effort with a pressure assist. A preselected pressure is held constant by gas flow from the ventilator for the duration of the patient's inspiratory effort. Passive exhalation ensues when the patient's inspiratory demand for flow diminishes to 25% of what the maximum flow was. Pressure support ventilation is designed principally to reduce the work of breathing in a spontaneously breathing patient (Brochard et al., 1989). This allows for a larger tidal volume at a given level of work. This particular type of assisted ventilation may be especially useful for patients who have a small diameter endotracheal tube in place and it helps reduce the fatigue often experienced with weaning from mechanical ventilation. Keep in mind that PSV differs from assist control ventilation in that there is no set machine rate of tidal volume. Since the patient decides the rate, and the tidal volume is determined by the amount of inflation pressure generated by the machine and the patient together, this modality may deliver a variable minute ventilation in a patient with an unreliable respiratory drive.

Proportional assist ventilation

Proportional assist ventilation (PAV) is a recent and promising development (Younes et al., 1987). As with PSV, inspiratory efforts from an awake patient are required. In contrast to PSV, PAV provides inspiratory assistance that is proportional to the

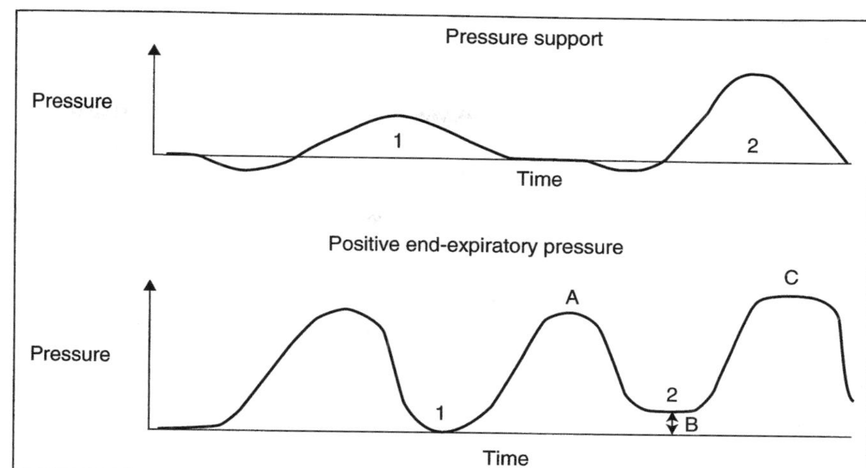

Fig. 8.4 *Pressure support*: 1, SIMV breath (pressure support off); 2, SIMV breath (pressure support on). *Positive end-expiratory pressure*: 1, PEEP off; 2, PEEP on; pressure at C = pressure A + pressure B (refer to text).

amount of patient effort. This should result in better and more comfortable patient–machine interaction.

High frequency ventilation

In an effort to minimize airway pressure during mechanical ventilation, several approaches employ rates much higher than those normally seen with spontaneous breathing. High frequency jet ventilation is the most extensively standardized mode of high frequency ventilation (Lunkenheimer et al., 1994). This form of mechanical ventilation is characterized by the administration of small tidal volumes (2–5 mL / kg) at rates of 100–200 jets / minute. The jet entrains gas from a secondary supply source of room air. There are some potential problems with this form of ventilation. The I : E ratio is altered from 1 : 4 to 1 : 2. The alteration in the I : E ratio may impair CO_2 removal. In addition, decreases in expiratory time can result in air stacking and volu-trauma can result if outflow is obstructed. An additional problem with the use of jet ventilation is that clinical experience is extremely limited and therefore there are not any typical reliable guidelines that can be used in the management of patients being ventilated with this modality applicable to pregnant patients (Lunkenheimer et al, 1994). There is only one report describing the use of high frequency jet ventilation in pregnancy, a patient who was managed with high frequency ventilation in late pregnancy secondary to respiratory failure from pneumonia and asthma. This patient, who had respiratory failure secondary to asthma and pneumonia, was managed with a combination of high frequency assist ventilation and intermittent positive pressure ventilation (Raphael & Bexton, 1993). The outcome in this particular case was good. However, high frequency ventilation should be employed with caution as reported experience in intensive care medicine has shown that jet ventilation is not consistently superior to conventional mechanical ventilation (Carlon et al., 1983).

Positive end-expiratory pressure

Critically ill patients with oxygenation problems, such as those with ARDS, frequently respond to the addition of positive end-expiratory pressure (PEEP) to a conventional method of ventilation, such as assist control (Shapiro et al., 1984) (Fig. 8.4). Increased end-expiratory pressure is produced by placing a threshold resistor in the exhalation limb of the breathing circuit. Expiratory flow is unimpeded so long as expiratory pressure exceeds an arbitrary limit. Gas flow ceases when pressure reaches the predetermined value, thereby resulting in maintenance of PEEP without impedance of expiratory gas flow (Shapiro et al., 1984).

PEEP enhances oxygenation in patients by alleviating the V/Q inequality (Ralph et al., 1985). This is accomplished principally by an increase in the functional residual capacity (FRC). PEEP may increase the FRC by lying direct increases in alveolar volume when PEEP up to 10 cmH_2O, is applied to normal alveoli. PEEP also recruits and re-expands alveoli that have previously collapsed (e.g. atelectasis) (Tyler & Cheney, 1979). PEEP may also restore V/Q matching by reducing cardiac output. Reduced pulmonary blood flow leads to a preferential reduction decrease in regional perfusion to areas of lung subjected to shunt during acute lung injury and may thereby enhance oxygenation (Dantzker et al., 1980).

Profound alterations in cardiovascular function may accompany PEEP therapy. Therefore, PEEP therapy should be instituted with care, and tailored to the needs of the patient. Low levels of PEEP (5–10 cmH_2O) can probably be used safely without invasive hemodynamic monitoring in most patients. However, at higher levels (>10 cmH_2O) adverse hemodynamic effects may occur and invasive monitoring of cardiac output and pulmonary capillary wedge pressure with a pulmonary artery catheter is recommended. The optimum level of PEEP (best "PEEP") is one that improves oxygenation without causing such adverse effects as reduced cardiac output and increased respiratory system compliance (Suter et al., 1975). This level is most effectively determined by performing a systemic PEEP trial, where respiratory parameters, such as arterial blood gases and respiratory system compliance, as well as cardiac parameters such as blood pressure and cardiac output are measured at successive levels of PEEP. Traditional criteria for administering PEEP include an arterial oxygen saturation of less than 90% with an $F_{I}O_2$ greater than 50%.

"Physiologic PEEP" is the theoretical amount of residual end-expiratory pressure produced during normal exhalation as a by-product of glottic closure. In an effort to reduce atelectasis, many clinicians will place ventilated patients using mechanical ventilators on 3–5 cmH_2O of baseline PEEP. Higher levels of PEEP have been used to promote airway recruitment in patients with significant pulmonary disease. Despite the potential disadvantages, the appropriate use of PEEP leads to airway recruitment, and reduction of intrapulmonary shunt, effecting an improvement in oxygenation (Suter et al., 1975).

Other methods of ventilation

Prone ventilation

Considerable published experience documents that oxygenation improves when patients with ARDS or acute lung injury (ALI) are turned from supine to prone. The degree of benefit varies. It is frequently of sufficient magnitude to allow a reduction in the fraction of inspired oxygen ($F_{I}O_2$), the level of PEEP, or both. Some patients respond well while others do not. The literature suggests that the response rate is somewhere between 50% and 75%. The initial reports demonstrating the prone position-induced improvement in oxygenation have hypothesized that it results from: (i) increases in the FRC; (ii) advantageous changes in diaphragm movement; (iii) a redirection of perfusion to better-ventilating, ventral lung regions; (iv) improvements in cardiac output and, accordingly, in mixed venous partial pressure of oxygen; and/or (v) better clearance of secretions (Piehl & Brown, 1976; Douglas et al., 1977).

Partial liquid ventilation

Liquid ventilation was developed as an outgrowth of advancements in underwater breathing equipment and semisynthetic blood products (Van Hook et al., 1995). This technique employs the oxygen-carrying capacity of perfluorochemicals. Perfluorocarbons (PFCs) are biologically inert compounds characterized by low surface tension, high density, and high respiratory gas solubility (Shaffer et al., 1992). The benefits of PLV appear to result primarily from a reduction in alveolar surface tension, recruitment of additional lung tissue for when there is ventilation/perfusion mismatch, and lavage of cellular debris (Leach et al., 1993; Hirschi et al., 1995; Overbeck et al., 1996; Gauger et al., 1998). Liquid ventilation involves the infusion of PFCs into the patient's airway in conjuction with low-pressure conventional ventilation. The perfluorochemical is instilled up to an amount estimated to comprise the patient's FRV. Total or complete liquid ventilation is much less frequently used and developed. The perfluorochemical promotes gas exchange directly, recruits otherwise atelectatic airways, and may serve as an anti-inflammatory lavage for the injured lung. Clinical trials are underway using partial liquid ventilation in adults (Hirschi et al., 1991, 1995, 1996). Its use in pregnancy is unclear.

Extracorporeal membrane oxygenation

Extracorporeal membrane oxygenation (ECMO) was first used successfully in the treatment of ARDS in 1972 (Hill et al., 1972). It evolved as a refinement of intraoperative cardiopulmonary bypass. Because ECMO involves perfusion as well as gas exchange, the term *extracorporeal life support* is probably a more apt description of the technique. This technique is administered in two broad categories: (i) venoarterial bypass which provides both cardiac output and oxygenation by removal of venous blood, which is then oxygenated and returned as arterial blood; and (ii) venovenous bypass provides respiratory support only (i.e. exchange of CO_2 but not O_2). To provide access, large-bore catheters are placed into the appropriate venous or arterial access sites. The internal jugular vein is the preferred venous site, while the common carotid artery is the preferred arterial site. In venovenous bypass, oxygenated blood is usually returned to the internal jugular, femoral, or iliac vein. In either method, full anticoagulation is required. The bypass circuit also can be used for ultrafiltration or hemodiafiltration (Prescenti et al., 1988).

The largest group to receive ECMO has been neonates with respiratory distress. Survival rates up to 90% have been reported by some investigators (ECMO Quarterly Report, 1994). The efficacy of ECMO in treatment of acute respiratory disease in adults is less clear. The National Institutes of Health sponsored a multicenter investigation of ECMO in the treatment of adult ARDS (Anderson & Bartlett, 1995). Compared with conventional mechanical ventilation methods in use at the time, ECMO offered no advantage. Some, however, still feel that advances in both ECMO itself and in the mechanical ventilation techniques used in patients who would require ECMO hold promise. The extracorporeal life support organization reports adult ARDS survival rates between 50% and 65% (Anderson et al., 1992). In one report, 62 out of 245 patients with ARDS were treated with ECMO (Mols et al., 2000). The survival rate was 55% in ECMO patients and 61% in non-ECMO patients. The author concluded that ECMO was a therapeutic option likely to increase survival; however, a randomized controlled study proving benefit is still needed.

Extracorporeal membrane oxygenation is an option for patients with potentially reversible pulmonary disease and who require significant ventilatory support based on specific parameters (compliance <0.5 mL/cmH_2O/kg, transpulmonary shunt >30% on $F_{I}O_2$ >0.6), and who have required mechanical ventilation less than a total of 10 days (Anderson & Bartlett, 1995). Advanced age, prolonged prior mechanical ventilation, absolute contraindication to anticoagulation, necrotizing pneumonia, or predicted poor quality of life are contraindications to the use of ECMO (Bartlett, 1990).

Nitric oxide

In recent years the use of inhaled nitric oxide (NO) therapy in adult intensive care units (ICUs) in the United Kingdom has become commonplace (Cuthbertson et al., 1997). The selective pulmonary vasodilatory effects of inhaled NO have been demonstrated in various models of ALI including endotoxin and oleic acid exposure, and smoke inhalation (McIntyre et al., 2000). Because NO is inhaled, it is an effective vasodilator of well-ventilated regions of the lung, thus reducing intrapulmonary shunt and improving arterial oxygenation. Furthermore, NO is rapidly bound to hemoglobin, which thereby inactivates it and prevents systemic vasodilation. The most common indication for inhaled NO is ALI/ARDS. Significant evidence suggests that inhaled NO improves oxygenation and reduces pulmonary artery pressure in the majority of patients with ALI/ARDS. Two randomized trials of inhaled NO therapy in ALI have recently been presented. In one European multicenter study 268 adult patients with early acute lung injury were evaluated for response to NO therapy. The investigators concluded that oxygenation was improved by inhaled NO but that the frequency of reversal of acute lung injury was not increased. Additionally, use of inhaled NO did not alter mortality, although it did reduce the frequency of severe respiratory failure in patients developing hypoxemia (Lundin, 1999). In another study, NO was noted to decrease shunt and pulmonary vascular resistance index and oxygenation. These findings suggested that inhaled NO improves oxygenation in critically hypoxemic patients (Baxter, 2002).

Complications of mechanical ventilation

Patients who undergo invasive mechanical ventilation experience complications caused by lung injury from oxygen toxicity; adverse effects from excessive ventilatory pressures, volumes, and flow rates; adverse effects from tracheal intubation; dangers from adjuvant drugs; stress-related sequelae; altered enzyme and hormone systems; nutritional problems; and psychologic trauma (Bezzant & Mortensen, 1994).

Oxygen toxicity

A variety of gross and histopathologic lesions have been described in human and experimental animal lung tissues that have been exposed to increased concentrations of oxygen in the airways (Bezzant & Mortensen, 1994). Free oxygen radicals generated by high concentrations of oxygen, in and along the airways and alveoli, attack intracellular enzyme systems, damage DNA, destroy lipid membranes, and increase microvascular permeability. The duration of exposure of the lungs to increased oxygen concentrations is directly related to the incidence and severity of any resultant lung injury. No definitive data are available to establish the upper limits of the concentration of oxygen in inspired air that can be considered safe (Bezzant Mortensen, 1994). However, the general consensus seems to be that oxygen concentrations greater than 50% in inspired air are undesirable and should be avoided if clinical circumstances permit. Therefore, one should institute measures to insure that the lowest possible concentration of oxygen is used during ventilatory support.

When oxygenation is inadequate, sedation, paralysis, and position change are possible therapeutic measures (Slutsky, 1994). Other factors in oxygen delivery, i.e. cardiac output and hemoglobin, should also be considered. In some clinical situations, when significant concerns over both elevated plateau pressure and high $F_{I}O_2$ exists, consideration for accepting an $S_{a}O_2$ slightly less than 90% is reasonable (permissive hypoxia) (Slutsky, 1994).

Baro-trauma

It has become increasingly evident that gas delivery into the lungs by a mechanical ventilator at excessive and inappropriate pressures, volumes, and flow rates can be a two-edged sword and can result in significant lung damage. In some cases, this produces additional injury and functional impairment instead of assisting the failing, sick lung (Kolobow, 1988). The most commonly reported adverse effect from excessive positive pressure mechanical ventilation is baro-trauma. Baro-trauma is generally defined as forceful escape of ventilatory gas from its contained airway–alveolar complex into adjacent tissue or compartment. The term is now also used in reference to cellular and ultrastructural pathologic changes in pulmonary parenchymal cells resulting from excessive intrapulmonary ventilatory gas pressures (Tsuno et al., 1990).

High PEEP has usually been reported as the leading cause of baro-trauma in patients with acute respiratory failure; however, more recent reports indicate that excessive peak inspiratory pressure may be more damaging to the lungs and produce baro-trauma lesions more commonly than high PEEP (Kolobow et al., 1987). Evidence separating the levels of airway pressures that can be considered safe from those that cause baro-trauma has not been established. However, there is general agreement that in most cases PEEP greater than 10 cmH_2O, mean airway pressure greater than 30 cmH_2O, and/or peak inspiratory pressure greater than 50 cmH_2O are all capable of producing baro-trauma lesions, particularly if continued for more than a few days. End-expiratory occlusion pressure (i.e. plateau pressure) is the best, clinically applicable estimate of average peak alveolar pressure (Slutsky, 1994). Therefore, it is the most important target pressure when trying to avoid alveolar over-distention. High plateau pressure (>35 cmH_2O) may be more harmful in most patients than high values of F_IO_2 (Slutsky, 1994).

Dynamic hyperinflation (gas trapping, auto-PEEP, intrinsic PEEP) also contributes to high airway pressure and alveolar over-distention. Auto-PEEP produces end-expiratory pressure through infraction of a new inspiration before all previous tidal volume is exhaled (Fig. 8.5). This often goes unnoticed and should be measured or estimated, especially in patients with airway obstruction. Management should include measures directed towards limiting the development of dynamic hyperinflation. Dynamic hyperinflation can be reduced by limiting total minute ventilation or decreasing the inspiratory to expiratory ratio (Slutsky, 1994).

Permissive hypercapnia

Hypercapnia has influences on brain function. Brain excitability decreases with inspired CO_2 concentrations up to 15%, and will increase accompanied by seizure activity at concentrations of 15–30%. Induction of anesthesia occurs at CO_2 concentrations of 40% (Shapiro et al., 1994). In addition, significant increases in cerebral blood flow with resultant increases in intracranial pressure, can be seen with acute hypercapnia. There are also significant circulatory hemodynamic responses to hypercapnia. The effect of CO_2 on the isolated heart muscle is one of temporary depression of function (Shapiro et al., 1994). There is also a depressant effect on the peripheral vascular smooth muscle of the precapillary resistant vessels. However, in the intact subject, elevation of circulating catecholamine levels secondary to the sympathetic stimulatory effects of hypercapnia overcome the direct depressant effect, and the result is an increase in cardiac output, a slight decrease in peripheral distance and a resultant tendency towards increased blood pressure. This stimulatory effect can be abolished by beta-adrenergic blockade (Walley et al., 1990). No definite data are available on the limits of tolerance to respiratory acidosis.

A recent case report documents survival after significant hypercapnia and respiratory acidosis when tissue anoxia and ischemia were prevented (Potkin & Swenson, 1992). A recent review of the subject of permissive hypercapnia concludes that deleterious effects of the associated hypercarbia in severe lung injury did not appear to be a significant limiting factor in preliminary human clinical trials (Shapiro et al., 1994). The avoidance of alveolar over-distention through pressure or volume limitation has significant support based on animal models and computer simulation. However, although current uncontrolled studies suggest benefit, controlled trials are urgently needed to confirm these findings before adoption of the treatment (permissive hypercapnia) can be endorsed (Shapiro et al., 1994). It should be remembered that in pregnancy this strategy may be harmful to the fetus and that if it is felt to be required, delivery of a mature fetus prior to instituting permissive hypercapnea should be considered.

Gastrointestinal hemorrhage

Critically ill patients who present with nongastrointestinal disease, such as acute respiratory failure, may develop gastrointestinal hemorrhage later in their intensive care course as a complication of critical illness (Lucas et al., 1971). Pathologically, stress ulcerations are erosions that are superficial to the muscularis mucosa. Stress ulcerations predominately involve the stomach and are usually found in the fundus with spearing of the antrum (Skillman et al., 1969). Stress ulcerations are present in the vast majority of the critically ill patients admitted to the ICU (Lucas et al., 1971). Severe or massive gastrointestinal bleeding occurs in about 5% of ICU patients. Risk factors for the development of upper GI hemorrhage include major trauma, severe hemorrhage, shock from any cause, sepsis, renal failure, jaundice, and acute respiratory failure. In one study, the most common respiratory disease associated with gastrointestinal bleeding was ARDS (Harris et al., 1977). Greater than 80% of 13 patients with ARDS bled, whereas only 9% of 44 patients with COPD bled. Duration of mechanical ventilation for more than 5 days is an important risk factor for upper GI hemorrhage (Schuster et al., 1984). Coagulaopathy is another risk factor associated with upper GI hemorrhage. In one study, 60% of 12 bleeding patients were thrombocytopenic (Harris et al., 1977). There is an increased risk of GI bleeding as the number of risk factors increases including evidence of multisystem failure, and especially when renal failure and jaundice are present (Skillman et al., 1969).

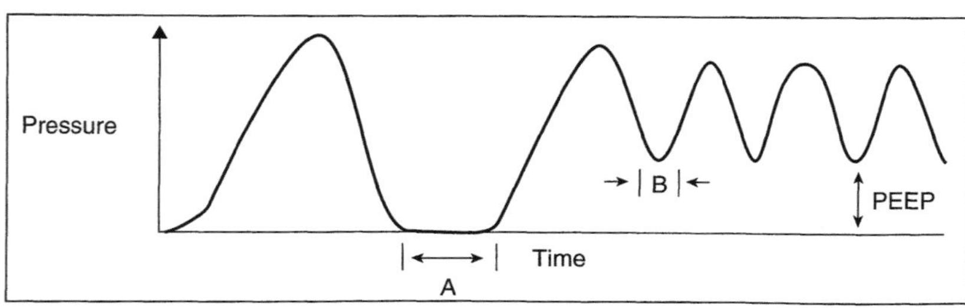

Fig. 8.5 Intrinsic positive end-expiratory pressure (PEEP). A, normal inspiratory time; B, shortened inspiratory time (refer to text).

Mucosal ischemia secondary to decreased gastric blood flow is one of the most important factors in stress ulceration. Increased concentrations of acid pepsin are not found in critically ill patients. The primary mechanism of ulceration is tissue acidosis or ischemia resulting in impaired mucosal handling of hydrogen ions that is already present (Kivilaakso & Silen, 1979). Initial therapy of stress ulceration should be directed at correcting hypotension, shock, and acidosis.

Prophylactic measures have centered primarily on neutralizing gastric acidity with antacids or decreasing gastric acid secretion with histamine receptor blockers such as cimetidine or ranitidine. Other prophylactic measures therapies include sucralfate, pirenzepine, pyridine, and secretin (Pingleton, 1988). Sucralfate is a basic aluminum salt of sucrose octasulfate that appears to provide stress ulcer protection without reducing levels of gastric acid. Available data suggest that sucralfate is as effective as antacids or cimetidine for prophylaxis of upper GI hemorrhage (Tryba et al., 1985). Antacids require excessive nursing time and additionally may of themselves result in complications including diarrhea, hypophosphatemia, hypomagnesemia, and metabolic alkalosis (Pingleton, 1988).

Cimetidine is associated with a larger number of and more diverse complications including acute renal failure, mental confusion, drug interactions, and thrombocytopenia (McGuigan, 1981). Both antacids and cimetidine are associated with gastric colonization caused by alkalinization of gastric pH. Resultant transmission of gastric organisms into the tracheal bronchial tree has been documented (DuMoulin et al., 1982). Gastric colonization and resultant nosocomial pneumonia may be lessened by the use of sucralfate. Nutrition may also be a useful prophylaxis against stress ulceration (Pingleton, 1988).

Thromboembolic complications

The actual frequency of pulmonary emboli complicating the course of patients with acute respiratory failure is unknown. Autopsy studies in respiratory ICU patients report an incidence of 8–27% (Pingleton, 1988). The source of pulmonary emboli in critically ill patients is primarily due to deep vein thrombosis. Critically ill patients present many risk factors for deep vein thrombosis including prolonged venous stasis caused by bed rest, right and left ventricular failure, dehydration, obesity, and advanced age. In one study, deep vein thrombosis occurred in 13% of respiratory ICU patients during the first week of intensive care (Moser et al., 1981). However, the precise risk of deep vein thrombosis in patients with acute respiratory failure is not known. Another source of pulmonary emboli in critically ill patients can be thrombosis associated with intravenous catheters (Pingleton, 1988). A recent study found that 66% of 33 consecutive patients monitored for a mean of 3 days with a pulmonary artery catheter had internal jugular thrombosis as detected venographically or on autopsy (Chastre et al., 1982). Recent autopsy data suggest that pulmonary emboli are present in patients with catheter-associated thrombosis (Connors et al., 1985). However, the relationship of pulmonary emboli to catheter-associated thrombosis is not clear.

The incidence of deep vein thrombosis is also increased during pregnancy and the postpartum period. The reported incidence varies between 0.018 and 0.29% during gestation and between 0.1 and 1% postpartum (Wessler, 1976). Although deep vein thrombosis can be seen at any stage of gestation, it appears to increase in frequency as pregnancy advances. The incidence of thromboembolic disease is increased in pregnancy secondary to several factors. There is increased vein distensibility during the first trimester and by the third trimester, the velocity of venous flow in the lower extremities is reduced by half. This happens in part because the gravid uterus provides a mechanical impediment to venous return (Wright et al., 1950). This tendency towards stasis is increased in the pregnant patient who requires prolonged bed rest for management of ventilatory failure. An additional problem is that fibrinogen, factor VIII, and other vitamin K dependent clotting factors are increased during pregnancy (Todd et al., 1965). There is also evidence of decreased fibrinolytic activity with reduced levels of available circulating plasminogen activator (Nilsson & Kullander, 1967). Overall the risk of thrombosis during pregnancy and the postpartum period for thrombosis may be up to 5.5 times greater than that for appropriately matched nonpregnant controls (Hathaway & Bonnar, 1987).

The incidence of pulmonary embolism in pregnancy and the postpartum period depends upon whether or not any underlying deep vein thrombosis is adequately treated. If untreated, as many as 24% of patients with antenatal deep vein thrombosis will have pulmonary emboli with a resultant mortality rate of approximately 15% (Wessler, 1976). However, if patients are treated with anticoagulants, embolization will occur in only 4.5% and the mortality rate will be less than 1% (Villasanta, 1965). It is obvious that the gravida suffers an extremely high risk of thromboembolic disease after suffering respiratory failure. Therefore, every attempt should be made to diagnose deep vein thrombosis and to administer agents to anticoagulate the patient prior to the development of pulmonary emboli (Laros, 1994).

Prevention of pulmonary emboli in populations at risk have centered on prophylaxis of deep vein thrombosis (Hull et al., 1986). These methods primarily include low-dose heparin, intermittent pneumatic leg compression devices, and combined prophylactic modalities (Hull et al., 1986). Both of these methods are safe when used in the pregnant patient with respiratory failure. It is important, however, to note that despite their safety, none of these prophylactic methods has been proven efficacious in patients with acute respiratory failure (Pingleton, 1988).

Treatment of established pulmonary emboli occurring in patients with acute respiratory failure includes systemic anticoagulation and fibrinolytic therapy. During pregnancy, the anticoagulant of choice is heparin (Laros, 1994). There are only a few case reports of use of fibrinolytic agents during pregnancy and thus conclusions about the safety of these agents during gestation must be withheld (Laros, 1994). Because of severe postpartum hemorrhage from the placental site, these agents should not be used for the first 10 postpartum days.

Renal complications

Acute renal failure and abnormalities of sodium and water excretion are frequent renal complications in critically ill patients with respiratory failure (Pingleton, 1988). The incidence of acute renal failure is about 10–20% in respiratory and surgical ICU patients. The development of renal failure in patients with respiratory failure is an ominous prognostic sign. In one study, there was an 80% mortality rate in patients with acute respiratory failure who developed renal failure (Kraman et al., 1979). Causes of renal failure in respiratory ICU patients include gastrointestinal bleeding with hemorrhagic shock, septic shock, aminoglycoside nephrotoxicity, and hypotension (Kraman et al., 1979). Additional data suggest that synergistic nephrotoxicity is exerted by Gram-negative bacteremia and aminoglycosides (Zager & Prior, 1986). Therapy of acute renal failure should be directed at its apparent cause.

Positive fluid balance

Alterations in renal hemodynamics and renal tubular function occur in patients with acute respiratory failure as a result of hypoxemia, acidosis, mechanical ventilation, and PEEP (Pingleton, 1988). Adverse consequences include positive water balance, edema, hyponatremia, and possible increased mortality. In addition, hormonal factors contribute to the positive fluid balance. Elevated antidiuretic hormone (ADH) was noted in almost half of 15 patients with acute respiratory failure admitted to the ICU (Szatalowicz et al., 1982). Recent data suggest that fluid balance may influence survival in ARDS. Data suggest that negative fluid balance (as reflected by weight loss and small cumulative intake–outputs) is an important variable of survival in ARDS (Simmons et al., 1987).

Infectious complications

Nosocomial pneumonia is a frequent complication with multiple adverse sequelae. It is associated with high mortality in patients with respiratory failure. In a recent analysis of patients with ARDS and pneumonia, only 12% survived (Seidenfeld et al., 1986). Mortality was directly related to infection and to the development of other additional complications. Factors increasing the risk of nosocomial pneumonia include coma, hypotension, prior respiratory disease, tracheal intubation, acidosis, azotemia, and leukopenia. Additional risk factors include the presence of an intracranial pressure monitor, treatment with cimetidine, hospitalization during the fall–winter season, and mechanical ventilator circuit changes every 24 hours (Montgomery et al., 1985). Diagnosis of nosocomial pneumonia is difficult, particularly in patients with respiratory failure showing with obvious radiographic infiltrates (Pingleton, 1988). These patients may also have other causes for their fever, leukocytosis, and positive blood cultures. In addition, the distinction between tracheal bronchial colonization and pneumonia is difficult (Johanson et al., 1972).

General strategies aimed at the prevention of nosocomial pneumonia include efforts to improve host defenses, as well as measures directed at decreasing airway colonization and bacterial inoculation into the lower airway.

Other infectious complications include bacteremia and sepsis. In one report, sepsis was the major and direct cause of death in 36% of patients who died within 72 hours after the onset of ARDS (Montgomery et al., 1985). Primary bacteremia originates most frequently from intravascular devices (Maki, 1981). In general, catheter infections are more common in catheters left in place for longer than 3 days (Pingleton, 1988). Bacteremia may also be a sign of infective endocarditis. Therefore, an echocardiogram is indicated to rule out intracardiac vegetations in unexplained bacteremia.

Nutritional complications

Nutritional complications in acute respiratory failure patients reflect the adverse effects of malnutrition upon the thoracic–pulmonary system, as well as complications associated with administration of nutritional support (Pingleton, 1988). Nutritionally associated complications can occur with both enteral and total parenteral nutrition (Bernard & Weser, 1984; Ang & Daly, 1986). Poor nutritional status does not appear to predispose the patient to the need for mechanical ventilation. However, malnourished patients who require mechanical ventilation have a significantly higher mortality rate than well-nourished patients requiring mechanical ventilation. Poor nutritional status can adversely affect thoracic–pulmonary function by impairment of respiratory muscle function, ventilatory drive and pulmonary defense mechanisms (Rochester & Esau, 1984).

The diaphragm is the critical respiratory muscle and malnutrition reduces diaphragmatic muscle mass (Pingleton, 1988). Respiratory muscle is impaired in poorly nourished humans. Underweight patients with reduction of diaphragmatic mass may have contractile force reductions out of proportion to the reduction in muscle mass (Pingleton, 1988). Hypophosphatemia or decreased inorganic phosphate precursors may also be responsible for respiratory muscle weakness. Nutritional repletion can improve altered respiratory muscle strength in some patients. Increase in maximal inspiratory pressure and body cell mass were noted in critically ill patients given parenteral nutrition for 2–4 weeks (Kelly et al., 1984). Malnutrition reduces ventilatory drive and influences the immune system. The systemic effects of malnutrition are most profound in cell-mediated immunity, as malnourished patients have suppressed delayed cutaneous hypersensitivity and impaired T-lymphocyte transformation in response to mitogens (Martin, 1987). Nutritional support can be instituted either by the enteral route or with total parenteral nutrition. Nutritionally associated hypercapnia can occur in patients receiving enteral feeding or total parenteral nutrition. This develops when excess carbohydrate calories are given (Pingleton, 1988). Carbon dioxide production is increased because calories in excess of energy needs result in lipogenesis and a markedly increased respiratory quotient (Pingleton, 1988). The respiratory quotient is defined as the ratio of carbon dioxide production to oxygen consumption during substrate utilization. Hypercapnia from increased CO_2 production is avoided in normal persons by a compensatory increase in ventilation. Patients with compromised ventilatory status may not be able to increase ventilation appropriately and hypercapnia may result (Pingleton, 1988). The practical significance of this potential complication is not entirely known.

Cardiovascular complications

Positive pressure ventilation often impairs cardiac output by disturbing the loading conditions of the heart. Blood returns to the thorax along pressure gradients from peripheral vessels to the right atrium. To the extent that intrathoracic pressures effect right atrial pressure, it may alter the gradient for venous return. Right ventricular output can also be affected by changes in right ventricular afterload. The latter is affected in a complex way by changes in lung volume. An increase in lung volume tends to increase the resistance of alveolar vessels while decreasing the resistance of extra alveolar vessels. The net effect on total resistance is unpredictable (Slutsky, 1994). Changes in intrathoracic pressure also affect left ventricular function; a higher intrathoracic pressure acts to reduce left ventricular afterload. Where poor left ventricular function is limiting cardiac output, an increase in thoracic pressure may result in better left ventricular emptying. This improved emptying may, under some circumstances have advantageous effects on right ventricular afterload and venous return. The effect of changes in ventricular settings on hemodynamics are complex. However, in general, cardiac output is adversely affected by increases in intrathoracic pressure.

Sedation/paralysis

Because of the discomfort inherent in receiving mechanical ventilation and intensive care, appropriate use of anxiolytics, analgesics, and sedatives is important to the welfare of the critically ill patient (Van Hook et al., 1995). Furthermore, pain relief may be necessary to render mechanical ventilation effectively. Conversely, inappropriate use of sedatives, anxiolytics, and/or analgesics may delay extubation, produce hemodynamic instability, or contribute to mental status abnormalities. Specific fetal side effects of these drugs have been referenced comprehensively (Rayburn & Zuspan, 1992; Briggs et al., 1994).

Narcotics are useful for pain relief, sedation, and anxiolysis (Balestrieri & Fisher, 1995). Morphine sulfate is used frequently as a primary agent for pain relief. In usually commonly administered dosages, morphine sulfate has relatively few adverse cardiovascular effects (Lowenstein et al., 1969). Intravenous administration is preferred over other parenteral routes, either intermittently or by continuous administration. Side effects relating to histamine release or cardiovascular interactions are uncommon. Potent synthetic narcotics such as fentanyl, alfentanil, and sufentanil are useful for continuous infusions as well. Ileus and tolerance are long-term side effects of narcotic administration.

Short- and intermediate-action benzodiazepines, such as midazolam, lorazepam, and diazepam, are useful anxiolytic/hypnotics in long-term mechanical ventilation. While not singularly effective at providing pain relief, the hypnotic effects of the agents are additive with the effects of narcotics. Midazolam is useful for acute events because of its relatively short half-life. Midazolam can produce delayed hypotension. Lorazepam carries the advantage of glucoronidase metabolism, which is well preserved and remains effective even in patients who have moderate degrees of liver disease. Diazepam has a rapid onset and a long half-life. For sporadic use, diazepam is an effective and inexpensive choice. For continued use, intermittent boluses or continuous infusions of midazolam or lorazepam are preferred (Balestrieri et al., 1995).

Because of haloperidol's relatively large margin of safety and minimal hemodynamic and sedating side effects, it is the antipsychotic of choice in chronically long-term mechanically ventilated patients. Agents such as haloperidol are useful for treatment of delirium and psychosis that is often a consequence of prolonged intensive care (Ayd, 1978).

For long-term sedation, which is often necessary for advanced modes of mechanical ventilation, propofol is in many ways an ideal agent. Given by continuous intravenous infusion, propofol has a very short single-dose half-life of 2–3 minutes. Rapid induction and emergence from anesthesia is possible with propofol. Because hypotension invariably occurs when sufficient doses are used to provide surgical anesthesia, propofol is not recommended for use in induction of anesthesia for delivery. In continuously infused doses necessary for mechanical ventilation, however, hypotension is less problematic. Propofol clearance is not appreciably altered in renal or hepatic disease states (Sebel & Lowdon, 1989).

Skeletal muscle paralysis is necessary under two broad circumstances. The first circumstance is when temporary paralysis is required for intubation. The second situation is when paralysis is a necessary addition to sedation for advanced mechanical ventilation methods (Van Hook et al., 1995). Intermittent or continuous doses of nondepolarizing muscle relaxants are generally employed. A nondepolarizing block is produced when the postjunctional membrane receptors are reversibly bound with the drug. The duration of the block depends on the rate at which the relaxant is redistributed. The relaxant effects of nondepolarizing drugs are reversed by anticholinergic-blocking drugs such as neostigmine (Cullen et al., 1994).

Of the several non-depolarizing agents available, pancuronium, vecuronium, and atracurium are most used. Pancuronium is effective for 60–90 minutes after an intubating dose is given. Anticholinergic effects of the drug may result in tachycardia and, rarely, hypotension (Duvaldstein et al., 1978; Cullen et al., 1994). Vecuronium produces a clinical effect for 30–60 minutes after an intubating dose. Hemodynamic effects are usually absent after typically used doses. Both vecuronium and pancuronium may have prolonged action in the presence of hepatic failure (Miller et al., 1984). Atracurium has a relatively short duration of action and is degraded nonenzymatically. It is, therefore, useful in patients with hepatic or renal failure. Any of the agents can be given by intermittent bolus or continuous infusion. Monitoring of the level for paralysis with nerve stimulator equipment ("twitch monitoring") is recommended during prolonged administration of paralytics. Because muscle relaxants paralyze without affording the patient any analgesia or sedation, appropriate monitoring for the adequacy of sedation is required any time a patient is pharmacologically paralyzed. None the less, because of the potential for paralysis while awake, muscle relaxants must be used only when clearly necessary (Ward et al., 1988; Cullen et al., 1994).

Table 8.9 lists agents commonly used for sedation, pain relief, and paralysis of the mechanically ventilated patient. Pain relief and sedation are very important components of the total care given to the ventilator "recipient." In many cases, otherwise difficult-to-ventilate patients have dramatically benefited from simple pain relief. Therefore, familiarity with the doses' interactions, side effects, and indications for analgesics, anxiolytics, nondepolarizing muscle relaxants, and antipsychotics is an important part of mechanical ventilation (Van Hook et al., 1995).

Table 8.9 Sedation and paralysis in mechanical ventilation

Narcotics
Morphine
Fentanyl
Anxiolytics
Midazolam
Diazepam
Anesthetics
Propofol
Nondepolarizing muscle relaxants
Vercuronium
Pancuronium
Atracurium

Thorough familiarity with any pharmacologic agent is necessary prior to its use.

ARDS

The criteria for ARDS include a $P_{A}O_2/F_{I}O_2$ ratio ≤200, bilateral pulmonary infiltrates, pulmonary capillary wedge pressure (PCWP) ≤18 mmHg, and no clinical evidence of elevated left atrial pressure (Slutsky, 1994). Recent work has provided compelling evidence that ARDS is a heterogeneous, not diffuse, lung injury, with areas of relatively normal lung interspersed with areas of alveolar and interstitial edema (Gattinoni et al., 1987). The result is a smaller physiologic lung volume. Exposure of relatively normal alveoli, with near normal compliance characteristics, to high distending pressures results in a larger delivered volume per lung unit, marked overdistention, and the possible increased risk of further lung injury (Shapiro et al., 1994). This scenario could conceivably occur regardless of which mode of ventilation generates the high inspiratory pressures used. These data, coupled with the persistent high mortality associated with ARDS, lead to the development of strategies to minimize potential injury, including permissive hypercapnia (Shapiro et al., 1994). The following guidelines for the management of mechanical ventilation for ARDS were developed at the Consensus Conference on Mechanical Ventilation, 1993 (Slutsky, 1994):

1 The clinician should choose a ventilator mode that has been shown to be capable of supporting oxygenation and ventilation in patients with ARDS and that the clinician has experience in using.
2 An acceptable $S_{a}O_2$ (usually ≥90%) should be targeted.
3 Based primarily on animal data, a plateau pressure ≥35 cmH_2O is of concern. We therefore recommend that when plateau pressure equals or exceeds this pressure, that tidal volume can be decreased (to as low as 5 mg/kg, or lower, if necessary). With clinical conditions that are associated with decreased chest wall compliance, plateau pressures somewhat greater than 35 cmH_2O may be acceptable.
4 To accomplish the goal of limiting plateau pressure, $P_{a}CO_2$ should be permitted to rise (permissive hypercapnia) unless the presence or risk of raised intracranial pressure or other contraindications exist which demand a more normal $P_{a}CO_2$ or pH. Rapid rises in $P_{a}CO_2$ should be avoided. In the presence of normal renal function, slow reduction of tidal volume may also allow renal-induced compensatory metabolic alkalosis and the potential for a higher pH at a given tidal volume.
5 PEEP is useful in supporting oxygenation. An appropriate level of PEEP may be helpful in preventing lung damage. The level of PEEP should however be minimized as PEEP may also be associated with deleterious effects. The level of PEEP required should be established by empirical trial and re-evaluated on a regular basis.

6 The current opinion is that F_IO_2 should be minimized. The trade-off, however, may be a higher plateau pressure and the relative risks of these two factors are not known. In some clinical situations when significant concerns over both elevated plateau pressure and high F_IO_2 exist, consideration for accepting an S_aO_2 slightly less than 90% is reasonable.

When oxygenation is inadequate, sedation, paralysis, and position change are possible therapeutic measures. Other factors in oxygen delivery (i.e. Q_v and hemoglobin) should also be considered.

Acute asthma

The patient with severe acute asthma who requires intubation and mechanical ventilation is also at risk of baro-trauma. Approximately 1–3% of patients with severe acute asthma attacks will require intubation and mechanical ventilation. The criteria for intubation of asthmatic patients include altered consciousness; apnea or severe respiratory distress; severe hypoxemia, hypercarbia, or respiratory acidosis; and arrhythmias (Soler et al., 1990). Intubation may worsen bronchospasm or precipitate laryngospasm in asthmatics, and therefore, the airway should be managed by highly skilled individuals. Since the basic pathophysiology of asthma involves air trapping, asthmatics should be ventilated with caution to avoid baro-trauma that may occur in the presence of elevated airway pressures (Soler et al., 1990). Failure to ventilate adequately or note clinical improvement in mechanically ventilated patients with status asthmaticus receiving maximum medical therapy should raise concern about severe extensive bronchial obstruction secondary to tenacious secretions. In this setting, flexible bronchoscopy by way of the endothracheal tube, for the removal of secretions via saline lavage may possibly be life saving (Einarsson et al., 1994). General anesthesia, helium/oxygen inhalation, or ketamine sedation also may be useful adjuncts in the treatment of life-threatening status asthmaticus not responsive to conventional therapy (Einarsson et al., 1994).

A recent report documents survival of a pregnant woman with unresponsive status asthmaticus after mechanical ventilation with a helium–oxygen mixture (George et al., 2001). Helium is an inert, nonflammable gas that possesses the lowest density of any gas other than hydrogen. Helium is an inert gas and has no direct harmful effect or interaction with human tissues. The beneficial effects of a helium–oxygen mixture derive from its lower density when compared to either 100% oxygen or any concentration of oxygen in air/nitrogen. Therapy for severe asthma is primarily directed at relieving bronchospasm and increasing the radius of the airways. Using traditional methods, this effect may take hours to days to accomplish. The effect of lowering the density of the inhaled gas with the use of helium–oxygen mixture can be achieved within minutes, thereby allowing for decreased resistance to gas flow, improved gas exchange, and decreased peak inflating pressures (George et al., 2001). In addition to decreasing resistance, administration of a gas mixture with a lower density and higher viscosity may improve gas flow by converting turbulent flow to laminar flow.

Weaning from mechanical ventilation

Weaning has been defined as the process whereby mechanical ventilation is gradually withdrawn and the patient resumes spontaneous breathing (Tobin & Yang, 1990). The outcome of a trial of weaning from mechanical ventilation depends on the patient's underlying condition and the aggressiveness of the physician. The weaning process can be a difficult one. In one study only 52% of 110 patients were successfully weaned on the first trial (Pardee et al., 1984). The major pathophysiologic determinants of weaning outcomes are hypoxemic respiratory failure, ventilator pump failure, cardiovascular performance, and psychological problems (Tobin & Yang, 1990; Slutsky, 1994). Systematic studies have never been conducted to determine the relative importance of these pathophysiologic mechanisms. However, many clinicians and investigators suspect that respiratory muscle dysfunction resulting from an imbalance, between respiratory neuromuscular capacity and load is the most important determinant (Slutsky, 1994).

Hypoxemic respiratory failure

Although mechanical ventilation is commonly instituted because of problems with oxygenation, this is rarely a cause of difficulty at the time that mechanical ventilation is being stopped. This is largely because ventilator discontinuation is not contemplated in patients who display significant problems with oxygenation. However, during a weaning trial, hypoxemia may occur as a result of hypoventilation, impaired pulmonary gas exchange, or decreased oxygen content of venous blood (Tobin & Yang, 1990). Impaired pulmonary gas exchange can be distinguished from pure hypoventilation by the presence of an elevated alveolar–arterial oxygen tension gradient. If the patient displays evidence of hypoxemic respiratory failure during weaning attempts, mechanical ventilation should be reinstituted until the cause of the hypoxemic respiratory failure has been identified and addressed. Impaired pulmonary gas exchange may be evidence of continuation of the initial precipitating illness or of other pathologic pulmonary processes such as pneumonia or pulmonary edema. These conditions should be treated prior to additional weaning attempts. Decreased oxygen content in venous blood may be secondary to a low hemoglobin. If this is the case, transfusion is indicated prior to additional weaning attempts. Hypoventilation may occur secondary to extensive sedation or respiratory muscle fatigue.

Respiratory muscle pump failure

As previously stated, respiratory muscle pump failure is probably the most common cause of failure to wean from mechanical ventilation. This may result from decreased neuromuscular capacity, increased respiratory muscle pump load, or both (Tobin & Yang, 1990) (Table 8.10). Decreased respiratory sensor output may result from neurologic structural damage, sedative agents, sleep deprivation, semi-starvation, and metabolic alkalosis (Tobin & Yang, 1990). In addition, mechanical ventilation in itself may decrease respiratory center output by a number of mechanisms: lowering of arterial CO_2 tension, with a consequent reduction in chemoreceptor stimulation; activation of pulmonary stress receptors; and stimulation of muscle spindles or joint receptors in the chest wall.

Of the conditions listed in Table 8.10, hyperinflation is one of the most important (Tobin & Yang, 1990). Alterations in the pattern of breathing during weaning may lead to the development of dynamic hyperinflation, which has a number of adverse effects on inspiratory muscle function (Swartz & Marino, 1985). The increase in lung volume causes the inspiratory muscles to shorten with consequent decrease in the force of contraction. In the hyperinflated chest, thoracic elastic recoil is directed inward which poses an additional elastic load. Finally, increased swings in trends of diaphragmatic pressure may impair diaphragmatic blood supply.

Malnutrition has a number of adverse effects on the respiratory system (Tobin & Alex, 1994). These adverse effects can interfere with weaning. It predisposes to nosocomial pneumonia and causes a decrease in the ventilatory response to hypoxia, decrease in diaphragmatic mass in thickness, and decrease in respiratory muscle strength and endurance. Malnutrition may be accompanied by metabolic abnormalities such as hypophosphatemia, hypokalemia, hypocalcemia, or hypomagnesemia that may adversely affect respiratory muscle function (Tobin & Yang, 1990). Corticosteroid therapy (Lewis & Belman, 1990) and thyroid disease (Laroche et al., 1989) may also impair respiratory muscle function. It should be remembered that respiratory muscle atrophy may result from the use of mechanical ventilation (Anzueto et al., 1987). Another possibility is that respiratory muscle fatigue may be a primary cause of failure to wean.

Increased ventilatory requirements may also lead to weaning failure. Factors that cause an increase in ventilatory requirements include increased CO_2 production, increased dead space ventilation, and an inappropriately elevated respiratory drive. Excessive administration of carbohydrate calories will cause an increase in the respiratory quotient (RQ) and increased CO_2 production and hypercapnia (Pingleton & Harmon, 1987).

Table 8.10 Causes of respiratory muscle pump failure

Decreased neuromuscular capacity
Decreased respiratory center output
Phrenic nerve dysfunction
Decreased respiratory muscle strength and/or endurance
Hyperinflation
Malnutrition
Decreased oxygen supply
Respiratory acidosis
Mineral and electrolyte abnormalities
Endocrinopathy
Disuse muscle atrophy
Respiratory muscle fatigue
Increased respiratory muscle pump load
Increased ventilatory requirements
Increased CO_2 production
Increased dead space ventilation
Inappropriately increased respiratory drive
Increased work of breathing

(Reproduced by permission from Tobin MJ, Yang K. Weaning from mechanical ventilation. Crit Care Clin 1990;6(3):725.)

Psychological problems

Dependence on mechanical ventilation can be associated with feelings of insecurity, anxiety, fear, agony, and panic (Bergbom-Enberg & Haljamae, 1989). Many patients develop a fear that they will remain dependent on mechanical ventilation and that discontinuation of ventilator support will result in sudden death. These psychologic factors are major determinants of outcome of weaning trials in some patients, especially those patients who require prolonged ventilator support (Holliday & Heyers, 1990).

Predicting weaning outcome

A wide variety of physiological indices have been proposed to guide the process of discontinuing ventilator support. The most commonly used indices are listed in Table 8.11. In general, these indices evaluate a patient's ability to sustain sponta-

Table 8.11 Variables used to predict weaning success

Gas exchange
P_aO_2 of ≤60 torr with F_IO_2 of ≥0.35
Alveolar–arterial PO_2 gradient of <350 torr
P_aO_2/F_IO_2 ratio of >200
Ventilatory pump
Vital capacity of >10–15 mL/kg body weight
Maximum negative inspiratory pressure <–30 cmH$_2$O
Minute ventilation <10 L/min
Maximum voluntary ventilation more than twice resting minute ventilation

(Reproduced by permission from Tobin MJ, Yang K. Weaning from Mechanical Ventilation. Crit Care Clin 1990;6(3):733.)

neous ventilation. The purpose of these indices is: (i) to identify the earliest time that ventilator support can be discontinued; and also (ii) to identify patients who are likely to fail a weaning trial and, thus, avoid cardiorespiratory and psychological distress or collapse (Tobin & Yang, 1990). Because these indices assess many different physiologic functions, they may also provide insight into the reasons for ventilator dependency in an individual patient and suggest an alteration in management (Tobin & Yang, 1990).

Weaning techniques

A variety of options for weaning from mechanical ventilation have been proposed and used over the past 25 years (Tobin & Alex, 1994). All of these methods are based on the progressive reduction in the contribution of the ventilator and the progressive increase in the patient's contribution to ventilation (Weinberger & Weiss, 1995).

A gradual T-tube weaning approach consists of sessions of spontaneous breathing of progressively increased duration, sessions through a T-tube circuit, of increasing duration interspersed between periods of mechanical ventilation (Nett et al., 1984). With the intermittent mandatory ventilation method, spontaneous breathing by the patient is assisted by a preset number of ventilatory-delivered breaths each minute. The intermittent mandatory ventilation rate is usually reduced in steps until a rate of zero or close to zero is reached. In the pressure support ventilation method of weaning, each breath is initiated by the patient but supported in part by positive pressure delivered by the ventilator. In this method, weaning involves a progressive decrease in the magnitude of the pressure delivered with each patient expired breath.

Recently an additional technique for weaning from mechanical ventilation has been proposed. This technique is called the "once-daily trial of spontaneous breathing." In this technique, patients are disconnected from the ventilator and allowed to breathe spontaneously through a T-tube circuit for up to 2 hours each day. If signs of intolerance develop, assist controlled ventilation is reinstituted for 24 hours, at which time another trial is attempted. Patients who tolerate a 2-hour trial without signs of distress are extubated. This method was recently compared to the intermittent mandatory ventilation, pressure support ventilation, and T-tube methods of weaning (Esteban et al., 1995). This study had two major findings. First, in a selected group of patients who were difficult to wean from mechanical ventilation, the rate of success of weaning depended on the technique employed; a once daily trial of spontaneous breathing led to extubation about three times more quickly than intermittent mandatory ventilation and about twice as quickly as pressure support ventilation. There were not significant differences in the rate of success between a once-daily trial and the multiple daily trial (T-tube trial) of spontaneous breathing, or between intermittent mandatory ventilation and pressure support ventilation.

The second important finding was that when ventilator support was discontinued without any special weaning techniques in about two-thirds of an unselected group of patients, only a small proportion of these patients required reintubation within 48 hours. Although the number of patients in each study group was small and the percentage of patients requiring reintubation (22.6%) could be considered high, one might infer from this study that no matter which method of weaning is used, a daily trial of unassisted breathing is justified to see whether the patient can tolerate the removal of ventilatory assistance (Weinberger & Weiss, 1995). No matter which method of weaning is used, careful attention must be paid to the large number of reversible factors that can adversely effect the process.

Conclusion

In summary, the management of the gravida with respiratory failure can be difficult. However, early recognition of respiratory failure and institution of ventilatory support, knowledge of the changes in the cardiorespiratory system that occurs in gestation, judicious therapy of underlying pathophysiologic aberrations, thoughtful measures to prevent known complications, and prudent attempts to release the patient from ventilator dependency may improve the outcome of pregnant patients who suffer respiratory failure.

References

ACOG. Pulmonary disease in pregnancy. ACOG Technical Bulletin 224:2. Washington, DC: ACOG, 1996.

Anderson GJ, James GB, Mathers NP, et al. The maternal oxygen tension and acid-base status during pregnancy. J Obstet Br Commonw 1969;76:17.

Anderson HL III, Bartlett RH. Extracorporeal and intravascular gas exchange devices. In: Ayres SM, Grenvik A, Holbrook PR, Shoemaker WC, eds. Textbook of critical care, 3rd edn. Philadelphia: WB Saunders, 1995:943–951.

Anderson HL III, Decius RE, Sinard JM, et al. Early experience with adult extracorporeal membrane oxygenation in the modern era. Ann Thorac Surg 1992;53:553–563.

Ang SD, Daly JM. Potential complications and monitoring of patients receiving total parenteral nutrition. In: Rombeau JL, Caldwell MD, eds. Parenteral nutrition. Philadelphia: WB Saunders, 1986:331.

Anzueto A, Tobin MJ, Moore G, et al. Effect of prolonged mechanical ventilation on diaphragmatic function: A preliminary study of a baboon model. Am Rev Respir Dis 1987;135:A201.

Ayd FJ Jr. Intravenous haloperidol therapy. Int Drug Ther Newslett 1978;13:20.

Balestrieri F, Fisher S. Analgesics. In: Chernow B, ed. The pharmacologic approach to the critically ill patient. Baltimore: Williams and Wilkins, 1995:640–650.

Barcroft J. On anoxemia. Lancet 1920;11:485.

Barron W, Lindheimer M. Medical disorders during pregnancy, 1st edn. St. Louis: Mosby-Year Book 1991:234.

Bartlett RH. Extracorporeal life support for cardio-pulmonary failure. Curr Probl Surg 1990;27:621–705.

Baudouin SV. Ventilator induced lung injury and infection in the critically ill. Thorax 2001;56(2):1150–1157.

Baxter FJ, Randall J, Miller JD, et al. Rescue therapy with inhaled nitric oxide in critically ill patients with severe hypoxemic respiratory failure (Brief report). Can J Anaesth 2002;49(3):315–318.

Belfort MA, Anthony J, Kirshon B. Respiratory function in severe gestational proteinuric hypertension: the effects of rapid volume expansion and subsequent vasodilatation with verapamil. Br J Obstet Gynaecol 1991;98(10):964–972.

Belfort MA, Anthony J, Saade GR, et al. The oxygen consumption: oxygen delivery curve in severe preeclampsia: evidence for a fixed oxygen extraction state. Am J Obstet Gynecol 1993;169(6): 1448–1455.

Bergbom-Enberg I, Haljamae H. Assessment of patient's experience of discomforts during respiratory therapy. Crit Care Med 1989; 17:1068–1072.

Bernard EA, Weser E. Complications and prevention. In: Rombeau JL, Caldwell MD, eds. Enteral and tube feeding. Philadelphia: WB Saunders, 1984:542.

Bezzant TB, Mortensen JD. Risks and hazards of mechanical ventilation: A collective review of published literature. Dis Monthly 1994;40:581–638.

Bidani A, Tzouanakis AE, Cardenas VJ, Zwischenbergr JB. Permissive hypercapnia in acute respiratory failure. JAMA 1994;272:957–962.

Biddle C. AANA Journal Course: Update for nurse anesthetists—Advances in ventilating the patient with severe lung disease. J Am Assoc Nurse Anesthetists 1993;61(2):170–174.

Briggs GG, Freeman RK, Yaffe SJ. Drugs in pregnancy and lactation, 4th edn. Baltimore: Williams and Wilkins, 1994.

Brochard L, Harf A, Lorino H, Lemaire F. Inspiratory pressure support prevents diaphragmatic fatigue during weaning from mechanical ventilation. Am Rev Respir Dis 1989;139:513–521.

Brower RG, Ware LB, Berthiaume Y, Matthay MA. Treatment of ARDS. Chest 2001;120:1347–1367.

Bryan-Brown CW, Baek SM, Makabali G, et al. Consumable oxygen: Oxygen availability in relation to oxyhemoglobin dissociation. Crit Care Med 1973;1:17–21.

Cain SM. Peripheral oxygen uptake and delivery in health and disease. Clin Chest Med 1983;4:139–148.

Carlon GC, Howland WS, Ray C, et al. High frequency jet ventilation —A prospective randomized evaluation. Chest 1983;84:551–559.

Carrey Z, Gottfried SB, Levy RD. Ventilatory muscle support in respiratory failure with nasal positive pressure ventilation. Chest 1990;97:150–158.

Chastre J, Cornud F, Bouchama A, et al. Thrombosis as a complication of pulmonary-artery catheterization via the internal jugular vein. Prospective evaluation by phlebography. N Engl J Med 1982;306: 278–281.

Cheek TG, Gutsche BB. Maternal physiologic alterations during pregnancy. In: Anesthesia for obstetrics. Baltimore: Williams & Wilkins, 1987:3.

Connors AF, Castele RJ, Farhaf NZ, Tomashefski JF. Complications of right heart catheterization. Chest 1985;88:567–572.

Cullen DJ, Bigatello LM, DeMonaco HJ. Anesthetic pharmacology and critical care. In: Chernow B, ed. The pharmacologic approach to the critically ill patient, 3rd edn. Baltimore: Williams and Wilkins, 1994:291–308.

Cuthbertson BH, Stott S, Webster NR. Use of inhaled nitric oxide in British intensive therapy units. Br J Anaesth 1997;78:696–700.

Dantzker DR, Lynch JP, Weg JC. Depression of cardiac output is a mechanism of shunt reduction in the therapy of acute respiratory failure. Chest 1980;77:636–642.

Deem S, Bishop MJ. Evaluation and management of the difficult airway. Crit Care Clin 1995;11:1–27.

Demling RH, Knox JB. Basic concepts of lung function and dysfunction: Oxygenation, ventilation, and mechanics. New Horiz 1993;1:362–370.

Douglas WW, Rehder K, Beynen FM, et al. Improved oxygenation in patients with acute respiratory failure: The prone position. Am Rev Respir Dis 1977;115:559–566.

Douglass JA, Tuxen DV, Horne M, et al. Myopathy in severe asthma. Am Rev Respir Dis 1992;146:517–519.

DuMoulin GC, Paterson DG, Hedley-Whyte J, et al. Aspiration of gastric bacteria in antacid-treated patients. Lancet 1982;1:242–245.

Duvaldstein P, Agoston S, Henzel D, et al. Pancouronium pharmacokinetics in patients with liver cirrhosis. Br J Anaesth 1978;50: 1131–1136.

ECMO Quarterly Report. Ann Arbor, MI: ECMO Registry of the Extracorporeal Life Support Organization (ELSO), May 1994.

Einarsson O, Rochester CL, Rosenbaum S. Airway management in respiratory emergencies. Clin Chest Med 1994;15(1):13–34.

Esteban A, Frutos F, Tobin MJ, et al. A comparison of our methods of weaning patients from mechanical ventilation. Spanish Lung Failure Collaborative Group. N Engl J Med 1995;332:345–350.

Freeman RK, Garite TJ, Nageotte MP. Fetal heart rate monitoring, 2nd edn. Baltimore: Williams & Wilkins, 1991.

Gattinoni L, Pesenti A, Avalli L, Rossi F, Bombino M. Pressure-volume curve of total respiratory system in acute respiratory failure: computed tomographic scan study. Am Rev Respir Dis 1987;136: 730–736.

Gauger PG, Overbeck MC, Chambers SD, et al. Partial liquid ventilation improves gas exchange and increases EELV in acute lung injury. J Appl Physiol 1998;84:1566–1572.

Gemzell CA, Robbe H, Strom G, et al. Observations on circulatory changes and muscular work in normal labor. Acta Obstet Gynecol Scand 1957;36:75–93.

George R, Berkenbosch JW, Fraser RF II, Tobias JD. Mechanical ventilation during pregnancy using a helium-oxygen mixture in a patient with respiratory failure due to status asthmaticus. J Perinatol 2001;21(6):395–398.

Gibbs CP, Banner TC. Effectiveness of Bicitra as a preoperative antacid. Anesthesiology 1984;61(1):97–99.

Gutierrez G, Brown SD. Gastric tonometry: a new monitoring modality in the intensive care unit. J Int Care Med 1995;10:34–44.

Harris SK, Bone RC, Ruth WE. Gastrointestinal hemorrhage in patients in a respiratory intensive care unit. Chest 1977;72(3): 301–304.

Hathaway WE, Bonnar J. Thrombotic disorders in pregnancy and the newborn. In: Hemostatic Disorders of the Pregnant Woman and Newborn. New York: Elsevier Scientific Publishing, 1987.

Hill JD, O'Brien TG, Murray JJ, et al. Prolonged extracorporeal oxygenation for acute post-traumatic respiratory failure (shock-lung syndrome): use of the Bramson membrane lung. N Engl J Med 1972;286:629–634.

Hinson JR, Marini JJ. Principles of mechanical ventilator use in respiratory failure. Annu Rev Med 1992;43:341–361.

Hirschi C, Kacmarek RM, Stanek K. Work of breathing CPAP and PSV imposed by the new generation mechanical ventilators: a long model study. Respir Care 1991;36:815.

Hirschi RB, Parent AB, Tooley R, et al. Liquid ventilation improves pulmonary function, gas exchange, and lung injury in a model of respiratory failure. Ann Surg 1995;221:79.

Hirschi RB, Pranikoff T, Wise C, et al. Initial experience with partial liquid ventilation in adult patients with acute respiratory distress syndrome. JAMA 1996;275:383–389.

Holliday JE, Heyers TM. The reduction of weaning time from mechanical ventilation using tidal volume and relaxation biofeed back. Am Rev Respir Dis 1990;141(5 Pt 1):1214–1220.

Hull RD, Raskedo GE, Hirsh J. Prophylaxis of venous thromboembolism. Chest 1986;89:374.

Johansen WG Jr, Pierce AK, Sanford JP, et al. Nosocomial respiratory infections with gram negative bacilli: the significance of colonization of the respiratory tract. Ann Intern Med 1972;77:701.

Katz VL, Dotters DJ, Droegemueller W. Perimortem Cesarean delivery. Obstet Gynecol 1986;68:571–576.

Kaunitz AM, Hughes JM, Grimes DA, et al. Causes of maternal mortality in the United States. Obstet Gynecol 1985;65:605–612.

Kelly SM, Rosa A, Field S, et al. Inspiratory muscle strength and body composition in patients receiving total parenteral nutrition therapy. Am Rev Respir Dis 1984;130:33–37.

Kivilaakso E, Silen W. Pathogenesis of experimental gastric-mucosal injury. N Engl J Med 1979;301:364–369.

Kollef MH, Schuster DP. The acute respiratory distress syndrome. N Engl J Med 1985;332:27–37.

Kolobow T. Acute respiratory failure. On how to injure healthy lungs (and prevent sick lungs from recovering). ASAIO Trans 1988;34:31–34.

Kolobow T, Moretti MP, Fumagalli R, et al. Severe impairment in lung function induced by high peak airway pressure during mechanical ventilation. Am Rev Respir Dis 1987;135:312–315.

Kraman S, Khan F, Patel S, Seriff N. Renal failure in the respiratory intensive care unit. Crit Care Med 1979;7:263–266.

Lain DC, DiBenedetto R, Morris SL, et al. Pressure control inverse ratio ventilation as a method to reduce peak inspiratory pressure and provide adequate ventilation and oxygenation. Chest 1989;95:1081–1088.

Laroche CM, Moxham J, Green M. Respiratory muscle weakness and fatigue. Q J Med 1989;71:373–397.

Laros RK Jr. Thromboembolic disease. In: Creasy RK, Resnik R, eds. Maternal Fetal Medicine; Principles and Practice. Philadelphia: WB Saunders Company, 1994.

Leach C, Fuhrman B, Morin F, et al. Perfluorocarbon-associated gas exchange (partial liquid ventilation) in respiratory distress syndrome: A prospective, randomized, controlled study. Crit Care Med 1993;21:1270–1278.

Lewis MI, Belman MJ. Respiratory muscle involvement in malnutrition. In: Tobin MJ (ed). The Respiratory Muscles. Philadelphia: JB Lippincott Company, 1990.

Lowenstein E, Hallowell P, Levine FH, et al. Cardiovascular response to large doses of intravenous morphine in man. N Engl J Med 1969;281:1389–1393.

Lucas CE, Sugawa C, Riddle J, Rector F, Rosenberg B, Walt AJ. Natural history and surgical dilemma of stress gastric bleeding. Arch Surg 1971;102:266–273.

Lundin S, Mang H, Smithies M, Stenqvist O, Frostell C. Inhalation of nitric oxide in acute lung injury: results of a European multicentre study. The European Study Group of Inhaled Nitric Oxide. Intens Care Med 1999;25(9):881–883.

Lunkenheimer PP, Salle BL, Whimster WF, et al. High-frequency ventilation: Reappraisal and progress in Europe and abroad. Crit Care Med (suppl) 1994;22:S19–23.

McGuigan JE. A consideration of the adverse effects of cimetidine. Gastroenterology 1981;80(1):181–192.

MacIntyre N, Nishimura M, Usada Y, Tokioka H, Takezawa J, Shimada Y. The Nagoya conference on system design and patient-ventilator interactions during pressure support ventilation. Chest 1990;97:1463–1466.

McIntyre RC, Pulido EJ, Bensard DD, Shames BD, Abraham E. Thirty years of clinical trials in acute respiratory distress syndrome. Crit Care Med 2000;28(9):3314–3331.

Maki DG. Nosocomial bacteremia: An epidemiologic overview. Am J Med 1981;70:719–732.

Martin TR. Relationship between malnutrition and lung infections. Clin Chest Med 1987;8(3):359–372.

Meyer TJ, Hill NS. Non-invasive positive pressure ventilation to treat respiratory failure. Ann Intern Med 1994;120:760–770.

Miller RD, Rupp SM, Fisher DM, et al. Clinical pharmacology of vecuronium and atracurium. Anesthesiology 1984;61:444–453.

Mols G, Loop T, Geiger K, Farthmann E, Benzing A. Extracorporeal membrane oxygenation: a ten-year experience. Am J Surg 2000; 180:144–154.

Montgomery BA, Stager MA, Carrico CJ, Hudson LD. Causes of mortality in patients with the adult respiratory distress syndrome. Am Rev Respir Dis 1985;132:485–489.

Moser KM, LeMoine JR, Nachtwey FJ, Spragg RG. Deep venous thrombosis and pulmonary embolism. JAMA 1981;246:1422–1424.

Nett LM, Morganroth M, Petty TL. Weaning from mechanical ventilation: A perspective and review of techniques. In: Bone RC, ed. Critical Care: A Comprehensive Approach. Park Ridge, Illinois, USA: American College of Chest Physicians 1984:171.

New W, Jr. Pulse oximetry. J Clin Monit 1985;1:126–129.

Nilsson I, Kullander S. Coagulation and fibrinolytic studies during pregnancy. Acta Obstet Gynecol Scand 1967;46:286–303.

Overbeck M, Pranikoff T, Yadao C, et al. Efficacy of perofluorocarbon partial liquid ventilation in a large animal model of acute respiratory failure. Crit Care Med 1996;24:1208–1214.

Pardee NE, Winterbauer RH, Allen JD. Bedside evaluation of respiratory distress. Chest 1984;85(2):203–206.

Pernoll ML, Metcalf J, Schlenker TL, et al. Oxygen consumption at rest and during exercise in pregnancy. Respir Physiol 1975;25:285–293.

Perutz MF. Hemoglobin structure and respiratory transport. Sci Am 1978;239:92–125.

Piehl MA, Brown RS. Use of extreme position changes in acute respiratory failure. Crit Care Med 1976;4:13–14.

Pingleton SK. Complications of acute respiratory failure. Am Rev Respir Dis 1988;137:1463–1493.

Pingleton SK, Harmon GS. Nutritional management in acute respiratory failure. JAMA 1987;257:3094–3099.

Pontoppidan H, Geffin B, Lowenstein E. Acute respiratory failure in the adult 2. N Engl J Med 1972;287:743–752.

Potkin RT, Swenson ER. Resuscitation from severe acute hypercapnia: determinants of tolerance and survival. Chest 1992;102:1742–1745.

Prescenti A, Gattinoni L, Kolobow T, et al. Extracorporeal circulation in adult respiratory failure. ASAIO Trans 1988;34:43–47.

Rackow EC, Astiz M. Pathophysiology and treatment of septic shock. JAMA 1991;266:548–554.

Ralph DD, Robertson HT, Weaver LJ, et al. Distribution of ventilation and perfusion during positive end-expiratory pressure in the adult respiratory distress syndrome. Am Rev Respir Dis 1985; 131:54–60.

Raphael JH, Bexton MDR. Combined high frequency ventilation in the management of respiratory failure in late pregnancy. Anaesthesia 1993;48:596.

Rasanen J, Cane RD, Downs JB, et al. Airway pressure release ventilation during acute lung injury: A prospective multicenter trial. Crit Care Med 1991;19:1234–1241.

Rayburn WF, Zuspan FP, eds. Drug Therapy in Obstetrics and Gynecology, 3rd edn. St. Louis: Mosby Year Book, 1992.

Rochester DF, Esau SA. Malnutrition and respiratory system. Chest 1984;85:411–415.

Schuster DP, Rowley H, Feinstein S, McGue MK, Zuckerman GR. Prospective evaluation of the risk of upper gastrointestinal bleeding after admission to a medical intensive care unit. Am J Med 1984; 76(4):623–630.

Sebel PS, Lowdon JD. Propofol: a new intravenous anesthetic. Anesthesiology 1989;71:260–277.

Segredo V, Caldwell JE, Matthay MA, et al. Persistent paralysis in critically ill patients after long-term administration of vecuronium. N Engl J Med 1992;327:524–528.

Seidenfeld JJ, Pohl DF, Bell RC, Harris GD, Johnason WG, Jr. Incidence, site and outcome of infections in patients with the adult respiratory distress syndrome. Am Rev Respir Dis 1986;134(1):12–16.

Sellick BA. Cricoid pressure to control regurgitation of stomach contents during induction of anesthesia. Lancet 1961;2:404.

Shaffer TH, Wolfson MR, Clark LC Jr. Liquid ventilation. Pediatr Pulmonol 1992;14:102–109.

Shapiro BA, Cane RD, Harrison RA. Positive end-expiratory pressure therapy in adults with special reference to acute lung injury: A review of the literature and suggested clinical correlations. Crit Care Med 1984;12:127–141.

Shapiro BA, Peruzzi WT, Kozelowski-Templin R. Clinical Application of Blood Gases, 5th edn. Chicago: Mosby Year Book, 1994.

Shibutani K, Komatsu T, Kubal K, et al. Critical level of oxygen delivery in anesthetized man. Crit Care Med 1983;11:640–643.

Shoemaker WC, Ayres S, Grenvik A, et al. Textbook of Critical Care, 2nd edn. Philadelphia: WB Saunders, 1989.

Simmons RS, Berdine GG, Seidenfeld JJ, et al. Fluid balance and the adult respiratory distress syndrome. Am Rev Respir Dis 1987; 135:924–929.

Skillman JJ, Bushnell LS, Goldman H, Silen W. Respiratory failure, hypotension, sepsis and jaundice: A clinical syndrome associated with lethal hemorrhage from acute stress ulceration of the stomach. Am J Surg 1969;117:523–530.

Slutsky AS. Consensus conference on mechanical ventilation—January 28–30, 1993 at Northbrook, Illinois, USA, Part 2. Int Care Med 1994;20:150.

Soler M, Imhof E, Perruchoud AP. Severe acute asthma. Pathophysiology, clinical assessment and treatment. Respiration 1990;57: 114–121.

Stock MC, Downs JB, Frolicher DA. Airway pressure release ventilation. Crit Care Med 1987;15:462–466.

Suter PM, Fairley HB, Isenberg MD. Optimum end-expiratory pressure in patients with acute pulmonary failure. N Engl J Med 1975;292:284–289.

Sutherland AD, Stock JG, Davies JM. Effects of preoperative fasting on morbidity and gastric contents in patients undergoing day-stay surgery. Br J Anaesth 1986;58:876–878.

Swartz MA, Marino PL. Diaphragmatic strength during weaning from mechanical ventilation. Chest 1985;85:736–739.

Szatalowicz VL, Goldberg JP, Anderson RJ. Plasma antidiuretic hormone in acute respiratory failure. Am J Med 1982;72:58–587.

Templeton A, Kelman GR. Maternal blood-gases, (P_AO_2-P_aO_2), physiologic shunt, and V_D/V_T in normal pregnancy. Br J Anaesth 1976; 48:1001–1004.

Tharratt RS, Allen RP, Albertson TE. Pressure controlled inverse ratio ventilation in severe adult respiratory failure. Chest 1988;94: 755–762.

Tobin MJ, Alex CG. Discontinuation of mechanical ventilation. In: Tobin MJ (ed.). Principles and Practice of Mechanical Ventilation. New York, McGraw-Hill, 1994:1177.

Tobin MJ, Yang K. Weaning from mechanical ventilation. Crit Care Clin 1990;6(3):725–747.

Todd ME, Thompson JH, Bowie EJW, et al. Changes in blood coagulation during pregnancy. Mayo Clin Proc 1965;40:370.

Tryba M, Zevounou F, Torok M, Zenz M. Prevention of acute stress bleeding with sucralfate, antacids, or cimetidine. A controlled study with pirenzepine as a basic medication. Am J Med 1985;79:55–61.

Tsuno K, Prato P, Kolobow T. Acute lung injury from mechanical ventilation at moderately high airway pressures. J Appl Physiol 1990; 69:956–961.

Tyler DC, Cheney FW. Comparison of positive end-expiratory pressure and inspiratory positive plateau in ventilation of rabbits with experimental pulmonary edema. Anesth Analg 1979;58:288–292.

Ueland K, Hansen JM. Maternal cardiovascular hemodynamics. II. Posture and uterine contractions. Am J Obstet Gynecol 1969; 103:1–7.

United States Public Health Service. Progress toward achieving the 1990 objectives for pregnancy and infant health. MMWR 1988; 37:405.

Van Hook JW, Ventilator therapy and airway management. Crit Care Obstet 1997;8:143.

Van Hook JW, Harvey CJ, Uckan E. Mechanical ventilation in pregnancy and postpartum minute ventilation and weaning. Am J Obstet Gynecol 1995;172:326(part 2). Abstract.

Villasanta U. Thromboembolic disease in pregnancy. Am J Obstet Gynecol 1965;93:142.

Ward ME, Corbeil C, Gibbons W, et al. Optimization of respiratory muscle relaxation during mechanical ventilation. Anesthesiology 1988;69:29–35.

Walley KR, Lewis TH, Wood LDH. Acute respiratory acidosis decreases left ventricular contractility but increases cardiac output in dogs. Circ Res 1990;67:628–635.

Weinberger SE, Weiss JW. Editorial: Weaning from ventilatory support. N Engl J Med 1995;332:388–389.

Wessler S. Medical management of venous thrombosis. Annu Rev Med 1976;27:313–319.

Woodley M, Whelan A (eds). The Washington Manual, Manual of Medical Therapeutics. St Louis: Little, Brown and Company, 1993.

Wright HP, Osborn SB, Edmonds DG. Changes in the rate of flow of venous blood in the leg during pregnancy, measured with radioactive sodium. Surg Gynecol Obstet 1950;90:481.

Younes M, Bilan D, Jung D, Kroker H. An apparatus for altering the mechanical load of the respiratory system. J Appl Physiol 1987;62:2491–2499.

Zager RA, Prior RB. Gentamicin and Gram-negative bacteremia. A synergism for the development of experimental nephrotoxic acute renal failure. J Clin Invest 1986;78:196–204.

9 Vascular access

Gayle Olson
Aristides Koutrouvelis

Introduction

Hemorrhage is one of the leading causes of death in the obstetric population; therefore, knowledge of central intravenous and arterial line insertions and maintenance is imperative. Arterial access affords advantages specifically in the critically ill gravida such as assured access for repeated arterial blood sampling and continuous arterial blood pressure monitoring. Central intravenous (IV) access allows for the rapid administration of fluid, blood products, and inotropes (for prompt resuscitation) as well as access for hemodynamic monitoring when indicated. Long-term central IV access may also be indicated for the gravida with coexisting disease (hyperemesis gravidarum, inflammatory bowel disease, cystic fibrosis, pancreatitis, and gastroparesis) who require access for the administration of parenteral nutrition, medication, hemodialysis, prolonged antibiotics for the treatment of resistant bacterial strains, chemotherapy, and intravenous prostacyclin for pulmonary hypertension as well as for other difficult intravenous access issues (Levine & Esser, 1988; Wolk & Rayburn, 1990; Korelitz, 1992; Wiedner et al., 1993; Stewart et al., 2001).

Establishing central venous and arterial access is often an acquired skill, requiring knowledge of catheter type, preparation techniques, and access routes.

Catheter types and placement sites

Choosing the venous catheter and the site for insertion is influenced by the indication (Table 9.1), duration of use, urgency of administration, and type of infusate (highly osmolar, sclerotic, thrombogenic) needed. Catheters with shorter lengths and larger diameters allow for more rapid flow rates. For example, doubling the tube diameter (0.71 mm or 22 gauge vs 1.65 mm or 16 gauge) results in almost a quadrupling of the flow rate (24.7 mL/min vs 96.3 mL/min) (De la Roche & Gauthier, 1993). Multilumen catheters are routinely used for central venous cannulation (Fig. 9.1). The more commonly used triple lumen catheter has an outside diameter of 2.3 mm (6.9 French) and provides three channels (three 18 gauge, or two 18 gauge plus one 16 gauge). The opening of each channel is separated from the other by 1 cm or more in order to reduce mixing of infusates.

Choosing a venous catheter

Depending on the route of insertion and duration of use, IV catheters are considered to be short-term transcutaneous, long-term transcutaneous, and implantable (Table 9.2). Catheters are considered to be either peripheral or central. A peripheral location is distal to a central vein and contains valves while a central location contains no valves and is considered to be at the level of the axillary or common femoral vein and all other veins oriented toward the heart from this level. The use of the terminology peripheral and central is also based on the peripheral or central location of insertion and the central location of the catheter tip. Central vein cannulation is required to accommodate the large-bore catheters necessary for high-volume administration rates. When administering highly osmolar, sclerotic, or thrombotic IV fluids, most clinicians agree that the catheter tip should be placed near the heart in the superior or inferior vena cava, although optimal placement has not been established in prospective human studies (McGee et al., 1993). Administration of potent vasoconstrictive agents such as norepinephrine and epinephrine mandate central venous access in order to minimize any potential adverse effects.

Short-term (days) transcutaneous catheters are constructed of polyethylene, polyurethane, polycarbonate, vinyl chloride, or silicone and are available in multiple lengths, diameters, and lumen numbers. Generally, they are used for periods of less than 2 weeks. These catheters are suitable for most obstetric patients in the "difficult access" group (history of IV drug abuse, IV chemotherapy, hypovolemia) and for others with rapidly resolvable conditions. Because of the intended

Table 9.1 Indications for prolonged venous access

Parenteral nutrition and drug therapy
Hyperemesis gravidarum
Inflammatory bowel disease
Gastroparesis
Pancreatitis
Cystic fibrosis
Short bowel syndrome
Heparin (heart valves, deep vein thrombosis)
Antibiotics (bacterial endocarditis, osteomyelitis)
Chemotherapeutic agents for malignancy
Magnesium sulfate
Lack of peripheral access
Previous intravenous drug abuse
Previous prolonged chemotherapy
Hemodialysis

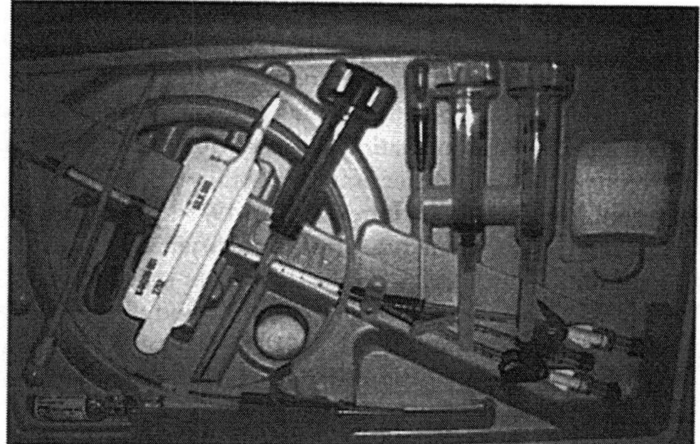

Fig. 9.1 Multilumen catheter insertion set up. Typically catheter kits are equipped with introducing needle, guidewire, dilating catheter, and triple-lumen catheter.

Table 9.2 Central venous catheter types

Type	Short term	Long term	Implantable
Location	Transcutaneous	Transcutaneous	Subcutaneous
Duration	<2 weeks	≥4 weeks	Months–years
Venous site	Peripheral	Central	Same as central
	Pedal	Subclavian	Long term
	Saphenous	External	Long term
	Femoral	Jugular	Huber point needle required for access to reservoir
		Internal jugular	
		Cephalic	
		Facial	
		Saphenous	
		Femoral	
Material	Polyethylene, polyurethane, vinyl chloride, silicone	Silicone	
Cuff	No cuff	Dacron	
Lumen	Varies		Single/double
Indication	Difficult access	Chronic illness	Chronic illness
Risks/benefits	Dislodgement of catheter Decreased patient mobility		Increased patient mobility
Tip	Open	Groshong valve	Reservoir

short duration of use, sites on the lower extremities, such as pedal, saphenous, and femoral veins, might be selected. Decreased patient mobility and the high risk of catheter dislodgement are among the generally accepted disadvantages of lower extremity access locations.

Long-term (weeks to months) transcutaneous catheters are usually constructed of more flexible and less thrombogenic derivatives of silicone and are passed through a subcutaneous tunnel between the points of venous insertion and exit from the skin (Ray et al., 1996; Marino, 1998). Frequently, these catheters incorporate a Dacron cuff just proximal to the skin exit site. Catheter tunneling and the Dacron cuff promote tissue ingrowth and fixation, and limit the spread of skin exit-site colonization or infection. Long-term catheters may incorporate a Groshong valve tip (Delmore et al., 1989; Pasquale et al., 1992). Such catheters are blind-ended but incorporate a side slit near the catheter tip. Positive pressure exerted through the catheter blows the slit walls open outwardly for fluid or medication administration, while negative pressure draws the slit walls inward for blood sampling. At rest, the catheter is closed, theoretically obviating the need for heparinization between periods of catheter use. Peripherally inserted central venous catheters (PICC), introduced in 1975 (Hoshal, 1975), are increasingly popular due to the ease of insertion compared with traditionally placed surgical catheters (Hickman and central venous ports), fewer complications, and the potential to decrease cost (Horattas et al., 2001). Implantable catheters attached to reservoirs placed into subcutaneous pockets are indicated for very long-term use (months to years), typically in patients requiring intermittent boluses or short infusions of parenteral medications (Andrews et al., 1990). Implantable catheters as well as implantable reservoir pumps (Blackshear et al., 1972) give patients maximal mobility, prevent catheter dislodgement, and eliminate external appliances inbetween periods of catheter use. Surgical cutdown for the insertion of implantable venous access devices has been shown to decrease early as well as late complications of venous access (Di Carlo et al., 2001). During catheter use, access to the reservoir is gained by transcutaneous placement of a special Huber-point needle that uses a noncoring tip. Vein sites commonly used for long-term catheter use include the subclavian, external and internal jugular, basilic, and greater saphenous veins. When the femoral, greater saphenous, or basilic veins are used, the catheter is tunneled to allow for port placement onto the lower chest, abdominal wall, thigh, or forearm (D'Angelo et al., 1997). Ideally, reservoirs for implantable catheters should be placed in a secure, flat, nonmobile area, preferably overlying a rib. As a result, abdominal wall placement is less desirable for these devices (Morris et al, 1991; Finney et al., 1992; Schuman & Ragsdale, 1995).

Choosing an arterial catheter

Arterial catheters should be used for specific purposes and for short time intervals. Arteries that are accessible to palpation and that can usually be cannulated include (in order of preference) the radial, dorsalis pedis, femoral, axillary, and brachial. In general, for an artery to be suitable for continuous monitoring of intraarterial pressures: (i) the diameter should be large enough to accommodate the catheter without occluding the lumen; (ii) there should be adequate collateral circulation; (iii) the site should be such that catheter care can be facilitated; and (iv) the site should not be prone to contamination.

Preparing for catheter insertion

Prior to cannulation of any vessel, it is necessary to assure patency of the vessel. In addition, arterial candidates should demonstrate good pulsation as well as adequate collateral flow. Contraindications to vessel cannulation include infection or inflammation at the site, arterial–venous or aneurysmal malformations, and arterial graft. Coagulopathy is a relative contraindication to cannulation. In the presence of coagulopathy, the use of a portable Doppler device affords easy visualization of the underlying vessels and minimizes the risk of carotid puncture and repetitive attempts. In an evaluation of catheter placement (subclavian vein, SCV, 96%; internal jugular vein, IJV, 4%) in 242 patients with corrected coagulopathy and 88 with uncorrected coagulopathy, only four bleeding complications significant enough to require intervention were identified. Three bleeding complications were easily controlled with a suture at the catheter insertion site, and the only variable significantly associated with a bleeding complication was a platelet count $<50 \times 10(9)/L$ ($P = 0.02$) (Mumtaz et al., 2000).

Skin preparation

Cutaneous antisepsis is paramount, as is hand washing, education of personnel, and use of the sterile technique to include large sterile drape, gown, and gloves (Puntis et al., 1990; Parras et al., 1994; Raad et al., 1994; O'Grady et al., 2002). Antiseptic agents that reduce skin microflora and are used for skin preparation include alcohol, iodine, chlorhexidine gluconate, and hexachlorophene. Alcohol has a broad spectrum of antibacterial activity but has no detergent action and therefore may not work well on dirty skin (Larson, 1988; Wyatt et al., 1990). The most popular antiseptic solution used is the povidone-iodine preparation Betadine. This is a water-soluble complex of iodine with a carrier molecule. Iodine is slowly released from the carrier molecule, thus reducing any irritating effects. Due to this slow release, the preparation should be left in contact with the skin for a least 2 min (Sheikh, 1986; Larson, 1988; Wyatt et al., 1990). Shaving at catheter insertion sites is not recommended as it abrades the skin and promotes bacterial colonization. If hair removal is necessary it should be clipped.

Catheterization techniques—general

The first technique described to place a catheter in a vessel is the direct approach. The direct approach involves palpation and direct needle puncture, usually with the advancement of a Teflon catheter over the needle and into the vessel. A second technique involves the use of a guidewire. This technique, originally described by Seldinger (1953), was for replacement of the needle during percutaneous arteriography. Once the vessel has been punctured and the return of blood flow (pulsatile in cases of arterial puncture) achieved, the needle is not advanced further, but rather a fine and flexible wire is inserted through the needle and into the lumen of the vessel. The sharp needle is then removed and a polyurethane-type catheter is threaded over the wire and into the vessel. Commercially produced catheters are available that incorporate an integral guidewire (a modified Seldinger technique). Beards and colleagues (1994) compared all three insertion techniques in 69 critically ill patients. The direct puncture technique was associated with the highest failure rate, followed by the modified and classic Seldinger techniques, respectively. The direct puncture technique also took significantly longer, used more catheters, and required more punctures per successful insertion than did the modified or classic Seldinger techniques. These authors also observed that polyurethane catheters were significantly less likely to block and require reinsertion than were the Teflon catheters. As a result, they strongly endorsed use of the classic Seldinger technique and polyurethane catheters.

Proper positioning is important for all venous and arterial cannulations. The patient should be in the Trendelenburg position and rolled slightly to the left in later stages of pregnancy when the inferior vena cava is susceptible to compression by the uterus. The legs can be raised if the patient is intolerant of the Trendelenburg position. If not accomplished previously, local anesthetic is infused into the region prior to enlarging the puncture site slightly with a scalpel in order to accommodate the catheter or dilators. Local anesthetic also is infiltrated into the sites of incisions or dissection for subcutaneous pockets for Dacron cuffs or reservoirs. After correct venous puncture, the syringe is removed carefully, while the operator covers the needle hub to prevent excessive bleeding and entry of air (for central venous punctures). In the Seldinger technique (used for most direct central venous punctures), a guidewire is placed through the needle, and the needle is withdrawn. A stiff dilator is then generally threaded over the wire and passed one or more times in order to dilate the tract to the vein. The dilator is then removed and is placed through the slightly larger catheter. The dilator-catheter assembly is then threaded over the wire into correct position, and the wire and dilator are removed. Correct placement is supported by confirming free aspiration of blood from the catheter and free flow (by gravity alone) of an appropriate crystalloid solution into the catheter.

Long-term transcutaneous catheters are generally placed using a peel-away sheath modification of Seldinger's technique. After dilation of the tract, a dilator-sheath assembly is advanced over the wire into the chosen vein, and the wire and dilator are removed. A silastic catheter is then threaded through the peel-away sheath. Upon proper positioning, the handles on the peel-away sheath are rotated perpendicular to its long axis until the sheath cracks. Pulling the sheath handles apart, the sheath is then simultaneously peeled in half along its long axis and removed while the catheter is carefully held in place.

Long-term transcutaneous, surgical cutdown, and implanted catheters are generally inserted following prophylactic antibiotic administration in an operating theater or outpatient surgical suite, thus maximizing sterility. Several authors have described utilizing real-time ultrasonography to facilitate venous location and puncture and to lessen the incidence of puncture-related complications (Denys et al., 1991; Sherer et al., 1993). Fluoroscopic guidance is used frequently to speed and simplify correct catheter positioning. Right atrial electrocardiography is also described for facilitating proper catheter tip placement (McGee et al., 1993).

The catheter-through-the-needle technique is also used, primarily for short-term transcutaneous catheterizations of central veins, and for PICC placement. Extreme caution must be taken never to pull the catheter back out through the needle; otherwise the catheter may be sheared, resulting in catheter embolus.

In cases of arterial cannulation, successful line placement can be confirmed by the appearance of pulsatile blood flow or, if any doubt exists, by blood gas analysis. For blood pressure monitoring, the catheter is connected to a transducer with a three-way stopcock and high-pressure tubing which is connected to a pressure bag containing normal saline and heparin (1,500 units/500 mL). The high-pressure tubing is necessary to prevent damping of blood pressure readings. The heparinized saline is administered through the pressurized bag at a rate of approximately 2–5 mL/hr in order to prevent the catheter from clotting off. It is critically important to purge all pressure lines and stopcocks prior to connecting the arterial line in order to prevent arterial air embolism. All set-ups should also have a purge or flush device that can be used to clear any blood that may back up into the pressure tubing as well as to clear the catheter itself and the stopcock after blood sampling.

Central venous and arterial lines should be sutured into place to prevent accidental disconnection or withdrawal. The catheter itself is then covered with a sterile, waterproof occlusive dressing after application of an antibiotic ointment at the skin puncture site. When withdrawing blood samples, the dead space in the system should be appreciated and a sufficient quantity of blood to account for this should be withdrawn and discarded prior to actual specimen collection. It is also very important to purge the system after specimen collection, lest the line clot off.

Venous access sites

Internal jugular vein

The IJV is a common central venous access route and its advantages include ease by which this vessel can be compressed in the case of hemorrhage, decreased risk for pneumothorax, and, when cannulated on the right side, avoidance of the thoracic duct. The IJV is located under the sternocleidomastoid muscle (SCM), and, at its junction with the SCV, helps form the brachiocephalic vein. Anatomic variation in the course of the IJV has been noted, and the relationship between the IJV and the carotid artery may be abnormal in 10% of the population (Fontes, 1998). Typically, when the head is turned away from the intended side of cannulation, the IJV forms a line from the pinna of the ear to the sternoclavicular joint and brings the IJV to a more anterior position relative to the carotid artery (Clemente, 1997; Marino, 1998). Both median and posterior approaches are possible for cannulation of the IJV, but irrespective of the approach, the right side is preferred because the thoracic duct is avoided and the IJV, innominate veins, and superior vena cava almost form a straight line resulting in a more direct course to the right atrium (Fontes, 1998).

In the median approach the head is turned *away* from the cannulation site with the body maintained in a 20–30° Trendelenburg position. This maintains the head in a "down" position, distending the IJV and minimizing air entrainment. A triangle region created by two heads of the SCM and the clavicle is then identified (Fig. 9.2). The carotid artery is palpated medial to the IJV and medial and posterior to the SCM and is retracted medially. An 18-gauge cannulating needle, attached to a syringe, is inserted at the apex of the triangle, bevel facing up, and at a 30–45° angle to the skin (Fig. 9.3). The needle is advanced toward the ipsilateral nipple. If the vein is not encountered by the time a depth of 5 cm is exceeded the needle should be withdrawn 4 cm and advanced again in a more lateral direction. When a vessel is entered a flash of blood is noted at the catheter hub. If the blood is bright red and pulsating, the carotid artery has been punctured. In this situation, remove the needle and apply pressure to the area for 5–10 minutes to encourage tamponade. When the carotid artery has been punctured, no further attempts should be made on either side because puncture of both arteries can have serious consequences.

To employ the posterior approach, the body position is the same but the physician should plan an insertion site 1 cm superior to the point where the external jugular vein (EJV) crosses over the lateral edge of the SCM. In the posterior approach, the needle is then inserted at the 3 o'clock position, bevel up, and is advanced along the underbelly of the SCM and then aimed toward the SCM at its sternal insertion and the suprasternal notch (Fig. 9.4). The IJV should be encountered 5–6 cm from the skin surface with this approach. If the advancing attempt does not produce a flash of blood in the hub of the needle, applying slow continuous negative pressure while withdrawing the needle potentiates identification of venous blood, thus identifying the vein. However, the absence of pulsatile blood flow does not necessarily ensure venous access has been achieved. Ideally, a pressure wave should be transduced to confirm a venous waveform (Ho & Lui, 1994; Fontes, 1998).

In addition to the above approaches, tunneled central venous catheters have also been described using the IJV versus the SCV. The IJV approach was easier to perform with fewer

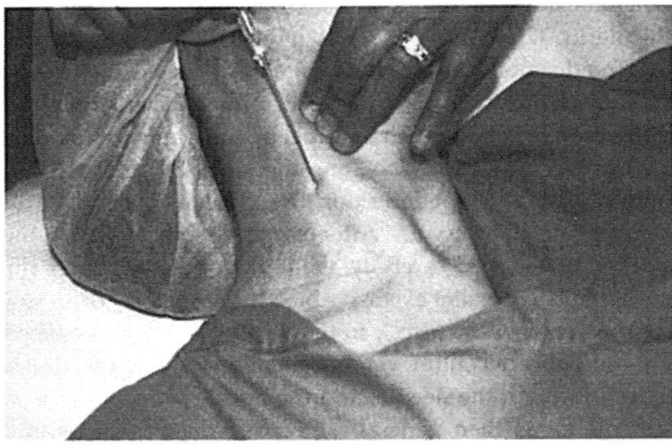

Fig. 9.3 Median approach to internal jugular vein cannulation. The carotid artery is palpated and retracted medially while the needle is inserted at the tip of the triangle and advanced toward the ipsilateral nipple.

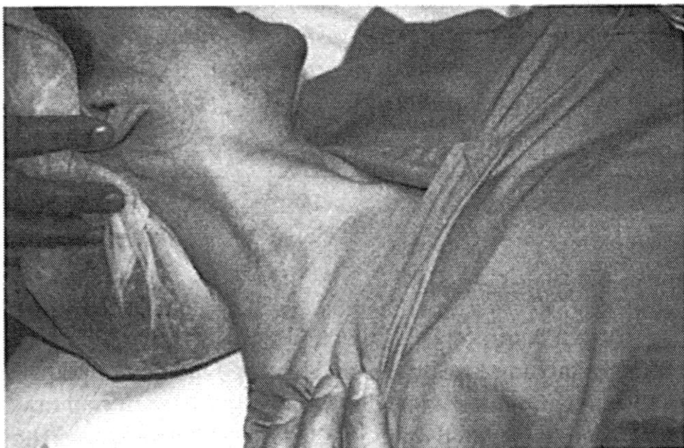

Fig. 9.2 Positioning for internal jugular vein cannulation. The head is turned away from the insertion site. A triangle is formed by the SCM and clavicle. (Model for demonstration only, sterile technique not used: in this and following photos (Figs 9.3–9.6).)

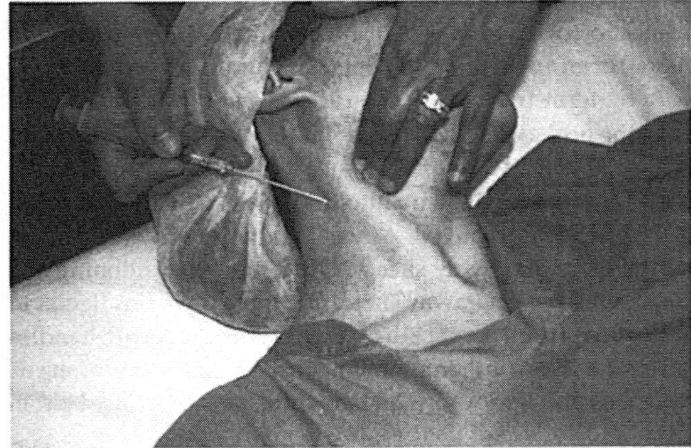

Fig. 9.4 Posterior approach to internal jugular vein cannulation. In the posterior approach the needle is advanced along the underbelly of the SCM aiming at the suprasternal notch.

complications (Macdonald et al., 2000). Complications of IJV cannulation include hematoma, carotid artery puncture, nerve damage, air embolus, and cardiac tamponade.

External jugular vein

The EJV is formed by the junction of the retromandibular and posterior auricular veins. It runs obliquely across the SCM along a line extending from the angle of the jaw to mid-clavicle. The EJV joins the SCV at an acute angle under the area of the clavicle (Clemente, 1997). The primary advantage of using the EJV for venous access is the decreased risk of pneumothorax. The disadvantages include difficulty in advancing a catheter, and vein perforation due to the acute angle with the SCV.

The patient is placed supine or in the Trendelenburg position and the head is turned *away* from the side of insertion. The vein can best be identified by applying pressure just above the clavicle and allowing the vein to engorge. Unfortunately, even under the best of conditions, 15% of patients will not have an identifiable EJV (Seneff, 1987). Once identified, the vein should be stabilized between the thumb and forefinger at a level midway between the clavicle and jaw and the catheter inserted with the bevel up. The length of the catheter should not exceed 15 cm. Undue force at the time of catheter insertion can result in perforation of the EJV at the angle in which it enters the SCV. Manipulation of the shoulder may facilitate passage of the J-wire past the clavicle without asserting undue pressure (Sparks et al., 1991). Another technique to maneuver a difficult EJV–SCV junction is described by Segura-Vasi and colleagues (1999). Upon meeting resistance at the EJV–SCV junction, the J-wire is withdrawn approximately 0.5 cm proximal to the junction. The triple-lumen catheter is then slowly advanced over the J-wire. The success of this maneuver may lie in the smaller diameter of the catheter tip (Belani et al., 1980; Segura-Vasi et al., 1999). Complications of EJV cannulation include thrombosis, superior vena cava perforation, and hydrothorax (Ho & Lui, 1994; Colomina et al., 2000).

Subclavian vein

The SCV is often used to gain central access. As a continuation of the axillary vein, the course of the SCV runs underneath the clavicle and along the outer surface of the anterior scalene muscle. At the level of the thoracic inlet, the SCV joins the IJV to form the brachiocephalic vein (Clemente, 1997; Marino, 1998). To cannulate the vein, the patient is placed in the supine position, maintaining a 15% Trendelenburg position, with the head *facing* the site of insertion and the arms pronated, slightly flexed, and down at the sides. We prefer placing a rolled towel under the spine and shoulder, and are of the opinion that this serves to widen the path between the first rib and the clavicle, but other clinicians may challenge that this is unnecessary. Next, the operator should visualize the path of the subclavian artery divided into medial, middle, and lateral thirds along the clavicular line (Fig. 9.5). Using this method, the junction of the medial and middle segment approximates the lateral aspect of the SCM insertion on the clavicle. Using this point for needle insertion may decrease the risk for pneumothorax. In the infraclavicular approach (Fig. 9.6), the skin puncture site is approximately 1 cm beneath the clavicle but should be further from the clavicle in order to lessen the risk of pneumothorax in patients with a thick chest wall. The bevel should initially be pointing upward. The catheter tip is "walked" along the underside of the clavicle touching the bone itself as needed, pointing toward the suprasternal notch and parallel to the patient's back. Upon entering the vein, the bevel is turned to the 3 o'clock position to facilitate passing the catheter. A supraclavicular approach has also been described, but it is generally less practiced (Young, 1978; Conroy et al., 1990). Immediate risks of SCV cannulation include pneumothorax,

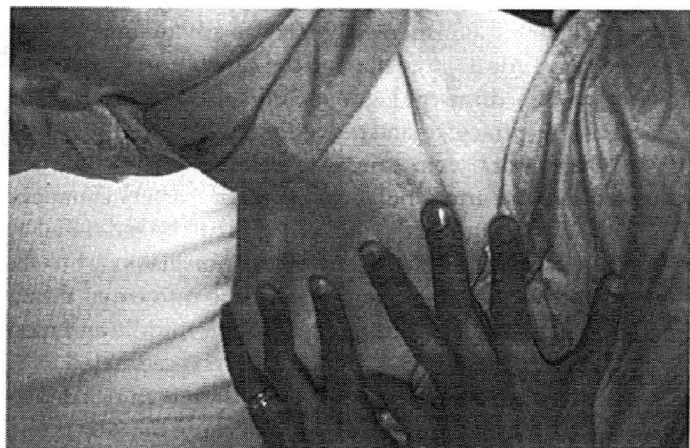

Fig. 9.5 Landmarks for subclavian vein cannulation. Using the clavicle, the subclavian vein is divided into thirds. The junction of the middle and medial third identifies the location for needle insertion.

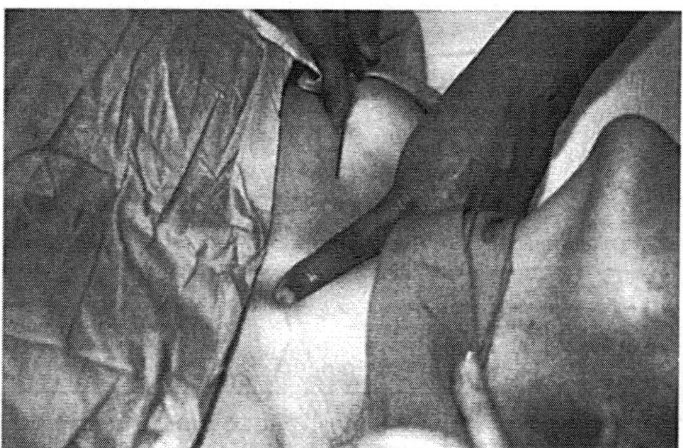

Fig. 9.6 Infraclavicular approach to subclavian vein cannulation. The head is turned toward the insertion site. The needle is inserted approximately 1 cm below the clavicle aimed at the suprasternal notch.

hemothorax, and catheter misplacement. A common location for misplacement of the catheter is in the ipsilateral IJV. Misplacement is most often detected by radiographic studies. Another technique has been described using the IJV occlusion test (Ambesh et al., 2001). In that study, the occlusion test was performed by applying external pressure on the IJV in the supraclavicular area for 10 seconds. During the application of pressure, the central venous pressure and waveform were observed. In all cases of catheter misplacement into the IJV, the central venous pressure increased 3–5 mmHg. If the misplaced catheter was in another vessel, the central venous pressure did not change with this maneuver. Thrombosis and subsequent pulmonary emboli have also been recognized (Harris et al., 1982).

Femoral vein

From lateral to medial, the femoral nerve, artery and vein traverse the femoral triangle by descending beneath the inguinal ligament (Clemente, 1997). The advantage of using the femoral vein is its large size and the absence of risk of pneumothorax. The disadvantages include venous thrombosis, femoral artery puncture, and reduction in hip mobility (Seneff, 1987). The femoral vein can be located 1–2 cm medial to a palpated femoral artery pulse. If the femoral artery cannot be palpated, the location of the femoral vein can be estimated by imagining a line from the anterior superior iliac crest to the public tubercle and then dividing the line into equal thirds. The femoral artery lies at the junction of the middle and most medial segment and the femoral vein can be estimated as 1–2 cm medial to this point (Fig. 9.7). The skin is punctured 2–3 cm caudal to the inguinal ligament to ensure the vein is cannulated in the area of the thigh. A catheter, at least 15 cm in length, can then be inserted into the femoral vein by directing the tip toward the vein at a 45° angle to the skin. Once in the vein, the angle of the catheter may be placed more parallel to the skin surface in order to align with the lumen of the vessel.

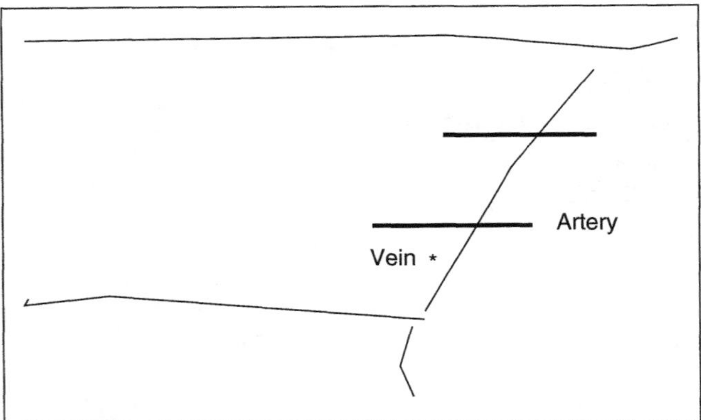

Fig. 9.7 Estimating femoral vein location. When the femoral arterial pulsations cannot be appreciated, the location of the femoral vein can be estimated. Draw a line from the anterior superior iliac crest to the pubic tubercle and divide into equal thirds. The junction of the medial and middle segment approximates the femoral artery and the vein will lie 2–3 cm more medial.

Femoral vein cannulation is generally not recommended for cardiopulmonary resuscitation or in cases of bleeding disorders (Marino, 1998). Complications of femoral vein cannulation include arterial puncture, hematoma, bleeding, local inflammation, malposition of catheter tip, and thrombosis (Durbec et al., 1997).

Cephalic vein

In its course away from the axillary vein, the cephalic vein travels below the clavipectoral fascia in the deltopectoral groove and descends down the lateral aspect of the arm (Clemente, 1997). The cephalic vein is most often used for central venous access via surgical cutdown.

Arterial access sites

Radial artery

The brachial artery divides into the radial and ulnar arteries in the forearm. The radial artery is a favored site for arterial cannulation due to its superficial location medial to the styloid process. The ulnar artery parallels the radial artery. Together, the radial and ulnar arteries form anastomosing palmar arches supplying blood to the hands (Clemente, 1997). Prior to cannulation of the radial artery, adequacy of collateral circulation must be established. The Allen test can be used in an attempt to document the adequacy of collateral flow. Even so, progressive delayed ischemia of the hand may occur, requiring amputation (Mangar et al., 1993).

Allen test

The Allen test evaluates the patency of the collateral circulation in the hand and is performed in the following manner: (i) the radial and ulnar arteries are occluded simultaneously; (ii) continuing this occlusion, the patient elevates the hand above his or her head; (iii) next, he or she repeatedly makes a fist until the hand blanches; and (iv) the pressure on the ulnar artery is then released. The palm should regain its normal color within 6 seconds. Delay of color from 7 to 15 seconds indicates that ulnar artery filling is slow. Persistent blanching for up to 15 seconds or more indicates an incomplete or occluded ulnar arch. Failure to regain normal color promptly is presumptive evidence of inadequate collateral flow, and the radial artery should thus not be cannulated. In performing this test, care is taken not to hyperextend the wrist, which could falsely compromise ulnar flow. In cases of radial-line-induced ischemia where perfusion to the hand has been compromised, we have successfully used a stellate ganglion block to promote vasodilation and return perfusion to near necrotic fingers.

Once adequate collateral circulation has been determined, preparation for cannulation of the radial artery can be undertaken. The wrist is dorsiflexed slightly to optimize exposure of the artery. This is best accomplished by use of an arm board and placement of a small gauze roll beneath the dorsal surface of the wrist, with tape placed across the patient's palm and upper forearm. When taping the upper forearm, care is taken not to constrict blood flow. Alternatively, an assistant may hold the patient's arm in place, but access to the puncture site is often obstructed in so doing. Once positioned, the area is prepped and anesthetized as described previously. We prefer using a 20- or 22-gauge Angiocath. The needle is advanced at a 30° angle to the artery until a flash of blood appears in the hub (Fig. 9.8). If using the direct puncture technique, the needle is then lowered and the catheter advanced while holding the needle stable. This can often be facilitated by rotating the catheter itself backward and forward, in a drilling motion. If the catheter fails to advance easily, it should not be forced, lest a traumatic pseudoaneurysm be produced. Often, both walls of the vessel will have been punctured and the catheter will lie posterior to the vessel. Once the catheter has been advanced beyond the tip of the metal needle, the needle should never be advanced, because the catheter is unlikely to be straight, and accordingly, its back wall is prone to being punctured by the needle, making further advancement of the catheter impossible. Instead, completely remove the needle and then slowly withdraw the catheter until pulsatile flow is established, at which point one can gently try to advance the catheter or pass a 25-gauge vascular wire through the catheter, followed by advancement over the wire. If neither of these maneuvers meets with success, the catheter should be removed and discarded. The procedure is then repeated with a new needle and catheter.

If the Seldinger technique (or a modification) is used, the needle is advanced until a flash of blood is observed in the hub of the catheter. After the flash is observed, the guidewire is advanced through the needle until it is 2–3 cm into the artery. The catheter can then be advanced over both guidewire and needle, or the needle can be removed and the catheter advanced over just the guidewire. Once the catheter has been advanced, the guidewire and/or needle is removed, pulsatile flow is established, and the line is secured and connected, as previously discussed.

Rarely, cutdown and direct visualization will be required for radial artery catheterization. A 2-cm transverse incision is made 2 cm proximal to the wrist fold, and the vessel is located by blunt dissection with small hemostats. The hemostats should separate the tissue in a plane parallel to the vessel in order to minimize vessel trauma. Skin hooks are helpful to hold the incision open. The dissection also is guided by intermittent palpation in order to maintain orientation to the vessel. Once exposed, a 1.0–1.5-cm length of vessel should be cleaned and mobilized, and 2-0 or 3-0 silk sutures are passed beneath the vessel with a right-angle clamp. We prefer using one suture proximal and one distal to the site of vessel puncture. The distal suture can be used to elevate the vessel for direct visual puncture. If vessel puncture is not initially successful, traction on the proximal suture will stop the bleeding, providing visualization of the puncture site and thus allowing the catheter to be inserted without the necessity of another puncture. Once catheterized, both sutures are removed (not tied) and the skin is closed. Pressure should be maintained on the cutdown site for 5 or 10 minutes in order to prevent hematoma formation.

Postcannulation radial arterial occlusion has been reported in up to 50% of patients in some data series (Bedford, 1977; Butt et al., 1987). Ischemic and necrotic complications are much less common, occurring in less than 1% of patients with radial artery cannulas. Fortunately, most thrombosed radial arteries recannalize within a few weeks (Hudson-Civetta & Caruthers-Banner, 1983).

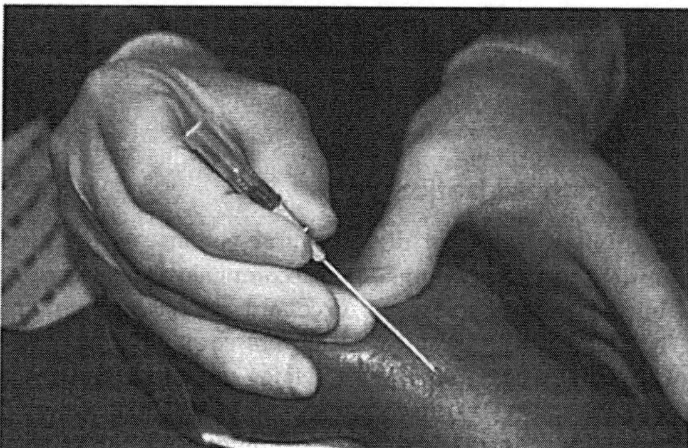

Fig. 9.8 Radial artery cannulation. The wrist is slightly dorsiflexed. The needle enters the skin at a 30° angle and advanced until a flash of blood appears in the hub. (Live insertion, sterile technique used.)

Brachial artery

The brachial artery is the continuation of the axillary artery. Collateral circulation is supplied by the ulnar collateral artery. This artery is best isolated just above the elbow crease medial to the biceps tendon. A 20-gauge, 2-inch catheter is inserted at a 30° angle to the skin until blood appears in the flash chamber. The vessel is then cannulated by either the direct or modified or classic Seldinger technique. Use of an arm board prevents flexion at the elbow and kinking of the catheter.

Use of the brachial artery entails greater risks than use of the radial artery, including the following: (i) adequacy of collateral circulation is much more difficult to assure; (ii) embolization could occlude either of the major arterial supplies to the hand; and (iii) bleeding in the area of the median nerve may result in neuropathy and Volkmann's contracture. Bleeding may require fasciotomy (Hudson-Civetta & Caruthers-Banner, 1983).

Cannulation of the brachial artery should not be attempted in patients with disorders of hemostasis.

Axillary artery

The axillary artery is the continuation of the subclavian artery. It enters the axilla from under the teres major and lies in the proximal groove between the biceps and triceps muscles medially in the arm. This artery is almost as large as the femoral artery and has significant collateral flow; axillary artery thrombosis does not lead to distal ischemia. Because the right axillary artery arises from the right brachiocephalic trunk in direct communication with the common carotid artery, air, clot, or particulate matter may embolize the brain during flushing. Thus, it may be safer to use the left axillary artery.

For cannulation, the patient can be positioned either with the hand beneath the head with the palm near the occiput or with the arm extended and externally rotated. The vessel is located by palpation, and an 18- or 20-gauge catheter, measuring at least 5 cm, is inserted into the artery until pulsatile blood is observed in the flash chamber. The needle is inserted initially at about a 30° angle to the skin, and once blood return is noted, is lowered for direct advancement or guidewire insertion. Location of the artery near the brachial plexus can result in nerve compression should a hematoma develop. Direct injury to the cords of the brachial plexus may occur during insertion attempts because the axillary artery, vein, and three cords of the brachial plexus form a neurovascular bundle within the axillary sheath. Similar to brachial cannulation, distal circulation should be checked regularly after axillary arterial line insertion.

Dorsalis pedis artery

The dorsalis pedis artery is located on the dorsal aspect of the foot and is usually easily palpated, but may be absent in 12% of the population. Collateral blood supply is usually good, and ischemia is uncommon following cannulation of this vessel. Collateral circulation, supplied by the lateral plantar artery, can be assessed by compression to occlusion of the dorsalis pedis artery, followed by pressure on the nail bed of the great toe until it blanches. On release of pressure on the nail bed, color should return within 2–3 seconds.

To facilitate cannulation of the dorsalis pedis, hold the patient's foot in a neutral position, and introduce a 20- or 22-gauge needle into the artery at a shallow angle to the skin. This is a vein where the use of guidewires is felt by many to be particularly useful for gaining access to the dorsalis pedis.

Femoral artery

The femoral artery is an extension of the external iliac artery. It lies just below the inguinal ligament midway along a line drawn from the superior iliac spine and symphysis pubis just lateral to the vein and medial to the nerve. The usual catheters employed range from 20 to 16 gauge, are 16 cm in length, and are attached to a 10-mL syringe. The needle is inserted about 2 cm below the inguinal ligament and at a 45° angle to the skin. The puncture of the vessel can often be felt by the operator and is heralded by the ability to rapidly aspirate bright red blood. Also, a gloved finger placed over the hub of the needle can usually feel the arterial pulsations. Once the vessel is punctured, the needle is lowered to between 15 and 30°, and a J-tipped guidewire is inserted. The needle is removed, and direct pressure is applied to the insertion site to prevent bleeding or hematoma formation. The catheter is placed over the guidewire, but it is not advanced until the distal (external) tip of the guidewire itself has been secured. Care is also taken to ensure the wire is straight, as any kinks will make passage of the catheter difficult. A scalpel nick of the skin may be required for ease of passage of the catheter through the skin. The wire is then removed and the catheter connected and secured.

A complication peculiar to femoral vessel cannulation is puncture of the back wall of the vessel above the inguinal ligament, where blood may dissect into the retroperitoneal area; this is capable of masking a hemorrhage of up to several liters. Because of the large size of the femoral artery and vein, the likelihood of an arteriovenons (AV) fistula is higher than with smaller vessels, should both vessels be penetrated with a single insertion. Risk of AV fistula formation also relates to the much larger catheters used for femoral arterial cannulation. Similarly, the larger puncture site makes bleeding at the time of line removal more problematic. Pressure should be applied to the femoral site for 10–20 minutes at removal.

Complications

A wide range of complications are associated with central venous and arterial catheters (Tables 9.3, 9.4). General catheter-use guidelines published by the Food and Drug Administration are directed at reducing catheter-related complications (FDA Drug Bulletin, 1989).

Failed catheterization

Ninety-five percent of direct central venous and surgical cutdown catheterizations are accomplished successfully, while EJV catheterization is successful only 70% of the time (Agee & Balk, 1992). Most reviewers site a low incidence of failed catheterizations for PICC lines, with a rare maximum incidence of 15.4% (Merrell et al., 1994). Ultrasound-guidance is an increasingly useful technique for the establishment of venous access in difficult cases (Hatfield & Bodenham, 1999).

Table 9.3 Complications of central venous catheters

Immediate	Delayed
Insertion failure	Venous thrombosis
Malposition	Pulmonary embolism
Air embolism	Superior vena caval syndrome
Catheter embolism	Venous stenosis
Cardiac arrhythmia	Arteriovenous fistula
Pneumothorax	Arterial pseudoaneurysm
Hemothorax	Catheter thrombosis
Hydrothorax/chylothorax	Catheter dislodgement/ breakage
Tracheal/esophageal injury	Catheter-related infection
Femoral nerve injury	Endocarditis
Brachial plexus injury	Cardiac perforation
Phrenic nerve injury	Cardiac tamponade
Vagus nerve injury	Suppurative thrombophlebitis
Recurrent laryngeal nerve injury	Clavicular osteomyelitis
Recurrent stellate ganglion injury	

Table 9.4 Complications of arterial catheters

Hematoma
Hemorrhage
Catheter occlusion
Catheter dislocation
Infection
Embolism
Ischemic injury
Thrombosis
Pseudoaneurysm
Arteriovenous fistula

Catheter malposition

Among the most devastating consequences of the malpositions is cardiac tamponade. This uncommon, yet, potentially catastrophic complication must be kept in mind after insertion of all central catheters. Optimal catheter tip location has not been established via prospective human study but most practitioners believe the superior vena cava, proximal to the right atrium, to be the ideal location (McGee et al., 1993). Catheter tips located in smaller, more proximal veins are more likely to be associated with venous thrombosis and stenosis while catheter tips positioned in the heart may be associated with cardiac arrhythmias, perforation, tamponade, valvular injury, or endocarditis. PICC catheter tip malpositioning from an antecubital approach is the most frequently seen with a rate of 21–55% (Goodwin & Carlson, 1993; McGee et al., 1993). Fluoroscopic guidance during insertion facilitates correct placement of all types of central venous catheters, as does right atrial electrocardiography (McGee et al., 1993), ultrasonography (Sherer et al., 1993), and electronic catheter tracking systems (McKee, 1991; Morris et al., 1991). Postinsertion chest radiographs are recommended universally with possibly the exception of the imaged-guided central venous catheter insertion (Agee & Balk, 1992; Baranowski, 1993; James et al., 1993; LaFortune, 1993; Nohr, 1994; Lucey et al., 1999). These radiographic studies should identify midline placement of the catheter tip in the center of the SVC, not abutting the atrial or ventricular wall.

Catheter dislodgement

Although little discussed, several PICC series report an incidence of accidental catheter dislodgement between 0.8% and 10.4% (Hoshal, 1975; Loughran et al., 1992; Goodwin & Carlson, 1993; Lam et al., 1994; Merrell et al., 1994). The method of catheter fixation utilized in the series with the highest accidental dislodgement rate was not specified (Lam et al., 1994), but the high overall incidence of this complication is a topic for concern and future research.

Pneumothorax

The risk of pneumothorax, 1–6%, is primarily associated with direct subclavian or jugular vein catheterization, is less following direct catheterization of other central veins, and is essentially eliminated with PICC and surgical cutdown techniques (Collin & Clarke, 1994; Nohr, 1994). Collin and Clarke (1994) reviewed the occurrence of delayed or late pneumothorax following central venous catheterization and recommended that postinsertion chest radiographs be expiratory and upright. Expiration results in a decreased volume of air in the lung but not in the pleural space thus magnifying the radiographic appearance of the pneumothorax (Tocino et al., 1985). Finally, repeat or delayed chest radiographs are indicated following catheterizations requiring multiple attempts, persistent (pleuritic or back) pain and respiratory symptoms. The standard treatment for pneumothorax has traditionally consisted of tube thoracostomy. However, in an investigation by Laronga and colleagues (2000), pneumothorax was managed by observation alone and/or the insertion of a pigtail catheter (8.5 French) with a Heimlich valve in the outpatient setting (Laronga et al., 2000). Also, in spontaneous-breathing patients who have developed a small pneumothorax, the use of 100% oxygen therapy for 60 minutes may denitrogenate and attenuate the pneumothorax and avert chest tube insertion.

Hemothorax and other bleeding complications

Hemothorax is an infrequent complication primarily of direct SCV catheterization. Because intrathoracic vascular structures are inaccessible for direct compression, subclavians, and, to a lesser degree, IJV direct venous catheterization is contraindicated in patients with a coagulopathy.

Extrapleural arterial puncture results in an extrapleural hematoma that may be visible on a chest radiograph. Erosion through the heart by a malpositioned catheter tip can result in life-threatening pericardial tamponade from bleeding or introducing an infusate. Arterial puncture or laceration during femoral venous catheterization, particularly above the inguinal ligament where recognition is limited, thus delaying compression may lead to retroperitoneal hemorrhage.

Thrombosis, stenosis, and occlusion

Thrombosis appears to be related to the relative diameters of the catheter and vessel (Kaye, 1983), the material and whether the catheter is tapered (Beards et al., 1994), and duration of insertion greater than 72 hours (Butt et al., 1987). The number of attempts before successful cannulation, low cardiac output, hypotension, use of vasopressors, peripheral vaso-occlusive processes, and Raynaud's disease all increase the risk of thrombosis. Generally, the smaller the catheter relative to the vessel, the lower the incidence of thrombosis.

Thrombosis of the great veins is frequently asymptomatic and therefore under-recognized and under-reported (Baranowski, 1993; Nohr, 1994). In SCV catheterization, the complication is clinically diagnosed with a frequency of less than 5% but is diagnosed in 20–40% of patients by contrast venography (Nohr, 1994). Although infrequent, pulmonary embolism from catheter-related venous thrombosis can occur (Leiby et al., 1989). Flushing protocols, with and without heparin, have been devised to reduce catheter thrombosis (Fry, 1992; Baranowski, 1993), and fibrinolytic agent administration through the catheter is frequently successful to reopen thrombosed catheters (Lawson et al., 1982; Bjeletich et al., 1987; Tschirhart & Rao, 1988; Atkinson et al., 1990; Haire et al., 1990; Wachs, 1990; Lawson, 1991). Additional treatment of catheter-related deep vein thrombosis may also involve catheter removal (Steed et al., 1986; Fraschini et al., 1987; Clarke & Raffin, 1990; Haire et al., 1990; Barclay et al., 1991; Baranowski, 1993; Nohr, 1994). Venous stenosis has been likewise detected in more than 20% of patients undergoing prolonged venous catheterization (Wanscher et al., 1988).

Catheter occlusion usually results from the formation of a fibrin plug at the catheter tip (Nohr, 1994). This is part of a fibrin sleeve that forms around essentially all IV catheters present for more than a week (Lowell & Bothe, 1991). Precipitate occlusions resulting from administering multiple incompatible medications via a catheter may be dissolved with 0.1 mol/L hydrochloric acid (Breaux et al., 1987; Shulman et al., 1988; Duffy et al., 1989), and lipid aggregation may be cleared with 70% ethyl alcohol (Pennington & Pithie, 1987).

The longer length and frequently the smaller diameter of PICCs may place these catheters at higher risk for thrombosis or occlusion. Keeping catheters scrupulously clean during insertion, using powderless or rinsed gloves, is advocated to reduce thrombogenicity (Hoshal, 1975). The reported incidence of PICC occlusion is between 1.0% and 8.2% (Loughran et al., 1992; Goodwin & Carlson, 1993; Merrell et al., 1994). Incorporation of a Groshong valve reduces catheter thrombosis or occlusion and the need for heparin flushes (Fry, 1992; Pasquale et al., 1992; Baranowski, 1993).

Thrombophlebitis

Mechanical phlebitis within the first week after catheterization is the most common complication seen with PICC lines (Baranowski, 1993), occurring in 4.7% to 11.4% of patients (Loughran et al., 1992; Goodwin & Carlson, 1993; James et al., 1993; Merrell et al., 1994). Most mechanical phlebitis will resolve with heat and elevation and do not require catheter removal.

Embolism

Clots adherent to the catheter tip, or even the vessel lumen, can be dislodged during flushing of the arterial line or at the time of removal. To reduce this risk, some have proposed that intermittent flushing be limited to 1–2 seconds, despite any basis in data. Flush solutions are heparinized for the purpose of reducing the risk of thrombosis and subsequent embolization.

Air embolism is a rare but potentially fatal complication associated with the insertion and maintenance of central venous catheters. Vesely (2001) reviewed complications for 11,583 central venous catheter insertions, 4,404 of which used a tunneled approach. Air embolism only occurred in 15 cases but all were in the tunneled group. Fourteen cases had undetectable, mild or moderate symptoms that resolved with supplemental oxygen, while one case was fatal. Air emboli may present as seizures, hemiparesis, or focal neurologic findings. Treatment is supportive and involves either the administration of 100% oxygen or the institution of hyperbaric chamber dives.

Nerve injury

Neurologic complications are rare, but have been documented in association with IJV catheterization. The close anatomic relationship of the lower brachial plexus to the IJV contribute to nerve damage especially during a traumatic cannulation attempt (DeMatteis, 1995).

Skin necrosis

Flow disturbances by the catheter in the small branches of any artery may produce ischemia and sloughing of the skin. Indeed, amputations of hands and feet have resulted from such complications. Blanching of the skin may occur with flushing of the catheter and indicate interference with skin circulation.

Bleeding

Any disturbances of the coagulation mechanism may result in oozing or frank bleeding at the site of arterial puncture. When such abnormalities exist, or are likely to exist, use of peripheral sites (radial and dorsalis pedis) is much preferred to the more central sites (axillary, brachial, femoral). Local pressure and use of topical thrombin spray may be sued to control bleeding, if peripheral. Ultimately, the goal is correction of the coagulopathy.

Catheter-related infection

Catheter-related infections (CRIs) include: exit-site and tunnel infections, catheter-associated bacteremia, catheter-associated sepsis, suppurative thrombophlebitis, endocarditis, and clavicular osteomyelitis. Both local site infection and septicemia increase with the duration of catheterization (Band & Maki, 1979). The rate of bacteremia with cutdowns is almost 10 times that with percutaneous cannulation. Catheter-associated bacteremia is the most serious of the CRIs as well as the leading cause of nosocomial infection (Brun-Buisson, 2001). It has been suggested that an estimated 80,000 cases of catheter-associated bacteremia occur annually in intensive care units (Brun-Buisson, 2001). Coagulase-negative staphylococci is the most common infectious agent noted in CRIs, while enterococci now rank as second. Unfortunately, many nosocomial pathogens, including those just mentioned, are exhibiting resistance to antibiotics.

Factors contributing to CRI include: multilumen catheters, repeated catheterization duration, type of dressing, experience of personnel inserting the catheter, and catheter location (Kruse & Shah, 1993; Egebo et al., 1996; Pearson et al, 1996).

CRI is often clinically diagnosed and is suspected upon recognizing local signs of infection (erythema, tenderness, purulent drainage) at the catheter exit site or systemic signs of infection (fever, rigors, fluid sequestration, rising WBC count), particularly in patients lacking another likely source of infection. Cultures are necessary only to define antibiotic treatment. Exit-site infections may be successfully treated with local care and antibiotics in many instances. Infections at tunneled sites, however, generally require catheter removal (Benezra et al., 1988; Clarke & Raffin, 1990; Nohr, 1994). CRI is excluded if culture of the catheter tip shows "no growth." Infection unrelated to the catheter is present if peripheral blood cultures have growth, but catheter tip cultures are without growth. Catheter colonization or infection exists if the catheter tip and/or aspirated blood cultures have growth, but peripheral blood cultures yield "no growth." Some authors would change nontunneled catheters over a wire in this instance, or administer specific antibiotics through tunneled catheters. Nohr and others recommend catheter removal should the involved organism be fungi, *S. aureus*, or other virulent bacteria (Benezra et al., 1988; Dugdale & Ramsey, 1990; Pizzo,1993; Rotstein et al., 1995). Finally, catheter-associated bacteremia or sepsis exits if peripherally drawn blood cultures and catheter tip and/or aspirated blood cultures yield the same organisms. In this instance, 10 or more days of appropriate antibiotic therapy and catheter removal are required. Catheter removal is also generally recommended in catheterized patients whose presumed catheter-unrelated infections fail to rapidly improve with appropriate treatment. Others have investigated the efficacy of thrombolytic therapy in treating catheter colonization or infection (Fishbein et al., 1990), a therapy that also may be necessary to medically treat septic thrombophlebitis (Clarke & Raffin, 1990). Still others have begun investigating the prophylactic use of antibiotics to reduce the incidence of CRIs (Hartman et al., 1989; Schwartz et al., 1990; Lim et al., 1991; Spafford et al., 1994). Given the absence of a clear consensus on the best method of diagnosing CRIs, developing and evaluating hospital-specific guidelines, giving consideration to the user population and catheter use patterns, seems appropriate (Bullard & Dunn, 1996; Civetta et al., 1996).

The Centers for Disease Contol (CDC) have issued guidelines for the prevention of intravascular device related infections (Pearson et al., 1996) which are further refined by investigators as knowledge of CRI grows (Brun-Buisson, 2001). Advances suggest CRI may be reduced by: reducing catheter manipulation, leaving unsoiled dressings in place for 7 days, not replacing tubing sooner than 96 hours, leaving peripherally inserted catheters in place for 96 hours, and not routinely replacing well-functioning central venous catheters (Brun-Buisson, 2001). In adults, peripheral arterial catheters are replaced and insertion site relocated no more frequently than every 4 days for infection control purposes (Pearson et al., 1996). The introduction of catheters impregnated with antimicrobials, both antiseptic and antibiotics, are available, and studies have documented the reduction of catheter-associated bacteremia with their use (Rafkin et al., 1990; Maki et al., 1991b; Bach et al., 1992; Dahlberg et al., 1995; Mimoz et al., 1996). Treating catheters with substances on both the luminal and external surfaces with agents such as triiododecylmethylammonium chloride and poly-*N*-vinylpyrrolidine allows binding with antibiotics (Jansen et al., 1992) and may reduce CRIs (Trooskin et al., 1985; Kamal et al., 1991; Thornton et al., 1996). When compared to nonimpregnated catheters, central venous catheters impregnated with minocycline and rifampin or chlorhexidine and silver sulfadiazine were associated with lower rates of catheter colonization and bloodstream infection (Darouiche et al., 1999). When the anti-infective catheters (minocycline and rifampin versus chlorhexidine and silver sulfadiazine) were compared with each other, the minocycline and rifampin combination was 1/3 as likely to be colonized ($P < 0.001$) (Darouiche et al., 1999). As with the use of any antibiotic, the perceived risk of inducing resistance through the use of antibiotic-impregnated catheters is considered. Therefore, the use of antimicrobial- or antiseptic-impregnated central venous catheters should only be considered if, after full adherence to other CRI control measures an unacceptably high rate of infection still exists (Pearson et al., 1996; Brun-Buisson, 2001). Finally, to insure that new technologies complement aseptic technique, hospital surveillance strategies should be implemented.

Catheter care

Although essentially all authors profess the value of catheter teams to insert and care for long-term and central venous catheters, there is little universal agreement on most other aspects of catheter use and care, including recommended length of use, catheter site care procedures, dressing type, catheter flushing protocols, treating the occluded catheter, catheter management in the patient with fever or suspected infection, or even how to define catheter-related infection. The confusion exists largely because of the paucity of prospective, randomized clinical trials and because of the differing populations studied in the available published studies. One of the best overall discussions is the very well referenced publication of Baranowski (1993). In the absence of a clear consensus on these aspects of catheter care, it is recommended that hospitals and practitioners establish practice guidelines and/or protocols that can be subsequently studied and modified within a quality improvement program.

Conclusion

Prolonged IV access is occasionally vital to the successful outcome of a pregnancy, particularly for the provision of TPN. A variety of IV devices are available, with more assuredly just over the horizon. The proper and safe use of these devices requires understanding of their indications, skill in their insertion, and competence in recognizing and treating their associated complications. Given evolving trends in the practice of medicine, it seems likely that more research will focus on the cost-effectiveness of IV catheters and practices and their adaptability for home use (Stokes & Irving, 1988; Boutin & Hagan, 1992; Kravitz, 1993; Mannel et al., 1994). Increasingly, health-care providers will require familiarity with these aspects of IV access.

References

Agee KR, Balk RA. Central venous catheterization in the critically ill patient. Crit Care Clin 1992;8:677–686.

Ambesh SP, Pandey JC, Dubey PK. Internal jugular vein occlusion test for rapid diagnosis of misplaced subclavian vein catheter into the internal jugular vein. Anesthesiology 2001;95(6):1377–1379.

Andrews JC, Walker-Andrews S, Ensminger WD. Long-term central venous access with a peripherally placed subcutaneous infusion port: initial results. Radiology 1990;176:45–47.

Atkinson JB, Bagnall HA, Gomperts E. Investigational use of tissue plasminogen activator (t-PA) for occluded central venous catheters. JPEN 1990;14:310–311.

Bach A, Bohrer H, Motsch J, et al. Prevention of catheter-related infections by antiseptic coating. Anesthesiology 1992;77:A259. Abstract.

Band JD, Maki DG. Infections caused by arterial catheters used for hemodynamic monitoring. Am J Med 1979;67:735–741.

Baranowski L. Central venous access devices: current technologies, uses, and management strategies. J Intraven Nurs 1993;16:167.

Barclay GR, Allen K, Pennington CR. Tissue plasminogen activator in the treatment of superior vena caval thrombosis associated with parenteral nutrition. Postgrad Med J 1991;66:398–400.

Beards SC, Doedens L, Jackson A, Lipman J. A comparison of arterial lines and insertion techniques in critically ill patients. Anaesthesia 1994;49:968–973.

Bedford RF. Radial arterial function following percutaneous cannulation with 18 and 20 gauge catheters. Anesthesiology 1977;47:37–39.

Belani KG, Buckley JJ, Gordon JR, Castaneda W. Percutaneous cervical central venous line placement: a comparison of the internal and external jugular vein routes. Anesth Analg 1980;59:40–44.

Benezra D, Kiehn TE, Gold JWM, et al. Prospective study of infections in indwelling central venous catheters using quantitative blood cultures. Am J Med 1988;85:495–498.

Bjeletich J, Hickman R, Stewart J, et al. Declotting central venous catheters with urokinase in the home by nurse clinicians. NITA 1987;Nov/Dec:428.

Blackshear PJ, Dorman FD, Blackshear PL Jr, Varco RL, Buchwald H. The design and initial testing of an implantable infusion pump. Surg Gynecol Obstet 1972;134:51–56.

Boutin J, Hagan E. Patients' preference regarding portable pumps. J Intravenous Nurs 1992;15:230–232.

Breaux CW, Duke D, Georgeson KE, et al. Calcium phosphate crystal occlusion of central venous catheters used for total parenteral nutrition in infants and children: prevention and treatment. J Pediatr Surg 1987;22:829–832.

Brun-Buisson C. New technologies and infection control practices to prevent intravascular catheter-related infections. Am J Respir Crit Care Med 2001;164(9):1557–1558.

Bullard KM, Dunn DL. Diagnosis and treatment of bacteremia and intravascular catheter infections. Am J Surg 1996;172:S13–19.

Butt W, Shann F, McDonnel G. Effect of heparin concentration and infusion rate of patency of arterial catheters. Crit Care Med 1987;15:230–232.

Civetta JM, Hudson-Civetta J, Bull S. Decreasing catheter-related infections and hospital costs by continuous quality improvement. Crit Care Med 1996;24:1660–1665.

Clarke DE, Raffin TA. Infectious complications of in-dwelling long-term central venous catheters. Chest 1990;97:966–972.

Clemente, CD. Anatomy: A regional atlas of the human body, 4th edn. Baltimore: Williams & Wilkins, 1997.

Collin GR, Clarke LE. Delayed pneumothorax: a complication of central venous catheterization. Surg Rounds 1994;17:589.

Colomina MJ, Godet C, Bago J, et al. Isolated thrombosis of the external jugular vein. Surg Laparosc Endosc Percutan Tech 2000;10(4):264–267.

Conroy JM, Rajagopalan PR, Baker JD III, et al. A modification of the supraclavicular approach to the central circulation. South Med J 1990;83:1178–1181.

Dahlberg PJ, Agger WA, Singer JR, et al. Subclavian hemodialysis catheter infections: a prospective, randomized trial of an attachable silver-impregnated cuff for prevention of catheter-related infections. Infect Control Hosp Epidemiol 1995;16:506–511.

D'Angelo FA, Ramacciato G, Aurello P, et al. Alternative insertion sites for permanent ventral venous access devices. Eur J Surg Oncol 1997;23(6):547–549.

Darouiche RO, Raad II, Heard SO, et al. A comparison of two antimicrobial-impregnated central venous catheters. Catheter Study Group. NEJM 1999;340:1–8.

De la Roche MR, Gauthier L. Rapid transfusion of packed red blood cells: effects of dilution, pressure, and catheter size. Ann Emerg Med 1993;22:1551–1555.

Delmore JE, Horbelt DV, Jack BL, et al. Experience with the Groshong long-term central venous catheter. Gynecol Oncol 1989;34:216–218.

DeMatteis J. Brachial plexus injury caused by internal jugular cannulation. Hospital Physician 1995:52.

Denys BG, Uretsky BF, Reddy PS, et al. An ultrasound method for safe and rapid central venous access. N Engl J Med 1991;324:566. Letter.

Di Carlo I, Cordio S, La Greca G, Privitera G, et al. Totally implantable venous access devices implanted surgically: a retrospective study on early and late complications. Arch Surg 2001;136(9):1050–1053.

Duffy LF, Kerzner B, Gebus V, et al. Treatment of central venous catheter occlusions with hydrochloric acid. J Pediatr 1989;114: 1002–1004.

Dugdale DC, Ramsey PG. *Staphylococcus aureus* bacteremia in patients with Hickman catheters. Am J Med 1990;89:137.

Durbec O, Viviand X, Potie F, et al. A prospective evaluation of the use of femoral venous catheters in critically ill adults. Crit Care Med 1997;25(12):1982–1985.

Egebo K, Toft P, Jakobsen CJ. Contamination of central venous catheters: The skin insertion wound is a major source of contamination. J Hosp Infect 1996;32:99–104.

Fraschini G, Jadeja J, Lawson M, et al. Local infusion of urokinase for the lysis of thrombosis associated with permanent central venous catheters in cancer patients. J Clin Oncol 1987;5:672–678.

FDA Drug Bulletin. Food and Drug Administration 1989;19:15.

Finney R, Albrink M, Hart M, et al. A cost-effective peripheral venous port system placed at the bedside. J Surg Res 1992;53:17–19.

Fishbein HD, Friedman HS, Bennett BB, et al. Catheter-related sepsis refractory to antibiotic treated successfully with adjunctive urokinase infusion. Pediatr Infect Dis J 1990;9:676–678.

Fontes M. Complications of central venous cannulation. Probl Anesth 1998;10(2):215–226.

Fry B. Intermittent heparin flushing protocols. A standardization issue. J Intraven Nurs 1992;15:160–163.

Goodwin ML, Carlson I. The peripherally inserted central catheter. J Intraven Nurs 1993;16:92–103.

Haire WD, Lieberman RP, Lund GB, et al. Obstructed central venous catheters. Restoring function with a 12-hour infusion of low-dose urokinase. Cancer 1990;66:2279–2285.

Harris JP, Calloway CA, Gordon BR. Subclavian vein thrombosis associated with central venous cannulation in head and neck surgery. Otolaryngol Head Neck Surg 1982;90(6):715–722.

Hartman LC, Urba WJ, Steis RG, et al. Use of prophylactic antibiotics for prevention of intravascular catheter-related infections in interleukin-2-treated patients (letter). JNCI 1989;81:1190.

Hatfield A, Bodenham A. Portable ultrasound for difficult central venous access. Br J Anaesth 1999;82(6):822–826.

Ho CM, Lui PW. Bilateral hydrothorax caused by left external jugular venous catheter perforation. J Clin Anesth 1994;6(3):243–246.

Holcombe BJ, Forloines-Lynn S, Garmhausen LW. Restoring patency of long-term central venous access devices. J Intraven Nurs 1992;15:36–41.

Horattas MC, Trupiano J, Hopkins S, et al. Changing concepts in long-term central venous access: catheter selection and cost savings. Am J Infect Control 2001;29(1):32–40.

Hoshal VL Jr. Total intravenous nutrition with peripherally inserted silicone elastomer central venous catheters. Arch Surg 1975;110: 644–646.

Hudson-Civetta J, Caruthers-Banner TE. Intra-vascular catheters: current guidelines for care and maintenance. Heart Lung 1983;12:466–476.

James L, Bledsoe L, Hadaway LC. A retrospective look at tip location and complications of peripherally inserted central catheter lines. J Intraven Nurs 1993;16:104.

Jansen B, Jansen S, Peters G, et al. In-vitro efficacy of a central venous catheter ("hydrocath") loaded with teicoplanin to prevent bacterial colonization. J Hosp Infect 1992;22:93–107.

Kamal GD, Pfaller MA, Rempe LE, et al. Reduced intravascular infection by antibiotic bonding. A prospective, randomized controlled trial. JAMA 1991;265:2364.

Kaye A. Invasive monitoring techniques: arterial cannulation, bedside pulmonary artery catheterization and arterial puncture. Heart Lung 1983;12:395–427.

Korelitz BI. Inflammatory bowel disease in pregnancy. Gastroenterol Clin North Am 1992;21:827–834.

Kravitz GR. Outpatient parenteral antibiotic therapy. Management of serious infections. Part I: Medical, socioeconomic, and legal issues. Advances in i.v. delivery. Hosp Pract 1993;28(suppl):21.

Kruse JA, Shah NJ. Detection and prevention of central venous catheter-related infections. Nutr Clin Pract 1993;8:163–170.

LaFortune S. The use of confirming x-rays to verify tip position for peripherally inserted catheters. J Intraven Nurs 1993;16: 246–250.

Lam S, Scannell R, Roessler D, et al. Peripherally inserted central catheters in an acute-care hospital. Arch Intern Med 1994;154:1833–1837.

Laronga C, Meric F, Truong M, et al. A treatment algorithm for pneumothoraces complicating central venous catheter insertion. Am J Surg 2000;180(6):523–526.

Larson E. Guidelines for use of topical antimicrobial agents. APIC Guidelines for Infection Control Practice. Am J Infect Control 1988;16:253–266.

Lawson M. Partial occlusion of indwelling central venous catheters. J Intraven Nurs 1991;14:157–159.

Lawson M, Bottino JC, Hurtubise MR, et al. The use of urokinase to restore the patency of occluded central venous catheters. Am J Intraven Ther Clin Nutr 1982;9:29–30,32–34.

Leiby JM, Purcell H, DeMaria JJ, et al. Pulmonary embolism as a result of Hickman catheter-related thrombosis. Am J Med 1989;86: 228–231.

Levine MG, Esser D. Total parenteral nutrition for treatment of severe hyperemesis gravidarum: maternal nutritional effects and fetal outcome. Obstet Gynecol 1988;72:102–107.

Lim SH, Smith MP, Salooja N, et al. A prospective randomized study of prophylactic teicoplanin to prevent early Hickman catheter-related sepsis in patients receiving intensive chemotherapy for haematological malignancies. J Antimicrob Chemother 1991;28:109–116.

Loughran SC, Edwards S, McClure S. Peripherally inserted central catheters. Guidewire versus nonguidewire use: a comparative study. J Intraven Nurs 1992;15:152–159.

Lowell JA, Bothe A Jr. Venous access: preoperative, operative, and postoperative dilemmas. Surg Clin North Am 1991;71:1231–1246.

Lucey B, Verghese JC, Haslam P, Lee MJ. Routine chest radiographs after central line insertion: mandatory postprocedural evaluation or unnecessary waste of resources. Cardiovasc Intervent Radiol 1999;22(5):381–384.

Macdonald S, Watt AJ, McNally D, Edwards RD, Moss JG. Comparison of technical success and outcome of tunneled catheters inserted via the jugular and subclavian approaches. J Vasc Interv Radiol 2000;11(2 Part 1):225–231.

McGee WT, Ackerman BL, Rouben LR, et al. Accurate placement of central venous catheters: a prospective, randomized, multicenter trial. Crit Care Med 1993;21:1118–1123.

McKee J. Future dimension in vascular access. Peripheral implantable ports. J Intraven Nurs 1991;14:387.

Maki DG, Wheeler SJ, Stolz SM, et al. Study of a novel antiseptic-coated central venous catheter. Crit Care Med 1991b;19(Suppl):S99. Abstract.

Mangar D, Laborde RS, Vu DN. Delayed ischaemia of the hand necessitating amputation after radial artery cannulation. Can J Anaesth 1993;40:247–250.

Mannel RS, Manetta A, Hickman RL Jr, et al. Cost analysis of Hickman catheter insertion at bedside in gynecologic oncology patients. J Am Coll Surg 1994;179:558–560.

Marino P. The ICU Book, 2nd edn. Baltimore: Williams and Wilkins, 1998.

Merrell SW, Peatross BG, Grossman MD, et al. Peripherally inserted central venous catheters. Low-risk alternatives for ongoing venous access. West J Med 1994;160:25–30.

Mimoz O, Pieroni L, Lawrence C, et al. Prospective randomized trial of two antiseptic solutions for prevention of central venous catheterization of arterial colonization and infection in intensive care unit patients. Crit Care Med 1996;24:1818–1823.

Morris P, Buller R, Kendall S, et al. A peripherally implanted permanent central venous access device. Obstet Gynecol 1991;78: 1138.

Mumtaz H, Williams V, Hauer-Jensen M, et al. Central venous catheter placement in patients with disorders of hemostasis. Am J Surg 2000;180(6):503–505.

Nohr C. Care of the surgical patient. Perioperative management and techniques. 2. Elective care. Vol 2. Surgical techniques, Supplement 3. Vascular access. Scientific American, Inc. Winter, 1994.

O'Grady NP, Alexander M, Dellinger EP, et al. Guidelines for the prevention of intravascular catheter-related infections. Centers for Disease Control and Prevention. MMWR 2002;51(RR-10):1–29.

Parras F, Ena J, Bouza E, et al. Impact of an educational program for the prevention of colonization of intravascular catheters. Infect Control Hosp Epidemiol 1994;15:239–242.

Pasquale MD, Campbell JM, Magnant CM. Groshong versus Hickman catheters. Surg Gynecol Obstet 1992;174:408–410.

Pearson ML, Hierholzer WJ Jr, Garner JS, et al. Guideline for prevention of intravascular device-related infections: Part I. Intravascular device-related infections; an overview. Ann J Infect Control 1996;24(4):262–277.

Pennington CR, Pithie AD. Ethanol lock in the management of catheter occlusion. JPEN 1987;11:507–508.

Pizzo PA. Management of fever in patients with cancer and treatment-induced neutropenia. N Engl J Med 1993;328:1323–1332.

Puntis JWL, Holden CE, Finkel Y, et al. Staff training: a key factor in reducing intravascular catheter sepsis. Arch Dis Child 1990;65: 335–337.

Raad II, Hohn DC, Gilbreath BJ, et al. Prevention of central venous catheter-related infections by using maximal sterile barrier precautions during insertion. Infect Control Hosp Epidemiol 1994;15:231–238.

Rafkin HS, Hoyt JW, Crippen DW. Prevention of certified venous catheter-related infection with a silver-impregnated cuff. Chest 1990;98:117S. Abstract.

Ray S, Stacey R, Imrie M, Filshie J. A review of 560 Hickman catheter insertions. Anesthesia 1996;51:981–985.

Rotstein C, Brock L, Roberts RS. The incidence of first Hickman catheter-related infection and predictors of catheter removal in cancer patients. Infect Control Hosp Epidemiol 1995;16:451–458.

Schuman E, Ragsdale J. Peripheral ports are a new option for central venous access. J Am Coll Surg 1995;180:456–460.

Schwartz C, Henrickson KJ, Roghmann K, et al. Prevention of bacteremia attributed to luminal colonization of tunneled central venous catheters with vancomycin-susceptible organisms. J Clin Oncol 1990;8:1591–1597.

Segura-Vasi AM, Suelto MD, Boudreaux AM. External jugular vein cannulation for central venous access. Anesth Analg 1999;88(3): 692–693.

Seldinger SI. Catheter replacement of the needle in percutaneous arteriography. Acta Radiol Diagn 1953;39:368–376.

Seneff MG. Central venous catheterization. A comprehensive review. Intensive Care Med 1987;2:163.

Sheikh W. Comparative antibacterial efficacy of Hibiclens and Betadine in the presence of pus derived from human wounds. Curr Ther Res 1986;40:1096.

Sherer DM, Abulafia O, DuBeshter B, et al. Ultrasonographically guided subclavian vein catheterization in critical care obstetrics and gynecologic oncology. Am J Obstet Gynecol 1993;169:1246–1248.

Shulman RJ, Reed T, Pitre D, et al. Use of hydrochloric acid to clear obstructed central venous catheters. JPEN 1988;12:509–510.

Spafford PS, Sinkin RA, Cox C, et al. Prevention of central venous catheter-related coagulase-negative staphylococcal sepsis in neonates. J Pediatr 1994;125:259–263.

Sparks CJ, McSkimming I, George L. Shoulder manipulation to facilitate central vein catheterization from the external jugular vein. Anaesth Intensive Care 1991;19(4):567–568.

Steed DL, Teodori MF, Peitzman AB, et al. Streptokinase in the treatment of subclavian vein thrombosis. J Vasc Surg 1986;4:28–32.

Stewart R, Tuazon D, Olson GL, Duarte AG. Pregnancy and primary pulmonary hypertension: Successful outcome with epoprostenol therapy. Chest 2001;119(3):973–975.

Stokes MA, Irving MH. How do patients with Crohn's disease fare on home parenteral nutrition? Dis Colon Rectum 1988;31:454–458.

Thornton J, Todd NJ, Webster NR. Central venous line sepsis in the intensive care unit: A study comparing antibiotic-coated with plain catheters. Anaesthesia 1996;51:1018–1020.

Tocino IM, Miller MH, Fairfax WR. Distribution of pneumothorax in the supine and semirecumbent critically ill adult. Am J Roentgenol 1985;144(5):901–905.

Trooskin SZ, Donetz AP, Harvey RA, et al. Prevention of catheter sepsis by antibiotic bonding. Surgery 1985;97:547–551.

Tschirhart JM, Rao MK. Mechanism and management of persistent withdrawal occlusion. Am Surg 1988;54:326–328.

Vesely TM. Air embolism during insertion of central venous catheters. J Vasc Interv Radiol 2001;12(11):1291–1295.

Wachs T. Urokinase administration in pediatric patients with occluded central venous catheters. J Intraven Nurs 1990;13:100–102.

Wanscher M, Frifelt JJ, Smith-Sivertsen C, et al. Thrombosis caused by polyurethane double-lumen subclavian vena cava catheter and hemodialysis. Crit Care Med 1988;16:624–628.

Wiedner LC, Fish J, Talabiska DG, et al. Total parenteral nutrition in pregnant patient with hyperemesis gravidarum. Nutrition 1993;9:446.

Wolk RA, Rayburn WF. Parenteral nutrition in obstetric patients. Nutr Clin Pract 1990;5:139–152.

Wyatt WJ, Beckett TA, Bonet V, Davis SM. Comparative efficacy of surgical scrub solutions on control of skin microflora. Infect Surg 1990;9:17–21.

Young J. How to insert a subclavian catheter. Internal jugular approach. Surgical Rounds 1978;28.

10 Blood component replacement therapy

David A. Sacks

Recent years have witnessed a decline in the frequency and volume of transfusions of blood products for emergency and urgent indications in obstetrics (Ekeroma et al., 1997). While largely speculative, the reasons for this trend include concerns about possible transfusion-related disease transmission, better understanding of the ability of pregnant women to tolerate acute blood loss and anemia, and cost concerns. With the recognition of its safety, the transition to typing and screening from typing and cross-matching red cell products has provided not only cost savings but also decreased wastage of this valuable resource (Ransom et al., 1998, 1999). This chapter will discuss the collection, separation, and storage of blood components. Indications for the transfusion of these products as well as complications of transfusions will be presented. Alternatives to allogeneic transfusions, including autologous transfusions, and both hemoglobin- and nonhemoglobin-containing synthetic products will also be discussed. Frequent references will be made to standards and suggestions of the American Association of Blood Banks (AABB) (Triulzi, 1999; Standards Program Committee, AABB, 2000; Petrides & Stack, 2001). The scope of this review will be limited to the use of blood products in obstetric critical care. The interested reader is referred to appropriate texts for discussions of the utilization of blood products for other indications in obstetrics (e.g. fetal alloimmunization, alloimmune thrombocytopenia, and chronic anemias).

Blood donation, collection, separation, and storage

Donor selection

A number of historical factors and laboratory tests are considered in an effort to assure the safety of the blood supply. In addition to those listed in Table 10.1, the prospective donor must be free of major organ disease, and not have received blood components or human tissue for the 12 months preceding donation. While those who received toxoids or killed viral, bacterial, or rickettsial vaccines are eligible to donate, those who received live attenuated vaccines (e.g. rubeola, polio, typhoid, rubella, varicella) must be deferred for 2–4 weeks following vaccination. Prospective donors who on questioning reveal behavior putting them at high risk for acquisition of human immunodeficiency virus (HIV), who are intoxicated, or have stigmata of alcohol habituation, or who have skin lesions at the venepuncture site are appropriately deferred. Routinely, qualifying recently pregnant women may donate if 6 or more weeks have passed beyond the date of pregnancy termination. If blood is intended for the infant of the mother, this temporal requirement may be waived with the consent of the woman's attending physician and the blood bank director. A "look-back" process must be in place in all blood banks for notification of physicians of recipients of blood from donors who subsequent to donation are found to be infected with HIV or hepatitis C virus (HCV) (Standards Program Committee, AABB, 2000).

Blood collection and component separation

Most blood is collected as whole blood, and then processed into red cells, plasma, and platelets. At the donor center, 450–500 mL are removed from a single donor, and initially collected in the first of three connected bags. To this bag has been added an anticoagulant/preservative solution, most commonly CPD (citrate phosphate dextrose) in a 1 : 7 volume ratio to the blood. The second is a satellite bag that contains an additive solution, whose purpose is to prolong red cell life (see components below). The third is an empty satellite bag, destined for receipt of platelet-rich plasma (Petrides & Stack, 2001). Although the temperature and duration of storage clearly influence the quality and function of blood components, this stage of blood processing is poorly standardized (Hogman & Merryman, 1999). Most often within 8 hours of donation, the triple bag is then centrifuged. This separates the unit into red cells and platelet-rich plasma. The latter is expressed mechanically into the third satellite bag. The red cell bag is then clamped, removed, and stored at 1–6°C. If an addi-

Table 10.1 Selected prerequisites and testing of prospective blood donors

Prerequisites
Age ≥17 years
Collection no more often than 8 weeks after whole blood; 4 weeks after infrequent apheresis
BP ≤180 mm systolic; ≤100 diastolic
Pulse 50–100 bpm; <50 if a healthy athlete
Temperature ≤37.5°
Hemoglobin ≥12 g/dL; hematocrit ≥38%
Testing of donated units for:
HIV antibody (anti-HIV-1 and -2); and antigen (p24 antigen)
Hepatitis B surface antigen (HbsAg) and core antibody (anti-HBc)
Hepatitis C antibody (anti-HCV)
Human T-cell lymphotropic virus antibody (anti-HTLV-I and -II)
Serologic test for syphilis
Deferrals
Indefinite
History of viral hepatitis after 11th birthday
HbsAg positive
Reactive anti-HBc on one or more occasions
Present or past clinical or laboratory infection with HCV, HTLV, or HIV
History of babesiosis or Chagas' disease
Evidence or stigmata of parenteral drug use
Use of a needle for nonprescription drugs
Those who spent ≥6 months in the UK between 1980 and 1996
For 3 years from the time of becoming asymptomatic after having had malaria, or after departing from an area where malaria is endemic
For 12 months from the time of:
Having had a tattoo
Skin penetration with an instrument contaminated with blood
Sexual contact with an individual who is positive for HIV or HbsAg
History of syphilis or gonorrhea

tive solution is to be used, it is expressed from the second bag into the first prior to clamping. The platelet-rich plasma is spun a second time. The supernatant plasma is removed, leaving a 50 mL solution of plasma in which platelets are concentrated. The latter are stored at room temperature (20–24°C) under constant gentle agitation for up to 5 days (Petrides & Stack, 2001).

To preserve labile coagulation factors V and VIII, the plasma from which the platelets have been separated must be frozen within 8 hours of phlebotomy. It is then stored at −18°C for up to 12 months, or at −65°C for up to 7 years. If cryoprecipitated AHF ("cryo") is to be made, the fresh frozen plasma (FFP) is kept frozen for 24 hours, then thawed to slush, spun, and the supernatant plasma removed. The now separated units of cryo and cryo-poor plasma are each refrozen at −18°C for up to 12 months (Petrides & Stack, 2001).

Blood storage

Blood components containing red cells or platelets must have their function as well as viability preserved, while components made of plasma must have only function preserved. For these reasons, their storage is somewhat different.

Storage of red blood cell (RBC) products

The RBC is a specialized cell which lacks a nucleus and which therefore cannot synthesize protein and enzymes. It also lacks mitochondria, and therefore must generate adenosine triphosphate (ATP) by metabolizing glucose to lactate. This route of intracellular energy synthesis is much less efficient than mitochondrial oxidation through the citric acid cycle (Hogman & Merryman, 1999). In a storage bag, the lactic acid produced within the RBC is buffered by bicarbonate in the surrounding extracellular fluid to form carbonic acid. Storing RBC products in gas-permeable plastic bags allows the CO_2 produced by the dissociation of carbonic acid to escape, thus slowing the lowering of pH within the storage bag (Hogman & Merryman, 1999).

The quality of RBC function is determined by the ability of these cells to provide O_2 to oxygen-poor tissues. Intracellular processes which decrease the affinity between hemoglobin and oxygen facilitate delivery of oxygen to oxygen-depleted peripheral cells. The peripheral cells which require oxygen produce CO_2, which is transported from them to the plasma and then to within the membrane of the RBC as the latter passes through the capillary. Within the RBC, the CO_2 and intracellular water are catalyzed by carbonic anhydrase to form H_2CO_3, which, in turn, is rapidly dissociated into H^+ and HCO_3^-. Under the influence of band 3 protein within the RBC, HCO_3^- is exchanged for Cl^- from the plasma (the "anion shift"). The RBC acidity resulting from the intracellular generation of HCl drives the dissociation of O_2 from hemoglobin, as deoxygenated hemoglobin buffers the H^+ ions (Bohr effect) and restores pH within the RBC. In addition, 2,3-diphosphoglycerate (2,3-DPG) within the RBC also binds to hemoglobin, and thus reduces its oxygen affinity. Any reduction in 2,3-DPG will decrease the ability of these cells to transfer O_2 to oxygen-depleted peripheral cells. The enzyme which depletes 2,3-DPG is activated at pH levels below 7.2 (Hogman, 1999). The lower the temperature of the RBC-containing product, the slower the production of lactate. Storage at a temperature of 4°C slows the progressive decline of pH, and thus also slows the decline in 2,3-DPG in stored RBCs. However, 2,3-DPG in banked cells is completely restored in vivo 1 week after transfusion (Hamasaki & Yamamoto, 2000). Because both platelet viability and factor VIII concentrations are decreased below room temperature, the separation of these components must take place prior to refrigeration of RBCs.

Storage solutions for RBCs

Acid citrate dextrose (ACD) is one of the simplest RBC storage solutions. An acid medium promotes RBC recovery in vivo, as well as preventing caramelization of the glucose-containing anticoagulant. The citrate is an anticoagulant, and is rapidly metabolized within the recipient upon transfusion. Dextrose serves as an energy source for the stored RBCs. The addition of inorganic phosphates, as in CPD facilitates synthesis of organic phosphates including ATP and 2,3-DPG necessary for RBC survival in storage. Adenine added to CPD (CPDA) helps maintain intracellular ATP levels and thus RBC viability (Hogman & Merryman, 1999; Petrides & Stack, 2001). RBC products may be stored up to 21 days in CPD and up to 35 days in CPDA-1 (Triulzi, 1999; Standards Programme Committee, AABB, 2000). The shelf life of a unit of RBCs is determined by the recovery rate of transfused cells 24 hours after transfusion; this rate must be ≥75% (Triutzi, 1999). Hypotonic additive solutions prolong shelf life by improving RBC morphology, decreasing storage hemolysis, and increasing 2,3-DPG (Hogman & Merryman, 1999). Additive solutions now in use which contain saline, adenine, glucose, and mannitol (e.g. AS-1) prolong the shelf life of RBCs to 42 days (Petrides & Stack, 2001). An experimental additive solution (EAS 61) which has a recovery of 84% of RBCs after 10 weeks of storage has been reported. The prolonged shelf life in this solution is attributed to its higher pH and adenine and phosphate concentrations, all of which drive ATP synthesis, and to the increased volume of the solution, which reduces RBC hemolysis (Hess et al., 2000).

Storage of RBCs for up to 10 years may be achieved by freezing them to temperatures of –65°C to –200°C (Triulzi, 1999). In the process of slow freezing the extracellular water freezes before the intracellular water does. The resultant intracellular dehydration results in cell deformation as well as tonic lysis on thawing. In contrast, rapid freezing results in intracellular ice crystal formation. To avoid cell damage, glycerol, a cryoprotective agent that rapidly penetrates the RBCs, is added during freezing. Because glycerol is hypertonic relative to RBCs, it must be added slowly, to allow osmotic equilibration between RBCs and surrounding fluid. For the same reason, on thawing, the cells must be washed with saline of progressively decreasing tonicity, beginning with 12% and ending with 0.9% (normal) saline (Petrides & Stack, 2001). Once thawed, at least 80% of the original RBCs must be recoverable (Standards Program Committee, AABB, 2000).

Rejuvenating solutions whose purpose is the restoration of ATP and 2,3-DPG in stored RBCs is available. They may be used to extend the shelf life of expiring units of RBCs (Hamasaki & Yamamoto, 2000; Petrides & Stack, 2001) and for thawed deglycerolized cells (Smith & Leitman, 2000; Valeri et al., 2000; Szymanski et al., 2001). The addition of a rejuvenating solution to RBCs which had been stored for 42 days just prior to glycerolization has been compared to not adding the solution. While there was no significant difference in the recovery of cells, those which had been exposed to the rejuvenating solution had higher 2,3-DPG and ATP concentrations than those which had not (Szymanski et al., 2001).

Leukocyte reduction

To be labeled "leukocyte reduced," a unit of RBCs must contain fewer than 5×10^6 white blood cells, and must retain 85% of the original RBCs (Triulzi, 1999; Standards Program Committee, AABB, 2000). Prestorage reduction of leukocytes from RBCs has many practical advantages. The transfusion-associated transmission of various obligate intracellular pathogens, including cytomegalovirus (CMV), human T-cell lymphotropic virus (HTLV), Epstein–Barr virus (EBV), and variant Creutzfeldt–Jacob virus (vCJD) is reduced. Reducing the white blood cell concentration of stored RBCs may decrease the incidence of a number of undesirable immune-mediated effects of RBC transfusions. Febrile nonhemolytic transfusion reactions are decreased with leukocyte reduction. Transmission of human leukocyte antigens (HLAs), the histocompatability antigens responsible for refractoriness, is also decreased, as may be the immunosuppressive effect of transfused mononuclear cells which affect tumor recurrence (Petrides & Stack, 2001).

Leukocyte filtration at the time of collection and in the laboratory has been utilized. In comparison with the former method, the latter offers the advantages of greater effectiveness in removal of leukocytes as well as quality control (Triulzi, 1999). In addition, leukocyte removal of blood stored at room temperature for 8 hours is more effective than that stored for 0–2 hours (Valeri et al., 2000). Prestorage and laboratory filtration both offer significant advantages over filtration at the time of transfusion. The latter does not eliminate activation products (cytokines) released from leukocytes which were stored with the RBCs, does not remove leukocytes as completely as the former, and, because of the delay in rate of transfusion necessitated by the use of a fine filter, may be contraindicated in situations requiring rapid blood replacement. There is currently a movement in the United States toward universal leukocyte depletion of RBC units. Such a policy is in effect in the United Kingdom and Canada (Petrides & Stack, 2001).

Storage of platelets

In the United States, platelets are collected as either platelet concentrates following blood collection, storage, and separation, or by apheresis. The latter is a process in which blood is withdrawn from a single donor, the platelets removed and stored, and the remainder of the blood retransfused into the donor. A unit of platelets prepared from whole blood must contain at least 5.5×10^{10} platelets at the time of use, while a unit of apheresed platelets must contain at least 3.0×10^{11} platelets (Standards Program Committee, AABB, 2000). Thus a unit obtained by apheresis contains approximately the same number of platelets as six units of platelet concentrates. By limiting the number of exposures to different donors, apheresed platelets offer the potential advantages of reduced exposure of the recipient to infectious disease agents as well as decreased exposure to donor antigens (Silberman, 1999).

However obtained, platelets must be properly stored to maintain both numbers and function. Like RBCs, platelets derive their energy from the metabolism of glucose to lactate. As with RBC storage, platelet storage in gas-permeable bags allows buffering of the lactate, and slows the accumulation of acids. Keeping the unit under constant gentle agitation facilitates gas exchange across the bag. Once the pH of the platelet product has dropped to 6.2, the unit is no longer usable, as this is the pH below which platelets irreversibly swell, agglutinate, and lyse (Standards Program Committee, AABB, 2000; Petrides & Stack, 2001). Because cold platelets lose their discoid shape and become spherical, they must be stored at room temperature, i.e. between 20°C and 24°C. Because the risk of bacterial contamination of platelet solutions stored at these temperatures increases after 5 days, the shelf life of a unit of platelets is limited to 5 days (Petrides & Stack, 2001).

Additive solutions for platelets are under development. It is hoped that by removing plasma surrounding the platelets and adding a platelet additive solution containing glucose, citrate, acetate, and phosphate the potential hazards which now attend platelet transfusions will be minimized, while the life and function of platelets will be prolonged (De Wildt-Eggen et al., 2000; Gulliksson, 2000; Rothwell et al., 2000).

Unlike with RBCs, attempts at cryopreservation of platelets have not met with success. However, the stated advantages of leukocyte depletion prior to transfusion that apply to RBCs also apply to platelets (Hogman, 1999; Silberman, 1999). Further reduction in febrile reactions following platelet transfusion has been reported when stored leukocyte-reduced platelets were washed in saline just prior to transfusion (Vo et al., 2001).

Storage of plasma

Because plasma can transmit pathogenic viruses, and because antibodies to some viruses may not yet be present in infected donors at the time of donation, two approaches have been added to the more conventional storage of frozen plasma. Fresh frozen plasma, donor-retested (FFP-DR) is prepared by quarantining the frozen unit for 112 days after the unit is collected. The donor is then retested for infectious viruses, and the unit released if the second set of tests is negative. The addition of this quarantine step allows detection of those donors who may have been infected but were in the seronegative window at the time of donation. The other approach is the treatment of pooled thawed plasma with solvent/detergent (SDP). The addition of these reagents inactivates lipid-enveloped viruses, including hepatitis B virus (HBV), HCV, HIV-1, and -2, and HTLV-I and -II. The success of a program in which FFP-DR supplemented by SDP was provided to 42 hospitals in one region as the only source of banked plasma has been reported (McCarthy et al., 2000).

Blood components and their indications

Whole blood

A unit of whole blood contains 450–500 mL of blood plus a volume of anticoagulant. The hematocrit of a typical unit is 36–44%. Transfusion of one unit will raise the recipient's hematocrit 3–4% or her hemoglobin concentration 1 g/dL. Whole blood is stored at 1–6°C. Because whole blood stored for ≥24 hours is deficient in platelets and labile clotting factors V and VIII, it is not a good source of clotting factors. The primary indication for whole blood is massive hemorrhage, i.e. loss of 25% of the blood volume accompanied by continued blood loss. Some blood banks reserve inventories of whole blood for those patients who have had replacement of ≥10 units of RBCs within 24 hours (Triulzi, 1999).

Red blood cells

The volume of a unit of RBCs equals that of a unit of whole blood from which 200–250 mL of plasma has been withdrawn. If only an anticoagulant (e.g. CPDA-1) has been added, the hematocrit of the unit is 70–80%. If stored in an additive solution, a typical unit has a hematocrit of 52–60%. Because a unit of RBCs contains the same number of cells as a unit of whole blood, it will raise the hematocrit and hemoglobin the same amount. Because the volume of the product is less than that of whole blood, it is indicated for those patients who require additional oxygen-carrying capacity but are normovolemic. It is also indicated for patients who tolerate volume expansion poorly, e.g. those in congestive heart failure (Triulzi, 1999).

Red blood cells, leukocyte reduced

Because of loss of RBCs during filtration, a leukocyte-reduced RBC unit will likely contain fewer RBCs than a unit of cells which has not been leukocyte reduced. As mentioned previously, while the USA has not as yet adopted a policy of universal leukocyte reduction of RBCs, other countries have (Petrides & Stack, 2001). Because alloimmunization to leukocyte antigens results in both refractoriness to platelet transfusions and recurrent febrile nonhemolytic transfusion reactions, this product is indicated for patients who have exhibited these complications following previous transfusions (Triulzi, 1999). It may also be used in transfusions to CMV-negative patients who are immunosuppressed in order to avoid transmission of CMV (Triulzi, 1999).

Red blood cells frozen , thawed, deglycerolized

There are currently two clear indications for long-term freezing of RBCs: preservation of RBCs of rare types and of autologous units. Because of the loss of RBCs during saline washing, more than one unit may have to be transfused to achieve the same in vivo hematocrit as would be achieved with a unit of RBCs that have not been glycerolized. Until recently, thawed cells had to be administered within 24 hours of saline washing, because the washing took place in an open system (Triulzi, 1999). An automated, closed, sterile system for washing frozen glycerolized cells opens the possibility of refrigeration of thawed RBCs to prolong shelf life following thawing (Hess et al., 2001).

Platelets

A consideration of the platelet concentration at which one or more units of this product should be transfused must first consider whether or not the patient is actively bleeding. Evidence from patients whose thrombocytopenia was associated with acute leukemia suggested that in the absence of active bleeding or fever patients need not receive platelet transfusions above a platelet count of 5,000/μL. Because bleeding is accompanied by platelet consumption and fever in a hypermetabolic state, the presence of either raises the platelet transfusion threshold to 10,000/μL. In the presence of massive bleeding and/or extensive vascular damage, especially in the face of a rapidly falling platelet count, transfusion at platelet counts of 100,000/μL may be appropriate. Finally, with normal platelet counts, bleeding in the face of platelet dysfunction such as may be found in patients taking nonsteroidal anti-inflammatory drugs or aspirin, and those with congenital platelet function defects (e.g. Glanzmann's thrombasthenia) platelet transfusion may help arrest ongoing bleeding (Petrides & Stack, 2001).

One unit of platelets usually raises the platelet count by 5000/μL. The typical platelet dose is 5–7 units of random donor platelets or one unit of apheresed platelets. Because naturally occurring antibodies in ABO-incompatible plasma which accompanies the platelets may rarely cause hemolysis of recipient cells and/or a positive direct antiglobulin test, it is best that transfused platelets be ABO compatible with the recipient. Because small quantities of whole RBCs and RBC fragments may be included in the platelet unit, it is best that Rh-negative girls, and women in their reproductive years receive platelets from Rh-negative donors. If such a recipient receives platelets from an Rh-positive donor, it is best that prophylactic Rh immune globulin be administered (Triulzi, 1999).

Plasma products (FFP, FFP-DR, SDP)

Plasma products are indicated for patients who have a deficiency in coagulation factors (e.g. liver failure) and who are about to undergo surgery, and those deficient in coagulation factors due to dilutional coagulopathy such as might be seen accompanying massive transfusion or disseminated intravascular coagulation. Coagulation factor deficiency is most commonly defined by the finding of a prothrombin time (PT) and/or a partial thromboplastin time (PTT) in excess of 1.5 times normal, or an internationally normalized ratio (INR) of 1.6 or greater. In an acute situation, the usual dose is an initial 3–4 units of frozen plasma, followed by additional units if the tests are still prolonged one-half hour after the initial transfusion. The plasma unit should be ABO compatible with the recipient. Once thawed, the plasma product should be used within 24 hours, as the thawed produce loses all of its labile factor content within that time period (Triulzi, 1999; Petrides & Stack, 2001).

Cryoprecipitated AHF (cryo)

Cryoprecipitated AHF contains factor VIII:C (procoagulant factor), factor VIII:vWF (von Willebrand factor), factor XIII, and fibrinogen. Most commonly it is used to replace fibrinogen in congenital and acquired fibrinogen deficiency. Its use is quite limited in obstetrics, as its parent product, FFP, contains all these clotting factors. One unit of FFP contains twice the amount of fibrinogen as is found in a unit of cryo. Prior to transfusion, a unit of cryo is thawed to 30–37°C. Once thawed, the unit must be administered within 6 hours (Triulzi, 1999; Petrides & Stack, 2001).

Transfusion practices

When to transfuse red blood cells

Determining that point at which red cell transfusion is life-saving in the nonpregnant patient is an exceedingly difficult task. This task is even more difficult during pregnancy, when shifts in oxygen carriage and cardiovascular changes unique to pregnancy must be considered. During acute blood loss a number of interrelated and temporally-sequenced physiologic changes occur in the body's attempt to maintain adequate tissue oxygenation. These changes may be summarized as those causing increased release of oxygen to vital tissues from RBCs and those increasing the supply of oxygen-bearing RBCs to these tissues.

The concentration of hemoglobin (hgb) is equal to the product to the hematocrit (the ratio of RBC volume to total blood volume) and the mean corpuscular hemoglobin content. In the absence of diseases altering the latter (e.g. thalassemia, folate deficiency) the ratio of hgb to hematocrit is fixed at approximately 1:3, and either measure may be used (Tan & Lim, 2001). A variety of consensus opinions have suggested that RBCs be administered when the hgb falls to levels of from 6 g/dL to 10 g/dL (Ekeroma et al., 1997; Simon et al., 1998; Blajchman & Hebert, 2001). These suggestions are based on animal data, anecdotal experience, and expert opinions (Blajchman & Hebert, 2001). Anecdotal reports in humans including those of patients who refuse transfusion suggest that in otherwise stable nonpregnant patients the risk of mortality increases below a hgb of 3.5 (Simon et al., 1998) to 5.0 g/dL (Tan & Lim, 2001). However, using these hgb concentrations as transfusion triggers fails to consider changes within the erythrocyte. The decline in hemoglobin below 9 g/dL is accompanied by a rapid right shift in the oxygen–hemoglobin dissociation curve due to the Bohr effect (Welch et al., 1992). Over 12–36 hours of declining hgb, an increase in erythrocyte 2,3-DPG occurs (Spence et al., 1993). Both mechanisms increase the dissociation between hemoglobin and oxygen, and thus increase the delivery of oxygen to oxygen-poor tissues.

Tissue oxygen extraction is contingent on oxygen delivery (Do_2) and oxygen consumption (Vo_2). The normal nonpregnant 70 kg individual has a Do_2 of 1,000 mL/min and a Vo_2 of 250 mL/min. The total body oxygen extraction ratio (ER) is therefore 25% (Table 10.2). It must be noted, however, that different organs extract oxygen at different rates. For instance, the ER for the heart is 55%, while that of the kidney is 10% (Stehling et al., 1994). As Do_2 falls due to decreased RBC mass, ER increases (Spence et al., 1993).

Because of the intravascular volume changes which occur during pregnancy, the application of suggestions for transfusion based exclusively on hemoglobin, hematocrit, or volume of blood loss derived from a nonpregnant population may lead to unnecessary administration of RBCs. In normal pregnancy both RBC and plasma volume expand, respectively, by 25% and 40%, with the rate of expansion of both blood components peaking near the end of the second trimester. This disproportionate expansion of plasma relative to red cell volume accounts for the "physiologic anemia of pregnancy." As opposed to the higher normal value in the nonpregnant state, anemia during pregnancy is defined as a hgb <10 g/dL (Simon et al., 1998). Because of the expansion in total blood volume, the loss of a large volume of whole blood by a pregnant woman may be better tolerated than the loss of an equivalent volume by a nonpregnant patient.

Table 10.2 Relationships between physiologic measurements and oxygen delivery

$CO = HR \times SV$
- CO = Cardiac output
- HR = Heart rate
- SV = Stroke volume

$C_ao_2 = (Hgb \times S_ao_2 \times 1.39) + (0.003 \times P_ao_2)$
- C_ao_2 = Oxygen content of arterial blood
- Hgb = Hemoglobin concentration
- S_ao_2 = Oxygen saturation of arterial blood
- P_ao_2 = Partial pressure of oxygen in arterial blood

$Do_2 = CO \times C_ao_2$
- Do_2 = Total amount of oxygen delivered to organs
- CO = Cardiac output
- C_ao_2 = Oxygen content of arterial blood

$Vo_2 = CO \times (C_ao_2 - C_vo_2)$
- Vo_2 = Oxygen consumption
- CO = Cardiac output
- C_ao_2 = Oxygen content of arterial blood
- C_vo_2 = Oxygen content of mixed venous blood

$ER = Vo_2/Do_2$
- ER = Oxygen extraction ratio
- Vo_2 = Oxygen consumption
- Do_2 = Total amount of oxygen delivered to organs

Another consideration unique to pregnancy is the effect of acute blood loss on the fetus. A case has been reported of a fetus who during fetomaternal hemorrhage demonstrated increased middle cerebral artery blood flow (Baschat et al., 1998). In another report, seven women underwent phlebotomies of 400 mL as autologous donations over 35 minutes each. A decrease in the middle cerebral artery pulsatility indices of their fetuses during phlebotomy was noted. In the latter report the absence of concomitant changes in maternal blood pressure and in fetal and maternal heart rates was also recorded (Suzuki et al., 2001). The authors of both reports postulated that the changes in the middle cerebral artery reflected compensatory changes in fetal cerebral blood flow attempting to maintain fetal cerebral oxygenation in the face of the loss of, respectively, fetal and maternal oxygen-carrying capacity (Baschat et al., 1998; Suzuki et al., 2001). Finally, while its relevance to fetal circulation and oxygenation is unclear, hemodilution in nonpregnant adults has been associated with decreased cerebral oxygen delivery despite increased cerebral blood flow (Tan & Lim, 2001).

The carriage of oxygen-bearing RBCs to tissues is dependent on a sequence of cardiovascular changes that accompany acute blood loss. The initial response is an adrenergically-mediated constriction of venules and small veins. This in turn results in increased venous return to the heart (increased preload). Systemic hypotension abruptly follows. The drop in capillary hydrostatic pressure resulting from the hypotension allows mobilization of fluid, which may restore up to 50% of the lost blood volume. Fluid mobilization also decreases the viscosity of blood, which in turn decreases the work the heart must perform to maintain circulatory adequacy (decreased afterload). The combination of increased preload and decreased afterload enables the heart to increase the volume of blood pumped with each contraction (stroke volume). Despite an increase in heart rate, the increase in stroke volume is the major contributor to the increase in cardiac output at this point (Table 10.2) (Welch et al., 1992; Stehling et al., 1994; Simon et al., 1998; Sibbald et al., 2000; Tan & Lim, 2001). With continued blood loss, selective arterial constriction occurs in the skin, skeletal muscle, and splanchnic organs, ultimately causing anaerobic metabolism and release of fixed acids. The metabolic acidosis stimulates hyperventilation as a means of respiratory compensation for a systemic fall in pH. The increased ventilatory rate is accompanied by increased negative intrathoracic pressure, which in turn serves to increase venous return to the heart. Selective vasoconstriction results in redistribution of blood flow to the brain and the coronary vessels (Welch et al., 1992; Stehling & Simon, 1994).

From the foregoing discussion, it should be clear that the delivery of oxygen to the tissues is a function of a variety of physiologic physiologic parameters, of which hgb concentration is only one (Simon et al., 1998; Sibbald et al., 2000; Tan & Lim, 2001). The mathematical relationships of these parameters is summarized in Table 10.2. In the presence of acute massive blood loss such as may be encountered in obstetrics, dynamic shifts may occur in oxygen loading, blood flow, RBC mass, oxygen affinity, and tissue demands (Simon et al., 1998). In addition, oxygen demand varies within and between different organs. It is not possible to either directly or indirectly measure oxygen delivery to all essential organs. However, some critical global physiologic measurements have been proposed (Table 10.3). Because these require invasive monitoring and because acute blood loss in obstetrics is frequently unpredictable and unanticipated the clinical utility of these measurements if limited.

Acute massive blood loss is an obstetric emergency that does not lend itself to consideration of a variety of physiological parameters prior to formulating a plan of management. Because oxygen delivery is dependent on both red cell mass and intravascular volume to transport that mass, replacement of the latter is a primary step in fluid resuscitation. An arbitrary, practical approach to acute blood loss is to first restore volume with crystalloid, and to then transfuse RBCs only if signs of oxygen deficiency persist (e.g. tachycardia, hypotension, tachypnea). An equally arbitrary though more quantitative plan for fluid replacement which is based on readily-accessible indirect indices of blood loss and accompanying hemodynamic changes is presented in Table 10.4. Of note is that replacement of fluids by isotonic crystalloids (e.g. normal saline, lactated Ringer's solution) is usually in a 3 : 1 ratio with estimated blood loss, as two-thirds of the volume of transfused crystalloids rapidly redistributes within the interstitial space (Petrides & Stack, 2001). Lower volumes of hypertonic saline are required for volume replacement because of this solution's ability to draw interstitial fluid into the intravascular space. Both natural (e.g. albumen) and synthetic (e.g. hetastarch, pentastarch) colloids also offer the advantages of requiring lesser volumes to restore intravascular osmotic pressure. However, colloids are more expensive than crystalloids. Pentastarch has the additional risks of exacerbating preexisting renal failure and of impaired coagulation. It has also been found to be embryocidal in rabbits and mice. No comparative study of any of these replacement fluids in pregnant women has been published (Acoa, 1998).

Red cell compatibility testing

Type and screen

Prior to an anticipated transfusion, the compatibility of the donor red cells with the potential recipient's serum must be ascertained. The initial step in this process is the determination of the potential recipient's ABO type. There follows a series of three tests. In the first of these, the immediate-spin phase, a drop of each of three type O reagent red cells which are known to contain clinically significant RBC antigens is mixed with two drops of potential recipient plasma or serum in a test tube at room temperature. The tube is then spun for 15 seconds, and the RBC button then resuspended. Any agglutination or hemolysis suggests the presence of "cold" (i.e. reacting at room, rather than body temperature) antibodies, most of which are of the IgM type. Because these "cold" antibodies are usually not responsible for transfusion-related hemolysis, some workers feel that this step in compatibility testing is unnecessary. The second step is the 37°C phase, during which the reagent RBC/recipient serum or plasma mixture, to which a potentiator such as low ionic strength saline (LISS) may have been added, is incubated at 37°C, spun, and read for hemolysis or agglutination. The final, or antiglobulin, phase of the antibody screen requires the washing of the RBC/recipient serum or plasma mixture with saline to remove unbound globulins, after which rabbit antihuman IgG is added to the test tube. The tube is spun and read. If in either of the prior phases IgG

Table 10.3 Critical physiologic measurements of tissue oxygen delivery

$P_{V}O_2$ <25 mmHg $P_{V}O_2$ = Pulmonary artery oxygen tension at completion of oxygen unloading
ER >50% ER = Oxygen extraction ratio
V_{O_2} <50% of baseline V_{O_2} = Oxygen consumption

(From Simon et al., 1998.)

Table 10.4 Fluid management in the face of acute blood loss

% blood volume lost	Sign(s)	Suggested replacement
<15%	No change	Crystalloid
30%	Tachycardia	Crystalloid
40%	Tachycardia + hypotension	Crystalloid and/or colloid; RBC if underlying disease
>40%	Tachycardia + severe hypotension	RBC, crystalloid and/or colloid

antibody to reagent red cells was present in the recipient serum or plasma and these antibodies adhered onto the corresponding antigens on the RBCs, the rabbit antihuman IgG should form a bridge between antibody-coated RBCs, detected as macroscopic or microscopic agglutination. The identity of any antibody which was detected during any of the three phases of antibody screening is then determined. Because of the theoretical possibility that a pregnant women previously found to not have antibodies may unpredictably develop antibodies to her fetus' RBC antigens, antibody screening must be performed within 3 days of transfusion (Petrides & Stack, 2001).

Type and cross-match

If the potential recipient has had no antibody detected during the antibody screen and has no prior history of having had an alloantibody detected, ABO and Rh-matched donor units may be selected. Then at room temperature a quick spin, as described above, using donor RBCs and recipient serum or plasma may be performed in anticipation of transfusion. The purposes of this abbreviated cross-match are to confirm ABO compatibility and to rule out the remote possibility that antibodies to antigens which were not present on the reagent RBCs and which are present on the donor RBCs are present in the recipient's serum or plasma. If, however, the patient has a history of alloimmunization and/or if antibodies were detected during screening, a complete cross-match consiting of the same three phases enumerated under type and screening but using donor RBCs is carried out prior to transfusion (Petrides & Stack, 2001).

Computer cross-matching

If the transfusion service has a computer system which meets FDA requirements and which has been validated for compatibility testing, that system may be used in lieu of an immediate spin cross-match to determine ABO compatibility of donor and potential recipient. The computer must contain logic to alert the blood bank to ABO incompatibility between the donor unit and the recipient (Standards Program Committee, AABB, 2000; Petrides & Stack, 2001). Because the FDA requirements for computer cross-matching are so stringent, this procedure is now in use in only a minority of blood banks in the United States.

Administration of blood products

Patient identification

The most common cause of fatal hemolytic transfusion reactions is the inadvertent transfusion of ABO-incompatible RBCs. For this reason the AABB enforces strict rules regarding patient identification at each step of the process (Standards Program Committee, AABB, 2000; Petrides & Stack, 2001). The patient must be positively identified at the time of specimen collection. A sample submitted for compatibility testing must contain the patient's name, unique identifying number, the date of drawing the specimen, and a means of identifying the person who drew it. Prior to release the unit is visually inspected. A unit that appears hemolyzed, contains clots or gas, or has a color different from that of the attached segments is quarantined and investigated for possible contamination. Immediately prior to transfusion the recipient's name and unique identification, both read from the patient's armband, are verified. The unit must contain the results of compatibility testing and the date of issue of the unit. Since major hemolytic reactions frequently occur during the first 10–15 minutes of blood administration, the patient is closely observed during this time period.

Blood warming

The administration of cold blood at a rate ≥100 mL/min may result in cold-induced changes in the conduction of the sinoatrial node, resulting in cardiac arrhythmias and arrest. Therefore blood administered at or in excess of this rate should first be warmed. Both warmers consisting of a coil of plastic tubing immersed in a temperature-controlled water bath and those made of an electrically heated plate in contact with a flat plastic blood bag are acceptable. Because of the risk of heat-induced hemolysis, warming a unit of blood by immersion in hot water or by using a microwave is not acceptable (Triulzi, 1999).

Duration of transfusion

A unit of blood that has been warmed to less than 10°C and that has not been out of the blood bank for more than 30 minutes may be returned to the bank for continued storage and later use. A unit which exceeds either of these parameters must be discarded. A unit of blood must be administered within 4 hours. These rules are designed to minimize the risk of bacterial contamination of blood that has been warmed above refrigeration temperatures (Triulzi, 1999; Standards Program Committee, AABB, 2000; Petrides & Stack, 2001).

Concurrent administration of intravenous fluids and medications

With the exception of normal saline, which is isotonic with blood, concurrent administration of other fluids is prohibited (Standards Program Committee, AABB, 2000). Hypotonic solutions (e.g. 5% dextrose) may induce hemolysis. The calcium found in lactated Ringer's solution may neutralize the citrate in the blood bag and result in clot formation. Administration of medications is also interdicted. The alkalinity of some medications may induce hemolysis of transfused blood.

Should a patient simultaneously receiving medication and a blood product have an adverse reaction, medical personnel will be unable to determine if the reaction is to the blood, the medication, or both. Furthermore, in such a circumstance only a portion of the medication dose will have been administered.

Filtration

Whether the product being transfused does or does not contain cells, it must be transfused through a line designed to retain particles that are potentially harmful to the recipient (Standards Program Committee, AABB, 2000). Standard blood administration sets contain filters whose pore size of 170–260 μm is sufficiently small to trap blood clots, fibrin strands, and other debris. While third-generation leukocyte-reduction filters are available, they may slow the rate of transfusion and become clogged. For those patients who require leukocyte-reduced blood products, prestorage leukocyte depletion is preferable (Triulzi, 1999).

Blood ordering practices for selected situations

Obstetric hemorrhage

However defined, obstetric hemorrhage is a rare but potentially lethal complication of pregnancy (ACOG, 1998; Alamia & Meyer, 1999; Bonnar, 2000). It is the third most common cause of maternal mortality in the United States, following thromboembolism and hypertensive disorders (ACOG, 1998). An estimate of the incidence of potentially life-threatening hemorrhage is 1 per 1,000 deliveries (Bonnar, 2000). Some obstetric diagnoses are associated with a more frequent requirement for transfusion, e.g. placenta previa (Frederiksen et al., 1999), placental abruption (Bonnar, 2000), and uterine rupture (Baskett & Kieser, 2001). However, the most common causes of obstetric hemorrhage (e.g. uterine atony (Ledee et al., 2001)) cannot be anticipated. Regardless of diagnosis, the number and type of blood products that must be transfused (Castaneda et al., 2000) are not predictable. Furthermore, the majority of women who suffer obstetric hemorrhages do not require blood transfusions (Alamia & Meyer, 1999). Therefore, establishing blood ordering policies and procedures which are at once protective of the patient but which do not waste a priceless resource is problematic.

Certain common-sense policies that incur little additional expense may save lives. A triennial review of maternal mortalities in the United Kingdom has repeatedly concluded that "haemorrhage drills" which serve to keep both labor and delivery and blood bank staff prepared to deal with this rare emergency be performed on a regular basis. It also recommends that an experienced operator participate in the management of all cases of placenta previa (Bonnar, 2000).

Given the unpredictable nature of obstetric hemorrhage, utilization of formulae such as the cross-match to transfusion (C/T) ratio (Triulzi, 1999; Petrides & Stack, 2001) are largely inapplicable in obstetric practice. Even when the patient's blood has undergone an antibody screen within the past 3 days and the results of that screen showed no antibodies, up to an additional 10–15 minutes are required to complete the cross-match on blood being held in the blood bank (Petrides & Stack, 2001). Waiting this amount of time may not be an option in the case of an acute, massive hemorrhage. For that reason, specific aspects of compatibility testing may be waived, depending upon the urgency of the situation (Standards Program Committee, AABB, 2000; Petrides & Stack, 2001). As noted in Table 10.5, in the absence of current, valid ABO typing on file in the blood bank, if immediate red cell transfusion is necessary, the patient should receive type O-negative blood. It must be borne in mind that a transfusion reaction, though unlikely, may still occur with transfusion of any type of uncross-matched blood, because among women who have never been pregnant or who have never received a transfusion, a small proportion (0.04%) will have non-ABO blood group antibodies (Petrides & Stack, 2001). Because O-negative blood is found in only 6% of the population, it is best to conserve RBCs of this type by transfusing type-compatible blood to recipients whose current, valid ABO and Rh typing is on file in the blood bank (Petrides & Stack, 2001). Given the rarity and unpredictability of sudden massive obstetric hemorrhage, some may prefer to have a clot tube drawn and held in the blood bank for compatibility testing should it prove necessary during the course of the patient's stay. Others may prefer to type and screen every parturient on admission to the labor suite. The human and financial costs for a routine type and screen policy have been reported. In one study, of 16,291 women who had a vaginal delivery, 76 (0.47%) required transfusion. All but four of the latter had identifiable risk factors (e.g. anemia, prior cesarean, prior postpartum hemorrhage, multiple pregnancy). The cost of a policy of universal typing and screening of all laboring women was estimated at $1 million; that of typing and screening only women with risk factors was $400,000 (Ransom et al., 1998). The requirement for transfusion for women undergoing cesarean delivery is also low. A review of 3,962 women who underwent both elective and emergency cesarean deliveries reported a transfusion rate of 3.3%. Three of the 132 transfused women had no risk factors (Ransom et al., 1999).

Massive transfusion is defined as the replacement of one blood volume within 24 hours, or the equivalent of the transfusion of 10 or more units of whole blood within 1 day (Triulzi, 1999; Standards Program Committee, AABB, 2000; Bonnar, 2000). Potential complications of massive transfusion include calcium depletion due to transfusion at a rate that exceeds the liver's ability to metabolize citrate, and cold-induced arrhythmias and coagulopathies due to rapid infu-

Table 10.5 Red blood cell testing scenarios for emergencies

Transfusion urgency	Compatibility testing status	ABO, Rh type	Antibody screen	Cross-match	Testing time* (min)
Lowest	Complete	ABO- and Rh-identical or -compatible	Yes	Yes	30–45
↓	Complete	ABO- and Rh-identical or -compatible	Yes†	Yes	10–15
	Incomplete; no cross-match	ABO- and Rh-identical or -compatible	Yes†	No	0
	Incomplete; no antibody screen	ABO- and Rh-identical or -compatible	No	Yes	10–15
	Incomplete; no antibody screen or cross-match	ABO- and Rh-identical or -compatible	No	No	0‡
Highest	Incomplete; no antibody screen or cross-match	Group O, Rh-negative	No	No	0

* Testing times assume that the cross-match is done at room temperature using an "immediate spin" only, which is ordinarily permissible only when there is no history of a blood group antibody and the current antibody screen is negative. Testing time does not include transportation times for specimens and blood components or all administrative steps.

† Assumes that ABO, Rh typing and antibody screen were performed earlier and found to be negative on a current valid scrum specimen (within 3 days of transfusion).

‡ Assumes a current, valid blood sample is available in the blood bank on which ABO typing has already been performed.

(Reproduced by permission from Petrides M, Stack G. Practical Guide to Transfusion Medicine. Bethesda, Maryland: American Association of Blood Banks, 2001, Table 7.1.)

sion of unwarmed bank blood (Triulzi, 1999; Petrides & Stack, 2001).

A major and difficult to diagnose complication is that of a transfusion-associated coagulopathy. This problem may be due to dilution of endogenous coagulation factors, or it may be multifactorial in origin (Petrides & Stack, 2001). Regardless of etiology, in the face of massive bleeding, the approach to diagnosis and treatment requires both clinical and laboratory observations. A coagulopathy seems likely in the presence of bleeding from nonsurgical sites (e.g. mucous membranes) or continued oozing from wounds and puncture sites (Triulzi, 1999; Bonnar, 2000). Blood for coagulation studies should be drawn as early following suspicion of a coagulopathy as is possible. These studies should include a prothrombin time, activated partial thromboplastin time, fibrinogen concentration, and platelet count. While waiting for laboratory results, the observation of a formed, retracted, stable clot in an unanticoagulated tube within 10 minutes of drawing suggests the absence of a coagulopathy.

In the face of massive hemorrhage, a platelet count of 50,000 or less seems a reasonable threshold at which to administer platelets (Alamia & Meyer, 1999; Bonnar, 2000; Standards Program Committee, AABB, 2000). One unit of apheresed platelets or 5–7 units of individual donor platelets is a reasonable starting dose. Abnormalities of the other coagulation studies may indicate administration of FFP, beginning with 4–6 units of the product (Triulzi, 1999). Only if coagulation tests are not available in a timely fashion, or if the bleeding is so profuse that waiting for laboratory results would not be prudent should a formulaic approach to transfusion of FFP be considered. Ratios of from 1–5 units of FFP for every 2–6 units of RBCs have been suggested (Bonnar, 2000; Petrides & Stack, 2001). Regardless of initial coagulation test results, it is advisable to recheck coagulation studies after allowing 15 minutes for equilibration following transfusion of FFP and/or platelets (Petrides & Stack, 2001).

Cesarean delivery

A patient undergoing a cesarean delivery will predictably lose an average of 1,000 mL, which is 500 mL greater than the average volume lost during a vaginal delivery (ACOG, 1998). One would therefore expect that cesarean deliveries would be associated with a greater frequency of transfusion than that reported in association with vaginal deliveries. Transfusion rates for cesareans of from 1.7% to 7.2% have been reported from institutions both in the United States (Cousins et al., 1996; Ransom et al., 1999) and abroad (Fenton, 1999; Cupitt & Raghavendra, 2000). The decision whether or not to transfuse frequently has a subjective component. One study examined 127 patients who had cesarean deliveries complicated by hemorrhage (defined as an intraoperative blood loss >1,500 mL, and/or a decrease in hematocrit of more than 10 points and/or a postoperative hematocrit <24%). There were no statistically significant differences in patient demographics, pre- or immediate postoperative hematocrit, estimated blood loss, hospital stay, infection rates or wound problems between those who received transfusions and those who did not. The only differences between transfused and nontransfused women were that those who were transfused had a higher mean hematocrit after stabilization (28% vs 23%) as well as a 6% incidence of transfusion-associated complications including hepatitis B and C and alloimmunization (Naef et al., 1995). Given the low probability of transfusion during or following a cesarean delivery, in those facilities in which blood is readily available a policy of either holding a clot tube in the blood bank (Cousins et al., 1996) or typing and screening the patient who is to undergo this procedure (Ransom et al., 1999) seems prudent.

Autologous blood

Autologous blood collection and transfusion is the use of blood donated by an individual for infusion back into the same individual. The three types of autologous donation pertinent to obstetrics, namely preoperative donation, acute normovolemic hemodilution, and intraoperative collection and reinfusion, will be discussed in that order.

Preoperative donation

Blood which is donated by and reinfused into the same individual has some theoretical benefits. Following donation, it usually takes 2–4 weeks for the body to restore red cells, whereas it takes only 3 days for it to restore plasma. Thus, the blood lost if surgery is performed within a month of donation will be more dilute than that circulating prior to donation, and fewer RBCs per unit volume will be lost (Petrides & Stack, 2001). Transfused autolgous blood should have no risks of disease transmission, transfusion reactions, or alloimmunization to foreign cellular antigens (Thomas et al., 1996; Triulzi, 1999). In practice, however, bacterial contamination of a stored unit remains an unlikely but real possibility, as is the possibility of inadvertently transfusing another donor's blood. Febrile transfusion reactions have been reported even with a proper autologous match. A postulated reason for these reactions is the infusion of cytokines or low levels of bacteria that may accumulate during storage (Petrides & Stack, 2001).

Prerequisites for and testing of autologous donors are less stringent than those for allogeneic donors. The prospective autologous donor must have a hemoglobin concentration of at least 11 g/dL or a hematocrit of at least 33%. She or he must be free of any evidence or risk of bacteremia at the time of donation. The last donation must precede the intended transfusion by at least 72 hours. Both units for transfusion and recipient's blood must be tested for ABO and Rh typing prior to transfusion (Standards Program Committee, AABB, 2000).

Given the theoretical risks and expense (Thomas et al., 1996; Toedt, 1999; Yeo et al., 1999; Suzuki et al., 2001) associated with preoperative donation, the indications and established benefits of autologous donations in obstetrics are few in number. Even in patients at high risk for indicated transfusions (e.g. placenta previa, placenta accreta) a minority of donors will ultimately be transfused. Those transfused may require additional allogeneic units besides the autologous units previously donated (Thomas et al., 1996). Particularly when the indication for transfusion was evidenced by recent blood loss, patients who are most likely to benefit from autologous donation may not meet the prerequisites for that donation. A review of 59 patients with placenta previa found that only 34% met criteria for autologous donation, and that 20% of the latter ultimately required transfusion (Toedt, 1999). The patient's candidacy for preoperative donation may be increased, however, by the administration of erythropoietin. A study of 26 women who had iron-deficiency anemia resistant to oral iron reported an increase in mean hemoglobin concentration of 3 g/dL within 3 weeks of treatment with a combination of parenteral iron and erythropoietin (Sifakis et al., 2001).

Acute normovolemic hemodilution (ANH)

Acute normovolemic hemodilution is a procedure in which one or more units of the patient's blood are withdrawn in the operating room just prior to initiating surgery. Simultaneously the whole blood removed is replaced with crystalloid or colloid. The number of units withdrawn are a function of the expected blood loss and the patient's tolerance to hemodilution. The blood removed is stored for up to 8 hours at room temperature, in the operating room, and then reinfused at the close of the procedure. The order in which the blood is reinfused is the last unit first, i.e. the units are given in the order of most to least dilute. The advantages of the procedure are that, as with preoperative donation, the blood lost at surgery will be dilute, and thus fewer RBCs than are ordinarily lost will be lost at surgery. In addition, the increase in venous return and decrease in resistance to flow following ejection from the left ventricle increases stroke volume and thus cardiac output (Petrides & Stack, 2001). Furthermore, the decrease in blood viscosity resulting from hemodilution increases oxygen delivery through the microvasculature. A unique advantage of ANH is that the whole blood that is reinfused contains both coagulation factors and viable platelets.

Prerequisites and testing for ANH are the same as those for autologous preoperative donation. Experience with this form of autologous donation and reinfusion in obstetrics is limited. One report of 38 women of whom 33 had placenta previa and who underwent cesarean delivery found that only one required homologous blood while 14 received additional previously donated autologous blood (Grange et al., 1998).

Intraoperative collection and reinfusion

Blood may be collected and reinfused from the surgical field. On removal through a suction device the aspirated blood is processed through a cell saver, in which the aspirate is centrifuged and filtered and the red cells washed (Waters et al., 2000). Washed cells held at room temperature must be reinfused within 6 hours (Petrides & Stack, 2001). The major advantage of this type of autologous transfusion procedure is that the blood does not leave the patient's side, thus minimizing the possibility of an administration error. Unlike preoperative donation and ANH, this procedure has no prerequisites. However, it is contraindicated in the presence of bacterial infection or malignancy. Rarely is enough blood salvaged to meet patient needs with this technique. In addition, the aspirated processed blood is deficient in coagulation factors and platelets (Petrides & Stack, 2001).

Potential complications of this procedure include bacterial contamination, metabolic acidosis, electrolyte imbalance, coagulopathy, and air embolism (Spahn & Casutt, 2000; Standards Program Committee, AABB, 2000). Additional concerns unique to its utilization during cesarean delivery include the possibility of transfusion to the mother of fetal cellular and acellular debris as well as the induction of an amniotic fluid embolism (Rebarber et al., 1998; Potter et al., 1999; Waters et al., 2000). Favorable clinical experience with intraoperative cell salvage at cesarean deliveries has been reported (Rebarber et al., 1998; Potter et al., 1999). One series found no increased incidence of disseminated intravascular coagulation, infectious morbidity, or requirement for ventilatory support in comparison with women who did not undergo cell salvage and reinfusion (Rebarber et al., 1998). A study that compared washed salvaged blood which had been passed through a 120 µm filter with that which had also been passed through a leukocyte-reduction filter found that after the latter procedure the blood contained significantly fewer bacteria and squamous cells. However, in comparison with central venous maternal blood, the fetal cell count was significantly greater in both filtered specimens (Waters et al., 2000). While the risk of maternal alloimmunization to all fetal antigens as a consequence of cell salvage and reinfusion at cesarean delivery cannot be eliminated, Rh-negative women whose babies are determined to be Rh positive should receive a dose of Rh-immune globulin commensurate with the volume of fetal blood found in their circulations postoperatively (Weiskopf, 2000).

Directed donation

The medical indications for designated, rather than anonymous, donations are few, and include patients with rare phenotypes or who require cellular blood products that are HLA compatible. The idea that blood from known donors is safer than that from volunteers is not supported by data (Triulzi, 1999). Furthermore, blood from genetically-related individuals carries a theoretically increased risk of graft-vs-host disease, and must therefore be irradiated prior to transfusion (Standards Program Committee, AABB, 2000).

Complications of blood transfusions

Immune-mediated complications

Any untoward response to transfusion of a blood product is defined as a transfusion reaction (Kopko & Holland, 2001). Such reactions are found in up to 10% of all blood recipients. Differentiating among the different types of reactions is extremely difficult, because of the similarity in symptoms among them (Table 10.6). However, attempting to make the distinction is necessary, as the severity and treatment of each type of reaction is unique. Fortunately, the three most common causes of transfusion-related mortality (acute intravascular hemolysis, bacterial sepsis, and transfusion-related acute lung injury) are the least common types of transfusion reactions (Kopko & Holland, 2001).

Acute transfusion reactions

Acute transfusion reactions are defined as those that occur within 24 hours of the completion of a transfusion. Five of the different types (Table 10.7) will be discussed.

Acute hemolytic transfusion reactions

There are two subtypes of acute hemolytic transfusion reactions. Of them, acute intravascular hemolysis (AIHTR) is the more lethal (Triulzi, 1999). The process is initiated by the transfusion of type A or B RBCs to a recipient who has preformed anti-A or anti-B antibodies. The most common reason for the transfusion of incompatible RBCs is patient/specimen misidentification. IgM or complement-fixing IgG antibodies initiate the complement cascade, ultimately binding the C5–9 component of complement (the membrane attack complex) onto the RBC. A pore in the RBC membrane then appears,

Table 10.6 Clinical findings associated with different types of transfusion reactions

Fever
Febrile nonhemolytic transfusion reaction
Hemolytic transfusion reaction, acute or delayed
Septic transfusion reaction
Transfusion-related acute lung injury—variably seen
Rash
Allergic and/or anaphylactic reactions
Hemolytic transfusion reaction
Shock
Acute hemolytic transfusion reaction (intravascular hemolysis)
Anaphylactic reaction
Septic
Transfusion-related acute lung injury—variably seen
Respiratory distress/dyspnea
Acute hemolytic transfusion reaction
Anaphylactic
Fluid overload, cardiogenic pulmonary edema
Transfusion-related acute lung injury

(Reproduced by permission from Petrides M, Stack G. Practical Guide to Transfusion Medicine. Bethesda, Maryland: American Association of Blood Banks, 2001, Table 7.1.)

Table 10.7 Acute transfusion reactions

Type	Signs and symptoms	Usual cause	Treatment	Prevention
Intravascular hemolytic (immune)	Hemoglobinemia and hemoglobinuria, fever, chills, anxiety, shock, DIC, dyspnea, chest pain, flank pain, oliguria	ABO incompatibility (clerical error) or other complement-fixing antibody causing antigen–antibody incompatibility	Stop transfusion; hydrate, support blood pressure and respiration; induce diuresis; treat shock and DIC, if present	Avoid clerical errors; ensure proper sample and recipient identification
Extravascular hemolytic (immune)	Fever, malaise, indirect hyperbilirubinemia, increased urine urobilinogen, falling hematocrit	IgG non-complement-fixing antibody often associated with delayed hemolysis	Monitor hematocrit, renal and hepatic function, coagulation profile; no acute treatment generally required	Avoid clerical errors; ensure proper sample and recipient identification
Febrile	Fever, chills, rarely hypotension	Antibodies to leukocytes or plasma proteins; hemolysis; passive cytokine infusion; sepsis. Commonly due to patient's underlying condition	Stop transfusion; give antipyretics; e.g. acetaminophen; for rigors in adults use meperidine 25–50 mg IV or IM	Pretransfusion antipyretic; leukocyte-reduced blood components, if recurrent
Allergic (mild to severe)	Urticaria (hives), rarely hypotension or anaphylaxis	Antibodies to plasma proteins; rarely antibodies to IgA	Stop transfusion; give antihistamine (PO or IM); if severe, epinephrine and/or steroids	Pretransfusion antihistamine; washed RBC components, if recurrent or severe; check pretransfusion IgA levels in patients with a history of anaphylaxis to transfusion
Hypervolemic	Dyspnea, hypertension, pulmonary edema, cardiac arrhythmias	Too rapid and/or excessive blood transfusion	Induce diuresis; phlebotomy; support cardiorespiratory system as needed	Avoid rapid or excessive transfusion
Transfusion-related acute lung injury (TRALI)	Dyspnea, fever pulmonary edema, hypotension, normal pulmonary capillary wedge pressure	HLA or leukocyte antibodies; usually donor antibody transfused with plasma in component	Support blood pressure and respiration (may require intubation)	Leukocyte-reduced RBCs if recipient has the antibody; notify transfusion service to quarantine remaining components from donor
Bacterial sepsis	Rigors, chills, fever, shock	Contaminated blood component	Stop transfusion; support blood pressure; culture patient and blood unil; give antibiotics; notify blood transfusion service	Care in blood collection and storage; careful attention to arm preparation for phlebotomy

DIC, disseminated intravascular coagulation; IM, intramuscular; IV, intravenous; PO, by mouth; RBC, red blood cells.
(Reproduced by permission from Triulzi DJ, ed. Blood Transfusion Therapy. A Physician's Handbook, 6th edn. Bethesda, Maryland: American Association of Blood Banks, 1999: 109–111, Table 5.)

which allows water to enter the cell. Osmotic intravascular lysis of the RBC ensues. Free hemoglobin may be detected in both blood and urine. Free hemoglobin binds the vasodilator nitric oxide. Unopposed endothelin then causes vasoconstriction of the renal vessels, with subsequent renal tubular necrosis and renal failure. The release of complement fragments, the anaphylotoxins C3a and C5a, and other inflammation mediators results in fever, shock, hypotension, and bronchospasm. The concomitant "cytokine storm" activates the coagulation system, and disseminated intravascular coagulation ensues (Triulzi, 1999; Petrides & Stack, 2001). While the most serious aspects of AIHTR (e.g. DIC, renal failure) occur infrequently, a positive association exists between the severity of the reaction and the volume of incompatible cells transfused as well as the rate of transfusion. Because of the potential life-threatening nature of this reaction, response must be swift (Table 10.8).

An acute extravascular hemolytic transfusion reaction (AEHTR) results when the intravascular IgG antibody either does not fix complement, or fixes only C3. The clinical picture of AEHTR is much less severe than that of AIHTR. Fever, a falling hematocrit, and a positive direct antiglobulin (Coombs) test are the more common findings (Petrides & Stack, 2001).

Table 10.8 Management of a suspected acute intravascular hemoloytic transfusion reaction

If an acute transfusion reaction occurs:

1 Stop blood component transfusion immediately
2 Verify the correct unit was given to the correct patient
3 Maintain IV access and ensure adequate urine output with an appropriate crystalloid or colloid solution
4 Maintain blood pressure, pulse
5 Maintain adequate ventilation
6 Notify attending physician and blood bank
7 Obtain blood/urine for transfusion reaction workup
8 Send blood bag and administration set to blood transfusion service immediately
9 Blood bank performs workup of suspected transfusion reaction as follows:
  A Check paper work to ensure correct blood component was transfused to the right patient
  B Evaluate plasma for hemoglobinemia
  C Perform direct antiglobulin test
  D Repeat other serologic testing as needed (ABO, Rh)

If intravascular hemolytic reaction is confirmed

10 Monitor renal status (BUN, creatinine)
11 Initiate a duresis
12 Analyze urine for hemoglobinuria
13 Monitor coagutation status (prothrombin time, partial thromboplastin time, fibrinogen, platelet count)
14 Monitor for signs of hemolysis (lactate dehydrogenase, bilirubin, haptoglobin, plasma hemoglobin)
15 Repeat compatibility testing (cross-match)
16 If sepsis is suspected, culture unit and patient, and treat as appropriate

(Reproduced by permission from Triulzi DJ, ed. Blood Transfusion Therapy. A Physician's Handbook, 6th edn. Bethesda, Maryland: American Association of Blood Banks, 1999: 108, Table 4.)

Febrile non-hemolytic transfusion reactions (FNHTR)

Fever commonly accompanies a variety of transfusion reactions (Table 10.6). Defined as a temperature elevation of 1°C or greater or a body temperature of 38°C within 4 hours of transfusion in the absence of hemolysis, a FNHTR is a diagnosis of exclusion (Triulzi, 1999; Petrides & Stack, 2001). Though a subject of controversy (Heddle, 1999; Sibinga, 1999), it is thought that, when accompanying RBC transfusions, these reactions are initiated by recipients' antibodies (cytotoxic antibodies and leukoagglutinins) against transfused leukocyte and platelet antigens. The antibody–antigen complexes contribute to the release of inflammatory cytokines (e.g. IL-1, IL-6, TNF-α) that mediate fever through the thermoregulatory center in the hypothalamus.

A FNHTR which accompanies a platelet transfusion is more likely due to transfusion of cytokines in the plasma accompanying the platelets (Heddle, 1999). That the cytokines accompanying the platelets may be derived at least in part from leukocytes stored with the platelets is suggested by the finding that the incidence of FNHTRs was positively associated with duration of storage for those receiving nonleukoreduced platelets, while no relationship was found between duration of storage and the incidence of FNHTR among recipients of platelets which had undergone prestorage leukoreduction (Patterson et al., 2000). Limiting the duration of exposure to donor leukocytes and the cytokines that accompany transfused pooled platelets has been proposed as the mechanism of the decreased incidence of FNHTRs found with shortened platelet storage (Kelley et al., 2000). That these inflammatory cytokines may not be the only substances accompanying transfused platelets that cause FNHTRs is suggested by the absence of difference in the incidence of these reactions between recipients of prestorage and bedside leukoreduced platelets (Kluter et al., 1999).

FNHTRs should be treated with antipyretics which do not contain aspirin because of concerns about inhibiting platelet adhesiveness with salicylates. For a patient who has had one prior FNHTR, the probability of recurrence with a subsequent transfusion is approximately 17% (Triulzi, 1999).

Allergic reactions

Allergic reactions are responses to allergens, the usual source of which is transfused plasma. Because all but washed RBCs and frozen, thawed, deglycerolized RBCs contain plasma, these reactions may occur in response to transfusion of virtually any blood product. Their severity runs the gamut from mild (urticarial) to severe (anaphylactoid). Urticarial reactions are usually mild and do not require discontinuation of the transfusion, but should be treated with antihistamines.

Anaphylactoid reactions are more severe, and may be seen in response to transfusion of donor plasma containing IgA to recipients who are deficient in IgA. Such recipients may have developed antibodies to IgA, because IgA-like substances are ubiquitous in the environment. For this reason, the IgA-deficient recipient may have an anaphylactoid response to her first transfusion. Anaphylactoid reactions are characterized by laryngospasm, bronchospasm, and hypotension. The first step in treatment is stopping the transfusion. As with anaphylactic (IgE-mediated) responses, they are treated with parenteral epinephrine, steroids, vasopressors, and intubation, as needed. If a patient who has a severe allergic reaction is demonstrated to be IgA deficient, an attempt should be made to obtain blood for future transfusion from IgA-deficient donors. If IgA deficiency is not the cause of the severe allergic reaction, subsequent transfusions should be with saline-washed cellular products. In addition, consideration should be given to pretransfusion steroids and antihistamines (Triulzi, 1999; Petrides & Stack, 2001).

Transfusion-related acute lung injury (TRALI)

The acute onset of respiratory distress and bilateral pulmonary edema possibly accompanied by fever and hypotension within 4 hours of transfusion of a blood product containing plasma should alert the clinician to the possibility of this complication. The most commonly proposed mechanism is the passive transfer of antiwhite cell (anti-HLA) antibodies from the donor that react with recipient neutrophils, causing aggregation and activation of the latter within the pulmonary vasculature. An alternative hypothesis is that recipient neutrophil activation is due to the passive transfer of lipid in donor plasma. Regardless of mechanism, the neutrophil activation and aggregation result in altered pulmonary vascular permeability and capillary leaks. The clinical syndrome is indistinguishable from adult respiratory distress syndrome (ARDS). As with ARDS, the treatment is supportive, incorporating ventilatory support and pressors. The recognition of TRALI is of importance, because the donors must be tested. If any are found to have antineutrophil antibodies in their plasma, they should be removed from the donor pool (Triulzi, 1999; Petrides & Stack, 2001).

Septic transfusion reaction

A temperature rise of 2°C or more, possibly accompanied by chills and/or shock during or shortly after transfusion of a blood product are signs of a possible septic transfusion reaction. These complicate the transfusions of up to 0.2% of RBC, 5% of apheresed platelet and 10% of random donor platelets (Kopko & Holland, 2001). The source of the bacterial infection is commonly contamination at the phlebotomy site. Because RBCs are stored at 1–6°C, and because Gram-negative bacteria (e.g. *Pseudomonas* species, *Yersinia enterocolitica*) proliferate at cold temperatures, Gram-negative sepsis is more common after RBC transfusions. In contrast, platelets, which are stored at room temperature, are more often associated with Gram-positive sepsis (e.g. *Staph. epidermidis*, *Bacillus* species) (Kopko & Holland, 2001). Mortality rates for RBC-associated sepsis approach 70%; those for platelet-associated sepsis, 25% (Petrides & Stack, 2001). Upon suspicion of a septic reaction, the blood should be immediately discontinued, and Gram stain and cultures of the donor units should be performed. Treatment of the infected recipient includes broad-spectrum antibiotics and aggressive supportive therapy, as needed. The supplier of the units should be notified, and other units from the same collection should be quarantined and tested for bacterial contamination (Triulzi, 1999; Kopko & Holland, 2001; Petrides & Stack, 2001).

Delayed transfusion reactions

Delayed hemolytic transfusion reactions

Delayed hemolytic reactions differ from acute hemolytic transfusion reactions in timing and mechanism. A delayed reaction will have its onset within days or weeks, but not hours of the transfusion. Unlike an AIHTR, the delayed reaction is either a primary or an anamnestic recipient response to transfused red cell antigens, usually of the Rh or Kell systems. Also unlike AIHTR, complement is rarely activated. Therefore red cell destruction is extravascular, and the hemoglobinemia, hemoglobinuria, and attendant systemic findings which characterize an AIHTR are either not present or present in a milder form. However, a delayed hemolytic reaction may be characterized by anemia, a positive direct antiglobulin test, and hyperbilirubinemia.

Delayed intravascular hemolytic reactions may also occur, particularly in response to transfusions of cells bearing Kidd (Jk^a, Jk^b) and Duffy (Fy^a, Fy^b) antigens. While complement fixation does occur, resulting in intravascular hemolysis, release of anaphylotoxins and cytokines is either absent or muted. While possible, the probability of a delayed intravascular hemolytic reaction being life-threatening is remote. The one procedure needed in response to both delayed extra- and intravascular hemolytic transfusion reactions is that the specific antibody must be identified, so that the recipient will receive blood which does not contain the corresponding antigen if transfusion is needed in the future (Triulzi, 1999; Petrides & Stack, 2001).

Transfusion-associated graft-vs-host disease (TA-GVHD)

Originally recognized in immunocompromised bone marrow recipients, graft-vs-host disease was subsequently reported in immunocompetent blood transfusion recipients (Williamson & Warwich, 1995; Hume & Preiksaitis, 1999). The disease results from the transfusion of T-lymphocytes to a recipient who has histocompatibility (e.g. HLA) antigens lacking in the donor. The donor lymphocytes then engraft, and mount an immunologic response against the host (Williamson & Warwich, 1995). The likelihood of engraftment of donor lymphocytes is increased when the donor and the recipient share other immunologic similarities. Cases of TA-GVHD have been reported when cells from donors who are homozygous for an HLA haplotype have been transfused to recipients who are heterozygous for that haplotype (Williamson & Warwich, 1995; Hume & Preiksaitis, 1999; Triulzi, 1999). The classic presentation of TA-GVHD is the development 1 or 2 weeks following transfusion of a maculopapular rash, diarrhea, and liver function abnormalities. A pancytopenia results because of antibody- and cytokine-mediated destruction of the bone marrow (Williamson & Warwich, 1995; Standards Program Committee, AABB, 2000; Petrides & Stack, 2001). There is no effective treatment, and death ensues in 90% of cases (Williamson & Warwich, 1995).

Gamma-irradiation of cellular products prior to transfusion eliminates the risk of TA-GVHD. While the standard dose of 25 Gy or more does not affect platelets, it does shorten the lifespan and increase potassium leakage of stored RBCs (Williamson & Warwich, 1995; Petrides & Stack, 2001). For this reason the US Food and Drug Administration recommends that irradiated units be used until either the date of expiration of the cells or 28 days beyond the date of irradiation of the cells. Because of the lethal nature of the disease, it is recommended that donor cells from blood relatives be irradiated prior to transfusion (Triulzi, 1999).

Post-transfusion purpura (PTP)

A decreasing platelet count, often accompanied by purpura within 3–10 days of transfusion of RBCs or platelets should raise suspicion of PTP. The platelet destruction is due to an anamnestically-produced alloimmune antibody to the high-frequency platelet antigen HPA-1. Those at risk must have had prior exposure to platelets, and therefore include those who have previously been transfused and women who have had prior pregnancies. A unique characteristic of this complication is that the antibody may destroy not only transfused HPA-1 platelets but also those of the recipient, the latter of which lack the HPA-1 antigen. This seeming autoimmune response may be due to the adsorption of the antigen from donor plasma onto the recipient's platelets. For this reason, for subsequent transfusions, persons who have exhibited PTP are advised to receive only washed RBCs, as this product should be free of platelet fragments and soluble platelet antigens. For those requiring subsequent platelet transfusion, the concomitant administration of IV-IgG and HPA-1-negative platelets may maintain an adequate post-transfusion platelet concentration (Petrides & Stack, 2001).

Blood-borne infectious disease

Minimizing the risk of disease transmission by cellular and acellular blood products is a task accomplished by donor selection, donor testing for infectious agents and their antibodies, and viral inactivation treatments (Eleftheriou et al., 1998; Burnouf & Radosevich, 2000; Dodd, 2000; Pamphilon, 2000). The latter are used primarily for pooled plasma products (Burnouf & Radosevich, 2000). A variety of viral, bacterial, protozoan, and spirochete infections may be transmitted by single-donor and pooled products (Petrides & Stack, 2001). Those blood-borne infections currently of greatest concern will be discussed.

Human immunodeficiency virus (HIV)

HIV, the causative agent of acquired immunodeficiency syndrome (AIDS), may be transmitted by any untreated blood product. Following transmission, the virus enters a latent period, during which time it continues to replicate. The period of latency may last up to several years, after which the virus invades and destroys T-helper (CD4) lymphocytes. Eventually the CD4 count drops, the viral load increases, and the immune system is impaired. Death results from opportunistic infections, complications of malignancies (e.g. Kaposi's sarcoma, central nervous system lymphoma), or both.

Limiting disease transmission has been accomplished by the development of tests designed to determine the presence of virus during the latency period in the potential donor's blood. The first tests detected anti-HIV antibody. These tests first become positive approximately 3 weeks after infection. A test for p24 antigen, the cell-free virion present early in HIV infection, shortened the window of detection to 16 days. Nucleic acid testing (NAT) for viral RNA has further shortened the detection window to 10 days (Tabor & Yu, 2000; Petrides & Stack, 2001). With the progressive shortening of the length of the window of detection, the incidence of transfusion-associated HIV infection has also decreased. In the USA, the per-unit risk with NAT testing is estimated at 0.9 : 1,000,000 (Dodd, 2000; Petrides & Stack, 2001). In the United Kingdom, the per-donation risk is estimated near 0.3 : 1,000,000 (Ekeroma et al., 1997; Pamphilon, 2000).

Human T-cell lymphotropic virus (HTLV-I, HTLV-II)

HTLV-I is the virus responsible for both adult T-cell leukemia/lymphoma (ATL) and tropical spastic paraparesis, also known as HTLV-associated myelopathy (HAM). HTLV-II is responsible for HAM but not ATL. The latency period of these viruses is quite long, and the lifetime probability of an antibody-positive individual developing either HAM or ATL is 4%. The per-unit probability of a transfusion recipient acquiring an HTLV infection during the latency window period is 1 : 641,000 (Dodd, 2000; Petrides & Stack, 2001).

Hepatitis C virus (HCV)

The genetic diversity of HCV likely accounts, at least in part, for differences in prevalence reported for this virus (Tanzi et al., 1997; Ebeling, 1998; Sfameni et al., 2000; Lauer & Walker,

2001). In contrast with other types of hepatitis, the course of the disease following infection is usually indolent. From 74 to 86% of those infected will have a persistent viremia. Eighty-five percent of those infected will progress to chronic hepatitis. Of those affected, most remain asymptomatic until the final stages of the disease, when cirrhosis and liver failure ensue. The annual risk of the development of hepatocellular carcinoma following the development of HCV cirrhosis is 1–4% per year (Lauer & Walker, 2001; Petrides & Stack, 2001). More sensitive tests for antiviral antibodies as well as NAT testing for HCV have reduced the per-unit risk of transfusion-associated HCV transmission to 1:103,000. Further refinement in HCV RNA testing will hopefully further decrease the incidence of transfusion-associated HCV. Insensitivity of antibody tests for anti-HCV has been postulated as being responsible for the transmission of HCV from quarantined FFP-DR (Humpe et al., 2000).

Hepatitis B virus (HBV)

Signs and symptoms which are characteristic of hepatitis, including icterus, nausea, and vomiting are found in over 50% of patients who have acute HBV infection. Of those infected approximately 10% will progress to chronic hepatitis, which may further progress to cirrhosis and hepatocellular carcinoma. A vaccine is available for HBV. The immunized individual develops antibodies to the hepatitis B surface antigen (anti-HBs). Because it is often unknown whether or not the prospective donor had been vaccinated in the past, anti-HBs is not used to test for the presence of the disease. The test which becomes positive earliest in the course of the disease, hepatitis B surface antigen (HbsAg) cannot be detected until 4–26 weeks following infection (Petrides & Stack, 2001). The likelihood of transfusion-associated infection during this window is 1:250,000 (Dodd, 2000).

Cytomegalovirus (CMV)

CMV is an obligate intracellular virus with a wide distribution and which is transmitted by infected leukocytes. CMV infection is usually asymptomatic, though immunocompromised (e.g. HIV+) individuals may have a fulminant course. Neonates who acquire CMV infection in utero, particularly those delivered preterm, are at risk for deafness and neurologic impairment (Petrides & Stack, 2001). For this reason, some (Ekeroma et al., 1997; Dodd, 2000) have suggested that all pregnant women receive either CMV-negative or leukoreduced blood, while others (Triulzi, 1999) have suggested reserving such units for only those women who are seronegative or whose CMV serological status is unknown.

Parvovirus B19

Parvovirus B19 is the cause of a self-limiting illness (erythema infectiosum, or fifth disease) that commonly affects children. Approximately 50% of adults exhibit antibodies to the virus. The virus proliferates in erythroid precursor cells, and also has an affinity for the P-antigen on the surface of RBCs (Prowse et al., 1997; Kailasam et al., 2001). A woman infected during pregnancy has a risk of 33% of transmission of the virus to the fetus. Approximately 4% of infected fetuses will develop nonimmune hydrops, which in turn is likely due to viral attack on erythroid precursor cells, viral myocarditis, or both. The fetal loss rate due to parvovirus B19 infection is 9% (Kailasam et al., 2001).

Parvovirus B19 may be transmitted by transfusion of infected blood products (Prowse et al., 1997; Dodd, 2000). The suggestion has been made that pregnant women who are the intended recipients of blood products should be tested for this virus, and those found to be seronegative should receive blood from seronegative donors (Prowse et al., 1997). Attempts to remove the virus from blood have also been reported. While solvent/detergent treatment of blood products does not remove the virus (Koenigbauer et al., 2000), filtration with a 15 nanometer filter was shown to reduce the viral load by a factor of 6 $\log_{10}$ (Abe et al., 2000).

Creutzfeldt–Jacob disease (CJD)

A rare fatal neurodegenerative disease, CJD is characterized clinically by progressive dementia, and pathologically by spongiform degeneration with neuronal loss but without associated inflammation. The agent responsible for the disease is an abnormal isoform (PrP^{SC}) of the prion protein PrP^{C} (Foster, 2000; Petrides & Stack, 2001). PrP^{C} is an intracellular protein which participates in synaptic transmission and which is degraded by cellular proteases. In contrast, PrP^{SC} resists protease degradation. Human disease following suspected transmission via corneal transplants, human growth hormone injections, and dura mater grafts has been reported to have a latency in excess of 30 years (Petrides & Stack, 2001).

First reported in the United Kingdom in 1996, vCJD may be related to ingestion of meat from animals who have bovine spongiform encephalopathy ("mad cow disease"). Variant CJD differs from classic CJD both clinically and pathologically. The clinical course is more rapid, with death ensuing within 2 years. The spongiform changes seen on pathological examination in vCJD surround plaques consisting of prion proteins. These plaques are an unusual finding in cases of classical CJD (Petrides & Stack, 2001).

There is no evidence that either CJD or vCJD are transmitted by blood or blood products (Vamvakas, 1999; Foster, 2000; Foster et al., 2000; Bessos et al., 2001; Petrides & Stack, 2001). However, the finding of prion proteins in the lymphoid tissue of patients infected with vCJD as well as in platelets and plasma (Vamvakas, 1999; Bessos et al., 2001) prompted a number of precautionary steps worldwide. In the United Kingdom a national policy of universal prestorage leukoreduction as well as a ban on all plasma products derived from donations made in the UK has been in effect since 1998 (Foster, 2000). Persons who resided for 6 or more months in the UK from 1980 to 1996 are permanently deferred as blood donors in the USA (Table 10.1), Canada, Austria, and New Zealand (Foster, 2000). It must be noted that there is no evidence that leukoreduction decreases the PrP^{SC} content of transfused blood. Furthermore, a theoretical concern has been expressed that these intracellular prions may be released as a consequence of leukocyte fragmentation during the filtration process (Petrides & Stack, 2001). It must also be noted that abnormal prions may be removed in the process of plasma fractionation (Foster et al., 2000).

Alternatives to transfusions of blood products

Patients who have religious proscriptions against the use of blood or blood products as well as those who fear the complications of transfusion may consider alternatives to these products. Erythropoietin, a glycoprotein that stimulates erythropoiesis, may have application in an obstetric setting. Oxygen-carriers such as perfluorocarbons (PFCs), hemoglobin solutions, and enzymatically-converted RBCs, though not now commercially available, may in the future have general application. With one exception, none of the products designed for oxygen carriage is licensed for human use in the United States. The one product is no longer being marketed (Petrides & Stack, 2001).

Recombinant human erythropoietin (rhEPO)

Erythropoietin is a naturally-occurring glycoprotein produced by the peritubular cells of the kidneys in adults. In both the nonpregnant and pregnant states, erythropoietin production increases in response to hypoxia and anemia (Vora & Gruslin, 1998; Petrides & Stack, 2001; Tan & Lim, 2001). In normal pregnancy, the concentration of erythropoietin increases to 2–4 times that of nonanemic nonpregnant controls (Vora & Gruslin, 1998). rhEPO has been available for use in humans for several years. Currently it must be stabilized in albumen to avoid adherence to glass or plastic tubing. Thus although the rhEPO is not itself a blood product, the solution in which it is administered contains a blood product (albumen). While this may limit its use in those who refuse any blood product, current research is directed at finding stabilizers for rhEPO that are not derived from blood (Petrides & Stack, 2001).

An adequate concentration of iron is necessary for rhEPO to stimulate erythropoiesis. With the administration of parenteral iron, an increase in RBC production is elicited within 3–4 days, and hemoglobin concentration is increased by 1 g/dL within a week (Petrides & Stack, 2001). rhEPO has been used during pregnancy to raise RBC concentrations in women who have end-stage renal disease and to increase RBC production for autologous donations (Vora & Gruslin, 1998). Hypertension is a potential side effect of rhEPO requiring vigilance during and following its use (Tan & Lim, 2001).

Substances which provide oxygen carriage

The synthesis of oxygen-carrying substances which may substitute for RBCs has been an elusive goal for several years. To date, a substitute which will mimic the physiologic behavior of the RBC within the cardiovascular system has not been developed. The hematocrit, viscosity, and shear forces of blood in the microvasculature are significantly lower than that those in large vessels (Winslow, 2000a,b). Oxygen extraction differs substantially within different organs (Stehling et al., 1994). The red cell substitutes which are now being studied do not have these adaptive properties (Winslow, 2000a,b). The ideal RBC substitute should have some of the properties of RBCs including similar oxygen and carbon dioxide transfer capabilities, reasonable shelf life, storage at room temperature, reasonable circulating life, and no toxicity to end-organs. They should also have certain advantages over RBCs, including the absence of disease transmission and the absence of incompatibility with all recipients (Winslow, 2000a,b; Coursin & Monk, 2001; Tan & Lim, 2001). While no RBC substitute has all of these properties, the benefits of selective use of some may ultimately prove to outweigh their shortcomings.

Perfluorocarbons (PFCs)

Perfluorocarbons are a class of halogenated hydrocarbons in which the hydrogen ion is replaced by fluoride ions, and which have the unique capability of carrying gases in solution. Because they are immiscible in water, they must be emulsified for use for intravascular oxygen carriage (ACOG, 1998; Lowe, 1999; Remy et al., 1999; Sibbald et al., 2000; Winslow, 2000a,b; Burris, 2001). The oxygen content of PFCs varies directly as the concentration of oxygen to which they are exposed and the concentration of the PFC in the plasma. Thus, unlike hemoglobin, whose binding and release of oxygen has a sigmoidal relationship with ambient oxygen tension, the relationship between a PFC of a given concentration and oxygen tension is linear (Fig. 10.1). This physical property clinically poses both challenges and advantages. Figure 10.1 shows that at standard ambient oxygen pressure nonanemic patients' hemoglobin would be saturated with oxygen whereas a 60% PFC concentrate would not. The tissue delivery of oxygen under those conditions for RBCs would be 5 mL/100 mL; that for the PFC would be 2 mL/100 mL. If, however, inspired oxygen concentration were to be increased to 90–100% and the consequent Po_2 to 400 torr, tissue oxygen delivery would be increased to 10 mL/100 mL (Lowe, 1999). At the level of the tissues, oxygen carried by PFCs is released from solution, whereas that carried by RBCs must traverse the red cell membrane. Oxygen carried

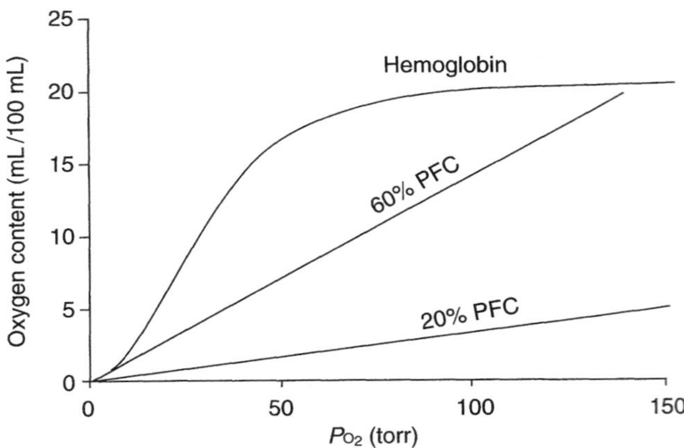

Fig. 10.1 The relationship between oxygen content and oxygen partial pressure (Po_2) for hemoglobin and emulsions containing 20 or 60% (w/v) of perfluorocarbon (PFC). (Reproduced by permission of the publisher Churchill Livingston from Blood Rev 1999;13:173. Lowe KC. Perfluorinated blood substitutes and artificial oxygen carriers.)

by PFCs is released at a rate twice that of oxygen released from RBCs (ACOG, 1998). PFCs are biologically inert, and are excreted as vapors from the lungs after passage through the reticuloendothelial system (Remy et al., 1999; Sibbald et al., 2000).

To date, controlled trials using PFCs for perioperative hemodilution and resuscitation from hemorrhagic shock have been conducted on orthopedic, urological, and gynecological patients (Lowe, 1999; Remy et al., 1999). Limited experience in pregnancy has been reported (Karn et al., 1985; Kale et al., 1993). A major limitation of these oxygen carriers are that to be effective, a high inspired oxygen tension must be maintained. Although the shelf life of a PFC at 5–10°C is up to 4 years, its intravascular half-life in animal studies is 4 days, and in humans 4 hours (Lowe, 1999; Petrides & Stack, 2001).

Hemoglobin-based oxygen carriers

As previously discussed, antibodies to antigens on RBC membranes necessitate transfusion of compatible blood. If that membrane could be removed with no deleterious effect on oxygen carriage, the need for compatibility testing would be obviated. However, in addition to bearing antigens, the RBC membrane preserves both the structure and the oxygen-delivery ability of its major component, hemoglobin (Stowell et al., 2001). Hemoglobin is a complex protein that consists of four chains, two α and two β. An α and a β chain form a stable dimer, and two such dimers are loosely held together to form a tetramer. Each of the four chains is attached to a heme moiety. The iron in the heme binds reversibly with oxygen. The 2,3-DPG within the RBC maintains its P_{50} (the partial pressure of oxygen at which 50% of the hemoglobin is saturated) at 27 torr. The average RBC has a lifespan of 120 days. Upon lysis of the RBC, the free hemoglobin is no longer in contact with the 2,3-DPG and its P_{50} drops to 10 torr, making it resistant to releasing oxygen to the tissues (Creteur et al., 2000). Furthermore, upon is release from the confines of the RBC membrane the hemoglobin tetramer rapidly dissociates into its component dimers. These dimers are rapidly cleared by the kidneys. Their precipitation in the proximal tubules may result in renal toxicity (Baron, 1999; Creteur et al., 2000; Winslow, 2000a,b). Stroma-(membrane-)free hemoglobin has other potentially undesirable characteristics. Hemoglobin exerts a high oncotic pressure (Palaparthy et al., 2000; Winslow, 2000a,b). While this may be a desirable trait in the management of hypovolemic shock, it may also limit the volume of free hemoglobin that may be infused. Because of its ability to bind nitrous oxide and to interact with endothelin, free hemoglobin also exerts a vasopressor effect (Habler & Messmer, 2000; Burris, 2001).

Three major sources of hemoglobin have been explored. Human hemoglobin derived from RBCs whose shelf life has expired has the advantage of limiting the risk of exposure of the recipient to foreign antigens (Baron, 1999). Certain undesirable effects, some of which have been attributed to stromal remnants, include complement, kinin, and coagulation system activation, histamine release, nephrotoxicity, and iron deposits (Remy et al., 1999). A limiting factor in the use of human hemoglobin is that only 5–10% of stored blood outdates (Stowell et al., 2001). In contrast, nonhuman sources of hemoglobin are readily available. Bovine hemoglobin does not contain 2,3-DPG, and has a P_{50} close to that of human hemoglobin (Remy et al., 1999). Its use in humans is hampered by theoretical concerns about its antigenicity and its potential for disease transmission (ACOG, 1998; Remy et al., 1999; Stowell et al., 2001). Recombinant hemoglobin is the result of site-directed mutagenesis of the globin gene, and is virtually free of risk of viral contamination (Palaparthy et al., 2000; Stowell et al., 2001). Clinical studies have found it to have a P_{50} of 30–33 torr, a plasma half-life four times greater than that of free hemoglobin, and indefinite storage half-life. However, its cost of production may be a limiting factor (ACOG, 1998).

Modifications of hemoglobin have been attempted in an effort to prevent its rapid clearance, preserve its capacity to efficiently deliver oxygen, and to avert its undesirable side effects. Modifications currently under investigation include cross-linking, polymerization, conjugation of hemoglobin with a macromolecule, and encapsulating hemoglobins. Intramolecular cross-linking by covalently attaching "bridges" to maintain the tetrameric structure of the hemoglobin molecule has been reported (Creuteur et al., 2000; Palaparthy et al., 2000; Winslow, 2000a,b; Stowell et al., 2001). In experimental animals, a dose-related increase in mean arterial pressure was reported with a diaspirin-linked compound (Palaparthy et al., 2000). A subsequent human trial found an increased mortality rate with this compound and the manufacturer withdrew it from investigation (Palaparthy et al., 2000; Burris, 2001). Either pure or cross-linked hemoglobin may undergo intermolecular cross-linking (polymerization) with a "bridge" such as glutaraldehyde (ACOG, 1998; Creuteur et al., 2000; Stowell et al., 2001). The products so produced have been shown to have a P_{50} higher than that of normal hemoglobin, a plasma half-life up to 30 hours, and high plasma concentrations without excessive oncotic pressure (Creuteur et al., 2000). Conjugation of pure, cross-linked, or polymerized hemoglobin with a macromolecule such as polyethylene glycol has been reported (ACOG, 1998; Creuteur et al., 2000; Stowell et al., 2001). The effects on P_{50} and half-life are similar to those reported for polymerized hemoglobin (Creuteur et al., 2000). Finally, encapsulation of hemoglobin in bilamellar spheres has been investigated in laboratory animals (Creuteur et al., 2000; Stowell et al., 2001). An intriguing potential for this oxygen-delivery vehicle is that of adding 2,3-DPG to the liposome envelope, thus improving the P_{50} and oxygen delivery of the product.

Major limitations of all hemoglobin-containing products are the costs of production and their short half-lives. Although some of the products mentioned in this section have been investigated in humans, none has been licensed in the United States. The only experience reported in pregnancy is in animals (Moon et al., 2001).

The woman who refuses blood transfusion

The numerous medical, legal, religious, and ethical issues surrounding the care of the pregnant and postpartum woman who categorically refuses a blood transfusion have been discussed in a number of publications (Sacks & Koppes, 1994; Liang & Ostheimer, 1995; Thomas, 1998; Schonholz, 1999; Harnett et al., 2000). Particularly for those refusing transfusion on religious grounds, the refusal of transfusion should not be interpreted as a death wish. In pregnancy, the preponderance of both common and statutory law has held that the patient's autonomous right to decline a transfusion supercedes the physician's duty to provide appropriate care (Sacks & Koppes, 1994; Liang & Ostheimer, 1995). The patient's signed refusal does not preclude the possibility of a civil action for either having given or withheld blood (Sacks & Koppes, 1994; Schonholz, 1999). Thus is behooves the attending obstetrician to have made appropriate inquiries and preparations in the event of such a patient experiencing massive blood loss. As some bleeding disorders may be treated with medication (e.g. von Willebrand's disease with desmopressin; Petrides & Stack, 2001), coagulation tests should be performed if indicated by personal or familial history of a possible bleeding disorder (Thomas, 1998). The patient's hemoglobin and/or hematocrit should be monitored during pregnancy. Iron and folate supplementation should be given routinely. Depending on the degree of anemia, patient compliance with medication, and proximity to delivery, iron deficiency may be treated with oral iron or a combination of oral or parenteral iron and erythropoietin. The patient should be made aware of the availability of intraoperative blood collection and reinfusion and acute normovolemic hemodilution. If she will accept these in a life-threatening emergency, the availability of the needed equipment and an anesthesiologist knowledgeable in the techniques should be arranged in advance of the delivery (Schonholz, 1999).

References

Abe H, Hirayama J, Ihara H, Ikeda H, Ikebuchi K. Removal of parvovirus B19 from hemoglobin solution by nanofiltration. Artif Cells Blood Substit Immobil Biotechnol 2000;28:375–383.

Alamia V, Meyer BA. Peripartum hemorrhage. Obstet Gynecol Clin North Am 1999;26:385–399.

American College of Obstetricians and Gynecologists. Postpartum Hemorrhage. ACOG educational bulletin no. 243. Washington, DC: American College of Obstetricians and Gynecologists, 1998.

Baron J-F. Blood substitutes. Haemoglobin therapeutics in clinical practice. Crit Care 1999;3:R99–102.

Baschat AA, Harman CR, Alger LS, Weiner CP. Fetal coronary and cerebral blood flow in acute fetomaternal hemorrhage. Ultrasound Obstet Gynecol 1998;12:128–131.

Baskett TF, Kieser KE. A 10-year population-based study of uterine rupture. Obstet Gynecol 2001;97:69S.

Bessors H, Drummond O, Prowse C, Turner M, MacGregor I. The release of prion protein from platelets during storage of apheresis platelets. Transfusion 2001;41:61–66.

Blajchman MA, Hebert PC. Red blood cell transfusion strategies. Transfus Clin Biol 2001;8:207–210.

Bonnar J. Massive obstetric haemorrhage. Baillieres Best Pract Res Clin Obstet Gynaecol 2000;14:1–18.

Burnouf T, Radosevich M. Reducing the risk of infection from plasma products: specific preventative strategies. Blood Rev 2000;14:94–110.

Burris D. Blood substitutes in surgery. Ann Chir Gynaecol 2001;90:76–80.

Castaneda S, Karrison T, Cibils LA. Peripartum hysterectomy. J Perinat Med 2000;28:472–481.

Coursin DB, Monk TG. Extreme normovolemic hemodilution: how low can you go and other alternatives to transfusion? Crit Care Med 2001;29:908–910.

Cousins LM, Teplick FB, Poeltler DM. Pre-cesarean blood bank orders: a safer and less expensive approach. Obstet Gynecol 1996;87:912–916.

Creteur J, Sibbald W, Vincent J-L. Hemoglobin solutions-not just red blood cell substitutes. Crit Care Med 2000;28:3025–3034.

Cupitt J, Raghavendra LP. Blood transfusion for cesarean section. Anaesthesia 2000;55:614–615.

De Wildt-Eggen J, Nauta S, Schrijver JG, Van Marwijk Kooy M, Bins M, Van Prooijen HC. Reactions and platelet increments after transfusion of platelet concentrates in plasma or and additive solution: a prospective, randomized study. Transfusion 2000;40: 398–403.

Dodd RY. Current viral risks of blood and blood products. Ann Med 2000;32:469–474.

Ebeling F. Epidemiology of the hepatitis C virus. Vox Sang 1998;74(Suppl 2):143–146.

Eleftheriou A, Kalakoutis G, Pavlides N. Transfusional transmitted viruses in pregnancy. J Pediatr Endocrinol Metab 1998;11:901–914.

Ekeroma AJ, Ansari, A, Stirrat GM. Blood transfusion in obstetrics and gynaecology. Br J Obstet Gynaecol 1997;104:278–284.

Fenton PM. Blood transfusion for caesarean section in Malawi: a study of requirements, amount given and effect on mortality. Anaesthesia 1999;54:1055–1058.

Foster PR. Prions and blood products. Ann Med 2000;32:501–513.

Foster PR, Welch AG, McLean C, et al. Studies on the removal of abnormal prion protein by processes used in the manufacture of human plasma products. Vox Sang 2000;78:86–95.

Frederiksen MC, Glassenberg R, Stika CS. Placenta previa: a 22-year analysis. Am J Obstet Gynecol 1999;180:1432–1437.

Grange CS, Douglas J, Adams TJ, Wadsworth LD. The use of acute hemodilution in parturients undergoing cesarean section. Am J Obstet Gynecol 1998;178:156–160.

Gulliksson H. Additive solutions for the storage of platelets for transfusion. Transfus Med 2000;10:257–264.

Habler OP, Messmer KF. Tissue perfusion and oxygenation with blood substitutes. Adv Drug Deliv Rev 2000;40:171–184.

Hamasaki N, Yamamoto M. Red blood cell function and blood storage. Vox Sang 2000;79:191–197.

Harnett MJ, Miller AD, Hurley RJ, Bhavani-Shankar K. Pregnancy, labour and delivery in a Jehovah's Witness with esophageal varices and thrombocytopenia. Can J Anesth 2000;47:1253–1255.

Heddle NM. Pathophysiology of febrile nonhemolytic transfusion reactions. Curr Opin Hematol 1999;6:420–426.

Hess JR, Rugg N, Knapp AD, Gormas JF, Silberstein EB, Greenwalt TJ. Successful storage of RBCs for 10 weeks in a new additive solution. Transfusion 2000;40:1012–1016.

Hess JR, Hill HR, Oliver CK, Lippert LE, Greenwalt TJ. The effect of two additive solutions on the postthaw storage of RBCs. Transfusion 2001;41:923–927.

Hogman CF. Storage of blood components. Curr Opin Hematol 1999;6:427–431.

Hogman CF, Meryman HT. Storage parameters affecting red blood cell survival and function after transfusion. Transf Med Rev 1999;13:275–296.

Hume HA, Preiksaitis JB. Transfusion associated graft-versus-host disease, cytomegalovirus infection and HLA alloimmunization in neonatal and pediatric patients. Transfus Sci 1999;21:73–95.

Humpe A, Legler TJ, Nubling CM, et al. Hepatitis C virus transmission through quarantine fresh-frozen plasma. Thromb Haemost 2000;84:784–788.

Kailasam C, Brennand J, Carneron AD. Congenital parvovirus B19 infection: experience of a recent epidemic. Fetal Diagn Ther 2001;16:18–22.

Kale PB, Sklar GE, Wesolowicz LA, DiLisio RE. Fluosol: therapeutic failure in severe anemia. Ann Pharmacother 1993;27:1452–1454.

Karn KE, Ogburn PL, Julian T, Cerra FB, Hammerschmidt DE, Vercellotti G. Use of a whole blood substitute, Fluosol-DA 20%, after massive postpartum hemorrhage. Obstet Gynecol 1985;65:127–130.

Kelley DJ, Mangini J, Lopez-Plaza I, Triulzi DJ. The utility of ≤3-day-old whole-blood platelets in reducing the incidence of febrile nonhemolytic transfusion reactions. Transfusion 2000;40:439–442.

Kluter H, Bubel S, Kirchner H, Wilhelm D. Febrile and allergic transfusion reactions after the transfusion of white cell-poor platelet preparations. Transfusion 1999;39:1179–1184.

Koenigbauer UF, Eastlund T, Day JW. Clinical illness due to parvovirus B19 infection after infusion of solvent/detergent-treated pooled plasma. Transfusion 2000;40:1203–1206.

Kopko PM, Holland PB. Mechanism of severe transfusion reactions. Transfus Clin Biol 2001;8:278–281.

Lauer GM, Walker BD. Hepatitis C virus infection. N Engl J Med 2001;345:41–52.

Ledee N, Ville Y, Musset D, Mercier F, Frydman R, Fernandez H. Management in intractable obstetric haemorrhage: an audit study on 61 cases. Eur J Obstet Gynecol Reprod Biol 2001;94:189–196.

Liang BA, Ostheimer GW. Legal issues in transfusing a Jehovah's Witness patient following cesarean section. J Clin Anesth 1995;7:522–524.

Lowe KC. Perfluorinated blood substitutes and artificial oxygen carriers. Blood Rev 1999;13:171–184.

McCarthy LJ, Danielson CFM, Rothernberger SS, et al. Completely converting a blood service region to the use of safer plasma. Transfusion 2000;40:1264–1267.

Moon PF, Bliss SP, Posner LP, Erb HN, Nathanielsz PW. Fetal oxygen content is restored after maternal hemorrhage and fluid replacement with polymerized bovine hemoglobin, but not with hetastarch, in pregnant sheep. Anesth Analg 2001;93:142–150.

Naef RW, Washburne JF, Martin RW, Magann EF, Scanlon PH, Morrison JC. Hemorrhage associated with cesarean delivery: when is transfusion needed? J Perinatol 1995;15:32–35.

Palaparthy R, Wang H, Gulati A. Current aspects in pharmacology of modified hemoglobins. Adv Drug Deliv Rev 2000;40:185–198.

Pamphilon D. Viral inactivation of fresh frozen plasma. Br J Haematol 2000;109:680–693.

Patterson BJ, Freedman J, Blanchette V, et al. Effect of premedication guidelines and leukoreduction on the rate of febrile nonhaemolytic platelet transfusion reactions. Transfus Med 2000;10:199–206.

Petrides M, Stack G. Practical Guide to transfusion medicine. Bethesda, Maryland: American Association of Blood Banks, 2001.

Potter PS, Waters JH, Burger GA, Mraovic B. Application of cell-salvage during cesarean section. Anesthesiology 1999;90:619–621.

Prowse C, Ludlam CA, Yap PL. Human parvovirus B19 and blood products. Vox Sang 1997;72:1–10.

Ransom SB, Fundaro G, Dombrowski MP. The Cost-effectiveness of routine type and screen admission testing for expected vaginal delivery. Obstet Gynecol 1998;92:493–495.

Ransom SB, Fundaro G, Dombrowski MP. Cost-effectiveness of routine blood type and screen testing for cesarean section. J Reprod Med 1999;44:592–594.

Rebarber A, Lonser R, Jackson S, Copel JA, Sipes S. The safety of intraoperative autologous blood collection and autotransfusion during cesarean section. Am J Obstet Gynecol 1998;179:715–720.

Remy B, Deby-Dupont G, Lamy M. Red blood cell substitutes: fluorocarbon emulsions and haemoblobin solutions. Br Med Bull 1999;55:277–298.

Rothwell SW, Maglasang P, Reid TJ, Gorogias M, Krishnamurti C. Correlation of in vivo and in vitro functions of fresh and stored human platelets. Transfusion 2000;40:988–993.

Sacks DA, Koppes RH. Caring for the female Jehovah's Witness: balancing medicine, ethics and the First Amendment. Am J Obstet Gynecol 1994;170:452–455.

Schonholz DH. Blood transfusion and the pregnant Jehovah's Witness patient: avoiding a dilemma. Mt Sinai J Med 1999;66:277–279.

Sfameni SF, Francis B, Wein P. Seroprevalence and assessment of risk factors for hepatitis C virus infection in pregnancy. Aust N Z J Obstet Gynaecol 2000;40:263–267.

Sibbald WJ, Messmer K, Fink MP. Roundtable conference on tissue oxygenation in acute medicine, Brussels, Belgium, 14–16 March 1998. Intensive Care Med 2000;26:780–791.

Sibinga CTS. Immune effects of blood transfusion. Curr Opin Hematol 1999;6:442–445.

Sifakis S, Angelakis E, Vardaki E, Koumantaki Y, Matalliotakis I, Koumantakis E. Erythropoietin in the treatment of iron deficiency anemia during pregnancy. Gynecol Obstet Invest 2001;51:150–156.

Silberman S. Platelets. Preparations, transfusion, modifications, and substitutes. Arch Pathol Lab Med 1999;123:889–894.

Simon TL, Alverson DC, AuBuchon J, et al. Practice parameter for the use of red blood cell transfusions. Arch Pathol Lab Med 1998;122:130–138.

Smith JD, Leitman SF. Filtration of RBC units: effect of storage time and temperature on filter performance. Transfusion 2000;40:521–526.

Spahn DR, Casutt M. Eliminating blood transfusion: new aspects and perspectives. Anesthesiology 2000;93:242–255.

Spence R, Cernaianu A, Carson J, DelRossi A. Transfusion and surgery. Curr Probl Surg 1993;30:1101–1180.

Standards Program Committee, American Association of Blood Banks. Standards for blood banks and transfusion services, 20th edn. Bethesda, Maryland: American Association of Blood Banks, 2000.

Stehling L, Simon TL. The red blood cell transfusion trigger. Arch Pathol Lab Med 1994;118:429–434.

Stehling L, Luban NL, Anderson KC, et al. Guidelines for blood utilization review. Transfusion 1994;34:438–448.

Stowell CP, Levin J, Spiess BD, Winslow RM. Progress in the development of RBC substitutes. Transfusion 2001;41:287–299.

Suzuki S, Tateoka S, Yagi S, et al. Fetal circulatory responses to maternal blood loss. Gynecol Obstet Invest 2001;51:157–159.

Szymanski IO, Teno RA, Lockwood WB, Hudgens R, Johnson GS. Effect of rejuvenation and frozen storage on 42-day-old AS-1 RBCs. Transfusion 2001;41:550–555.

Tabor E, Yu M-YW. Summary of a workshop on the imlementation of NAT to screen donors of blood and plasma for viruses. Transfusion 2000;40:1273–1275.

Tan IKS, Lim JMJ. Anaemia in the critically ill—the optimal haematocrit. Ann Acad Med Singapore 2001;30:293–299.

Tanzi M, Bellelli E, Benaglia G, et al. The prevalence of HCV infection in a cohort of pregnant women, the related risk factors and the possibility of vertical transmission. Eur J Epidemiol 1997;13:517–521.

Thomas JM. The treatment of obstetric haemorrhage in women who refuse blood transfusion. Br J Obstet Gynaecol 1998;105:127–128.

Thomas MJG, Gillon J, Desmond MJ. Consensus conference on autologous transfusion. Preoperative autologous donation. Transfusion 1996;36:633–639.

Toedt ME. Feasibility of autologous blood donation in patients with placenta previa. J Fam Pract 1999;48:219–221.

Triulzi DJ, ed. Blood transfusion therapy. A physician's handbook, 6th edn. Bethesda, Maryland: American Association of Blood Banks, 1999.

Valeri CR, Pivacek LE, Cassidy GP, Ragno G. The survival, function, and hemolysis of human RBCs stored at 4°C in additive solution (AS-1. AS-3, or AS-5) for 42 days and then biochemically modified, frozen, thawed, washed, and stored at 4°C in sodium chloride and glucose solution for 24 hours. Transfusion 2000;40: 1341–1345.

Vamvakas EC. Risk of transmission of Creutzfeldt–Jacob disease by transfusion of blood, plasma, and plasma derivatives. J Clin Apheresis 1999;14:135–143.

Vo TD, Cowles J, Heal JM, Blumberg N. Platelet washing to prevent recurrent febrile reactions to leucocyte-reduced transfusions. Transfus Med 2001;11:45–47.

Vora M, Gruslin A. Erythropoietin in obstetrics. Obstet Gynecol Surv 1998;53:500–508.

Waters J, Biscotti C, Potter PS, Phillipson E. Amniotic fluid removal during cell salvage in the cesarean section patient. Anesthesiology 2000;92:1531–1536.

Weiskopf RB. Erythrocyte salvage during cesarean section. Anesthesiology 2000;92:1519–1522.

Welch HG, Meehan KR, Goodnough LT. Prudent strategies for elective red blood cell transfusion. Ann Intern Med 1992;116:393–402.

Williamson LM, Warwich RM. Transfusion-associated graft-versus-host disease and its prevention. Blood Rev 1995;9:251–261.

Winslow RM. Blood substitutes. Adv Drug Deliv Rev 2000a;40:131–142.

Winslow RM. Blood substitutes: refocusing an elusive goal. Br J Haematol 2000b;111:387–396.

Yeo M, Tan HH, Choa LC, Ong YW, Liauw P. Autologous transfusion in obstetrics. Singapore Med J 1999;40:631–634.

11 Hyperalimentation

Jeffrey P. Phelan

Pregnancy represents one of the most profound physiologic stresses that a woman will experience. The length of pregnancy as well as the unique nature of the fetomaternal unit requires that significant adaptation be made by the mother to assure optimal fetal and maternal outcomes (Table 11.1). Most women adapt physiologically with a minimal need for supplementation other than with a few minerals and vitamins. In rare circumstances, the mother may be unable to meet this nutritional challenge, thereby necessitating medical intervention to overcome nutritional deficiencies. Often, the deficiency is brief and readily ameliorated by dietary adjustment and/or pharmacotherapy. When these measures fail, or in a prolonged critical illness, nutritional support by the enteral or parenteral route will become obstetrically necessary.

In 1972, Lakoff and Feldman published the first report of parenteral feeding during pregnancy in a woman with anorexia nervosa (Lee et al., 1986). Since then, there have been several case reports of successful use of enteral, and central venous (CVN) and peripheral venous (PVN) nutrition in pregnancy for various indications (Hamaoui & Hamaoui, 1998).

Normal nutrition in pregnancy

Our understanding of the crucial relationship between maternal nutritional status and perinatal outcome has improved substantially in the last three decades. Maternal prepregnancy weight and weight gain during pregnancy are important determinants of fetal growth and perinatal mortality. Low prepregnancy weight and poor weight gain during pregnancy are associated with a lower average birth weight, and higher perinatal morbidity (Taffel, 1986; Abrams et al., 1989; Institute of Medicine, 1990; Abrams & Newmann, 1991).

In the normal singleton pregnancy, the average total extra energy necessary to meet the metabolic demands of the fetus, placenta, and uterus is about 80,000 kcal or about 300 kcal/day in addition to maternal basal needs (National Research Council, 1989). In the pregnant adolescent, slightly more calories are required (National Research Council, 1989). This should result in a total weight gain of about 11–14 kg. Caloric requirements increase but not uniformly throughout pregnancy (Fig. 11.1). For example, the first half of pregnancy is under the predominant influence of progesterone and aldosterone, and is referred to as the anabolic phase. Here, the maternal accumulation and storage of fat, protein, minerals, and fluid, accounts for most of the maternal weight gain (Dunnihoo, 1990). The latter half of pregnancy is characterized by the catabolic phase. This phase is under the influence of human placental lactogen (HPL) cortisol, estrogen, and deoxycorticosterone. This leads to the depletion of maternal glycogen, fat, and protein stores to provide glucose, free fatty acids, and free amino acids for the fetal accumulation of fat and protein and placental growth (Dunnihoo, 1990). Fetal fat depots are important storage sites for high-calorie density tissue, fat-soluble vitamins, and essential fatty acids, necessary for brain growth and metabolism in the perinatal period. In contrast, amino acids are fundamental building blocks for organ development and enzyme synthesis. Any aberration of this process may affect fetal growth.

The placenta plays a crucial role in fetomaternal nutrition and is more than a biologic pipeline passively directing nutrients from the mother to fetus. For example, placental human chorionic gonadotropin (HCG) is important for the maintenance of the corpus luteum in early pregnancy; and progesterone, produced from the corpus luteum, induces a glucose-sparing effect in the placenta, and makes more glucose available to the developing embryo. By stimulating lipolysis, HPL stimulates free fatty acid release into the maternal circulation to serve as a caloric source. As a result, free fatty acids spare amino acids and glucose to be passed transplacentally to the actively growing fetus. Protein synthesis for uterine growth is stimulated by placental estrogen, and stimulates systematic vasodilation to help maintain uteroplacental blood flow.

Additionally, the placenta has well-developed mechanisms to control passage of substrate to the fetus (Table 11.2). The effectiveness of the passage of any substance across the syncytiotrophoblast depends on a number of factors listed in Table 11.3.

Malnutrition in pregnancy

Our knowledge of the effects of nutritional deprivation in pregnancy are based primarily on animal studies and unfortunate human circumstance. Although several well-designed experiments studying the effects of starvation in pregnant rats are available, the suitability of using the rodent model for studying the primate pregnancy has been questioned (Payne & Wheeler, 1968). One would expect, intuitively, that the consequences of nutritional deprivation to the mother or fetus in a multifetal gestation of short duration (the typical rodent gestation) should differ from one of a singleton gestation of long duration (the typical human pregnancy). Pond and colleagues (1969), following their experiments in swine, concluded the following: "All gravidas fed protein-deficient diets lost weight. The earlier the protein deficiency began, the more

Table 11.1 Changes in pregnancy that relate to nutrition

Weight gain (11–14 kg)
Fetal and placental growth
Increased fat stores
Increased total body water (6–9 L)
Increased extracellular volume
Vascular space increased 40–55%
RBC mass increased 25%
Dilutional anemia and normal MCV (normal hemoglobin >10 g/dL, hct >30%)
Dilutional hypoalbuminemia
Increased clotting factor production
Retention of sodium (1,000 mEq) and potassium (350 mEq)
Increased cardiac output (50%), heart rate (20%), stroke volume (25–40%) with reduced systemic vascular resistance (20%)
Increased renal blood flow (50%) and glomerular filtration rate (50%) with increased clearance of glucose urea and protein
Creatinine clearance increased (100–180 mL/min)
Increased serum lipids
Increased total iron-binding capacity (40%)
Increased serum iron (30%)
Hypomotility of gastrointestinal tract
Delayed gastric emptying
Gastroesophageal reflux
Constipation

hct, hematocrit; MCV, mean corpuscular volume.

Table 11.2 Substances that cross the placenta and currently accepted mechanisms of transport

Transport mechanism	Substances transported
Passive diffusion	Oxygen Carbon dioxide Fatty acids Steroids Nucleosides Electrolytes Fat-soluble vitamins
Facilitated diffusion	Sugars/carbohydrates
Active transport	Amino acids Some cations Water-soluble vitamins
Solvent drag	Electrolytes
Pinocytosis, breaks in membrane	Proteins

(Reproduced by permission from Martin R, Blackburn G. Hyperalimentation in pregnancy. In: Berkowitz R, ed. Critical care of the obstetric patient. Churchill Livingstone, New York, 1983.)

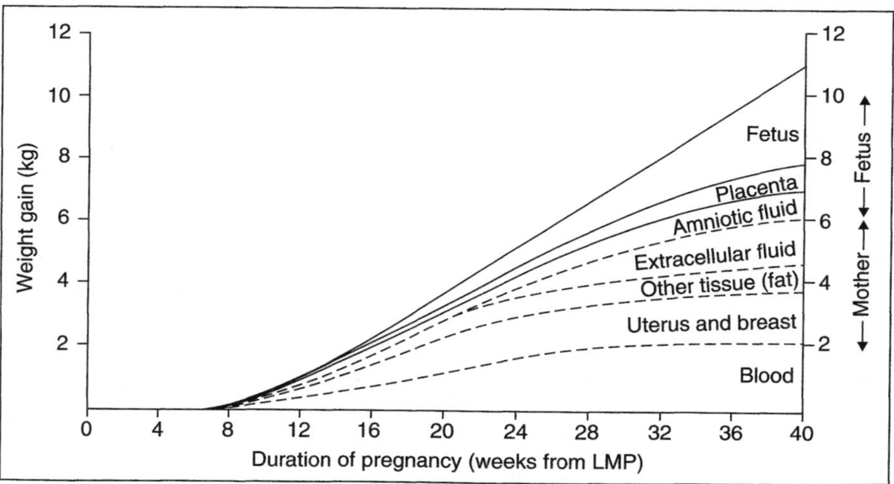

Fig. 11.1 Patterns and components of maternal weight gain during pregnancy. (From Pitkin, RM. Obstetrics and gynecology. In: Schneider HA, Anderson CE, Cousin DB, eds. Nutritional support of medical practice, 2nd edn. Hagerstown, MD: Harper & Row, 1983 pp. 491–506.)

Table 11.3 Factors responsible for the transport of substrates between the maternal–fetal units

Maternal–fetal concentration gradient
Physical properties of the substrate
Placental surface area
Uteroplacental blood flow
Nature of transport mechanism (passive vs. active transport)
Specific binding or carrier proteins in maternal or fetal circulation
Placenta metabolism of the substance

severe the adverse effects." Protein deficiency during periods of fetal growth may affect DNA/RNA synthesis in vital organs (brain, liver) or enzyme systems. Maternal prepregnant labile protein reserve may mitigate the effect of protein deprivation in pregnancy. Riopelle and colleagues (1975) made the following observations of the rhesus monkey: "Although protein deficiency tends to increase fetal morbidity and mortality, the precise effect is dependent on several interacting factors. The improvement in metabolic efficiency in response to starvation is greater in the pregnant than the nonpregnant monkey." Antonov (1947) reported that birth weight was reduced by 400–600 g when pregestational nutrition was poor during the war in Leningrad. Reporting on undernourished women during a famine in Holland, Smith and Stein and Susser (Smith, 1947; Stein, 1975) observed that birth weight declined 10% and placental weight 15% when poor nutrition occurred in the third trimester with caloric intake less than 1,500 g/day.

Generalized caloric intake reduction, as well as specific deficiencies like protein, zinc, folate, and oxygen, have been implicated in the etiology of fetal growth restriction (Neggars et al., 1991; Goldenburg et al., 1992). Winick's hypothesis is particularly helpful in understanding the effect of maternal malnutrition on fetal growth (Winick, 1971). There are three phases of fetal growth: cellular hyperplasia, followed by both hyperplasia and hypertrophy, and then predominantly hypertrophy. Fetal malnutrition early in pregnancy is likely to cause a decrease in cell size and number, resulting in symmetric growth failure, while a later insult affects only cell size and not number, resulting in an asymmetric growth failure. This difference is of prognostic importance because postnatal catch-up growth is more likely with asymmetric rather than symmetric intrauterine growth impairment. Even when low total fetal body weight suggests growth retardation, the severity varies with the organ system. The adrenals and heart are more severely affected than the brain or skeleton (Lafever et al., 1979).

Nutritional assessment during pregnancy

Several protocols have been proposed to evaluate the nutritional status of women during pregnancy. Some are based on parameters including maternal morphometry, serum biochemistry, and provoked immune responses (Martin & Blackburn, 1983; Wolk & Rayburn, 1990). In practice, however, such techniques have limited utility for the following reasons:

1 Normal values obtained in nonpregnant women cannot be readily extrapolated to the hemodiluted pregnant patient.
2 Immune function is impaired in normal pregnancy.
3 Nutritional supplementation is initiated in pregnant patients whose food intake is inadequate before these observations can be made.
4 Although nitrogen balance and creatinine clearance may be effective methods to assess protein status in the nonpregnant patient, both are altered markedly by the increased glomerular filtration rate in normal pregnancy.

Routes for nutritional support

The decision whether a given patient requires nutritional support is best determined by a multidisciplinary team composed of the obstetrician, intensivist, clinical nutritionist, and the patient. Once the decision for nutritional support has been made, two routes of hyperalimentation are available. These are enteral and parenteral hyperalimentation. The enteral route should be the first consideration unless it is impractical, ineffective, or intolerable. Enteral hyperalimentation is associated with fewer complications than CVN or PVN and is more physiologic. Enteral, in contrast with parenteral, helps maintain bowel function, causes fewer maternal metabolic derangements, is more cost-effective, and is easier to monitor maternal health. When using enteral hyperalimentation, delayed gastric emptying typical of pregnancy should be taken into account. The maternal risks of regurgitation and aspiration can be reduced by simply adjusting the feeding solution delivery rates.

Parenteral hyperalimentation or total parenteral nutrition (TPN) may be given in a peripheral (PVN) or a central (CVN) vessel for nutritional support. For example, Watson and colleagues (1990) reported favorably on the tolerance and efficacy of hypercaloric, hyperosmotic 3-in-1 PVN in pregnant patients. While the precise indications and potential side effects had not been elucidated satisfactorily by 1990 (Watson et al., 1990), CVN carries a greater risk than PVN. Most of those risks are related to the mechanical risks associated with central venous access. Nevertheless, PVN cannot be continued for more than 1–2 weeks because of the risk of phlebitis (Hamaoui & Hamaoui, 1998). If, as pointed out by Hamaoui and Hamaoui, PVN does meet the nutritional needs of the pregnant woman, CVN may not be medically justifiable due to the greater maternal risks (Turrentine et al., 1994; Hamaoui & Hamaoui, 1998).

The majority of pregnant patients requiring nutritional support receive CVN. Some of the more common indications for its use in pregnant patients are shown in Table 11.4. CVN is

Table 11.4 Possible criteria for consideration of pregnant patients for total parenteral nutrition

Inaccessible or inadequate gastrointestinal nutritional route for any reason
Maternal malnutrition
- Weight loss greater than 1 kg/week for 4 weeks consecutively
- Total weight loss of 6 kg or failure to gain weight
- Underlying chronic disease that increases basal nutritional demands and/or precludes enteral feedings such as inflammatory bowel disease, unremitting pancreatitis
- Prepregnancy malnutrition
- Biochemical markers of malnutrition
  - Severe hypoalbuminemia less than 2.0 g/dL
  - Persistent ketosis
  - Hypocholesterolemia
  - Lymphocytopenia
  - Macrocytic anemia: diminished folic acid
  - Microcytic anemia and decreased serum Fe
  - Negative nitrogen balance
- Anthropometric markers of malnutrition
  - Weight and height
  - Growth rate
    - Poor weight gain
    - Delayed growth of adolescent
  - Skin fold thickness
  - Head, chest, waist, and arm circumference
- Intrauterine growth retardation of the fetus

(Reprinted by permission from the American College of Obstetricians and Gynecologists Obstetrics and Gynecology 1982; 59: 660–664.)

generally well tolerated by the pregnant woman and is convenient for the medical staff. CVN delivers a precise mixture of nutrients directly into the maternal bloodstream, and at the same time, allows the parenteral administration of necessary medications such as insulin and heparin. The disadvantages include the necessity for central venous access, the possibility of maternal metabolic derangements, a costlier delivery system and a more complicated method of maternal monitoring.

Calculation of nutritional requirements

To determine the untritional needs of a pregnant woman, the first step is to estimate the woman's total caloric needs. Maintenance needs, described as basal energy expenditure (BEE), can be calculated using Wilmore's normogram (Wilmore, 1980) or the Harris–Benedict equation for women (Harris & Benedict, 1919), and adjusted slightly for pregnancy (Driscoll & Blackburn, 1990).

$$\text{BEE(kcal)} = 655 + 9.563(W) + 1.85(H) - 4.676(A)$$

where W = weight in kg, H = height in cm, and A = age in years.

During pregnancy this value is then multiplied by the "stress factor" of 1.25 to account for the caloric demands of pregnancy (Badgett & Feingold, 1997).

Table 11.5 Sample calculation of total parenteral nutrition requirements for a 60-kg patient

Total protein requirements	= 1.5 g/kg = 1.5 × 60
	= 90 g/day
Total caloric requirements	= 36 kcal/kg = 36 × 60
	= 2,160 kcal/day
If calories are provided in a ratio of 70% : 30%, dextrose : lipid:	
Daily dextrose requirement	= (2,160 × 0.7) (3.4 kcal/g)
	= 445 g
Daily lipid requirement	= (2,160 × 0.3) (9 kcal/g)
	= 72 g

Infusion is usually begun at about 50% of total estimated needs and increased gradually to target values at a rate that minimizes maternal metabolic derangement.

$$\text{Maintenance therapy: BEE(kcal)} \times 1.2 + 300\,\text{kcal for singleton pregnancies or } 500\,\text{kcal for twins}$$

Anabolic therapy:

$$\text{Parenteral: BEE(kcal)} \times 1.75$$
$$\text{Enteral: BEE(kcal)} \times 1.50$$

The estimation of caloric requirements should be individualized and tailored to the patient's current metabolic rate. Commercially available metabolic carts, which base estimation of caloric requirement on oxygen consumption and carbon dioxide production, have recently become available for clinical use. These systems are generally quite accurate except at very high F_iO_2 values (≥60%). The recommended dietary allowance is an additional 300 kcal/day in singleton or 500 kcal/day in twin pregnancies in the second and third trimesters. A nutritionally deficient pregnant woman may require more than 300 kcal/day for supplementation in a singleton pregnancy.

A useful but imprecise rule to help a patient maintain a positive nitrogen balance (Oldham & Shaft, 1957) is 36 kcal/kg/day. The effectiveness of maternal nutritional support is monitored by plotting maternal weight gain against standard charts and serial sonographic estimates of fetal growth. The American Academy of Pediatrics and the American College of Obstetrics and Gynecology recommend a weight gain of 1–2 kg for the first trimester, with 0.4 kg/week and 0.35 kg/week in the second and third trimesters, respectively (Little & Frigoletto, 1988). Fetal growth can be evaluated against appropriate normograms. A sample calculation of CVN requirements for a 60-kg pregnant patient is described in Table 11.5.

Amino acids

When the intake of other nutrients are adequate, nitrogen and energy intake are the dominant factors influencing positive nitrogen balance. Protein catabolism rises with an increase in the maternal metabolic rate; whereas, protein need is dependent on the woman's previous nutritional status, the provision of nonprotein energy, and the rate of desired replacement. With the expansion of the maternal circulating blood volume and growth of the uterus, fetus, and placenta, maternal requirements for protein intake are increased during pregnancy. The minimum daily protein requirement throughout pregnancy is approximately 1 g/kg to meet maternal and fetal nutritional needs. The adequacy of maternal protein intake can be assessed by measuring maternal serum protein levels and urea nitrogen excretion. Also, most commercially available amino acid products have been used successfully to maintain normal fetal growth. In certain situations such as maternal renal failure, protein and caloric requirements are increased significantly, and frequent dialysis may require higher amounts. Under these circumstances, survival rates appear to correlate with the adequacy of maternal caloric intake. For example, the protein requirements may reach 2 g/kg to maintain a normal nitrogen balance.

Carbohydrates

Dextrose, the most common energy source, is easily metabolized, promotes nitrogen retention, is readily miscible with other additives, is available in many strengths, and is relatively inexpensive. The disadvantages may include increased oxygen consumption, increased carbon dioxide production, and hyperglycemia. But, the low caloric potency of dextrose (3.4 kcal/kg) precludes its use as the sole source of energy. Dextrose in concentrations greater than 10% (600 mosm) should not be administered peripherally to avoid osmolarity-induced phlebitis and venospasm. To infuse hyperosmolar solutions and utilize alternative energy/substrates, central venous access is medically necessary. Although infusion rates of 4–6 mg/kg/min reduce the severity and the likelihood of maternal complications, insulin may be necessary to maintain maternal euglycemia. Assuming maternal euglycemia can be maintained, no adverse fetal effects have been described.

Fat emulsions

Lipids are an important component of TPN in the pregnant patient for the following reasons:

1 They are an excellent energy source (approximately 9 kcal/g).
2 Essential fatty acids are utilized for fetal fat depot forma-

Table 11.6 Recommended daily allowances for pregnant and nonpregnant women

Nutrients (units)	Nonpregnant	Pregnant	% increase
Energy (kcal)	2,200	2,500	14
Protein (g)	44–45	60	20
Calcium (mg)	1,200*	1,200	50
Phosphorus (mg)	800	1,200	50
Iron (mg)	15	30	100
Magnesium (mg)	280	320	14
Iodine (μg)	150	175	17
Zinc (mg)	12	15	25
Selenium (μg)	55	65	18
Vitamin A (μg RE)	800	800	0
Vitamin D (μg)	10†	10	0
Vitamin E (mg and TE)	8	10	25
Vitamin K (μg)	55	55	0
Vitamin C (mg)	60	70	17
Thiamine (mg)	1.1	1.5	36
Riboflavin (mg)	1.3	1.6	23
Niacin (mg NE)	15	17	13
Folate (μg)	180	400	122
Vitamin B_6 (mg)	1.6	2.2	38
Vitamin B_{12} (μg)	2.0	2.2	10

* Above age 24, RDA is 800 mg (no further bone growth).
† Above age 24, RDA is 5 μg (no further bone growth).
RDA, recommended dietary allowance.
(Reproduced by permission from Hamaoui E, Hamaoui M. Nutritional assessment and support during pregnancy. Gastroenterology Clinics of North America. W.B. Saunders, Philadelphia, PA 1998; 27(1): 90.)

Table 11.7 Monitoring during total parenteral nutrition

Daily weights
Strict I/O
Urine sugar and ketones
Serum glucose monitoring (every 6–12 hr)
Daily electrolytes
Liver function assessment, calcium
PO_4, magnesium, albumin (2–3 times/week)
Weekly nitrogen balance
Fetal growth assessment (every 2–4 weeks)

I/O, input/output.

tion, brain development and myelination, and lung surfactant synthesis.

3 Fatty-acid metabolism requires less oxygen and produces less carbon dioxide than glucose metabolism.

Most commercially available solutions are a suspension of chylomicrons of arachidonic acid precursors and essential fatty acids in a base of safflower or soybean oil. Emulsions are available in concentrations of 10% and 20%. Infusion is usually limited to 12 hours a day, both because chylomicrons may remain in maternal circulation for up to 8–10 hours after administration and due to concern about possible bacterial contamination of the solution when infusion is prolonged. Since the placental transport of fatty acids is primarily by passive diffusion, a high maternal–fetal concentration gradient is necessary to ensure adequate lipid transfer. Essential fatty-acid deficiency usually requires 4 weeks or more of nutritional depletion to become clinically manifested (Parenteral and Enteral Nutrition Team, 1988). Maternal serum hypertriglyceridemia and ketosis are important complications of lipid use that should be sought and corrected. Initial concerns about preterm labor and placental infarction from fat embolism (Heller, 1968) have failed to materialize with the concentrations of lipid commonly used for TPN (i.e. 30–40% of total caloric requirements) (Elphick et al., 1978).

Fluids and electrolytes

Maternal fluid requirements over the course of a singleton term pregnancy are increased dramatically as total body water increases by about 8–9 L. This 8–9 L requirement for water is to compensate for the expansion of extracellular and intravascular volumes, fetal needs, and amniotic fluid formation. Inadequate plasma volume expansion adversely affects fetal well-being (Daniel et al., 1989; Rosso et al., 1992). An additional 30 mL/day over standard maintenance fluids is considered sufficient to satisfy maternal fluid requirements (National Research Council, 1989).

Care should be taken to match any additional losses (e.g. gastrointestinal fluid from hyperemesis) with the appropriate solutions. Fluid replacement should be separate from the hyperalimentation solution to prevent complications due to changes in rate and contents of the TPN delivered. Suggested recommended dietary allowance for electrolytes and vitamins for pregnant and nonpregnant women are displayed in Table 11.6. These are based on estimates of oral recommended dietary allowances actually absorbed. Commercially available intravenous vitamin preparations have proven to be adequate for normal fetal growth.

Table 11.8 Complications of total parenteral nutrition in the obstetric patient

Catheter related
Pneumothorax
Arterial laceration
Mediastinal hematoma
Malposition
Brachial plexus/phrenic nerve palsy
Catheter sepsis
Subclavian vein thrombosis/right atrial thrombosis
Hydro/chylothorax
Metabolic
Deficiencies of vitamins, minerals, electrolytes, trace metals, or essential fatty acids
Hyperglycemia
Hepatic dysfunction and fatty infiltration
Carbon dioxide retention
Over/underhydration
Other
Bowel atrophy
Cholecystitis
Heparin-related complications (e.g. hemorrhage, thrombocytopenia, or osteopenia)
Neonatal
Maternal diabetes syndrome (e.g. macrosomia, postnatal hypoglycemia)
Growth retardation

Monitoring and complications

A suggested protocol for monitoring the pregnant patient receiving TPN is outlined in Table 11.7. Commonly encountered complications of nutritional therapy (Turrentine et al., 1994; Hamaoui & Hamaoui, 1998) are detailed in Table 11.8.

References

Abrams B, Newmann V. Small for gestational age birth: maternal predictors and comparison with risk factors of spontaneous preterm delivery in same cohort. Am J Obstet Gynecol 1991;164:785–790.

Abrams B, Newman V, Key T, Parker J. Maternal weight gain and preterm delivery. Obstet Gynecol 1989;74:577–583.

Antonov AN. Children born during siege of Leningrad in 1942. J Pediatr 1947;30:250–259.

Badgett T, Feingold M. Total parenteral nutrition in pregnancy. Case review and Guidelines for calculating requirements. J Matern-Fetal Med 1997;6:215–217.

Daniel SS, James LS, Stark RI, et al. Prevention of the normal expansion of maternal plasma volume: a model for chronic fetal hypoxemia. J Dev Physiol 1989;11:225–228.

Driscoll DF, Blackburn GL. Total parenteral nutrition 1990. A review of its current status in hospitalized patients and the needs for patient-specific feeding. Drugs 1990;40:346–363.

Dunnihoo D. Fundamentals of gynecology and obstetrics. Philadelphia: JB Lippincott, 1990:164–176.

Elphick MC, Filshie GM, Hull D. The passage of fat emulsion across the human placenta. Br J Obstet Gynaecol 1978;85:610–618.

Goldenberg RL, Tamura T, Cliver SP, et al. Serum folate and fetal growth retardation: a matter of compliance? Obstet Gynecol 1992;79:719–722.

Hamaoui E, Hamaoui M. Nutritional Assessment and support during pregnancy. Gastroenterol Clin N Am 1998;27(1):89–121.

Harris J, Benedict F. Biometric studies of basal metabolism in man. Washington, DC: Carnegie Institute of Washington, 1919, publication no. 279.

Heller L. Clinical and experimental studies in complete parenteral nutrition. Scand J Gastroenterol 1968;4(suppl):4–7.

Institute of Medicine, Committee on Nutritional Status During Pregnancy and Lactation. National Academy of Sciences. Nutrition during pregnancy. Washington, DC: National Academy Press, 1990.

Lafever HN, Jones CT, Rolph TP. Some of the consequences of intrauterine growth retardation. In: Visser HKA, ed. Nutrition and metabolism of the fetus and infant. The Hague: Martinus Nijhoff, 1979:43.

Lakoff KM, Feldman JD. Anorexia nervosa associated with pregnancy. Obstet Gynecol 1972;36:699–701.

Lee R, Rodger B, Young C, et al. Total parenteral nutrition in pregnancy. Obstet Gynecol 1986;68:563–571.

Little G, Frigoletto F, eds. Guidelines for perinatal care, 2nd edn. Washington, DC: American College of Obstetrics and Gynecologists, 1988.

Martin R, Blackburn G. Hyperalimentation in pregnancy. In: Berkowitz R, ed. Critical care of the obstetric patient. New York: Churchill Livingstone, 1983:133–163.

National Research Council. Subcommittee on the Tenth Edition of the RDA's Food and Nutrition Board. Commission on Life Sciences. Washington, DC: National Academy Press, 1989.

Neggars YH, Cutter GR, Alvarez JO, et al. The relationship between maternal serum zinc levels during pregnancy and birthweight. Early Hum Dev 1991;25:75–85.

Oldham H, Shaft B. Effect of caloric intake on nitrogen utilization during pregnancy. J Am Diet Assoc 1957;27:847.

Parenteral and Enteral Nutrition Team. Parenteral and enteral nutrition manual, 5th edn. Ann Arbor, MI: University of Michigan Hospitals, 1988.

Payne PR, Wheeler EF. Comparative nutrition in pregnancy and lactation. Proc Nutr Soc 1968;27:129–138.

Pitkin RM. Obstetrics and gynecology. In: Schneider HA, Anderson CE, Coursin DB, eds. Nutritional support of medical practice, 2nd edn. Hagerstown, MD: Harper & Row, 1983:491–506.

Pond WG, Strachan DN, Sinha YN, et al. Effect of protein deprivation of the swine during all or part of gestation on birth weight, postnatal growth rate, and nucleic acid content of brain and muscle of progeny. J Nutr 1969;99:61–67.

Riopelle AJ, Hill CW, Li SC. Protein deprivation in primates versus fetal mortality and neonatal status of infant monkeys born of deprived mothers. Am J Clin Nutr 1975;28:989–993.

Rosso P, Danose E, Braun S, et al. Hemodynamic changes in underweight pregnant women. Obstet Gynecol 1992;79:908–912.

Smith CA. Effects of maternal undernutrition upon newborn infants in Holland: 1944–1945. J Pediatr 1947;30:229–243.

Smith C, Refleth P, Phelan J, et al. Long-term hyperalimentation in the pregnant woman with insulin-dependent diabetes: a report of two cases. Am J Obstet Gynecol 1981;141:180–183.

Stein Z, Susser M. The Dutch famine 1944–1945, and the productive process. I. Effects on six indices at birth. Pediatr Res 1975;9:70–76.

Taffell SM, National Center of Health Services. Maternal weight gain and the outcome of pregnancy: United States; 1980. Vital and Health Statistic Series 21-No.44. DHHS (PHS) 86, Public Health Service, Washington, DC: US Government Printing Office, 1986.

Turrentine MA, Smalling RW, Parisi V. Right atrial thrombus as a complication of total parenteral nutrition in pregnancy. Obstet Gynecol 1994;84:675–677.

Watson LA, Bermarilo AA, Marshall JF. Total peripheral parenteral nutrition in pregnancy. JPEN 1990;14:485–489.

Wilmore D. The metabolic management of the critically ill. New York: Plenum, 1980.

Winick M. Cellular changes during placental and fetal growth. Am J Obstet Gynecol 1971;109:166-176.

Wolk RA, Rayburn WF. Parenteral nutrition in obstetric patients. Nutr Clin Pract 1990;5:139–152.

12 Dialysis

Gail L. Seiken

The need for dialytic support in pregnancy, while uncommon, is by no means a rarity. There are many case reports throughout the literature of dialysis during pregnancy. Dialysis may be required in the setting of acute renal failure (ARF), end-stage renal disease (ESRD), or deterioration of chronic renal failure (CRF) during pregnancy. In fact, pregnant women who experience progressive loss of renal function represent approximately 20% of women undergoing dialysis (Hou, 1999). Furthermore, prophylactic dialysis has been instituted in the setting of CRF in the hopes of improving maternal and fetal outcomes.

Overview of dialysis

Dialysis refers to renal replacement therapy designed to correct electrolyte abnormalities and remove excess fluids and toxic products of protein metabolism. In the setting of CRF, dialysis is usually initiated when the glomerular filtration rate (GFR), as determined by the 24-hour urine creatinine clearance, reaches 5–10 mL/min. At this level of renal function, biochemical abnormalities such as hyperkalemia and metabolic acidosis are likely to develop, as are fluid overload and uremic complications (Table 12.1). In patients with diabetes who often have other end-organ damage, including autonomic neuropathy and vascular disease, dialytic support may be required even earlier, when GFR reaches 15 mL/min.

The physiology of dialysis is based on diffusive and convective transport. Diffusion refers to the random movement of a solute down its concentration gradient. It is by this means that the majority of urea and solute clearance is achieved. Convection is that solute movement that occurs by means of solvent drag as water is removed, either by hydrostatic or osmotic force. A lesser degree of clearance is obtained during fluid removal by ultrafiltration.

Modes of dialysis

Options for dialysis include hemodialysis and peritoneal dialysis, with the latter consisting of continuous ambulatory peritoneal dialysis (CAPD), continuous cycling peritoneal dialysis (CCPD), and nocturnal intermittent peritoneal dialysis (NIPD).

Hemodialysis

Hemodialysis requires a vascular access for extracorporeal therapy. This is usually a surgically created artificial arteriovenous (AV) shunt or a native AV fistula, although dual-lumen central venous catheters can be used temporarily (Fig. 12.1). Products of protein metabolism, such as urea nitrogen, potassium, and phosphate, are removed by both diffusion and convection across a semipermeable dialyzer membrane, while ions such as bicarbonate and calcium diffuse into the blood. Fluid removal is accomplished by applying hydrostatic pressure across the dialyzer membrane. The dialysis prescription for nonpregnant patients generally consists of 3–4 hours of hemodialysis thrice weekly, depending on urea generation rate and dialyzer solute clearance. Heparinization is generally employed throughout the dialysis treatment.

Peritoneal dialysis

The various forms of peritoneal dialysis have in common the removal of these same metabolites and excess fluid, albeit by diffusion and convective flow across the peritoneal membrane. Surgical placement of a peritoneal catheter allows repeated access to the peritoneal cavity (Fig. 12.2). Removal of fluid by osmotic force is achieved by instilling a hypertonic dialysate such as dextrose solution into the peritoneal cavity. Urea and other ions present in high concentrations diffuse from the peritoneal vasculature into the dialysate, while calcium and a bicarbonate source such as lactate move in the opposite direction. Depending on the mode of peritoneal

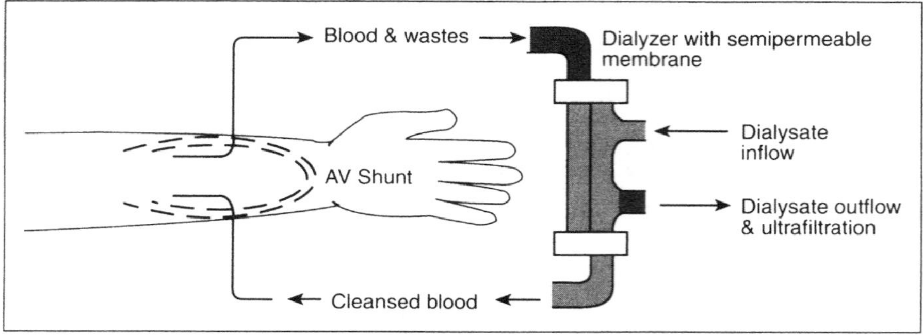

Fig. 12.1 Hemodialysis.

Table 12.1 Indications for initiation of dialysis

Hyperkalemia
Metabolic acidosis
Volume overload
Uremic pericarditis
Uremic encephalopathy
GFR 5–10 mL/min

GFR, glomerular filtration rate.

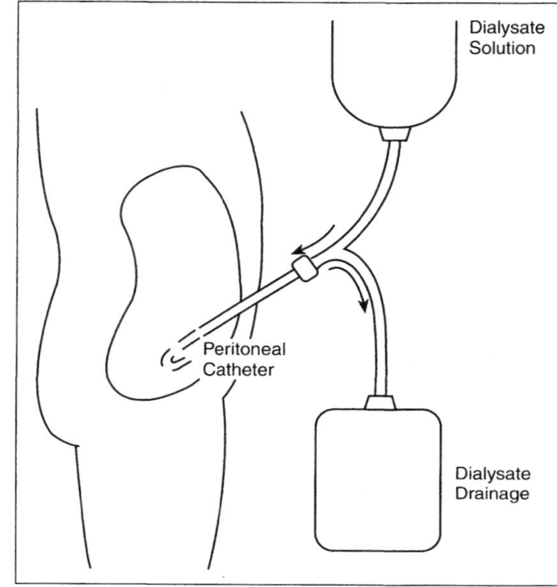

Fig. 12.2 Peritoneal dialysis.

dialysis selected, dialysate is instilled and drained either manually or automatically at repeated intervals throughout the day. CAPD consists of approximately four manual exchanges per day; the peritoneum is filled with several liters of dialysate with each exchange, and the fluid is drained 4–6 hours later. Both CCPD and NIPD utilize an automated cycler to repeatedly fill and drain the peritoneum at shorter intervals throughout the night. CCPD differs in that it also includes a daytime dwell for added clearance.

Dialysis and pregnancy

Hemodialysis vs peritoneal dialysis

Both hemodialysis and peritoneal dialysis have been used successfully in pregnancy, although randomized prospective trials to determine the optimal therapy have not been done. Early reports favored peritoneal dialysis, demonstrating greater fetal survival than with hemodialysis, although these studies were limited by small numbers of patients and the use of historical controls in some: 67% vs. 20% (Gadallah, 1992), 83% vs. 42% (Hou, 1994b), and 63% vs. 20% (Redrow et al., 1988). Furthermore, this benefit has not been borne out in more recent analyses and likely reflects improvement in outcome for pregnant patients on dialysis as a whole. The National Registry for Pregnancy in Dialysis Patients (NPDR) documented virtually identical fetal survival rates among 184 pregnancies for hemodialysis (39.5%) vs. peritoneal dialysis (37%) (Okundaye et al., 1998). Similar data are described by Chan and colleagues (82% vs. 72%) in their review of all pregnancies in dialysis patients at their institution since 1965 (Chan et al., 1998), although nearly one-third of their patients conceived prior to the onset of dialysis.

There are many theoretical reasons to utilize peritoneal dialysis in pregnancy, most notably of which is the steady-state removal of uremic toxins (Table 12.2). This, coupled with easier fluid removal, should minimize episodes of hypotension and thus placental insufficiency. Additional advantages of peritoneal dialysis often include less severe anemia, as well as better blood pressure control and more liberal dietary restrictions due to the continuous nature of the therapy. Furthermore, peritoneal dialysis obviates the need for systemic anticoagulation. In diabetic patients, the use of intraperitoneal insulin can facilitate strict glycemic control. There have also been several case reports of successful intraperitoneal magnesium administration for the treatment of preeclampsia, maintaining a steady-state magnesium serum level of ap-

Table 12.2 Mode of dialysis: advantages in pregnancy

Hemodialysis	Peritoneal dialysis
Less work intensive for patient	Stable biochemical environment
No risk of peritoneal catheter-related complications	Continuous fluid removal avoids hypotension
Adequate clearances late in gestation readily obtained	Allows liberal fluid intake
No interruption in therapy needed after cesarean section	Permits continuous insulin administration in diabetes mellitus
	No anticoagulation necessary
	Permits administration of intraperitoneal $MgSO_4$ in preeclampsia
	Hypertension easier to control
	Less severe anemia

proximately 5 mEq/L, although generally, alternative therapy may be recommended in renal failure to avoid magnesium toxicity (Redrow et al., 1988; Elliott et al., 1991). Despite these apparent advantages of peritoneal dialysis, several unique complications exist, including catheter-related complications such as laceration of the uterine vessels (Hou, 1993) and peritonitis. Hou reported precipitation of preterm labor and delivery in two of three patients secondary to peritonitis. Peritoneal dialysis catheters have been placed as late as 29 weeks' gestation. In some patients, however, difficulties with catheter obstruction and failure to drain necessitate placement of multiple catheters or conversion to hemodialysis. It is difficult to determine whether either method of dialysis actually precipitates preterm labor, because preterm labor has been described in the setting of both hemodialysis and peritoneal dialysis, as well as in CRF alone.

Intensive dialysis

Generally, modification of the dialysis prescription in pregnancy has been recommended for patients treated with both hemodialysis and peritoneal dialysis. Although there are no firm guidelines, it is the belief of most nephrologists that a more intensive dialysis regimen is required during pregnancy to minimize fetal exposure to uremic toxins and improve outcome. This is based in part on the fact that pregnancy outcome appears to be better in those women who require initiation of dialysis due to a deterioration of renal function during pregnancy, as well as among women with significant residual renal function who require dialysis prior to conception (Hou, 1994b). Infant survival as reported by the NPDR was 73% in the former group of women, although only 40% in those women who were already on dialysis at the time of pregnancy (Okundaye et al., 1998). Similar pregnancy success rates in dialysis patients were reported by Bagon and colleagues based on a review of all pregnancies in Belgium extending beyond the first trimester (Bagon et al., 1998). Furthermore, pregnancy appears to be most common during the first year of dialysis, presumably related to the greater residual renal function often present at the initiation of renal replacement therapy. However, there are reports of successful pregnancies in severely uremic patients and patients on dialysis for more than 10 years, as well as pregnancy failures in women treated with intensive dialysis.

Intensive dialysis corresponds to initiation of dialysis at levels of BUN and creatinine approximately 60–70 mg/dL and 6–7 mg/dL, respectively, maintaining levels less than 50 mg/dL and 5 mg/dL, respectively (Hou, 1994b). To maintain such low levels of azotemia in pregnancy, dialysis patients may require a significant increase in total treatment time. This is especially true in the third trimester when fetal urea production increases and may account for as much as 540 mg/day (Hou & Grossman, 1990), a 10% increase. For women on hemodialysis, daily treatments of 5 or more hours may be necessary to obtain adequate clearances late in gestation. As with hemodialysis, a patient's treatment requirements may increase markedly with peritoneal dialysis as well, especially because women in the latter half of gestation may be unable to tolerate the standard dwell volumes due to abdominal fullness. A switch to CCPD with an increased frequency of small volume exchanges and supplemental manual exchanges is often required late in gestation to obtain adequate clearance. A combination of hemodialysis and peritoneal dialysis may even be indicated.

Although the ideal dialysis prescription has yet to be established, the National Registry data suggests a trend towards greater infant survival and more advanced gestational age in those women receiving more than 20 hours of hemodialysis weekly (Okundaye et al., 1998). Others have confirmed this finding, although no benefit was found in those women prescribed a higher dose of peritoneal dialysis (Chan et al., 1998). Surprisingly, however, the number of weekly hemodialysis treatments had no effect, despite the theoretical advantages. No guidelines exist with regard to evaluating the adequacy of dialysis, although a minimum combined renal and dialytic clearance of 15 mL/min is recommended.

An additional benefit of intensive dialysis is that a low level of azotemia should minimize the risk of polyhydramnios, although it is not known if this will lead to improved outcome or a decreased incidence of preterm labor. Polyhydramnios, seen in a high percentage of pregnancies, has been ascribed to the urea diuresis that normally occurs in utero due to high fetal levels of urea nitrogen, as well as to fluid shifts that accompany intermittent hemodialysis (Nageotte & Grundy, 1988; Hou, 1994a). An increased frequency of hemodialysis in particular limits the large interdialytic weight gains often seen in hemodialysis patients, thus avoiding hypotension and enabling better blood pressure control by minimizing that component of hypertension that is volume mediated.

Modification of the dialysis prescription

With respect to hemodialysis, certain parameters of the dialysis prescription may warrant adjustment. Specifically, a lower sodium dialysate of 134 mEq/L is recommended due to the mild physiologic hyponatremia of pregnancy. Similarly, a bicarbonate concentration as low as 25 mEq/L may be necessary to avoid alkalemia, due to the repeated exposure to a bicarbonate dialysate and the concomitant respiratory alkalosis seen in pregnancy. Acetate dialysis is not generally recommended because it has been associated with an increased frequency of hypotension, although there are no data in pregnancy. A standard calcium dialysate can be used with both hemodialysis and peritoneal dialysis, thus ensuring a net positive calcium balance sufficient to meet fetal requirements. Due to placental production of calcitriol, however, there is augmented gastrointestinal absorption of calcium from calcium-containing antacids; thus, serum calcium levels must be monitored to avoid hypercalcemia (Grossman & Hou, 1994). With both methods of dialysis, one must also monitor closely for hypokalemia, which may develop with frequent dialysis.

Changes in the efficacy of peritoneal dialysis have not been noted during pregnancy. In one patient studied there was no apparent change in peritoneal physiology or peritoneal blood flow as assessed by the standard peritoneal equilibration test of glucose and creatinine (Lew & Watson, 1992). Similarly, Redrow and colleagues reported excellent ultrafiltration in all patients throughout pregnancy, and less than a one-third decrease in peritoneal solute clearance in three patients studied (Redrow et al., 1988).

Dialysis and uteroplacental perfusion

Doppler flow velocity measurements have been performed during and after hemodialysis in an attempt to assess the effect of hemodialysis on uteroplacental blood flow. Results have been conflicting, with studies reporting unchanged, worsened, and improved perfusion during dialysis as assessed by the systolic–diastolic ratio or resistance index (Weiner et al., 1991; Jakobi et al., 1993; Krakow et al., 1993). In those patients studied, however, there was no evidence of uterine irritability or fetal distress as measured by external fetal monitoring during hemodialysis.

Mode of delivery

There are no data to support preference for any particular mode of delivery in pregnant dialysis patients. Rates of cesarean section range from 24% to more than 60% (Registration Committee of the EDTA, 1980; Yasin, 1988; Hou, 1993a; Bagon, 1998; Chan, 1998). Cesarean delivery should be performed for standard obstetric indications. In peritoneal dialysis patients requiring cesarean section, both standard and extraperitoneal approaches have been utilized (Redrow, 1988; Hou, 1990b). In either case, it may be necessary to interrupt peritoneal dialysis for several days to allow healing of the abdominal wall and prevent dialysate leak or hernia formation. Peritoneal dialysis can be reinitiated using smaller dwell volumes initially, with a progressive increase in volume as tolerated. If necessary, temporary hemodialysis can be performed in the interim.

Incidence of pregnancy in end-stage renal disease

The exact incidence of pregnancy in ESRD is unknown, although the National Registry documented a conception rate of 2.2% over a 4-year period, based on a survey of approximately 40% of all US dialysis units between 1992 and 1995 (Okundaye et al., 1998). Among more than 6,000 women of childbearing age, 73% of whom received hemodialysis, 135 pregnancies were reported (109 in hemodialysis patients, 18 in peritoneal dialysis patients, and eight pregnancies in which the mode of dailysis was unknown). A comparable conception rate of 0.44% was described among nearly 40,000 women undergoing renal replacement therapy in Japan in 1997 (Toma et al., 1998). Previously, the European Dialysis and Transplant Association (EDTA) had reported on 115 pregnancies in approximately 8,500 women on dialysis between the ages of 15 and 44 through 1978 (Registration Committee of the EDTA, 1980). Similarly, Gadallah and colleagues reported an incidence of 3.6% in hemodialysis patients (Gadallah et al., 1992) and a retrospective survey of pregnancy in hemodialysis patients in Saudi Arabia between 1985 and 1990 revealed an incidence of less than 1% (Souqiyyeh et al., 1992). These statistics, however, are likely to underestimate the true incidence of conception in ESRD because many pregnancies in dialysis patients end in early miscarriage and therefore remain undetected, and many groups fail to report unsuccessful outcomes. Additionally, the true number of women who are sexually active and do not use contraception is unknown.

Women with CRF or ESRD are often uninformed of the potential for conception and the need for birth control. Similarly, many physicians remain unaware of this possibility as well. Amenorrhea or irregular menses along with a markedly decreased fertility are often seen in CRF, in part related to hyperprolactinemia. With administration of erythropoietin and correction of anemia, menses as well as fertility may be

Table 12.3 Signs and symptoms of uremia

Organ involvement	Subjective complaints	Objective findings
Neurologic	Cognitive difficulties Sleep–wake reversal Dysesthesias	Hyperreflexia, asterixis Seizures, encephalopathy Peripheral neuropathy
Hematopoietic	Easy bruising and bleeding Fatigue	Anemia Prolonged bleeding time
Gastrointestinal	Metallic taste Constipation Nausea	Angiodysplasia
Musculoskeletal	Weakness Bone pain	Carpal tunnel syndrome Bone fractures Myopathy
Cardiovascular	Dyspnea Chest pain	Hypertension Pulmonary edema Pericarditis
Dermatologic	Pruritus	Cutaneous calcifications
Endocrine	Decreased libido	Decreased fertility Dysmenorrhea, amenorrhea

restored. Symptoms of early pregnancy may be confused with uremia, thus delaying the diagnosis (Table 12.3). Furthermore, laboratory tests including serum pregnancy tests may be difficult to interpret in this population due to impaired excretion of human chorionic gonadotropin in renal failure (Schwarz et al., 1985). Thus, confirmation of pregnancy and assessment of gestational age will rely upon ultrasound. The mean gestational age at diagnosis of pregnancy is 16.5 weeks in women with ESRD (Hou et al., 1993). There is little information regarding fertility differences among women utilizing peritoneal vs. hemodialysis for ESRD, although registry data suggested a higher rate of conception in women receiving the latter (Okundaye et al., 1998).

Maternal complications

In the past, women with severe renal disease were often advised to terminate pregnancies due to the belief that pregnancy carried a high risk of maternal complications and a low success rate. Potential complications include an accelerated decline in renal function, accelerated hypertension, an increased risk of superimposed preeclampsia, worsened anemia often requiring transfusion, hemodialysis access thrombosis, and an increased incidence of abruptio placentae (Table 12.4). The latter cannot be ascribed solely to the use of heparin during hemodialysis because it has been seen with greater than normal frequency in patients on peritoneal dialysis as well.

Pregnancy has been associated with a permanent decline in renal function in a relatively small percentage of patients with mild renal failure, defined by a serum creatinine of <1.4 mg/dL. This risk may be increased significantly in those women with moderate or severe renal failure, especially in the setting of uncontrolled hypertension. It is always important to rule out readily reversible causes of declining renal function, such as volume depletion, pyelonephritis, and obstruction. One report of 37 pregnant women with moderate or severe renal failure, defined as a serum creatinine greater than 1.4 mg/dL, demonstrated a deterioration in renal function, defined as greater than a 50% rise in creatinine, in 16% (Cunningham et al., 1990). Five of these six women also suffered from poorly controlled chronic hypertension, and a clinical diagnosis of superimposed preeclampsia was established in nearly 60% overall. Similarly, a more recent review encompassing more than 80 pregnant women with renal failure demonstrated accelerated hypertension in nearly 50% and an accelerated decline in renal function in more than one-third

Table 12.4 Renal failure and pregnancy: maternal complications

Accelerated decline in renal function
Accelerated hypertension
Superimposed preeclampsia
Preterm labor
Worsened anemia
Hemodialysis access thrombosis
Abruptio placentae
Spontaneous abortion and second-trimester fetal loss

(Imbasciati & Ponticelli, 1991). Hou reviewed these studies along with five others, all of which confirmed the increased incidence of accelerated renal failure in women with a serum creatinine greater than 1.4 mg/dL at the time of conception (Hou, 1999). Severe hypertension and proteinuria were predictive of an accelerated course in more than 20% of patients with moderate to severe renal failure due to a wide range of primary glomerular diseases (Jungers et al., 1997). Preterm delivery was seen in more than half of these cases, with a high incidence of intrauterine growth retardation as well. Of interest, a review of pregnancy in patients with diabetic nephropathy, defined as nephrotic-range proteinuria and severe hypertension failed to describe an accelerated loss of renal function during pregnancy, although nearly one-third of women had reached ESRD or died during the 3-year follow-up period (Reece et al., 1998). Three maternal deaths have been reported to date, one of which was the result of lupus cerebritis (Okundaye et al., 1998).

Fetal complications

The likelihood of fetal survival beyond the neonatal period is better than previously believed (Table 12.5). Surveys conducted by the EDTA (Registration Committee of the EDTA, 1980), the American Nephrology Nursing Association (Hou, 1994b), as well as a group in Saudi Arabia (Souqiyyeh et al., 1992) reported a fetal viability of 20–30% in those pregnancies that were not electively terminated. The EDTA survey revealed that greater than 50% of pregnancies resulted in spontaneous abortion (Registration Committee of the EDTA, 1980). Hou, in a more recent US survey, noted a comparable incidence of 54% fetal loss, including spontaneous abortion, stillbirth, and neonatal death (Hou, 1994a). Furthermore, virtually all infants delivered were premature, and approximately 20% were growth-restricted. When stratified according to year, however, survival was greater than 50% in those pregnancies occurring since 1990. The increased frequency of CAPD in recent years did not account for this difference, because survival was improved in hemodialysis patients. As noted previously, polyhydramnios attributed to the fetal urea diuresis is seen with greater frequency in renal failure and may contribute to the high incidence of prematurity. Additionally, a urea-induced diuresis following delivery may result in volume depletion in the neonatal period. Early reports failed to identify an increased incidence in congenital anomalies (Registration Committee of the EDTA, 1980; Hou, 1994b). However, the NPDR reported on 11 infants with congenital anomalies among 55 live births (Okundaye et al., 1998). Not surprisingly, there was also a high proportion of infants with developmental delays or long-term medical problems documented at follow-up, the latter possibly attributable to problems often encountered with premature birth. Unfortunately, there is little additional long-term follow-up on infants exposed to azotemia in utero with regards to physical and intellectual development.

Table 12.5 Renal failure and pregnancy: fetal complications

Spontaneous abortion and fetal loss (50%)
Preterm delivery (>90%)
Intrauterine growth restriction (20%)
Polyhydramnios

Anemia

Anemia develops during pregnancy largely due to an increase in plasma volume without a corresponding increase in red cell mass. In renal failure, the picture is complicated by a relative deficiency in erythropoietin production by the diseased kidneys, as well as shortened red cell survival, bone marrow suppression by uremic toxins, and possible superimposed nutritional deficiencies. The severe anemia that was typical of ESRD in the past is now treated successfully in most cases with recombinant human erythropoietin (rHuEpo). Furthermore, correction of the anemia of ESRD may result in return of regular menses due to resolution of hyperprolactinemia (Hou et al., 1993).

Recombinant human erythropoietin has been studied in pregnant animals at doses used clinically without apparent complications. Hou reported on 11 patients with CRF treated with rHuEpo in whom no congenital anomalies were seen and no rHuEpo could be detected in the cord blood (Hou, 1994b). All of the women required an increase in their dose of rHuEpo, compared with prepregnancy, and three still required blood transfusions during pregnancy. Only one woman experienced severe hypertension complicating therapy, although several required additional antihypertensive medications. Additional reports have yielded similar results (Barth et al., 1994; Scott et al., 1995; Bagon et al., 1998; Okundaye et al., 1998). It is accepted by most obstetricians that a hemoglobin less than 6 g/dL is associated with increased perinatal mortality and maternal morbidity secondary to high-output failure. Given this fact, as well as the increased risk of bleeding complications in uremia due to platelet dysfunction, and the overwhelming likelihood of preterm delivery, the recommendation for women with renal disease is an empirical 50% increase in rHuEpo dose once the pregnancy is detected, with a goal of maintaining the hemoglobin at more than 10 g/dL (Hou, 1994b). Most patients require oral iron supplementation or intermittent intravenous iron, because iron deficiency eventually develops in most patients successfully treated with rHuEpo. Although intravenous iron has been used without incident in at least 20 patients, it is generally recommended only if iron deficiency persists despite oral therapy.

Dietary guidelines

Dietary restrictions in renal failure generally consist of modest protein restriction, as well as restrictions of potassium, phosphate, and sodium intake. Fluids are restricted to 1 L daily, with more liberal intake permitted in those with substantial residual urine output. In pregnancy, however, protein intake is liberalized to allow for normal fetal development. The recommended protein intake is 1 g/kg/day in hemodialysis and 1.5 g/kg/day in peritoneal dialysis, with an additional 20 g/day allowed for pregnancy (Hou, 1994b). Increasing delivery of dialysis is recommended for worsening azotemia rather than strict protein restriction. Supplementation of water-soluble vitamins, which are removed during dialysis, is recommended, as well as supplementation with folate, zinc, and iron. Standard prenatal vitamins, which may contain excess vitamin A, are best avoided.

Pregnancy and acute renal failure

Most of the literature pertaining to dialysis in pregnancy concerns those women with CRF or ESRD. There are, however, a number of case reports of dialysis for ARF in pregnancy. Hemodialysis has been the primary form of dialysis utilized, both for ARF and acute ingestion of toxic substances (Trebbin, 1979; Kleinman et al., 1991; Devlin, 1994). Because the incidence of ARF itself has fallen to less than 1% of pregnancies in developed countries, the need for acute dialysis is rare (Krane, 1988).

Summary

Although pregnancy remains uncommon in women with severe CRF or ESRD, it is nevertheless a possibility, especially with modern treatment. With intensive management by the obstetrician and nephrologist, the likelihood of a favorable outcome can be maximized. This may entail early initiation of dialysis in women with CRF or intensified dialytic therapy in those already requiring renal replacement therapy. It is not clear whether either mode of dialysis offers a true advantage in terms of better fetal outcome. While most nephrologists do not advocate a change to peritoneal dialysis in those patients already receiving hemodialysis, there is a tendency to recommend peritoneal dialysis as first-line therapy in those patients who develop a need for chronic dialysis during pregnancy.

References

Bagon JA, Vernaeve H, de Muylder X, et al. Pregnancy and dialysis. Am J Kidney Dis 1998;31:756–765.

Barth W, Lacroix L, Goldberg M, Greene M. Recombinant human erythropoietin (rHEpo) for severe anemia in pregnancies complicated by renal disease. Am J Obstet Gynecol 1994;170:329A.

Chan WS, Okun N, Kjellstrand CM. Pregnancy in chronic dialysis: a review and analysis of the literature. Int J Artif Organs 1998; 21:259–268.

Cunningham FG, Cox SM, Harstad TW, et al. Chronic renal disease and pregnancy outcome. Am J Obstet Gynecol 1990;163: 453–459.

Devlin K. Pregnancy complicated by acute renal failure requiring hemodialysis. Anna J 1994;27:444–445.

Elliot JP, O'Keeffe DF, Schon DA, Cherem LB. Dialysis in pregnancy: a critical review. Obstet Gynecol Surv 1991;46:319–324.

Gadallah MF, Ahmad B, Karubian F, Campese VM. Pregnancy in patients on chronic ambulatory peritoneal dialysis. Am J Kidney Dis 1992;20:407–410.

Grossman S, Hou S. Obstetrics and gynecology. In: Daugirdas JT, Ing TS, eds. Handbook of dialysis. New York: Little, Brown, 1994:649–661.

Hou SH. Peritoneal dialysis and haemodialysis in pregnancy. Bailliere's Clin Obstet Gynaecol 1987;1:1009–1025.

Hou SH. Pregnancy in continuous ambulatory peritoneal dialysis (CAPD) patients. Perit Dial Int 1990;10:201–204.

Hou SH. Pregnancy and birth control in CAPD patients. Adv Perit Dial 1993;9:173–176.

Hou SH. Pregnancy in women on haemodialysis and peritoneal dialysis. Bailliere's Clin Obstet Gynaecol 1994a;8:481–500.

Hou SH. Frequency and outcome of pregnancy in women on dialysis. Am J Kidney Dis 1994b;23:60–63.

Hou S. Pregnancy in chronic renal insufficiency and end-stage renal disease. Am J Kidney Dis 1999;33:235–252.

Hou SH, Grossman SD. Pregnancy in chronic dialysis patients. Semin Dial 1990;3:224–229.

Hou SH, Orlowski J, Pahl M, et al. Pregnancy in women with end-stage renal disease: treatment of anemia and premature labor. Am J Kidney Dis 1993;21:16–22.

Imbasciati E, Ponticelli C. Pregnancy and renal disease: predictors for fetal and maternal outcome. Am J Nephrol 1991;11:353–362.

Jakobi P, Weiner Z, Geri R, Zaidise I. Umbilical and arcuate uterine artery flow velocity measurements during acute hemodialysis. Gynecol Obstet Invest 1993;37:247–248.

Jungers P, Chauveau D, Choukroun G, et al. Pregnancy in women with impaired renal function. Clin Nephrol 1997;47:281–288.

Kleinman GE, Rodriquez H, Good MC, Caudle MR. Hypercalcemic crisis in pregnancy associated with excessive ingestion of calcium carbonate antacid (milk-alkali syndrome): successful treatment with hemodialysis. Obstet Gynecol 1991;78:496–499.

Krakow D, Castro LC, Schwieger J. Effect of hemodialysis on uterine and umbilical artery Doppler flow velocity waveforms. Am J Obstet Gynecol 1993;170:1386–1388.

Krane NK. Acute renal failure in pregnancy. Arch Intern Med 1988;148:2347–2357.

Lew SQ, Watson JA. Urea and creatinine generation and removal in a pregnant patient receiving peritoneal dialysis. Adv Perit Dial 1992;8:131–135.

Nageotte MP, Grundy HO. Pregnancy outcome in women requiring chronic hemodialysis. Obstet Gynecol 1988;72:456–459.

Okundaye I, Abrinko P, Hou S. Registry of pregnancy in dialysis patients. Am J Kidney Dis 1998;31:766–773.

Redrow M, Lazaro C, Elliot J, et al. Dialysis in the management of pregnant patients with renal insufficiency. Medicine 1988;67:199–208.

Reece EA, Leguizamon G, Homko C. Pregnancy performance and outcomes associated with diabetic nephropathy. Am J Perinatol 1998;15:413–421.

Registration Committee of the European Dialysis and Transplant Association. Successful pregnancies in women treated by dialysis and kidney transplantation. Br J Obstet Gynaecol 1980;87:839–845.

Schwarz A, Post KG, Keller F, Molzahn M. Value of human chorionic gonadotropin measurements in blood as a pregnancy test in women on maintenance hemodialysis. Nephron 1985;39:341–343.

Scott LL, Ramin SM, Richey M, et al. Erythropoietin use in pregnancy: two cases and a review of the literature. Am J Perinatol 1995;12:22–24.

Souqiyyeh MZ, Huraib SO, Saleh AG, Aswad S. Pregnancy in chronic hemodialysis patients in the Kingdom of Saudi Arabia. Am J Kidney Dis 1992;19:235–238.

Toma H, Tanabe K, Tokumoto T, et al. A nationwide survey on pregnancies in women on renal replacement therapy in Japan. Nephrol Dial Transpl 1998;31:A163.

Trebbin WM. Hemodialysis and pregnancy. JAMA 1979;241: 1811–1812.

Weiner Z, Thaler I, Ronen N, Brandes JM. Changes in flow velocity waveforms in umbilical and uterine artery following haemodialysis. Br J Obstet Gynaecol 1991;98:1172–1173.

Yasin SY, Bey Doun SN. Hemodialysis in pregnancy. Obstet Gynecol Surv 1988;43:655–668.

13 Cardiopulmonary bypass

Audrey S. Alleyne
Peter L. Bailey

Cardiopulmonary bypass (CPB), a commonly used and often necessary technique during cardiac surgery, results in significant alterations in patient physiology. Virtually every organ system is affected by CPB. Some of the prominent adverse effects include: (i) profound alterations in coagulation (dilution of all clotting factors, intense heparinization, platelet dysfunction); (ii) disturbances in cardiovascular function (hypotension, nonpulsatile blood flow, myocardial ischemia and cardiac stunning, arrhythmias); and (iii) a significant generalized systemic inflammatory response. Systemic embolization of particulate material occurs, including marrow and fat spilled into the chest when the sternum is split. Air embolization also frequently occurs. Embolic phenomena are thought to be major contributors to the significant risk of cerebrovascular accident (2–6%) and neurocognitive dysfunction (20–60%) (Shaw et al., 1987; Murkin et al., 1995; Roach et al., 1996). In addition, the management of patients requiring CPB frequently includes the use of hypothermic techniques, invasive monitoring, and the administration of a variety of cardiovascular drugs. Not infrequently, complications involving one or more major organ systems are experienced.

The application of "off-pump" coronary artery bypass for patients with coronary artery disease has become popular to a great degree because of the inherent risks of CPB (Plomondon et al., 2001). However, off-pump approaches are not available for patients with cardiac valvular surgical disease, the cardiac pathology that most often affects the pregnant patient. Minimally invasive cardiac surgical approaches and techniques, which are practiced selectively in some centers, reduce surgical incision length, may allow for more rapid recovery, and have preferred cosmetic outcomes. Minimally invasive approaches do not, however, avoid the need for CPB.

The first reports of cardiac surgery during pregnancy were published in 1952 and involved 11 closed mitral commissurotomies performed during pregnancy (Brock, 1952; Cooley & Chapman, 1952; Logan & Turner, 1952; Mason et al., 1952). In 1961, Harken and Taylor published a review of 394 published cases of cardiac surgery during pregnancy. In this series, a maternal mortality rate of 1.8% and a fetal mortality rate of 9% were reported. This reported maternal mortality was not different from that seen in nonpregnant patients undergoing similar procedures.

Valve repair procedures

Most available reports of cardiac surgery during pregnancy involve valve repair or replacement. Early collective experience in over 500 patients undergoing closed mitral valvotomy prior to 1965 was associated with maternal mortality of under 2% and fetal mortality under 10% (Ueland, 1965). In 1968, Knapp and Arditi presented data on 27 additional pregnant patients undergoing this procedure. These investigators found no maternal mortality, but a 15% perinatal mortality rate. In 1983, Becker published results from a survey of 600 members of the Society of Thoracic Surgeons. One hundred and one cases of closed mitral commissurotomy during pregnancy were described, mostly from centers outside the United States and performed during the second trimester of pregnancy due to progressive congestive failure. No maternal deaths were reported, and the perinatal mortality rate was 3%. Bernal and Miralles (1986), in a review of the literature, reported maternal and fetal mortalities of less than 2% and 10%, respectively, in 394 patients undergoing closed commissurotomy. In 1987, Vosloo and Reichart described 41 patients undergoing closed mitral commissurotomy during pregnancy. As with most previous studies, no maternal mortality was seen; however, overall fetal wastage was 12%. Fetal wastage increased to 17% for procedures performed in the third trimester. Today, with the availability of continuous electronic fetal heart rate monitoring during surgery and the possibility of simultaneous cesarean section should severe fetal compromise be detected, such losses might be significantly less.

Percutaneous balloon mitral commissurotomy has been safely performed in pregnant women with severe mitral stenosis (Ben Farhat et al., 1997; Gupta et al., 1998; Mangione et al., 2000; Fawzy et al., 2001; Uygur & Beksac, 2001). Abouzied and co-workers (Abouzied et al., 2001) reported improved hemodynamics and symptoms in 16 pregnant women with severe mitral stenosis who underwent balloon mitral commissurotomy. There were no immediate detrimental effects of radiation exposure related to fluoroscopy on the fetuses and 14 of the 16 women successfully continued their pregnancies to or near term delivering healthy infants. Mishra and colleagues (2001) report similar results in 85 severely symptomatic pregnant women with critical mitral stenosis. They noted that although the procedure was safe and generally effective, suboptimal results occurred in four of the 85 patients while mitral regurgitation increased by 1–2 grades in 18 of the 85 patients.

Despite the potential advantages of closed commissurotomy during pregnancy, this approach is associated with a significant likelihood of patients requiring additional surgery at a later date. Mangione and co-workers (2000) published favorable results with only 9% of their 23 patients requiring repeat valvuloplasty after 8 years of follow-up while Fawzy and colleagues (2001) reported that 16% of their patients undergoing mitral balloon valvuloplasty developed restenosis over a follow-up period of 9 years. In the series of Vosloo and Reichart (1987), 22% of patients receiving closed commissurotomy required an additional cardiac surgery during a follow-up period lasting from 5 to 17 years.

Most surgeons in the United States advocate open valvuloplasty in pregnant patients (Chambers & Clark, 1994). In nonpregnant patients, open commissurotomy also may be performed as safely as closed procedures, with both better short- and long-term results (Roe et al., 1971). Such procedures, however, require CPB, a technique that introduces an entirely different and greater set of risks to the fetus compared to closed procedures.

The body of literature describing the experiences of pregnant patients undergoing cardiac operations with CPB is comprised of case reports and surveys with no one institution or team of individuals having a large experience (Chambers & Clark, 1994). Historically, with regard to risk assessment, it has been thought that pregnancy does not necessarily increase maternal morbidity and mortality of cardiovascular surgical procedures. In 1969, Zitnik and co-workers reported a maternal mortality of 5% and a fetal mortality of 33% in open heart operations performed during pregnancy. A review of reported cases from 1958 to 1991 found a 2.9% maternal mortality and a 20.2% embryo–fetal mortality (Pomini et al., 1996). A subsequent analysis by Parry and Westaby (1996) found similar results and suggested that the maternal mortality was comparable to that in a nonpregnant cardiac surgical population. A review of the period 1984–1996 revealed a fetal–neonatal mortality of 30% and a maternal mortality of 6% for cardiovascular procedures performed during pregnancy (Weiss et al., 1998). In this same review the maternal mortality increased to 12% while the fetal mortality decreased to 5% for maternal cardiovascular surgery performed immediately after delivery. Overall, these results suggest that the maternal risk of mortality associated with cardiovascular procedures performed during pregnancy should be at most only modestly greater than in otherwise similar but nonpregnant females. Delaying maternal cardiovascular surgery until shortly after delivery may improve fetal outcome, but likely introduces a significant increase in maternal mortality.

Coronary artery bypass grafting

The performance of coronary artery bypass grafting (CABG) without CPB ("off-pump" CABG, beating heart CABG) will avoid the risks to the mother and fetus, which are intrinsic to CPB. Silberman and co-workers (1996) describe a case of coronary artery bypass performed on a beating heart without the use of CPB on a patient at 22 weeks' gestation who had intractable angina due to spontaneous dissection of the left anterior descending artery. She subsequently gave birth to a healthy term baby. Although this report is promising, long-term (10 years) results of beating heart CABG are not yet known to be equal to that of traditional CABG techniques which rely on CPB. In addition, beating heart CABG requires particular skill and expertise and is not easily performed by all cardiac surgeons.

For obvious reasons, no well-controlled studies have been reported assessing the impact of CPB on the pregnant patient, the fetoplacental unit, or fetal outcome. In addition, many of the existing case series reports date back to the late 1950s (Dubourg et al., 1959) and early 1960s. Current approaches and techniques that cardiac patients receive have changed significantly over time. Thus, many conclusions regarding maternal care and fetal outcome must be regarded as tentative.

Uteroplacental perfusion and CPB physiology

Uteroplacental blood flow (UPBF) is the major determinant of oxygen and other essential nutrient transport to the fetus. A direct correlation between uterine blood flow (UBF) and fetal oxygenation has been demonstrated in both animal models and humans (Skillman et al., 1985; Bilardo et al., 1990). UPBF is derived primarily from uterine arteries, with a smaller contribution (of unknown significance) coming from the ovarian arteries. The uterine arteries are branches of the internal iliac arteries. Uterine artery blood flow (UABF) increases two- to threefold in pregnancy and can represent up to 12% of the cardiac output. Increases in UBF during pregnancy are due to both physical (increased diameter of the uterine artery) and physiological (decreased responsiveness of the uterine artery to endogenous circulating vasoconstrictors) mechanisms. Selective uterine artery relaxation during pregnancy may be the result of vasodilators released from its endothelium, such as PGI2 or nitric oxide, or local hormonal actions, which diminish the activity of certain intracellular enzymes that mediate vasoconstriction.

UBF is related to perfusion pressure and vascular resistance according to the formula:

$$\text{UBF} = \frac{\text{Uterine arterial pressure} - \text{Uterine venous pressure}}{\text{Uterine vascular resistance}}$$

Under normal circumstances during pregnancy, the uterine arteries are maximally dilated. Thus, significant systemic hypotension will not stimulate an autoregulatory response to cause further uterine artery vasodilatation and thus, there is no mechanism for UABF to increase. Although in the ovine model, placental blood flow and fetal perfusion changes do not always parallel alterations in UABF (Landauer et al., 1986), in the human it is generally considered axiomatic that any significant fall in systemic pressure will result in a corresponding decrease in uterine and placental perfusion, with resultant fetal hypoxia. During CPB various factors can affect placental circulation, such as, poor placental perfusion during nonpulsatile flow, uterine arteriovenous shunts, uterine artery spasm, and particulate and gas embolism (Mahli et al., 2000). In light of the real potential for hypotension and flow alterations associated with CPB, it is obvious that fetal perfusion can easily be compromised.

Anesthesia

Although in experimental models some anesthetic agents may produce teratogenic effects, especially after prolonged administration, modern anesthetics are considered to be safe for use in the pregnant surgical patient (Smith, 1963; Shnider & Webster, 1965; Brodsky et al., 1980; Duncan et al., 1986; Mazze & Kallen, 1989, 1991). However, there may be an increased risk of fetal loss with first-trimester exposure to general anesthesia, which can be accentuated by the trauma of surgery, especially with surgical procedures on or around the uterus (Brodsky et al., 1980; Duncan et al., 1986).

In the pregnant cardiac surgery patient, it is more likely that the immediate cardiovascular depressant actions of anesthetic agents indirectly constitute a greater threat to the fetus. Cardiac surgery patients in general are often unable to tolerate the depressant hemodynamic effects of many anesthetic agents. The propensity for the pregnant cardiac surgery patient to experience compromised hemodynamic function during anesthesia and surgery as well as during CPB can compromise uteroplacental perfusion. Other factors, such as maternal anemia, respiratory alkalosis, and the administration of catecholamines or vasoactive drugs, also can contribute to impaired uterine artery pressure or resistance and uteroplacental perfusion and exacerbate fetal hypoxia and acidosis. Anesthetic techniques and agents should be chosen after careful consideration of maternal cardiac pathology and cardiovascular status in an attempt to minimize adverse hemodynamic effects in the mother in order to maintain uteroplacental perfusion (Figs 13.1, 13.2, 13.3).

Ventilation

Mechanical positive-pressure ventilation is instituted routinely in patients undergoing cardiac surgery, and various degrees of hyperventilation are frequently produced, either intentionally or inadvertently. Blood gas disturbances can effect sympathetic activity and thus indirectly effect UBF. In addition, hyperventilation may decrease uteroplacental perfusion either through mechanical means by increasing intrathoracic pressure and decreasing cardiac output, or through the induction of hypocapnia, which decreases UBF. Thus, hyperventilation should be minimized or avoided in the pregnant surgical patient unless specifically indicated (see later discussion).

Patient positioning

Lateral uterine displacement during cardiac surgery is essential to avoid aortocaval compression, decreased cardiac output, and uteroplacental perfusion (Clark, 1991). A lateral tilt of at least 30–40° has been recommended during CPB (Nazarian et al., 1976; Becker, 1983). This is especially crucial because CPB often results in hypotension, even in the nonpregnant patient. A combination of a wedge and table tilt is generally adequate to achieve appropriate lateral uterine displacement.

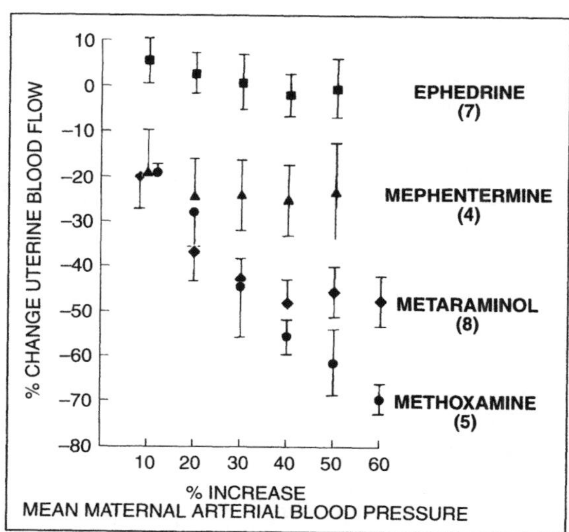

Fig. 13.1 Mean changes in uterine blood flow at equal elevations of mean arterial blood pressure following vasopressure administration. (Reproduced by permission from Ralston DH, Snider SM, Delorimer AA. Effects of equipotent ephedrine, metaraminol, mephentermine and methoxamine on uterine blood flow in the pregnant ewe. Anesthesiology 1974;40:354. Copyright © 1974 Williams & Wilkins Co.)

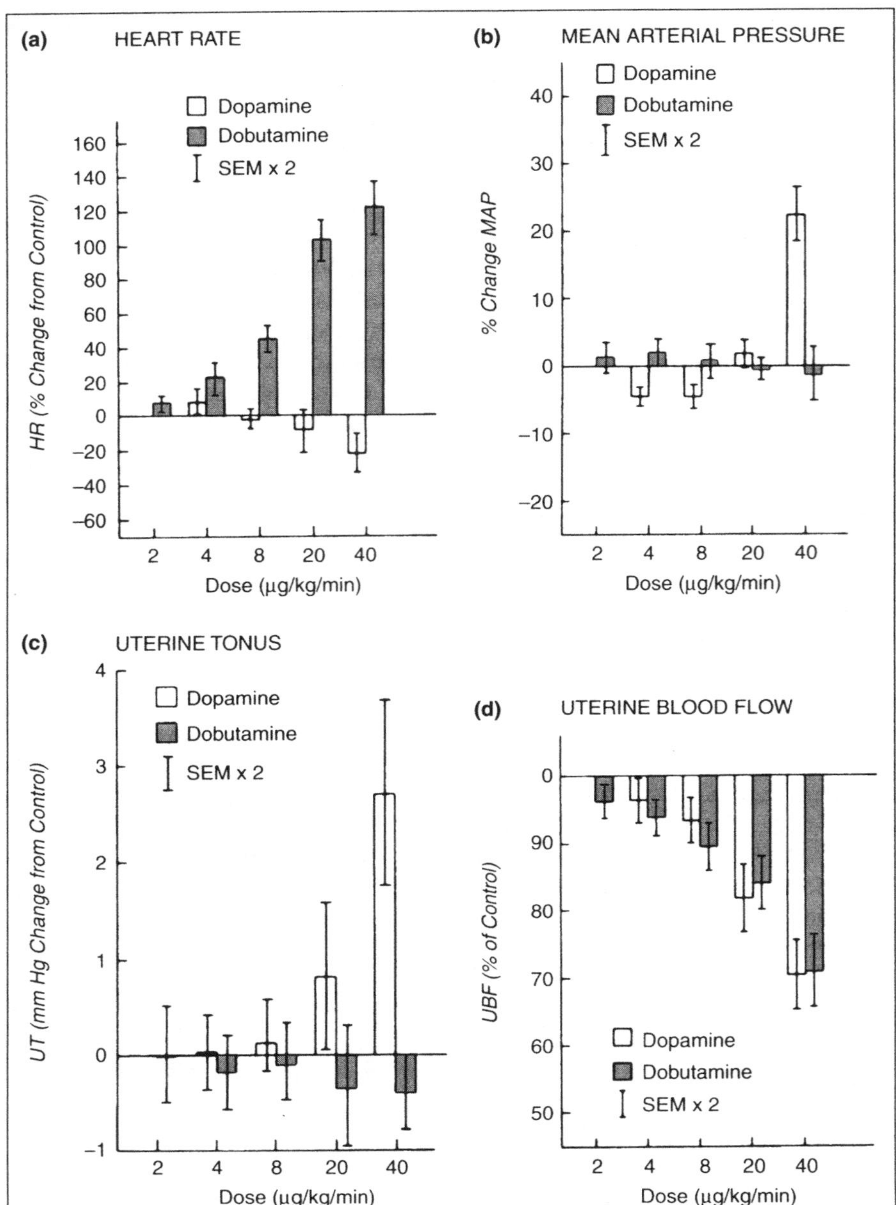

Fig. 13.2 Comparison of average changes in (a) HR, (b) MAP, (c) UT, and (d) UBF at various rates of dopamine and dobutamine infusion in pregnant ewes. HR, heart rate; MAP, mean arterial pressure; UT, uterine tonus; UBF, uterine blood flow. (Reproduced by permission from Fishburne JI, Meis PJ, Urban RB, et al. Vascular and uterine responses to dobutamine and dopamine in the gravid ewe. Am J Obset-Gynecol 1980;137:944.)

Cannulation

Cannulation of the inferior vena cava might partially obstruct blood flow in this vessel. While it is unlikely that such obstruction would lead to severe problems for either mother or fetus, it could potentially impair uteroplacental perfusion due to increased uterine venous pressure or to decreased blood return to the right heart with resultant diminished cardiac output (Meffert & Stansel, 1968).

Cardiopulmonary bypass prime

The various components of the CPB apparatus (e.g. tubing) require approximately 2 L of priming solution in most adult circuits. Priming of the CPB circuit produces hemodilution which is an important element of CPB for many patients. It decreases blood product utilization and its attendant costs and risks. Hemodilution also improves the rheology of blood by decreasing its viscosity, resulting in a lower arterial resistance

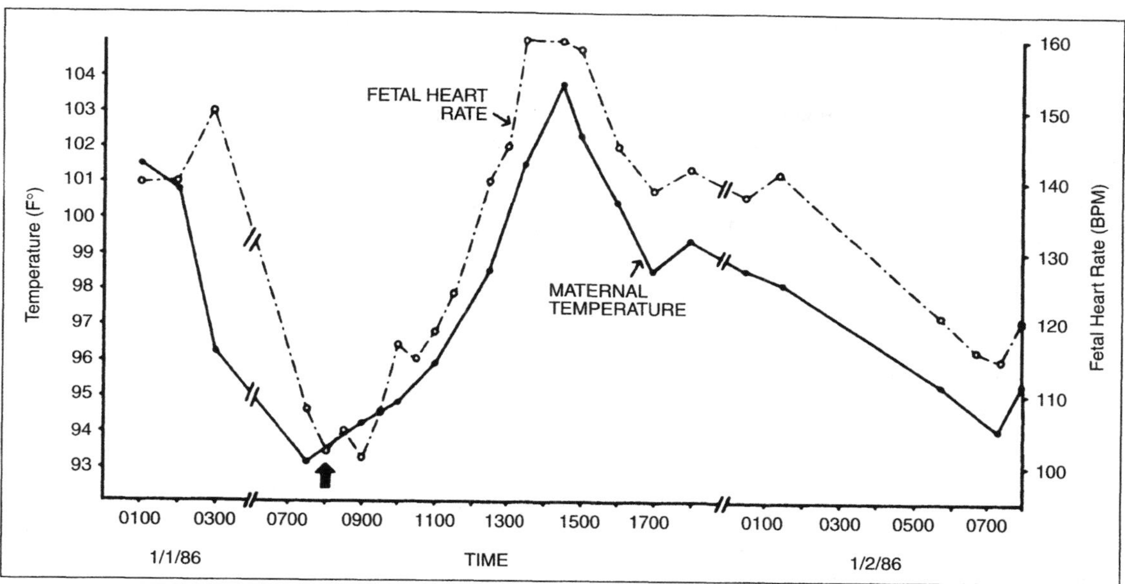

Fig. 13.3 Maternal temperature and fetal heart rate (FHR). The FHR plot directly parallels the maternal temperature. The arrow at 0800, 1/1/86, represents the nadir of maternal BP: 87/46 mmHg (mean arterial pressure, 69). Within 20 minutes the BP was 94/57 mmHg (mean arterial pressure, 69). The mean arterial pressure during the rest of the illustrated time ranged from 64 to 76. Previous and subsequent pressures during this pregnancy ranged from 90/50 to 110/65 mmHg (mean arterial pressure, 63–80). BPM, beats per minute. (Reproduced by permission from Jadhon ME, Main EK. Fetal bradycardia associated with maternal hypothermia. Obstet Gynecol 1988;72:496.)

and improved peripheral perfusion (Cooper & Slogoff, 1993). Other purported benefits of hemodilution during CPB include decreases in major organ complications, such as cerebral vascular accident, and renal and pulmonary dysfunction. In the pregnant cardiac surgical patient, or any anemic patient for that matter, CPB associated hemodilution may result in severe anemia. This can compromise the oxygen-carrying capacity of blood as well as oxygen delivery. Anemic patients with poor cardiac function may not tolerate severe hemodilution. Whole blood or RBCs can be added to the prime of the CPB circuit so that the resultant hematocrit is no less than 21–26% (Eilen et al., 1981). Hemodilution and subsequent changes in hormone concentrations, such as a decrease in progesterone, may play a role in triggering uterine contractions (Korsten et al., 1989). Korsten and co-workers (1989) suggested that the addition of progesterone to the prime may be helpful in avoiding preterm uterine activity, but this approach requires further investigation before incorporation into clinical practice.

Oxygenator type

Because bubble oxygenators may be associated with a greater incidence of embolic phenomena, membrane oxygenators are recommended for the conduct of CPB in the gravid patient.

Hypothermia

Hypothermia was considered an important component of CPB for many years in order to decrease systemic and vital organ oxygen consumption and minimize organ damage. As mentioned above, hypothermia has been used with acceptable maternal–fetal outcomes (Plunkett et al., 2000). However, its use is now deemed less beneficial and perhaps unnecessary. While hypothermia can cause alterations in acid–base status and can lead to coagulation disorders, completely normothermic or even mildly hyperthermic conditions may exacerbate neurological deficits (McLean & Wong, 1996). Hypothermia can also influence uterine tone.

In pregnant dogs, cooling to 28°C is associated with an increase in uterine tone (Assali & Westin, 1962). However, this did not result in any demonstrable effect on fetal survival, and pregnant ewes cooled to 29°C did not exhibit fetal distress as long as maternal acidosis and hypoxia were avoided (Matsuki & Oyama, 1972). In fetal lamb studies, hypothermia interfered with placental function, impairing respiratory gas transfer and transplacental flow to the fetal organs. This suggests that the placenta exposed to hypothermia in vivo is not a good fetal oxygenator (Adzick et al., 1984; Bradley et al., 1989; Hawkins et al., 1991). Fetal heart rate has been reported to decrease in parallel with maternal temperature (see Fig. 13.3), and serious fetal arrhythmias may occur at temperatures of 32°C or less (Kawkabani et al., 1999). However, pregnant patients have been subjected to cardiac and noncardiac surgery and cooled as low as 25°C (Boatman & Bradford, 1958; Matsuki & Oyama, 1972; Koh, et al., 1975; Levy et al., 1980; Lamb et al., 1981; Mora & Grunewald, 1987; Korsten et al., 1989) with no reportable adverse fetal effects. In other reported cases fetal heart tones became undetectable during surgery, only to once again become audible postoperatively (Buffolo et al., 1994; Mahli et al., 2000). Although the risk of fetal arrhythmia and cardiac arrest is increased at temperatures below 35°C (Hess & Davis, 1964; Nagy et al., 1988; Johnson & Saltzman, 1991; Pomini et al., 1996; Mahli et al., 2000), mild hypothermia can often be tolerated because of fetal autoregulation (Rossouw et al., 1993) and has been suggested to protect the fetus by reducing fetal oxygen requirements.

Rewarming is associated with increased frequency of uterine contractions (Becker, 1983). Furthermore, many reports of fetal heart rate decelerations have been reported in association with rewarming. Mahli and co-workers (2000) suggest that these fetal decelerations may be secondary to deficient delivery of heat to the fetus during rewarming as a result of vasoconstriction of the umbilical vessels. Current knowledge and practice has been to avoid aggressive rewarming strategies, which were more often practiced in the past. Aggressive rewarming targets or rates can be associated with increased CNS adverse effects (Grigore et al., 2002).

While the actual risks of hypothermia are probably controllable if aortic clamp times are not prolonged, minimal (34–35°C) to mild (32°C) hypothermic perfusion is likely to be the most rational approach in the pregnant patient. Because hypothermia is of little incremental benefit to patients below 32–34°C, unless circulatory arrest is required during CPB for surgical repair, pregnant patients can either "drift" to 34°C or be cooled to mild hypothermic degrees.

Pulsatility

Nonpulsatile flow is most commonly employed during CPB. It can be argued that pulsatile flow would be superior, providing a more normal physiologic milieu and better tissue and organ perfusion than nonpulsatile blood flow. For example, differences in vascular resistance, oxygen delivery, and myocardial lactate production indicate the superiority of pulsatile CPB (Trimakas et al., 1979; Philbin, 1993; Vedrinne et al., 2000). However, clinical application of pulsatile flow during CPB is uncommon. In a pregnant patient receiving nonpulsatile CPB described by Farmakides and colleagues (Farmakides et al., 1987), Doppler velocimetry suggested the presence of pulsatile uterine artery flow, although these findings may have been affected by pump artifact (Strickland et al., 1991). Tripp and co-workers (1999) report the use of pulsatile bypass during the aortic valve replacement of a 25-year-old female at 14 weeks' gestation. She subsequently delivered a healthy infant at term. The use of pulsatile perfusion holds some promise of improving maternal and fetal survival but further investigation is needed.

Flow rate

Because normal cardiac output in pregnant women is often greater than 6 L/min (Clark et al., 1989), the usual flows (~2.5 L/m^2) employed during CPB may be too little. Changes in baseline fetal heart rate have been identified after initial flow rates as high as 80 mL/kg/min, even in the absence of maternal hypotension (Chambers & Clark, 1994). Increases in CPB flows to 3.0–4.0 L/m^2 have been successfully (if only temporarily) employed during surgery in the pregnant patient, especially in response to fetal bradycardia (Lamb et al., 1981; Becker, 1983; Chambers & Clark, 1994). For example, Koh and associaties (Koh et al., 1975) were the first to describe improvement in fetal bradycardia by increasing flow rate by 16%. Other investigators have since confirmed the value of increasing pump flow rate to improve fetal bradycardia (Veray et al., 1970; Werch et al., 1977; Trimakas et al., 1979; Lamb et al., 1981; Bernal & Miralles, 1986; Korsten et al., 1989).

Pressure

The ideal mean arterial pressure (MAP) during CPB is not firmly established for cardiac surgical patients in general. In the pregnant patient, the use of moderate to high arterial pressures during CPB is recommended. MAP should initially be maintained at a level of 70 mmHg or greater. It is preferable to produce elevations in MAP with fluid volume administration and high flow rates as opposed to vasopressor administration, which could have an adverse effect on UPBF. It should be anticipated that on institution of CPB, transient but significant hypotension occurs and frequently produces fetal bradycardia (Koh, 1975; Trimakas et al., 1979; Levy, 1980; Lamb, 1981). This is generally correctable by appropriate manipulations of pump flow and pressure.

Anticoagulation

Anticoagulation is essential during CPB. It is generally accomplished with heparin therapy and in general poses no risks to the fetus. Such anticoagulation is typically reversed with protamine sulfate following successful weaning and separation from CPB. There are no available data concerning the use of antifibrinolytics in the pregnant cardiac patient to improve hemostasis and decrease perioperative blood loss.

Cardioplegia

Myocardial protection during CPB is essential to reduce perioperative cardiac morbidity. Both cold and warm blood cardioplegia have been shown to reduce cardiac morbidity (Fremes et al., 2000). The application of cardioplegia may need to be more frequent with the maintenance of high flows during CPB, especially if normothermia or only mild hypothermia is employed. Normothermic perfusion often results in early rewarming of the left ventricle leading to difficulties with myocardial protection (Parry & Westaby, 1996). Cardiac activity may return as frequently as every 10 minutes under these circumstances. In one study, 3.5 L of cardioplegia was required to adequately suppress cardiac activity (Korsten et al., 1989). The use of cold cardioplegia has been associated with fetal bradycardia (Garry et al., 1996) and continuous cold pericardial irrigation or warm blood cardioplegia has been suggested as effective alternatives (Lichtenstein et al., 1991). Concomitant tocolytic therapy may potentially also increase the need for cardioplegia and it is generally avoided as an elective prophylactic measure.

Acid–base status

Acid–base status may vary significantly during CPB. The most common approaches to the management of acid–base status during CPB are called alpha STAT and pH STAT. Briefly, alpha STAT management attempts to maintain a normal enzymatic milieu. This is accomplished by targeting normocarbia, as determined by blood gas analysis of a blood sample at a temperature of 37°C. pH STAT management attempts to maintain a pH of 7.4, no matter what the patient's temperature. This usually involves the addition of carbon dioxide to the CPB oxygenator to maintain a calculated patient blood $P\text{CO}_2$ of 40 mmHg at the patient's temperature during hypothermic CPB. While commonly practiced in the past, pH STAT approaches have become less popular in the adult cardiac surgical patient population.

The management of arterial carbon dioxide partial pressures has particular relevance for the pregnant patient undergoing CPB, because maternal hyperventilation can impair fetal oxygenation (Motoyama et al., 1967; Levinson et al., 1974). Levinson and colleagues (Levinson et al., 1974) reported that in the unanesthetized pregnant ewe, mechanical hyperventilation with normocarbia maintained by the addition of carbon dioxide impaired UBF because of the intrathoracic effects of positive pressure on cardiac output. These authors found that respiratory alkalosis additionally impaired fetal oxygenation. On the other hand, after studying anesthetized ewes, Motoyama and co-workers (1967) attributed impairment of fetal oxygenation solely to the respiratory alkalosis produced by huperventilation and not the negative hemodynamic effects of positive pressure. Maternal metabolic alkalemia also impaired fetal oxygenation, while maternal hypercapnia with acidemia was associated with an increase in fetal oxygenation. These changes were due to a combination of alterations in oxygen transfer within the placenta and changes in umbilical blood flow. As summarized by Motoyama and associates (1967) reports in humans support the notion that the fetal effects of maternal hyperventilation can be deleterious. Based on available information, avoidance of significant disturbances in acid–base balance, especially respiratory alkalosis, is recommended.

Cardiopulmonary bypass duration

The technical proficiency and speed of the cardiac surgical team are two of the primary determinants of outcome in cardiac surgery. With regards to the pregnant cardiac patient, fetal morbidity and mortality also appear to increase with CPB duration. Thus, it is essential that CPB time be minimized in the pregnant patinet.

Fetal monitoring during cardiopulmonary bypass

Open heart operations have been performed on pregnant women at various stages of pregnancy. Younger gestational age has been associated with a higher fetal morbidity (Strickland et al., 1991) leading many to suggest that cardiac surgery is best done between 24 and 28 weeks' gestation after the completion of organogenesis and attainment of fetal viability. If neonatal intensive care facilities are available, a cesarean delivery just before CPB may be an option (Zitnik et al., 1969; Parry & Westaby, 1996). In the previable fetus (<24 weeks), cesarean delivery would generally not be indicated, even if fetal compromise were detected during CPB. Even in the 24–26-week gestational age range, the potential risks of an additional major abdominal operation during the perioperative period in patients undergoing open heart surgery must be carefully weighed against the likelihood of improved neonatal survival. Emergency use of CPB for cesarean delivery may become necessary, however, if the maternal status deteriorates (Penning et al., 2001). Because neonatal morbidity and mortality statistics change, and can be influenced by the level of care any one center can provide, consultation with a neonatologist is recommended. However, even if nonintervention is elected, careful fetal monitoring is important, because in the presence of bradycardia, alterations in pump flow and pressure may often improve fetal status and outcome without the need to resort to operative delivery. Such monitoring is often most easily performed with continuous external electronic fetal heart rate monitoring, assuming fetal size and maternal habitus do not preclude such a technique. Otherwise, intermittent auscultation may allow the obstetric attendant to detect significant decreases in fetal heart rate and suggest the need for interventions (Liu et al., 1985).

Fetal bradycardia during CPB has been frequently reported in the literature (Koh et al., 1975; Eilen et al., 1981; Farmakides et al., 1987; Korsten et al., 1989; Mahli et al., 2000). Resolution of the bradycardia often occurs after separation from bypass but occasionally can persist (Chambers & Clark, 1994) lasting several hours postoperatively (Burke et al., 1990; Mahli et al., 2000). Mahli and associates (Mahli et al., 2000), discuss several possible etiologies for this observed fetal bradycardia in their case report of a 32-week parturient undergoing mitral commissurotomy for severe mitral stenosis secondary to rheumatic valve disease. Fetal hypoxia and acidosis, maternal hypothermia, and administration of drugs which cross through the placenta are suggested as possible causes. Fetal hypoxia can be due to reduced oxygen content of maternal blood, reduced uterine perfusion pressure, and/or increased uterine arterial resistance (Strickland et al., 1991). Koh and colleagues (1975) report the occurrence of fetal bradycardia seen during CPB which subsided in response to improved maternal blood flow. Other authors have also noted restoration of normal (Veray et al., 1970; Trimakas et al., 1979; Korsten et al., 1989; Westaby et al., 1992; Chambers & Clark, 1994; Pomini et al., 1996) and even elevated fetal heart by increasing perfusion pressure to the uteroplacental bed and by increasing maternal blood flow (Koh et al., 1975; Werch et al., 1977).

A decrease in maternal blood pressure can occur at various stages of cardiac surgery and is common during cannulation of the inferior or superior vena cava, right atrium, or aorta just before initiating CPB. Significant hypotension also occurs shortly after onset of CPB (Mahli et al., 2000). Hemodilution is thought to play a role, while the release of vasoactive substances has also been postulated as an etiologic factor (Lees et al., 1971; Gordon et al., 1975; Mooij et al., 1988; Pomini et al., 1996). Other fetal heart rate features, such as diminished variability, fetal tachycardia and a sinusoidal-like pattern, have also been described in association with decreased perfusion during CPB and may be amenable to pump manipulation, as described previously (Koh et al., 1975; Levy et al., 1980; Korsten et al., 1989; Burke et al., 1990). Fetal decelerations or diminished variability occurring despite increased CPB flow in normothermic patients with normal acid–base status are thought to be secondary to fetal exposure to many of the drugs administered during the conduction of anesthesia (Katz et al., 1976; Trimakas et al., 1979; Eilen et al., 1981; Mahli et al., 2000).

If technically feasible, uterine activity also should be monitored during CPB. Uterine contractile activity should be anticipated especially during periods of reduced flow during and after CPB. Uterine contractions occur frequently, especially during cooling and rewarming (Becker, 1983). It has been suggested that these contractions create a temporary oxygen deficit to the fetus in a manner similar to a "stress test" (Pomini et al., 1996) and can be an important predictor of fetal death (Bernal & Miralles, 1986). The mechanism(s) responsible for these uterine contractions have not been clearly delineated. The dilutional effect of CPB has been postulated to reduce the hormonal levels of progesterone resulting in increased uterine excitability (Becker, 1983; Korsten et al., 1989; Parry & Westaby, 1996). Sabik and co-workers (1992) have implicated the production of vasoactive prostaglandins. In 1992, using the fetal lamb model, they administered indomethacin to inhibit prostaglandin synthesis and found that it prevented the increase in placental vascular resistance frequently observed during CPB (Sabik et al., 1992). In 1994, they examined fetal lambs treated with either indomethacin or high-dose steroids before undergoing CPB and calculated placental vascular resistance and placental blood flow (Sabik et al., 1994). They found placental vascular resistance decreased and placental blood flow increased when compared to controls and suggested that the production of a placental vasoconstrictive prostaglandin is one mechanism responsible for decreased placental blood flow seen after CPB (Sabik et al., 1994). Nitric oxide release and other factors have also been postulated to have a role (Champsaur et al., 1997; Vedrinne et al., 1998).

If regular contractions do appear, they should be treated promptly to avoid placental insufficiency and fetal hypoxia. Treatments include increased perfusion pressure and pump flow and consideration may be given to tocolysis. Korsten and colleagues (1989) reported uterine contractions that appeared shortly after the initiation of CPB and were decreased with the intravenous infusion of ritodrine hydrochloride. Terbutaline or magnesium sulfate may be appropriate alternative agents. However, caution should be exercised in administering drugs with potent cardiovascular effects to a patient with significant cardiac disease undergoing CPB. Some advocate prophylactic tocolytic administration (Kawkabani et al., 1999) while others consider tocolytic therapy only appropriate given firm evidence of preterm labor (chambers & Clark, 1994). During the postoperative period, careful fetal and uterine activity monitoring should be continued.

Fetal survival

Actual fetal risks of CPB are difficult to establish, because evidence exists almost exclusively from compilations of case report data (Zitnik et al., 1969; Rossouw, et al., 1993). Becker's survey of 68 CPB procedures performed during pregnancy by members of the Society of Thoracic Surgery suggested an overall fetal death rate of 16% (Becker, 1983) (Table 13.1). Westaby and associates (1992) compiled a summary of reported cases of CPB during pregnancy between 1959 and 1990, with a cumulative fetal death rate of 17.4% (Table 13.2). Such figures may best serve as a starting point for discussion of mortality risks involved. For the patient who has reached a stage of viability, where cesarean delivery may be considered, fetal death rate can be controlled, because ominous fetal heart rate pat-

Table 13.1 Summary of cardiac procedures performed during pregnancy*

Procedure	Total	Indication for operation	Maternal survivors	Fetal survivors	Fetal deaths
Closed mitral commissurotomy	101	CHF (96), emboli (3), hemoptysis	101	98	3
Open mitral commissurotomy	23	CHF (23)	23	22	1
Mitral valve replacement	19	CHF (14), endocarditis (1), thrombosed prothesis (4)	18	15	4
Aortic valve replacement	10	Aortic stenosis (7), endocarditis (3)	10	6	4
Pulmonary embolectomy	3	Shock (3)	3	2	1
Closure of atrial or ventricular septal defect	8	CHF (4), elective operation (4)	8	7	1
Coronary bypass	3	Unstable angina (3)	3	3	0
Myxoma removal	2		2	2	0

* Includes cardiopulmonary bypass (CPB) and non-CPB procedures.
CHF, congestive heart failure.
(From Becker RM. Intracardiac surgery in pregnant women. Ann Thorac Surg 1983;36:453–458.)

Table 13.2 Summary of reported cases of cardiac surgery performed with cardiopulmonary bypass during pregnancy, 1959–1990*

Procedure	No. of patients	Indication for operation	Maternal deaths	Fetal deaths
Open mitral commissurotomy	33	CHF (27)*	0	2
Mitral valve replacement	29	CHF (21); endocarditis (1); thrombosed prosthesis (7)	1	6
Aortic valve replacement	15	Aortic stenosis (9); endocarditis (6)	0	5
Pulmonary embolectomy	4	Shock (4)	0	1
Closure of ASD or VSD	22	CHF (8)*	1	6
Coronary bypass	4	Unstable angina (4)	0	0
Myxoma removal	4	—		
Repair of thoracic aorta	3	Leaking/ruptured aneurysm (3)	0	0
Tetralogy of Fallot	1	—	0	0
Total (%)	115		2 (1.7)	20 (17.4)

* Data in literature were incomplete.
ASD, atrial septal defect; CHF, congestive heart failure; VSD, ventricular septal defect.
(Reproduced by permission from Westaby S, Parry AJ, Forfar JC. Reoperation for prosthetic valve endocarditis in the third trimester of pregnancy. Ann Thorac Surg 1992;53:263.)

terns not promptly corrected by alterations in flow rate or pressure can be recognized and simultaneous cesarean performed (Martin et al., 1981). For patients with fetuses younger than 24–26 weeks, a 10–15% fetal mortality rate with heart surgery and CPB appears to be a reasonable figure. For the term or near-term fetus, pre-CPB delivery would also be an appropriate option to avoid the potential need for concomitant cardiac and obstetric surgery.

Postoperative course

The most common problems cardiac surgery patients experience in the immediate postoperative period involve hemostasis, and cardiovascular and respiratory function. Less commonly, but not rarely, renal function may deteriorate and renal failure significantly worsens the prognosis. In the pregnant patient, such problems, if severe, may necessitate postoperative emergency cesarean section (Baraka et al., 2000).

Patients undergoing CPB can suffer significant neurologic complications after heart surgery. Deficits can occur in up to 50% of patients, with a much smaller (2–3%) percent experiencing permanent focal or cognitive problems (Shaw et al., 1987; Murkin et al., 1995; Roach et al., 1996). In pregnant patients, these problems also are likely to be of concern for several reasons. Emergency procedures, and especially open heart operations, will increase neurological complication rates. Systemic embolization and stroke will also be increased in pregnant patients if their condition includes rheumatic valvular disease with bacterial endocarditis and the presence of vegetations. Obviously, any disability will add significant burdens to a new mother and family.

Once postoperative bleeding has resolved, and depending on the type of valvular prosthesis employed, mothers may require continued and consistent anticoagulation postoperatively. The complex issues surrounding the use of heparin versus warfarin derivatives in these patients is discussed elsewhere in this text.

Delivery of the fetus may take place several months after cardiac operation. At the time of delivery, the cardiac team should be made aware and complete evaluation of the mother's cardiovascular status should be undertaken even if maternal outcome after cardiac surgery has been excellent. The team should be prepared for treatment of any cardiac problems (e.g. hemorrhage) that may arise during or after delivery.

References

Abouzied AM, Al Abbady M, Al Gendy MF, et al. Percutaneous balloon mitral commissurotomy during pregnancy. Angiology 2001;52:205–209.

Adzick NA, Harrison MR, Slate RK, Glick PL, Villa RI. Surface cooling and rewarming the fetus: a technique for experimental fetal cardiac operation. Surg Forum 1984;35:313–316.

Assali NS, Westin B. Effects of hypothermia on uterine circulation and on the fetus. Proc Soc Exp Biol Med 1962;109:485–488.

Baraka A, Kawkabani N, Haroun-Bizri S. Hemodynamic deterioration after cardiopulmonary bypass during pregnancy: resuscitation by postoperative emergency Cesarean section. J Cardiothorac Vasc Anesth 2000;14:314–315.

Becker RM. Intracardiac surgery in pregnant women. Ann of Thorac Surg 1983;36:453–458.

Ben Farhat M, Gamra H, Betbout F, et al. Percutaneous balloon mitral commissurotomy during pregnancy. Heart 1997;77:564–567.

Bernal JM, Miralles PJ. Cardiac surgery with cardiopulmonary bypass during pregnancy. Obstet Gynecol Surv 1986;41:1–6.

Bilardo CM, Nicolaides KH, Campbell S. Doppler measurements of fetal and uteroplacental circulations: relationship with umbilical venous blood gases measured at cordocentesis. Am J Obstet Gynecol 1990;162:115–120.

Boatman KK, Bradford VA. Excision of an internal carotid aneurysm during pregnancy employing hypothermia and a vascular shunt. Ann Surg 1958;148:271–275.

Bradley SM, Verrier ED, Duncan BW. Cardiopulmonary bypass in the fetal lamb. Effect of sodium nitroprusside. Circulation 1989; 80(Suppl 2):220.

Brock R. Valvulotomy in pregnancy. Proc R Soc Med 1952;45:538.

Brodsky JB, Cohen EN, Brown BW, Jr., Wu ML, Whitcher C. Surgery during pregnancy and fetal outcome. Am J Obstet Gynecol 1980;138:1165–1167.

Buffolo E, Palma JH, Gomes WJ, et al. Successful use of deep hypothermic circulatory arrest in pregnancy. Ann Thorac Surg 1994;58: 1532–1534.

Burke AB, Hur D, Bolan JC, Corso P, Resano FG. Sinusoidal fetal heart rate pattern during cardiopulmonary bypass. Am J Obstet Gynecol 1990;163:17–18.

Chambers CE, Clark SL. Cardiac surgery during pregnancy. Clin Obstet Gynecol 1994;37:316–323.

Champsaur G, Vedrinne C, Martinot S, et al. Flow-induced release of endothelium-derived relaxing factor during pulsatile bypass: experimental study in the fetal lamb. J Thorac Cardiovasc Surg 1997;114:738–744.

Clark SL. Cardiac disease in pregnancy. Crit Care Clin 1991;7: 777–797.

Clark SL, Cotton DB, Lee W, et al. Central hemodynamic assessment of normal term pregnancy. Am J Obstet Gynecol 1989;161:1439–1442.

Cooley DA, Chapman DW. Mitral commissurotomy during pregnancy. JAMA 1952;150:1113.

Cooper JRJ, Slogoff S. Hemodilution and priming solutions for cardiopulmonary bypass. Baltimore: Williams and Wilkins, 1993:124–137.

Dubourg G, Broustet P, Brigaud H, et al. Correction complete d'une Triade de Fallot, en circulation extra-corporelle, chez une femme enceinte. Arch Mal Coeur 1959;52:1389–1391.

Duncan PG, Pope WD, Cohen MM, Greer N. Fetal risk of anesthesia and surgery during pregnancy. Anesthesiology 1986;64:790–794.

Eilen B, Kaiser IH, Becker RM, Cohen MN. Aortic valve replacement in the third trimester of pregnancy: case report and review of the literature. Obstet Gynecol 1981;57:119–121.

Farmakides G, Schulman H, Mohtashemi M, Ducey J, Fuss R, Mantell P. Uterine-umbilical velocimetry in open heart surgery. Am J Obstet Gynecol 1987;156:1221–1222.

Fawzy ME, Kinsara AJ, Stefadouros M, et al. Long-term outcome of mitral balloon valvotomy in pregnant women. J Heart Valve Dis 2001;10:153–157.

Fremes SE, Tamariz MG, Abramov D, et al. Late results of the Warm Heart Trial: the influence of nonfatal cardiac events on late survival. Circulation 2000;102:19(Suppl 3):339–345.

Garry D, Leikin E, Fleisher AG, Tejani N. Acute myocardial infarction in pregnancy with subsequent medical and surgical management. Obstet Gynecol 1996;87:802–804.

Gordon RJ, Ravin M, Daicoff GR, Rawitscher RE. Effects of hemodilution on hypotension during cardiopulmonary bypass. Anesth Analg 1975;54:482–488.

Grigore AM, Grocott HP, Mathew JP, et al., the Neurologic Outcome Research Group of the Duke Heart Center. The rewarming rate and increased peak temperature alter neurocognitive outcome after cardiac surgery. Anesth Analg 2002;94:4–10.

Gupta A, Lokhandwala YY, Satoskar PR, Salvi VS. Balloon mitral valvotomy in pregnancy: maternal and fetal outcomes. J Am Coll Surg 1998;187:409–415.

Harken DE, Taylor WJ. Cardiac surgery during pregnancy. Clin Obstet Gynecol 1961;4:697.

Hawkins JA, Paape KL, Adkins TP, Shaddy RE, Gay WA. Extracorporeal circulation in the fetal lamb. Effects of hypothermia and perfusion rate. J Cardiovasc Surg 1991;32:295–300.

Hess OW, Davis CD. Electronic evaluation of the fetal and maternal heart rate during hypothermia in a pregnant woman. Am J Obstet Gynecol 1964;89:801–807.

Johnson MD, Saltzman DH. Cardiac Disease. St. Louis: Mosby Year Book, 1991:210–259.

Katz JD, Hook R, Barash PG. Fetal heart rate monitoring in pregnant patients undergoing surgery. Am J Obstet Gynecol 1976;125: 267–269.

Kawkabani N, Kawas N, Baraka A, Vogel T, Mangano CM. Case 3—1999. Severe fetal bradycardia in a pregnant woman undergoing hypothermic cardiopulmonary bypass. J Cardiothorac Vasc Anesth 1999;13:346–349.

Knapp RC, Arditi LI. Closed mitral valvulotomy in pregnancy. Clin Obstet Gynecol 1968;11:978–991.

Koh KS, Friesen RM, Livingstone RA, Peddle LJ. Fetal monitoring during maternal cardiac surgery with cardiopulmonary bypass. Can Med Assoc J 1975;112:1102–1104.

Korsten HH, Van Zundert AA, Mooij PN, De Jong PA, Bavinck JH. Emergency aortic valve replacement in the 24th-week of pregnancy. Acta Anaesth Belg 1989;40:201–205.

Lamb MP, Ross K, Johnstone AM, Manners JM. Fetal heart monitoring during open heart surgery. Two case reports. Br J Obstet Gynaecol 1981;88:669–674.

Landauer M, Phernetton TM, Rankin JH. Maternal ovine placental vascular responses to adenosine. Am J Obstet Gynecol 1986;154: 1152–1155.

Lees MH, Herr RH, Hill JD, et al. Distribution of systemic blood flow of the rhesus monkey during cardiopulmonary bypass. J Thorac Cardiovasc Surg 1971;61:570–586.

Levinson G, Shnider SM, Delorimier AA, Steffenson JL. Effects of maternal hyperventilation on uterine blood flow and fetal oxygenation and acid-base status. Anesthesiology 1974;40:340–347.

Levy DL, Warriner RA, III, Burgess GE, III. Fetal response to cardiopulmonary bypass. Obstet Gynecol 1980;56:112–115.

Lichtenstein SV, Abel JG, Panos A, Slutsky AS, Salerno TA. Warm heart surgery: experience with long cross-clamp times. Ann Thorac Surg 1991;52:1009–1013.

Liu PL, Warren TM, Ostheimer GW, Weiss JB, Liu LM. Foetal monitoring in parturients undergoing surgery unrelated to pregnancy. Can Anaesth Soc J 1985;32:525–532.

Logan A, Turner RWD. Mitral valvulotomy during pregnancy. Lancet 1952;1:1286.

McLean RF, Wong BI. Normothermic versus hypothermic cardiopulmonary bypass: central nervous system outcomes. J Cardiothorac Vasc Anesth 1996;10:45–52.

Mahli A, Izdes S, Coskun D. Cardiac operations during pregnancy: review of factors influencing fetal outcome. Ann Thorac Surg 2000;69:1622–1626.

Mangione JA, Lourenco RM, dos Santos ES, et al. Long-term follow-up of pregnant women after percutaneous mitral valvuloplasty. Catheter Cardiovasc Interv 2000;50:413–417.

Martin MC, Pernoll ML, Boruszak AN, Jones JW, LoCicero J, III. Cesarean section while on cardiac bypass: report of a case. Obstet Gynecol 1981;57:(Suppl 6):41S–45S.

Mason J, Stable FE, Szekely PJ. Cardiac disease in pregnancy. J Obstet Gyn Brit Em 1952;59:569.

Matsuki A, Oyama T. Operation under hypothermia in a pregnant woman with an intracranial arteriovenous malformation. Can Anaesth Soc J 1972;19:184–191.

Mazze RI, Kallen B. Reproductive outcome after anesthesia and operation during pregnancy: a registry study of 5405 cases. Am J Obstet Gynecol 1989;161:1178–1185.

Mazze RI, Kallen B. Appendectomy during pregnancy: a Swedish registry study of 778 cases. Obstet Gynecol 1991;77:835–840.

Meffert WG, Stansel HC, Jr. Open heart surgery during pregnancy. Am J Obstet Gynecol 1968;102:1116–1120.

Mishra S, Narang R, Sharma M, et al. Percutaneous transseptal mitral commissurotomy in pregnant women with critical mitral stenosis. Indian Heart J 2001;53:192–196.

Mooij PNM, De Jong PA, Bavinck JH, Korsten HHM, Bonnier JJR, Berendes JN. Aortic valve replacement in the second trimester of pregnancy: a case report. Eur J Obstet Gyn Reprod Biol 1988;29: 347–352.

Mora CT, Grunewald KE. Reoperative aortic and mitral prosthetic valve replacement in the third trimester of pregnancy. J Cardiothorac Anesth 1987;1:313–317.

Motoyama EK, Rivard G, Acheson F, Cook CD. The effect of changes in maternal pH and P-CO2 on the P-O2 of fetal lambs. Anesthesiology 1967;28:891–903.

Murkin JM, Martzke JS, Buchan AM, Bentley C, Wong CJ. A randomized study of the influence of perfusion technique and pH management strategy in 316 patients undergoing coronary artery bypass surgery. II. Neurologic and cognitive outcomes. J Thorac Cardiovasc Surg 1995;110:349–362.

Nagy Z, Aranyosi J, Komaromy B, Peterffy A. Open mitral commissurotomy in pregnancy. Scand J Thorac Cardiovasc Surg 1988; 22:17–18.

Nazarian M, McCullough GH, Fielder DL. Bacterial endocarditis in pregnancy: successful surgical correction. J Thorac Cardiovasc Surg 1976;71:880–883.

Parry AJ, Westaby S. Cardiopulmonary bypass during pregnancy. Ann Thorac Surg 1996;61:1865–1869.

Penning S, Thomas N, Atwal D, Nageotte M, McConnell D. Cardiopulmonary bypass support for emergency cesarean delivery in a patient with severe pulmonary hypertension. Am J Obstet Gynecol 2001;184:225–226.

Philbin DM. Pulsatile blood flow. Baltimore: Williams and Wilkins, 1993:323–337.

Plomondon ME, Cleveland JC, Jr., Ludwig ST, et al. Off-pump coronary artery bypass is associated with improved risk-adjusted outcomes. Ann Thorac Surg 2001;72:114–119.

Plunkett MD, Bond LM, Geiss DM. Staged repair of acute type I aortic dissection and coarctation in pregnancy. Ann Thorac Surg 2000; 69:1945–1947.

Pomini F, Mercogliano D, Cavalletti C, Caruso A, Pomini P. Cardiopulmonary bypass in pregnancy. Ann Thorac Surg 1996;61:259–268.

Roach GW, Kanchuger M, Mangano CM, et al. Adverse cerebral outcomes after coronary bypass surgery. Multicenter Study of Perioperative Ischemia Research Group and the Ischemia Research and

Education Foundation Investigators. New Engl J Med 1996;335: 1857–1863.

Roe BB, Edmunds LH, Jr., Fishman NH, Hutchinson JC. Open mitral valvulotomy. Ann Thorac Surg 1971;12:483–491.

Rossouw GJ, Knott-Craig CJ, Barnard PM, Macgregor LA, Van Zyl WP. Intracardiac operation in seven pregnant women. Ann Thorac Surg 1993;55:1172–1174.

Sabik JF, Assad RS, Hanley FL. Prostaglandin synthesis inhibition prevents placental dysfunction after fetal cardiac bypass. J Thorac Cardiovasc Surg 1992;103:733–741.

Sabik JF, Heinemann MK, Assad RS, Hanley FL. High-dose steroids prevent placental dysfunction after fetal cardiac bypass. J Thorac Cardiovasc Surg 1994;107:116–124.

Shaw PJ, Bates D, Cartlidge NE, et al. Neurologic and neuropsychological morbidity following major surgery: comparison of coronary artery bypass and peripheral vascular surgery. Stroke 1987;18: 700–707.

Shnider SM, Webster GM. Maternal and fetal hazards of surgery during pregnancy. Am J Obstet Gynecol 1965;92:891–900.

Silberman S, Fink D, Berko RS, Mendzelevski B, Bitran D. Coronary artery bypass surgery during pregnancy. Eur J Cardiothorac Surg 1996;10:925–926.

Skillman CA, Plessinger MA, Woods JR, Clark KE. Effect of graded reductions in uteroplacental blood flow on the fetal lamb. Am J Physiol 1985;249:H1098–1105.

Smith BE. Fetal prognosis after anesthesia during gestation. Anesth Analg 1963;42:521–526.

Strickland RA, Oliver WC, Jr., Chantigian RC, Ney JA, Danielson GK. Anesthesia, cardiopulmonary bypass, and the pregnant patient. Mayo Clin Proc 1991;66:411–429.

Trimakas AP, Maxwell KD, Berkay S, Gardner TJ, Achuff SC. Fetal monitoring during cardiopulmonary bypass for removal of a left atrial myxoma during pregnancy. Johns Hopkins Med J 1979;144: 156–160.

Tripp HF, Stiegel RM, Coyle JP. The use of pulsatile perfusion during aortic valve replacement in pregnancy. Ann Thorac Surg 1999; 67:1169–1171.

Ueland K. Cardiac surgery and pregnancy. Am J Obstet Gynecol 1965;92:148.

Uygur D, Beksac MS. Mitral balloon valvuloplasty during pregnancy in developing countries. Eur J Obstet Gyn Reprod Biol 2001;96: 226–228.

Vedrinne C, Tronc F, Martinot S, et al. Effects of various flow types on maternal hemodynamics during fetal bypass: is there nitric oxide release during pulsatile perfusion? J Thorac Cardiovasc Surg 1998; 116:432–439.

Vedrinne C, Tronc F, Martinot S, et al. Better preservation of endothelial function and decreased activation of the fetal renin-angiotensin pathway with the use of pulsatile flow during experimental fetal bypass. J Thorac Cardiovasc Surg 2000;120:770–777.

Veray FX, Hernandez CJJ, Raffucci F, Pelegrina IA. Pregnancy after cardiac surgery. Conn Med 1970;34:496–499.

Vosloo S, Reichart B. The feasibility of closed mitral valvotomy in pregnancy. J Thorac Cardiovasc Surg 1987;93:675–679.

Weiss BM, von Segesser LK, Alon E, Seifert B, Turina MI. Outcome of cardiovascular surgery and pregnancy: a systematic review of the period 1984–1996. Am J Obstet Gynecol 1998;179:1643–1653.

Werch A, Lambert HM, Cooley D, Reed CC. Fetal monitoring and maternal open heart surgery. Southern Med J 1977;70:1024.

Westaby S, Parry AJ, Forfar JC. Reoperation for prosthetic valve endocarditis in the third trimester of pregnancy. Ann Thorac Surg 1992;53:263–265.

Zitnik RS, Brandenburg RO, Sheldon R, Wallace RB. Pregnancy and open-heart surgery. Circulation 1969;39:5(Suppl 1):257–262.

14 Noninvasive monitoring

John Anthony
Michael A. Belfort

The appropriate management of critically ill patients requires frequent observation of biophysical variables. The most important of these variables describe the delivery of oxygenated blood to the peripheral tissues. Peripheral oxygen saturation and markers of hemodynamic function are essential prerequisites in the provision of intensive care, the development of which was initially based upon the accuracy and utility of pulmonary artery catheters as an investigative tool. While this technology has remained synonymous with critical care practice it is now recognized that the invasive nature of this monitoring is associated with a range of complications. Newer, noninvasive technologies have been developed that now provide similar, or more extensive data with fewer risks.

Noninvasive hemodynamic assessment has permitted the collection of diagnostic and research data beyond the arena of critical care. Information derived from the use of echocardiography in particular has helped to expand our understanding of many conditions including the physiological events of normal pregnancy, the pathogenesis of preeclampsia, the abnormalities characteristic of various forms of heart disease, and a variety of medical disorders. In some circumstances, echocardiography has become an integral part of the prepregnancy and antenatal assessment of women with heart disease.

This chapter will review some aspects of this technology and the clinical issues associated with the use of noninvasive monitoring that may be encountered in obstetric practice.

The measurement of cardiac output

An adequate cardiac output is essential to deliver oxygenated blood to the peripheral tissues. Low output will reflect either hypovolemia or ventricular failure. Knowledge of the cardiac output will determine management and will also allow calculation of other derived hemodynamic values including vascular resistance and oxygen delivery and consumption indices.

In the past, cardiac output was measured using the Fick principle. This principle states that the amount of a substance taken up by the body per unit time equals the difference between the arterial and venous levels multiplied by the blood flow. Hence, oxygen consumption by the body divided by the arteriovenous oxygen difference equals the cardiac output. This principle has been modified to use other markers including dye dilution techniques and the thermodilution principle of the pulmonary artery catheter. In the latter case, iced water is the marker injected into the right atrium with a probe measuring the temperature of the blood flowing through the pulmonary artery thus allowing the derivation of the cardiac output from the area under the curve. This technique, although clinically robust, may produce results that are confounded by variations in catheter position, variations in injectate temperature and volume, as well as differences in the rate of saline injection.

These technologies have nevertheless contributed to our understanding of physiology and pathophysiology and remain the gold standard against which newer techniques are assessed. The need to cannulate peripheral and central vessels has been associated with some risk of injury and justified the search for safer technology.

Ultrasound in the form of echocardiography allows estimation of cardiac output by measuring changes in left ventricular dimensions during systole measured in the plane below the level of the mitral valve. By assuming that the ventricle is ellipsoid in shape and that the long axis is double the short axis, stroke volume can be calculated from the cube of the change in left ventricular dimension. This measurement is inaccurate when the assumptions upon which it is based are no longer true. Hence, the dilated ventricle and the pregnant woman with an increased volume and end-diastolic dimensions violate these assumptions and may overestimate stroke volume and cardiac output.

Doppler ultrasound has added to the utility of echocardiography by allowing an estimation of blood velocity. The Doppler principle measures the frequency of a reflected ultrasound beam striking moving erythrocytes where the change in frequency detected is proportional to the velocity of the red cells moving in the axis of the beam. The velocity of a column of red cells multiplied by the period of ejection provides a measure of the distance travelled by a column of blood during systole. The use of ultrasound to measure the diameter of the vessels containing the blood will allow calculation of cross-sectional area with subsequent derivation of stroke volume and cardiac output. The velocity of blood flow can also be related to the pressure gradient down which the blood is moving providing a way of calculating intracardiac pressure gradients and pulmonary artery pressures.

Doppler probes may be range-gated (pulsed) to allow the measurement of a signal from a given depth of tissue. The pulsed Doppler signal usually allows simultaneous ultrasound imaging and estimation of the angle of insonation between the Doppler probe and the vessel. This latter measurement is important because the calculation of velocity from the reflected Doppler signal requires a knowledge of the angle between the ultrasound beam and the column of blood from which the signal is being reflected. Where the signal is perpendicular to the moving column of blood, no movement will be detected, and the closer the beam moves to being parallel to the vessel, the more completely the reflected vector represents the velocity of the cells in the path of the beam.

The combination of cross-sectional echocardiography and Doppler measurement of flow velocity at specific points in the heart and great vessels allows the determination of volumetric flow. The mitral and aortic valve orifices and the root or arch of the aorta have all been studied using both suprasternal and intraesophageal Doppler probes. Potential for error exists in these techniques both in the calculation of the insonation angle and the measurement of the cross-sectional area of the vessel. Of the different sites studied, the best correlation between the Doppler technique and thermodilution studies was documented in the aortic valve orifice measurements. Although transthoracic Doppler studies are the most widely accessible tool, transesophageal Doppler allows the posterior structures of the heart to be more clearly imaged with more accurate diagnosis of cardiac pathology and precise alignment to the aortic valve in both the long and short axis as well as providing long axis views of the ascending aorta (Flachskampf et al., 1992). The use of multiplanar transesophageal echocardiography allows precise measurements of asymmetric ventricles that cannot be reliably imaged using a transthoracic probe (Krebs et al., 1996). The probe has particular utility in the diagnosis of aortic dissection and thromboembolism (Lee et al., 1992) although the need for esophageal endoscopy limits the application of this technology to specific situations including intraoperative and postoperative care.

Other techniques of measuring cardiac output include impedance cardiography based upon changes in transthoracic electrical resistance associated with the ejection of blood into the pulmonary circulation. This technique has been shown to overestimate low cardiac output with the opposite error in high cardiac output states.

Doppler ultrasound and the physiology of pregnancy

Doppler techniques have confirmed the increased cardiac output and stroke volume of pregnancy associated with progressive increases in left atrial dimension and function.

Both filling phases of the left ventricle show increased filling velocities (E- and A-wave velocity). The increase in early wave velocity occurs by the end of the first trimester whereas the peak A-wave velocity changes occur in the third trimester. The E/A ratio increases in the first trimester but falls again as the A-wave velocity increases and is accompanied by decreasing left ventricular isovolumetric relaxation time (Mesa et al., 1999; Valensise et al., 2000).

Left ventricular mass increases significantly while fractional shortening and velocity of shortening diminish throughout pregnancy (Mone et al., 1996). Systolic function is preserved by falling systemic (including uterine artery) resistance (Mesa et al., 1999; Valensise et al., 2000). Peak left ventricular wall stress, an indicator of afterload, has been demonstrated in early pregnancy and normalizes as ventricular mass increases in the mid-trimester (Mone et al., 1996). Geva et al. (1997) similarly report a 45% increase in cardiac output in normal pregnancy accompanied by an increase in left ventricular end-diastolic volume and increased end-systolic wall stress accompanied by transient left ventricular hypertrophy. These authors also report a reversible decline in left ventricular function during the second and third trimesters.

Systemic arterial vascular compliance is thought to diminish because of reduced vascular tone (Poppas et al., 1997).

The pulmonary circulation shows increased flow during pregnancy with some reduction in vascular resistance without any significant alteration in blood pressure. These changes are evident by 8 weeks' gestation without any subsequent alteration and return to prepregnancy values by 6 months' postpartum (Robson et al., 1991).

Doppler ultrasound and critical care

There are few studies that address this issue and noninvasive techniques for the routine estimation of stroke volume and ventricular filling pressures have only been recently reported in the obstetric literature. Validation studies have, however, been conducted and show reliable correlation between noninvasive techniques and values derived by the use of pulmonary artery catheters. Two-dimensional and Doppler echocardiography was used to demonstrate this in a group of 11 critically ill obstetric patients. The findings of this study showed a high correlation between invasive and noninvasive techniques in the measurement of stroke volume and cardiac output. Ventricular filling pressures and pulmonary artery pressures also showed a similar significant correlation with invasive techniques (Belfort et al., 1994).

The specific choice of echocardiographic technique for estimating stroke volume and ejection fraction was explored in the same group of patients. Comparisons between M-mode and two-dimensional Doppler techniques revealed similar findings although M-mode echocardiography was not possible in two out of 11 subjects. This study also allowed calculation of the ejection fraction by dividing the stroke volume by the end-diastolic volume. Using this equation, similar results were obtained by all the methods employed (Rokey et al., 1995).

Belfort et al. have reported a series of 14 patients with an indication for invasive hemodynamic monitoring in whom Doppler ultrasound was used as a guide to clinical management. These 14 women had a spectrum of pathologies ranging from intractable hypertension to complex cardiac lesions and included women with oliguria and pulmonary edema. This pilot study concluded that the monitoring had facilitated management and only two patients went on to have invasive monitoring in order to allow continuous monitoring. Large volumes of fluid were administered to some of these patients (up to 8 L of crystalloid) without fluid overload or pulmonary edema developing. To date this is the only study that has indicated the potential utility of routine rapid echocardiographic assessment of left ventricular function in critically ill obstetric patients (Belfort et al., 1997).

Doppler ultrasound and preeclampsia

Doppler echocardiography has provided a ready means of studying women at risk of developing hypertensive complications during pregnancy. Longitudinal studies have demonstrated that women with nonproteinuric or gestational hypertension maintain a hyperdynamic circulation with a high cardiac output throughout pregnancy. By contrast women destined to develop preeclampsia have significantly elevated cardiac output without any change in systemic resistance in the preclinical phase of the disease. This is followed by a fall in cardiac output and increasing resistance co-incident with the onset of clinical disease (Bosio et al., 1999).

More recently, studies have focused on echocardiographically described cardiac structure and function in preeclampsia, especially in relation to levels of atrial and brain natriuretic peptide (ANP, BNP). Initial work had related elevated ANP levels to increased left atrial dimensions following delivery in normal pregnancies. These increased ANP levels did not lead to any demonstrable diuresis in normal postpartum women. Women with preeclampsia had bigger atria and higher ANP levels in the early puerperium and these changes were associated with natriuresis and diuresis. The hypothesis related by these findings was that increased atrial distension in preeclampsia triggered a diuretic response.

These data have been contested. The most detailed study, to date, by Borghi et al. described detailed cardiac findings among 40 women with mild preeclampsia compared to a control cohort of pregnant women and nonpregnant controls. This study showed a progressive rise in left ventricular mass between nonpregnant women compared to normal pregnancy with a further increase in mass among women with preeclampsia. Ejection fraction and fractional shortening decreased in normal pregnancy while not reaching statistical significance. However, women with preeclampsia had a significant reduction in both these parameters in comparison to nonpregnant women. In addition, left ventricular end-diastolic volume rose significantly in preeclampsia. Together with a fall in cardiac output in the preeclamptic group, these findings suggest a compensatory increase in ventricular size to maintain cardiac output against an elevated systemic vascular resistance.

The latter study also showed changes in the peak filling velocities of the left ventricle during diastole. The E/A ratio fell significantly during pregnancy, partly reflecting increased preload. In preeclamspsia further augmentation of the A-wave peak velocity resulted in further significant reduction in the ratio. Collectively these data support the notion of changes in both cardiac systolic and diastolic function. The authors also measured ANP levels. In keeping with previous studies elevated levels of ANP were found in pregnancy with further increments occurring in preeclampsia. These could not be accounted for by differences in atrial size although a significant correlation was found between left ventricular mass and volume in women with preeclampsia (Borghi et al., 2000).

Doppler ultrasound and cardiomyopathy

Doppler ultrasound has an important role in the management and evaluation of women with impaired ventricular function.

Echocardiography is used to delineate impaired left ventricular systolic function in women with suspected peripartum cardiomyopathy. It plays a further role in the ongoing evaluation of women once this diagnosis has been made. Specifically the prognosis has been related to the normalization of left ventricular size and function within 6 months of delivery (Pearson et al., 2000). Currently accepted opinion is that approximately 50% of affected women will recover normal function. Those who have persistently impaired function face a significant risk of mortality (Pearson et al., 2000).

Subsequent pregnancies in women with a prior diagnosis of cardiomyopathy demand careful echocardiographic assessment. Although no clear agreement exists regarding risk, those with persistently abnormal left ventricular function have been advised against pregnancy. Conflicting reports have been made concerning those who become pregnant. De Souza et al. report on the evaluation of seven women who became pregnant after developing peripartum cardiomyopathy in a previous pregnancy. All pregnancies were well tolerated without significant change in symptomatology. Echocardiographic studies showed no change in left ventricular end-diastolic diameters with an increase occurring in left ventricular fractional shortening (De Souza et al., 2001). Other studies have reported similarly successful pregnancies (Sutton et al., 1991). However, there are papers suggesting a risk of recurrent cardiomyopathy and impaired contractile reserve, even in those with apparently normal left ventricular function prior to pregnancy (Demakis et al., 1971; Lampert et al., 1997).

Doppler ultrasound and other medical disorders

Echocardiocardiography is an essential investigation in women with structural heart disease due to valvular damage or congenital malformation (Gultekin et al., 1994; Ben Farhat et al., 1997; Martinez Reding et al., 1998; Niwa et al., 1999; Wilansky et al., 1999; Barbosa et al., 2000; Mangione et al., 2000). Although not a frequent occurrence, echocardiography will also contribute to the diagnosis of Libman Sacks endocarditis that occurs among women suffering from systemic lupus erythematosus, with or without antiphospholipid antibodies (Gleason et al., 1993; Hojnik et al., 1996).

The management of Marfan's syndrome also requires echocardiographic assessment because of the risk of catastrophic aortic dissection. Transesophageal echocardiography is the preferred method for evaluating the ascending aorta. The risk of dissection correlates with an aortic root diameter greater than 4 cm (Elkayam et al., 1995). Aortic dissection may also occur under other circumstances and may follow the use of crack cocaine (Ecknauer et al., 1999; Madu et al., 1999).

The role of transesophageal Doppler

Esophageal Doppler monitoring of hemodynamic data has been carried out in adult intensive care units and found to be equivalent to data derived from pulmonary artery catheter measurements (Singer et al., 1989). Pregnancy data are few and only one study has reported the use of transesophageal Doppler monitoring in pregnancy compared to pulmonary artery catheters. This study showed that the Doppler consistently underestimated cardiac output by 40% in women under the age of 35 years (Penny et al., 2000). This error may be due to the assumptions implicit in the algorithm used to calculate output. These assumptions include a fixed aortic diameter during systole and a fixed percentage of blood perfusing upper and lower parts of the body Pregnancy physiological changes probably invalidate these assumptions. The authors nevertheless conclude that esophageal Doppler may contribute to the estimation of trends over time.

Oximetry in the intensive care environment

Spectrophotometry is the detection of specific light frequencies reflected by a range of molecules. Specific molecules reflect specific frequencies and their reflective properties differ with changes in molecular conformation. Oximetry is the detection of oxygenated and deoxygenated blood. The oxygenated hemoglobin reflects more light at 660 nm whereas at 940 nm deoxyhemoglobin reflects infrared light more strongly. This allows the simultaneous acquisition of peripheral signals from which the ratio of oxy- to deoxyhemoglobin can be calculated and expressed as a percentage of oxyhemoglobin saturation.

Oximetry may be based on transcutaneous measurements or can be derived from mixed venous blood via a probe located in a pulmonary artery catheter. The peripheral pulse oximetry devices rely on detection of pulsed alterations in light transmitted between transmitter and a photodetector. This filtered signal is necessary to eliminate the signal arising from venous blood that would contain more deoxyhemoglobin.

Although oximetry is regarded as an effective method of monitoring oxygenation, some limitations are recognized. They include the assumptions that methemoglobin and carboxyhemoglobin are not present in significant concentrations. Mixed venous oxygen saturation monitoring is less frequently used than peripheral oxygen saturation monitoring. It also shows greater spontaneous variation than peripheral monitors but has a clinical role to play in determining the balance between peripheral oxygen delivery and peripheral oxygen consumption. This is a robust measurement that will reflect changes in cardiac output, hemoglobin concentration, arterial and venous hemoglobin oxygen saturation. This provides useful clinical information in many clinical circumstances. A number of the determinants of the ultimate mixed venous oxygen saturation value have the potential to change at any given moment (hemoglobin, oxygen saturation, and cardiac output). It is therefore important to understand that it is only when all other parameters remain stable that changes in the mixed venous oxygen saturation reflect changes in cardiac output.

Capnometery

Exhaled gas can be evaluated using an infrared probe and a photodetector set to detect carbon dioxide. This is usually found in the expiratory limb of a ventilator circuit. Expired gas shows a pattern of increasing carbon dioxide concentration related to the sequential expiration of air in the upper airway followed by air from the alveoli. The end-expiratory (or end-tidal) carbon dioxide concentration should approximate the partial pressure of carbon dioxide in arterial blood. The development of a gradient between these measurements reflects an increase in anatomical or physiological dead space. In the latter event, low cardiac output and pulmonary embolism may both affect the measurement. Changes in end-tidal partial pressure of carbon dioxide have been correlated to changes in cardiac output and may be used as a means of monitoring the efficacy of resuscitation.

Transcranial Doppler ultrasound

The normal cerebral blood flow changes of pregnancy are poorly documented compared with the physiologic alterations in other vascular beds during gestation. This is due, partly, to technical difficulties associated with in vivo studies of blood flow in the human brain. Angiography, the gold standard in the evaluation of the cerebral vasculature, is an invasive test and presents obvious ethical concerns for its use in normal pregnant women. Very few data on the physiologic adaptations of the brain to pregnancy are available in the current literature and most texts dealing with the changes of pregnancy do not address this issue at all. There are also ethical problems with using angiography and other methodologies involving radiation, as well as magnetic resonance imaging during pregnancy. The advent of Doppler ultrasound, and in particular transcranial Doppler (TCD) ultrasound, has changed this. It is now possible to acquire Doppler-derived velocity information from most of the basal brain arteries (including almost all of the Circle of Willis branches) with a noninvasive technique. Using these data, it is possible to diagnose arterial malformations, functional abnormalities, and physiological changes in brain blood velocity. One can detect direction and velocity of blood flow, and from this infer the presence of distal or proximal arterial constriction or dilatation. In addition, TCD can be used to determine real-time changes over very short time intervals and to continuously monitor cerebral blood velocity during surgical procedures, or experimental drug protocols. TCD has been extensively used in the clinical scenario by neurologists and neurosurgeons to detect and follow cerebral vasospasm in patients with subarachnoid hemorrhage (Aaslid et al., 1984). Investigators are beginning to use TCD to define pregnancy-induced/associated changes in the cerebral circulation.

Belfort et al. (2001) have recently defined the hemodynamic changes, specifically velocity, resistance indices, and cerebral perfusion pressure, in the middle cerebral artery distribution of the brain during normal pregnancy. TCD, ultrasound was used to determine the systolic, diastolic, and mean blood velocities in the middle cerebral arteries in non-laboring women studied longitudinally (at 4-week intervals) during normal gestation. The resistance index (RI), pulsatility index (PI), and cerebral perfusion pressure (CPP) were calculated using the velocity and blood pressure data. The mean value, and the 5% and 95% percentiles, were defined and it was noted that the middle cerebral artery (MCA) velocities and the resistance and pulsatility indices decrease, while the CPP increases, during normal pregnancy. Figure 14.1 shows the CPP change during normal pregnancy. This study defined the normative ranges for middle cerebral artery velocity, resistance indices, and cerebral perfusion pressure during normal human pregnancy using longitudinally collected data.

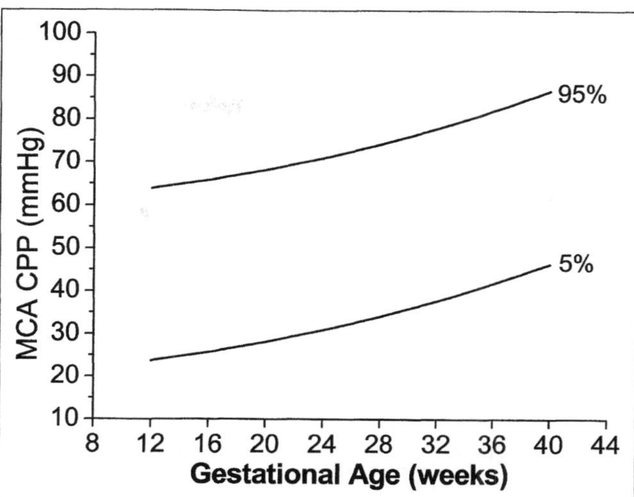

Fig. 14.1 Cerebral perfusion pressure (CPP) changes during a normal pregnancy.

Doppler ultrasound, bias and confounders

There are a number of confounding influences that can affect the interpretation of Doppler cerebral velocity data. These include any factors that may: (i) increase the CO_2 or H^+ tension in the cerebral circulation; (ii) decrease or increase the hemoglobin concentration; (iii) independently alter the diameter of the vessel being studied at the point of insonation; and (iv) introduce error, such as cigarette smoking and changes in posture. In pregnant women: (v) gestational age is another important factor that requires consideration, since as the pregnancy progresses there are significant hemodynamic changes.

Increased CO_2 tension leads to cerebral vasodilation, as does acidosis. Patients undergoing cerebral Doppler studies should, ideally, be studied in a steady state or should have their end-tidal CO_2 tension measured in order to control for fluctuations. Even the minimal increases in tidal volume and respiratory rate associated with labor contractions may be of importance. Labor itself has been shown to be associated with decreases in mean middle cerebral artery flow velocity.

Hemoconcentration and hemodilution are also important and attention should be paid to the hematocrit level in studies where blood loss or volume infusion may have altered the hemoglobin content of the blood during the study period.

The segmental nature of the vasospasm seen in some conditions, notably preeclampsia, is of concern as well since the same segment of artery can show completely different velocity profiles depending on its state of contraction. Thus, if the region of vessel being insonated is apt to change, its diameter velocity readings may be inaccurate, particularly if some indication of downstream vascular condition is being extrapolated. In this regard, the M1 portion of the middle cerebral artery has been shown to be unlikely to change diameter (Gibo et al., 1981), since it is well supported by alveolar tissue in its bony canal. The angle of insonation is critical since the velocity is related to the cos of the angle of insonation (q). If q is less than 10° the error involved is almost negligible and quite acceptable for most purposes. Because of the anatomy of the bony canal through which the M1 portion of the MCA runs, the angle of insonation very rarely exceeds 10°. This ensures that, in almost all cases, once the optimum signal is obtained the angle of insonation is less than 10°.

The effect of maternal cigarette smoking on middle cerebral artery blood flow velocities during normal pregnancy was described by Irion et al. (1996). They found that the systolic, diastolic, and mean velocities of the middle cerebral artery, detected in both the left lateral decubitus and sitting positions, were significantly higher at 18 and 26 weeks' gestation in women who smoked cigarettes. They determined that the number of cigarettes smoked positively correlated with increased middle cerebral artery velocities. This factor must be taken into account when studying women known to smoke, and is an important confounding factor in some of the earlier studies published. Posture should be taken into account when studying pregnant, and in particular, preeclamptic pregnant women. A change from lying to sitting has been shown to significantly increase both systolic and diastolic velocities in the middle cerebral artery in such patients.

Another important variable that must be taken into account when studying pregnant women is the gestational age. As pregnancy advances there is a reduction in middle cerebral artery velocity which should be controlled for when comparing women of different gestational ages.

Cerebral perfusion pressure

Under normal conditions, the arterioles in the cerebrovascular system are responsible for about 80% of the vascular resistance. Because arterioles have active smooth muscle tone, they do not behave simply like tubes of variable dimension. Smooth muscle tone in the arterioles reduces their diameter when systolic pressure is transmitted into them via the arteries. In addition, this tone also tends to close the arterioles when pressure falls during the pulse cycle. Under conditions of low vascular resistance, the arterioles remain open throughout the pulse cycle and the active smooth muscle tone never causes them to close completely. However, even a slight increase in arteriolar tone will narrow the diameter of open arterioles and, in some cases, cause them to close completely when the pressure within them falls at the end of the pulse cycle. The pressure at which an arteriole closes is called its "critical closing pressure" (Dewey et al., 1974; Aaslid et al., 1984). Critical closing pressure explains why arterioles close as pressure falls during the pulse cycle and why fewer arterioles are open at the end of the pulse cycle than earlier, when pressure is at its systolic maximum. Thus, pressure at the end of a pulse cycle is less effective in perfusing the capillary bed than that early in the cycle. In the brain, CPP is reduced as arteriolar resistance rises abruptly due to more and more arterioles reaching their critical closing pressure. Another feature of arteriolar tone is its effect in delaying the flow of blood from arteries to capillaries. When arteriolar tone is high it reduces the rate of blood flow from arteries to capillaries. This maintains the arterial blood pressure at a higher level for a longer portion of the pulse cycle than if the arteriolar tone was low and there was a rapid runoff of blood. Blood pressure distends the arterial segments and blood is effectively stored in the arteries while the pressure decays during the pulse cycle. The amount stored in each segment depends on the compliance of the artery and the pressure gradient between the lumen and the region outside the artery. The result of storing blood in the arteries and reducing the rate of flow through arterioles is to slow the deceleration of blood flow during the pulse cycle. The more compliant the arterial segment, the slower the deceleration during the pulse cycle. This feature of arteriolar tone interacting with arterial pressure and arterial compliance affects the shape of the velocity profile during the pulse cycle. When arteriolar tone is low, blood velocity rapidly rises to a maximum and falls quickly to a minimum. In contrast, when arteriolar tone is high, the blood flow velocity falls more slowly. The area under the pulsatile amplitude of the velocity waveform, and the height of the pulse velocity wave, may be used to estimate the proportion of blood flow stored in arterial segments during the peak of the pulse cycle and released when pressure falls during the cycle.

One of the major problems with the currently used Doppler indices is that they were initially developed for use in peripheral vascular examination of large diameter arteries such as the femoral, dorsalis pedis, and brachial arteries. Indices such as the PI and RI focus on the systolic component of the velocity profile. The traditional Doppler indices of hemodynamics (i.e. the RI and PI) provide limited data regarding arteriolar tone when applied to the cerebral circulation. Both the RI defined as $(\text{velocity}_{\text{systolic}} - \text{velocity}_{\text{diastolic}})/(\text{velocity}_{\text{systolic}})$ and the PI defined as $(\text{velocity}_{\text{systolic}} - \text{velocity}_{\text{diastolic}})/(\text{velocity}_{\text{mean}})$ are significantly influenced by the systolic velocity which reflects large-caliber arterial constriction. These indices were originally developed using older technology and larger diameter arteries (femoral artery and aorta). The typical waveform shape from such arteries has a tall peaked systolic component, a steep diastolic slope, and a low/nonexistent diastolic component. The smaller diameter arteries that are now easily visualized with modern equipment provide completely different waveforms from those seen in the larger diameter, higher velocity, and higher resistance vessels. Using indices that focus on the systolic velocity tends to ignore aspects of waveform shape peculiar to lower resistance vascular beds. Specifically, the typical waveform seen in low resistance, low velocity, smaller diameter arteries has a low systolic velocity, flatter diastolic downslope, and a proportionately higher diastolic velocity, than that seen in high resistance, high velocity arteries.

A further deficiency of the current cerebral Doppler assessment techniques is that they fail to take into account the systemic arterial pressure, a vital component of the cerebral perfusion pressure. In 1986 Aaslid et al. validated a Doppler method of estimating CPP. They measured velocity in the middle cerebral artery (Doppler ultrasound), and intraventricular pressure and radial arterial blood pressure (direct strain gauge transducers) in 10 patients undergoing a supratentorial shunt procedure. They estimated CPP using the following ratio: (mean flow velocity)/(pulsatile amplitude of flow velocity) multiplied by the arterial blood pressure. To increase the accuracy, Fourier analysis was used and only the amplitude of the first harmonic of the pulsatility in both flow-velocity and arterial blood pressure recordings were used. They expressed their calculations as:

$$\mathrm{CPP} = \frac{V_0}{V_1} \times \mathrm{ABP}_1$$

where V_0 is the mean and V_1 is the amplitude of the first harmonic of the velocity waveform, and ABP_1 is the first harmonic of the arterial pressure wave. Their experimental results confirmed the validity of the method. The standard deviation between estimated CPP (CPP_e) and measured CPP (CPP_m) was 8.2 mmHg at a CPP of 40 mmHg, and the mean deviation was only 1 mmHg.

Belfort et al. (2000) have adapted the method of Aaslid et al. (1986) by altering the formula to reflect the area under the pulsatile amplitude of the flow velocity and arterial blood pressure waveforms rather than the first harmonic. Their equation, using areas under pulsatile amplitudes, is as follows (Belfort et al., 2000):

$$\mathrm{CPP} = \frac{\mathrm{Velocity}_{\mathrm{mean}}}{\mathrm{Velocity}_{\mathrm{mean}} - \mathrm{Velocity}_{\mathrm{diastolic}}} \times (\mathrm{BP}_{\mathrm{mean}} - \mathrm{BP}_{\mathrm{diastolic}})$$

Recently Belfort et al. (2002) have suggested that elevated CPP, rather than decreased CBF, is the key determinant of cerebral injury in preeclampsia/eclampsia. Since this technology is still in its infancy as a noninvasive monitoring tool in severe preeclamptics routine use of this modality is not recommended until further research has confirmed the findings. However, in those cases of refractory seizure activity unresponsive to conventional therapy, TCD may offer another diagnostic option. In those cases where CPP is shown to be significantly elevated, drug therapy can be tailored to lowering the CPP (i.e. with labetalol) versus those rare cases where there is a low CPP and presumably cerebral ischemia from underperfusion, a cerebral vasodilator such as nimodipine can be used.

Conclusion

Noninvasive techniques of monitoring will become increasingly utilized as an alternative to the invasive techniques currently practiced in most intensive care units. This technology, however, requires expertise in the application and interpretation of data. Even correctly interpreted data are of unknown utility and stringent evaluation is necessary before this (often) expensive technology is incorporated into routine clinical practice.

References

Aaslid R, Huber P, Nornes H. Evaluation of cerebrovascular spasm with transcranial Doppler ultrasound. J Neurosurg 1984;60(10): 37–41.

Aaslid R, Lundar T, Lindegaard KF, Nornes H. Estimation of cerebral perfusion pressure from arterial blood pressure and transcranial Doppler recordings. In: Miller JD, Teasdale GM, Rowan JO, Galbraith SL, Mendelow AD, eds. Intracranial Pressure VI. Berlin Heidelberg: Springer-Verlag, 1986:226–229.

Barbosa PJ, Lopes AA, Feitosa GS, et al. Prognostic factors of reheumatic mitral stenosis during pregnancy and puerperium. Arq Bras Cardiol 2000;75(3):215–224.

Belfort MA, Rokey R, Saade GR, Moise KJ Jr. Rapid echocardiographic assessment of left and right heart hemodynamics in critically ill obstetric patients. Am J Obstet Gynecol 1994;171(4):884–892.

Belfort MA, Mares A, Saade GR, Wen T, Rokey R. Two-dimensional echocardiography and Doppler ultrasound in managing obstetric patients. Obstet Gynecol 1997;90(3):326–330.

Belfort MA, Tooke-Miller C, Varner M, et al. Evaluation of a noninvasive transcranial Doppler and blood pressure bases method for the assessment of cerebral perfusion pressure in pregnant women. Hypertens Pregnancy 2000;19(3):331–340.

Belfort MA, Tooke-Miller C, Allen JC, et al. Changes in flow velocity, resistance indices, and cerebral perfusion pressure in the maternal middle cerebral artery distribution during normal pregnancy. Acta Obstet Gynecol Scand 2001;80:104–112.

Belfort MA, Varner MC, Dizon-Townson DS, Grunewald C, Nisell H. Cerebral perfusion pressure, and not cerebral blood flow, may be the critical determinant of intracranial injury in preeclampsia: a new hypothesis. Am J Obstet Gynecol 2002;187:626–634.

Ben Farhat M, Gamra H, Betbout F, et al. Percutaneous balloon mitral commissurotomy during pregnancy. Heart 1997;77(6):564–567.

Borghi C, Esposti DD, Immordino V, et al. Relationship of systemic hemodynamics, left ventricular structure and function, and plasma natriuretic peptide concentrations during pregnancy complicated by preeclampsia. Am J Obstet Gynecol 2000;183(1):140–147.

Bosio PM, McKenna PJ, Conroy R, O'Herlihy C. Maternal central hemodynamics in hypertensive discorders of pregnancy. Obstet Gynecol 1999;94(6):978–984.

De Souza JL, de Carvalho Frimm C, Nastari L, Mady C. Left ventricular function after a new pregnancy in patients with peripartum cardiomyopathy. J Card Fail 2001;7(1):30–35.

Demakis JG, Rahimtoola SH, Sutton GC, et al. Natural course of peripartum cardiomyopathy. Circulation 1971;44:1053–1061.

Dewey RC, Pieper HP, Hunt WE. Experimental cerebral hemodynamics. Vasomotor tone, critical closing pressure, and vascular bed resistance. J Neurosurg 1974;41(5):597–606.

Ecknauer E, Schmidlin D, Jenni R, Schmid ER. Emergency repair of incidentally diagnosed ascending aortic aneurysm immediately after caesarean section. Br J Anaesth 1999;83(2):343–345.

Elkayam U, Ostrzega E, Shotan A, Hehra A. Cardiovascular problems in pregnant women with the Marfan syndrome. Ann Intern Med 1995;123(2):117–122.

Flachskampf FA, Hoffmann R, Verlande M, Schneider W, Ameling W, Hanrath P. Initial experience with a multiplane transoesophageal echo-transducer: assessment of diagnostic potential. Eur Heart J 1992;13(9):120–126.

Geva T, Mauer MB, Striker L, Kirshon B, Pivarnik JM. Effects of physiologic load of pregnancy on left ventricular contractility and remodelling. Am Heart J 1997;133:53–59.

Gibo H, Carver CC, Rhoton AL, Jr., Lenkey C, Mitchell RJ. Microsurgical anatomy of the middle cerebral artery. J Neurosurg 1981; 54(2):151–169.

Gleason CB, Stoddard MF, Wagner SG, Longaker RA, Pierangeli S, Harris EN. A comparison of cardiac valvular involvement in the primary antiphospholipid syndrome versus anticardiolipin-negative systemic lupus erythematosus. Am Heart J 1993;125(4):1123–1129.

Gultekin F, Baskin E, Gokalp A, Dogan K. A pregnant woman with Ebstein's anomaly. A case report. Mater Med Pol 1994;26(4): 149–151.

Hojnik M, George J, Ziporen L, Shoenfeld Y. Heart valve involvement (Libman-Sacks endocarditis) in the antiphospholipid syndrome. Circulation 1996;93(8):1579–1587.

Irion O, Moutquin JM, Williams K, Forest JC. Reference values and influence of smoking on maternal middle cerebral artery blood flow. Am J Obstet Gynecol 1996;174:367A.

Krebs W, Klues HG, Steinert S, et al. Left ventricular volume calculations using a multiplanar transoesophageal echoprobe; in vitro validation and comparison with biplane angiography. Eur Heart J 1996;17(8):1279–1288.

Lampert M, Weinert L, Hibbard J, Korcarz C, Lindheimer M, Lang RM. Contractile reserve in patients with peripartum cardiomyopathy and recovered left ventricular function. Am J Obstet Gynecol 1997;176(1 pt 1):189–195.

Lee LC, Black IW, Hopkins A, Walsh WF. Transoesophageal echocardiography in heart disease—old technologies, new tricks. Aust N Z J Med 1992;22(5 Suppl):527–531.

Madu EC, Shala B, Baugh D. Crack-cocaine-associated aortic dissection in early pregnancy—a case report. Angiology 1999;50(2): 163–168.

Mangione JA, Lourenco RM, dos Santos ES, et al. Long-term follow-up of pregnant women after percutaneous mitral valvuloplasty. Catheter Cardiovasc Interv 2000;50(4):413–417.

Martinez Reding J, Cordero A, Kuri J, Martinez Rios MA, Salazar E. Treatment of severe mitral stenosis with percutaneous balloon valvotomy in pregnant patients. Clin Cardiol 1998;21(9):659–663.

Mesa A, Jessurun C, Hernandez A, et al. Left ventricular diastolic function in normal human pregnancy. Circulation 1999;99(4):511–517.

Mone SM, Sanders SP, Colan SD. Control mechanisms for physiological hypertrophy of pregnancy. Circulation 1996;94(4):667–672.

Niwa K, Perloff JK, Kaplan S, Child JS, Miner PD. Eisenmenger syndrome in adults: ventricular septal defect, truncus arteriosus, univentricular heart. J Am Coll Cardiol 1999;34(1):223–232.

Pearson GD, Veille JC, Rahimtoola S, et al. Peripartum cardiomyopathy: National Heart, Lung, and Blood Institute and Office of Rare Diseases (National Institutes of Health) workshop recommendations and review. JAMA 2000;283(9):1183–1188.

Penny JA, Anthony J, Shennan AH, de Swiet M, Singer M. A comparison of hemodynamic data derived by pulmonary artery flotation catheter and the esophageal Doppler monitor in preeclampsia. Am J Obstet Gynecol 2000;183:658–661.

Poppas A, Shroff SG, Korcarz CE, et al. Serial assessment of the cardiovascular system in normal pregnancy. Role of arterial compliance and pulsatile arterial load. Circulation 1997;95(10):2407–2415.

Robson SC, Hunter S, Boys RJ, Dunlop W. Serial changes in pulmonary haemodynamics during human pregnancy: a non-invasive study using Doppler echocardiography. Clin Sci (Colch) 1991:80(2): 113–117.

Rokey R, Belfort MA, Saade GR. Quantitative echocardiographic assessment of left ventricular function in critically ill obstetric patients: a comparative study. Am J Obstet Gynecol 1995;173(4): 1148–1152.

Singer M, Clarke J, Bennet ED. Continuous hemodynamic monitoring by esophageal Doppler. Crit Care Med 1989;17:447–452.

Sutton MS, Cole P, Plappert M, Saltzman D, Goldhaber S. Effects of subsequent pregnancy on left ventricular function in peripartum cardiomyopathy. Am Heart J 1991;121(6 Pt 1):1776–1778.

Valensise H, Novelli GP, Vasapollo B, et al. Maternal cardiac systolic and diastolic function: relationship with uteroplacental resistances. A Doppler and echocardiographic longitudinal study. Ultrasound Obstet Gynecol 2000;15(6):487–497.

Wilansky S, Phan B, Adam K. Doppler echocardiography as a predictor of pregnancy outcome in the presence of aortic stenosis: A case report. J Am Soc Echocardiogr 1999;12:324–325.

15 Pulmonary artery catheterization

Gary A. Dildy III
Steven L. Clark

Since its introduction into clinical medicine three decades ago, the pulmonary artery catheter has come to play an indispensable role in the management of critically ill patients in a number of specialties, including obstetrics (Swan et al., 1970; Clark et al., 1985; Clark & Cotton, 1988; European Society, 1991). Several prospective trials demonstrate the benefits of pulmonary artery catheterization in select critically ill patients. Such benefits include a reduction in operative morbidity and mortality in certain complicated surgical patients and a significant mortality reduction in patients in shock in whom catheter-obtained parameters lead to changes in therapy (Sola & Bender, 1993; Mimoz et al., 1994). In one study, management recommendations changed as a direct result of knowledge obtained by pulmonary artery catheter placement in 56% of patients admitted to an intensive care unit (Coles et al., 1993). In patients with major burn injuries, survival is predicted by early response to pulmonary artery catheter-guided resuscitation (Schiller et al., 1995). This technique, however, is not without its critics (Cruz & Franklin, 2001). In a nonrandomized observational study, Califf and colleagues (1996) demonstrated increased mortality and cost associated with pulmonary artery catheterization, and suggested that a randomized trial aimed at better patient selection is needed. One recent randomized controlled trial (n = 201) of the pulmonary artery catheter in critically ill patients concluded that its use is not associated with increased mortality (Rhodes et al., 2002).

In response to concerns of increased morbidity and mortality associated with the pulmonary catheter in observational studies, the National Heart, Lung, and Blood Institute (NHLBI) and the US Food and Drug Administration (FDA) conducted the Pulmonary Artery Catheterization and Clinical Outcomes workshop in 1997 to develop recommendations to improve pulmonary artery catheter utility and safety (Bernard et al., 2000). They concluded that a "need exists for collaborative education of physicians and nurses in performing, obtaining, and interpreting information from the use of pulmonary artery catheters. This effort should be led by professional societies, in collaboration with federal agencies, with the purpose of developing and disseminating standardized educational programs. Areas given high priority for clinical trials were pulmonary artery catheter use in persistent/refractory congestive heart failure, acute respiratory distress syndrome, severe sepsis and septic shock, and low-risk coronary artery bypass graft surgery."

This chapter provides an overview of placement techniques and complications; indications for the use of this diagnostic tool in the obstetric patient are examined in more detail in the ensuing chapters.

Catheter placement

The procedure for catheter placement involves two phases. The initial phase of pulmonary artery catheterization is establishing venous access with a large-bore sheath. Access is most commonly obtained via the internal jugular or subclavian veins; however, under certain circumstances (e.g. where access to the neck or thoracic region is difficult or in a patient with a coagulopathy where bleeding from a major artery could be hazardous), peripheral veins—including cephalic or femoral—can be used (Findling & Lipper, 1994). Insertion of the introducer sheath via the right internal jugular vein is described here.

Insertion of the sheath

To catheterize the internal jugular vein, the patient is placed supine in a mild Trendelenburg position with the head turned to the left. The landmark for insertion is the junction of the clavicular and sternal heads of the sternocleidomastoid muscle. When this junction is indistinct, its identification can be facilitated by having the patient raise her head slightly. When the landmark has been identified, 1% lidocaine is infiltrated into the skin and superficial subcutaneous tissue.

The internal jugular vein is entered first with a finder needle, consisting of a 21-gauge needle on a 10-mL syringe. The skin is punctured at the junction of the two clavicular heads, and the needle is directed with constant aspiration toward the ipsilateral nipple at an angle approximately 30° superior to the plane of the skin. Free flow of venous blood confirms the position of the internal jugular vein. Next, the needle is withdrawn and the vein once again entered with a 16-gauge needle and syringe. Then a guidewire is placed through the needle and into the jugular vein. This placement is perhaps the most crucial part of the entire procedure, and it is vital that the guidewire passes freely without any resistance whatsoever. Free passage confirms entrance into the vein.

Next, the needle is removed with the guidewire left in place. The incision is widened with a scalpel, and the introducer sheath-vein dilator apparatus is introduced over the guidewire. During introduction of the introducer sheath-vein dilator, it is crucial that the proximal tip of the guidewire be visible at all times, to avoid inadvertent loss of the guidewire into the central venous system. The introducer sheath-vein dilator apparatus is advanced with a slight turning motion along the guidewire. In general, the point of entry into the vein is felt clearly by a sudden decrease in resistance. The sheath apparatus then is advanced to the hilt. The conscious patient is instructed to hold her breath to prevent negative intrathoracic pressure and air embolism, and the guidewire and trocar are quickly removed with the sheath left in place. Occasionally, portable real-time sonography may be helpful in guiding central venous cannulation (Lee et al., 1989; Sherer et al., 1993).

Most current introducer systems contain an accessory port, which attaches to the proximal end of the introducer sheath and includes a one-way valve that prevents air introduction into the central venous system during removal of the guidewire and trocar. To keep the line open, the sheath then is infused with a crystalloid solution containing 1 unit of heparin per milliliter and secured in place with a suture.

Insertion of the catheter

Phase two involves the actual placement of the pulmonary artery catheter (Fig. 15.1). Careful attention must be paid to maintaining sterile technique as the catheter is removed from the package. The distal and proximal ports are flushed to assure patency. The balloon then is tested with 1 mL of air. When the catheter has been attached to the physiologic monitor and the air completely flushed from the system, minute movements in the catheter tip should produce corresponding oscillations on the monitor. The catheter tip is introduced through the sheath and advanced approximately 20 cm. At this point, the balloon is inflated and the catheter advanced through the introducer sheath into the central venous system. Occasionally, portable real-time sonography may be helpful in guiding central venous cannulation (Sherer et al., 1993).

Waveforms and catheter placement

Once within the superior vena cava, the balloon on the tip of the catheter will advance with the flow of blood into the heart. Characteristic waveforms and pressures are observed. Entrance into the right ventricle is signaled by a high spiking waveform with diastolic pressures near zero. This is the time of maximum potential complications during catheter placement, because most arrhythmias occur as the catheter tip impinges on the interventricular septum. For this reason, the catheter must be advanced rapidly through the right ventricle and into the pulmonary artery. If premature ventricular contractions occur during this process and the catheter does not advance promptly out of the right ventricle, the balloon should be deflated and the catheter withdrawn to the right atrium.

As soon as the catheter enters the pulmonary artery, the waveform has two notable characteristics. First, and most important, is the rise in diastolic pressure from that seen in the right ventricle. Second, a notching of the peak systolic waveform often is seen and represents closure of the pulmonic valve. After entrance into the pulmonary artery has been confirmed (in most pregnant women, this occurs between 40 and 45 cm of catheter length), the catheter is advanced farther until the tip reaches a point within the pulmonary vasculature

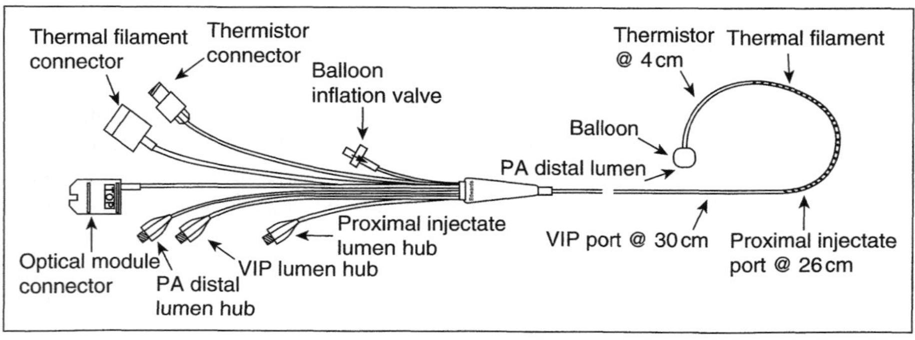

Fig. 15.1 Pulmonary artery catheter. (Reproduced by permission from American Edwards Laboratories.)

where the balloon diameter exceeds that of the corresponding pulmonary arterial branch. At this point, a wedge tracing is observed. If the balloon is deflated, the tracing should return to a pulmonary artery pattern.

Following catheter placement, it is essential that health-care personnel skilled in the interpretation of these waveforms continuously monitor the waveforms for evidence of catheter migration (spontaneous advancement), which may lead to pulmonary infarction. This may be manifest by the appearance of a spontaneous "wedge" tracing at the distal port, rather than the pulmonary artery waveform, which should be continuously manifest on the display monitor. Alternately, the appearance of a pulmonary artery waveform in the central venous pressure port will alert the attendant to distal catheter migration and the need for adjustment (Santora et al., 1991). Komadina et al. described disturbingly high interobserver variability in the interpretation of waveform tracings, although agreement on numerical wedge pressure readings was high (Komadina et al., 1991). In a similar manner, Iberti et al. reported a wide variation in the understanding of pulmonary artery catheter waveforms and techniques among critical care nurses using this device (Iberti et al., 1994). It would appear that graphic recording at end expiration is the most reliable means of measuring hemodynamic pressures (Johnson & Schumann, 1995). Clearly, continuous training and credentialing programs are essential for health-care providers utilizing these techniques.

Caution also is advised during pulmonary artery catheter removal; techniques to avoid complications have been described (Wadas, 1994).

Cardiac output determination

Once in place, cardiac output is obtained with the use of a cardiac output computer connected to a terminal on the pulmonary artery catheter. This instrument derives cardiac output from thermodilution curves created by the injection of cold or room-temperature saline into the proximal central venous port of the catheter. The resultant flow-related temperature changes detected at the distal thermistor are converted into cardiac output by the computer and correlate well in pregnant women with those obtained by the more precise, but clinically cumbersome, oxygen extraction (Fick) technique (Clark et al., 1989). Nevertheless, it should be emphasized that cardiac output determinations are of most value in following trends in individual patients; caution is advised in relying on absolute cardiac output values, and sound clinical judgment is essential in data interpretation (Vender, 1993). One study suggests that the thermodilution technique may overestimate cardiac output, especially with very low values (Espersen et al., 1995). In addition, meticulous attention must be paid to technique if reliable information regarding cardiac output is to be obtained. The exact injectate temperature must be known, the proximal injectate port must have advanced beyond the introducer sheath, and the introducer sheath sidearm must be closed (Boyd et al., 1994). If the central venous port line becomes nonfunctional, room-temperature thermodilution cardiac outputs can be used with saline injection into the sideport, with the understanding that a slight overestimation of cardiac output will occur (Pesola & Pesola, 1993). Additional issues that affect the validity of cardiac output measurements include the rate of injection, the timing of injection during the respiratory cycle, the position of the patient, and the presence of other, concurrent infusions (Sommers et al., 1993). More recently, techniques have been evaluated for continuous cardiac output measurement, both by thermodilution and with the use of a special flow-directed Doppler pulmonary artery catheter (Segal et al., 1991; Mihaljevic et al., 1994).

With appropriate modification of technique, right ventricular ejection fraction measurements also may be obtained with the pulmonary artery catheter (Cockroft & Withington, 1993; Safcsak & Nelson, 1994). Specially designed fiberoptic catheters allow continuous assessment of mixed venous oxygen saturation in critically ill patients. Newer techniques for continuous thermodilution measurement compare well with conventional methods (Inomata et al., 1994; Lefrant et al., 1995).

Complications

Most complications encountered in patients undergoing pulmonary artery catheterization are a result of obtaining central venous access. Such events include pneumothorax and insertion site infection and occur in 1–5% of patients undergoing this procedure (Patel et al., 1986; Scott, 1988; Gilbert et al., 2000). Potential complications of pulmonary artery catheterization per se include air embolism, thromboembolism, pulmonary infarction, catheter-related sepsis, direct trauma to the heart or pulmonary artery, postganglionic Horner's syndrome, and catheter entrapment (Lanigan & Cornwell, 1991; Vaswani et al., 1991; Yellin et al., 1991; Manager et al., 1993; Bernardin et al., 1994; Soding et al., 1994). Such complications occur in 1% or less of patients. More recently, a pressure release balloon has been described to limit overinflation and potentially reduce the risk of vessel rupture (Shevde et al., 1994). Arrhythmias, consisting of transient premature ventricular contractions, occur during catheter insertion in 30–50% of patients and are generally of no clinical consequence.

The remaining complications can be minimized or eliminated by careful attention to proper insertion maintenance and removal techniques (Wadas, 1994). In patients with right-to-left shunts, the use of this catheter is hazardous; when its placement is deemed mandatory, the use of carbon dioxide instead of air for balloon inflation may minimize the risk or systemic air embolism (Moorthy et al., 1991). An FDA task force has summarized recommendations regarding methods to minimize complications of central venous catheterization procedures (US Food and Drug Administration, 1989).

Numerous studies have documented the frequent discrepancy between measurements of pulmonary capillary wedge pressure and central venous pressure during pregnancy (Benedetti et al., 1980; Cotton et al., 1985; Clark & Cotton, 1988; Bolte et al., 2000). In such circumstances, clinical use of the central venous pressure would be misleading. For these reasons, in a modern perinatal intensive care unit, central venous monitoring is seldom, if ever, indicated. Where proper equipment and personnel exist, the vast amount of additional information obtainable by pulmonary artery catheterization far outweighs the slight potential increase in risk attributable to catheter placement. Pulmonary artery catheterization is nearly always preferable.

Noninvasive techniques

Despite the small risks associated with properly managed pulmonary artery catheterization, the search continues for noninvasive methods of central hemodynamic assessment of the critically ill patient. Such techniques generally focus on sonographic or bioimpedance techniques to estimate cardiac output, and have been described in both pregnant and nonpregnant patients (Easterling et al., 1987; Belfort et al., 1991, 1996; Clark et al., 1994; Weiss et al., 1995). In addition, investigation continues into techniques to allow noninvasive central pressure determination (Ensing et al., 1994). These techniques appear to be useful in a research setting or in patients requiring only a single evaluation of hemodynamics in order to classify their disease and initiate appropriate therapy. Invasive techniques, however, remain the mainstay of long-term management of complex, critically ill obstetric patients.

References

Belfort MA, Rokey R, Saade GR, et al. Rapid echocardiographic assessment of left and right heart hemodynamics in critically ill obstetric patients. Am J Obstet Gynecol 1991;171:884–892.

Belfort MA, Mares A, Saade G, et al. A re-evaluation of the indications for pulmonary artery catheters in obstetrics: the role of 2-D echocardiography and Doppler ultrasound. Am J Obstet Gynecol 1996; 174:331.

Benedetti TJ, Cotton DB, Read JC, et al. Hemodynamic observations in severe preeclampsia with a flow-directed pulmonary artery catheter. Am J Obstet Gynecol 1980;136:465.

Bernard GR, Sopko G, Cerra F, et al. Pulmonary artery catheterization and clinical outcomes: National Heart, Lung, and Blood Institute and Food and Drug Administration Workshop Report. Consensus Statement. JAMA 2000 May 17;283(19):2568–2572.

Bernardin G, Milhaud D, Roger PM, et al. Swan-Ganz catheter related pulmonary valve infective endocarditis: a case report. Intensive Care Med 1994;20:142–144.

Bolte AC, Dekker GA, van Eyck J, van Schijndel RS, van Geijn HP. Lack of agreement between central venous pressure and pulmonary capillary wedge pressure in preeclampsia. Hypertens Pregnancy 2000;19(3):261–271.

Boyd O, Mackay CJ, Newman P, et al. Effects of insertion depth and use of the sidearm of the introducer sheath of pulmonary artery catheters in cardiac output measurement. Crit Care Med 1994; 22:1132–1135.

Califf RM, Fulkerson WJ, Jr, Vidaillet H, et al. The effectiveness of right-heart catheterization in the initial case of critically ill patients. JAMA 1996;18:889.

Clark SL, Cotton DB. Clinical opinion: clinical indications for pulmonary artery catheterization in the patient with severe preeclampsia. Am J Obstet Gynecol 1988;158:453–458.

Clark SL, Horenstein JM, Phelan JP, et al. Experience with the pulmonary artery catheter in obstetrics and gynecology. Am J Obstet Gynecol 1985;152:374–378.

Clark SL, Cotton DB, Lee W, et al. Central hemodynamic assessment of normal term pregnancy. Am J Obstet Gynecol 1989;161:1439–1442.

Clark SL, Southwick J, Pivarnik JM, et al. A comparison of cardiac index in normal term pregnancy using thoracic electrical bioimpedance and oxygen extraction (Fick) technique. Obstet Gynecol 1994;83:669–672.

Cockroft S, Withington PS. The measurement of right ventricular ejection fraction by thermodilution. A comparison of values obtained using differing injectate ports. Anaesthesia 1993;48:312–314.

Coles NA, Hibberd M, Russell M, et al. Potential impact of pulmonary artery catheter placement on short term management decisions in the medical intensive care unit. Am Heart J 1993;126:815–819.

Cotton DB, Gonik B, Dorman K, et al. Cardiovascular alterations in severe pregnancy induced hypertension: relationship of central venous pressure to pulmonary capillary wedge pressure. Am J Obstet Gynecol 1985;151:762–764.

Cruz K, Franklin C. The pulmonary artery catheter: uses and controversies. Crit Care Clin 2001 Apr;17(2):271–291.

Easterling T, Watts D, Schmucker B, et al. Measurement of cardiac output during pregnancy: validation of Doppler technique and clinical observations in preeclamplsia. Obstet Gynecol 1987;69:845–850.

Ensing G, Seward J, Darragh R, et al. Feasibility of generating hemodynamic pressure curves from noninvasive Doppler echocardiographic signals. J Am Coll Cardiol 1994;23:434–442.

Espersen K, Jensen EW, Rosenberg D, et al. Comparison of cardiac output techniques: Thermodilution, Doppler, CO_2 rebreathing and the direct Fick method. Acta Anaesthesiol Scand 1995;39:245–251.

European Society of Intensive Care Medicine. Expert panel: the use of the pulmonary artery catheter. Intensive Care Med 1991;17:I–VIII.

Findling R, Lipper B. Femoral vein pulmonary artery catheterization in the intensive care unit. Chest 1994;105:874–877.

Gilbert WM, Towner DR, Field NT, Anthony J. The safety and utility of pulmonary artery catheterization in severe preeclampsia and eclampsia. Am J Obstet Gynecol 2000;182(6):1397–1403.

Iberti TJ, Daily EK, Leibowitz AB. Assessment of critical care nurses' knowledge of the pulmonary artery catheter. Crit Care Med 1994;22:1674–1678.

Inomata S, Nishikawa T, Taguchi M. Continuous monitoring of mixed venous oxygen saturation for detecting alterations in cardiac output after discontinuation of cardiopulmonary bypass. Br J Anaesth 1994;72:11–16.

Johnson MK, Schumann L. Comparison of three methods of measurement of pulmonary artery catheter readings in critically ill patients. Am J Crit Care 1995;4:300–307.

Komadina KH, Schenk DA, LaVeau P, et al. Interobserver variability in the interpretation of pulmonary artery catheter pressure tracings. Chest 1991;100:1647–1654.

Lanigan C, Cornwell E. Pulmonary artery catheter entrapment. Anaesthesia 1991;46:600–601.

Lee W, Leduc L, Cotton DB. Ultrasonographic guidance for central venous catheterization. Am J Obstet Gynecol 1989;161:1012–1013.

Lefrant JY, Bruelle P, Ripart J, et al. Cardiac output measurement in critically ill patients: Comparison of continuous and conventional thermodilution techniques. Can J Anesth 1995;42:972–976.

Manager D, Connell GR, Lessin JL. Catheter induced pulmonary artery haemorrhage resulting from a pneumothorax. Can J Anaesth 1993;40:1069–1072.

Mihaljevic T, von Segesser LK, Tonz M, et al. Continuous thermodilution measurement of cardiac output: in-vitro and in-vivo evaluation. Thorac Cardiovasc Surg 1994;42:32–35.

Mimoz O, Rauss A, Rekik N, et al. Pulmonary artery catheterization in critically ill patients: a prospective analysis of outcome changes associated with catheter-prompted changes in therapy. Crit Care Med 1994;22:573–579.

Moorthy SS, Tisinai KA, Speiser BS, et al. Cerebral air embolism during removal of a pulmonary artery catheter. Crit Care Med 1991;19:981–983.

Patel C, Laboy V, Venus B, et al. Acute complications of pulmonary artery catheter insertion in critically ill patients. Crit Care Med 1986;14:195–197.

Pesola HR, Pesola GR. Room temperature thermodilution cardiac output. Central venous vs side port. Chest 1993;103:339–341.

Rhodes A, Cusack RJ, Newman PJ, Grounds RM, Bennett ED. A randomised, controlled trial of the pulmonary artery catheter in critically ill patients. Intensive Care Med 2002;28(3):256–264.

Safcsak K, Nelson LD. Thermodilution right ventricular ejection fraction measurements: room temperature versus cold temperature injectate. Crit Care Med 1994;22:1136–1141.

Santora T, Ganz W, Gold J, et al. New method for monitoring pulmonary artery catheter location. Crit Care Med 1991;19:422–426.

Schiller WR, Bay RC, McLachlan JG, et al. Survival in major burn injuries is predicted by early response to Swan-Ganz-guided resuscitation. Am J Surg 1995;170:696–699.

Scott WL. Complications associated with central venous catheters. A survey. Chest 1988;91:1221–1224.

Segal J, Gaudiani V, Nishimura T. Continuous determination of cardiac output using a flow directed Doppler pulmonary artery catheter. J Cardiothorac Vasc Anesth 1991;5:309–315.

Sherer DM, Abulafia O, DuBeshter B, et al. Ultrasonically guided subclavian vein catheterization in critical care obstetrics and gynecologic oncology. Am J Obstet Gynecol 1993;169:1246–1248.

Shevde K, Raab R, Lee P. Decreasing the risk of pulmonary artery rupture with a pressure relief balloon. J Cardiothorac Vasc Anesth 1994;8:30–34.

Soding PF, Klinck JR, Kong A, et al. Infective endocarditis of the pulmonary valve following pulmonary artery catheterization. Intensive Care Med 1994;20:222–224.

Sola JE, Bender JS. Use of the pulmonary artery catheter to reduce operative complications. Surg Clin North Am 1993;73:253–264.

Sommers MS, Woods SL, Courtade MA. Issues in methods and measurement of thermodilution cardiac output. Nurs Res 1993;42:228–233.

Swan JHC, Ganz W, Forrester J, et al. Catheterization of the heart in man with use of a flow-directed balloon-tipped catheter. N Engl J Med 1970;283:447–451.

US Food and Drug Administration. Precautions necessary with central venous catheters. FDA Drug Bulletin, July 1989;15.

Vaswani S, Garvin L, Matuschak GM. Postganglionic Horner's syndrome after insertion of a pulmonary artery catheter through the internal jugular vein. Crit Care Med 1991;19:1215–1216.

Vender JS. Clinical utilization of pulmonary artery catheter monitoring. Int Anesthesiol Clin 1993;31:57–85.

Wadas TM. Pulmonary artery catheter removal. Crit Care Nurse 1994;14:63–72.

Yellin LB, Filler JJ, Barnette RE. Nominal hemoptysis heralds pseudoaneurysm induced by a pulmonary artery catheter. Anesthesiology 1991;74:370–373.

Weiss S, Calloway E, Cairo J, et al. Comparison of cardiac output measurements by thermodilution and thoracic electrical bioimpedance in critically ill vs. noncritically ill patients. Am J Emerg Med 1995;13:626–631.

IV Disease processes

16 Seizures and status epilepticus

Tawnya Constantino
Michael W. Varner

Epilepsy is a common clinical disorder seen in women of reproductive age. The prevalence in developed countries is estimated at 5–10 per 1,000, with an annual incidence of 50 per 100,000 and a lifetime incidence of a single seizure of 110 per 1,000 (Hauser et al., 1993). There is no evidence to suggest that this distribution should be any different for women of reproductive age, making this condition among the more common neurologic disorders seen in pregnant women.

Etiology

Epilepsy is a predisposition to recurrent seizures based on identified or suspected dysfunction of the central nervous system. The occurrence of seizures may represent a myriad of etiologies (Table 16.1). Because optimum treatment of seizures should be directed at their underlying etiology(ies), confirmation of the underlying etiology(ies) is important. Irrespective of etiology, generalized convulsive seizures, because of the potential for maternal physical injury, prolonged apnea and/or an unguarded airway, and for fetal injury and/or hypoxia–ischemia, require immediate and urgent attention. Partial seizures, unless followed by secondary generalized tonic–clonic seizures, pose much lower risks for mother and baby and thus require less emergent responses.

It is not clear that pregnancy increases seizure frequency. Engel and Perley (1998) report that 22% of pregnant women had decreased seizure frequency, 24% had increased seizure frequency and 54% had no change. Of those women with increased seizure frequency, the most likely time for exacerbation was the first trimester. This most commonly reflects subtherapeutic anticonvulsant levels secondary to pregnancy-associated pharmacokinetic changes and/or decreased medication ingestion because of concerns about teratogenesis.

Seizure prophylaxis

The development of effective anticonvulsant medications has revolutionized the lives and prognoses of individuals with epilepsy. The options for treatment have expanded rapidly in recent years although effects of these medications during pregnancy are still not well known. An extensive review of these options is beyond the scope of this chapter and recent reviews are available (Pschirrer & Monga, 2001; Yerby, 2001). Pregnancy registries are available through the pharmaceutical companies for many of the newer anticonvulsant medications and patients should be encouraged to enroll with these registries voluntarily.

If the patient desires to discontinue the anticonvulsant medication, it ideally should be accomplished preconceptionally as the greatest risk to the fetus is during the first trimester of the pregnancy. In addition, it is optimal to determine if seizures are going to recur or worsen after stopping the medication before the patient becomes pregnant. It is not recommended that the anticonvulsant medication be discontinued if the patient has a history of recurrent seizures in the past, even if they have been seizure free on medication for over a year. In some instances, if the patient discontinues the medication and loses complete seizure control, she may never again be able to completely control the seizures with medication. If the patient still desires to try and stop the medication before or during the pregnancy, consultation with a neurologist or epileptologist is recommended for further counseling.

Because of the increases in maternal blood volume and hepatic metabolism during pregnancy, total levels of anticonvulsants decline in almost all pregnant women. Free drug levels also decline during pregnancy because anticonvulsants are highly protein bound and serum albumin decreases during pregnancy, but the percentage decline is much less than for total drug levels. Monitoring total drug levels will be sufficient if the patient is clinically well controlled. However, free (e.g. nonprotein-bound) drug levels should be obtained and monitored if the woman is having recurrent or persistent seizures or side effects.

In women whose seizures have been well controlled for at least the preceding year and whose therapeutic free and total anticonvulsant levels have been determined preconceptionally, anticonvulsant drug levels need only be determined

Table 16.1 International classification of seizures by mode of onset and spread*

Type/subtype	Characteristics	Medication(s)
Partial		
Simple partial	Electrical abnormality confined to one localized area of the brain. The person remains conscious and fully aware	Carbamazepine, lamotrigine, oxcarbazepine, topiramate, levetiracetam, zonisamide
Complex partial	Impaired consciousness, often exhibiting automatisms. The electrical abnormality usually starts in the temporal lobes. May spread to the rest of the brain and result in secondary generalized tonic–clonic seizures	As above
Generalized		
Generalized tonic–clonic	Initial stiffness (tonic) and collapse followed by generalized jerking (clonic) movements, averaging several minutes in duration. Often apneic and involuntarily incontinent. Thereafter followed by relaxation and deep unconsciousness. Postictal confusion and fatigue may last for hours. Also known as 'grand mal' seizures	Carbamazepine, oxcarbazepine, valproic acid, lamotrigine, phenytoin, topiramate, zonisamide, levetiracetam
Absence	Brief episodes of unconsciousness, sometimes with fluttering of the eyelids. Rapid recovery. Also known as 'petit mal' seizures	Valproic acid, lamotrigine, topiramate
Myoclonic	Sudden symmetrical shock-like limb movements with or without loss of consciousness	Valproic acid, lamotrigine, topiramate, zonisamide, levetiracetam
Tonic	Stiffening of the whole body with or without loss of consciousness	
Atonic	Momentary loss of limb muscle tone causing sudden collapse, head drooping, etc.	

* (From Commission on Classification and Terminology of the International League Against Epilepsy. Proposal for revised clinical and electroencephalographic classification of epileptic seizures. Epilepsia 1981;22:489.)

every trimester. However, if the woman has had uncontrolled seizures within the year prior to conception, recurrent seizure activity during the pregnancy, develops troublesome side effects, or is suspected of noncompliance, then monthly free anticonvulsant levels should be monitored. If total drug levels decrease by more than 60%, or if free drug levels decrease by more than 30% and values fall out of the recommended therapeutic range, the dosage should be increased.

All anticonvulsant drugs have folic acid antagonist properties. As a result, women taking anticonvulsant medications are at a relative increased risk for having fetuses with a number of structural abnormalities, including cleft lip and palate, congenital heart defects, and neural tube defects (Kelly, 1984; Rosa, 1991; Omtzigt et al., 1992). It is generally acknowledged that anticonvulsants double the risk of teratogenicity from baseline and that multiple anticonvulsants increase the risk still further. Of the anticonvulsant drugs that are currently widely utilized, valproic acid has the highest risk of neural tube defects and thus is not recommended in women planning a pregnancy unless an alternative drug cannot be used. Although it is not completely clear how much supplementation is needed in this population, all women of reproductive age should now be advised to ingest at least 4 mg of folic acid per day for at least several months preconceptionally and through the first few months of pregnancy in order to reduce the fetal risk of neural tube defect.

Beyond the first few months, pregnant women on anticonvulsants should be continued on at least 400 µg/day of folic acid. They should also receive vitamin K (10 mg po qd) beginning 4 weeks before expected delivery until birth in order to minimize the risk of neonatal hemorrhage (Deblay et al., 1982).

Because of the rapid postpartum changes in maternal blood volume, women receiving anticonvulsant medications during pregnancy should have free and total drug levels assessed at 2 weeks postpartum. Serum levels commonly rise in the first few weeks after delivery in association with resolution of the hormonally-mediated effects of pregnancy. If medication doses were increased during the pregnancy, the patient may develop symptoms of medication toxicity if doses are not appropriately lowered again in the postpartum period.

Evaluation of new-onset seizures in pregnancy

While most seizure disorders manifest themselves prior to pregnancy, the initial onset of seizures and epilepsy can occur during pregnancy (Table 16.2). Acute etiologies (hemorrhage, thrombosis, etc.) must be ruled out and any underlying predisposing factors treated appropriately. A careful history is often very helpful in establishing a diagnosis. Witnesses, family members, and the patient should be questioned. The onset, duration and characteristics of the seizure should be described. The setting in which the episode occurred should be defined. The possibility of precipitating factors must be pursued, including:

- infection (recent history of febrile illness ± change in mental status, history of parenteral drug use, recent dental work, heart murmur, or valvular heart disease);
- alcohol and/or drugs (consider cocaine, or amphetamine withdrawal) or toxin exposure;
- eclampsia (hypertension, proteinuria);
- mass lesions (history of malignancy, focal findings on examination);
- intracranial hemorrhage (sudden onset of "worst headache of my life");
- intracranial thrombosis (fluctuating neurologic deficits); and
- trauma.

For much of the history witnesses are better sources than patients, but patients are the best source for presence and type of aura. The health-care provider should determine whether the patient completely lost consciousness and whether incontinence of bowel or bladder occurred. Determining whether there was an aura and whether there was antigrade amnesia or postictal confusion is also important.

Vital signs should be promptly assessed and patients evaluated for orthostatic hypotension. Fetal heart rate monitoring should be undertaken if the fetus is within the realm of potential viability. A complete physical examination should be performed, with particular attention to the neurologic (fundoscopy, cranial nerves, speech, mental status, neck, motor, sensory and deep tendon reflexes) and cardiovascular (heart murmur, arrhythmia) systems.

Initial laboratory evaluation should include a complete blood count, chemistry profile, liver function testing, toxicology screen, and urinalysis.

Even if the patient has a normal neurologic examination, an electroencephalogram (EEG) and brain imaging study are still indicated. If intracranial hemorrhage is suspected a computed tomography (CT) scan should be considered, as the CT scan is the procedure of choice for detection of acute intracranial hemorrhage. If time is not a factor, a magnetic resonance imaging (MRI) study would be preferable as MRI technology is more sensitive for intracranial anatomy than is the CT scan. If intracranial infection is suspected, a lumbar puncture should be performed. For patients in whom cerebral emboli are suspect-

Table 16.2 Differential diagnosis of initial seizure(s) during pregnancy

Condition	Clinical presentation	Diagnostic considerations
Brain tumor	Most likely to become symptomatic in the first trimester. Rare	Papilledema should be prominent with supratentorial tumors
Intracranial hemorrhage	Sudden severe headache or loss of consciousness. May have been preceded by a 'sentinel' bleed	Arteriovenous malformations are more likely in younger, nonhypertensive women. Aneurysms are more likely in older, parous, hypertensive women
Cerebral venous thrombosis	Fluctuating deficits and/or consciousness	Most common in late pregnancy and the first few weeks after delivery
Gestational epilepsy	Variable. Very rare	A diagnosis of exclusion
Eclampsia	Usually preceded by generalized headache, visual disturbances and/or abdominal pain	Associated with hypertension, proteinuria and other symptoms and laboratory abnormalities (elevated liver function studies, decreased platelet counts)

ed, electrocardiogram, and electrocardiogram examinations are recommended. A diagnosis of cerebral thrombosis should prompt a hypercoaguability evaluation.

The most common differential diagnosis of a seizure is syncope. In contradistinction to seizures, syncope is *not* associated with incontinence, tongue biting, or confusion (before and/or after the episode).

Treatment of seizures

As previously emphasized, optimum treatment should be based on the known or presumed diagnosis. Although this information is often historical and available either from the patient, her friends or family, or her medical records, the diagnoses outlined in Tables 16.1 and 16.2 must be considered, particularly in the seizing or postictal patient for whom a medical history is not available.

Consultation with a neurologist is particularly important in the setting of an initial seizure (unless the diagnosis of eclampsia is reasonably certain), particularly if the neurologic examination is abnormal, the seizure is focal, or the EEG is abnormal.

The prenatal care provider should be familiar with the anticonvulsants that are considered the most effective for the individual seizure classifications (Table 16.1).

Alternate treatment options for patients with medically refractory epilepsy include vagal nerve stimulation therapy, which has no known or suspected adverse effects on pregnancy, and epilepsy surgery. Surgical options, in general, should be addressed before or after pregnancy.

Status epilepticus

While uncommon (less than 1% of all pregnant epileptic women), major motor status epilepticus requires immediate intervention to prevent permanent brain damage or death to both mother and fetus. Although treatment will be administered to both mother and fetus, primary attention should be directed towards the mother since maternal resuscitation and stabilization will optimally resuscitate her fetus. Initial attention must be paid to the maternal airway. As soon as the airway is secured, maternal oxygen saturation should be assessed and sufficient oxygen administered to return these values to normal, with intubation if necessary. Concurrent assessments should evaluate maternal blood pressure as well as forebrain and brain stem status.

Additional key initial evaluation should include a medical history (if available from accompanying persons) and baseline laboratory studies (CBC, glucose, calcium, electrolytes, phosphorus, arterial blood gases, urinalysis, and anticonvulsant levels when appropriate). Fetal well-being in the form of fetal heart rate monitoring (if the pregnancy has reached a viable gestational age) should then be undertaken. If there is any question of recent exposure, serum or urine screens for substances of abuse should also be performed (within the informed consent guidelines of the individual jurisdiction).

The patient must be admitted to an intensive care area, the maternal airway must be secured and intravenous access established for administration of normal saline, glucose, thiamine, and anticonvulsant medication.

Included in the differential diagnosis of status epilepticus are two conditions that respond dramatically to therapeutic, and therefore diagnostic, IV infusions. These conditions are hypoglycemia and Wernicke's encephalopathy. Eclampsia must also be considered in the diagnosis, particularly if the pregnancy is beyond 20 weeks' gestation and hypertension and proteinuria are present.

A glucose bolus should be initially administered, usually 50 mL of D50, even before a blood glucose level is checked. If the woman is seizing because of hypoglycemia this administration can be life-saving. If the woman is hyperglycemic, the additional amount of glucose will not significantly worsen her condition.

Although Wernicke's encephalopathy (thiamine, or vitamin B_1, deficiency) is rare in women of reproductive age, the dramatic improvement that can be seen with thiamine administration warrants administration of thiamine, 100 mg IV, followed by 50–100 mg IM/IV qd if a significant response is seen.

If the woman is not responsive to these initial therapeutic measures, specific medical therapy should be promptly undertaken. This should consist of an intravenous benzodiazepine (10 mg diazepam or 4 mg lorazepam) which can be repeated in 10–15 minutes if seizure activity continues, followed by administration of an appropriate anticonvulsant (fosphenytoin or phenytoin) (Table 16.3). These medications are all short acting, allowing the patient to regain consciousness more rapidly and be more thoroughly assessed from a neurologic perspective.

If seizures still persist at this point (≥60 minutes), the patient should be intubated and sedated, usually with phenobarbital (20–25 mg/kg, not to exceed 100 mg/min; Table 16.3). If seizures still persist, the patient should be anesthetized using a general anesthetic while continuous EEG monitoring is performed under the supervision of a neurologist.

Subsequent management and prognosis

With control of the seizures attention must be directed to the treatment of any underlying or predisposing conditions and to the prevention of recurrence. The most common cause of status epilepticus in the epileptic population is noncompliance with medication. Therefore it is critical to ascertain if the patient was taking the medication. If the patient forgets doses, then a pill-box or other memory aids should be suggested. Medication dosing must be optimized. Ideally, preconcep-

Table 16.3 Treatment of status epilepticus in pregnancy

1 *Initial stabilization*
- A Secure the airway
- B Establish intravenous access
- C Admit to intensive care unit

2 *Therapeutic trials* (to be administered sequentially)

Medication	Dosage	Intent
Glucose	50 ml of D50 IV	Correct hypoglycemia
Thiamine (vitamin B_1)	100 mg IV, followed by 50–100 mg IM/IV qd	Correct Wernicke's encephalopathy

3 *Initiate first-line anticonvulsants* (*one* from *each* drug class)

Drug class/ Specific drug	Dosage	Therapeutic levels	Precautions
Benzodiazepine			
Diazepam	5–10 mg IV q 10–15 min		Max. dosage 30 mg
Lorazepam	4 mg IV; may repeat × 1 in 10–15 min		Max. dosage 8 mg/12 hr
Anticonvulsant			
Fosphenytoin	15–20 mg phenytoin equivalents/kg IV × 1; begin maintenance dose 12 hr after loading dose	Total = 10–20 µg/mL Free = 1–2 µg/mL	Continuous EKG and blood pressure monitoring recommended during IV infusions. Use nonglucose-containing IV fluids
Phenytoin	15–20 mg/kg IV q 30 min prn; begin maintenance dose 12 hr after loading dose	Total = 10–20 µg/mL Free = 1–2 µg/mL	Continuous EKG and blood pressure monitoring recommended during IV infusions. Use nonglucose-containing IV fluids

4 *Intubation and sedation*
- A Intubation
- B Intravenous sedation
  - Phenobarbital (20–25 mg/kg, administration not to exceed 100 mg/min)
  - Midazolam (0.02–0.10 mg/kg/hr)
  - Propofol (5–50 µg/kg/min, start at 5 µg/kg/min IV × 5 min, then increase 5–10 µg/kg/min q 5–10 min until desired effect)

5 *General anesthesia*
- A If seizures still persist, institute general anesthesia with halothane and NMJ blockade

EKG, electrocardiogram; NMJ, neuromuscular junction.

tional total and free anticonvulsant levels would be available so that medication dosage can be readjusted accordingly.

Establishment or resumption of a supportive lifestyle must also be emphasized. Women should be encouraged to eat regular meals, get adequate rest, nutrition, and sleep as well as avoid stress whenever possible. They should be counseled to avoid hazardous situations as well as alcohol and other sedatives.

Well-controlled epilepsy is not a contraindication to breast-feeding. While most anticonvulsants do cross into breast milk, they achieve much lower levels than in the maternal serum, ranging between 10 and 40% for phenytoin and carbamazepine, respectively. Contraindications to breast feeding would be increased seizure activity due to sleep deprivation or infant sedation from medication effect (most commonly a concern with phenobarbital).

References

Deblay FM, Vert P, Andre M, et al. Transplacental vitamin K prevents hemorrhagic disease of infants of epileptic mothers. Lancet 1982;1:1247.

Engel J, Perley T. Pregnancy and the mother. Epilepsy: A Comprehensive Textbook. Philadelphia, PA: Lippincott; 1998:2029–2030.

Hauser AW, Annegers JF, Hurland LT. Incidence of epilepsy and unprovoked seizures in Rochester, Minnesota 1935–84. Epilepsia 1993;34:453–468.

Kelly TE. Teratogenicity of anticonvulsant drugs. I. Review of the literature. Am J Med Genet 1984;19:413–434.

Omtzigt JCG, Los FJ, Grobbee DE, et al. The risk of spina bifida aperta after first-trimester exposure to valproate in a prenatal cohort. Neurology 1992;42:119–125.

Pschirrer ER, Monga M. Seizure disorders in pregnancy. Obstet Gynecol Clin North Am 2001;28:601–611.

Rosa F. Spina bifida in infants of women treated with carbamazepine during pregnancy. N Engl J Med 1991;324:674–677.

Yerby MS. The use of anticonvulsants during pregnancy. Semin Perinatol 2001;25:153–158.

17 Acute spinal cord injury

Sheryl Rodts-Palenik
James N. Martin, Jr

The loss of physical and personal independence that can occur with spinal cord injury (SCI) is a catastrophe that impacts the lives of approximately 7–10,000 Americans each year. A significant number of these patients are women (20–30%) (NSCISC, 2000; Blackwell, 2001). The average age at which SCI occurs is somewhere between 16 and 45 years (Blackwell, 2001), and therefore many women incurring these injuries do so during their reproductive years. Loving and caring for a child may have always been part of their life plans, and many may wish to bear children despite the disruption resulting from their injury. The obstetrician thus may become involved as part of the team working to stabilize the pregnant patient in the critical first hours after an acute spinal cord injury, or managing the pregnancy, labor, and delivery of a patient years later when the sequelae of chronic spinal cord damage are present. Competent care in either setting requires the physician to be knowledgeable about the common, predictable, complications specific to the acute and chronic forms of SCI.

Acute care of the pregnant patient with spinal cord injury

The primary goal of emergent care of a pregnant patient with acute spinal cord trauma is to diagnose and treat life-threatening injuries, while preventing any unnecessary traction or motion of the spinal column (Table 17.1). As with any trauma patient, insuring the survival of the pregnant patient and her fetus begins with a primary survey and prompt attention to the ABCs: Airway management, Breathing, and Circulation. The physiologic adaptations of the mother to her pregnancy and the autonomic dysfunction of neurogenic shock can obscure the detection of shock originating from other traumatic injuries. Thus, the contributions of the obstetric consultant are fundamental in elucidating the true clinical scenario.

In the patient with a SCI, the manner in which the spine is stabilized is of critical importance to prevent secondary extension of the damage. The medical care provided by those first to arrive on the accident scene can have long-reaching implications for the future neurologic integrity of the patient. In acute trauma, the necessity for immediate airway management often precludes the feasibility of a complete neurologic assessment (Table 17.2). The most common level of injury to the spinal cord is at the level of C5, followed by C4 and C6. (Marotta, 2000). As such, cervical spine immobilization is key prior to any attempts to intubate patients suspected of having cervical spine trauma. Several authors have shown that a common error in initial management is in providing cervical spine *traction* instead of *immobilization* (Bivins et al., 1988; Holley & Jorden, 1989).

Orotracheal intubation employing rapid sequence induction using the jaw-thrust maneuver instead of head-tilt is considered by some to be the procedure of choice in SCI patients (Ward, 2001). However, utilizing video fluoroscopy in cadavers with C5–6 instability, Donaldson and co-workers, demonstrated that indirect nasal intubation techniques produced less spinal motion than direct oral intubation techniques (Donaldson et al., 1993). Chin lift/jaw thrust and cricoid pressure caused more motion than some of the blind nasal intubation techniques. With instability at the level of C1–2, no difference in motion was detected between oral or nasal techniques, while the chin-lift/jaw-thrust maneuvers caused the most motion associated with intubation (Donaldson et al., 1997). Ideally intubation procedures should be performed by a minimum of three people in concert, one to perform the intubation, one to assist and provide cricoid pressure, and a third to insure in-line immobilization of the spine (Ward, 2001). While all trauma patients should be considered to have a full stomach, the pregnant patient in late gestation has the additional risk of aspiration due to her reduced gastric sphincter tone compounded by the mechanical effects of increased gastric pressure from her gravid uterus. Consequently, appropriately applied cricoid pressure is essential to prevent reflux of gastric content into the trachea. The importance of spinal immobilization cannot be overemphasized. The institution of tracheal protective procedures such as jaw-thrust, bag-valve-mask ventilation, and cricoid pressure, while necessary, can inadvertently cause movement of the cervical spine and subsequent damage if meticulous stabilization is not practiced (Donaldson et al., 1993; Ward, 2001).

The evaluation of the circulatory system in a pregnant trauma patient with acute SCI can be very difficult. The typical assessment parameters may be obscured by the altered hemodynamics of pregnancy, the autonomic derangements of neurogenic shock, and cardiovascular instability from acute hemorrhage. The presence of hypotension, a common component of both hemorrhagic and neurogenic shock, can be confused with the normal reduction in blood pressure associated with pregnancy itself. Supine hypotension can further complicate assessment of trauma patients as aortocaval compression stimulates sympathetic output, increasing both blood pressure and heart rate. Even the normal dilutional anemia of pregnancy can be misinterpreted as a sign of acute blood loss.

If the patient has a cervical or high thoracic injury, the presence of neurogenic shock may obfuscate the assessment of circulatory status. The presenting signs and symptoms of spinal neurogenic shock are typically the exact opposite of those expected with hypovolemia. While both disorders present with hypotension, the classic stigmata of hypovolemia result from enhanced sympathetic output. Reflex sympathetic stimulation maximizes cardiac function and increases peripheral vasoconstriction, resulting in tachycardia, delayed capillary refill, and cool, clammy extremities. Conversely, spinal neurogenic shock is due to an acute *loss* of sympathetic input from below the injury. Subsequently, there is no shunting of blood from the periphery back toward the heart and other critical organs. In addition to warm, dry skin and preserved capillary refill, such patients exhibit a "paradoxical bradycardia" (Mahoney, 2001) when sympathetic input to the heart is lost,

Table 17.1 Acute spinal cord injury

Goals of therapy
To stabilize the patient
To immobilize the spine in an attempt to prevent further injuries
To evaluate and treat other injuries
To achieve early recognition, prevention, and management of frequently encountered complications

Management protocol
Initial stabilization should be achieved, including stabilization of the patient's neck, airway management, circulatory system assessment, and fetal monitoring
Methylprednisolone should be considered within 8 hours of the SCI and given as a bolus dose of 30 mg/kg, followed by infusion at 5.4 mg/kg/hr for 23–48 hours
Central hemodynamic monitoring may be required for optimum fluid management of neurogenic shock
Adequate fluid and pressor support may be necessary during the period of neurogenic shock
Delivery may be indicated for obstetric indications, to facilitate maternal resuscitation, or in conjunction with surgery for other injuries

Table 17.2 Innervation of spinal segments and muscles* and grading scale for evaluation of motor function

Spinal segment	Muscle	Action
C5, C6	Deltoid	Arm abduction
C5, **C6**	Biceps	Elbow flexion
C6, C7	Extensor carpi radialis	Wrist extension
C7, C8	Triceps	Elbow extension
C8, T1	Flexor digitorum profundus	Hand grasp
C8, **T1**	Hand intrinsics	Finger abduction
L1, **L2**, **L3**	Iliopsoas	Hip flexion
L2, **L3**, **L4**	Quadriceps	Knee extension
L4, **L5**, **S1**, S2	Hamstrings	Knee flexion
L4, **L5**	Tibialis anterior	Ankle dorsiflexion
L5, S1	Extensor hallucis longus	Great-toe extension
S1, S2	Gastrocnemius	Ankle plantar flexion
S2, S3, S4	Bladder, anal sphincter	Voluntary rectal tone
Grade	*Muscle strength*	
5	Normal strength	
4	Active power against both resistance and gravity	
3	Active power against gravity but not resistance	
2	Active movement only with gravity eliminated	
1	Flicker or trace of contraction	
0	No movement or contraction	

* The predominant segments of innervation are shown in boldface type.
(Reproduced by permission from Chiles BW III, Cooper PR. Acute spinal injury. N Engl J Med 1996;334:514.)

and vagal control predominates. Preserved vasodilation in the periphery promotes heat loss, leading to hypothermia and further exacerbation of the bradycardia.

Thus, the emergency team must be alert to the contradictory influences of pregnancy, hypovolemia, and neurogenic autonomic disruption while evaluating and stabilizing the pregnant trauma patient. Because of time constraints in deciphering these various factors, the presence of significant hypotension should be considered and treated as hypovolemia until safely proven otherwise. The primary survey should be accompanied by simultaneous intravenous fluid resuscitation through two large-bore IVs, serial vital sign measurements, and the placement of a Foley catheter (Mahoney, 2001). Conventional *wedging* of the patient's back to avoid caval compression can result in exacerbation of spinal trauma. However, these same benefits may be achieved by a 15° tilt of the backboard if the patient is immobilized, or by simple manual displacement of the gravid uterus to the left. Obvious external bleeding is controlled, and a search is initiated for evidence of internal hemorrhage.

Ultrasound provides rapid assessment for fluid in the cul de sac, abdominal cavity, renal gutters, perisplenic, perihepatic, pericardial, and retroplacental areas and, if negative, may allow avoidance of peritoneal lavage and its associated risks (Gilson et al., 1995; Goodwin et al., 2001). If ultrasound is not immediately available (or the study is equivocal), there is no other explanation for the patient's shocked state, or there is obvious severe abdominal/thoracic trauma, peritoneal lavage is required to rule out intra-abdominal hemorrhage. An open entry technique is recommended during the late second and third trimesters to minimize risk to the gravid uterus (Gilson et al., 1995; ACOG, 1998). This is best performed with sharp dissection at or above the umbilicus while elevating the anterior wall away from the uterus. The anterior abdominal peritoneum can then be opened under direct visualization. The procedure is considered diagnostic if either greater than 100,000 RBCs per mL are detected or bowel contents are present in the effluent.

The status of the fetus is not only important in its own right, but also serves as a marker of changes in maternal hemodynamics. A previously normal fetus can tolerate a remarkable diminution in uterine blood flow before abnormalities supervene in the fetal heart tracing (Lucas, et al., 1965). The onset of tachycardia, late decelerations, bradycardia, or a sinusoidal pattern can herald a deleterious change in maternal oxygenation, acid–base, or hemodynamic status. Likewise, adequate correction of maternal metabolic or hemodynamic derangements may be signaled by a return to a reassuring fetal heart rate tracing.

Whether or not concurrent hypovolemia is present, placement of a pulmonary artery catheter and an arterial line may be advantageous in guiding fluid and pressor administration in the pregnant patient with neurogenic shock. Cardiac output and mean arterial pressure must be carefully monitored to prevent the cardiopulmonary complications that often accompany spinal cord injury (Marotta, 2000). If an initial search for subclinical bleeding (chest and pelvic X-rays, pericardial and abdominal ultrasound, peritoneal lavage, or CT) fails to reveal evidence of hemorrhage, neurogenic shock is presumed to be the cause of the patient's hypotension (Ward, 2001). Attention should then be directed toward countering the cardiopulmonary dysfunction associated with neurogenic shock, and measures to maximally preserve residual spinal cord function should be instituted. To this end, intravenous fluid administration is decreased to maintenance rates and therapy with pressor agents (dopamine and dobutamine) is started. The period of neurogenic shock can last weeks. During this time, sympathomimetics and occasionally atropine sulfate are essential to counter parasympathetic dominance and to facilitate restoration of vascular tone and cardiac performance. Maintaining perfusion of injured spinal tissue and oxygen supplementation reduces the threat of secondary ischemic damage to traumatized tissue. Consultation with an expert in blood pressure management under these circumstances is important.

In patients with blunt spinal cord injury, the administration of high-dose methylprednisolone early in treatment has been recommended as a proactive measure to reduce the extent of paralysis in the long term (Gilson et al., 1995; Marotta, 2000; Mahoney, 2001). This recommendation is based on findings from two multicenter, double-blind, randomized trials in which patients received placebo, naloxone, or very high-dose methylprednisolone therapy within 8 hours of their injury. The methylprednisolone group experienced significantly greater improvement in sensation and motor function up to 1 year after injury (Bracken et al., 1990, 1992). Theorized mechanisms by which methylprednisolone improves neurological outcome include blocking PGF-2α induced membrane lipid peroxidation (Liu et al., 2001), potentiating the neuroprotective/regenerative effects of taurine in the damaged cord (Benton et al., 2001), and suppressing expression of neurotropin receptors involved in secondary cell death (Brandoli et al., 2001). Follow-up multicenter randomized trials by the same investigators verified efficacy and refined treatment protocols (Bracken et al., 1997, 1998). In the recommended regimens, all patients less than 8 hours from the occurrence of blunt spinal trauma receive a 30 mg/kg loading dose of methylprednisolone over 15 minutes. If the initial bolus was administered within 3 hours of injury, a continuous drip of 5.4 mg/kg/hr methylprednisolone is infused for 23 hours. Patients loaded between 3 and 8 hours after injury receive the same post-bolus infusion but it is extended over a longer interval (48 hours). There is no proven benefit to initiating high-dose steroid therapy to any patient beyond 8 hours from their injury.

Although high-dose steroid therapy is approved by the Food and Drug Administration (FDA) and considered by many as standard of care, the dosages employed are some of the highest used in any clinical scenario. Patients receiving steroids have an increased incidence of pneumonia and require more ventilation and intensive care nursing (Gerndt et al., 1997). Those receiving the 48-hour regimen are also more likely to have more severe sepsis and severe pneumonia than patients who receive the 24-hour regimen (Bracken et al., 1998). Recently, valid concern has been expressed regarding the statistical methods, randomization, and conclusions of the original National Acute Spinal Cord Injury Studies (Nesathurai, 1998; Coleman et al., 2000; Hurlbert, 2000; Short et al., 2000). Thus, if steroids are administered, vigilance for, and prophylaxis of, anticipated steroid-related complications (infections, gastrointestinal bleeding, wound disruption, steroid myopathy, avascular necrosis, and glucose intolerance) are necessary.

The secondary survey of the pregnant patient with an acute SCI focuses on more precisely defining the nature and extent of the lesion and determining the status of the fetus. A thorough neurological exam is required and complete documentation is important so that improvement or deterioration of the lesion can be monitored with serial examinations. Once the lesion has been clinically identified a number of radiological studies may become necessary to futher define it and help with planning for appropriate treatment. X-rays of the cervical spine are the standard initial studies used to assess the injury and dictate what further modalities may be needed. CT is best for bony detail and may become necessary to clarify fractures revealed by X-rays, when: (i) neurologic injury is present; (ii) more extensive injury is clinically apparent than is seen on the X-ray; or (iii) injury detected on the X-ray suggests instability. If a neurologic lesion appears to be progressing, CT myelography may be required to exclude spinal cord compression by an extrinsic mass such as a hematoma (Ward, 2001). As will be discussed later, ionizing radiation can have adverse fetal consequences. The input of the obstetrician may be helpful in minimizing fetal radiation exposure.

Fetal concerns during acute spinal cord injury

While it is important to remember that there are at least two individuals to be cared for in every pregnant trauma patient, initial efforts should be focused primarily on the stabilization of the mother. Care should not be withheld, delayed, or attenuated because of the pregnancy, since the welfare of the fetus depends on the well-being of the mother. There are two exceptional circumstances where it may be more appropriate to attend to the fetus first and these are: (i) a viable fetus in a dying mother; or (ii) a dying viable fetus in a stabilized mother. In either case, prompt cesarean delivery is indicated. Because 48% of SCI patients die as a result of their injuries (Marrota, 2000), the possibility of perimortem cesarean delivery is very real in these patients. The procedure should be initiated if there is no response to CPR within 4 minutes, with the intent to complete delivery by 5 minutes (Katz et al., 1986). Delivery relieves caval compression and also allows for a large autotransfusion of blood back into the circulation when the uterus is evacuated and contracts down. These events, together with maintaining a leftward tilt, increase venous return, the efficacy of chest compressions, and ultimately survival. Direct access to the maternal aorta via the abdominal incision may also allow its compression above the renal arteries and optimization of blood flow to the brain and heart.

If the mother is stable, cesarean delivery should also be performed as a rescue procedure for a stressed/distressed but viable fetus. Documentation of the fetal heart rate should ideally be included as part of the primary survey on a pregnant trauma patient ascertained to be in the third trimester of her pregnancy (Morris et al., 1996). Fetal heart rate monitoring should begin with completion of the primary survey in patients with a viable and potentially salvageable baby. When immediate delivery for fetal indications is necessary and no anesthesia is available, cesarean section without anesthesia has been reported in patients with neurogenic shock and a lesion above T10 (Gilson et al., 1995). However, anesthesia is generally required and recommended for all SCI patients undergoing cesarean delivery. The clinician should anticipate the possibility of uterine atony if dopamine is being used to treat neurogenic shock, because of its uterine relaxant effect (Gilson et al., 1995).

The pregnant woman with SCI may require many examinations involving radiation, both acutely and later in her care. Currently, a cumulative radiation exposure of up to 5 rad or less is regarded as unlikely to have significant teratogenic effects (ICRP, 1982; Brent, 1989). With the exception of CT, individual diagnostic procedures typically deliver radiation in the millirad range (Table 17.3) and will not subject the fetus to enough ionizing radiation to inflict harm. However, the cumu-

Table 17.3 Estimated radiologic doses for common trauma radiographs

Cervical spine	<1 mrad
Chest (two views)	0.02–0.07 mrad
Abdomen (one view)	100 mrad
Pelvis	200–500 mrad
Lumbar spine	600–1,000 mrad
Hip (one view)	200 mrad
CT head/chest (shielded)	<1,000 mrad
CT abdomen/lumbar spine	3,500 mrad
CT pelvis	3,000–9,000 mrad

(From Jagoda A, Kessler SG. Trauma in pregnancy. In: Harwood-Nuss A, ed. The Clinical Practice of Emergency Medicine, 3rd edn. Philadelphia, PA: Lippincott, Williams and Wilkins; 2001 and American College of Obstetricians and Gynecologists Committee Opinion. Guidelines for diagnostic imaging during pregnancy. Number 158, Sept. 1995.)

lative dose of the studies required to define and treat an SCI may approach the critical threshold. The radiation exposure from numerous higher-dose studies, such as abdominal or pelvic CT scans, barium studies, and intravenous pyelography, may quickly add up to more than 5 rad (Damilakis et al., 2000). In a study involving 114 pregnant patients admitted to a trauma center between 1995 and 1999, the mean *initial* radiation exposure was 4.5 rad. Cumulative radiation exposure exceeded 5 rad in 85% of patients (Bochicchio et al., 2001). Minimizing fetal exposure is a fundamental component of patient care. While there should be no hesitation to perform necessary radiological studies in patients with an acute SCI, one should insure that only those studies that are truly indicated are obtained. Whenever possible, the number of views obtained should be minimized and radiologic techniques employed to diminish the dose absorbed per view (International Commission on Radiological Protection, 1982). Monitoring devices such as personal radiation monitors or thermoluminescent dosimeters can be used to provide an accurate measure of cumulative radiation exposure (Goldman & Wagner, 1999). Whenever possible, lead sheets should be used to limit maternal abdominal and pelvic exposure.

Long-term antepartum/intrapartum concerns

Long-term care of the pregnant patient with SCI requires cognizance of the specific, predictable medical complications that may occur in such pregnancies. The acute care of the SCI patient revolves around treatment of neurogenic shock and minimizing secondary injury to the cord. Of primary importance in managing the chronic SCI patient is the prevention, prompt recognition of, and treatment of, autonomic hyperreflexia (AH). This potentially life-threatening complication occurs in up to 85% of patients with lesions at or above T5–6 (although it has been reported with lesions as low as T10; (Gimovsky et al., 1985) following the resolution of spinal shock (Westgren et al., 1993; Baker & Cardenas, 1996)). Reflex activity generally returns within 6 months of injury, at which time those patients with damage above the region of splanchnic sympathetic outflow (T6 to L2) become susceptible to the development of AH (Colachis, 1992). With this complication, noxious stimuli create impulses that enter the cord at different levels and progress upward until they are blocked by the lesion. Unable to ascend further, afferent impulses are channeled instead by interneurons to synapse with sympathetic nerves, resulting in an extensive, multilevel dispersal of sympathetic activity (Colachis, 1992). This explosive autonomic discharge can manifest suddenly and dramatically. The patient typically develops an intense, pounding headache, profuse sweating, facial flushing, and nausea. Nasal congestion, piloerection and a blotchy rash above the level of the lesion are also frequently present.

Impressive signs accompany the physical expressions of sympathetic discharge. In a matter of seconds, blood pressure may increase threefold to reach malignant levels. Systolic blood pressures as high as 260 mmHg and diastolic pressures in excess of 200 mmHg have been reported (Colachis, 1992). Left untreated, such hypertensive crises can quickly lead to retinal hemorrhage, cerebrovascular accidents, intracranial hemorrhage, seizures, encephalopathy, and death (Abouleish, 1980).

The same spinal cord lesion that blocks the ascent of sensory impulses that trigger sympathetic discharge, also prevent the descent of central supraspinal inhibitory impulses. Intense compensatory reflex parasympathetic output is thus channeled outside of the spinal system via the vagus nerve. Consequently, the patient with autonomic hyperreflexia can present with paradoxical bradycardia and cardiac dysrhythmias in synchrony with the manifestations of unrestrained sympathetic activity.

Recognition and prevention are paramount in avoiding the potentially lethal consequences of AH. AH can occur in response to virtually any sensory stimulus below the level of the lesion, during any stage of pregnancy. It has been reported in conjunction with cervical examination, bladder and bowel distention, catheterization, rectal disimpaction, breastfeeding, and episiotomy (Baker & Cardenas, 1996). Hence any potentially noxious stimuli should be consciously avoided or minimized by employing topical anesthetic jelly for digital exams, catheterization, and fecal disimpaction (Greenspoon & Paul, 1986).

While bladder distention is the most common precipitant of AH overall (Lindan et al., 1980), labor is a potent stimulus for the pregnant SCI patient. In susceptible patients, it should be anticipated and differentiated from preeclampsia. Maternal death secondary to intracranial hemorrhage has been reported when AH was misdiagnosed as preeclampsia (Abouleish, 1980). The hypertension of preeclampsia usually persists into the immediate puerperium, often resolving slowly in the first days postpartum. In contrast, the hypertension of AH crescendos with each contraction and subsides in the interim between contractions, with occasional patients actually becoming hypotensive between contractions. It abates abruptly with removal of the noxious stimulus. Patient familiarity and experience with AH is also helpful for rapid differentiation between these disease entities.

Immediate management of AH is oriented towards identifying the inciting stimulus and normalization of blood pressure. The patient should be assessed for bladder distention from lack or obstruction of drainage, uterine contractions, perineal distention, and fecal impaction. Tight clothing, footwear, or external fetal monitoring straps can also cause AH. Blood pressure can be lowered quickly simply be changing the maternal position from supine to erect. Short-acting pharmacologic agents such as nifedipine or hydralazine are also useful for lowering the blood pressure until more definitive therapy with regional anesthesia is feasible. Short-acting agents are preferable to longer acting drugs since they allow avoidance of prolonged hypotension between contractions once the stimulus is removed or suppressed.

Prophylactic and therapeutic administration of regional anesthesia is the cornerstone of labor management of the SCI patient at risk for AH. Epidural anesthesia effectively disrupts the propagation of sympathetic afferent impulses through the spine. Although obtaining a good regional block in patients with prior neurologic damage or back surgery can be technically difficult, it is nearly universally successful in preventing or aborting an episode of AH (Greenspoon & Paul, 1986; Crosby et al., 1992; Baker & Cardenas, 1996). Failure of regional anesthesia to arrest ongoing AH is one of the few unique indications for cesarean section in a patient with SCI. The depth of general anesthesia typically required to suppress AH often results in neonatal suppression. Thus, when feasible, supplemental regional anesthesia should be employed for cesarean section patients with high spinal lesions (Baker & Cardenas, 1996). Alternatively, if general anesthesia is used, adequate neonatal resuscitation expertise and equipment should be immediately available at the time of delivery.

Given the potential for serious maternal morbidity and death, the possibility of AH should be anticipated in patients with SCI, and a plan for care should be established well in advance of labor. Early antepartum anesthesia consultation is mandatory, not only for those parturients at risk for AH, but for all SCI patients. This allows for the risks and benefits of regional anesthesia to be discussed in a controlled setting, and alerts the patient to the possibility, and consequences, of AH in labor. It is recommended that an epidural be placed as soon as the patient presents in labor, as well as prior to induction or augmentation of labor (Crosby et al., 1992). Meticulous and frequent blood pressure monitoring is essential. Placement of an arterial line and continuous cardiac monitoring for dysrhythmia are recommended (Greenspoon & Paul, 1986). Continuous bladder drainage is also advisable. An early anesthesia consult also provides an opportunity for pulmonary function assessment. Patients with cervical or high thoracic lesions can have compromised pulmonary capacity secondary to debilitated intercostal muscle function as well as an attenuated cough reflex. Patients with SCI often have baseline vital capacities measuring less than 2 L, predisposing them to atelectesis, pneumonia, and diminishing their capacity to satisfy oxygen requirements (Baker & Cardenas, 1996). The burden of pregnancy-related decrements in functional reserve capacity and expired reserve volume, as well as increased oxygen consumption, can culminate in the need for assisted ventilation in SCI patients. Thus, ventilatory function should be monitored with serial vital capacity measurements (Greenspoon & Paul, 1986) and ventilatory support initiated when the VC falls below 15 mL/kg (Macklem, 1986).

In summary, care of the acute spinal cord patient requires an awareness of commonly occurring serious or life-threatening complications. Immediate care consists of initial stabilization, treatment of neurogenic shock, and the avoidance of secondary cord damage by minimizing physical manipulation and cord hypoxia. Extended antepartum and intrapartum care is focused on prevention, recognition, and expeditious management of AH. Comprehensive management of pregnant SCI patients necessitates attention to the multitude of medical complications that accompany chronic SCI including urinary hygiene, pressure sores, thromboembolic surveillance, and pulmonary toilet, and the potential for unattended delivery secondary to unperceived labor. The reader is referred to the comprehensive reviews by Hughes and Baker (Hughes et al., 1991; Baker & Cardenas, 1996).

References

Abouleish E. Hypertension in a paraplegic parturient. Anesthesiology 1980;53(4):348.

American College of Obstetrics and Gynecology. Obstetric aspects of trauma management. Educational Bulletin Number 251, September 1998.

Baker ER, Cardenas DD. Pregnancy in spinal cord injured women. Arch Phys Med Rehabil 1996;77(5):501–507.

Benton RL, Ross CD, Miller KE. Spinal taurine levels are increased 7 and 30 days following methylprednisolone treatment of spinal cord injury in rats. Brain Res 2001;893(1–2):292–300.

Bivins HG, Ford S, Bezmalinovic Z, Price HM, Williams JL. The effect of axial traction during orotracheal intubation of the trauma victim with an unstable cervical spine. Ann Emerg Med 1988;17(1): 25–29.

Blackwell TL, Krause JS, Winkler T, Stiens S. Spinal Cord Injury: Guidelines for Life Care Planning and Case Management. Appendix A: Demographic Characteristics of Spinal Cord Injury. New York: Demos Medical Publishing, Inc.;2001:133–138.

Bochicchio GV, Napolitano LM, Haan J, Champion H, Scalea T. Incidental pregnancy in trauma patients. J Am Coll Surg 2001;192(5): 566–569.

Bracken MB, Shepard MJ, Collins WF, et al. A randomized, controlled trial of methylprednisolone or naloxone in the treatment of acute spinal-cord injury. Results of the Second National Acute Spinal Cord Injury Study. N Engl J Med 1990;322(20):1405–1411.

Bracken MB, Shepard MJ, Collins WF Jr, et al. Methylprednisolone or naloxone treatment after acute spinal cord injury: 1-year follow-up data. Results of the second National Acute Spinal Cord Injury Study. J Neurosurg 1992;76(1):23–31.

Bracken MD, Shepard MJ, Holford TR, et al. Administration of methylprednisolone for 24 or 48 hours or tirilazad mesylate for 48 hours in the treatment of acute spinal cord injury. Results of the Third National Acute Spinal Cord Injury Randomized Controlled Trial. National Acute Spinal Cord Injury Study. JAMA 1997;277(20): 1597–1604.

Bracken MB, Shepard MJ, Holford TR, et al. Methylprednisolone or tirilazad mesylate administration after acute spinal cord injury: 1-year follow up. Results of the third National Acute Spinal Cord Injury randomized controlled trial. J Neurosurg 1998;89(5):699–706.

Brandoli C, Shi B, Pflug B, Andrews P, Wrathall JR, Mocchetti I. Dexamethasone reduces the expression of p75 neurotrophin receptor and apoptosis in contused spinal cord. Brain Res Mol Brain Res 2001;87(1):61–70.

Brent RL. The effect of embryonic and fetal exposure to x-ray, microwaves, and ultrasound: counseling the pregnant and nonpregnant patient about these risks. Semin Oncol 1989;16(5):347–368.

Colachis SC III. Autonomic hyperreflexia with spinal cord injury. J Am Paraplegia Soc 1992;15(3):171–186.

Coleman WP, Benzel D, Cahill DW, et al. A critical appraisal of the reporting of the National Acute Spinal Cord Injury Studies (II and III) of methylprednisolone in acute spinal cord injury. J Spinal Disord 2000;13(3):185–199.

Crosby E, St-Jean B, Reid D, Elliot RD. Obstetrical anaesthesia and analgesia in chronic spinal cord-injured women. Can J Anaesth 1992;39(5 Pt 1):487–494.

Cross LL, Meythaler JM, Tuel SM, Cross AL. Pregnancy, labor and delivery post spinal cord injury. Paraplegia 1992;30(12):890–902.

Damilakis J, Perisinakis K, Voloudaki A, Gourtsoyiannis N. Estimation of fetal radiation dose from computed tomography scanning in late pregnancy: depth-dose data from routine examinations. Invest Radiol 2000;35(9):527–533.

Donaldson WF III, Towers JD, Doctor A, Brand A, Donaldson VP. A methodology to evaluate motion of the unstable spine during intubation techniques. Spine 1993;18(14):2020–2023.

Donaldson WF III, Heil BV, Donaldson VP, Silvaggio VJ. The effect of airway maneuvers on the unstable C1–C2 segment. A cadaver study. Spine 1997;22(11):1215–1218.

Gerndt SJ, Rodriguez JL, Pawlik JW, et al. Consequences of high-dose steroid therapy for acute spinal cord injury. J Trauma 1997;42(2): 279–284.

Gilson GJ, Miller AC, Clevenger FW, Curet LB. Acute spinal cord injury and neurogenic shock in pregnancy. Obstet Gynecol Surv 1995;50(7):556–560.

Gimovsky ML, Ojeda A, Ozaki R, Zerne S. Management of autonomic hyperreflexia associated with a low thoracic spinal cord lesion. Am J Obstet Gynecol 1985;153(2):223–224.

Goldman SM, Wagner LK. Radiologic ABCs of maternal and fetal survival after trauma: when minutes may count. Radiographics 1999;19(5):1349–1357.

Goodwin H, Holmes JF, Wisner DH. Abdominal ultrasound examination in pregnant blunt trauma patients. J Trauma 2001;50(4): 689–693.

Greenspoon JS, Paul RH. Paraplegia and quadriplegia: special considerations during pregnancy and labor and delivery. Am J Obstet Gynecol 1986;155(4):738–741.

Holley J, Jorden R. Airway management in patients with unstable cervical spine fractures. Ann Emerg Med 1989;18(11):1237–1239.

Hughes SJ, Short DJ, Usherwood MM, Tebbutt H. Management of the pregnant woman with spinal cord injuries. Br J Obstet Gynaecol 1991;98(6):513–518.

Hurlbert RJ. Mehylprednisolone for acute spinal cord injury: an inappropriate standard of care. J Neurosurg 2000;93(Suppl 1):1–7.

International Commission on Radiological Protection. Protection of the patient in diagnostic radiology ICRP Publication 34. Oxford, England: Pergamon, 1982.

Katz VL, Dotters DJ, Droegemueller W. Perimortem cesarean delivery. Obstet Gynecol 1986:68(4):571–576.

Lindan R, Joiner B, Freehafer AA, Hazel C. Incidence and clinical features of autonomic dysreflexia in patients with spinal cord injury. Paraplegia 1980;18(5):285–292.

Liu D, Li L, Augustus L. Prostaglandin release by spinal cord injury mediates production of hydroxyl radical, malondialdehyde and cell death: a site of the neuroprotective action of methyprednisolone. J Neurochem 2001;77(4):1036–1047.

Lucas W, Kirschbaum T, Assali NS. Spinal shock and fetal oxygenation. Am J Obstet Gynecol 1965;93(4):583–587.

McGregor JA, Meeuwsen J. Autonomic hyperreflexia: a mortal danger for spinal cord-damaged women in labor. Am J Obstet Gynecol 1985;151(3):330–333.

Macklem PT. Muscular weakness and respiratory function. N Engl J Med 1986;314(12):775–776.

Mahoney BD. Spinal cord injuries. In: Harwood-Nuss A, ed. The Clinical Practice of Emergency Medicine, 3rd edn, Philadelphia, PA: Lippincott Williams and Wilkins, 2001;495–500.

Marotta JT. Spinal injury. In: Rowland, LP, ed. Merritt's Neurology, 10th edn, Philadelphia, PA: Lippincott Williams and Wilkins, 2000:416–423.

Morris JA Jr, Rosenbower TJ, Jurkovich GJ, et al. Infant survival after cesarean section for trauma. Ann Surg 1996;223(5):481–491.

National Spinal Cord Injury Statistic Center. Spinal Cord Injury: Facts and figures at a glance. January, 2000. Birmingham, Alabama.

Nesathurai S. Steroids and spinal cord injury: revisiting the NASCIS 2 and NASCIS 3 trials. J Trauma 1998;45(6):1088–1093.

Nunn CR, Bass JG, Eddy VA. Management of the pregnant patient with acute Spinal cord injury. Tenn Med 1996;89(9):335–337.

Short DJ, El Masry WS, Jones PW. High dose methylprednisolone in the management of acute spinal cord injury—a systematic review from a clinical perspective. Spinal Cord 2000;38(5):273–286.

Ward KR. Trauma Airway Management. In: Harwood-Nuss A, ed. The Clinical Practice of Emergency Medicine, 3rd edn. Philadelphia, PA: Lippincott Williams and Wilkins, 2001:433–441.

Westgren N, Hultling C, Levi R, Westgren M. Pregnancy and delivery in women with a traumatic spinal cord injury in Sweden, 1980–1991. Obstet Gynecol 1993;81(6):926–930.

18 Cerebrovascular accidents

Mark W. Tomlinson
Bernard Gonik

Cerebral vascular accidents in the pregnant patient are a rare but frequently catastrophic event. The uncommon occurrence in young women often makes the diagnosis and subsequent management a challenge. Stroke is classified as either hemorrhagic or ischemic. Anatomically, intracranial hemorrhage (ICH) can be divided into intracerebral hemorrhage and subarachnoid hemorrhage (SAH). Ischemic stokes can result from thromboembolic events, severe hypertension, or significant hypotension. Typically, SAH during pregnancy is due to ruptured cerebral aneurysms or arteriovenous malformations (AVM), while intracerebral hemorrhage is primarily associated with hypertension, although there is often pathologic overlap depending on the location of the lesion. Other less common conditions that can be associated with ICH include moyamoya disease, dural venous sinus thrombosis, mycotic aneurysm, choriocarcinoma, vasculitides, brain tumors, and coagulopathies (Enomoto & Got, 1987; Isla et al., 1997). Cocaine and phenylpropanolamine also have been associated with ICH in pregnant patients (Maher, 1987; Henderson & Torbey, 1988; Iriye et al., 1995).

Regulation of cerebral blood flow

Human cerebral blood flow averages approximately 50 ml/min/100 g of brain tissue and is normally regulated to maintain constant flow over a wide range of systemic BPs (Kety & Schmidt, 1948; Lassen, 1959). In addition, cerebral blood flow is markedly affected by levels of systemic oxygen and carbon dioxide; elevation of $P\text{co}_2$ by as little as 15 mmHg results in a 75% increase in cerebral blood flow (Kety & Schmidt, 1948). Similarly, a reduction in arterial $P\text{o}_2$ to 50 mmHg results in a 100% increase in cerebral blood flow. On the other hand, elevation of the normal arterial $P\text{o}_2$ by the inhalation of pure oxygen results in a 15% decrease in cerebral blood flow, and hyperventilation with a decrease in $P\text{co}_2$ by 15 mmHg results in a 33% decrease (Kety & Schmidt, 1948). In the previously normotensive patient, the process of cerebral blood flow autoregulation is not reliably maintained at levels of mean arterial pressure in excess of 140 mmHg; this level is somewhat higher for patients with longstanding chronic hypertension. Pressures in excess of these levels can result in SAH, even in the absence of underlying vascular defects.

Subarachnoid hemorrhage

Aneurysms and AVMs are believed to develop secondary to congenital defects in cerebral vasculature formation. Aneurysms are sacular dilations of the vessel generally located at an angle of bifurcation in or near the circle of Willis. AVMs are an interconnected complex of arteries and veins lacking an intervening capillary bed. In contrast to aneurysms, AVMs can be found throughout the brain but are most commonly seen in the frontoparietal and temporal regions. As many as 60% of patients with AVMs may also have aneurysms which can be located within the AVM itself or in other uninvolved vessels (Redekop et al., 1998). The usual anatomic distribution of both vascular abnormalities in pregnancy is similar to that in the nongravid population (Dias & Sekhar, 1990). Figure 18.1 displays the most common locations of aneurysms in the pregnant patient.

The natural history of intracranial aneurysms in the nonpregnant patient varies, depending on several clinical factors. Asymptomatic lesions account for 95% of intracranial aneurysms and are usually identified incidentally. Cerebral angiography has identified aneurysms incidentally in approximately 1% of individuals, and autopsy series reported their presence in between 1% and 6% of patients (Schievink, 1997). These asymptomatic lesions rupture at a rate of 1–2% per year (Jane et al., 1985; Barrow & Reisner, 1993). Activities reported to precede aneurysmal rupture include emotional strain, heavy lifting, coughing, coitus, urination, and defecation. All of these activities may increase intracranial pressure (ICP) and alter hemodynamics. Symptomatic aneurysms present a greater risk. Their annual risk of rupture is 6% (Barrow & Reisner, 1993). Once bleeding has occurred morbidity and

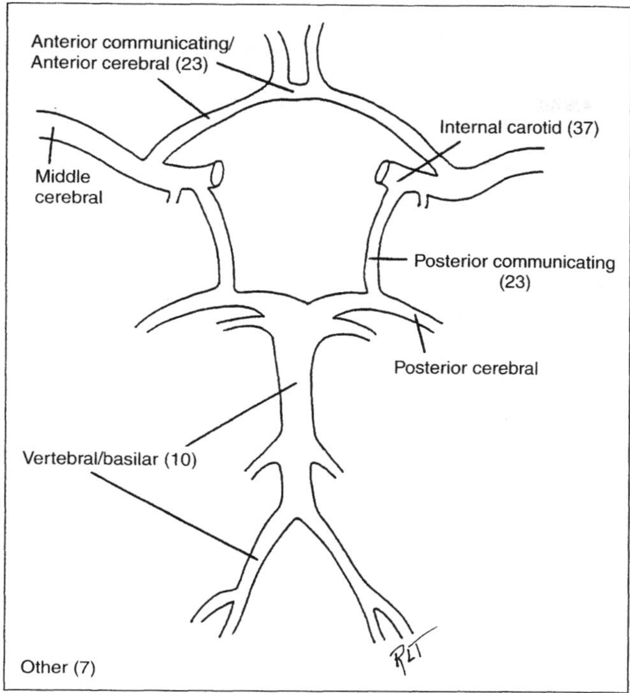

Fig. 18.1 Location of cerebral aneurysms in pregnancy (%).

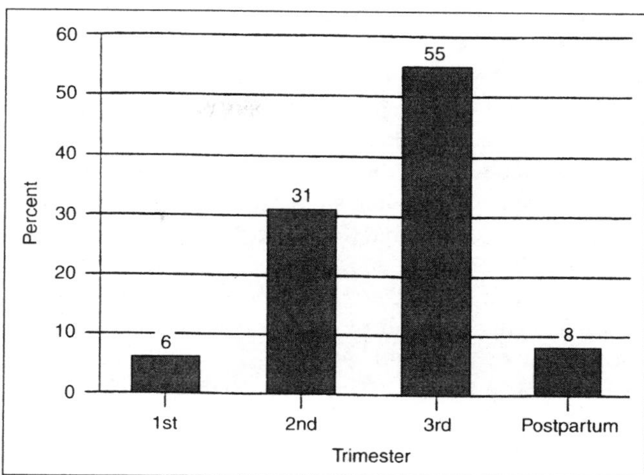

Fig. 18.2 Gestational age distribution of aneurysmal SAH.

mortality rates are high. More than 10% of patients will die before reaching the hospital. Of those patients hospitalized, 40% will die within the first 30 days after the event. More than 30% of survivors will have significant neurologic morbidity (Schievink, 1997). Significant factors affecting the patient's ultimate outcome include the patient's clinical condition upon presentation, the occurrence of rebleeding, and the development of secondary vasospasm (Barrow & Reisner, 1993). In addition, patients who have bled from an aneurysm are at risk of developing new aneurysms at a rate of approximately 2% per year (Juvela et al., 1993).

In the United States, AVMs may be present in approximately 0.1% of the population (Arteriovenous Malformation Study Group, 1999). The natural history of these lesions in the non-pregnant population is variable with some malformations enlarging, while others may stay the same or even regress (Abdulrauf et al., 1999). Outcomes of patients with AVMs are influenced by presenting symptoms and subsequent treatment. Spontaneous bleeding is the most common presentation accounting for between 30 and 80% of all cases. These patients have the worst prognosis with a mortality rate of 1–15%. Seizures without hemorrhage may be the first symptom in 16–53% of patients, while headache is the initial complaint in 7–48%. Focal neurologic deficit without bleeding is seen in 1–40% of patients. Patients with untreated AVMs have an annual risk of bleeding of 2–4%, with a mortality rate of 1% (Barrow & Reisner, 1993; Arteriovenous Malformation Study Group, 1999). Autopsy data suggest that as many as 12% of patients with AVMs may remain asymptomatic throughout life (Arteriovenous Malformation Study Group, 1999).

During pregnancy, the incidence of SAH is 1–5 per 10,000 pregnancies. Maternal mortality is 30–40%, but rates as high as 80% have been reported (Dias & Sekhar, 1990; Wilterdink & Feldmann, 1994). Fetal outcome parallels that of the mother and reflects the maternal condition as well as the gestational age at delivery (Dias & Sekhar, 1990). Because the condition is rare, pregnancy's effect on cerebral aneurysms and AVMs is controversial. Most episodes of SAH occur later in pregnancy (Wilterdink & Feldmann, 1994; Reichman & Karlman, 1995). The timing of SAH during pregnancy is shown in Fig. 18.2. Several physiologic changes occurring during pregnancy may theoretically predispose these cerebrovascular abnormalities to bleed. These factors include increases in blood volume, stroke volume, and cardiac output (Cunningham et al., 1997). Although labor and delivery would seem to be a particularly high-risk time, Williams et al. (1998) demonstrated a decrease in middle cerebral artery flow velocity at the peak of contractions during active labor and second stage pushing in 15 normotensive women. There was no significant difference in flow between the two events. The decreased flow velocity in the middle cerebral artery was postulated to result from an autoregulatory, vasodilation of downstream intracranial arteries due to increased ICP. Cerebral perfusion pressure, as estimated using transcranial Doppler, is also decreased during epidural anesthesia (Williams & Wilson, 1999).

Despite the theoretical concern, pregnancy does not appear to increase the incidence of SAH, and bleeding during labor and delivery is infrequent (Cannell & Botterell, 1956; Copelan & Mabon, 1962; Amias, 1970; Robinson et al., 1972, 1974; Wiebers & Whisnant, 1985; Wiebers, 1988; Dias & Sekhar, 1990; Forster et al., 1993). Most pregnancies complicated by SAH are preceded by unaffected gestations. In a review of 154 patients prepared by Dias and Sekhar (1990), only 25% were nulliparous, and the mean parity of patients with aneurysmal and AVM ruptures was 2.0 and 1.4, respectively. Barno and Freeman (1976) reviewed 24 years of maternal mortality in Minnesota resulting from SAH. The mean parity among the 37 deaths was 2.9. In Forster et al.'s (1993) report on AVMs in reproductive-age women, the annual rate of hemorrhage was higher in women when they were pregnant than when they were not (9.3% vs 4.5%), but the rate in pregnancy was no different from the 9.6% annual rate in reproductive-age women who never became pregnant. Horton et al. (1990) found no difference in the rate of hemorrhage between their pregnant and nonpregnant patients with AVMs (3.5% vs 3.1%) and thus concluded that pregnancy was not a risk factor for bleeding.

The maternal mortality associated with aneurysmal bleeding is not increased due to pregnancy (Cannell & Botterell, 1956; Pedowitz & Perrell, 1957; Amias, 1970; Dias & Sekhar, 1990). Conversely, AVM-associated mortality appears to be increased in gravid compared with nongravid patients. This likely is related to the poor neurologic condition of these patients at presentation.

Major complications associated with SAH include vasospasm, recurrent hemorrhage, and hydrocephalus. Vasospasm is seen in up to 70% of patients with aneurysm and is a significant factor in subsequent morbidity and mortality (Al-Yamany & Wallace, 1999; Treggiari-Venzi et al., 2001). Vasospasm is seen less commonly in those patients with AVM bleeds (Kassell et al., 1985; Wilterdink & Feldmann, 1994). This complication is caused, at least in part, by the release of several vasoactive products of hemoglobin breakdown in the subarachnoid space; the degree of vasospasm appears to correlate with the amount and distribution of subarachnoid blood (Giannotta et al., 1977; Fisher et al., 1980; Heros et al., 1983; Adams, 1987; Grolimund et al., 1988). The resultant ischemia is a major cause of permanent disability and death (Giannotta et al., 1986). Angiographically, vasospasm appears as cerebral arterial narrowing, sometimes with a beaded pattern. Vasospasm is associated with decreased cerebral blood flow as measured by transcranial Doppler and radioactive tracers such as xenon 133 and transcranial Doppler (Kassell et al., 1985).

Recurrent hemorrhage is a particularly morbid complication and is especially likely in patients with ruptured aneurysm. In the untreated patient, the risk of rebleeding is 6% during the first 48 hours. The risk of rebleeding continues to occur at a rate of 1.5% per day for the remainder of the first 2 weeks. By the end of 6 months, 30–40% will have had a subsequent hemorrhage (Barrow & Reisner, 1993). Mortality increases with each successive bleed, with a rate of 64% and 80% after the first and second rebleed, respectively (Adams et al., 1976). Although few data are available that specifically address the pregnant patient, the risk of recurrent bleeding appears to be similar in this population (Wilterdink & Feldmann, 1994).

Acute hydrocephalus is a very poor prognostic factor in SAH. It has received relatively little attention in pregnant and nonpregnant patients alike. In a large prospective series of nonobstetric patients reported by van Gijn et al. (1985), the incidence of acute hydrocephalus was 20%. The accompanying mortality rate was significantly higher when ventricular dilation was present. Ventricular drainage did not decrease overall mortality despite an initial clinical improvement.

Clinical presentation

Pregnancy does not significantly alter the clinical presentation of SAH. Signs and symptoms of aneurysmal or AVM bleeding are indistinguishable. Intracerebral bleeding associated with severe preeclampsia may also have similar findings. The presenting symptom is usually a sudden-onset severe headache. Frequently, other signs and symptoms accompany the headache. These may include nausea and vomiting, meningeal signs, ocular hemorrhages, decreased level of consciousness, hypertension, focal neurologic signs, and seizures (Giannotta et al., 1986; Schievink, 1997). In addition to the stiff neck resulting from meningeal irritation, patients may complain of severe low back and redicular leg pain as the bloody CSF moves into the spinal column. Up to half of patients with SAH report a severe headache several days before the acute bleeding episode (Schievink, 1997). Specific findings are dependent on the size, location, and rapidity of the bleed. When the hemorrhage is massive, the patient may be moribund at presentation.

One of the most important prognostic indicators of outcome is the patient's condition at presentation. A number of scales have been developed to categorize the severity of the clinical condition in order to guide management and determine prognosis. The Hunt and Hess (1968) scale (Table 18.1) is the most widely used and grades the patient's condition based on level of consciousness, presence of meningeal signs, and focal neurologic signs. This scale has been criticized due to significant intra-observer and inter-observer variation, as well as poor correlation of the meningeal signs with outcome in the presence of normal consciousness (van Gijn et al., 1994). To remedy

Table 18.1 Hunt and Hess clinical grading scale

Grade	Criteria
I	Asymptomatic, or minimal headache and slight nuchal rigidity
II	Moderate to severe headache, nuchal rigidity, no neurologic deficit other than cranial nerve palsy
III	Drowsiness, confusion, or mild focal deficit
IV	Stupor, moderate to severe hemiparesis, early decerebrate rigidity and vegetative disturbances
V	Deep coma, decerebrate rigidity, moribund

Table 18.2 World Federation of Neurological Surgeons (WFNS) SAH scale

WFNS grade	Glasgow Coma Scale	Motor deficit
I	15	Absent
II	13–14	Absent
III	13–14	Present
IV	7–12	Present or absent
V	3–6	Present or absent

Table 18.3 Glasgow Coma Scale

Behavior	Patient response	Component score
Eye opening (E)	Spontaneous	4
	To speech-loud voice	3
	To pain	2
	None	1
Best verbal response (V)	Oriented	5
	Confused, disoriented	4
	Inappropriate words	3
	Incomprehensible	2
	Sounds—none	1
Best motor response (M)	Obeys	6
	Localizes	5
	Flexion (withdraws)	4
	Abnormal flexion posturing	3
	Extension posturing	2
	None	1

Coma score = E + V + M. Patients scoring 3 or 4 have an 85% chance of dying or remaining vegetative, while scores above 11 indicate only a 5–10% likelihood of death or vegetative state and 85% chance of moderate disability or good recovery. Intermediate scores correlate with proportional chances of recovery.

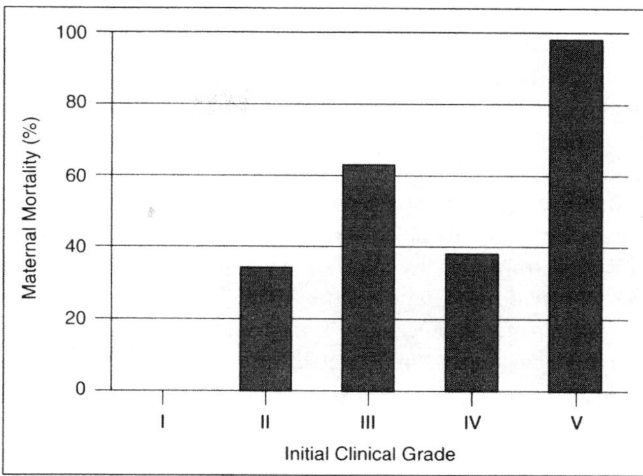

Fig. 18.3 Maternal mortality versus initial clinical grade after aneurysmal hemorrhage.

Table 18.4 Comparison of subarachnoid hemorrhage (SAH) and eclampsia

	SAH	Eclampsia
Headache	Explosive–severe	Insidious–dull
Nausea and vomiting	Common	Uncommon
Loss of consciousness	2/3	All (seizure)
Nuchal rigidity	90%	Uncommon
Seizures	15%	All
Hypertension	30–50%	All
Proteinuria	Uncommon	Common
Focal motor weakness	20%	Rare

(Adapted by permission from Giannotta SL, Daniels J, Golde SH, et al. Ruptured intracranial aneurysms during pregnancy: a report of four cases. J Reprod Med 1986;31:139.)

these limitations, a committee of the World Federation of Neurologic Surgeons proposed the more objective WNFS Scale (Table 18.2) that combined the Glasgow Coma Scale (Teasdale & Jennett, 1974) with the presence or absence of motor deficits (Drake, 1988). The Glasgow Coma Scale is presented in Table 18.3. Despite its advantages, the WNFS scale has yet to be widely incorporated into practice (van Gijn et al., 1994). Maternal mortality in relation to initial clinical grade of aneurysmal hemorrhage is shown in Fig. 18.3 (Dias, 1990).

Diagnosis

It is imperative that the clinician maintains a high index of suspicion due to the rarity and life-threatening nature of the condition. Frequently, SAH is confused with eclampsia, resulting in diagnostic delays (Gianotta et al., 1986; Witlin et al., 1997). Table 18.4 compares clinical findings of SAH and eclampsia. All abnormal neurologic signs and symptoms in the gravida should be evaluated thoroughly. A team approach, with appropriate maternal–fetal medicine, neurology, and neurosurgery consultation should be sought to guide the diagnostic work-up. A computed tomography (CT) scan of the brain, lumbar puncture (if necessary) and cerebral angiography is the common sequence of testing. The CT scan can predict, with a high degree of accuracy, the type of hemorrhage and its site of origin. In addition, cerebral CT can be useful in determining the presence of life-threatening hematomas that require surgical evacuation, as well as the development of hydrocephalus (Schievink, 1997). The ability of the CT scan to detect blood in the subarachnoid space decreases from up to 95% within 24 hours of an acute hemorrhage to 50% 1 week after (van Gijn & van Fongen, 1982). If the CT scan is normal and there is a high index of suspicion, the CSF should be examined for blood or xanthochromia. Nonclearing bloody CSF found at lumbar puncture supports the diagnosis of SAH, but it is not diagnostic. It may be seen with a traumatic tap and occasionally with other conditions, such as preeclampsia. Cerebral angiography, including magnetic resonance angiography, remains the best diagnostic tool for identifying any vascular abnormality. In addition, important anatomic (and therefore prognostic) information is usually obtained with these invasive techniques. However, angiography may fail to visualize the cause of SAH in 20% of patients (Gianotta et al., 1986). In these cases, a repeat angiogram may be necessary to rule out false-negative results secondary to vasospasm or clot filling of the aneurysm. A magnetic resonance imaging (MRI) scan lacks sensitivity in detecting acute SAH (Schievink, 1997), but it may be helpful in situations where the initial angiogram fails to identify the lesion. This technique also can identify vascular lesions in the spinal cord (Wilterdink & Feldmann, 1994). Abdominal shielding should be considered during any radiologic examination of the gravid patient.

Identifying patients at risk for having an asymptomatic intracranial aneurysm has been advocated due to the significant morbidity and mortality associated with rupture and the relatively low risk associated with aneurysmal surgery. Patients likely to benefit from this approach are those with two or more affected first-degree relatives or those with autosomal dominant polycystic kidney disease. When screened, 9% of the former group (Ronkainen et al., 1995) and 5–10% of the latter group were found to have asymptomatic aneurysms (Chapman et al., 1992; Ruggieri, 1994). Ideally this screening and indicated treatment would be completed preconceptually.

Management

Standard neurologic management of SAH is only slightly altered during pregnancy. The clinical goals of preventing neurologic complications and treating them when they occur remain the same. Neurosurgical principles should guide therapy. In all patients thought to be viable, immediate management involves evacuation of any life-threatening hematoma (Giannotta & Kindt, 1979; Sadasivan et al., 1990). A number of considerations have led neurosurgeons to perform early aneurysm clipping in the post-SAH period (4 days) for patients with grades I–III. These considerations include the disastrous consequences of rebleeding and the decreased vasospasm with early removal of cisternal blood. Advances in neurosurgery and neuroanesthesia have aided the early surgical approach (Giannotta & Kindt, 1979; Kassell et al., 1981; Ljunggren et al., 1982, 1984; Taneda, 1982; Kassell & Torner, 1984; Giannotta et al., 1986). Early operation also allows for therapies such as induced hypertension and volume expansion to be instituted to combat vasospasm without increasing the risk of rebleeding (Giannotta & Kindt, 1979; Kassell et al., 1981, 1982, 1985; Buckland et al., 1988; Schievink & Zabramski, 1998). Improved outcomes for both the mother and the fetus have been realized with early surgical intervention in pregnant patients (Dias & Sekhar, 1990). Patients with significant neurologic deficits (grades IV and V) are less likely to undergo early aneurysm clipping due to an extremely high operative mortality. Rather, such patients receive medical therapy until their condition improves. The proper timing for resection of AVMs is more controversial due to the smaller number of cases reported. No clear benefit to surgery in these patients has been found, with some surgeons advocating operative intervention in AVMs only to remove clinically significant hematomas (Grenvik & Safar, 1981; Dias & Sekhar, 1990). One alternative is embolization of the AVM under angiographic control prior to surgical excision (Aminoff, 1994).

Endovascular occlusion therapy is a relatively new and promising therapeutic option. It involves delivering occlusive devices to the aneurysm or AVM through intravascular catheters. One method is the placement of metal coils within the lesion, which lead to thrombosis and occlusion. Recently the successful use of endovascular occlusion therapy has been reported in two pregnant patients with aneurysmal SAH (Piotin et al., 2001). The first patient was delivered by cesarean section at 32 weeks during the acute event followed immediately by embolization. In the second case treatment occurred at 22 weeks. The remainder of the pregnancy was uncomplicated and the patient was delivered vaginally at term (Piotin et al., 2001). Other devices used in nonpregnant patients have included sclerosing drugs, balloons, and glue. These modalities can be used when the lesion is inoperable or as an initial therapy in conjunction with more defintive surgery. Despite the promise, long-term outcome is not yet known (Schievink, 1997; Bendok et al, 1998; Arteriovenous Malformation Study Group, 1999).

Adjunctive medical therapy for SAH is directed toward reducing the risks of cerebral ischemia due to vasospasm and rebleeding. Patients are generally confined to bed rest in a dark, quiet room. They are administered stool softeners, sedatives, and analgesics. Hypertension, hypervolemia, and hemodilution, often referred to as "triple-H" therapy are used to prevent and treat vasospasm and improve cerebral perfusion. Colloid solutions are frequently chosen for volume expansion. Vasopressors or inotropic agents are used to elevate the systolic blood pressure to between 150 and 200 mmHg (Awad et al., 1987; Soloman et al., 1988; Levy & Giannotta, 1990).

Nimodipine, a dihydropyridone calcium-channel blocker, has been used since the early 1980s to combat vasospasm following aneurysmal SAH. Its use has been associated with significant decreases in severe neurologic deficits and death (Allen et al., 1983; Al-Yamany & Wallace, 1999; Treggiari-Venzi et al., 2001). The usual initial dose of nimodipine is 60 mg orally every 4 hours (Al-Yamany & Wallace, 1999; Treggiari-Venzi et al., 2001). Nimodipine has been used in pregnancy for the treatment of cerebral vasospasm associated with severe preeclampsia or eclampsia (Horn et al., 1990; Belfort et al.,

1993, 1999b; Anthony et al., 1996). Like other calcium-channel blockers, nimodipine will also affect the fetal vasculature (Belfort et al., 1994, 1995). Belfort et al. (1999a) reviewed the use of nimodipine compared with magnesium sulfate for seizure prophylaxis in preeclampsia in a trial involving more than 800 women. There was no difference in adverse fetal outcomes between the two treatments. During the initial stages of the trial there was an increased incidence of eclamptic seizures in the nimodipine group when a dose of 30 mg every 4 hours was used. This difference disappeared when the dose was increased to that typically used for the prevention of vasospasm in SAH.

A complete discussion of the neurosurgical and anesthetic principles of craniotomy for aneurysm clipping is beyond the scope of this chapter. However, there are two intraoperative therapies—hypotension and hypothermia—commonly instituted to reduce complications, which raise special concerns in the pregnant patient. Hypotension is sometimes instituted to reduce the risk of rupture of the aneurysm during dissection. Although maternal hypotension may pose a threat to fetal well-being, it has been successfully induced with sodium nitroprusside or isoflurane in a number of cases (Donchin et al., 1978; Rigg & McDonogh, 1981; Willoughby, 1984; Newman & Lam, 1986). Based on experimental evidence, administration of sodium nitroprusside in pregnant patients has raised concerns regarding potential fetal cyanide toxicity. Thus, if surgery is to be performed during pregnancy, it is recommended that infusion rates not exceed 10 μg/kg/min (Willoughby, 1984). The fetal effects of maternal hypotension should be evaluated throughout the perianesthetic period with electronic fetal heart rate monitoring. Adverse changes in fetal cardiac activity suggest the need for elevation in maternal BP if safe and feasible from the maternal standpoint. Many of the drugs used in anesthesia may decrease fetal heart rate variability, thereby complicating fetal heart rate monitor interpretation (van Buul et al., 1993). Excessive hyperventilation has been shown to further decrease uterine blood flow during sodium nitroprusside administration and should be avoided (Levinson et al., 1974). Because of the potential fetal risks of maternal hypotension, some authors recommend cesarean delivery immediately prior to intracranial surgery in term or near-term gestation (Kassell et al., 1981).

Hypothermia is instituted during cerebral aneurysm clipping as a means of cerebral protection from potential ischemia due to aneurysm rupture, retractor injury, or hypotension. This protective effect is due at least in part to decreased cerebral metabolism with a 7% drop in cerebral oxygen consumption for every 10°C drop in body temperature. Other possible mechanisms include decreases in free radical formation, lipid peroxidation, and release of excitatory neurotransmitters (Connolly & Solomon, 1998; Schievink & Zabramski, 1998). Stange and Hallidin (1983) have suggested that hypothermia is well tolerated by the mother and fetus, provided that other confounding variables (e.g. respiratory exchange, acidosis, and electrolyte balance) are controlled. The majority of experience with hypothermia and hypotension in pregnancy, however, is anecdotal. Regardless of the neurosurgical technique employed, maternal outcome remains the most important predictor of eventual fetal outcome.

After a successful repair of an aneurysm or AVM, the most frequent obstetric concern relates to mode of delivery. Earlier authors routinely recommended elective cesarean section for these patients. This was particularly true along with consideration of sterilization if an AVM was responsible for the SAH (Robinson et al., 1974). More recent data and reanalysis of some older studies suggest that labor and vaginal delivery pose no additional risk to mother or fetus (Copelan & Mabon, 1962; Fleigner et al., 1969; Robinson et al., 1972; Minielly et al., 1979; Parkinson & Bachers, 1980; Dias & Sekhar, 1990; Horton et al., 1990; Forster et al., 1993). It has been suggested that these recommendations probably also hold true for the patient who begins labor before surgical correction is attempted or in the case in which the intracranial lesion is inaccessible to surgical intervention (Young et al., 1983; Dias & Sekhar, 1990). The number of cases on which such recommendations are based, however, is small. In the review by Dias and Sekhar (1990), involving 53 patients with uncorrected AVM or aneurysm, those delivering vaginally had almost twice the mortality rate of those undergoing cesarean section. Nevertheless, this difference did not reach statistical significance, possibly due to small sample size. Moreover, even those authors suggesting vaginal delivery for such women generally hedge their bets by recommending shortening of the second stage of labor with forceps delivery, recommendations not entirely consistent with the presumed safety of the labor and delivery process. We suggest that the available data be discussed with the patient in planning route of delivery. Ultimate management decisions should be based primarily on the maternal condition, with modifications for fetal intervention based on gestational age. Figure 18.4 summarizes the management of the pregnant patient with SAH.

Preecalmpsia-associated intracerebral hemorrhage

Pathophysiology

Intracerebral hemorrhage is the most common cause of death in the eclamptic patient; it is identified in up to 60% of all deaths associated with this condition (Table 18.5). Intracerebral hemorrhage is more likely to occur in the older parturient and is correlated better with advancing maternal age and hypertension than with seizure activity. When hemorrhage does occur, it often does not coincide with the onset of seizures but rather may be manifested as long as 6 hours or more after the onset of convulsions (Sheehan & Lynch, 1973). The pathology of preeclampsia-related intracerebral hemorrhage has been

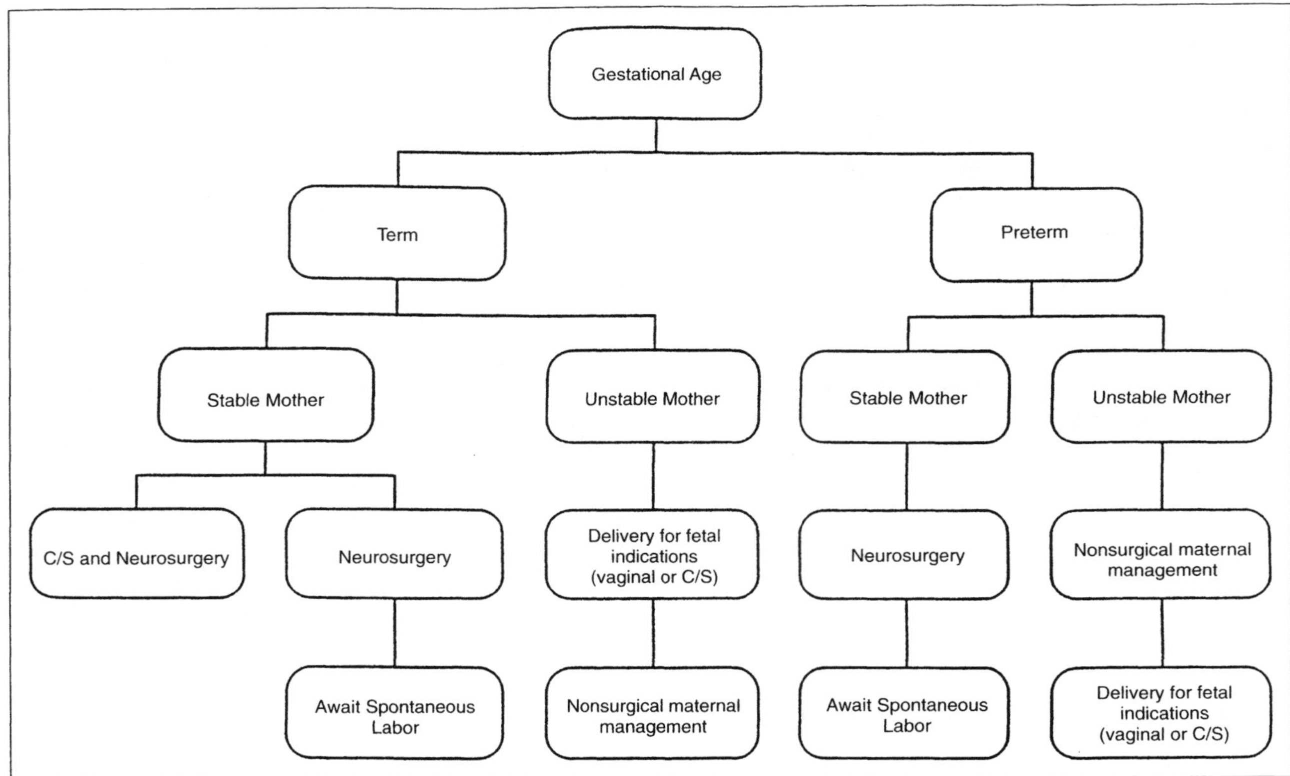

Fig. 18.4 Management scheme for subarachnoid hemorrhage due to cerebral aneurysm or arteriovenous malformation during pregnancy. C/S, cesarean

Table 18.5 Causes of death in patients with preeclampsia/eclampsia

	Donnelly & Lock (1954)	Hibbard (1973)	Lopez-Llera (1982)	Evan et al. (1983)
Cerebral				
Hemorrhage	180	21	62	14
Edema	—	13	—	6
Pulmonary				
Edema	133	3	—	3
Insufficiency	29	4	10	—
Hepatic				
Rupture	30	—	1	3
Necrosis	—	10	—	2
Renal				
Failure	—	2	—	7
Necrosis	—	5	1	—
Coagulopathy	39	6	7	6
Anesthesia	12	—	—	—
Sepsis	18	—	2	—
Drug overdose	—	—	2	—
Undetermined	92	1	3	8
Total	533	67	86	49

(From Evan S, Frigoletto FD, Jewett JF. Mortality of eclampsia: a case report and the experience of the Massachusetts Maternal Mortality Study. N Engl J Med 1983;309:1644.)

reviewed by Sheehan and Lynch (1973). They described a variety of pathologic findings ranging from cortical petechiae possibly due to ischemia resulting from severe vasospasm to a single large intracerebral hemorrhage near a large vessel in the white matter. The clinical report of flashes of light and other fluctuating neurologic signs and symptoms in these patients supports the concept of intermittent ischemia as a factor, although the definitive pathologic events involved still remain to be elucidated.

Clinical presentation

A detailed presentation on the clinical aspects of eclampsia has been reviewed elsewhere in this text. In brief, the eclamptic patient traditionally presents with hypertension and tonic–clonic convulsions. The occurrence of seizure activity, however, does not usually result in the subsequent development of intracerebral hemorrhage, even if a transient neurologic deficit is identified in the postictal period. When small intracerebral hemorrhages do occur, the patient may present initially with only drowsiness or complaints of flashes of light. If the disease progresses, stupor and focal neurologic deficits will worsen. Hemiplegia or rapidly progressive coma and cerebral death may be identified when a more massive cerebral bleed occurs (Donnelly & Lock, 1954; Hibbard, 1973; Lopez-Llera, 1982; Evan et al., 1983). It is important to consider the fact that a sudden increase in blood pressure may be a result of, rather than a cause of, intracranial bleeding (Witlin et al., 1997).

Diagnosis

The diagnosis of preeclampsia is a common activity in the obstetrician's daily practice. The clincian, however, may not always be alert to the fact that a variety of subtle neurologic abnormalities, such as lethargy, visual disturbances, and even acute psychosis, can herald the onset of an intracerebral hemorrhage. With modern CT scanners, abnormal radiologic findings that correlate with the pathologic findings described by Sheehan and Lynch are being detected more frequently (Brown et al., 1988; Milliez et al., 1990). Despite these findings, CT and MRI scans are not recommended as a routine part of the evaluation for uncomplicated eclamptic patients, because management is rarely altered. These diagnostic tools should be employed early in the evaluation when atypical presentations, focal neurologic signs, or a prolonged coma are encountered (Brown et al., 1988; Milliez et al., 1990; Digre et al., 1993).

Management

Acute surgical intervention, even for the removal of a large intracerebral hematoma, is rarely of benefit (Heros & Morcos, 2000). Control of seizure activity and severe hypertension, however, is always indicated. Thrombocytopenia is not an uncommon complication of preeclampsia and may aggravate the intracerebral bleeding process. Appropriate management requires monitoring of coagulation indices and replacement therapy as indicated. If the patient's outcome appears to be grave, consideration of perimortem cesarean delivery should be made.

Adjunctive approaches

Potent glucocorticoids such as dexamethasone have been used widely for the treatment of cerebral edema and ischemia. Support for their use comes not only from laboratory evidence of steroid-induced membrane stabilization but also from the often dramatic clinical improvement of patients with brain tumors (Fishman, 1982). Little clinical evidence exists, however, for the efficacy of steroids, in any dose, in altering the progress and outcome in the presence of elevated ICP (Dearden et al., 1986). Cerebral edema can result in elevated ICP. The neurosurgeon may wish to invasively monitor this variable in some patients to avoid severe intracranial hypertension. In patients with SAH, monitoring usually is done with a ventriculostomy so that CSF can be drained if hydrocephalus is present. The ventriculostomy may be connected to a transducer for continuous monitoring. ICP elevations resulting from cerebral edema may be treated with mannitol, an osmotic diuretic. The mechanism of action for mannitol is felt to be primarily by extraction of both intracellular and extracellular fluid from brain tissue (Nath & Galbraith, 1986). However, mannitol may also produce vasoconstriction, alter blood viscosity, and effect local oxygen delivery (Muizelaar et al., 1984). Mannitol is a nonmetabolized sugar that is available in 20% and 25% solutions. Typically, 12.5–50.0 g are administered intravenously, as needed, to keep the ICP below 20 mmHg. The development of hyperosmolality is a potential hazard of mannitol therapy and can be monitored by serum osmolality determinations. Normal values are 280–300 mosmol/L; the drug should be withheld when a level of 315–320 mosmol/L or a serum sodium of 150 mEq/dL is reached. Evidence exists to suggest that the combination of mannitol and furosemide may result in a greater and more sustained reduction in ICP than either agent given alone (Pollay et al., 1983; Wilkinson & Rosenfeld, 1983). Care must be taken to prevent hypovolemia resulting from the accompanying diuresis, which could aggravate placental and cerebral hypoperfusion. Barbiturate therapy also may be useful in otherwise refractory intracranial hypertension. Pentobarbital is administered slowly in a dose of 5–10 mg/kg actual body weight and may be continued in doses of 2–4 mg/kg/hr. Patients who do not respond to these pharmacologic measures require intubation and hyperventilation to a $P\text{CO}_2$ of 25–30 mmHg to reduce ICP.

In the presence of either ICH or cerebral edema, rapid initiation of diagnostic procedures and therapy is essential. Although pregnancy may complicate the diagnosis, once this life-threatening condition is recognized, pregnancy should not slow or alter appropriate therapy.

Ischemic stroke

Ischemic stroke is uncommon in reproductive-aged women, but pregnancy has traditionally been believed to increase the risk compared to nonpregnant women (Wiebers, 1985). The incidence is reported at 1 in 10,000 (Simolke et al., 1991; Kittner et al., 1996). More recent population-based data has suggested that pregnancy does not increase the risk of ischemic stroke after controlling for confounding variables. During the postpartum period, however, there was more than a twofold increase in the relative risk of cerebral infarction (Kittner et al., 1996). Although ischemic stroke is associated with significant neurologic morbidity, the maternal mortality appears to be less than that seen with hemorrhagic stroke (Witlin et al., 1997, 2000).

A variety of medical conditions are associated with ischemic strokes. A simple classification scheme divides the conditions into ateriopathies, hematologic disorders, and cardioembolic phenomena. Significant atherosclerosis is uncommon in women of reproductive age but can be seen in patients with longstanding diabetes, hypertension, hyperlipidemia, and tobacco use. Cerebral arteritis occurring in patients with systemic lupus may also lead to ischemic stroke. The risk of thrombosis in pregnancy is increased with acquired or inherited thrombophilias such as antiphospholipid antibody syndrome, protein C, S, and antithrombin III deficiency, and the factor V Leiden mutation leading to activated protein C resistance. Elevated levels of homocysteine and a mutation in the prothrombin gene have also been implicated in an increased risk of thrombosis. Sickle cell disease with frequent crisis can lead to generalized vascular damage that may include the cerebral vessels. Aortic or mitral valve disease, atrial fibrillation, peripartum cardiomyopathy, and bacterial endocarditis may give off emboli that can occlude segments of the cerebral circulation (Wiebers, 1985; Donaldson & Lee, 1994).

The presenting symptoms of ischemic strokes are nonspecific and commonly seen in preeclampsia. As with ICH, this can lead to a delay in diagnosis. Headache is the most common presenting symptom, with focal neurologic deficits, seizures and visual changes also occurring frequently. Hypertension is frequently but not universally present. New onset hypertension may occur after the acute event (Witlin et al., 1997, 2000).

The diagnostic evaluation begins with a CT scan whenever there are any atypical neurologic symptoms. An MRI may also be necessary if the clinical setting is suspicious and the CT scan is nondiagnostic (Witlin et al., 2000). If thrombosis is identified, maternal blood studies should include lupus anticoagulant and anticardiolipin antibody, and the factor V Leiden mutation. Blood for homocysteine levels and the prothrombin variant mutation may also be obtained. Protein C, S, and antithrombin III levels should be deferred until after anticoagulation is stopped. Both the acute event and anticoagulation can affect these levels. Protein S levels are also decreased during pregnancy and postpartum (Comp et al., 1986). If an embolic episode is suspected, an electrocardiogram and echocardiogram are indicated (Donaldson & Lee, 1994).

Treatment is based on the underlying etiology. In thrombotic or embolic conditions, anticoagulation is often required. Heparin is the drug of choice during pregnancy because it does not cross the placenta. Low molecular weight heparins have been increasingly used during pregnancy when anticoagulation is required. Advantages include more predictable anticoagulant effect, less frequent dosing, and possibly a decreased risk of thrombocytopenia and osteoporosis when compared to unfractionated heparin (American College of Obstetrics and Gynecology, 2000). Coumadin can be used after delivery and while breastfeeding (American Academy of Pediatrics, 1994).

Cerebral vascular accidents associated with pregnancy are rare events with most obstetricians caring for at most one or two such patients in an entire career. Due to the frequently tragic outcomes and the common overlap of clinical presentation with preeclampsia, it is essential for the clinician to consider stroke as part of the initial differential diagnosis. The diagnostic work-up can then proceed in a timely fashion when any atypical findings are present thus minimizing delays in diagnosis and subsequent treatment.

References

Abdulrauf SI, Malik GM, Awad IA. Spontaneous angiographic obliteration of cerebral arteriovenous malformations. Neurosurgery 1999;44:280–287.

Adams EBT, Loach AB, O'Laoire SA. Intracranial aneurysms: analysis of results of microneurosurgery. Br Med J 1976;2:607–609.

Adams HP, Kassell NF, Torner JC, et al. Predicting cerebral ischemia after aneurysmal subarachnoid hemorrhage: influences of clinical condition, CT results, and antifibrinolytic therapy. Neurology 1987;37:1586–1591.

Allen GS, Ahn HS, Preziosi TJ, et al. Cerebral arterial spasm: a controlled trial of nimodipine in patients with subarachnoid hemorrhage. N Engl J Med 1983;308:619–624.

Al-Yamany M, Wallace MC. Management of cerebral vasospasm in patients with aneurysmal subarachnoid hemorrhage. Intensive Care Med 1999;25:1463–1466.

American Academy of Pediatrics, Committee on Drugs. Transfer of drugs and other chemicals into human milk. Pediatrics 1994;93:137.

American College of Obstetrics and Gynecology Practice Bulletin. Thromboembolism in pregnancy. Compendium of Selected Publications 2000;19:1096.

Amias AG. Cerebral vascular disease in pregnancy. I. Haemorrhage. J Obstet Gynaecol Br Commonw 1970;77:100–120.

Aminoff MJ. Maternal neurologic disorders. In: Creasy RK, Resnik R, eds. Maternal-fetal medicine. Philadelphia: WB Saunders, 1994.

Anthony J, Mantel G, Johanson R, Dommisse J. The haemodynamic and respiratory effects of intravenous nimodipine used in the treatment of eclampsia. Br J Obstet Gynaecol 1996;103:518–522.

Arteriovenous Malformation Study Group. Arteriovenous malformation of the brain in adults. NEJM 1999;340:1812.

Awad IA, Carter LP, Spetzler RF, et al. Clinical vasospasm after subarachnoid hemorrhage: response to hypervolemic hemodilution and arterial hypertension. Stroke 1987;18:365–372.

Barno A, Freeman DW. Maternal deaths due to spontaneous subarachnoid hemorrhage. Am J Obstet Gynecol 1976;125:384–392.

Barrow DL, Reisner A. Natural history of intracranial aneurysms and vascular malformations. Clin Neurosurg 1993;40:3–39.

Belfort MA, Carpenter RJ Jr., Kirshon B, Saade GR, Moise KJ Jr. The use of nimodipine in a patient with eclampsia: color flow Doppler demonstration of retinal artery relaxation. Am J Obstet Gynecol 1993;169:204–206.

Belfort MA, Saade GR, Moise KJ Jr., et al. Nimodipine in the management of preeclampsia: maternal and fetal effects. Am J Obstet Gynecol 1994;171:417–424.

Belfort MA, Saade GR, Suresh M, Johnson D, Vedernikov YP. Human umbilical vessels: responses to agents frequently used in obstetric patients. Am J Obstet Gynecol 1995;172:1395–1403.

Belfort MA, Anthony J, Saade GR. Prevention of eclampsia. Semin Perinatol 1999a;23:65–78.

Belfort MA, Saade GR, Yared M, et al. Change in estimated cerebral perfusion pressure after treatment with nimodipine or magnesium sulfate in patients with preeclampsia. Am J Obstet Gynecol 1999b; 181:402–407.

Bendok BR, Getch CC, Malisch TW, et al. Treatment of aneurysmal subarachnoid hemorrhage. Semin Neurol 1998;18:521.

Brown CEL, Purdy P, Cunningham FG. Head computed tomographic scans in women with eclampsia. Am J Obstet Gynecol 1988;159: 915–920.

Buckland MR, Batjer HH, Giesecke AH. Anesthesia for cerebral aneurysm surgery: use of induced hypertension in patients with symptomatic vasospasm. Anesthesiology 1988;69:116–119.

van Buul BJA, Nijhuis JG, Slappendel R, et al. General anesthesia for surgical repair of intracranial aneurysm in pregnancy: effects on fetal heart rate. Am J Perinatol 1993;10:183–186.

Cannell DE, Botterell EH. Subarachnoid hemorrhage and pregnancy. Am J Obstet Gynecol 1956;72:844.

Chapman AB, Rubinstein D, Hughes R, et al. Intracranial aneurysms in autosomal dominant polycystic kidney disease. N Engl J Med 1992;327:916–920.

Comp PC, Thurnau GR, Welsh J, Esmon CT. Functional and immunologic protein S levels are decreased during pregnancy. Blood 1986;68:881–885.

Connolly ES, Solomon RA. Hypothermic cardiac standstill for cerebral aneurysm surgery. Neurosurg Clin N Am 1998;9:681–695.

Copelan EL, Mabon RF. Spontaneous intracranial bleeding in pregnancy. Obstet Gynecol 1962;20:373.

Cunningham FG, MacDonald PC, Gant NF, et al., eds. Maternal adaptation to pregnancy. In: Williams Obstetrics, 20th edn. Stamford, CT: Appleton & Lange, 1997;191.

Dearden NM, Gibson JS, McDowall DG, et al. Effect of high-dose dexamethasone on outcome from severe head injury. J Neurosurg 1986;64:81–88.

Dias M, Sekhar L. Intracranial hemorrhage from aneurysms and arteriovenous malformations during pregnancy and the puerperium. Neurosurg 1990;27:855–865.

Digre KB, Varner MW, Osborn AG, Crawford S. Cranial magnetic resonance imaging in severe preeclampsia vs eclampsia. Arch Neurol 1993;50:399–406.

Donchin Y, Amirav B, Yarkoni S. Sodium nitroprusside for aneurysm surgery in pregnancy. Br J Anaesth 1978;50:849–851.

Donaldson JO, Lee NS. Arterial and venous stroke associated with pregnancy. Neurol Clin 1994;12:583–599.

Donnelly JF, Lock FR. Causes of death in five hundred thirty-three fatal cases of toxemia of pregnancy. Am J Obstet Gynecol 1954; 68:184.

Drake CG. Report of World Federation of Neurological Surgeons Committee on a universal subarachnoid hemorrhage grading scale. J Neurosurg 1988;68:985.

Enomoto H, Goto H. Moyamoya disease presenting as intracerebral hemorrhage during pregnancy: case report and review of the literature. Neurosurgery 1987;20:33–35.

Evan S, Frigoletto FD, Jewett JF. Mortality of eclampsia: a case report and the experience of the Massachusetts Maternal Mortality Study, 1954–1982. N Engl J Med 1983;309:1644–1647.

Fisher CM, Kistler JP, Davis JM. Relation of cerebral vasospasm to subarachnoid hemorrhage visualized by computerized tomographic scanning. Neurosurgery 1980;6:1–9.

Fishman RA. Steroids in the treatment of brain edema. N Engl J Med 1982;306:359–360.

Fleigner JR, Hooper RS, Kloss M. Subarachnoid hemorrhage and pregnancy. J Obstet Gynaecol Br Commonw 1969;76:912–917.

Forster DMC, Kunkler IH, Hartland P. Risk of cerebral bleeding from arteriovenous malformations in pregnancy: the Sheffield experience. Stereotact Funct Neurosurg 1993;61(Suppl 1):20–22.

Giannotta SL, Kindt GW. Total morbidity and mortality rates of patients with surgically treated intracranial aneurysms. Neurosurgery 1979;4:125–128.

Giannotta SL, McGillicuddy JE, Kindt GW. Diagnosis and treatment of postoperative cerebral vasospasm. Surg Neurol 1977;8:286–290.

Giannotta SL, Daniels J, Golde SH, et al. Ruptured intracranial aneurysms during pregnancy: a report of four cases. J Reprod Med 1986;31:139–147.

van Gijn J, van Dongen KJ. The time course of aneurysmal haemorrhage on computed tomograms. Neuroradiology 1982;23:153–156.

van Gijn J, Hijdra A, Wijdicks EFM, et al. Acute hydrocephalus after aneurysmal subarachnoid hemorrhage. J Neurosurg 1985;63: 355–362.

van Gijn J, Bromerg JEC, Lindsay KW, Hasan D, Vermeulen M. Definition of initial grading, specific events, and overall outcome in patients with aneurismal subarachnoid hemorrhage. Stroke 1994; 25:1623–1627.

Grenvik A, Safar P. Brain Failure and Resuscitation. New York: Churchill Livingstone, 1981.

Grolimund P, Weber M, Seiler RW, et al. Time course of cerebral vasospasm after severe head injury. Lancet 1988;ii:1173.

Henderson CE, Torbey M. Rupture of intracranial aneurysm associated with cocaine use during pregnancy. Am J Perinatol 1988;5:142–143.

Heros RC, Morcos JJ. Cerebrovascular surgery: past, present, and future. Neurosurgery 2000;47:1007–1033.

Heros RC, Zervas NT, Varsos V. Cerebral vasospasm after subarachnoid hemorrhage: an update. Ann Neurol 1983;14:599–608.

Hibbard LT. Maternal mortality due to acute toxemia. Obstet Gynecol 1973;42:263–270.

Horn EH, Filshie M, Kerslake RW, Jaspan T, Worthington BS, Rubin PC. Widespread cerebral ischaemia treated with nimodipine in a patient with eclampsia. BMJ 1990;301:794.

Horton JC, Chambers WA, Lyons SL, et al. Pregnancy and the risk of hemorrhage from cerebral arteriovenous malformations. Neurosurgery 1990;27:867–871.

Hunt WE, Hess RM Surgical risk as related to time of intervention in the repair of intracranial aneurysms. J Neurosurg 1968;28:14–20.

Iriye BK, Asrat T, Adashek JA, Carr MH. Intraventricular haemorrhage and maternal brain death associated with antepartum cocaine abuse. Br J Obstet Gynaecol 1995;102:68–69.

Isla A, Alvarez F, Gonzalez A, et al. Brain tumor and pregnancy. Obstet Gynecol 1997;89:19–23.

Jane JA, Kassell NF, Torner JC, Winn RH. The natural history of aneurysms and arteriovenous malformations. J Neurosurg 1985;62: 321–323.

Juvela S, Porras M, Heiskanen O. Natural history intracranial aneurysms: a long-term follow-up study. J Neurosurg 1993;79:174–182.

Kassell NF, Torner JC. The International Cooperative Study on Timing Aneurysm Surgery: an update. Stroke 1984;15:566–570.

Kassell NF, Boarini DJ, Adams HP, et al. Overall management of ruptured aneurysm: comparison of early and later operation. Neurosurgery 1981;9:120–128.

Kassell NF, Peerless SJ, Durward QJ, et al. Treatment of ischemic deficits from vasospasm with intravascular volume expansion and induced arterial hypertension. Neurosurg 1982;11:337–343.

Kassell NF, Sasaki T, Colohan ART, et al. Cerebral vasospasm following aneurysmal subarachnoid hemorrhage. Stroke 1985;16:562–572.

Kety SS, Schmidt CF. The nitrous oxide method for the quantitative determination of cerebral blood flow in man: theory, procedure and normal values. J Clin Invest 1948;27:476.

Kittner SJ, Stern BJ, Feeser BR, et al. Pregnancy and the risk of stroke. N Engl J Med 1996;335:768–774.

Lassen NA. Cerebral blood flow and oxygen consumption in man. Physiol Rev 1959;39:183.

Levinson G, Shnider SM, DeLorimier AA, et al. Effects of maternal hyperventilation on uterine blood flow and fetal oxygenation and acid-base balance. Anesthesiology 1974;40:340–347.

Levy ML, Giannotta SL. Induced hypertension and hypervolemia for treatment of cerebral vasospasm. Neurosurg Clin North Am 1990;1: 357–365.

Ljunggren B, Brandt L, Sunbarg G, et al. Early management of aneurysmal subarachnoid hemorrhage. Neurosurgery 1982;11: 412–418.

Ljunggren B, Brandt L, Saveland H, et al. Outcome in 60 consecutive patients treated with early aneurysm operation and intravenous nimodipine. J Neurosurg 1984;61:864.

Lopez-Llera M. Complicated eclampsia: fifteen years' experience in a referral medical center. Am J Obstet Gynecol 1982;142:28–35.

Maher LM. Postpartum intracranial hemorrhage and phenylpropanolamine use. Neurology 1987;37:1686.

Milliez J, Dahoun A, Boudraa M. Computed tomography of the brain in eclampsia. Obstet Gynecol 1990;75:975–980.

Minielly R, Yuzpe AA, Drake CG. Subarachnoid hemorrhage secondary to ruptured cerebral aneurysm in pregnancy. Obstet Gynecol 1979;53:64–70.

Muizelaar JP, Lutz HA, Becker DP. Effect of mannitol on ICP and CBF and correlation with pressure autoregulation in severely head-injured patients. J Neurosurg 1984;61:700–706.

Nath F, Galbraith S. The effect of mannitol on cerebral white matter content. J Neurosurg 1986;65:41–43.

Newman B, Lam AM. Induced hypotension for clipping of a cerebral aneurysm during pregnancy: a case report and brief review. Anesth Analg 1986;65:675–678.

Parkinson D, Bachers G. Arteriovenous malformations: summary of 100 consecutive supratentorial cases. J Neurosurg 1980;53:285–299.

Pedowitz P, Perrell A. Aneurysm complicated by pregnancy. Am J Obstet Gynecol 1957;73:736.

Piotin M, de Souza Fiho CBA, Kothimbakam R, Moret J. Endovascular treatment of acutely ruptured intracranial aneurysms in pregnancy. Am J Obstet Gynecol 2001;185:1261–1262.

Pollay M, Fullenwider C, Roberts PA, et al. Effect of mannitol and furosemide on blood-train osmotic gradient and intracranial pressure. J Neurosurg 1983;59:945–950.

Redekop G, TerBrugge K, Montanera W, Willinsky R. Arterial aneurysms associated with cerebral arteriovenous malformations: classification, incidence, and risk of hemorrhage. J Neurosurg 1998;89:539–546.

Reichman OH, Karlman RL. Berry aneurysm. Surg Clin North Am 1995;75:115–121.

Rigg D, McDonogh P. Use of sodium nitroprusside in deliberate hypotension during pregnancy. Br J Anaesth 1981;53:985–987.

Robinson JL, Hall CJ, Sedzimir CB. Subarachnoid hemorrhage in pregnancy. J Neurosurg 1972;36:27–33.

Robinson JL, Hall CS, Sedzimir CB. Arteriovenous malformations, aneurysms, and pregnancy. J Neurosurg 1974;41:63–70.

Ronkainen A, Puranen MI, Hernesniemi JA, et al. Intracranial aneurysms: MR angiographic screening in 400 asymptomatic individuals with increased familial risk. Radiology 1995;195:35–40.

Ruggieri PM, Poulos N, Masaryk TJ, et al. Occult intracranial aneurysms in polycystic kidney disease: screening with MR angiography. Radiology 1994;191:33–39.

Sadasivan B, Malik G, Lee C, Ausman J. Vascular malformations and pregnancy. Surg Neurol 1990;33:305–313.

Schievink W. Intracranial aneurysms. N Engl J Med 1997;336:28–40.

Schievink W, Zabramski JM. Brain protection for cerebral aneurysm surgery. Neurosurg Clin North Am 1998;9:661–671.

Sheehan HL, Lynch JB. Pathology of toxemia of pregnancy. Baltimore: Williams and Wilkins, 1973.

Simolke GA, Cox SM, Cunningham FG. Cerebrovascular accidents complicating pregnancy and the puerperium. Obstet Gynecol 1991;78:37–42.

Solomon RA, Fink ME, Lennihan L. Early aneurysm surgery and prophylactic hypervolemic hypertensive therapy for the treatment of aneurysmal subarachnoid hemorrhage. Neurosurgery 1988;23: 699–704.

Stange K, Hallidin M. Hypothermia in pregnancy. Anesthesiology 1983;58:460.

Taneda M. Effect of early operation for ruptured aneurysms on prevention of delayed ischemic symptoms. J Neurosurg 1982;57: 622–628.

Teasdale G, Jennett B. Assessment of coma and impaired consciousness. Lancet 1974;2:81–84.

Treggiari-Venzi MM, Suter PM, Romand JA. Review of medical prevention of vasospasm after aneurysmal subarachnoid hemorrhage: a problem of neurointensive care. Neurosurgery 2001;48:249–261.

Wiebers D, Whisnant J. The incidence of stroke among pregnant women in Rochester, Minn., 1955 through 1979. JAMA 1985;254: 3055–3057.

Wiebers DO. Ischemic cerebrovascular complications of pregnancy. Arch Neurol 1985;42:1106–1113.

Wiebers DO. Subarachnoid hemorrhage in pregnancy. Semin Neurol 1988;8:226–229.

Wilkinson HA, Rosenfeld S. Furosemide and mannitol in the treatment of acute experimental intracranial hypertension. Neurosurgery 1983;12:405–410.

Williams KP, Wilson S. Evaluation of cerebral perfusion pressure changes in laboring women: effects of epidural anesthesia. Ultrasound Obstet Gynecol 1999;14:393–396.

Williams KP, Galerneau F, Wilson S. Effect of labor on maternal cerebral blood flow velocity. Am J Obstet Gynecol 1998;178:59–61.

Willoughby JS. Sodium nitroprusside, pregnancy and multiple intracranial aneurysms. Anaesth Intensive Care 1984;12:358–360.

Wilterdink JL, Feldmann E. Cerebral hemorrhage. In: Devinsky O, Feldman E, Hainline B, eds. Neurological complications of pregnancy. New York: Raven, 1994;13.

Witlin AG, Friedman SA, Egerman RS, Frangieh AY, Sibai B. Cerebrovascular disorders complicating pregnancy—beyond eclampsia. Am J Obstet Gynecol 1997;176:1139–1145.

Witlin AG, Mattar F, Sibai B. Postpartum stroke: A twenty-year experience. Am J Obstet Gynecol 2000;183:83–88.

Young DC, Leveno KJ, Whalley PS. Induced delivery prior to surgery for ruptured cerebral aneurysm. Obstet Gynecol 1983;61:749–752.

19 Cardiac disease

Michael R. Foley

Although cardiac disease complicates only 1–4% of all pregnancies in the United States, such conditions continue to account for up to 10–25% of maternal mortality (Koonin et al., 1991; DeSwiet, 1993; Hogberg et al., 1994; Berg et al., 1996; Jacob et al., 1998). Until the past decade, rheumatic heart disease was the most prevalent form of cardiac disease in the obstetric population. Because of advances in the treatment of congenital heart disease in newborns and children, more young women with corrected defects are reaching reproductive age and attempting pregnancy. As a consequence, congenital heart disease is now the most common form of heart disease complicating pregnancy in North American women. On the other end of the spectrum, more women are postponing pregnancy until the fourth or fifth decade of life—a time where underlying medical conditions such as hypertension and diabetes, coupled with advancing maternal age, may exacerbate the incidence of acquired heart disease complicating pregnancy. This chapter, therefore, will focus on the precarious interaction between cardiac disease and pregnancy.

Counseling the pregnant cardiac patient

Prior to 1973, the Criteria Committee of the New York Heart Association (NYHA) recommended a classification of cardiac disease based on clinical function (classes I–IV). Table 19.1 outlines the specifics of the NYHA classification system. Such a classification is useful in discussing the pregnant cardiac patient, although patients who begin pregnancy as functional class I may develop congestive heart failure and pulmonary edema during the course of gestation.

This functional classification system, although somewhat antiquated, remains most useful when comparing the performance of individuals with uniform etiologic and anatomic defects. In general, most women who begin pregnancy as a functional class I or II have an improved outcome as compared with those classified as class III or IV (Hsieh et al., 1993).

Counseling the pregnant cardiac patient regarding her prognosis for successful pregnancy is further complicated by recent advances in medical and surgical therapy, fetal surveillance, and neonatal care. Such advances render invalid many older estimates of maternal mortality and fetal wastage. Table 19.2 represents a synthesis of maternal risk estimates for various types of cardiac disease that was initially developed for the first edition of this text in 1987. Counseling of the pregnant cardiac patient, as well as general management approaches, were based on this classification (Clark, 1987). Category I included conditions that, with proper management, were associated with negligible maternal mortality (1%). Cardiac lesions in category II traditionally carried a 5–15% risk of maternal mortality. Patients with cardiac lesions in group III were, and probably remain, subject to a mortality risk exceeding 25%. In all but exceptional cases, this risk is unacceptable, and prevention or interruption of pregnancy is generally recommended.

Currently available data suggest that today maternal mortality is almost exclusively seen in patients with pulmonary hypertension, endocarditis, coronary artery disease, cardiomyopathy, and sudden arrhythmia. DeSwiet, reporting on maternal mortality from heart disease in the United Kingdom between 1985 and 1987, stated that all deaths occurred due to endocarditis (22%), pulmonary hypertension (30%), coronary artery disease (39%), and cardiomyopathy or myo-

Table 19.1 New York Heart Association (NYHA) functional classification system

Class I	No limitations of physical activity, ordinary physical activity does not precipitate cardiovascular symptoms such as dyspnea, angina, fatigue, or palpitations
Class II	Slight limitation of physical activity. Ordinary physical activity will precipitate cardiovascular symptoms. Patients are comfortable at rest
Class III	Less than ordinary physical activity precipitates symptoms that markedly limit activity. Patients are comfortable at rest
Class IV	Patients have discomfort with any physical activity. Symptoms are present at rest

Table 19.2 Maternal risk associated with pregnancy

Group I: Minimal risk of complications (mortality <1%)
Atrial septal defect*
Ventricular septal defect*
Patent ductus arteriosus*
Pulmonic/tricuspid disease
Corrected tetralogy of Fallot
Bioprosthetic valve
Mitral stenosis, New York Heart Association (NYHA) classes I and II
Marfan syndrome with normal aorta
Group II: Moderate risk of complications (mortality 5–15%)
Mitral stenosis with atrial fibrillation†
Artificial valve*†
Mitral stenosis, NYHA classes III and IV
Aortic stenosis
Coarctation of aorta, uncomplicated
Uncorrected tetralogy of Fallot
Previous myocardial infarction
Group III: Major risk of complications or death (mortality >25%)
Pulmonary hypertension
Coarctation of aorta, complicated
Marfan syndrome with aortic involvement

* If unassociated with pulmonary hypertension.
† If anticoagulation with heparin, rather than coumadin, is elected.

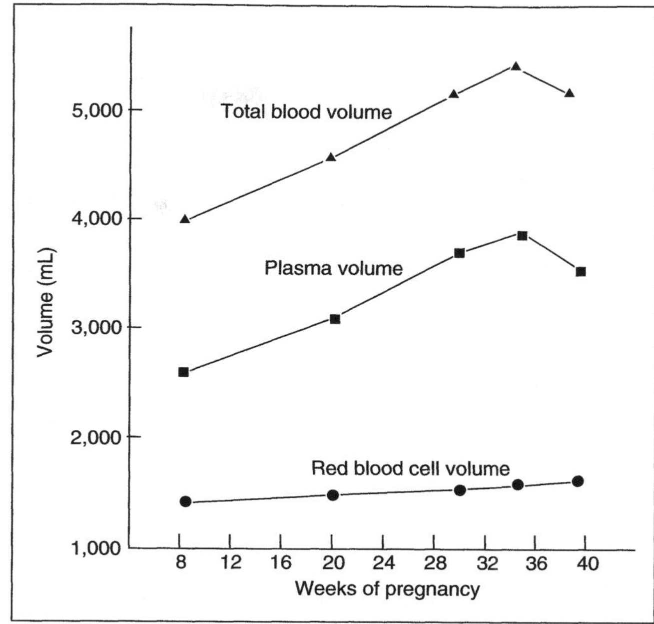

Fig. 19.1 Changes in total blood volume, plasma volume, and red cell volume in normal pregnancy (Reproduced by permission from Shnider SM, Levinson G. Anesthesia for Obstetrics, 3rd edn. Lippincott, Williams & Wilkins, 1993.)

carditis (9%) (DeSwiet, 1993). Similarly, a review of maternal mortality in Utah from 1982 to 1994 revealed 13 cardiac deaths, four (31%) due to pulmonary hypertension, four secondary to cardiomyopathy (31%), two due to coronary artery disease (15%), and three (23%) due to sudden arrhythmia (Varner, 1997). In a smaller series of maternal deaths from West Virginia between 1985 and 1989, the two cardiac deaths described were due to cardiomyopathy (Dye et al., 1992).

In a study of 252 pregnancies in women with cardiac disease the following independent predictors of cardiac events (congestive heart failure, arrhythmia, and stroke) were identified (Siu et al., 1997):

- NYHA functional class III or IV.
- Maternal cyanosis.
- History of prior arrhythmia.
- Pulmonary vascular disease.
- Myocardial dysfunction (ejection fraction <40%).
- Left heart obstruction.

In a study by Presbitero et al. (1994), looking at the outcome of the mother and the fetus in pregnancies complicated by cyanotic congenital heart disease, the adverse impact of low maternal oxygen saturation was clearly illustrated. The likelihood of a live birth was less frequent (12%) if the mother's resting oxygen saturation was below 85% as compared to a resting oxygen saturation of greater than 85% (63%). It would appear, however, that with appropriate obstetric care, the presence or absence of the aforementioned secondary complications of cardiomyopathy, pulmonary hypertension, endocarditis, and sudden arrhythmias play a much more important role in determining ultimate maternal outcome, than the primary structural nature of the cardiac lesion itself.

Physiologic considerations

The unique problems encountered by the pregnant woman with cardiac disease are secondary to four principal physiologic changes (ACOG, 1992).

1 *A 50% increase in intravascular volume* is seen in normal pregnancy be early to mid-third trimester. Figure 19.1 illustrates the changes in total blood volume, plasma volume, and red cell volume during normal pregnancy. In patients whose cardiac output is limited by intrinsic myocardial dysfunction, valvular lesions, or ischemic cardiac disease, volume overload will be poorly tolerated any may lead to congestive failure or worsening ischemia. In patients with an anatomic predisposition, such volume expansion may result in aneurysm formation or dissection (e.g. Marfan syndrome). Even in women with multiple pregnancies, the heart is able to withstand repetitive episodes of gestational volume overload without lasting detrimental structural or functional changes (Sandaniantz et al., 1996).

2 *Decreased systemic vascular resistance* (SVR) becomes especially important in patients with the potential for right-to-left shunts, which will invariably be increased by a falling

Table 19.3 Central hemodynamic changes associated with normal term pregnancy

	Nonpregnant	Pregnant	Percent change*
Cardiac output (L/min)	4.3 ± 0.9	6.2 ± 1.0	+43
Heart rate (bpm)	71 ± 10.0	83 ± 1.0	+17
Systemic vascular resistance (dyne/cm/sec^5)	1,530 ± 520	1,210 ± 266	−21
Pulmonary vascular resistance (dyne/cm/sec^5)	119 ± 47.0	78 ± 22	−34
Colloid oncotic pressure (mmHg)	20.8 ± 1.0	18.0 ± 1.5	−14
COP – PCWP (mmHg)	14.5 ± 2.5	10.5 ± 2.7	−28
Mean arterial pressure (mmHg)	86.4 ± 7.5	90.3 ± 5.8	–NSC
Pulmonary capillary wedge pressure (mmHg)	6.3 ± 2.1	7.5 ± 1.8	–NSC
Central venous pressure (mmHg)	3.7 ± 2.6	3.6 ± 2.5	NSC
Left ventricular stroke work index (g/m/m^2)	41 ± 8	48 ± 6	+NSC

* NSC = no statistically significant change.
COP – PCWP = colloid oncotic pressure – pulmonary capillary wedge pressure (mmHg).
(Reproduced by permission from Clark SL, et al: Central hemodynamic assessment of normal term pregnancy. Am J Obstet Gynecol 1989;161:1439.)

SVR during pregnancy. Such alterations in cardiac afterload also complicate adaption to pregnancy in patients with certain types of valvular disease. Table 19.3 summarizes the central hemodynamic changes associated with normal term pregnancy.

3 *The hypercoagulability associated with pregnancy* heightens the need for adequate anticoagulation in patients at risk for arterial thrombosis (artificial valves and some subsets of atrial fibrillation) at a time when optimum anticoagulation with coumarin derivatives may have adverse fetal consequences. Table 19.4 outlines the relative changes in the coagulation factors and inhibitors associated with normal pregnancy. For women receiving any type of therapeutic anticoagulation, the risk of serious postpartum hemorrhage is also increased.

4 *Marked fluctuations in cardiac output* normally occur in pregnancy, particularly during labor and delivery (van Oppen et al., 1996). Such changes increase progressively from the first stage of labor, reaching, in some cases, an additional 50% by the late second stage. The potential for further dramatic volume shifts occurs around the time of delivery, both secondary to postpartum hemorrhage and as the result of an "autotransfusion" occurring with release of vena caval obstruction and sustained uterine contraction. Such volume shifts may be poorly tolerated by women whose cardiac output is highly dependent on adequate preload (pulmonary hypertension) or in those with fixed cardiac output (mitral stenosis). Figure 19.2 illustrates the marked fluctuations in cardiac output associated with normal labor, delivery, and postpartum (Clark et al., 1989).

The risk classification presented in Table 19.2 assumes clean delineation of various cardiovascular lesions. Unfortunately, in actual practice this is only rarely the case. Optimal management of a patient with any specific combination of lesions requires a thorough assessment of the anatomic and functional capacity of the heart, followed by an analysis of how the physiologic changes described previously will impact on the specific anatomic or physiologic limitations imposed by the intrinsic disease. Such an analysis will allow a prioritization of often conflicting physiologic demands and greatly assist the clinician in avoiding or managing potential complications.

Table 19.4 Coagulation factors and inhibitors during normal pregnancy

Factor	Nonpregnant	Late pregnancy
Factor I (fibrinogen)	200–450 mg/dL	400–650 mg/dL
Factor II (prothrombin)	75–125%	100–125%
Factor V	75–125%	100–150%
Factor VII	75–125%	150–250%
Factor VIII	75–150%	200–500%
Factor IX	75–125%	100–150%
Factor X	75–125%	150–250%
Factor XI	5–125%	50–100%
Factor XII	75–125%	100–200%
Factor XIII	75–125%	35–75%
Antithrombin III	85–110%	75–100%
Antifactor Xa	85–110%	75–100%

(Reprinted by permission from Hathaway WE, Bonnar J. Coagulation in pregnancy. In: Hathaway WE, Bonnar J, eds. Perinatal Coagulation. New York: Grune & Stratton, 1978.)

Certain management principles generally apply to most patients with cardiac disease. These include the judicious use of antepartum bed rest and meticulous prenatal care. Intrapartum management principles include laboring in the lateral position; the use of epidural anesthesia, which will minimize intrapartum fluctuations in cardiac output (although the use of epidural narcotic rather than epidural local anesthesia may be more appropriate for patients with certain types of cardiac lesions); the administration of oxygen; and endocarditis prophylaxis. Positional effects on maternal cardiac output during labor with epidural analgesia have recently been

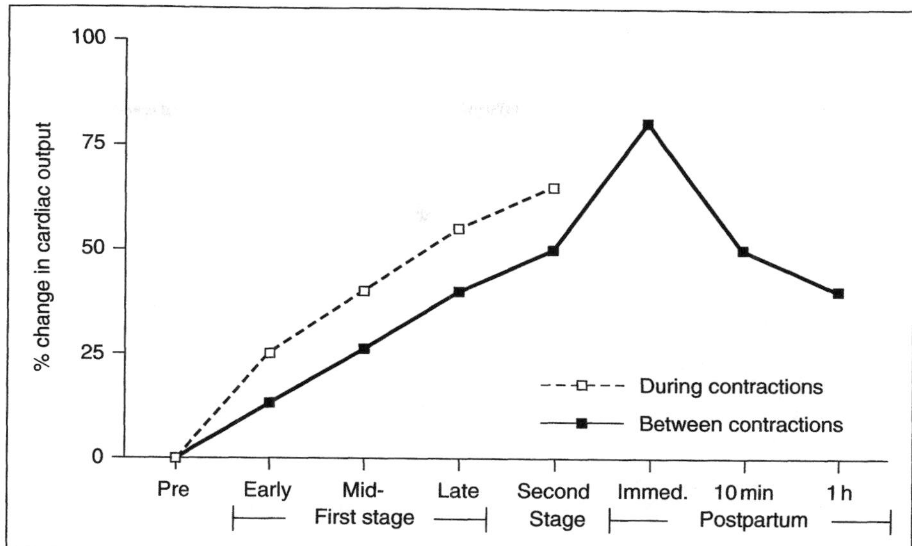

Fig. 19.2 Fluctuations in cardiac output associated with normal labor, delivery, and postpartum. (Reproduced by permission from Bonica JJ, McDonald JS. Principles and Practice of Obstetrics Analgesia and Anesthesia, 2nd edn. Lippincott, Williams & Wilkins, 1994.)

detailed (Danilenko-Dixon et al., 1996). Additional management recommendations may vary according to the specific lesion present. For patients with significant cardiac disease, management and delivery in a referral center is recommended. In many cases, management with peripheral pulse oximetry is replacing invasive hemodynamic monitoring.

Congenital cardiac lesions

As previously discussed, the relative frequency of congenital as opposed to acquired heart disease is changing (Ullery, 1954; Szekely et al., 1973; DeSwiet, 1993; Hsieh et al., 1993). Rheumatic fever is less common in the United States, and more patients with congenital cardiac disease now survive to reproductive age. In a review in 1954, the ratio of rheumatic to congenital heart disease seen during pregnancy was 16:1; by 1967, this ratio had changed to 3:1 (Ullery, 1954; Niswander et al., 1967; Szekely et al., 1973). A more recent report from Taiwan suggested a rheumatic–congenital cardiac ratio of 1:1.5 during pregnancy (Hsieh et al., 1993). Similarly, in the United Kingdom between 1973 and 1987, the number of deaths from congenital heart disease has doubled, whereas the number of deaths from acquired heart disease has halved (DeSwiet, 1993). In the subsequent discussion of specific cardiac lesions, no attempt will be made to duplicate existing comprehensive texts regarding physical diagnostic, electrocardiographic, and radiographic findings of specific cardiac lesions. Rather, the discussion presented here focuses on aspects of cardiac disease that are unique to pregnancy.

Atrial septal defect

Atrial septal defect (ASD) is the most common congenital lesion seen during pregnancy, and, in general, it is asymptomatic (Veran et al., 1968; Etheridge & Pepperell, 1971; Rush et al., 1979). The two significant potential complications seen with ASD are arrhythmias and heart failure. Although atrial arrhythmias are not uncommon in patients with ASD, their onset generally occurs after the fourth decade of life; thus, such arrhythmias, however unlikely, are becoming more of a concern with the recent prevalence of delayed childbearing. In patients with ASD, atrial fibrillation is the most common arrhythmia encountered; however, supraventricular tachycardia and atrial flutter also may occur. Initial therapy is with digoxin; less commonly, propranolol, quinidine, or even cardioversion may be necessary. The hypervolemia associated with pregnancy results in an increased left-to-right shunt through the ASD, and, thus, a significant burden is imposed on the right ventricle. Although this additional burden is tolerated well by most patients, congestive heart failure and death with ASD have been reported (Schaefer et al., 1968; Neilson et al., 1970; Hibbard, 1975). In contrast to the high-pressure–high-flow state seen with ventricular septal defect (VSD) and patent ductus arteriosus (PDA), ASD is characterized by high pulmonary blood flow associated with normal pulmonary artery pressures. Because pulmonary artery pressures are low, pulmonary hypertension is unusual. An unusual potential complication that exists with ASD is "paradoxical embolization." Thromboemboli from leg or pelvic veins may be directed across the ASD into the systemic circulation, "paradoxically," resulting in ischemic neurologic complications. The vast majority of patients with ASD, however, tolerate pregnancy, labor, and delivery without complication. Neilson et al. (1970) reported 70 pregnancies in 24 patients with ASD; all patients had an uncomplicated ante- and intrapartum course. During labor, avoidance of fluid overload, oxygen administration, labor in the lateral recumbent position, and pain

Table 19.5 Recommendations of AHA/ACC task force on antibiotic prophylaxis for selected valve lesions

Valve lesion (endocarditis risk)	Need for prophylaxis	
	Uncomplicated vaginal delivery*	**Cesarean section**
High risk for endocarditis		
Prosthetic cardiac valve (includes bioprosthetic and homograph valves)	Optional	Not recommended
Prior bacterial endocarditis		
Complex cyanotic congenital heart disease†		
Surgically constructed systemic pulmonary shunts or conduits		
Moderate risk for endocarditis		
Other congenital cardiac malformations		
Acquired valvular dysfunction (e.g. rheumatic heart disease)	Not recommended	Not recommended
Hypertrophic cardiomyopathy		
Mitral valve prolapse with leaflet thickening and/or regurgitation		
Negligible risk for endocarditis		
Mitral valve prolapse without regurgitation	Not recommended	Not recommended
Physiologic, functional, or innocent murmurs		
Previous rheumatic fever without valvular dysfunction		

* Vaginal delivery not involving vaginal or rectal lacerations or manual exploration of the uterus.

† Includes single ventricle states, transposition of the great arteries, tetralogy of Fallot.

AHA/ACC = American Heart Association/American College of Cardiology.

(From Dajani AS, Taubert KA, Wilson W, et al. Prevention of Bacterial Endocarditis. Recommendations by the American Heart Association. Circulation 1997;96:358–366.)

relief with epidural anesthesia, as well as prophylaxis against bacterial endocarditis, are the most important considerations (Table 19.5 provides a review of the American Heart Association and the American College of Cardiology Joint Task Force on antibiotic prophylaxis for selected valve lesions (Dajani et al., 1997)). A more detailed discussion regarding the prevention of bacterial endocarditis is found later in this chapter.

Ventricular septal defect

Ventricular septal defect may occur as an isolated lesion or in conjunction with other congenital cardiac anomalies, including tetralogy of Fallot, transposition of the great vessels, and coarctation of the aorta. The size of the septal defect is the most important determinant of clinical prognosis during pregnancy. Small defects are tolerated well, while larger defects are associated more frequently with congestive failure, arrhythmias, or the development of pulmonary hypertension. In addition, a large VSD often is associated with some degree of aortic regurgitation, which may add to the risk of congestive failure. Pregnancy, labor, and delivery are generally well tolerated by patients with an uncomplicated VSD. Schaefer et al. (1968) compiled a series of 141 pregnancies in 56 women with VSD. The only two maternal deaths were in women whose VSD was complicated by pulmonary hypertension (Eisenmenger's syndrome). Because of the high risk of death associated with unrecognized pulmonary hypertension, echocardiography or cardiac catheterization is essential in any adult patient in whom persistent VSD is suspected, or in whom the quality or success of the previous repair is uncertain (Gilman, 1991; Jackson et al., 1993).

The primary closure of a moderately restrictive or nonrestrictive VSD in early childhood usually prevents the subsequent development of secondary pulmonary vascular hypertension and therefore permits an uneventful pregnancy. Fortunately, significant postoperative electrophysiologic conduction abnormalities are rarely encountered.

Although very rarely indicated, successful primary closures of VSDs during pregnancy have been reported. Intrapartum management considerations for patients with uncomplicated VSD or PDA are similar to those outlined for ASD. In general, invasive hemodynamic monitoring is usually unnecessary.

Patent ductus arteriosus

Although PDA is one of the most common congenital cardiac anomalies, its almost universal detection and closure in the newborn period makes it uncommon during pregnancy (Szekely & Julian, 1979). As with uncomplicated ASD and VSD, most patients are asymptomatic, and PDA is generally well tolerated during pregnancy, labor, and delivery. As with a large VSD, however, the high-pressure–high-flow left-to-right shunt associated with a large, uncorrected PDA can lead to pulmonary hypertension. In such cases, the prognosis becomes much worse. In one study of 18 pregnant women who died of congenital heart disease, three had PDA; however, all of these patients had severe secondary pulmonary hypertension (Hibbard, 1975). In most circumstances, however, an asymptomatic young woman with a small or moderate-sized PDA, without pulmonary hypertension, will have a relatively uncomplicated pregnancy. Apart from a single case report of a spontaneous postpartum rupture of a PDA, in a patient with normal pulmonary pressure and without ductal aneurysm (Jayakrishnan, 1921), the risks are minimal. Antibiotic prophylaxis against infective endarteritis during delivery is an important consideration.

Eisenmenger's syndrome/pulmonary hypertension

Eisenmenger's syndrome develops when, in the presence of congenital left-to-right shunt, progressive pulmonary hypertension leads to shunt reversal or bidirectional shunting. Although this syndrome may occur with ASD, VSD, or PDA, the low-pressure–high-flow shunt seen with an ASD is far less likely to result in pulmonary hypertension and shunt reversal than is the condition of high-pressure and high-flow symptoms seen with the VSD and PDA. Whatever the etiology, pulmonary hypertension carries a grave prognosis during pregnancy. During the antepartum period, the decreased SVR associated with pregnancy increases the likelihood or degree of right-to-left shunting. Pulmonary perfusion then decreases; this decrease results in hypoxemia and deterioration of maternal and fetal condition. In such a patient, systemic hypotension leads to decreased right ventricular filling pressures; in the presence of fixed pulmonary hypertension, such decreased right heart pressures may be insufficient to perfuse the pulmonary arterial bed. This insufficiency may result in sudden, profound hypoxemia. Such hypotension can result from hemorrhage or complications of conduction anesthesia and may result in sudden death (Knapp & Arditi, 1967; Gleicher et al., 1979; Pirlo & Herren, 1979; Sinnenberg, 1980). Avoidance of such hypotension is the principal clinical concern in the intrapartum management of patients with pulmonary hypertension of any etiology.

Maternal mortality in the presence of Eisenmenger's syndrome is reported as 30–50% (Gleicher et al., 1979; Pirlo & Herren, 1979; Gilman, 1991; Jackson et al., 1993). In a review of the subject, Gleicher et al. (1979) reported a 34% mortality associated with vaginal delivery and a 75% mortality associated with cesarean section. In a more recent report, Weiss et al. (1998) reviewed the published literature from 1978 to 1996 investigating Eisenmenger's syndrome, primary pulmonary hypertension and secondary pulmonary hypertension during pregnancy. Despite advances in maternal and cardiac care during this interval, the overall composite mortality rate for Eisenmenger's syndrome during pregnancy remained 36%—relatively unchanged for the last two decades (Meyer et al., 1994; Saha et al., 1994; Smedstad et al., 1994; Avila et al., 1995; Presbitero et al., 1995). In this series, however, there appeared to be little difference in mortality when comparing vaginal delivery (48%) to cesarean section (52%). These investigators also concluded that maternal prognosis depended on the early diagnosis of pulmonary vascular disease during pregnancy, early hospital admission, and individually tailored treatment during pregnancy with specific attention focused on the postpartum period. Table 19.6 reviews the management and outcome of pregnant women with Eisenmenger's syndrome (Weiss, 1998). In addition to the previously discussed problems associated with hemorrhage and hypovolemia, thromboembolic phenomena have been associated with up to 43% of all maternal deaths in Eisenmenger's syndrome (Gleicher et al., 1979). In the more recent report by Weiss et al. (1998), however, pulmonary thromboembolism accounted for only three of the 26 (12%) maternal deaths in this composite analysis. Sudden delayed postpartum death, occurring 4–6 weeks after delivery, also has been reported (Gleicher et al., 1979; Clark, 1985a; Weiss et al., 1998). Such deaths may involve a rebound worsening of pulmonary hypertension associated with the loss of pregnancy-associated hormones, which leads to decreased pulmonary vascular resistance during gestation (Clark et al., 1989).

Caution should be exercised when evaluating for the presence of pulmonary hypertension with noninvasive techniques such as Doppler/echocardiogram. These techniques have a clear tendency to significantly overestimate the degree of pulmonary hypertension during pregnancy and may incorrectly diagnose the presence of pulmonary hypertension in up to 32% of cases when compared with cardiac catheterization (Penning et al., 2001). If any question exists regarding the presence of pulmonary hypertension, pulmonary artery catheterization with direct measurement of pulmonary artery pressures may be performed on an outpatient basis in early pregnancy. Where significant pulmonary hypertension exists, pregnancy termination in either the first or second trimester appears to be safer than allowing the pregnancy to progress to term (Elkayam & Gleicher, 1984). Dilation and curettage in the first trimester or dilation and evacuation in the second trimester are the methods of choice. Hypertonic saline and F-series prostaglandins are contraindicated, the latter due to arterial oxygen desaturation seen with the use of this agent (Hankins et al., 1988). Prostaglandin E2 suppositories appear to be safe under these circumstances.

For the patient with a continuing gestation, hospitalization for the duration of pregnancy is highly recommended. Continuous administration of oxygen, the pulmonary vasodilator of choice, is suggested and may improve perinatal outcome. In cyanotic heart disease of any etiology, fetal outcome correlates well with maternal hemoglobin, and successful pregnancy is unlikely with a hemoglobin greater than 20 g/dL (Presbitero et al., 1994). Maternal P_ao_2 should be maintained at a level of 70 mmHg or above (Sobrevilla et al., 1971). Third-trimester fetal surveillance with antepartum testing is important because at

Table 19.6 Management and outcome of pregnant women with Eisenmenger's syndrome ($n = 73$)

	Maternal survival	Maternal mortality
Number (%)	47 (64%)	26 (36%)
Age (years)	26.4 ± 4.8	24.9 ± 4.5
Hospital admission (weeks of pregnancy)	26.7 ± 6.5	31.4 ± 5.9
Toxemia of pregnancy	2 (4%)	3 (12%)
Delivery (weeks of pregnancy)	35.1 ± 3.5	34.4 ± 4.4
Vaginal delivery	27 (57%)	11 (48%)
Operative delivery	20 (43%)	12 (52%)
Monitoring		
Noninvasive, not reported	24 (51%)	15 (63%)
Invasive SAP and/or CVP	23 (49%)	9 (37%)
Invasive PAP	8 (17%)	6 (25%)
Anesthesia/analgesia		
Not reported	13 (28%)	5 (22%)
Regional techniques	22 (47%)	8 (35%)
General anesthesia	12 (25%)	7 (30%)
Local anesthesia/analgesia	0	3 (13%)
Oxytocic drugs	14 (30%)	4 (17%)
Antithrombotic therapy	28 (60%)	12 (46%)
Neonatal survival	43 (96%)*	20 (77%)
Maternal death, days postpartum	—	5 (0–30)

Data presented are mean value ± SD, number (%) of patients, or median (range).

* In two cases neonatal outcome was not reported. Three patients died before delivery and 23 died after delivery.

CI, confidence interval; CVP, central venous pressure; PAP, pulmonary artery pressure; SAP, systemic arterial pressure.

(From Weiss BM, Zemp L, Burkhardt S, Hess O. Outcome of pulmonary vascular disease in pregnancy: a systemic overview from 1978 through 1996. J Am Coll Cardio 1998;31:1650–1657.)

least 30% of the fetuses will suffer growth restriction (Gleicher et al., 1979). Although the overall fetal wastage with Eisenmenger's syndrome is reported to be up to 75%, more recent information suggests a more favorable outcome. Weiss et al. reported a neonatal survival rate of nearly 90% in cases of Eisenmenger's syndrome. Unfortunately, since only late pregnancy cases were reviewed, no conclusions can be drawn about the rate of early fetal wastage.

Pulmonary artery catheterization may be useful to monitor preload and cardiac output during the intrapartum period, although many clinicians now believe the risk of this technique may outweigh its benefits in patients with cyanotic heart disease (Weiss & Atanassoff, 1993). During labor, uterine contractions are associated with a decrease in the ratio of pulmonary to systemic blood flow (Q_pQ_s) (Midwall et al., 1978). Pulmonary artery catheterization and serial arterial blood gas determinations allow the clinician to detect and treat early changes in cardiac output, pulmonary artery pressure, and shunt fraction. In many cases, pulse oximetry may offer appropriate guidance in the intrapartum management of these patients without the need for and/or the associated risks of, pulmonary artery catheterization. Because the primary concern in such patients is the avoidance of hypotension, any attempt at preload reduction (i.e. diuresis) must be undertaken with great caution, even in the face of initial fluid overload. We prefer to manage such patients on the "wet" side, maintaining a preload margin of safety against unexpected blood loss, even at the expense of mild pulmonary edema. Recently, the use of inhaled nitric oxide and intravenous prostacyclin therapy have shown promise as potentially helpful agents in reducing the pulmonary vascular resistance while relatively sparing the systemic vascular resistance (Sitbon et al., 1995; Shapiro et al., 1997).

Anesthesia for patients with pulmonary hypertension is controversial. Theoretically, conduction anesthesia, with its accompanying risk of hypotension, should be avoided. However, there are several reports of its successful use in patients with pulmonary hypertension of different etiologies (Spinnato et al., 1981; Abboud et al., 1983). The use of epidural or intrathecal morphine sulfate, a technique devoid of effect on systemic BP, represents perhaps the best approach to anesthetic management of these difficult patients.

Ebstein's anomaly

Because it accounts for only 1% of all congenital cardiac disease, Ebstein's anomaly is uncommonly encountered during pregnancy (Waickman et al., 1984; Donnelly et al., 1991; Connolly & Warnes, 1994). This anomaly consists of apical displacement of the tricuspid valve, with secondary tricuspid regurgitation and enlargement of both the right atrium and ventricle. Paroxysmal atrial arrhythmias have been reported to occur in up to one-third of nonpregnant women with Ebstein's anomaly and represent a potential concern during pregnancy. The Wolff–Parkinson–White syndrome is frequently associated with Ebstein's anomaly and may represent a risk factor for excessively rapid ventricular rates in response to the increased incidence of atrial arrhythmias that are associated with Ebstein's anomaly (Kounis et al., 1995). Despite these concerns, in a review of 111 pregnancies in 44 women, no serious maternal complications were noted. Seventy-six percent of pregnancies ended in live births, with a 6% incidence of congenital heart disease in the offspring of these women (Connolly & Warnes, 1994).

Coarctation of the aorta

Coarctation of the aorta accounts for approximately 10% of all congenital cardiac disease. The most common site of coarctation is the origin of the left subclavian artery. Associated anomalies of the aorta and left heart, including VSD and PDA, are common, as are intracranial aneurysms in the circle of Willis (Taylor & Donald, 1960). Coarctation is often asymptomatic. Its presence is suggested by hypertension confined to the upper extremities, although Goodwin (1961) cites data suggesting a generalized increase in peripheral resistance throughout the body. Resting cardiac output may be increased; however, increased left atrial pressure with exercise suggests occult left ventricular dysfunction. Aneurysms also may develop below the coarctation or involve the intercostal arteries and may lead to rupture. In addition, ruptures without prior aneurysm formation have been reported (Barrett et al., 1982).

Over 400 patients with coarctation have been reported during pregnancy, with maternal mortality ranging from 0% to 17% (Schaefer et al., 1968; Deal & Wooley, 1973; Barrett et al., 1982). In a 1940 review of 200 pregnant women with coarctation of the aorta, Mendelson (1940) reported 14 maternal deaths and recommended routine abortion and sterilization of these patients. Deaths in this series were from aortic dissection and rupture, congestive heart failure, cerebral vascular accidents, and bacterial endocarditis. Six of the 14 deaths occurred in women with associated lesions. In contrast to this dismal prognosis, a more recent series by Deal and Wooley (1973) reported 83 pregnancies in 23 women with uncomplicated coarctation of the aorta. All were NYHA class I or II prior to pregnancy. In these women, there were no maternal deaths or permanent cardiovascular complications. In one review, aortic rupture was more likely to occur in the third trimester, prior to labor and delivery (Barash et al., 1975). Thus, it appears that today, patients having coarctation of the aorta uncomplicated by aneurysmal dilation or associated cardiac lesions who enter pregnancy as class I or II have a good prognosis and a minimal risk of complications or death. Even if uncorrected, uncomplicated coarctation has historically carried with it a risk of maternal mortality of only 3–4% (Goodwin, 1961). Surgical repair of the coarctation, often accomplished in early childhood, usually results in long-term normalization of blood pressure. Weakness in the aortic wall, both proximal and distal to the repair, is histologically similar (cystic medial necrosis) to the aortic weakness exhibited in Marfan syndrome. Despite these concerns, most patients with a successfully repaired coarctation of the aorta have a relatively unremarkable pregnancy. Saidi et al. (1998) followed 18 pregnancies in women who had undergone a successful repair of their aortic coarctations. All 18 women had uneventful pregnancies. Interestingly, the incidence of preeclampsia in this series was no different than that reported in the normal population. Maternal risk, however, is clearly increased if preeclampsia develops (Shime et al., 1987). In the presence of aortic or intervertebral aneurysm, known as aneurysm of the circle of Willis, or associated cardiac lesions, the risk of death may approach 15%; therefore, termination of pregnancy should be strongly considered.

Tetralogy of Fallot

Tetralogy of Fallot refers to the cyanotic complex of VSD, overriding aorta, right ventricular hypertrophy, and pulmonary stenosis. Most cases of tetralogy of Fallot are corrected during infancy or childhood. Several published reports attest to the relatively successful outcome of pregnancy in patients with corrected tetralogy of Fallot (Loh & Tan, 1975; Shime, 1987). In a review of 55 pregnancies in 46 patients, there were no maternal deaths among nine patients with correction prior to pregnancy; in patients with an uncorrected lesion, however, maternal mortality has traditionally ranged from 4% to 15%, with a 30% fetal mortality due to hypoxia (Meyer et al., 1964; Shime, 1987). In patients with uncorrected VSD, the decline in SVR that accompanies pregnancy can lead to worsening of the right-to-left shunt. This condition can be aggravated further by systemic hypotension as a result of peripartum blood loss. A poor prognosis for successful pregnancy has been related to several prepregnancy parameters, including a hemoglobin exceeding 20 g/dL, a history of syncope or congestive failure, electrocardiographic evidence of right ventricular strain, cardiomegaly, right ventricular pressure in excess of 120 mmHg, and peripheral oxygen saturation below 85%.

Transposition of the great vessels

Transposition of the great vessels is uncommon during pregnancy. A series of pregnant patients who were followed subsequent to the Mustard (atrial switch) operation reported 12 of 15 live births and no maternal deaths (Clarkson et al., 1994). In a similar series of seven patients with transposition having undergone the Mustard or Rastelli procedure, no maternal deaths were reported (Lao et al., 1994). In one case, however, pregnancy termination was necessary due to maternal deterioration. The arterial switch operation (Jatene) is now most frequently used to repair D-transposition of the great arteries (Jatene et al., 1982). This procedure appears to reduce the late morbidity rates that are often described with the atrial repairs (Gutgesell et al., 1994; Losay & Hougen, 1997). Women that have had successful arterial switch procedures are now entering reproductive ages.

Pulmonic stenosis

Pulmonic stenosis is a common congenital defect. Although obstruction can be valvular, supravalvular, or subvalvular, the degree of obstruction, rather than its site, is the principal determinant of clinical performance. A transvalvular pressure gradient exceeding 60 mmHg in a symptomatic patient is generally considered severe and may suggest the need for percutaneous valvoplasty or formal surgical correction. Maternal well-being is rarely significantly affected by pulmonic stenosis. Even 20 years ago, a compilation (totaling 106 pregnancies) of three series of patients with pulmonic stenosis revealed no maternal deaths (Schaefer et al., 1968; Neilsen et al., 1970; Hibbard, 1975). With severe stenosis, right heart failure can occur; fortunately, this is usually less clinically severe than is the left heart failure associated with mitral or aortic valve lesions. The incidence of fetal congenital heart disease in patients with pulmonic valve stenosis appears to be approximately 20% with a 55% concordance rate (Teerlink & Foster, 1998).

Fetal considerations

Perinatal outcome in patients with cyanotic congenital cardiac disease correlates best with hematocrit; successful outcome in patients with a hematocrit exceeding 65% or hemoglobin exceeding 20 g/dL is unlikely. Presbitero and associates (1994) described outcome in 96 pregnancies complicated by cyanotic congenital heart disease. Patients with Eisenmenger's syndrome were excluded from this analysis. Although only one maternal death was seen (from endocarditis 2 months postpartum), the pregnancy loss rate was 51%. Functional class III or IV, hemoglobin greater than 20 g/dL, and a prepregnancy oxygen saturation less than 85% all were associated with a high risk for poor pregnancy outcome. Such patients have an increased risk of spontaneous abortion, intrauterine growth restriction, and stillbirth. Maternal P_aO_2 below 70 mmHg results in decreased fetal oxygen saturation; thus, P_aO_2 should be kept above this level during pregnancy, labor, and delivery. In the presence of maternal cardiovascular disease, the growth-restricted fetus is especially sensitive to intrapartum hypoxia, and fetal decompensation may occur more rapidly (Block et al., 1984; Hsieh et al., 1993). During the antepartum period, serial antepartum sonography for the detection of growth restriction and antepartum fetal heart rate testing are recommended in any patient with significant cardiac disease.

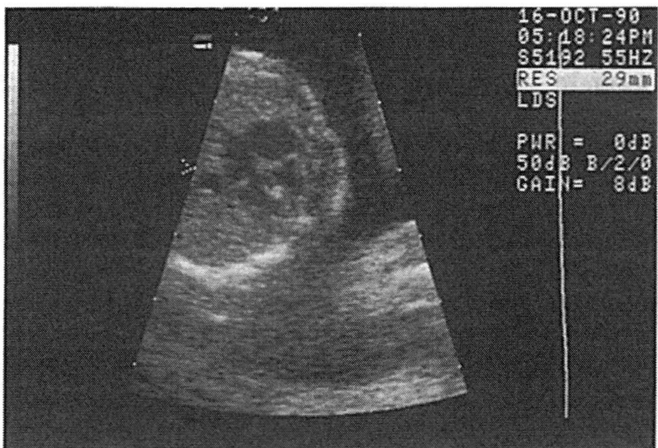

Fig. 19.3 Echocardiographic image of a fetus at 19 weeks in a mother with a VSD. A similar VSD is demonstrated in this fetus.

Fetal activity counting also may be of value in patients with severe disease (Simon et al., 1986). In a series of six patients with cyanotic cardiac disease, every pregnancy was eventually delivered secondary to fetal, rather than maternal, deterioration (Patton et al., 1990).

Of equal concern in patients with congenital heart disease is the risk of fetal congenital cardiac anomalies. This risk appears to be on the order of 5%, although one older study suggested that the actual risk may be as high as 10%, or even higher in women whose congenital lesion involves ventricular outflow obstruction (Whittemore et al., 1982; Driscoll et al., 1993; Presbitero et al., 1994; Teerlink & Foster, 1998) (see Fig. 19.3). In such patients, fetal echocardiography is indicated for prenatal diagnosis of congenital cardiac defects (Allan et al., 1994). Of special interest is that affected fetuses appear to be concordant for the maternal lesion in approximately 50% of cases. The genetics and embryologic development of congenital cardiac defects have been reviewed by Clark (1996).

Acquired cardiac lesions

Many common complaints associated with normal pregnancy including dyspnea, fatigue, orthopnea, palpitations, presyncope and pedal edema mimic the symptoms of valvular heart disease making the clinical diagnosis difficult. Jugular venous distention, brisk and collapsing pulses, and a diffuse and laterally displaced left ventricular impulse, all normal physiologic adaptations to pregnancy, further confound the clinical assessment. On auscultation of the normal heart during pregnancy, it is not unusual to hear an accentuated first heart sound (S1) or a systolic flow murmur that peaks in mid-systole and is best appreciated along the left sternal border. A third heart sound (S3), a fourth heart sound (S4), or a diastolic murmur are uncommon in normal pregnancy and require an echocardiographic assessment.

Doppler echocardiography in normal pregnancy reflects the physiologic consequences of the increased intravascular volume and blood flow on the cardiac chambers and valves. There is an increase in the left ventricular end-diastolic dimension and a decrease in the left ventricular end-systolic dimension representing an increase in both the stroke volume and ejection fraction. The aortic root dimension, as well as the mitral and tricuspid annuli, are slightly increased. The left ventricular mass increases by as much as 30% with minimal changes in wall thickness (Otto, 1997). Flow velocities across the aortic valve are minimally increased but rarely exceeded 1.5 m/sec by Doppler assessment. Campos et al. (1993) studied 18 pregnant women longitudinally throughout pregnancy utilizing Doppler echocardiogram. Mild valvular regurgitation was detected consistently throughout pregnancy. Aortic regurgitation was rarely detected; however, mitral (0–28%) tricuspid (39–94%), and pulmonic regurgitation (22–94%) were found to increase substantially from early to late gestation. Table 19.7 reviews the effect of pregnancy on the clinical and echocardiographic findings associated with cardiac valvular abnormalities (Teerlink & Foster, 1998).

Acquired valvular lesions generally are rheumatic in origin, although endocarditis secondary to intravenous drug abuse may occasionally occur, especially with right heart lesions. During pregnancy, maternal morbidity and mortality with such lesions result from congestive failure with pulmonary edema or arrhythmias. Szekely et al. (1973) found the risk of pulmonary edema in pregnant patients with rheumatic heart disease to increase with increasing age and with increasing length of gestation. The onset of atrial fibrillation during pregnancy carries with it a higher risk of right and left ventricular failure (63%) than does fibrillation with onset prior to gestation (22%). In addition, the risk of systemic embolization after the onset of atrial fibrillation during pregnancy appears to exceed that associated with onset in the nonpregnant state. In counseling the patient with severe rheumatic cardiac disease on the advisability of initiating or continuing pregnancy, the physician must also consider the long-term prognosis of the underlying disease. Chesley (1980) followed 134 women who had functionally severe rheumatic heart disease and who had completed pregnancy for up to 44 years. He reported a mortality of 6.3% per year but concluded that in patients who survived the gestation, maternal life expectancy was not shortened by pregnancy. Thus, in general, pregnancy does not appear to introduce long-term sequelae for patients who survive the pregnancy (Elkayam & Gleicher, 1984).

Pulmonic and tricuspid lesions

Isolated right-sided valvular lesions of rheumatic origin are uncommon; however, such lesions are seen with increased frequency in intravenous drug abusers, where they are secondary to valvular endocarditis. Pregnancy-associated hypervolemia is far less likely to be symptomatic with right-sided lesions than with those involving the mitral or aortic valves. In a review of 77 maternal cardiac deaths, Hibbard (1975) reported no deaths associated with isolated right-sided lesions. In a more recent review, congestive heart failure

Table 19.7 The effect of pregnancy on the clinical and echocardiographic findings associated with cardiac valvular abnormalities

	Heart sounds	Murmur	Other	Doppler echocardiography
Aortic stenosis (AS)	Diminished or single S2—unchanged	Increase in intensity and duration	Systolic ejection click unchanged	Increase in Doppler gradient; AVA unchanged
Aortic insufficiency (AI)	Diminished S2—unchanged	Decreased or unchanged	Wide pulse pressure—increased or unchanged	LV dimensions may increase secondary to pregnancy not AI
Mitral stenosis (MS)	Loud 1—increased; P2—increased	Increased	S2–OS interval decrease or unchanged	Increase in Doppler gradient, decrease in pressure half-time and increase in calculated MVA
Mitral regurgitation (MR)	Diminished S1—unchanged	Decreased or unchanged	S3—unchanged	LV dimensions may increase secondary to pregnancy not MR
Pulmonic stenosis (PS)	Diminished P2—unchanged	Increase in intensity and duration	Systolic ejection click unchanged	Increase in Doppler gradient
Pulmonic insufficiency (PI)	Diminished P2—unchanged	Decreased or unchanged	N/A	RV dimensions may increase secondary to pregnancy not PI
Tricuspid stenosis (TS)	N/A	Increased	N/A	N/A
Tricuspid regurgitation (TR)	N/A	Decreased or unchanged	N/A	RV dimensions may increase secondary to pregnancy not TR

AVA, arteriovenous anastomosis; LV, left ventricle; MVA, mitral valve anastomosis; RV, right ventricle.

occurred in only 2.8% of women with pulmonic stenosis (Whittemore et al., 1982). Even following complete tricuspid valvectomy for endocarditis, pregnancy, labor, and delivery are generally well tolerated. Cautious fluid administration is the mainstay of labor and delivery management in such patients. In general, invasive hemodynamic monitoring during labor and delivery is not necessary. A successful pregnancy has been reported following Fontan repair of congenital tricuspid atresia (Hess et al., 1991).

Mitral stenosis

Mitral stenosis is the most common rheumatic valvular lesion encountered during pregnancy (Clark et al., 1985a). It can occur as an isolated lesion or in conjunction with aortic or right-sided lesions. When mitral stenosis is significant (valve area <1.5 cm^2) the principal hemodynamic aberration involves a left ventricular diastolic filling obstruction, resulting in a relatively fixed cardiac output. Marked increases in cardiac output accompany normal pregnancy, labor, and delivery. If the pregnant patient is unable to accommodate such volume fluctuations, atrial arrhythmias and/or pulmonary edema may result.

Ideally it is best to treat significant mitral stenosis prior to pregnancy with balloon and/or surgical commissurotomy. Often the diagnosis of mitral stenosis will be discovered for the first time during pregnancy illustrating what is frequently referred to as "occult" mitral stenosis. The hemodynamic changes accompanying normal pregnancy may represent the first time the patient's cardiovascular system has been significantly stressed. These patients may present with "acute" pulmonary edema and/or atrial fibrillation as the initial diagnostic clue to the presence of mitral stenosis. When clinical symptoms persist despite attentive medical management, interventional therapy may be prudent. Percutaneous balloon mitral valvuloplasty during pregnancy has become increasingly prevalent. More than 100 pregnant women have undergone percutaneous balloon mitral valvuloplasty without periprocedural maternal or fetal mortality. Multiple case reports (Palacios et al., 1988; Smith et al., 1989; Glantz et al., 1993) and case series (Esteves et al., 1991; BenFarhat, 1992; Chow et al., 1992; Gangbar et al., 1992; Ribeiro et al., 1992; Patel et al., 1993; Iung et al., 1994; Kalra et al., 1994) support the relative safety of this procedure during pregnancy. Procedural complications include cardiac tamponade, maternal arrhythmias, transient uterine contractions, and systemic thromboembolism. Transesophageal echocardiography can be used as the sole imaging modality thereby eliminating the undesired radiation exposure associated with fluoroscopy.

Cardiac output in patients with mitral stenosis is largely dependent on two factors. First, these patients are dependent on adequate diastolic filling time. Thus, while in most patients tachycardia is a clinical sign of underlying hemodynamic instability, in patients with mitral stenosis, the tachycardia itself, regardless of etiology, may contribute significantly to hemodynamic decompensation. During labor, such tachycardia may accompany the exertion of pushing or be secondary to pain or anxiety. Such a patient may exhibit a rapid and dramatic fall in cardiac output and BP in response to tachycardia. This fall compromises maternal as well as fetal well-being. To avoid hazardous tachycardia, the physician should consider intravenous beta-blocker therapy for any patient with severe mitral stenosis who enters labor with a pulse exceeding 90–100 bpm. A short acting beta-blocker, such as esmolol, is ideal in that minute-to-minute heart rate control can be achieved without the undesired prolonged beat-blockade that is associated with more conventional agents such as propranolol. In patients who are not initially tachycardic, acute control of tachycardia with an intravenous beta-blocking agent is only rarely necessary (Clark et al., 1985a).

A second important consideration in patients with mitral stenosis is left ventricular preload. In the presence of mitral stenosis, pulmonary capillary wedge pressure is not an accurate reflection of left ventricular filling pressures. Such patients often require high-normal or elevated pulmonary capillary wedge pressures to maintain adequate ventricular filling pressure and cardiac output. Any preload manipulation (i.e. diuresis), therefore, must be undertaken with extreme caution and careful attention to maintenance of cardiac output.

Potentially dangerous intrapartum fluctuations in cardiac output can be minimized by using epidural anesthesia (Ueland et al., 1972); however, the most hazardous time for these women appears to be the immediate postpartum period. Such patients often enter the postpartum period already operating at maximum cardiac output and cannot accommodate the volume shifts that follow delivery. In a series of patients with severe mitral stenosis, Clark and colleagues found that a postpartum rise in wedge pressure of up to 16 mmHg could be expected in the immediate postpartum period (Fig. 19.4) (Clark et al., 1985a). Because frank pulmonary edema is infrequent with wedge pressures below 28–30 mmHg (Forrester & Swan, 1974), it follows that the optimal predelivery wedge pressure for such patients is approximately 14 mmHg or lower, as indicated by pulmonary artery catheterization (Clark et al., 1985a). Such a preload may be approached by cautious intrapartum diuresis and with careful attention to the maintenance of adequate cardiac output. Active diuresis is not always necessary in patients who enter labor with evidence of only mild fluid overload. In such patients, simple fluid restriction and the associated sensible and insensible fluid losses that accompany labor can result in a significant fall in wedge pressure prior to delivery.

Previous recommendations for delivery in patients with cardiac disease have also included the liberal use of midforceps to shorten the second stage of labor. In cases of severe disease, cesarean section with general anesthesia also has been advocated as the preferred mode of delivery (Ueland et al.,

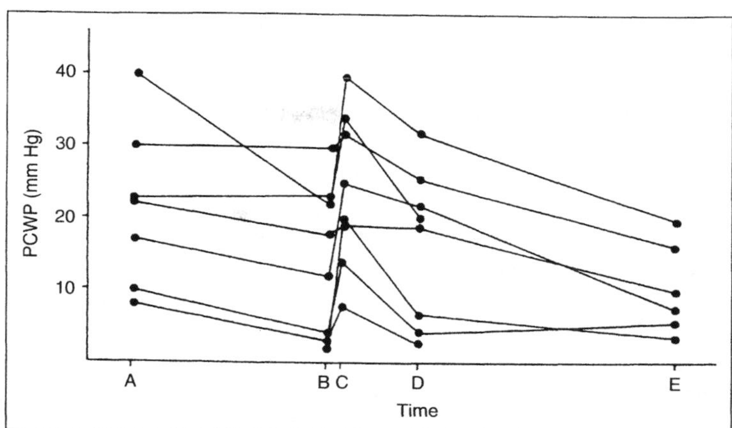

Fig. 19.4 Intrapartum alterations in pulmonary capillary wedge pressure (PCWP) in eight patients with mitral stenosis. (A) First-stage labor. (B) Second-stage labor, 15–30 minutes before delivery. (C) Five to 15 minutes postpartum. (D) Four to 6 hours postpartum. (E) Eighteen to 24 hours postpartum. (Reproduced by permission from Clark SL, Phelan JP, Greenspoon J, et al. Labor and delivery in the presence of mitral stenosis: central hemodynamic observations. Am J Obstet Gynecol 1985b;152:986.)

1970). If intensive monitoring of intrapartum cardiac patients cannot be carried out in the manner described here, such recommendations for elective cesarean delivery may be valid. With the aggressive management scheme presented, however, our experience suggests that vaginal delivery is safe, even in patients with severe disease and pulmonary hypertension. Midforceps deliveries are rarely appropriate in modern obstetrics (ACOG, 1994) and should be reserved for standard obstetric indications only.

Mitral insufficiency

Hemodynamically significant mitral insufficiency is usually rheumatic in origin and most commonly occurs in conjunction with other valvular lesions. This lesion generally is well tolerated during pregnancy, and congestive failure is an unusual occurrence. A more significant risk is the development of atrial enlargement and fibrillation. There is some evidence to suggest that the risk of developing atrial fibrillation may be increased during pregnancy (Szekely et al., 1973). In Hibbard's review of 28 maternal deaths associated with rheumatic valvular lesions, no patient died with complications of mitral insufficiency unless there was coexisting mitral stenosis (Hibbard, 1975).

Mitral valve prolapse

Congenital mitral valve prolapse is much more common during pregnancy than is rheumatic mitral insufficiency and can occur in up to 17% of young healthy women. This condition is generally asymptomatic (Markiewicz et al., 1976). The midsystolic click and murmur associated with congenital mitral valve prolapse are characteristic; however, the intensity of this murmur, as well as that associated with rheumatic mitral insufficiency, may decrease during pregnancy because of decreased SVR (Haas, 1976). Endocarditis prophylaxis during labor and delivery is recommended for rheumatic mitral insufficiency as well as for the more common mitral valve prolapse syndrome, if associated with a regurgitant murmur or evidence of valvular insufficiency by echocardiography.

Aortic stenosis

Aortic stenosis is most commonly of rheumatic origin and usually occurs in conjunction with other lesions. Less often it occurs congenitally (bicuspid valve) and represents 5% of all congenital cardiac lesions. In several series of pregnancies in women with cardiac disease, no maternal deaths due to aortic stenosis have been observed (Shime et al., 1987; DeSwiet, 1993; Jacob et al., 1998). In contrast to mitral valve stenosis, aortic stenosis generally does not become hemodynamically significant until the orifice has diminished to one-third or less of normal. Patients with a valvular peak gradient less than 50 mmHg or an aortic valve area greater than 1.5 cm^2 are considered to have mild disease and are unlikely to require any medical or surgical intervention. Moderate disease is diagnosed when the peak gradient increases to 50–75 mmHg or the aortic valve area is between 1.0 and 1.5 cm^2. These patients can be managed medically with frequent echocardiographic assessments to evaluate for worsening disease. Should the valvular peak gradient exceed 75 mmHg, the ejection fraction measure less than 55%, or the aortic valve area measure less than 1.0 cm^2, however, patients are considered to have severe disease and surgical correction should be entertained.

The major problem experienced by patients with valvular aortic stenosis is maintenance of cardiac output. Because of the relative hypervolemia associated with gestation, such patients generally tolerate pregnancy well. With severe disease, however, cardiac output will be relatively fixed, and during exertion it may be inadequate to maintain coronary artery or cerebral perfusion. This inadequacy can result in angina, myocardial infarction, syncope, or sudden death. Thus, marked limitation of physical activity is vital to patients with severe disease. If activity is limited and the mitral valve is competent, pulmonary edema will be rare during pregnancy.

Delivery and pregnancy termination appear to be the times

of greatest risk for patients with aortic stenosis (Arias & Pineda, 1978). The maintenance of cardiac output is crucial; any factor leading to diminished venous return will cause an increase in the valvular gradient and diminished cardiac output. Hypotension resulting from blood loss, ganglionic blockade from epidural anesthesia, or supine vena caval occlusion by the pregnant uterus may result in sudden death. Such problems are similar to those encountered in patients with pulmonary hypertension, discussed previously.

The cardiovascular status of patients with aortic stenosis is complicated further by the frequent coexistence of ischemic heart disease; thus, death associated with aortic stenosis often occurs secondary to myocardial infarction rather than as a direct complication of the valvular lesion itself (Arias & Pineda, 1978). The overall reported mortality associated with aortic stenosis in pregnancy has been as high as 17%. Today, it would appear that with appropriate care and in the absence of coronary artery disease, however, the risk of death is minimal (DeSwiet, 1993; Lao et al., 1993; Jacob et al., 1998). Pulmonary artery catheterization, particularly with the availability of continuous cardiac output and mixed venous oxygen monitoring, may allow more precise hemodynamic assessment and control during labor and delivery. Because hypovolemia is a far greater threat to the patient than is pulmonary edema, the wedge pressure should be maintained in the range of 15–17 mmHg to maintain a margin of safety against unexpected peripartum blood loss.

Aortic insufficiency

Aortic insufficiency is most commonly rheumatic in origin and as such is associated almost invariably with mitral valve disease. The aortic insufficiency generally is well tolerated during pregnancy because the increased heart rate observed with advancing gestation decreases time for regurgitant flow during diastole. In Hibbard's series of 28 maternal rheumatic cardiac deaths, only one was associated with aortic insufficiency in the absence of concurrent mitral stenosis (Hibbard, 1975). Endocarditis prophylaxis during labor and delivery is indicated.

Peripartum cardiomyopathy

Peripartum cardiomyopathy is defined as cardiomyopathy developing in the last month of pregnancy or the first 5 months postpartum in a woman without previous cardiac disease and after exclusion of other causes of cardiac failure (Demakis et al., 1971; Lampert & Lang, 1995; Hibbard et al., 1999; Pearson et al., 2000) (Table 19.8). It is, therefore, a diagnosis of exclusion that should not be made without a concerted effort to identify valvular, metabolic, infectious, or toxic causes of cardiomyopathy. Much of the current controversy surrounding this condition is the result of many older reports in which these causes of cardiomyopathy were not investigated adequately. Other peripartum complications, such as amniotic fluid embolism, severe preeclampsia, and corticosteroid or sympathomimetic-induced pulmonary edema, also must be considered before making the diagnosis of peripartum cardiomyopathy. Sympathomimetic agents also may unmask underlying peripartum cardiomyopathy (Blickstein et al., 1988).

Table 19.8 Criteria for diagnosis of peripartum cardiomyopathy

Classic

1 Development of cardiac failure in the last month of pregnancy or within 5 months of delivery
2 Absence of an identifiable cause for the cardiac failure
3 Absence of recognizable heart disease prior to the last month of pregnancy

Additional

4 Left ventricular systolic dysfunction demonstrated by classic echocardiographic criteria, such as depressed shortening fraction (less than 30%), ejection fraction (less than 45%), and a left ventricular end-diastolic dimension of more than 2.7 cm per m^2 of body surface area (Hibbard et al., 1999)

The incidence of peripartum cardiomyopathy is estimated to be between 1 in 3,000 and 1 in 4,000 live births, which would translate to 1,000–1,300 women affected each year in the United States (Homans, 1985; Lampert & Lang, 1995; Ventura et al., 1997). An incidence as high as 1% has been suggested in women of certain African tribes; however, idiopathic heart failure in these women may be primarily a result of unusual culturally mandated peripartum customs involving excessive sodium intake and may represent, as such, simple fluid overload (Seftel & Susser, 1961; Veille, 1984; Homans, 1985). In the United States, the peak incidence of peripartum cardiomyopathy occurs in the second postpartum month, and there appears to be a higher incidence among older, multiparous black females (Veille, 1984; Witlin et al., 1997). Other suggested risk factors include twinning and pregnancy-induced hypertension (Veille, 1984; Cunningham et al., 1986). In rare cases, a familial recurrence pattern has been reported. The condition is manifest clinically by the gradual onset of increasing fatigue, dyspnea, and peripheral or pulmonary edema. Physical examination reveals classic evidence of congestive heart failure, including jugular venous distention, rales, and an S3 gallop. Cardiomegaly and pulmonary edema are found on chest X-ray, and the ECG often demonstrates left ventricular and atrial dilatation and diminished ventricular performance. In addition, up to 50% of patients with peripartum cardiomyopathy may manifest evidence of pulmonary or systemic embolic phenomena. Overall mortality ranges from 25% to 50% (Veille, 1984; Homans, 1985).

The histologic picture of peripartum cardiomyopathy involves nonspecific cellular hypertrophy, degeneration, fibrosis, and increased lipid deposition. Many reports have documented the presence of a diffuse myocarditis and currently more evidence exists for myocarditis as a cause of peripartum cardiomyopathy than for any other purported etiology (Pearson, 2000). Because of the nonspecific clinical and pathologic nature of peripartum cardiomyopathy, however, its existence as a distinct entity has been questioned (Cunningham et al., 1986). Its existence as a distinct entity is supported primarily by epidemiologic evidence suggesting that 80% of cases of idiopathic cardiomyopathy in women of child-bearing age occur in the peripartum period. Such an epidemiologic distribution also could be attributed to an exacerbation of underlying subclinical cardiac disease related to the hemodynamic changes accompanying normal pregnancy. Because such changes are maximal in the third trimester of pregnancy and return to normal within a few weeks postpartum, however, such a pattern does not explain the peak incidence of peripartum cardiomyopathy occurring, in most reports, during the second month postpartum. The National Heart, Lung and Blood Institute and Office of Rare Diseases (National Institute of Health) Workshop Recommendation and Review on peripartum cardiomyopathy currently supports the disease as a distinct entity (Pearson et al., 2000). Nevertheless, the diagnosis of peripartum cardiomyopathy remains primarily a diagnosis of exclusion and cannot be made until underlying conditions, including chronic hypertension, valvular disease, and viral myocarditis, have been excluded.

Therapy includes digitalization, diuretics, sodium restriction, and afterload reduction. Angiotensin-converting enzyme inhibitors should be avoided prenatally, but are a mainstay of therapy otherwise. Early endomyocardial biopsy to identify a subgroup of patients who have a histologic picture of inflammatory myocarditis and who may be responsive to immunosuppressive therapy has been suggested. Immunosuppressive therapy should also be considered if the patient shows inadequate improvement after 2 weeks of standard heart failure therapy. Therapeutic anticoagulation should be considered when the ejection fraction is less than 35% to prevent thrombosis and emboli. A notable feature of peripartum cardiomyopathy is its tendency to recur with subsequent pregnancies. Several older reports have suggested that a prognosis for future pregnancies is related to heart size. Patients whose cardiac size returned to normal within 6–12 months had an 11–14% mortality in subsequent pregnancies; those patients with persistent cardiomegaly had a 40–80% mortality (Demakis et al., 1971). Lampert (1997), however, demonstrated persistent decreased contractile reserve even in women who had regained normal resting left ventricular size. Witlin (1997), in a series of 28 patients with peripartum cardiomyopathy, reported that only 7% had regression; in those undertaking subsequent pregnancy, two-thirds decompensated earlier than in the index pregnancy. Thus, while a subsequent pregnancy is absolutely contraindicated in all patients with persistent cardiomegaly, the substantial risk of maternal decompensation in patients with normal heart size would seem, in most cases, to be unacceptable as well.

Idiopathic hypertrophic subaortic stenosis (asymmetric septal hypertrophy)

Idiopathic hypertrophic subaortic stenosis (IHSS) or asymmetric septal hypertrophy (ASH), which the defect is also referred to, is an autosomal dominantly inherited condition with variable penetrance. It most commonly becomes clinically manifest in the second or third decade of life; thus, it often may be first manifest during pregnancy. Detailed physical and echocardiographic diagnostic criteria have been described elsewhere. Primarily, IHSS involves asymmetric left ventricular hypertrophy, typically involving the septum to a greater extent than the free wall. The hypertrophy results in obstruction to left ventricular outflow and secondary mitral regurgitation, the two principal hemodynamic concerns of the clinician (Kolibash et al., 1975). Although the increased blood volume associated with normal pregnancy should enhance left ventricular filling and improve hemodynamic performance, this positive effect of pregnancy is counterbalanced by a fall in systemic vascular resistance and an increase in heart rate and myocardial contractility. In addition, tachycardia resulting from pain or anxiety during labor further diminishes left ventricular filling and aggravates the relative outflow obstruction, an effect also resulting from the second-stage Valsalva maneuver.

The keys to successful management of the peripartum period in patients with IHSS involve avoidance of hypotension (resulting from conduction anesthesia or blood loss) and tachycardia, as well as conducting labor in the left lateral recumbent position. The use of forceps to shorten the second stage also has been recommended. As with most other cardiac disease, cesarean section for IHSS patients should be reserved for obstetric indications only. General management principles for these patients have been reviewed by Spirito et al. (1997).

Despite the potential hazards, maternal and fetal outcomes in IHSS patients are generally good. In a report of 54 pregnancies in 23 patients with IHSS, no maternal or neonatal deaths occurred (Oakley et al., 1979). Although beta-blocking agents once were used routinely in patients with IHSS, currently they are reserved for patients with angina, recurrent supraventricular tachycardia, or occasional beta-blocker-responsive arrhythmias. Although fetal bradycardia and growth restriction have been reported in patients receiving beta-blockers, a cause-and-effect relationship is not clear; in general, the benefits of such therapy outweigh potential fetal effects. Subacute bacterial endocarditis antibiotic prophylaxis is recommended.

Marfan syndrome

Marfan syndrome is an autosomal dominant disorder characterized by generalized weakness of connective tissue; the weakness results in skeletal, ocular, and cardiovascular abnormalities. The increased risk of maternal mortality during pregnancy stems from aortic root and wall involvement, which may result in aneurysm formation, rupture, or aortic dissection. Fifty percent of aortic aneurysm ruptures in women under age 40 occur during pregnancy (Barrett et al., 1982). Rupture of splenic artery aneurysms also occurs more frequently during pregnancy. Sixty percent of patients with Marfan syndrome have associated mitral or aortic regurgitation (Pyeritz & McKusick, 1979). Although some authors feel pregnancy is contraindicated in any woman with documented Marfan syndrome, prognosis is best individualized and should be based on echocardiographic assessment of aortic root diameter and postvalvular dilation. It is important to note that enlargement of the aortic root is not demonstrable by chest X-ray until dilation has become pronounced.

Women with an abnormal aortic valve or aortic dilation may have up to a 50% pregnancy-associated mortality; women without these changes and having an aortic root diameter less than 40 mm have a mortality less than 5% (Pyeritz, 1984). Such patients do not appear to have evidence of aggravated aortic root dilatation over time (Rossiter et al., 1995). Even in patients meeting these echocardiographic criteria, however, special attention must be given to signs or symptoms of aortic dissection, since serial echocardiographic assessments may not be predictive of complications (Rosenblum et al., 1983). In counseling women with Marfan syndrome, the genetics of this condition and the shortened maternal lifespan must be considered, in addition to the immediate maternal risk. The routine use of oral beta-blocking agents to decrease pulsatile pressure on the aortic wall has been recommended (Slater & DeSanctis, 1979). If cesarean section is performed, retention sutures should be considered because of generalized connective tissue weakness.

Myocardial infarction

Coronary artery disease is uncommon in women of reproductive age; therefore, myocardial infarction in conjunction with pregnancy is rare (Hankins et al., 1985; Scheikh & Harper, 1993; Badui et al., 1994). In the most recent comprehensive review of acute myocardial infarction associated with pregnancy, 125 well-documented cases of myocardial infarction in 123 pregnancies were identified (Roth & Elkayam, 1996) (Table 19.9). It appears from this retrospective review that myocardial infarction most often occurred during the third trimester in multigravidas older than 33 years of age. The most common anatomic location for the infarct was the anterior wall and the overall maternal death rate was 21%. Maternal death most often occurred at the time of the infarct or within 2 weeks of the infarct, often associated with the labor and delivery process. The fetal death rate was 13% and was clearly associated with maternal deaths. Fifty-four percent of the patients in this review had a morphologic assessment of their coronary arteries. Coronary atherosclerosis with or without intracoronary thrombus was detected in 43% of patients, coronary thrombus without atherosclerotic disease in 21%, coronary dissection in 16%, and normal coronary arteries in 29%. In a concurrent review of myocardial infarction during pregnancy and the puerperium the overall findings were remarkably similar (Badui et al., 1996). Thus, it appears that the increased hemodynamic burden imposed on the maternal cardiovascular system in late pregnancy may unmask latent coronary artery disease in some women and worsen the prognosis for patients suffering infarction.

Women with class H diabetes mellitus face risks beyond those imposed by their cardiac disease alone. Although successful pregnancy outcome may occur, maternal and fetal risks are considerable. Extensive and comprehensive counseling for these women is extremely important (Gast & Rigg, 1985).

Antepartum care of women with prior myocardial infarction should include bed rest to minimize myocardial oxygen demands. Diagnostic radionucleotide cardiac imaging during pregnancy results in a fetal dose of no more than 0.8 rad and, thus, does not carry a significant risk of teratogenesis (Elkayam & Gleicher, 1984). If cardiac catheterization becomes necessary, the simultaneous use of contrast echocardiography may reduce the need for cineangiography and, thus, reduce radiation exposure to the fetus (Elkayam et al., 1983). In women with angina, nitrates have been used without adverse fetal effects. Schumacher et al. (1997) reported success for treatment of acute myocardial infarction during pregnancy with tissue plasminogen activator. Although minor electrocardiographic changes are often seen in pregnant women, evaluation of the electrocardiogram in women with suspected ischemic heart disease should not vary significantly because of pregnancy (Veille et al., 1996). Delivery within 2 weeks of infarction is associated with increased mortality; therefore, if possible, attempts should be made to allow adequate convalescence prior to delivery. If the cervix is favorable, cautious induction under controlled circumstances after a period of hemodynamic stabilization is optimal. Labor in the lateral recumbent position, the administration of oxygen, pain relief with epidural anesthesia, and, in selected cases, hemodynamic monitoring with a pulmonary artery catheter are important management considerations.

In two prospective American studies, having six or more pregnancies was associated with a small but significant increase in the risk of subsequent coronary artery disease (Ness et al., 1993).

Table 19.9 Selected data in 123 pregnancies complicated by 125 myocardial infarctions

Variable	Antepartum group (*n*=78)*	Peripartum group (*n*=17)†	Postpartum group (*n*=30)‡	All groups (*n*=125)
Maternal age (years)	33±6	34±5	29±6	32±6
Age range (years)	16–45	23–44	17–42	16–45
Anterior MI location (%)§	50/77 (65)	14/16 (87)	25/29 (86)	89/122 (73)
Multiparous (%)§	64/73 (88)	13/16 (81)	16/22 (73)	93/111 (84)
Hypertension (%)	21	24	17	19
Diabetes mellitus (%)	6	0	3	5
Ischemic heart disease (%)	10	0		7
Smoking (%)	32	12		26
Family history of MI (%)	12	0		8
Hyperlipidemia (%)	1	0		2
Preeclampsia (%)	10	18		11
Elective cesarean (%)	15	6		14
Semiselective or emergency cesarean (%)	14	12		12
CHF after MI (%)	12 (15)	7 (41)	6 (20)	25 (19)
Coronary anatomy available (%)	36 (46)	8 (47)	24 (80)	68 (54)
Stenosis	21 (58)‖	1 (12)	7 (29)¶	29 (43)
Thrombus	8 (22)	1 (12)	5 (21)	14 (21)
Dissection	3 (8)	0 (0)	(33)	11 (16)
Aneurysm	2 (6)	0 (0)	1 (4)	3 (4)
Spasm	1 (3)	0 (0)	0 (0)	1 (1)
Normal	9 (25)	6 (75)		20 (29)
Death				
Mothers (%)	11 (14)	6 (35)	9 (30)	26 (21)
Infants (%)	12 (15)	3 (18)	1 (3)	16 (13)
Infant death associated with maternal death (%)	8/12 (67)	1/3 (33)	1/1 (100)	10/16 (62)

CHF, congestive heart failure; MI, myocardial infarction.

* Includes patients who had myocardial infarctions that occurred 24 hours or more before labor.

† Includes patients who had myocardial infarctions that occurred within 24 hours before or after labor.

‡ Includes patients who had myocardial infarctions that occurred between 24 hours before and 3 months after labor.

§ The number in the denominator is the number of relevant patients.

‖ Associated thrombus in seven cases.

¶ Associated thrombus in one case.

(Reproduced by permission from Roth A, Elkayam U. Acute myocardial infarction associated with pregnancy. Annals of Internal Medicine 1996;125(9):751–762.)

Anticoagulation

Anticoagulation in the patient with an artificial heart valve and/or atrial fibrillation during pregnancy is controversial (Ginsberg & Barron, 1994). The key issue involves our lack of an ideal agent for anticoagulation during pregnancy. Warfarin (coumadin) is relatively contraindicated at all stages of gestation due to its association with fetal warfarin syndrome in weeks 6–9 and its relationship to fetal intracranial hemorrhage and secondary scarring at later stages (Hall et al., 1980; Briggs et al., 1994). On the other hand, there is some evidence to suggest that for arterial thrombosis prevention with artificial valves (unlike the situation with venous thromboembolic disease), heparin may be less effective than warfarin (Oakley & Doherty, 1976; Antunes et al., 1984; Golby et al., 1992).

In 1984, Salazar et al. (1984) described 227 pregnancies in 156 women with cardiac valve prostheses. Women treated with warfarin throughout gestation had a 28% incidence of spontaneous abortion, 7% stillbirths, and 2% neonatal deaths. Eight percent of the fetuses had features of the fetal warfarin syndrome. In contrast, no spontaneous abortions, stillbirths, or neonatal deaths were observed in women receiving heparin before and warfarin after the 13th week of gestation. A subsequent series of pregnancies revealed a 30% incidence of fetal warfarin syndrome in patients treated with warfarin throughout gestation, with no cases when heparin was given prior to week 12, coumadin until week 38, and then heparin until delivery.

One deficiency in these studies is a lack of detailed neonatal neurologic evaluation and follow-up; thus, while the risk of fetal warfarin syndrome when warfarin derivatives are taken between weeks 6 and 9 is between 8% and 30%, the frequency of intracranial hemorrhage in fetuses whose mothers receive warfarin after week 12 is unknown. Several more recent series from outside the United States have reported on the use of warfarin in pregnant patients with prosthetic valves. In patients receiving warfarin, spontaneous abortion rates of 7–37% have been reported, with a 2% incidence of embryopathy (Vitali et al., 1986; Sareli et al., 1989; Born et al., 1992; Hanania et al., 1994; Lee et al., 1994; Sbarouni & Oakley, 1994). On the other hand, two series comparing maternal thromboembolic events in patients receiving heparin versus warfarin showed a two- to threefold increase of this potentially devastating complication in the heparin group (Hanania et al., 1994; Sbarcuni & Oakley, 1994).

Thus, a choice between fetal and maternal risks must be made, and neither choice is ideal. Two approaches, however, appear to be acceptable. One involves substitution of heparin for warfarin from the time pregnancy is diagnosed until 12 weeks' gestation, followed by warfarin until 38 weeks, at which time heparin is reinstituted until delivery. The second approach involves using adjusted-dose subcutaneous heparin throughout pregnancy (Deviri et al., 1985; Dalen & Hirsh, 1986). The patient must be involved in this choice and thoroughly informed of the risks and benefits of either approach (Vongpatanasin et al., 1996). A patient who requires anticoagulation when not pregnant should be treated during pregnancy, although the medication used may be different. Pregnant women having prosthetic heart valves should be treated with one of the aforementioned regimens from conception until delivery. During the postpartum period, warfarin may be reinstituted.

The adjusted-dose regimen employs sodium heparin given subcutaneously in doses of 8,000–14,000 units every 8–12 hours in a dose sufficient to prolong the activated partial thromboplastin time (aPTT) obtained at 8–12 hours after the dose (trough) to 1.5–2.0 times control. This heparin regimen should provide plasma heparin levels of 0.2–0.4 units/mL if measured by the protamine heparin assay. Although conclusive data in absent, low molecular weight heparin may also provide a viable alternative method for anticoagulation during pregnancy.

There have been small series of patients with nonbiologic prosthetic heart valves who have been treated during pregnancy with antiplatelet agents, including aspirin and dipyridamole. Although maternal outcome was good, a high rate of spontaneous abortion was encountered in one study. The small size of these series, however, makes it difficult to draw conclusions about the safety and efficacy of these regimens (Biale et al., 1980; Nunez et al., 1983; Deviri et al., 1985).

Patients with bioprosthetic or xenograft valves usually are not treated with anticoagulants (Vongpatanasin et al., 1996). This fact makes the bioprosthetic valve the ideal choice of prosthesis for young women of childbearing age (Starr & Grunkemeier, 1984). Patients with a bioprosthetic valve who are in atrial fibrillation or have evidence of thromboembolism, however, should be anticoagulated.

Prevention of bacterial endocarditis

The American Heart Association recommendations for endocarditis prophylaxis are outlined in Table 19.10, and the recommendations of the American Heart Associations/American College of Cardiology Task Force on antibiotic prophylaxis for selected cardiac valve lesions are reviewed in Table 19.5. Controversy persists regarding the need for prophylaxis with vaginal delivery. One approach is to administer the high-risk regimen to patients with systemic-pulmonary shunts, artificial valves, or a history of endocarditis, reserving the low-risk regimen for pregnant patients with other structural abnormalities. There appear to be two major problems with the current suggestion by the American Heart Association that uncomplicated vaginal delivery does not require endocarditis prophylaxis. First, to be most effective, antibiotic administration is recommended from one-half to 1 hour prior to the anticipated bacteremia; we have yet to meet the clinician who can reliably predict, one-half to 1 hour prior to birth, that the delivery will

Table 19.10 Bacterial endocarditis prophylaxis drug regimens

Standard regimen (ampicillin, gentamicin, and amoxicillin)
IV or IM administration of ampicillin, 2 g, plus gentamicin, 1.5 mg/kg (not to exceed 120 mg), 30 min before procedure; followed by amoxicillin, 1.0 g, orally 6 hr after initial dose; alternatively, the parenteral regimen (1 g) may be repeated once 6 hr after initial dose

Ampicillin/amoxicillin/penicillin-allergic patient regimen (vancomycin and gentamicin)
IV administration of vancomycin, 1 g over 1 hr plus IV or IM administration of gentamicin, 1.5 mg/kg (not to exceed 120 mg), 1 hr before procedure. Complete infusion within 20 min of procedure onset

Alternate low-risk patient regimen (amoxicillin/ampicillin)
2 g orally 1 hr before procedure; or ampicillin 50 mg/kg within 30 min of procedure onset

(Modified by permission from Dajani AS, Taubert KA, Wilson W, et al. Prevention of bacterial endocarditis: recommendations of the American Heart Association. JAMA 1997;277:1794–1801. Copyright 1990, American Medical Association.)

be "uncomplicated" and not involve vaginal or rectal lacerations or the need for manual exploration of the uterus. Second, as outlined at the beginning of this chapter, a review of recent maternal cardiac deaths in Western countries reveals that postpartum endocarditis is one of the leading causes of mortality. Thus, most clinicians involved in the day-to-day management of pregnant cardiac patients recommend one of the aforementioned regimens for most patients (Table 19.10).

Dysrhythmias

While minor ECG changes are commonly seen during pregnancy, significant dysrhythmias are rare (Veille et al., 1996). The use of antiarrhythmic therapy has been reviewed extensively by Rotmensch et al. (1987). Many of these medications have been used to treat fetal dysrhythmias as well (Kleinman et al., 1985). Digoxin, procainamide, and quinidine may be used for the usual indications and in therapeutic doses have not been shown to be harmful to the fetus. A digoxin-like immunoreactive substance appears in some normal and preeclamptic patients during the second trimester and can be identified in many patients during the third trimester (Phelps et al., 1988). If serum monitoring of digoxin levels is anticipated, a pretreatment level should be obtained to improve interpretation of results.

The use of beta-blockers is appropriate in some tachyarrhythmias, in IHSS, and for the control of hyperthyroid symptoms. In a critical review, Frishman and Chesner (1988) concluded that beta-blocker therapy is not associated with adverse neonatal outcome. Neonatal hypoglycemia and bradycardia may occur, although they are usually not serious. Intrauterine growth restriction may be a consequence of the disease for which the beta-blockers are prescribed rather than a complication of therapy itself. Beta-blockers such as atenolol and acebutolol have lower degrees of plasma binding and are excreted in breast milk at higher concentrations, sufficient to cause bradycardia, hypotension, and poor perfusion in the infant. Verapamil is a calcium-entry-blocking drug that is effective in the conversion of a supraventricular tachycardia to sinus rhythm. Although there are no reports of its adverse effect on the fetus, there is little experience with it in pregnancy.

Women with life-threatening arrhythmias should have an evaluation prior to conception to determine whether: (i) surgical or catheter ablation; (ii) an antitachycardia pacemaker; or (iii) an automatic implantable cardiovert-defibrillator is appropriate. The issue of anticoagulation for atrial fibrillation in pregnancy has not been addressed specifically. It seems reasonable, however, to anticoagulate a pregnant patient if she meets the criteria described for nonpregnant patients. These include atrial fibrillation with a history of thromboembolic complications, atrial fibrillation in the presence of valvular disease such as mitral stenosis or regurgitation, atrial fibrillation in cardiomyopathy, or atrial fibrillation with thyrotoxic heart disease. Anticoagulation is recommended for 3 weeks prior to cardioversion of atrial fibrillation and for 4 weeks after conversion to sinus rhythm. Anticoagulation should be considered in the patient with atrial fibrillation and congestive heart failure.

Cardioversion appears safe for the fetus (Schroeder & Harrison, 1971). The presence of an artificial pacemaker, similarly, does not affect the course of pregnancy (Jaffe et al., 1987).

Pregnancy after cardiac transplantation

The number of pregnant women who have undergone cardiac transplantation is small; nevertheless, from a compilation of 47 pregnancies from 35 heart transplant recipients generalizations can be made (Scott et al., 1993; Branch et al., 1998). First, most patients are maintained on cyclosporine and azathioprine; often, prednisone is added to the regimen. While theoretic concerns may exist regarding potential teratogenesis of these agents, limited experience with heart transplant patients and more extensive experience with patients having undergone renal transplant suggest that such fears are unfounded (Kossoy et al., 1988; Key et al., 1989). Patients should be counseled that these agents appear to pose minimal, if any, risk of adverse fetal effects.

Second, with regard to maternal risk, patients with cardiac transplants who have no evidence of rejection and have normal cardiac function at the onset of pregnancy appear to tolerate pregnancy, labor, and delivery well (Lowenstein et al., 1988; Key et al., 1989; Hedon et al., 1990; Camann et al., 1991; Scott et al., 1993; Branch et al., 1998). The denervated heart retains normal systolic function and contractile reserve (Borrow et al., 1985; Greenberg et al., 1985; Kim et al., 1996). Such patients undergo the normal hemodynamic response to pregnancy, as well as the expected intrapartum hemodynamic changes (Key et al., 1989; Kim et al., 1996). Central hemodynamic changes associated with pregnancy in a stable cardiac transplant recipient were described by Kim et al. (1996), and were not significantly different from those expected during normal pregnancy.

To date, no reported cases exist of maternal death during pregnancy in cardiac transplant recipients. While three cases have been reported of delayed death following pregnancy, in two of these, voluntary withdrawal from the immunosuppressive agents and/or inappropriate medical care was implicated; there is no evidence that the antecedent pregnancy was related to the death of these women.

During pregnancy, meticulous prenatal care is essential, as is careful cardiology follow-up with frequent ECGs, cardiac catheterizations, and heart biopsies, as would be indicated in the nonpregnant state. Close attention must be paid to symptoms or signs of transplant rejection, which generally may be successfully managed by adjustments in medication. There appears to be an increased risk of pregnancy-induced hypertension, preterm delivery and low-birth-weight babies in these patients. Serial sonography to assess for adequate fetal growth and third-trimester antepartum fetal testing are recommended. There is no convincing evidence that the use of a pulmonary artery catheter will favorably influence the intrapartum management of these patients. Cesarean section and all but outlet instrumental vaginal deliveries should be reserved for standard obstetric indications.

References

Abboud JK, Raya J, Noueihed R, et al. Intrathecal morphine for relief of labor pain in a parturient with severe pulmonary hypertension. Anesthesiology 1983;59:477–479.

Allan LD, Sharland GK, Milburn A, et al. Prospective diagnosis of 1006 consecutive cases of congenital heart disease in the fetus. J Am Coll Cardiol 1994;23:1452–1458.

American College of Obstetricians and Gynecologists. Cardiac disease in pregnancy. Technical Bulletin 168, June 1992.

American College of Obstetricians and Gynecologists. Operative vaginal delivery. Technical Bulletin 196, August 1994.

Antunes MJ, Myer IG, Santos LP. Thrombosis of mitral valve prosthesis in pregnancy: management by simultaneous caesarean section and mitral valve replacement. Case report. Br J Obstet Gynaecol 1984;91:716–718.

Arias F, Pineda J. Aortic stenosis and pregnancy. J Reprod Med 1978;20:229–232.

Avila WS, Grinberg M, Snitcowsky R, et al. Maternal and fetal outcome in pregnant women with eisenmenger's syndrome. Eur Heart J 1995;16:460–464.

Badui E, Rangel A, Enciso R. Acute myocardial infarction during pregnancy and puerperium in athletic women. Two case reports. Angiology 1994;45:897–902.

Badui E, Rangel A, Enciso R. Acute myocardial infarction during pregnancy and puerperium review. Angiology 1996;47,8:739–756.

Barash PG, Hobbins JC, Hook R, et al. Management of coarctation of the aorta during pregnancy. J Thorac Cardiovasc Surg 1975;69: 781–784.

Barrett JM, VanHooydonk JE, Boehm FH. Pregnancy-related rupture of arterial aneurysms. Obstet Gynecol Surv 1982;37:557–566.

BenFarhat M, Maatouk F, Betbout F, et al. Percutaneous balloon mitral valvuloplasty in eight pregnant women with severe mitral stenosis. Eur Heart J 1992;13:1659–1664.

Berg CJ, Atrash HK, Koonin LM, et al. Pregnancy related mortality in the United States, 1987–1990. Obstet Gynecol 1996;88:161–167.

Biale Y, Cantor A, Lewenthal H, et al. The course of pregnancy in patients treated with artificial heart valves treated with dipyridamole. Int J Gynaecol Obstet 1980;18:128–132.

Blickstein I, Zalel Y, Katz Z, et al. Ritodrine-induced pulmonary edema unmasking underlying peripartum cardiomyopathy. Am J Obstet Gynecol 1988;159:332–333.

Block BSB, Llanos AJ, Creasy RK. Responses of the growth-retarded fetus to acute hypoxemia. Am J Obstet Gynecol 1984;148:878–885.

Born D, Martinez EE, Almeida P, et al. Pregnancy in patients with prosthetic heart valves: the effects of anticoagulation on mother, fetus and neonate. Am Heart J 1992;124:413–417.

Borrow KM, Neumann A, Arensman FW, et al. Left ventricular contractility and contractile reserve in humans after cardiac transplantation. Circulation 1985;71:866–872.

Branch KR, Wagoner LE, et al. Risks of subsequent pregnancies on mother and newborn in female heart transplant recipients. J Heart Lung Transplant 1998;17:698–702.

Briggs GB, Bodendorfer JW, Freeman RK, Yaffe SJ, eds. Drugs in pregnancy and lactation. Baltimore: Williams and Wilkins, 1994.

Brown CS, Bertolet BD. Peripartum cardiomyopathy: A comprehensive review. Am J Obstet Gynecol 1998;178:409–414.

Camann WR, Goldman GA, Johnson MD, et al. Cesarean delivery in a patient with a transplanted heart. Anesthesiology 1989;71:618.

Camann WR, Jarcho J, Mintz KJ, et al. Uncomplicated vaginal delivery 14 months after cardiac transplantation. Am Heart J 1991;121:939–941.

Campos O, Andrade JL, Bocanegra J, et al. Physiologic multivalvular regurgitation during pregnancy: a longitudinal Doppler echocardiographic study. Int J Cardiol 1993;40:265–272.

Chesley LC. Severe rheumatic cardiac disease and pregnancy: the ultimate prognosis. Am J Obstet Gynecol 1980;126:552–558.

Chow WH, Chow TC, Wat MS, et al. Percutaneous balloon mitral valvotomy in pregnancy using the inoue balloon catheter. Cardiology 1992;81:182–185.

Clark EB. Pathogenic mechanisms of congenital cardiovascular malformations revisited. Semin Perinatol 1996;20:465–472.

Clark SL. Structural cardiac disease in pregnancy. In: Clark SL, Cotton DB, Phelan JP, eds. Critical care obstetrics. Oradell, NJ: Medical Economics Books, 1987:92.

Clark SL, Phelan JP, Greenspoon J, et al. Labor and delivery in the presence of mitral stenosis: central hemodynamic observations. Am J Obstet Gynecol 1985a;152:984–988.

Clark SL, Horenstein JM, Phelan JP, et al. Experience with the pulmonary artery catheter in obstetrics and gynecology. Am J Obstet Gynecol 1985b;152:374–378.

Clark SL, Cotton DB, Lee W, et al. Central hemodynamic assessment of normal term pregnancy. Am J Obstet Gynecol 1989;161:1439–1442.

Clarkson PM, Wilson NJ, Neutze JM, et al. Outcome of pregnancy after the Mustad operation for transposition of the great arteries with intact ventricular septum. J Am Coll Cardiol 1994;24:190–193.

Connolly HM, Warnes CA. Ebstein's anomaly: outcome of pregnancy. J Am Coll Cardiol 1994;23:1194–1198.

Cunningham FG, Pritchard JA, Hankins GD, et al. Peripartum heart failure: idiopathic cardiomyopathy or compounding cardiovascular events? Obstet Gynecol 1986;67:157–168.

Dajani AS, Taubert KA, Wilson W, et al. Prevention of bacterial endocarditis: recommendations of the American Heart Association. JAMA 1997;277:1794–1801.

Dalen E, Hirsh J, co-chairmen. American College of Chest Physicians and the National Heart, Lung, and Blood Institute National Conference on Antithrombotic Therapy. Chest 1986;89(Suppl 2): 1S–106S.

Danilenko-Dixon DR, Tefft L, Cohen RA, et al. Positional effects on maternal cardiac output during labor with epidural analgesia. Am J Obstet Gynecol 1996;175:867–872.

Deal K, Wooley CF. Coarctation of the aorta and pregnancy. Ann Intern Med 1973;78:706–710.

Demakis JG, Rahimtoola SH, Sutton GC, et al. Natural course of peripartum cardiomyopathy. Circulation 1971;44:1053–1061.

DeSwiet M. Maternal mortality from heart disease in pregnancy. Br Heart J 1993;69:524.

Deviri E, Levinsky L, Yechezkel M, et al. Pregnancy after valve replacement with porcine xenograft prosthesis. Surg Gynecol Obstet 1985;160:437–443.

Donnolly JE, Brown JM, Radford DJ. Pregnancy outcome and Ebstein's anomaly. Br Heart J 1991;66:368–371.

Douglas PS, Ginsberg GS. The evaluation of chest pain in women. N Engl J Med 1996;334:1311.

Driscoll DJ, Michels VV, Gesony WM, et al. Occurrence risk for congenital heart defects in relatives of patients with aortic stenosis, pulmonary stenosis, or ventricular septal defect. Circulation 1993;87(Suppl 2):I114–120.

Dye TD, Gordon H, Held B, et al. Retrospective maternal mortality case ascertainment in West Virginia. Obstet Gynecol 1992; 167:72–76.

Elkayam U, Kawanishi D, Reid CL, et al. Contrast echocardiography to reduce ionizing radiation associated with cardiac catheterization during pregnancy. Am J Cardiol 1983;52:213–214.

Elkayam V, Gleicher N. Cardiac problems in pregnancy, I. Maternal aspects: the approach to the pregnant patient with heart disease. JAMA 1984;251:2838–2839.

Esteves CA, Ramos AI, Braya SL, et al. Effectiveness of percutaneous balloon mitral valvotomy during pregnancy. Am J Cardiol 1991;68:930–934.

Etheridge MJ, Pepperell RJ. Heart disease and pregnancy at the Royal Women's Hospital. Med J Aust 1971;2:277–281.

Forrester JS, Swan HJC. Acute myocardial infarction: a physiological basis for therapy. Crit Care Med 1974;2:283–292.

Frishman WH, Chesner M. Beta-adrenergic blockers in pregnancy. Am Heart J 1988;115:147–152.

Gangbar EW, Watson KR, Howard RJ, et al. Mitral balloon valvuloplasty in pregnancy: Advantages of a unique balloon. Cathet Cardiovasc Diagn 1992;25:313–316.

Gast MJ, Rigg LA. Class H diabetes and pregnancy. Obstet Gynecol 1985;66:S5–7.

Gilman DH. Cesarean section in undiagnosed Eisenmenger's syndrome. Report of a patient with a fatal outcome. Anesthesia 1991;46:371–373.

Ginsberg JS, Barron WM. Pregnancy and prosthetic heart valves. Lancet 1994;344:1170–1172.

Glanz JC, Pomerantz RM, Cunningham MJ, et al. Percutaneous balloon valvuloplasty for severe mitral stenosis during pregnancy: A review of therapeutic options. Obstet Gynecol Surv 1993;48:503–508.

Gleicher N, Midwall J, Hochberger D, et al. Eisenmenger's syndrome and pregnancy. Obstet Gynecol Surv 1979;34:721–741.

Golby AJ, Bush EC, DeRook FA, et al. Failure of high-dose heparin to prevent recurrent cardioembolic strokes in a pregnancy patient with a mechanical heart valve. Neurology 1992;42:2204–2206.

Goodwin JF. Pregnancy and coarctation of the aorta. Clin Obstet Gynecol 1961;4:645.

Greenberg ML, Uretsky BF, Reddy PS, et al. Long-term hemodynamic follow-up of cardiac transplant patients treated with cyclosporin and prednisone. Circulation 1985;71:487–494.

Gutgesell HP, Massaro TA, Kron IL. The arterial switch operation for transposition of the great arteries in a consortium of university hospitals. Am J Cardiol 1994;74:959–960.

Haas JM. The effect of pregnancy on the midsystolic click and murmur of the prolapsing posterior leaflet of the mitral valve. Am Heart J 1976;92:407–408.

Hall JG, Pauli RM, Wilson KM. Maternal and fetal sequelae of anticoagulation during pregnancy. Am J Med 1980;68:122–140.

Hanania G, Thomas D, Michel PL, et al. Pregnancy and prosthetic heart valves: a French cooperative retrospective study of 155 cases. Eur Heart J 1994;15:1651–1658.

Hankins GDV, Wendel GD, Leveno KJ, et al. Myocardial infarction during pregnancy: a review. Obstet Gynecol 1985;65:139–146.

Hankins GDV, Berryman GK, Scott RT, et al. Maternal arterial desaturation with 15 methyl prostaglandin F2 alpha for uterine atony. Obstet Gynecol 1988;72:367–370.

Hedon B, Montoya F, Cabrol A. Twin pregnancy and vaginal birth after heart transplantation. Lancet 1990;335:476–477.

Hess DB, Hess LW, Heath BJ, et al. Pregnancy after Fontan repair of tricuspid atresia. South Med J 1991;84:532–534.

Hibbard LT. Maternal mortality due to cardiac disease. Clin Obstet Gynecol 1975;18:27–36.

Hibbard JU, Lindheimer M, Lang RM. A modified definition for peripartum cardiomyopathy and prognosis based on echocardiography. Obstet Gynecol 1999;94:311–316.

Hogberg U, Innala E, Sandstrom S. Maternal mortality in Sweden, 1980–1988. Obstet Gynecol 1994;84:240–244.

Homans DC. Peripartum cardiomyopathy. N Engl J Med 1985;312: 1432–1437.

Hsieh TT, Chen KC, Soong JH. Outcome of pregnancy in patients with organic heart disease in Taiwan. Asia Oceania J Obstet Gynecol 1993;19:21–27.

Hunt SA. Pregnancy in heart transplant patients: a good idea? J Heart Lung Transplant 1991;10:499.

Iung B, Cormier B, Elias J, et al. Usefulness of percutaneous balloon commissurotomy for mitral stenosis during pregnancy. Am J Cardiol 1994;73:398–400.

Jackson GM, Dildy GA, Varner MW, et al. Severe pulmonary hypertension in pregnancy following successful repair of ventricular septal defect in childhood. Obstet Gynecol 1993;82(Suppl):680–682.

Jacob S, Bloebaum L, Shah G, Varner MW. Maternal martality in Utah. Obstet Gynecol 1998;91:187–191.

Jaffe R, Gruber A, Fejgin M, et al. Pregnancy with an artificial pacemaker. Obstet Gynecol Surv 1987;42:137–139.

Jatene AD, Fontes VF, Souza LC, et al. Anatomic correction of transposition of the great arteries. J Thorac Cardiovasc Surg 1982;83:20–26.

Jayakrishnan AG, Loftus B, Kelly P, et al. Spontaneous postpartum rupture of a patent ductus arteriosus. Histopathology 1921;21: 383.

Kalra GS, Arora R, Khan JA, et al. Percutaneous mitral commissurotomy for severe mitral stenosis during pregnancy. Cathet Cardiovasc Diagn 1994;33:28–30 discussion 31.

Key TG, Resnik R, Dittrich HC, et al. Successful pregnancy after cardiac transplantation. Am J Obstet Gynecol 1989;160:367–371.

Kim KM, Sukhani R, Slogoff S, Tomich PG. Central hemodynamic changes associated with pregnancy in a long term cardiac transplant recipient. Am J Obstet Gynecol 1996;174:1651–1653.

Kleinman CS, Copel JA, Weinstein EM, et al. In-utero diagnosis and treatment of fetal supraventricular tachycardia. Semin Perinatol 1985;9:113–129.

Knapp RC, Arditi LI. Pregnancy complicated by patent ductus arteriosus with reversal of flow. NY J Med 1967;67:573.

Koh KS, Friesen RM, Livingstone RA, et al. Fetal monitoring during maternal cardiac surgery with cardiopulmonary bypass. Can Med Assoc J 1975;112:1102.

Kolibash AJ, Ruiz DE, Lewis RP. Idiopathic hypertrophic subaortic stenosis in pregnancy. Ann Intern Med 1975;82:791.

Koonin LM, Atrash HK, Lawson HW, et al. Maternal mortality surveillance, United States 1979–1986. MMWR CDC Surveill Summ 1991;40:1–13.

Kossoy LR, Herbert CM, Wentz AC. Management of heart transplant recipients: guidelines for the obstetrician gynecologist. Am J Obstet Gynecol 1988;159:490–499.

Kounis NG, Zavras GM, Papadaki PJ, et al. Pregnancy induced increase of supraventricular arrhythmias in Wolff-Parkinson-White syndrome. Clin Cardiol 1995;18:137–140.

Kultursay H, Turkoglu C, Akin M, et al. Mitral balloon valvuloplasty with transesophageal echocardiography without using fluroscopy. Cathet Cardiovasc Diagn 1992;27:317–321.

Lampert MB, Weinert L, Hibbard J, et al. Contractile reserve in patients with peripartum cardiomyopathy and recovered left ventricular function. Am J Obstet Gynecol 1997;176:189–195.

Lampert MD, Lang RM. Peripartum cardiomyopathy. Am Heart J 1995;180:860–870.

Lao TT, Sermer M, MaGee L, et al. Congenital aortic stenosis and pregnancy—a reappraisal. Am J Obstet Gynecol 1993;169:540–545.

Lao TT, Sermer M, Colman JM. Pregnancy following surgical correction for transposition of the great arteries. Obstet Gynecol 1994;83:665–668.

Lee CN, Wu CC, Lin PY, et al. Pregnancy following cardiac prosthetic valve replacement. Obstet Gynecol 1994;83:353–356.

Loh TF, Tan NC. Fallot's tetralogy and pregnancy: a report of a successful pregnancy after complete correction. Med J Aust 1975;2:141.

Losay J, Hougen TJ. Treatment of transposition of the great arteries. Curr Opin Cardiol 1997;12:84–90.

Loscalzo J. Paradoxical embolization: Clinical presentation, diagnostic strategies and therapeutic options. Am Heart J 1986;112:141.

Lowenstein BR, Vain NW, Perrone SV, et al. Successful pregnancy and vaginal delivery after heart transplantation. Am J Obstet Gynecol 1988;158:589–590.

Mangione JA, Zuliani MF, DelCastillo JM, et al. Percutaneous doulbe balloon mitral valvuloplasty in pregnant women. Am J Cardiol 1989;64:99–102.

Markiewicz W, Stoner J, London E, et al. Mitral valve prolapse in one hundred presumably healthy young females. Circulation 1976;53:464–473.

Mendelson CL. Pregnancy and coarctation of the aorta. Am J Obstet Gynecol 1940;39:1014.

Meyer EC, Tulsky AS, Sigman P, et al. Pregnancy in the presence of tetralogy of Fallot. Am J Cardiol 1964;14:874.

Meyer NL, Mercer B, Khoury A, Sibai B. Pregnancy complicated by cardiac disease: Maternal and perinatal outcome. J Maternal Fetal Med 1994;3:31–36.

Midwall J, Jaffin H, Herman MV, et al. Shunt flow and pulmonary hemodynamics during labor and delivery in the Eisenmenger syndrome. Am J Cardiol 1978;42:299–303.

Neilson G, Galea EG, Blunt A. Congenital heart disease and pregnancy. Med J Aust 1970;30:1086–1088.

Ness RB, Harris T, Cobb J, et al. Number of pregnancies and the subsequent risk of cardiovascular disease. N Engl J Med 1993;328: 1528–1533.

Niswander KR, Berendes H, Dentschberger J, et al. Fetal morbidity following potential anoxigenic obstetric conditions: V. Organic heart disease. Am J Obstet Gynecol 1967;98:871–876.

Nunez L, Larrea JL, Aguado MG, et al. Pregnancy in 20 patients with bioprosthetic valve replacement. Chest 1983;84:26–28.

Oakley CM, Doherty P. Pregnancy in patients after heart valve replacement. Br Heart J 1976;38:1140–1148.

Oakley GDG, McGarry K, Limb DG, et al. Management of pregnancy in patients with hypertropic cardiomyopathy. Br Med J 1979;1: 1749–1750.

van Oppen ACC, Stigter RH, Bruinse HW. Cardiac output in normal pregnancy: A critical review. Obstet Gynecol 1996;87: 310–318.

Otto CM, Easterling TR, Beneditti TJ. Role of echocardiography in the diagnosis and management of heart disease in pregnancy. In: Otto CM, ed. The Practice of Clinical Echocardiography. Philadelphia: WB Saunders, 1997:495–519.

Palacios IF, Block PC, Wilkins GT, et al. Percutaneous mitral balloon valvotomy during pregnancy in a patient with severe mitral stenosis. Cathet Cardiovasc Diagn 1988;15:109–111.

Patel JJ, Mitha AS, Hussen F, et al. Percutaneous mitral valvotomy in pregnant patients with tight pliable mitral stenosis. Am Heart J 1993;125:1106–1109.

Patton DE, Lee W, Cotton DB, et al. Cyanotic maternal heart disease in pregnancy. Obstet Gynecol Surv 1990;45:594–600.

Pearson GD, Veille JC, Rahimtoola S, Hsia J, et al. Peripartum cardiomyopathy—National Heart, Lung and Blood Institute and Office of Rare Diseases (National Institute of Health) workshop recommendations and review. JAMA 2000;283:1183–1188.

Penning S, Robinson D, Major C, Garite. A comparison of echocardiography and pulmonary artery catheterization for evaluation of pulmonary artery pressure in pregnant patients with suspected pulmonary hypertension. Am J Obstet Gynecol 2001;18:1568–1570.

Perloff JK, Child JS, Edwards JE. New guidelines for the clinical diagnosis of mitral valve prolapse. Am J Cardiol 1986;57:1124–1129.

Phelps SJ, Cochran EC, Gonzalez-Ruiz A, et al. The influence of gestational age and preeclampsia on the presence and magnitude of serum endogenous digoxin-like immunoreactive substance(s). Am J Obstet Gynecol 1988;158:34–39.

Pirlo A, Herren AL. Eisenmenger's syndrome and pregnancy. Anesth Rev 1979;6:9.

Presbitero P, Somerville J, Stone S, et al. Pregnancy in cyanotic congenital heart disease. Outcome of mother and fetus. Circulation 1994;89:2673–2676.

Presbitero P, Rabajoli F, Somerville J. Pregnancy in patients with congenital heart disease. Schweiz Med Wochenschr 1995;125:311–315.

Pyeritz RE. Maternal and fetal complications of pregnancy in the Marfan syndrome. Am J Med 1984;71:784–790.

Pyeritz RE, McKusick VA. The Marfan syndrome: diagnosis and management. N Engl J Med 1979;300:772–777.

Rand RJ, Jenkins DM, Scott DG. Maternal cardiomyopathy of pregnancy causing stillbirth. Br J Obstet Gynecol 1975;82:172.

Ribeiro PA, Fawzy ME, Awad M, et al. Balloon valvotomy for pregnant patients with severe pliable mitral stenosis using the Inoue technique with total abdominal and pelvic shielding. Am Heart J 1992;124:1558–1562.

Rosenblum NG, Grossman AR, Gabbe SG, et al. Failure of serial echocardiographic studies to predict aortic dissection in a pregnant patient with Marfan's syndrome. Am J Obstet Gynecol 1983; 146:470–471.

Rossiter JP, Repke JT, Morales AJ, et al. A prospective, longitudinal evaluation of pregnancy in the Marfan syndrome. Am J Obstet Gynecol 1995;173:1599–1606.

Roth A, Elkayam U. Acute myocardial infarction associated with pregnancy. Ann Intern Med 1996;125:751–762.

Rotmensch HH, Rotmensch S, Elkayam U. Management of cardiac arrhythmias during pregnancy: current concepts. Drugs 1987;33:623–633.

Rush RW, Verjans M, Spraklen FH. Incidence of heart disease in pregnancy. A study done at Peninsula Maternity Services hospitals. S Afr Med J 1979;55:808–810.

Saha A, Balakrishnan KG, Jaiswal PK, et al. Prognosis for patients with Eisenmenger syndrome of various aetiology. Int J Cardiol 1994;45:199–207.

Saidi AS, Bezold LI, Altman CA, et al. Outcome of pregnancy following intervention for coarctation of the aorta. Am J Cardol 1998; 82:786–788.

Salazar E, Zajarias A, Gutierrez N, Iturbe I. The problem of cardiac valve prostheses, anticoagulants, and pregnant women. Circulation 1984;70(Suppl I):I-169–I-177.

Sandaniantz A, Saint Laurent L, Parisi AF. Long-term effects of multiple pregnancies on cardiac dimensions and systolic and diastolic function. Am J Obstet Gynecol 1996;174:1061–1064.

Sareli P, England MJ, Berk MR, et al. Maternal and fetal sequelae of anticoagulation during pregnancy in patients with mechanical heart valve prostheses. Am J Cardiol 1989;63:1462–1465.

Sbarouni E, Oakley CM. Outcome of pregnancy in women with valve prostheses. Eur Heart J 1994;15:1651.

Schaefer G, Arditi LI, Solomon HA, et al. Congenital heart disease and pregnancy. Clin Obstet Gynecol 1968;11:1048–1063.

Scheikh AU, Harper MA. Myocardial infarction during pregnancy: management and outcome of two pregnancies. Am J Obstet Gynecol 1993;169:279–283.

Schroeder JS, Harrison DC. Repeated cardioversion during pregnancy. Treatment of refractory paroxysmal atrial tachycardia during three successive pregnancies. Am J Cardiol 1971;27:445–446.

Schumacher B, Belfort MA, Card RJ. Successful treatment of acute myocardial infarction during pregnancy with tissue plasminogen activator. Am J Obstet Gynecol 1997;176:716–719.

Scott JR, Wagoner LE, Olsen SL, et al. Pregnancy in heart transplant recipients: management and outcome. Obstet Gynecol 1993;82:324–327.

Seftel H, Susser M. Maternity and myocardial failure in African women. Br Heart J 1961;23:43.

Shapiro SM, Oudiz RJ, Cao T, et al. Primary pulmonary hypertension: improved long term effects and survival with continuous intravenous epoprostenol infusion. J Am Coll Cardiol 1997;30:343–349.

Shime J, Mocarski EJM, Hastings D, et al. Congenital heart disease in pregnancy: short- and long-term implications. Am J Obstet Gynecol 1987;156:313–322.

Simon A, Sadovsky E, Aboulatia Y, et al. Fetal activity in pregnancies complicated by rheumatic heart disease. J Perinat Med 1986;14:331.

Sinnenberg RJ. Pulmonary hypertension in pregnancy. South Med J 1980;73:1529–1531.

Sitbon O, Brenot F, Denjean A, et al. Inhaled nitric oxide as a screening vasodilator agent in primary pulmonary hypertension: A dose-response study and comparison with prostacyclin. Am J Respir Crit Care Med 1995;151:384–389.

Siu SC, Sermer M, Harrison DA, et al. Risk and predictors for pregnancy-related complications in women with heart disease. Circulation 1997;96:2789–2794.

Slater EE, DeSanctis RW. Dissection of the aorta. Med Clin North Am 1979;63:141–154.

Smedstad K, Cramb R, Morison DH. Pulmonary hypertension and pregnancy: A series of eight cases. Can J Anaesth 1994;41:502–512.

Smith R, Brender D, McCredie M. Percutaneous transluminal balloon dilation of the mitral valve in pregnancy. Br Heart J 1989;61:551–553.

Snabes MC, Poindexter AN. Laparoscopic tubal sterilization under local anethesia in women with cyanotic heart disease. Obstet Gynecol 1991;78:437.

Sobrevilla LA, Cassinelli MT, Carcelen A, et al. Human fetal and maternal oxygen tension and acid–base status during delivery at high altitude. Am J Obstet Gynecol 1971;111:1111–1118.

Spinnato JA, Kraynack BJ, Cooper MW. Eisenmenger's syndrome in pregnancy: epidural anesthesia for elective cesarean section. N Engl J Med 1981;304:1215–1217.

Spirito P, Seidman CE, McKenna WJ, Maron BJ. The management of hypertrophic cardiomyopathy. N Engl J Med 1997;336:775–785.

Starr A, Grunkemeier GL. Selection of a prosthetic valve. JAMA 1984;251:1739–1742.

Szekely P, Julian DG. Heart disease and pregnancy. Curr Probl Cardiol 1979;4:1–74.

Szekely P, Turner R, Snaith L. Pregnancy and the changing pattern of rheumatic heart disease. Br Heart J 1973;35:1293–1303.

Taylor SH, Donald KW. Circulatory studies at rest and during exercise in coarctation, before and after correction. Br Heart J 1960;22:117.

Teerlink JR, Foster E. Valvular heart disease in pregnancy: A contemporary perspective. Cardiol Clin 1998;16:573–598.

Ueland K, Hansen J, Eng M, et al. Maternal cardiovascular dynamics. V. Cesarean section under thiopental, nitrous oxide and succinylcholine anesthesia. Am J Obstet Gynecol 1970;108:615–622.

Ueland K, Akamatsu TJ, Eng M, et al. Maternal cardiovascular dynamics: VI: Cesarean section under epidural anesthesia without epinephrine. Am J Obstet Gynecol 1972;114:775–780.

Ullery JC. Management of pregnancy complicated by heart disease. Am J Obstet Gynecol 1954;67:834.

Veille JC. Peripartum cardiomyopathies: a review. Am J Obstet Gynecol 1984;148:805–818.

Veille JC, Kitzman DW, Bacevice AE. Effects of pregnancy on the electrocardiogram in healthy subjects during strenuous exercise. Am J Obstet Gynecol 1996;175:1360–1364.

Ventura SJ, Peters KD, Martin JA, Maurer JD. Births and deaths: united states, 1996. Mon Vital Stat Rep 1997;46(1 Suppl 2):1–40.

Veran FX, Cibes-Hernandez JJ, Pelegrina I. Heart disease in pregnancy. Obstet Gynecol 1968;34:424.

Vitali E, Donatelli R, Quanini E, et al. Pregnancy in patients with mechanical prosthetic heart valves. J Cardiovasc Surg 1986;27: 221–227.

Vongpatanasin W, Hillis LD, Lange RA. Prosthetic heart valves. N Engl J Med 1996;335:407–416.

Waickman LA, Skorton DJ, Varner MW, et al. Ebstein's anomaly and pregnancy. Am J Cardiol 1984;53:357–358.

Weiss BM, Atanassoff PG. Cyanotic congenital heart disease and pregnancy: natural selection, pulmonary hypertension and anesthesia. J Clin Anesth 1993;5:332.

Weiss BM, Zemp L, Seifert B, Hess O. Outcome of pulmonary vascular disease in pregnancy: A systemic overview from 1978 through 1996. J Am Coll Cardiol 1998;31:1650–1657.

Whittemore R, Hobbins JC, Engle MA. Pregnancy and its outcome in women with and without surgical treatment of congenital heart disease. Am J Cardiol 1982;50:641–651.

Witlin AG, Mabie WC, Sibai BM. Peripartum cardiomyopathy: An ominous diagnosis. Am J Obstet Gynecol 1997;176:182–188.

20 Thromboembolic disease

Donna Dizon-Townson
Shailen S. Shah
Jeffrey P. Phelan

Pulmonary embolism (PE), albeit a rare event, remains the leading cause of maternal mortality in the United States (Berg et al., 1996). The maternal mortality rate from pulmonary embolism has shown little change over time (Bonnar, 1999). Furthermore, deep venous thrombosis (DVT) can cause significant morbidity. Pregnancy-related venous thromboembolism (VTE) has been reported to occur in approximately 0.5–3.0 per 1,000 pregnancies based on studies using radiographic documentation (Toglia & Weg, 1996; Gherman et al., 1999; Lindqvist et al., 1999). Clinical symptomatology can be confirmed with objective testing in most cases because almost 75% of patients who present with suspected thromboembolic disease and are then subjected to testing such as Doppler ultrasound or venography do not have the condition (Ginsberg, 1996). When DVT is diagnosed and heparin treatment instituted, the incidence of PE and maternal mortality can be decreased by 3- and 18-fold, respectively. The goal of this review is to facilitate the recognition of the clinical signs and symptoms of VTE disorders, describe a rational approach to a the work-up of suspected hypercoagulable state, and review the use of various diagnostic and treatment modalities.

Incidence and risk factors

Although many studies about maternal mortality cite PE as the leading cause, they do not distinguish VTE from amniotic fluid or air embolism (Rochat et al., 1988; Franks et al., 1990; Lawson et al., 1990). At least half of these deaths are due to thrombotic embolism (Barbour & Pickard, 1955; McLean et al., 1979; Kaunitz et al., 1985; Gabel, 1987; Sachs et al., 1988; Franks, 1990). The overall maternal mortality rate in the United States between 1980 and 1985 was 14.1 of 100,000 live births. Of these, 14.3% were due to embolism (Rochat et al., 1988). As illustrated in Fig. 20.1, from 1970 to 1985, maternal mortality rates from PE declined by 50% (Franks, 1990).

The traditionally held view is that the maternal risk for VTE is greater in the immediate puerperium, especially following cesarean delivery. Postpartum DVT has been reported to occur 3–5 times more often than antepartum DVT, and 3–16 times more frequently after cesarean as opposed to vaginal delivery (Bergqvist et al., 1983; Letsky, 1985). In contrast, Rutherford and associates (1991) found that the highest incidence of pregnancy-related VTE was not in the puerperium but in the first trimester of pregnancy (Fig. 20.2). These authors also found that the risk of DVT did not increase with advancing gestational age but stayed relatively constant (Fig. 20.2). In contrast, PE (Fig. 20.2) was almost twice as likely to occur in the postpartum patient (Rutherford et al., 1991) and appeared to be related to the route of delivery (Fig. 20.3). More recently, Gerhardt and colleagues reported on 119 women with a pregnancy-related VTE (Gerhardt et al., 2000). Approximately half (62 women) experienced a DVT during pregnancy: 14 (23%) in the first trimester, 13 in the second trimester, and 35 (56%) in the third trimester. The other half (57 woman) experienced a DVT in the immediate puerperium: 38 (68%) following vaginal delivery and 19 (32%) following cesarean section. In summary, pregnancy-related VTE may occur at any time during pregnancy or the immediate puerperium. Therefore, regardless of gestational age, the clinician should have a heightened awareness for the diagnosis when a gravid or postpartum woman presents with clinical symptomatology suspicious for VTE.

The most important risk factors during pregnancy are immobility and bed rest. "Bed rest" is often recommended for a variety of obstetric disease such as threatened preterm labor or preeclampsia. The clinician should keep in mind the increased risk for VTE when making recommendations for limited maternal physical activity or long distance travel. Traveling long distances by air may also increase a pregnant woman's risk of a pulmonary embolus. Additional risk factors in the gravid woman include surgery, trauma, or a prior history of superficial vein thrombosis (Danilenko-Dixon et al., 2001).

Ethnic background and maternal age are important risk factors for PE. The overall mortality rate for Black woman was 3.2 times higher than for White women. In addition, women 40 years or older were at a 10 times greater risk of mortality than

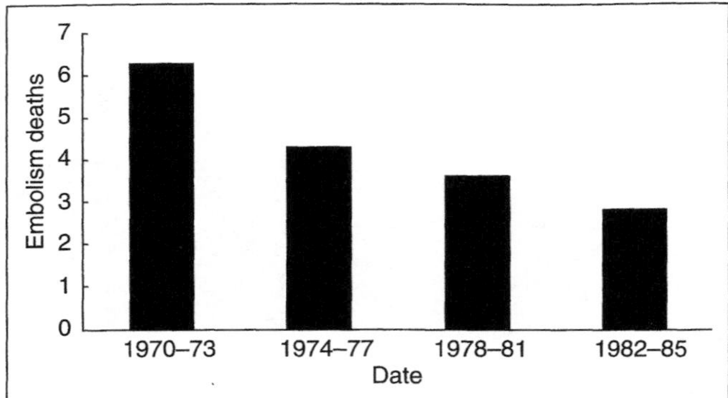

Fig. 20.1 Maternal deaths due to pulmonary embolism per 100,000 births from 1970 to 1985. (Reproduced by permission from Franks AL, Atrash HK, Lawson HW et al. Obstetrical pulmonary embolism mortality, United States, 1970–985. Am J Public Health 1990;80:720–722.)

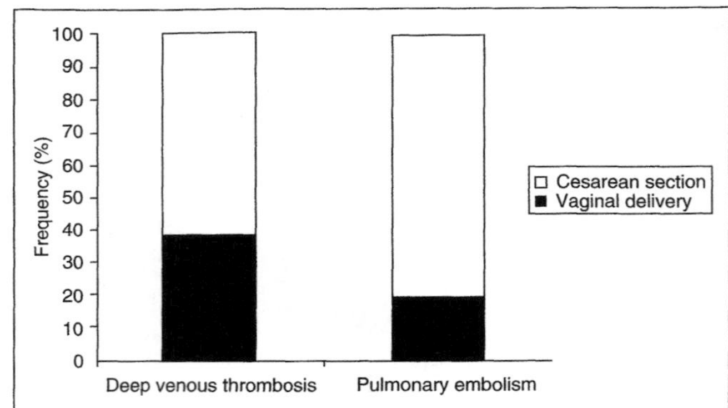

Fig. 20.3 The frequency of postpartum deep venous thrombosis and pulmonary embolism according to route of delivery. (Reproduced by permission from Rutherford SE, Montoro M, McGehee W et al. Thromboembolic disease associated with pregnancy: an 11-year review. Am J Obstet Gynecol 1991;164:286.)

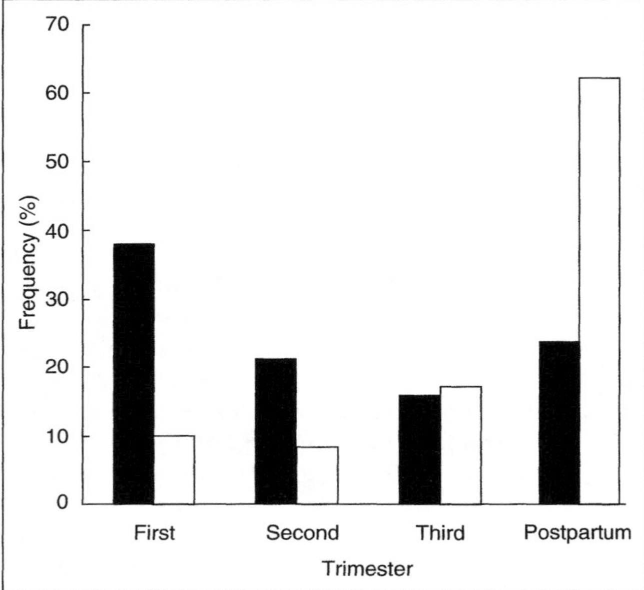

Fig. 20.2 Distribution of deep venous thrombosis and pulmonary embolism during each trimester of pregnancy and the postpartum period. (Reproduced by permission from Rutherford SE, Montoro M, McGehee W et al. Thromboembolic disease associated with pregnancy: an 11-year review. Am J Obstet Gynecol 1991;164:286.)

women under 25 for both ethnic groups (Franks et al., 1990) (Fig. 20.4).

A prior history of a VTE confers a greater risk for recurrence especially if the initial event was idiopathic or associated with a hereditary or acquired thrombophilia (Brill-Edwards et al., 2000). In a prospective cohort study investigating the risk of recurrence of pregnancy-related VTE in 125 women who had a history of VTE, heparin was withheld antepartum but administered 6 weeks postpartum in all women. Two out of eight patients (20%; 95% CI 2.5–55.6%) whose initial event was idiopathic (no temporary risk factor) and who had an identified thrombophilia had a recurrence of a pregnancy-related VTE. It is assumed that the risk of recurrence diminishes as the time from initial event increases. The mean time from initial event to enrollment in the study was 4 years. Both acquired and inherited thrombophilias are now beginning to be studied in a systematic fashion. The inherited thrombophilias that used to be the most commonly investigated were deficiencies of protein C, protein S, and antithrombin III. More recently, studies relating to the prevalence of the factor V Leiden, prothrombin G20210A, and the 5,10-methylenetetrahydrofolate reductase mutations have been reported (Brill-Edwards et al., 2000). The most commonly investigated acquired thrombophilia is the antiphospholipid syndrome.

In summary, the risk of VTE varies between pregnant women, therefore individualization of management must be emphasized. This risk will depend not only on the gestational age of the pregnancy, but also on additional clinical factors such as a prior history of thromboembolism, mode of delivery, prolonged immobilization, age, and ethnicity. In the presence of a personal or familial history of VTE, testing for thrombophilia should be accomplished to better define the specific risk (Table 20.1). A comprehensive thrombophilia work-up should include testing for functional deficiencies of protein C, protein S, and antithrombin III. These tests should be performed preferably when the patient is not pregnant and prior to anticoagulation. In addition, molecular tests for factor V Leiden and the prothrombin G20210A mutation which are unaffected by pregnancy or anticoagulation should also be performed. To complete the evaluation, testing for antiphospholipids such as anticardiolipin antibodies and lupus anticoagulant should be included. A positive test for antiphospholipid syndrome appears to carry the greatest impact on maternal and fetal outcome in subsequent pregnancies.

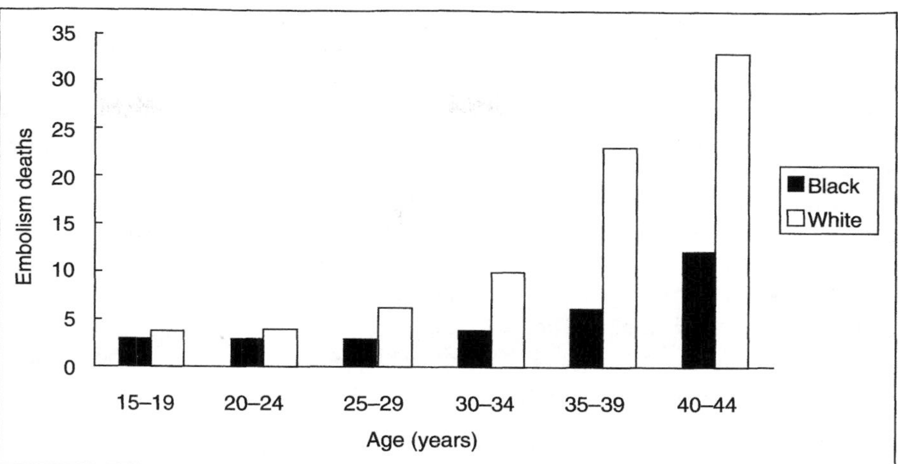

Fig. 20.4 Maternal death per 100,000 births by maternal age and race. (From Franks AL, Atrash HK, Lawson HW et al. Obstetrical pulmonary embolism mortality, United States, 1970–985. Am J Public Health 1990;80:720–722; and reproduced by permission from Rutherford SE, Phelan JP. Clinical management of thromboembolic disorders in pregnancy. Crit Care Clin 1991;7:809–828.)

Table 20.1 Factors associated with a higher risk of pulmonary embolism

Maternal age
Ethnic background
Operative delivery
Prior thromboembolism
Prolonged immobilization
Inherited coagulation disorders
Trauma

Normal hemostasis

The hemostatic system is a delicate balance between procoagulation and anticoagulation. Individuals with abnormalities promoting coagulation are considered to have thrombophilia. In comparison, individuals with abnormalities favoring bleeding have hemophilia. Few systems are more complex than hemostasis. Interactions among the vessel wall, platelets, and soluble molecules in the vicinity of an injury work to repair the vessel defect without sacrificing nearby vessel patency. The key processes are: (i) vasoconstriction; (ii) formation of a platelet plug; (iii) formation of a stable "seal" by coagulation factors; (iv) prevention of spread of the clot along the vessel wall; (v) prevention of occlusion of the vessel by clots when possible; and (vi) remodeling and gradual degradation of the clot after it is no longer needed.

The maintenance of normal blood flow requires intact, patent blood vessels. After an injury, the hemostatic and fibrinolytic systems work together to protect vascular integrity and assist in repair. Vessel wall integrity, platelet aggregation, normal function of the coagulation cascade, and fibrinolysis are all vital to this process. The initial response to injury is vasoconstriction, which reduces local blood flow and limits the size of the thrombus needed to seal a defect (Stead, 1985). After platelets begin to adhere to the exposed vessel wall, they change shape and secrete the contents of their granules. This action leads to further platelet accumulation or aggregation, and results in the formation of a platelet plug.

The numerous substances released by platelets include thromboxane A_2 (TxA_2), a potent vasoconstrictor and pre-aggregatory agent (Needleman et al., 1976; Thompson & Harker, 1983); serotonin, a vasoconstrictor (Thompson & Harker, 1983); and adenosine diphosphate (ADP), which enhances platelet aggregation. Platelets also produce vascular permeability factor and platelet growth factor, which stimulate fibroblasts and vascular smooth muscles (Letsky, 1985; Stead, 1985). Released platelet factor 4 (PF_4) and beta-thromboglobulin are used as markers of platelet activity (Files et al., 1981; Kaplan & Owen, 1981). The platelet contractile protein, thrombasthenin, enables secretion of these substances and also enhances clot retraction (Letsky, 1985). A platelet surface phospholipoprotein, platelet factor 3 (PF_3), becomes available to bind factor V to catalyze the formation of thrombin. Thrombin, in turn, potentiates platelet aggregation (Kaplan & Owen, 1981).

Whereas TxA_2 is the result of platelet arachidonic acid metabolism, arachidonic acid in endothelial cells is metabolized to prostacyclin (PGI_2). Prostacyclin inhibits aggregation and stimulates vasodilation, and thus counteracts TxA_2 by increasing cyclic adenosine monophosphate (AMP) (Stead, 1985). Because PGI_2 is concentrated within the vessel wall, the greater the distance from the lumen, the lower the concentration of PGI_2 and the higher the concentration of proaggregatory substances. As platelets begin to seal a vascular defect, the coagulation cascade produces fibrin, which is polymerized as clot and incorporated into the platelet plug.

Proteolytic cleavage or conformational changes activate the circulating clotting factors at the site of injury. Factors II, VII, IX, and X require a vitamin K-dependent reaction in the liver in which gamma-carboxyglutamic acid residues are attached to the protein structure. This action provides a location to form a complex with calcium ion and phospholipid receptors on the platelet or endothelial cell membranes. Subsequent steps in the clotting cascade occur at those sites and include the formation of thrombin. Once formed, this is released into the fluid phase.

The intrinsic and extrinsic pathways lead to the final common clotting pathway. Both pathways are activated by components of the vessel wall and lead to activation of progressive exponential increase in subsequent factors. In the intrinsic pathway, high-molecular-weight kininogen and kallikrein are cofactors for the initial step of the process, the activation of factor XII (XIIa). By catalyzing the formation of kallikrein from prekallikreins, factor XIIa also helps to initiate fibrinolysis, activate the complement system, and produce kinins (Stead, 1985). Factor XI is activated by XIIa and then cleaves factor IX to form IXa. The extrinsic pathway is so named because this pathway relies on tissue thromboplastin as a cofactor. Tissue thromboplastin is released into the circulation following membrane damage or proteolysis (Stead, 1985). Factor VII is then activated to VIIa which, with tissue thromboplastin, can activate factors IX or X. The common pathway begins with activation of factor X by either VIIa or IXa, in combination with the protein cofactor VIII:C (the antihemophilic factor) and the calcium ion, on the platelet surface (to form PF_3). Factor Xa, assisted by cofactor Va, enzymatically divides prothrombin into thrombin and a peptide activation fragment, F_{1+2}. Separation from this fragment liberates thrombin into the fluid phase. Thrombin catalyzes the formation of fibrin monomers from fibrinogen and, thus, releases fibrinopeptides A and B and facilitates activation of V, VIII:C, and XIII. A fibrin gel is created by the hydrophobic and electrostatic interactions of the fibrin alpha and gamma chains. Subsequently, factor XIIIa forms covalent bonds linking nearby alpha and gamma chains to form a stable polymerized fibrin clot into which water is also incorporated.

Trapped within the clot are proteins that contribute to the enzymatic digestion of the fibrin matrix: plasminogen and plasminogen activators. A variety of substances can activate plasminogen. Plasma plasminogen activator is activated by factor XIIa. Release of tissue activators (tissue plasminogen activator) from blood vessel epithelium (especially venous) is stimulated by exercise, emotional stress, trauma, surgery, hypotensive shock, pharmacologic agents, and activated protein C (Comp & Esman, 1981; Letsky, 1985; Stead, 1985). The fibrinolytic enzymes streptokinase and urokinase also activate plasminogen (Robbins, 1982). Having been activated from plasminogen, plasmin cleaves arginyl-lysine bonds in many substrates, including fibrogen, fibrin, factor VIII, and complement (Bonnar et al., 1970; Robbins, 1982). The result of plasmin action on fibrin and fibrinogen is release of protein fragments, referred to as fibrinogen degradation products (or fibrin split products). The larger fragments, which may have slow clotting activity, are further divided by plasmin. These fragments have anticoagulant activity, in that they inhibit the formation and cross-linking of fibrin (Stead, 1985). Measurement of fibrin degradation products provides an indirect measurement of fibrinolysis. Alpha-2 antiplasmin, a specific plasmin inhibitor that binds to fibrin and fibrinogen, is found in serum, platelets, and within the clot, along with other inhibitors of plasmin or plasminogen activity (Robbins, 1982).

As a potent inhibitor of thrombin, antithrombin III (AT III) is important in the regulation of hemostasis. In decreasing affinity, AT III binds and inactivates factors IXa, Xa, XIa, and XIIa. AT III acts as a substrate for these serine proteases but forms stable intermediate bonds with the active portion and, thus, neutralizes the respective enzyme (Brandt, 1985). Heparin binds to AT III and induces a conformational change that increases the affinity of AT III for thrombin. The otherwise slow inactivation of thrombin by AT III is accelerated greatly by even small amounts of heparin. After a stable thrombin–AT III complex is formed, heparin is released and available for repetitive catalysis. Excess amounts of AT III are normally present in the circulation, and some are bound to endothelial cell membranes via heparan, a sulfated mucopolysaccharide with a function similar to heparin. The presence of heparan on intact endothelial cell surfaces and its binding to AT III, which neutralizes thrombin, help to prevent local extension of the thrombus beyond the sites of vessel injury (Comp & Clouse, 1985). Deficiency of AT III leads to a substantially higher incidence of thrombotic events (Megha et al., 1990).

Protein C and S are normally part of the protein C anticoagulant system. Like certain clotting factors, their synthesis depends on vitamin K and involves addition of gamma-carboxyglutamic acid residues that enable binding, via calcium ions, to cell surfaces. Protein C is attached to endothelial cells, and protein S is attached to endothelial and platelet membranes. Endothelial cell surfaces also have a specific protein receptor for thrombin, thrombomodulin. The binding of thrombin to thrombomodulin, in the presence of protein S, activates protein C (APC) and promotes anticoagulation. Complexes of APC and adjacently bound protein S cofactor proteolyze the phospholipid-bound factors VIII:Ca and Va. This action results in a second mechanism to prevent extension of the thrombus beyond the area of vessel injury (Comp & Clouse, 1985). Deficiencies of either protein C or S are associated with an increase in thromboembolic events (Broekmans et al., 1985; Comp & Clouse, 1985). Homozygosity of protein C deficiency leads to fatal neonatal purpura fulminans (Marciniak et al., 1985).

Changes in hemostasis in pregnancy

Almost a century ago, Virchow described the triad of blood hypercoagulability, venous stasis, and vascular damage conferring an increased risk for thrombosis. All of these conditions occur during pregnancy thus conferring an increased risk for pregnancy-related VTE (Table 20.2). Estrogen stimulation of hepatic synthesis of several procoagulant proteins increases

Table 20.2 Hemostatic changes during pregnancy

Hemostatic changes promoting thrombosis
Increased factor levels V, VII, VIII, IX, X, XII, fibrinogen
Placental inhibitors of fibrinolysis
Tissue thromboplastin released into the circulation at placental separation
Venous stasis of the lower extremities
Endothelial damage associated with parturition
Hemostatic changes countering thrombosis
Decreased factor levels XI, XIII
Pregnancy-specific protein neutralizing AT III

with pregnancy. Levels of factors V, VII, VIII, IX, X, XII, and fibrinogen increase. Venous stasis secondary to progesterone-mediated smooth muscle vascular relaxation and mechanical compression by the gravid uterus occurs. Placental separation and operative delivery can cause endothelial vascular damage.

Compensatory mechanisms such as concomitant rise in fibrinolytic activity help to maintain coagulation equilibrium (Woodhams et al., 1980). As pregnancy progresses, a low-grade chronic intravascular coagulation results in fibrin deposition in the internal elastic lamina and smooth muscle cells of the spiral arteries of the placental bed (Hathaway & Bonnar, 1978). Increased fibrin split products and D-dimers during this period suggest ongoing increased fibrinolytic activity (Hathaway & Bonnar, 1978). Within an hour of delivery, this fibrinolytic potential decreases and returns to normal. These changes are believed to contribute to the hypercoagulability of the puerperium (Rutherford et al., 1991). Levels of factors XI and XIII decrease. Plasma fibrinolytic activity decreases as a result of placental inhibitors but can return to normal within 1 hour after delivery (Bonnar et al., 1969). When the placenta separates, tissue thromboplastin is released into the circulation increasing the chance for thrombosis (Bonnar, 1981). Additional factors balancing the increased tendency toward coagulation may be a pregnancy-specific protein (PAPP-A) which, like heparin, facilitates neutralization of thrombin by AT III (Brandt, 1985). Platelet counts appear to remain in the normal range during pregnancy, but have been documented to be significantly higher than predelivery on days 8 and 12 after vaginal delivery, and continued to rise 16 days after a cesarean delivery (Atalla et al., 2000). The platelet count remained significantly higher than predelivery values for 24 days after cesarean delivery (Atalla et al., 2000).

Hereditary thrombophilias

Approximately half of the women who have a pregnancy-related VTE possess an underlying congenital or acquired thrombophilia (Grandone et al., 1998). In almost 50% of patients with a hereditary thrombophilia, the initial thrombotic event occurs in the presence of an additional risk factor such as pregnancy, oral contraceptive use, orthopedic trauma, immobilization, or surgery (De Stefano et al., 1994; Middeldorp et al., 1998).

Antithrombin III deficiency, although the most rare of the congenital thrombophilias, is the most thrombogenic conferring a 50% lifetime and pregnancy-related risk for thrombosis (Eldor, 2001). AT III deficiency occurs in approximately 0.02–0.17% of the general population and 1.1% of individuals with a history of VTE. Deficiencies of protein C and protein S, although less thrombogenic than AT III deficiency, are more common (Eldor, 2001). Carrier rates for deficiencies of protein C and S are 0.14–0.5% in the general population. In individuals who have had a history of VTE, 3.2% will have either protein C or protein S deficiency.

As a result of the Human Genome Project and major advances in gene identification, common genetic predispositions to thrombophilia, including factor V Leiden, and the prothrombin G20210A mutation, have been described. Resistance to activated protein C (APC) is now known to be the most common genetic predisposition to thrombosis (Bertina et al., 1994; Dahlback, 1994; Zoller & Dahlback, 1994). Eighty to 100% of cases of resistance to APC are due to the factor V Leiden mutation. This mutation is a missense mutation (single base nucleotide substitution) in the gene encoding factor V protein. Individuals carrying the factor V Leiden mutation have an abnormal factor V protein which fails to undergo the normal conformation change required for the proteolytic degradation by APC. Individuals with factor V Leiden have normal levels of factor V protein, but this protein is resistant to the normal degradation by APC. Heterozygous carriers have a sevenfold increase in the risk for venous thrombosis, whereas homozygous carriers have an 80-fold increased risk. Carrier rates for factor V Leiden are 6–8% in northern Europeans and 4–6% in US Caucasians (Dizon-Townson et al., 1997; Ridker, et al. 1997). Another mutation in the 3′ untranslated region of the prothrombin gene, prothrombin G20210A, leads to elevated prothrombin levels (>155%) and a 2.1-fold increase in the risk for thrombosis. The prevalence of the mutation in the Caucasian population is 2%. The prevalence of the mutation is 6% among unselected patients with thrombosis and about 18% in families with unexplained thrombophilia.

Deep venous thrombosis

Clinical diagnosis

In the gravid patient, DVT appears to occur more often in the deep proximal veins and has a predilection for the left leg (Dahlman et al., 1989; Barbour & Pickard, 1995). The clinical diagnosis of DVT (Barnes et al., 1975) is difficult and requires objective testing. Of those patients with clinically suspected

Table 20.3 Clinical symptoms and signs of lower extremity deep venous thrombosis

Unilateral pain, swelling, tenderness, and/or edema
Limb color changes
Palpable cord
Positive Homan's sign
Positive Löwenberg test
Limb-size difference > 2 cm

DVT, half will not be confirmed by objective testing. Due to the long-term implications of anticoagulant therapy and the expense of a hypercoagulable workup, clinical symptomatology of VTE should usually be confirmed with objective testing before a diagnosis is rendered.

Symptoms and signs of DVT are illustrated in Table 20.3. Swelling is considered whenever there is at least a 2-cm measured difference in circumference between the affected and normal limbs. Homan's sign is present when passive dorsiflexion of the foot in a relaxed leg leads to pain, presumably in the calf or popliteal areas. The Lowenberg test is positive if pain occurs distal to a BP cuff rapidly inflated to 180 mmHg. The presence of marked swelling, cyanosis or paleness, a cold extremity, or diminished pulses signals the rare obstructive iliofemoral vein thrombosis. DVT has also significant long-term implications, and a prior history of DVT may affect the patient's symptomatology. Years after a severe obstructive DVT, patients may experience postphlebitic syndrome (skin stasis dermatatitis or ulcers). An investigation of 104 women with a median postthrombosis interval of 11 years revealed that 4% had ulceration, and only 22% were without complaints (Bergqvist et al., 1990). Finally, it is important to remember that pregnant patients commonly complain of swelling and leg discomfort and, as such, do not require objective testing in every instance. It is important to remember that the first sign of DVT may be the occurrence of a PE. In a similar manner, silent DVT has been found in 70% of patients with angiographically proven PE (Hull, 1983).

During the initial evaluation in a pregnant patient with clinical symptomatology suspicious for a pregnancy-related VTE, risk factors as described above should be sought. Again "bed rest" or limited physical activity, which is frequently recommended for a variety of obstetric diseases, is a common risk factor for VTE events. As always, clinical signs and symptoms of DVT should be corroborated with objective testing.

Diagnostic studies

Ultrasound

Noninvasive testing is usually the first step in confirming the diagnosis of DVT. Real-time imaging with compression ultrasound (CUS), including duplex Doppler, is the method of choice. CUS uses firm compression with the ultrasound transducer probe to detect an intraluminal defect. Experience is required for accurate interpretation, and the affected leg should be compared with the unaffected one. Maneuvers such as Valsalva (which distends the vein the slows the proximal flow), release of pressure over a distal vein (which causes a rapid proximal flow of blood), and squeezing of the muscles all cause changes in Doppler shift. Real-time imaging in the presence of DVT may detect a mass in the vessel lumen, a failure of the lumen diameter to increase with Valsalva, or a failure of the vein to compress with pressure (Raghavendra et al., 1984). Alternatively, imaging may identify a hematoma, popliteal cyst, or other pathology to explain the patient's symptoms. In a symptomatic nonpregnant individual, CUS has a sensitivity of 95% for proximal DVT (73% for distal DVT) and specificity of 96% for detecting all DVT, with a negative predictive value of 98% and a positive predictive value for 97% (Douketis & Ginsberg, 1995). At least 50% of small calf thrombi are missed due to collateral venous channels (PIOPED Investigators, 1990; Gottlieb et al., 1999). Repeating the examination within 2–3 days may reveal a previously latent clot.

During pregnancy, the iliac vessels are especially difficult to image. This is due to pressure from the gravid uterus on the inferior vena cava. As a result, Doppler findings must be interpreted cautiously. In the puerperal patient, imaging may visualize a clot in the iliac vessels as well as in pelvic thrombophlebitis or ovarian vein thrombosis. The use of computed tomography (CT) or magnetic resonance imaging (MRI), however, may be more helpful in these latter conditions. MRI is now being used more frequently for the diagnosis of DVT in the pregnant patient and may eventually become the imaging modality of choice (Spritzer et al., 1995).

Ascending venography

Venography is the gold standard for the diagnosis of DVT in pregnancy. With the patient at an approximate 40° incline and bearing weight on her unaffected leg, radiographic contrast dye is injected into a dorsal vein of the involved foot. This position allows for the gradual and complete filling of the leg veins without layering of the dye and reduces the likelihood of a false-positive test. Nonetheless, false-positive tests may result from poor technique, poor choice of injection site, contraction of the leg muscles, or extravascular pathology such as a Baker's (popliteal) cyst, hematoma, cellulites, edema, or muscle rupture. In addition, the larger diameter of the deep femoral and iliac veins can lead to incomplete filling with the dye and unreliable results. Positive identification of a thrombus requires visualization of a well-defined filling defect in more than one radiography view (Fig. 20.5). Suggestive signs of a DVT include abrupt termination of a vessel, absence of opacification, or diversion of blood flow.

Unlike ultrasonography and Doppler procedures, venography is associated with significant side effects. Twenty-four percent of patients will experience minor side effects of muscle

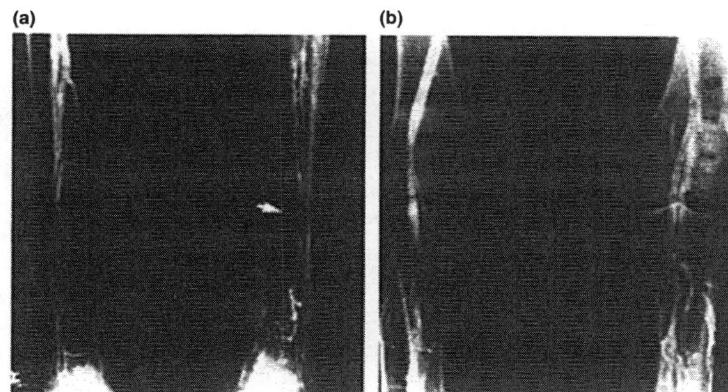

Fig. 20.5 A contrast venogram shows each of two legs: (a) a cut-off sign in the posterior tibial vein and filling defects in the popliteal vein in one leg; (b) a normal study in the other leg.

pain, leg swelling, tenderness, or erythema (Bettman & Paulin, 1977). These side effects can be reduced by 70% by lowering the concentration of contrast medium (PIOPED investigators, 1990). Using a heparinized saline flush after dye injection and the concomitant use of corticosteroids can minimize the risks of phlebitis and clot formation. Radiation exposure to the fetus has been estimated at less than 1.0 rad for unilateral venography including fluoroscopy and spot films without an abdominal shield (Ginsberg et al., 1980a). This is well below the minimum level of radiation exposure considered teratogenic (ACOG, 1997).

Impedance plethysmography

Though infrequently used during pregnancy, other methods for diagnosis of DVT include impedance plethysmography (IPG), thermography, iodine 125 fibrinogen scanning, and radionuclide venography. To assess blood flow in the lower extremities, IPG uses changes in electrical resistance in response to changes in fluid volume. It is highly sensitive to proximal thrombosis but frequently fails to detect those below the knee. With inflation of a thigh cuff, blood is retained in the leg. In the absence of venous obstruction, sudden deflation results in immediate outflow of blood and a concomitant sudden increase in electrical resistance. A much slower change is associated with impaired outflow, which indirectly implies venous thrombosis (Markisz, 1985). In the symptomatic nonpregnant patient, IPG has a sensitivity of 83% and specificity of 92% for detecting proximal DVT. Because DVT confined to the calf rarely results in PE, anticoagulation for such DVT is not mandatory. In patients with suspected calf vein thrombosis, IPG may allow the clinician to avoid anticoagulation or venography by excluding extension of the clot above the knee over a 2-week period while the presumed calf thrombosis is treated with heat and elevation (Moser & LeMoine, 1981; Huisman et al., 1986; Kohn et al., 1987; Monreal et al., 1987; Mohr et al., 1988). In pregnancy, compression of the inferior vena cava by the gravid uterus can yield falsely positive results (Nicholas et al., 1985), and confirmation of DVT with venography may be necessary.

Thermography

Thermography detects DVT by an increase in skin temperature. Infrared radiation emission is increased when blood flow is diverted to superficial collaterals or when inflammation is present. Changes are more likely to occur with extensive disease. False-negative results can occur with early or limited thrombosis.

Iodine 125 fibrinogen scanning

This technique is contraindicated during pregnancy because unbound radioactive iodine 125 (^{125}I) crosses the placental barrier (Kakkar, 1972; Bentley & Kakkar, 1979). Unbound ^{125}I also enters breast milk. In both instances, ^{125}I can be concentrated in the fetal or neonatal thyroid and produce goiter. Because ^{125}I has a half-life of 60.2 days (PIOPED Investigators, 1990), temporary interruption of lactation is impractical. Thus, the preferred approach, if this radiographic technique is medically necessary, is to avoid breastfeeding. To avoid the small risk of hypothyroidism, nonradioactive iodine should be administered orally for 24 hours prior to and for 2 weeks after the procedure.

In nonlactating postpartum patients, ^{125}I-labeled fibrinogen can be used to identify DVT. Iodine 125 has a longer half-life and gives a smaller radiation dose than the previously used ^{131}I. After intravenous (IV) injection, ^{125}I fibrinogen is incorporated like normal fibrinogen into developing thrombi. Sequential scintillation scanning is performed at any time between 4 and 72 hours. With each scan, radioactivity is compared with background precordial values in the search for a hot spot. For the lower thigh and calf, accuracy can be as high as 92% (Kakkar, 1972). Higher background counts in the femoral artery, bladder, and overlying muscle mass make detection of thrombi in the common femoral and pelvic veins difficult. False-positives can be due to hematoma, inflammation, or surgical wound uptake. Alternatively, if an old thrombus is no longer taking up fibrinogen or forms after the ^{125}I has been cleared from the circulation, a false-negative study may result.

Radionuclide venography

Radionuclide venography using technetium 99m (^{99m}Tc) particles is of low risk to the fetus and can be used to obtain leg studies as well as perfusion lung scans. When performed with rapid sequence gamma camera, which may not be available in many institutions, this technique is more than 90% accurate for DVT above the knee (Kakkar, 1972; Bentley & Kakkar, 1979). Sequential, staged imaging using BP cuffs on the legs to delay flow is an alternative. Correlations with conventional venography of 95% in the thigh and 100% in the pelvis have been reported (Bentley & Kakkar, 1979).

Pulmonary embolus

Clinical diagnosis

The sudden onset of unexplained dyspnea and tachypnea are the most common clinical findings that suggest a PE (Table 20.4) (Rosenow et al., 1981; Kohn et al., 1987; Leclerc, 1994). Other signs and symptoms include cough, pleuritic chest pain, apprehension, atelectatic rales, hemoptysis, fever, diaphoreses, friction rub, cyanosis, and changes in the heart sounds (accenuated second heart sound, gallop, or murmur). The clinical manifestations of PE are influenced primarily by the number, size, and location of the emboli. Preexisting health problems, such as pneumonia, congestive heart failure, or cancer, may also confuse the clinical interpretation. If an infarction of the lung occurs after a PE, the patient will typically complain of pleuritic chest pain and hemoptysis and will have a friction rub.

Table 20.4 Clinical symptoms and signs associated with pulmonary thromboembolism

Symptoms	
Tachypnea	90%
Tachycardia	40%
Hemoptysis	Less common
Diaphoresis	Less common
Fever	Less common
Rales	Less common
Wheezing	Less common
Syncope	Less common
Signs	
Dyspnea	80%
Pleuritic chest pain	70%
Apprehension	60%
Nonproductive cough	50%

(From Leclerc JR. Pulmonary embolism. In: Rake RE, ed. Conn's current therapy—1994. Philadelphia: WB Saunders, 1994:199–205; Rosenow EC III, Osmundson PJ, Brown ML. Pulmonary embolism. Mayo Clin Proc 1981;56:161–178; and Kohn H, Konig B, Mostbeck A. Incidence and clinical feature of pulmonary embolism in patients with deep venous thrombosis. A prospective study. Eur J Nucl Med 1987;13:S11–S13.)

Signs of right-sided heart failure, such as jugular venous distention, liver enlargement, left parasternal heave, and fixed splitting of the second heart sound, can be seen when at least 50% of the pulmonary circulation has been obstructed. This may be caused by large emboli or multiple small ones, and is termed *massive pulmonary embolism* (Bell et al., 1977). Of note, while multiple small pulmonary emboli can mimic massive pulmonary emboli, they can also present with no symptoms at all or resemble common pregnancy discomforts.

Not only does silent DVT sometimes lead to symptomatic PE, some patients with clinical DVT can develop silent PE. In a group of 105 patients with objectively confirmed DVT, 60 (57%) were felt to have PE by lung scanning; 59% of these were asymptomatic (Kohn et al., 1987). In 49 patients with proximal DVT and no symptoms of PE, 35% had high-probability lung scans (Dorfman et al., 1987). Thus, although noninvasive tests for DVT have been proposed as screening tools for PE, sensitivity and negative predictive values are poor (38% and 53%, respectively) (Schiff et al., 1987). Once DVT diagnosis is confirmed, the occurrence of silent PE is of diminished clinical importance because the treatment in pregnancy is similar.

Diagnostic studies

Laboratory studies

In addition to clinical examination, an arterial blood gas reading obtained on room air is the first step in confirming the diagnosis. An arterial P_ao_2 greater than 85 mmHg is reassuring but does not exclude PE. In one study (Robin, 1977), 14% of 43 patients with angiographically proven PE had a P_ao_2 greater than or equal to 85 mmHg. If the P_ao_2 is low and PE is suspected, anticoagulation should be considered while definitive diagnostic tests are performed (Table 20.5).

Electrocardiogram

The most common ECG finding is tachycardia. Unfortunately, this sign is often transient and may not be observed. In cases of

Table 20.5 Commonly used laboratory and radiographic techniques for assisting in the diagnosis of pulmonary embolism

Arterial blood gas	$P_ao_2 < 85$ mmHg
Electrocardiogram	Sinus tachycardia Right axis shift S1 Q3 T3 pattern
Chest X-ray	Focal oligemia Atelectasis Pleural effusion Hemidiaphragm elevation

massive PE, the ECG signs of acute cor pulmonale may be seen. These include a right axis shift with an S1 Q3 T3 pattern and nonspecific T-wave inversion. The "classic" S1 Q3 T3 pattern is encountered in only 10% of patients with confirmed PE (Leclerc, 1994).

Chest X-ray

Chest radiographs are abnormal in 70% of patients with PE (Rosenow et al., 1981) but are mostly useful in excluding other causes for pulmonary embarrassment. Elevation of the hemidiaphragm, atelectasis, and pleural effusion are the most common radiographic abnormalities. Focal oligemia (an area of increased radiolucency and decreased vascular marking) is seen in 2% of cases (Moses et al., 1974). Massive PE can lead to a change in cardiac size or shape, increased filling of a pulmonary artery, or a sudden termination of a vessel. Infiltrates or plural effusion are later signs of pulmonary infarction. In summary, the primary role of the chest radiograph is to eliminate other causes of the patient's symptoms and to assist in the interpretation of the lung scans.

Alveolar–arterial oxygen gradient

Pulmonary embolism causes decreased perfusion and increases mismatching and shunting. In cases of PE, the disparity between alveolar and arterial oxygen is often exaggerated. As such, alveolar–arterial oxygen gradient has been suggested as a simple screening test to exclude a pulmonary embolus. An alveolar–arterial oxygen gradient of 15 mmHg or greater is considered abnormal. In nonpregnant patients, few patients with documented PE had a normal alveolar–arterial oxygen gradient (PIOPED Investigators, 1990; McFarlane & Imperiale, 1994). However, studies in pregnant patients by Powrie et al. (1998) concluded that the alveolar–arterial gradient should not be used because more than 50% of women with a documented pulmonary embolus would have been missed. Thus, the role of the alveolar–arterial oxygen gradient as a screening test for PE may be limited to nonpregnant adults.

Ventilation-perfusion lung scan

The gold standard for the diagnosis of PE remains pulmonary arteriography. However, either ventilation perfusion (V/Q) lung scan or spiral CT, two noninvasive methods for diagnosis of PE, may be considered prior to invasive pulmonary arteriography. The costs of both tests are similar. The advantage of the V/Q scan is the accumulation of research establishing sensitivities and specificities for results of the procedure. The V/Q scan is useful in the presence of very low probability scan result and low clinical suspicion or high probability scan result and high clinical suspicion. Unfortunately, 40–60% are intermediate and therefore additional testing is required.

The lung perfusion scan is performed by IV injection of ^{99m}Tc-labeled albumin microspheres or macroaggregates. These particles are trapped within the pulmonary precapillary arteriolar bed and occlude less than 0.2% of the vessels (Gold & McCormack, 1966). Pulmonary function does not change, except in patients with severe pulmonary hypertension (Vincent et al., 1968; Mills et al., 1980). Injection is performed with the patient supine in order to increase apical perfusion; imaging is performed with the patient upright to better visualize the lung bases. The following views should be obtained: anterior, posterior, right and left lateral, and right and left posterior oblique. Perfusion lung scans are highly sensitive, and a normal study virtually excludes PE (Kipper et al., 1982; Rutherford & Phelan, 1991). Altered pulmonary perfusion from any source, such as pneumonia, tumor, atelectasis, or effusion, can result in a false-positive scan. For example, separate investigations revealed normal pulmonary arteriograms in 38% of patients with segmental perfusion defects (Markisz, 1985) and in 83% of those with a high probability of PE by perfusion lung scan (Urokinase Pulmonary Embolism Trial, 1973).

In the Prospective Investigation on Pulmonary Embolism Diagnosis (PIOPED) study, 755 individuals had both V/Q scan and pulmonary angiogram. Two hundred and fifty-one of the 755 (33%) had a PE confirmed by angiogram. When a high probability scan was reported 102/116 (88%) had a PE confirmed by angiogram. For an intermediate, low probability, normal to near normal scan 33%, 12%, and 4% respectively had a PE confirmed on angiogram. The overall sensitivity was 98% and specificity was 10%. When chest X-ray opacification corresponds with perfusion defects, the scan is considered nondiagnostic. Subsequent angiography has shown that the likelihood of PE is low with isolated subsegmental defects or matching ventilation/perfusion defects and high in the presence of ventilation/perfusion mismatching or multiple defects (Fig. 20.6). Chronic obstructive pulmonary disease, though infrequent during pregnancy, is the most common confounding factor in evaluation of the scans. In such cases, arteriography is often recommended.

No adverse fetal effects of xenon 133 (^{133}Xe) or ^{99m}Tc lung scanning have been reported, and the exposure dose has been estimated to be significantly less than that received with pulmonary arteriography (Henkin, 1982). The absorbed radiation dose to the lung is approximately 50–75 mrad with ^{99m}Tc aerosol versus 300 mrad with ^{133}Xe (the highest does of the ventilation agents mentioned) (Alderson, 1987). Even if both V/Q scanning and pulmonary angiography are performed, the total dose (<0.1 rad) will be far less than the lowest dose associated with a teratogenic effect in the human fetus (National Council on Radiation Protection and Measurements, 1977).

Nevertheless, oxygen-15 (^{15}O)-labeled carbon dioxide inhalation may, in the future, be useful in pregnancy, due to an even lower radiation dose. The ^{15}O is incorporated rapidly in $H_2{}^{15}O$, which fails to clear the pulmonary circulation in areas of underperfusion. Resulting hot spots are visualized scintigraphically. The major disadvantage is the requirement for a

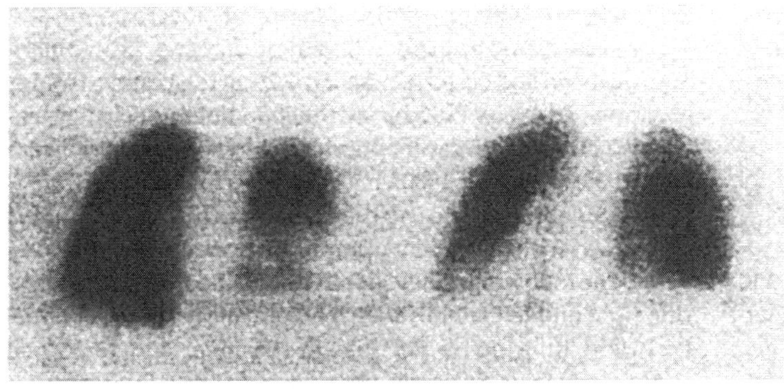

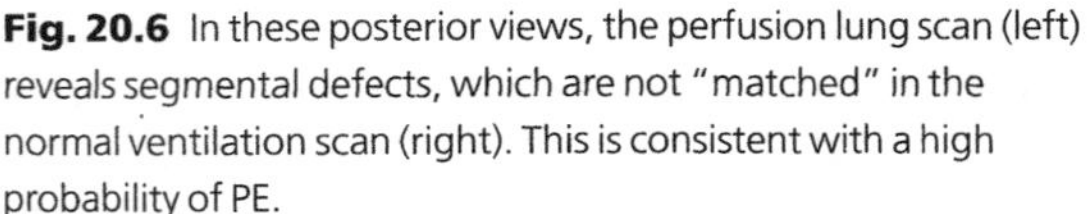

Fig. 20.6 In these posterior views, the perfusion lung scan (left) reveals segmental defects, which are not "matched" in the normal ventilation scan (right). This is consistent with a high probability of PE.

cyclotron in order to produce the ^{15}O, which has a half-life of 2.1 minutes (Nichols et al., 1980).

Spiral CT

The spiral CT is an alternative to the V/Q scan. This procedure is a chest CT scan with contrast administered via a peripheral IV. The chest CT is performed with narrow collimation during rapid administration of IV contrast. The examination is completed in approximately 15–20 minutes. Both sensitivity and specificity of spiral CT in nonpregnant patients for central pulmonary embolus are approximately 94%. The primary advantage of spiral CT is that it is noninvasive, and provides direct visualization of an embolus at a segmental level or higher, as well as visualization of other disease pathology (pleural effusions, consolidation, emphysema, pulmonary masses) which may cause similar respiratory symptomatology (Cross et al., 1998; Lipchik & Goodman, 1999; Kim et al., 1999). In comparison to the V/Q scan only 5% are indeterminate requiring additional testing. The disadvantage is that the procedure is operator dependent and is often done only in tertiary care centers.

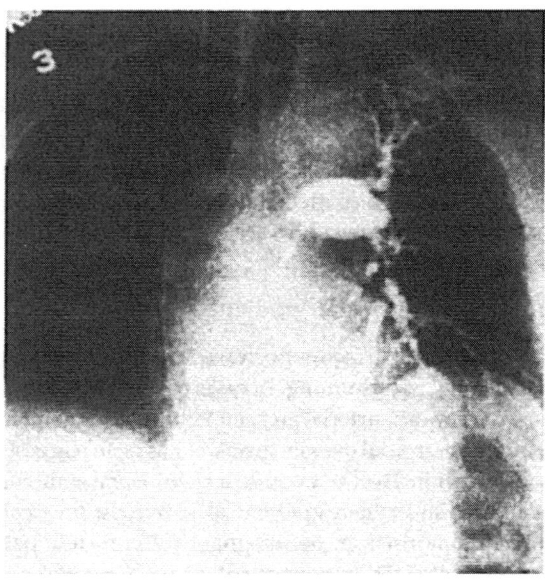

Fig. 20.7 Arteriogram of the left pulmonary artery shows filling defects and an unperfused segment of lung as shown by the absence of contrast dye.

Pulmonary artery catheterization

A number of findings can suggest PE on pulmonary artery catheterization. Failure to wedge or the inability to obtain the appropriate waveform can occur in the case of completely occlusive embolism distal to the catheter tip. If the failure to wedge is combined with pulmonary hypertension, further investigation to rule out PE is warranted (Traeger, 1985). Using a minimal amount of contrast material, in conjunction with fluoroscopy, can be useful. Occlusion of the distal port of the catheter (Fairfax et al., 1984) or inability to measure cardiac output because of embedding of the catheter tip in the clot (Lewis et al., 1982) are also clues to the presence of a PE. Elevated central venous pressures (>10 mmHg) may suggest a massive PE (Dalen et al., 1969).

Pulmonary arteriography

Pulmonary arteriography is the definitive technique for confirming the diagnosis of PE, but can be indeterminate. Injection of contrast medium selectively into lobar or segmental branches of the pulmonary artery yields clear visualization of vessels greater than 2.5 mm in diameter (Hull et al., 1983). A clot may be seen as a filling defect that does not obstruct flow or as an abruptly terminated vessel, possibly with a trailing edge of dye where the clot incompletely fills the lumen (Fig. 20.7). Multiple views may be needed to exclude PE. Risks are related to the use of catheterization and contrast dye. With pulmonary arteriography, morbidity has been reported to be as high as 4–5%, and mortality rates are 0.2–0.3% (Dalen et al., 1979; Mills et al., 1980). Most serious complications, however, occur in patients with underlying pulmonary hypertension and right ventricular end-diastolic pressure exceeding 20 mmHg (Mills et al., 1980).

Pulmonary arteriography is recommended when initial noninvasive lung scanning is indeterminate, does not correlate with clinical suspicion, or indicates moderate probability of PE. The physician should take into account corresponding V/Q defects and/or chest X-ray findings (PIOPED Investigators, 1996). The risks of thrombolytic therapy (e.g. streptokinase) or surgical interruption of the vena cava necessitate angiographic confirmation prior to consideration of these measures.

Digital subtraction pulmonary angiography

This relatively noninvasive tool involves the injection of a contrast medium into a peripheral vein and computerized subtraction of the preinjection chest X-ray from the postinjection film. Theoretically, an image of the pulmonary arterial vasculature, as exemplified by contrast filling, is obtained. However, poor imagining often results from respiratory and cardiac motion, and resolution with this technique is not as good as the conventional arteriography. In addition, it is difficult to obtain multiple projection views, and nonselective filling can cause vessel overlap. Digital subtraction angiography may be promising, given continued technologic improvement.

Indium 111 platelet imaging

This technique is not yet available for widespread clinical use but shows promise in the diagnosis and management of patients with thromboembolic disease. Platelets are extracted from venous blood, labeled, and reinjected into the donor. The platelets then accumulate at sites of active thrombosis. Heparin blocks the incorporation of these platelets into an established nonexpanding thrombus. Images are obtained with gamma camera scintigraphy. For DVT, sensitivity is 90–95%, and specificity is 95–100% (Ezekowitz et al., 1985). Hematomas, wound infection, and prostheses can give false-positive results. Little data are available regarding the usefulness of this technique in PE. Since this technique relies on the presence of active thrombosis, it may permit anticoagulation to be monitored more effectively.

Anticoagulant therapy

Heparin therapy

Heparin (Hirsch, 1991) is a heterogeneous acidic mucopolysaccharide with a high molecular weight, a property that prevents it from crossing the placenta (Table 20.6). The molecular weight in commercial preparations ranges from 4,000 to 40,000 daltons, and biologic activities of the different fractions also vary. Recent reports have suggested that the separation and use of the lower-molecular-weight molecules (4,000–6,000 daltons) may provide a preparation of higher, more uniform activity (Bratt et al., 1985; Samama, 1986; Gillis et al., 1992; Fejgin & Lourwood, 1994; Rasmussen et al., 1994; Sturridge & Letsky, 1994; Ginsberg & Hirsh, 1995; Lensing et al., 1995; Koopman et al., 1996; Levine et al., 1996). Low-molecular-weight heparin (LMWH) differs slightly in its anticoagulant activity from standard unfractionated heparin (S-heparin), and has a greater bioavailability and longer anti-factor Xa activity (Samama, 1986; Koopman et al., 1996; Levine et al., 1996).

Heparin exerts its primary anticoagulant activity by binding to plasma AT III. Once bound, the configuration of AT III is changed. This facilitates binding to and neutralization of factor Xa and thrombin primarily, and to a lesser extent factors IXa, XIa, and XIIa. Its antifactor Xa activity is inversely proportional to the molecular weight of the heparin fragment (Fejgin & Lourwood, 1994). Once released, heparin can then interact similarly with other AT III molecules. Small amounts of heparin can inhibit the initial steps of the clotting cascade. After a thrombus has been formed, however, much more heparin is needed to neutralize the larger amounts of already formed thrombin and prevent extension of the clot (White et al., 1979). As thrombin production diminishes, the heparin dose needed may decrease.

A disadvantage of heparin is the need for parenteral

Table 20.6 The distinguishing pharmacologic features of heparin and warfarin

	Heparin	Warfarin
Molecular weight (daltons)*	12,000–15,000	1,000
Mechanism of action	Binds AT III	Vitamin K-dependent factors
Administration	Intravenous, subcutaneous	Oral
Half-life	1.0–2.5 hr	2.5 days
Anticoagulant effect	Immediate	36–72 hr
Laboratory monitoring	Heparin levels, aPTT antifactor Xa	Prothrombin time, INR
Reversal	Protamine sulfate	Vitamin K
Placental transfer	None	Crosses

* Mean molecular weight.
INR, international normalized ratio.

administration via an IV or a subcutaneous route. Heparin is not absorbed via the gastrointestinal tract, and intramuscular injections result in erratic absorption and carry a risk of hematoma formation. The half-life of heparin varies with the dose, the type of heparin, and the extent of active thrombosis. For example, higher doses result in both a higher peak and a longer half-life (DeSwart et al., 1982). Half-lives of less than 1 hour to more than 2.5 hours have been found. Moreover, heparin levels may become abnormally elevated in cases of hepatic or renal failure (Perry et al., 1974). Continuous IV infusion has been shown to result in more consistent levels and fewer hemorrhagic events than does administration via intermittent IV boluses. Subcutaneous administration also gives a steadier effect, but slower absorption results in a 2–4 hours delay in peak levels.

Another difficulty associated with heparin is adequate monitoring of its bioeffect in order to ensure an adequate yet safe dose. Laboratories vary in the type of tests they can offer, partly because the procedures are technique-sensitive, and skill is required for consistent results. The activated partial thromboplastin time (aPTT) is the most commonly available test. Prolongation of the aPTT to 1.5–2.5 times the control value has been shown to be useful in monitoring patients (Basu et al., 1972; Hyers et al., 1986). There is a significant increase in clot extension with aPTT levels below 1.5, but no increase in bleeding complications as 2.5 is approached. Thus, anticoagulation in the upper range of 1.5–2.5 times control appears to be ideal.

Although no single laboratory test appears clearly superior in predicting bleeding, heparin assay may be the most helpful (Holm et al., 1985). Heparin levels are measured indirectly using the protamine sulfate neutralization test in which the amount of protamine sulfate needed to reverse the effects of heparin on the thrombin clotting time is measured. Plasma heparin levels of 0.2–0.5 IU/mL are desirable for full therapeutic anticoagulation. In some institutions, measurement of inhibition of factor Xa has been developed as a monitoring tool for heparin anticoagulation.

Low-molecular-weight heparin

Low-molecular-weight heparin is distinguishable pharmacologically from S-heparin by its preferential inactivation of factor Xa (Table 20.7). Antifactor Xa activity is inversely related to the molecular weight of the fragment. This means that LMWH has a greater anti-Xa activity than S-heparin. While any heparin will inactivate factor Xa by binding to AT III, S-heparin, by virtue of its longer saccharide chain and pentasaccharide sequence, also inactivates thrombin by forming a ternary complex with AT III and thrombin. In this way, S-heparin inhibits the activity of both factor Xa and thrombin. Because LMWH lacks the longer saccharide chains, this agent does not inhibit thrombin, and its associated potential for bleeding is, therefore, less.

LMWH offers additional advantages over S-heparin (Fejgin & Lourwood, 1994; Lensing et al., 1995). For example, LMWH has a plasma half-life 2–4 times longer and a more predictable anticoagulant response than S-heparin. LMWH has less pronounced effects on platelet function and vascular permeability (with significantly less risk of heparin-induced thrombocytopenia). Unlike S-heparin, LMWH can resist inhibition by PF_4.

LMWH and S-heparin are similar in that neither crosses the placenta and both are administered either IV or subcutaneously. Protamine sulfate is used to reverse both heparins, although LMWH is less affected by the action of protamine sulfate (Fejgin & Lourwood, 1994). Further, LMWH is administered as a weight-dependent dose, and because of its predictable effect, no monitoring of levels is necessary.

LMWH has been shown to be effective when administered

Table 20.7 The distinguishing pharmacological features of standard (unfractionated) heparin (S-heparin) and low-molecular-weight heparin (L-heparin)

	S-heparin	L-heparin
Molecular weight (daltons)*	12,000–15,000	4,000–6,000
Mechanism of action	Binds ATP III	Binds ATP III
Inhibitory activity	Factor Xa	Factor Xa
	Thrombin	
Administration	IV	IV
	SQ	SQ
Half-life (hr)	1	4
	3	4
Laboratory monitoring	APTT	None needed; may be measured by antifactor Xa
	Heparin levels	
	Antifactor Xa	
Reversal	Protamine sulfate	Protamine sulfate
Placental transfer	None	None

* Mean molecular weight.
IV, intravenous; SQ, subcutaneous.

on an outpatient basis for the treatment of DVT (Lepercq et al., 2001; Brown, 2002). Thus, the higher initial cost of the drug may be outweighed by the absence of need for hospitalization. However, caution should be exercised when using outpatient anticoagulation for the acute treatment of VTE during pregnancy (Lepercq et al, 2001). Numerous studies have demonstrated equivalence or superiority of LMWH to S-heparin for a variety of prophylactic and therapeutic indications (Clagett et al., 1995; Berqvist et al., 1996; Geerts et al., 1996; Koopman et al., 1996; Levine et al., 1996). Although not yet approved for therapeutic anticoagulation in pregnancy, this agent is increasingly prescribed for this indication, and most authorities believe LMWH will soon completely replace S-heparin for the prophylaxis and treatment of thromboembolic disorders. Although the ideal dosage for the pregnant patient has not been established, standard doses in nonpregnant women are enoxaparin 1 mg/kg subcutaneously twice a day for therapeutic purposes, and 30–40 mg subcutaneously twice a day for prophylaxis.

Heparin side effects

The primary risk of heparin anticoagulation (Table 20.8) is bleeding, which occurs in approximately 5–10% of patients (Hall et al., 1978; Walker & Jick, 1980; Bonnar, 1981) but can affect as many as one-third (Holm, 1985). Prior to initiating anticoagulation, the physician should request a baseline clotting profile to identify those patients with an underlying coagulation defect. The number of bleeding episodes appears to relate to the total daily dose of heparin and the prolongation of the aPTT. Unlike continuous infusion or subcutaneous injection, bolus infusion is associated with a higher total dose of heparin and a much greater risk of bleeding. When needed, as in the case of overdose or to prevent bleeding at the time of emergency surgery, rapid reversal of heparinization with either S-heparin or LMWH can be accomplished with protamine sulfate.

Because the primary hemostatic defense in heparinized patients is platelet aggregation, drugs such as nonsteroidal anti-inflammatory agents or dextran, which interfere with platelet number or function, may induce bleeding. For example, patients receiving aspirin have twice the risk of bleeding (Walker & Jick, 1980). Because heparin is an acidic molecule and incompatible with many solutions containing medications (e.g. aminoglycosides), heparin activity may be affected. However, there should be no loss of heparin activity when such drugs are administered at separate sites (Hirsch, 1991).

Another side effect of heparin therapy is thrombocytopenia. Estimates of the incidence of thrombocytopenia for S-heparin vary from 1% to 30% (Chong et al., 1982; Barbour & Pickard, 1995) and are around 2% for LMWH (Fejgin & Lourwood, 1994). However, according to Fausett et al. (2001), heparin-induced thrombocytopenia during pregnancy is rare when compared with nonpregnant women. Thrombocytopenia typically occurs, if at all, within hours to 15 days after the initiation of full-dose heparin therapy (Hirsch, 1991; Barbour & Pickard, 1995). Clinically, the thrombocytopenia may be mild (platelet count >100,000/mm^3). With the mild form, treatment can be continued without an undue risk of bleeding. The severe form, however, requires discontinuation of heparin therapy and is reversible. In the latter circumstance, heparinoids have been found to be 93% efficacious (Magnani, 1993). For patients receiving heparin therapy, maternal platelet counts should be determined in the first 2–3 weeks of therapy. Thereafter, platelet counts are probably unnecessary (Barbour & Pickard, 1995).

The mechanism involved in the thrombocytopenia is incompletely understood but appears to involve platelet clumping and sequestration, immune-mediated destruction, and consumption through low-grade disseminated intravascular coagulation. While heparin-associated thrombocytopenia is most frequently encountered in patients receiving high-dose heparin, patients on prophylactic low-dose heparin, have a lower risk of this condition (Galle et al., 1978; Phillips et al., 1983; Hirsch et al., 1992). Patients on LMWH have been noted to occasionally experience thrombocytopenia (Ginsberg & Hirsh, 1995; Lepercq et al., 2001). Heparin derived from bovine lung rather than porcine gut is more often associated with thrombocytopenia (Rao et al., 1989).

Hypersensitivity to heparin therapy can result in chills, fever, and urticaria. Rarely, anaphylactic reactions to heparin have occurred.

Osteoporosis and symptomatic fractures are another side effect of prolonged heparin therapy (Griffith, 1965; de Swiet et al., 1983; Zimran et al., 1986; Dahlman et al., 1990, 1994; Dahlman, 1993). These changes in bone density have ranged from demineralization changes observed in the spine, hip, and femur radiographs to overt fractures (de Swiet et al., 1983; Dahlman et al., 1990, 1994; Dahlman, 1993) and occur in patients who receive both S-heparin and LMWH. In 184 women given long-term heparin prophylaxis during pregnancy, symptomatic vertebral fractures occurred in four postpartum. The mean dose in those with symptomatic vertebral fractures ranged from 15,000 to 30,000 units/day. In one such patient, the mean dose received was as little as 15,000 units/day for 7 weeks (Dahlman, 1993). Radiographic changes have been observed in up to one-third of women receiving heparin therapy

Table 20.8 Side effects of heparin anticoagulation

Side effect	Incidence (%)
Bleeding	5–10
Thrombocytopenia	5–10
Osteoporotic changes	2–17
Anaphylaxis	Rare

for longer than a month (Ginsberg & Hirsh, 1995). Reversal after discontinuing therapy can be slow (de Swiet et al., 1983; Zimran et al., 1986), but there is reassuring evidence that reversal of osteopenia does occur and that treatment in consecutive pregnancies may not increase a woman's risk of this complication (Dahlman et al., 1990). Pregnant women receiving heparin therapy should be advised to take at least one additional gram (should not exceed 2 g total per day) of supplemental calcium and encouraged to perform daily weight-bearing exercises.

The careful administration of subcutaneous heparin prevents erratic absorption and local bruising. Preferably, the subcutaneous fat of the anterior flank (lateral abdominal wall) should be used rather than sites in the arms and legs. These latter sites are more painful and are subject to rapid absorption of heparin in association with movement. A small needle is fully inserted vertically into a raised fold of skin and withdrawn atraumatically after injection. Patients should be advised against massaging the injection sites as this increases absorption. Overall, heparin is safe for use in pregnancy; the perinatal outcome among heparin users is comparable to nonusers (Ginsberg et al., 1988).

Warfarin

Warfarin, a coumarin derivative, is the most commonly used oral anticoagulant (see Table 20.6). It inhibits regeneration of active vitamin K in the liver. Vitamin K is required to carboxylate the glutamic acid residues on factors II, VII, IX, and X and protein C. These factors are otherwise inactive and unable to complex normally with calcium and phospholipid receptors.

Except in the rare situation in which heparin cannot or should not be used, warfarin is contraindicated in pregnancy (Table 20.9). With a molecular weight of 1,000 daltons, warfarin easily crosses the placenta. Administration in the first 6–9 weeks of gestation has been associated with warfarin embryopathy. This syndrome may include nasal hypoplasia, depression of the bridge of the nose, and epiphyseal stippling, such as is seen in Conradi-Hunermann chondrodysplasia punctata (Hall et al., 1978; Ginsberg et al., 1989b; Ginsberg & Hirsh, 1992; Colvin et al, 1993). Exposure during the second and third trimesters is associated with a variety of CNS and ophthalmologic abnormalities. It is suspected that some of these abnormalities are related to fetal hemorrhage and scar tissue formation. In a retrospective review of published reports, abnormal live-born infants occurred in 13% of pregnancies in which warfarin or related substances were used. Approximately 4% resulted in infants with warfarin embryopathy. Of patients with warfarin embryopathy, approximately 30% may be developmentally retarded (Hall et al., 1978). In those infants with CNS abnormalities, dorsal midline dysplasia (e.g. agenesis of the corpus callosum), Dandy-Walker malformation, midline cerebellar atrophy and ventral midline dysplasia (e.g. optic atrophy) have been described (Stevenson et al., 1980). Such literature reviews, however, may be skewed in favor of abnormal outcomes. A review of 22 children of mothers who took warfarin during pregnancy revealed no significant difference when compared with controls; this outcome suggests that the incidence of abnormalities may be lower than previously reported (Chang et al., 1984). Because of the anticoagulant effect in the fetus, there is also a higher risk of fetal hemorrhage at delivery. Thus, women who are treated with coumarin derivatives and contemplate pregnancy should be switched to heparin prior to conception. In select patients with cardiac disease at risk of arterial thromboembolic events, the apparent increased effectiveness of warfarin may justify the associated fetal risks. There appears, however, to be little justification for the use of coumarin derivatives in the treatment or prophylaxis of venous thromboembolism.

Table 20.9 Maternal and fetal side effects of warfarin therapy during pregnancy

Maternal
Bleeding
Skin necrosis/gangrene
Purple toes syndrome
Hypersensitivity
Fetal
Hemorrhage
Warfarin embryopathy
CNS abnormalities
Optic atrophy
Mental retardation

The major maternal complication (see Table 20.9) of warfarin use is bleeding, which occurs more often with warfarin than with subcutaneous heparin (Hull et al., 1982). Warfarin anticoagulation is also more sensitive to fluctuations in clotting factors and plasma volume and requires more frequent monitoring and adjustments. Numerous medications (Standing Advisory Committee, 1982), including some antibiotics, can augment or inhibit warfarin (coumarin derivative) activity (Table 20.10).

Less common side effects of warfarin therapy are skin necrosis and gangrene (Horn et al., 1981). Once an underlying disease is excluded as a cause of such dermatologic changes, warfarin should be discontinued and appropriate medical and/or surgical therapy instituted. The purple toes syndrome (Lebsack & Weibert, 1982; Park et al., 1993), an infrequent complication of warfarin therapy, is characterized by dark, purplish, mottled toes and occurs 3–10 weeks after the initiation of coumarin therapy. In most instances, this condition is reversible, but a few patients will progress to necrosis or gangrene. In rare circumstances, amputation may be necessary.

Table 20.10 Selected drugs that interact with coumarin derivative anticoagulants

May potentiate oral anticoagulants	May antagonize oral anticoagulants
Alcohol, dose-dependent	Antacids
Chlorpromazine	Antihistamines
Cimetidine	Barbiturates
Danocrine	Carbamazepine
Metronidazole	Corticosteroids
Neomycin	Oral contraceptives
Nonsteroidal antiinflammatory drugs	
Salicylates, large doses	Primidone
Thyroxine	Rifampin
Trimethoprim	Vitamin K
Phenytoin	

(Reproduced by permission from Standing Advisory Committee for Haematology of the Royal College of Pathologists. Drug interaction with coumarin derivative anticoagulants. Br Med J 1982;185:274–275.)

Measurement of the prothrombin time (PT) is used to monitor the anticoagulant effect of warfarin. Therapeutic levels can be reached after 3–5 days and should yield a PT of 1.5–2.5 times control (international normalized ratio, INR) (Hirsch, 1988). In a study of 266 nonpregnant patients with PE, early treatment with warfarin (begun during days 1–3) was found to be as effective as continuous IV heparin in preventing recurrences, with similar rates of bleeding complications. The major advantage with warfarin was a 30% decrease in hospital time (Gallus et al., 1986).

Reversal of anticoagulation depends on regeneration of clotting factors and is slow. Administration of parenteral vitamin K can lead to reversal in 6–12 hours. In an acute situation, fresh frozen plasma can be given to provide clotting factors.

Antepartum management

Patients at high risk for thromboembolic disease require consideration for anticoagulation or prophylactic therapy during pregnancy and the puerperium. Such patients are those with hereditary thrombophilia, prior history of VTE, mechanical heart valve, atrial fibrillation, trauma/prolonged immobilization/major surgery, other familial hypercoagulable states, and antiphospholipid syndrome (ACOG, 2000). Patients with the following conditions are at highest risk and should be considered for therapeutic heparin anticoagulation: artificial heart valves, AT III deficiency, history of rheumatic heart disease with current atrial fibrillation, homozygosity for factor V Leiden or prothrombin G20210A, and receiving chronic anticoagulation for recurrent thromboembolism (ACOG, 2000).

If the patient's clinical picture strongly suggests VTE, anticoagulation with heparin should be considered prior to diagnostic studies to minimize the risk of an embolic event while awaiting confirmation of the diagnosis. After obtaining a baseline clotting profile and a complete hypercoagulable evaluation, the physician can most easily achieve rapid anticoagulation by using an initial IV bolus of 70–100 units/kg or 5,000–10,000 units (Hirsch, 1991). For massive PE, an initial IV bolus as high as 15,000 units has been recommended (Moser & Fedullo, 1983). Initial continuous infusion rates can be calculated at 15–20 units/kg/hr. Doses that prolong the aPTT 1.5–2.5 times normal or give a plasma heparin level of 0.2–0.5 units/mL are considered therapeutic. Adequate and rapid initial anticoagulation is essential to minimize the risk of PE. The heparin dose is ideally adjusted every 4 hours until adequate anticoagulation has been achieved. Excessive doses that prolong the aPTT beyond 2.5 times normal or result in plasma heparin levels above 0.5 units/mL are associated with a greater likelihood of maternal bleeding (Bonnar et al., 1969; Hirsch, 1991). In pregnancy, the required dose is related more closely to the maternal circulating blood volume than to maternal body weight (Ellison et al., 1989). To ensure accurate results, blood samples should be drawn remote from the site of heparin infusion. After initial adjustment and stabilization of the heparin dose, once daily laboratory testing is sufficient. The infusion dose required may change as active thrombosis abates. A useful protocol for the adjustment to the dose of IV heparin is presented in Table 20.11 (Toglia & Weg, 1996).

There is no difference between patients with DVT and PE as to the amount of heparin required to achieve therapeutic anticoagulation (Tenero et al., 1989). However, recommendations for duration of IV infusion vary. A *minimum* of 2 days with DVT and 5 days with PE are suggested (Bonnar, 1981; Letsky, 1985). Most authors recommend IV therapy for 5–7 days. Historically, the goal was to continue IV heparin until: (i) active thrombosis has stopped; (ii) thrombi are firmly attached to the vessel wall; and (iii) organization has begun (Bonnar, 1981; Letsky, 1985).

The period of continuous IV infusion is followed in pregnancy by therapeutic subcutaneous heparin for the duration of the pregnancy (Anderson et al., 1982). Postpartum anticoagulation will need to be continued for 6–12 weeks in most patients. According to Schulman and associates (1995), 6 months, not 6 weeks, of prophylactic anticoagulation after a first episode of venous thromboembolism may be required to lower the recurrence rate. In contrast, Hirsch (1995) suggests that duration of anticoagulant therapy depends on whether the patient has a reversible risk factor for DVT, such as DVT after surgery or trauma, or a permanent risk factor, such as idiopathic DVT (the absence of any risk factors). With the Hirsch classification (Barbour et al., 1995), prolonged anticoagulant therapy would be 6 weeks for the reversible group and 6 months for idiopathic DVT.

Monitoring of therapy in patients receiving adjusted-dose (therapeutic) subcutaneous heparin is more complex than

Table 20.11 Protocol for adjustment of the dose of intravenous heparin*

Activated partial thromboplastin time (sec)†	Repeat bolus?	Stop infusion?	New rate of infusion	Repeat measurement of activated partial thromboplastin time
<50	Yes (5,000 IU)	No	+3 mL/hr (+2,880 IU/24 hr)	6 hr
50–59	No	No	+3 mL/hr (+2,880 IU/24 hr)	6 hr
60–85‡	No	No	Unchanged	Next morning
86–95	No	No	−2 mL/hr (−1,920 IU/24 hr)	Next morning
69–120	No	Yes (for 30 min)	−2 mL/hr (−1,920 IU/24 hr)	6 hr
>120	No	Yes (for 60 min)	−4 mL/hr (−3,840 IU/24 hr)	6 hr

* A starting dose of 5,000 IU is given as an intravenous bolus, followed by 31,000 IU per 24 hours, given as a continuous infusion in a concentration of 40 IU per milliliter. The activated partial thromboplastin time is first measured 6 hours after the bolus injection, adjustments are made according to the protocol, and the activated partial thromboplastin time is measured again as indicated. Adapted from Hirsch J. Heparin. N Engl J Med 1991;324:1565.
† The normal range, measured with the Dade-Actin-FS reagent, is 27–35 seconds.
‡ The therapeutic range of 60–85 seconds is equivalent to a heparin level of 0.2–0.4 IU per milliliter by protamine titration or 0.35–0.7 IU per milliliter according to the level of inhibition of factor Xa. The therapeutic range varies with the responsiveness of the reagent used to measure the activated partial thromboplastin time to heparin.
(Reproduced by permission from Toglia MR, Weg JG. Venous thromboembolism during pregnancy. N Engl J Med 1996;335:108.)

with the IV route. With respect to the timing of aPTT in relationship to intermittent injection, some authorities recommend monitoring the mid-dose aPTT (i.e. drawn at 6 hr for patients receiving 12-hr injections), while an increasing number of physicians favor adjusting the heparin dose to achieve a level near 2.5 times control just prior to the next dose. Data to document the superiority of the approach are lacking; it is hoped that the use of LMWH will, in the near future, make such discussion moot.

Reported alternatives to long-term intermittent injections in pregnancy have included continuous infusions of heparin via a Hickman catheter (Nelson et al., 1984) or subcutaneous pump (Barss et al., 1985). In one series, six patients received continuous subcutaneous infusion to reach therapeutic PTTs of 1.5–2.0 times controls. Although there were no recurrences of thrombosis, five of the patients experienced major or minor bleeding complications (Barss et al., 1985).

A goal for antepartum care should also be to maximize a pregnant woman's candidacy for regional anesthesia. The American Society of Anesthesia has recommended that patients receiving higher doses of LMWH (specifically enoxaparin, 1 mg/kg twice daily) should not receive neuraxial blocks for 24 hours from the last dose (American Society of Regional Anesthesia, 1998). Furthermore, obtaining an antifactor Xa level before placing the block was not recommended since it did not adequately predict the risk of bleeding. No specific recommendations were made regarding low-dose prophylactic LMWH heparin (enoxaparin 30–40 mg twice daily). Consideration for switching to S-heparin at approximately 37 weeks should be made due to the shorter half-life. A normal aPTT usually is sufficient to ensure the safety of epidural anesthesia in a patient anticoagulated with S-heparin, as long as the platelet count is normal.

Intrapartum management

The risk of significant hemorrhage is small for patients on anticoagulations who deliver vaginally, as long as the platelet count and function are normal and uterine atony is avoided. Regional anesthetics (epidural and spinal), however, are not recommended in a fully anticoagulated patient because of the potential risk of epidural or spinal cord hematoma formation. For patients requiring cesarean delivery, therapeutic anticoagulation becomes more complex. On admission to labor and delivery, a clotting profile and hematocrit should be drawn. There are three basic choices in the approach to anticoagulant management is such patients:

1 *Continue therapeutic anticoagulation.* This approach is recommended for particularly high-risk patients, such as those with recent PE, iliofemoral thrombosis, or mechanical heart valve prostheses. Because a more uniform therapeutic heparin level is desirable, the patient may be changed from subcutaneous injection to continuous IV infusion. A heparin level of 0.4 units/mL or a low therapeutic aPTT (close to 1.5 time normal) may be desirable in these surgical patients.
2 *Reduce the subcutaneous heparin dose.* In patients at lower risk of thromboembolism, the heparin dose can be reduced to a prophylactic level (5,000 units every 12 hours); this dose is not associated with increased surgical bleeding.
3 *Stop or withhold heparin administration.* For patients at increased risk for operative bleeding (i.e. suspected placenta accreta) and at relatively low risk of clot propagation, heparin may be temporarily withheld or its effects reversed with protamine sulfate. Nonpharmacologic prophylaxis (e.g. pneumatic compression stockings) may be substituted during the intraoperative period.

With patients who are anticoagulated and in whom rapid reversal is deemed essential, protamine sulfate can be used to reverse either S-heparin or LMWH heparin. One milligram of protamine sulfate neutralizes 100 units of heparin. To determine the proper dose of protamine, several approaches are available. One is to calculate the amount of circulating heparin by estimating the plasma volume at 50 mL/kg of body weight and multiplying the plasma volume by the heparin concentration (Letsky, 1985). In most institutions, however, this procedure may not be technically feasible. If heparin level is not available, the amount of protamine sulfate to give should be underestimated or slowly titrated to the whole-blood clotting time because of the short half-life (rapid metabolism) of heparin and the irreversible anticoagulant effect of excess protamine. No single dose should exceed 50 mg. A 50-mg dose is almost never needed because it would neutralize 5,000 units of circulating heparin, an amount of heparin highly unlikely to be present. Protamine sulfate should be administered IV over 20–30 minutes to prevent hypotension. In patients receiving adjusted-dose subcutaneous heparin, a dose of 5–10 mg of protamine sulfate is often sufficient; further doses may be given, depending on the aPTT value. It should be emphasized that for vaginal delivery, even significantly prolonged aPTT values rarely results in clinical hemorrhage, and thus do not require protamine sulfate therapy.

Patients who present for delivery on warfarin anticoagulant are at heightened risk for bleeding with either vaginal or operative delivery. Parental vitamin K can help to regenerate the clotting factors within 12 hours. If there is little time, or reversal is not adequate, fresh frozen plasma can be given to supply clotting factors. Regardless, the pregnant woman should be stabilized and be sufficiently able to clot before operative delivery is initiated.

Postpartum management

Conversion from heparin to warfarin anticoagulation should be initiated postpartum in the hospital to minimize the maternal risk of complications. Once the patient has delivered and is sufficiently stable, full heparin anticoagulation should be resumed. Then, oral warfarin therapy should be started with 10–15 mg orally per day for 2–4 days, followed by 2–15 mg/day as indicated by the INR or PT (Hirsch, 1991). One approach is to give the warfarin sodium at 6 p.m., then draw an INR or PT at 6 a.m. the following day, adjusting the dose for the subsequent day's warfarin according to that morning's results. Once the patient is therapeutically anticoagulated, heparin is discontinued. Postpartum suppression of lactation with estrogen is associated with a much higher incidence of thromboembolic complications and is contraindicated (Daniel et al., 1967; Jeffcoate et al., 1968).

Prophylaxis of thromboembolism

Dosage of heparin needed during pregnancy appears to increase because of increases in heparin-binding proteins, plasma volume, renal clearance, and heparin degradation by the placenta. All contribute to a decreased bioavailability of heparin. Due to lack of adequate prospective trials, a number of different prophylactic regimens have been proposed. Low-dose prophylaxis with S-heparin may be administered via 5,000–7,500 units every 12 hours during the first trimester, 7,500–10,000 units every 12 hours during the second trimester, followed by 10,000 units every 12 hours during the third trimester unless the aPTT is elevated. Alternatively, LMWH may be used. For low-dose prophylaxis, dalteparin 5,000 units once or twice daily, or enoxaparin 40 mg once or twice daily may be used. Adjusted-dose prophylaxis may be accomplished with either dalteparin 5,000–10,000 units every 12 hours, or enoxaparin, 30–80 mg every 12 hours (ACOG, 2000). An increase from 5,000 units to 7,500–10,000 units in the third trimester (Bonnar, 1981) is often recommended (Howell et al., 1983). Except for doses exceeding 8,000 units, laboratory monitoring is not usually required (Bonnar, 1981). Caution should be used in the patient with diminished renal function, which may elevate heparin levels.

Employing only perioperative (cesarean) prophylaxis may be considered for certain patients, such as those with obesity or unusually reduced ambulation. Conservative mechanical methods, such as intermittent pneumatic compression boots or graduated elastic compression stockings, may also be helpful. Early postoperative ambulation is also important in preventing thromboembolism. Low-dose heparin is accepted as prophylaxis for a variety of surgical procedures (Collins et al., 1988). Although in some general surgical or orthopedic patients dihydroergotamine in combination with heparin is felt to be more effective than heparin alone (Kakkar et al., 1979; Salzman & Hirsh, 1987), its use in pregnant or parturient women has not been studied. Thus, its use cannot be recommended. The combination of mechanical methods, especially pneumatic compression, and low-dose heparin may be the optimal approach for high-risk patients (Stringer & Kakkar, 1989; Clark-Pearson et al., 1993). LMWH has been found useful in abdominal surgery; one dose is given preoperatively, followed by additional doses once very 24 hours (European Fraxiparin Study Group, 1988; Hirsch & Barrowcliffe, 1988).

Therapeutic anticoagulation is necessary during pregnancy for those patients with mechanical heart valves (Salazar et al., 1984) or inherited deficiency of a natural anticoagulant such as AT III (Nelson et al., 1985). In women with AT III deficiency, successful outcomes have been achieved with the use of subcutaneous and IV heparinization, accompanied by infusion of AT III concentrate at the time of abortion or delivery (Nelson et al., 1985). AT III deficiency should be considered when heparin requirements increase beyond typical dosages. Without such therapy, maternal morbidity or mortality and fetal loss are extremely high. Deficiencies of proteins C and S are also associated with thrombotic tendency (De Stefano et al., 1988). In patients with medical histories remarkable for VTE, a systematic comprehensive approach to thrombophilic screening should be pursued. Knowledge of an individual's thrombophilic status can be used to better predict VTE recurrence risk (Brill-Edwards et al., 2000).

Antiplatelet agents such as aspirin and dipyridamole may be helpful in preventing thrombosis in the arterial circulation and with some prosthetic heart valves. There is no known role for these agents in the prevention of pregnancy-associated VTE disease. Perioperative prophylaxis with dextran appears beneficial in some surgical patients, but the risk of bleeding is higher than with heparin, and dextran's usefulness in pregnant patients has not been established (Salzman & Hirsh, 1987).

A potential but yet unproven approach in pregnancy for intrapartum prophylaxis in patients without an active thrombotic process is ultra-low-dose IV heparin (Negus et al., 1980). In a randomized study to prevent postoperative DVT in nonpregnant patients, a dose of 1 IU/kg/hr reduced the incidence of DVT from 22% to 4%.

Thrombolytic therapy

Defibrinating agents may be indicated in case of life-threatening thromboembolism (Urokinase–Streptokinase Pulmonary Emoblism Trial, 1974; Sharma et al., 1985; Moran et al., 1989; Turrentine et al., 1995). Streptokinase, urokinase, and tissue plasminogen activator activate plasminogen, which sets in motion the body's natural fibrinolytic system. Although helpful in early management of massive PE, thrombolysis plus heparin may not yield improved mortality over heparin alone (Urokinase–Streptokinase, 1974). Because of the potential risk of bleeding, thrombolytic therapy has not been recommended within 10 days of surgery or parturition (Moran et al., 1989). Recommended treatment schedules vary, but all consist of an IV loading dose followed by continuous infusion for 12–72 hours, depending on the clinical situation (Sharma et al., 1985). Thrombolytic therapy is followed by anticoagulant therapy to prevent recurrence. A review of 172 patients by Turrentine et al. (1995) demonstrated that thrombolytic therapy could be used relatively safely during pregnancy in selected clinical situations (Table 20.12) and that these agents were partially or completely successful in 86–90% of recipients. Nonetheless, the authors suggested that traditional therapies should be used first, and, if unsuccessful, thrombolytic agents should be reserved for life- or limb-threatening VTE with the understanding of the increased risk of bleeding complications.

Table 20.12 Maternal and perinatal outcome in 172 patients who received thrombolytic therapy during pregnancy

	N	%
Hemorrhage	14	8
Preterm birth	10	6
Perinatal deaths	10	6
Maternal deaths	2	1

(Reproduced by permission from Turrentine MA, Braeems G, Ramirez MM. Use of thrombolytics for the treatment of thromboembolic disease during pregnancy. Obstet Gynecol 1995;50:534–541.)

Ancrod, derived from Malayan pit viper venom, is contraindicated in pregnancy. Animal studies have shown a high incidence of fetal death. Postpartum hemorrhage from the placental site also occurs at a greater frequency.

Surgical intervention

With pregnancy, surgical intervention may be indicated in some clinical situations, such as replacement of a thrombosed cardiac valve prosthesis, thrombectomy for acute iliofemoral thrombosis, embolectomy of a life-threatening massive PE, or vena cava interruption for recurrent venous emboli despite adequate anticoagulation or when anticoagulation is absolutely contraindicated. Embolectomy is a heroic measure, which may occasionally be life-saving. Transvenous catheter embolectomy has been performed successfully for expeditious management of massive PE with cardiovascular collapse (Kramer et al., 1986). There are a variety of methods for interruption of the vena cava. These methods include complete ligation, Teflon clips, and devices inserted transvenously, such as the umbrella filter or the Greenfield filter (Hux et al., 1986).

Special considerations

Antithrombin III deficiency

The first evidence of an inherited AT III defect is frequently a thromboembolic event (Megha et al., 1990). Pregnant patients with inherited AT III deficiency often require therapeutic anticoagulation through the pregnancy and the puerperium (Brandt, 1981; Hellgren et al., 1982; Samson et al., 1984; Nelson et al., 1985; Leclerc et al., 1986; De Stefano et al., 1988; Schwartz et al., 1989; Conrad et al., 1990). In addition to heparin therapy throughout pregnancy (Brandt, 1981; Samson et al., 1984; Leclerc et al., 1986; Conrad et al., 1990), IV administration of AT III concentrate may be necessary (Nelson et al., 1985; De Stefano et al., 1988) to minimize the patient's risk of a thromboembolism. This can be accomplished with fresh frozen plasma, but AT III concentrate is preferable (Brandt, 1981;

Samson et al., 1984; Leclerc et al., 1986). The loading dose of AT III is 50–70 units/kg. This is followed by 20–30 units/kg/day to maintain an AT III level of 80% of normal (Hellgren et al., 1982). The higher the AT III level, the less heparin will be required for therapeutic anticoagulation. If these patients remain untreated during pregnancy, 68% will develop thromboembolism (Hellgren et al., 1982; Nelson et al., 1985; Schwartz et al., 1989; Conrad et al., 1990). In patients who require high doses of heparin to achieve anticoagulation, prophylactic biweekly doses of AT III concentrate may be necessary (Schwartz et al., 1989). Many patients require lifelong anticoagulation, which is best achieved by oral anticoagulants when not pregnant and heparin throughout pregnancy.

Protein C or S deficiencies

In contrast to patients with AT III deficiency, patients with protein C or S deficiency carry a lower risk of antepartum thrombosis (Broekmans et al., 1985; Compt & Clouse, 1985; Marciniak et al., 1985; Rose et al., 1986; Malm et al., 1988; Lac et al., 1989, 1990; Conrad et al., 1990; Tharakan et al., 1993; Faught et al., 1995; Goodwin et al., 1995). The incidences of antepartum thrombosis in the untreated patient with protein C and protein S deficiency in one series was 17% and 0% respectively. The postpartum risks, however, were similar (Conrad et al., 1990). While there is a split of opinion regarding heparin prophylaxis during pregnancy, there is uniform agreement that anticoagulant therapy is warranted in the puerperium (Broekmans et al., 1985; Comp & Clouse, 1985; Marciniak et al., 1985; Rose et al., 1986; Malm et al., 1988; Lao et al., 1989, 1990; Conrad et al., 1990; Tharakan et al., 1993; Faught et al., 1995; Goodwin et al., 1995). For patients with recurrent thromboembolism or a family history of these deficiencies, prenatal screening for AT III, protein C, and protein S appears reasonable.

References

Alderson PO. Scintigraphic evaluation of pulmonary embolism. Eur J Nucl Med 1987;13:S6–S10.

American College of Obstetricians and Gynecologists Education Bulletin Number 233 Teratology. Washington, DC, February 1997.

American College of Obstetricians and Gynecologists Education Bulletin Number 19, August 2000.

American Society of Regional Anesthesia (ASRA). Recommendations for neuraxial anesthesia and anticoagulation. VA:ASRA, 1998.

Anderson G, Fagrell B, Holmgren K, et al. Subcutaneous administration of heparin: a randomized comparison with intravenous administration of heparin to patients with deep-vein thrombosis. Thromb Res 1982;27:631–639.

Atalla RK, Thompson JR, Oppenheimer CA, Bell SC, Taylor DJ. Reactive thrombocytosis after caesarean section and vaginal delivery: implications for maternal thromboembolism and its prevention. Br J Obstet Gynaecol 2000;107(3):411–414.

Barbour LA, Pickard J. Controversies in thromboembolic disease during pregnancy: a critical review. Obstet Gynecol 1995;86:621–633.

Barbour LA, Smith JM, Marar RA. Heparin levels to guide thromboembolism prophylaxis during pregnancy. Am J Obstet Gynecol 1995;173:1869–1873.

Barnes RW, Wu KK, Hoak JC. Fallibility of the clinical diagnosis of venous thrombosis. JAMA 1975;234:605–608.

Barss VA, Schwartz PA, Greene MF, et al. Use of the subcutaneous heparin pump during pregnancy. J Reprod Med 1985;30:899–901.

Basu D, Gallus A, Hirsh J, et al. A prospective study of the value of monitoring heparin treatment with the activated partial thromboplastin time. N Engl J Med 1972;287:324–327.

Bell WR, Simon TL, DeMets DL. The clinical features of submassive pulmonary emboli. Am J Med 1977;62:355–360.

Bentley PG, Kakkar VV. Radionuclide venography for the demonstrations of the proximal deep venous system. Br J Surg 1979;66: 687–690.

Berg CJ, Atrash HK, Koonin LM, Tucker M. Pregnancy-related mortality in the United States, 1997–1990. Obstet Gynecol 1996;88:161–167.

Bergqvist A, Bergqvist D, Hallbook T. Acute deep vein thrombosis (DVT) after cesarean section. Acta Obstet Gynecol (Scand) 1983;62:473–477.

Bergqvist A, Bergqvist D, lindhagen A, et al. Late symptoms after pregnancy-related deep vein thrombosis. Br J Obstet Gynaecol 1990;97:338–344.

Bergqvist D, Benoni G, Bjorgell O, et al. Low molecular-weight heparin (enoxaparin) as prophylaxis against venous thromboembolism after total hip replacement. N Engl J Med 1996;335:696–700.

Bertina RM, Koeleman BPC, Koster T, et al. Mutation in blood coagulation factor V associated with resistance to activated protein C. Nature 1994;396:64–67.

Bettman MA, Paulin S. Leg phlebography: the incidence, nature and modifications of undesireable side effects. Radiology 1977;122: 101–108.

Bonnar J. Venous thromboembolism and pregnancy. Clin Obstet Gynecol 1981;8:445–473.

Bonnar J. Can more be done in obstetric and gynecologic practice to reduce morbidity and mortality associated with venous thromboemblism. Am J Obstet Gynecol. 1999;180(4):784–791.

Bonnar J, McNichol GP, Douglas AS. Fibrinolytic enzyme system and pregnancy. Br Med J 1969;3:387–389.

Bonnar J, McNichol GP, Douglas AS. Coagulation mechanisms during and after normal childbirth. Br Med J 1970;2:200–203.

Brandt JT. Current concepts of coagulation. Clin Obstet Gynecol 1985;28:3–14.

Brandt P. Observations during the treatment of antithrombin III deficient women with heparin and antithrombin concentrate during pregnancy, parturition, and abortion. Thromb Res 1981;22: 15–24.

Bratt G, Tornebohm E, Lockner D, et al. A human pharmacological study comparing conventional heparin and a low molecular weight heparin fragment. Thromb Haemost 1985;53:208–211.

Brill-Edwards P, Ginsberg J, Gent M, et al. For the recurrence of clot in this pregnancy study group. N Engl J Med 2000;343:1439–1444.

Broekmans AW, Bertina RM, Reinalda-Poot J, et al. Hereditary protein-S deficiency and venous thromboembolism. Thromb Haemost 1985;53:273–277.

Chang MKB, Harvey D, deSwiet M. Follow-up study of children whose mothers were treated with warfarin during pregnancy. Br J Obstet Gynaecol 1984;91:70–73.

Chong BH, Pitney WR, Castaldi PA. Heparin-induced thrombocytopenia: association of thrombotic complications with heparin-dependent IgG antibody that induces thromboxane synthesis and platelet aggregation. Lancet 1982;2:1246–1249.

Clagett GP, Anderson FA, Heit J, et al. Prevention of venous thromboembolism. Chest 1995;108 (Suppl 4):S312–334.

Clark-Peterson DL, Synan IS, Dodge R, et al. A randomized trial of low-dose heparin and intermittent pneumatic calf compression for the prevention of deep venous thrombosis after gynecologic oncology surgery. Am J Obstet Gynecol 1993;168:1146–1154.

Collins R, Scrimgeour A, Peto R. Reduction in fatal pulmonary embolism and venous thrombosis by perioperative administration of subcutaneous heparin. N Engl J Med 1988;318:1162–1173.

Colvin BT, Barrowcliff TW. The British Society from Haematology guidelines on the use and monitoring of heparin 1992: second revision. J Clin Pathol 1993;46:97–103.

Colvin BT, Machin SJ, Barrowcliffe TW, et al. Audit of oral anticoagulant treatment. The BCHS British Haemostasis and Thrombosis Task Force of the British Society for Haematology. J Clin Pathol 1993;46(12):1069–1070.

Comp PC, Clouse L. Plasma proteins C and S: the function and assay of two natural anticoagulants. Lab Management 1985;23:29–32.

Comp PC, Esman CT. Generation of fibrinolytic activity by infusion of activated protein C in dogs. J Clin Invest 1981;68:1221–1228.

Conrad J, Horellou MH, Van Dredan P, et al. Thrombosis and pregnancy in congenital deficiencies in antithrombin III, protein C or protein S: study of 78 women. Thromb Haemost 1990;63:319–320.

Cross JJ, Kemp PM, Walsh CG, Flower CD, Dixon AK. A randomized trial of spiral CT and ventilation perfusion scintigraphy for the diagnosis of pulmonary embolism. Clin Radiol 1998;53:177–182.

Dahlback B. Inherited resistance to activated protein C, a major cause of venous thrombosis, is due to a mutation in the factor V gene. Haemostasis 1994;24:139–151.

Dahlman TC. Osteoporotic fractures and the recurrence of thromboembolism during pregnancy and the puerperium in 184 women undergoing thromboprophylaxis with heparin. Am J Obstet Gynecol 1993;168:1265–1270.

Dahlman TC, Hellgren M, Blomback M. Thrombosis prophylaxis in pregnancy with use of subcutaneous heparin adjusted by monitoring heparin concentration in plasma. Am J Obstet Gynecol 1989;161:420–425.

Dahlman T, Lindvall N, Hellgren M. Osteopenia in pregnancy during long-term heparin treatment: a radiologic study postpartum. Br J Obstet Gynaecol 1990;97:221–224.

Dahlman TC, Sjoberg HE, Ringertz H. Bone mineral density during long-term prophylaxis with heparin in pregnancy. Am J Obstet Gynecol 1994;170:1315–1320.

Dalen JE, Banas JS, Brooks HC, et al. Resolution rate of acute pulmonary embolism in man. N Engl J Med 1969;280:1194–1199.

Dalen JE, Brooks HL, Johnson LW, et al. Pulmonary angiography in acute pulmonary embolism: indications, techniques, and results in 367 patients. Am Heart J 1971;81:175–185.

Daniel DG, Campbell H, Turnbull AC. Puerperal thromboembolism and suppression of lactation. Lancet 1967;2:287–289.

Danilenko-Dixon DR, Heit JA, Silverstein MD, et al. Risk factors for deep vein thrombosis and pulmonary embolism during pregnancy or post partum: a population-based, case control study. Am J Obstet Gynecol 2001;184(2):104–110.

De Stefano V, Leone G, DeCarolis S, et al. Management of pregnancy in women with antithrombin III congenital defect: report of four cases. Thromb Haemost 1988;59:193–196.

De Stefano V, Leone G, Mastrangelo S, et al. Clinical manifestations and management of inherited thrombophilia: retrospective analysis and follow-up after diagnosis of 238 patients with congenital deficiency of antithrombin III, protein C, protein S. Thromb Haemost 1994;72:352–358.

DeSwart CAM, Nijmeter B, Roelofs JMM, et al. Kinetics of intravenously administered heparin in normal humans. Blood 1982;60:1251–1258.

de Swiet M, Ward PD, Fidler J, et al. Prolonged heparin therapy in pregnancy causes bone demineralization. Br J Obstet Gynaecol 1983;90:1129–1134.

Dizon-Townson DS, Nelson LM, Jang H, Varner MW, Ward K. The incidence of the factor V Leiden mutation in an obstetric population and its relationship to deep vein thrombosis. Am J Obstet Gynecol 1997;176:883–886.

Dorfman GS, Cronan JJ, Tupper TB, et al. Occult pulmonary embolism: a common occurrence in deep venous thrombosis. AJR 1987;148: 263–267.

Douketis JD, Ginsberg JS. Diagnostic problems with venous thromboembolic disease in pregnancy. Haemostasis 1995;25:58–71.

Eldor A. Thrombophilia, thrombosis and pregnancy. Thromb Haemost 2001;86:104–111.

Ellison MJ, Sawyer WT, Mills TC. Claculation of heparin dosage in a morbidly obese woman. Clin Pharm 1989;8:65–68.

European Fraxiparin Study (EFS) Group. Comparison of a low molecular weight heparin and unfractionated heparin for the prevention of deep vein thrombosis in patients undergoing abdominal surgery. Br J Surg 1988;75:1058–1063.

Ezekowitz MD, Pope CF, Smith EO. Indium-111 platelet imaging. In: Goldhaber SE, ed. Pulmonary embolism and deep vein thrombosis. Philadelphia: WB Saunders, 1985;261–267.

Fairfax WR, Thomas F, Orme JF. Pulmonary artery catheter occlusion as an indication of pulmonary embolism. Chest 1984;86:270–272.

Faught W, Garner P, Jones G, Ivey B. Changes in protein C and protein S levels in normal pregnancy. Am J Obstet Gynecol 1995;172: 147–150.

Fausett MB, Vogtlander M, Lee RM, et al. Heparin-induced thrombocytopenia is rare in pregnancy. Am J Obstet Gynecol 2001;185(1): 148–152.

Fejgin MD, Lourwood DL. Low molecular weight heparins and their use in the obstetrics and gynecology. Obstet Gynecol Surv 1994; 49:424–431.

Files JC, Malpass TW, Yee EK, et al. Studies of human platelet alpha-granule release in vivo. Blood 1981;58:607–618.

Franks AL, Atrash HK, Lawson HW, et al. Obstetrical pulmonary embolism mortality, United States, 1970–85. Am J Public Health 1990;80:720–722.

Gabel HD. Maternal mortality in South Carolina from 1970 to 1984: an analysis. Obstet Gynecol 1987;69:307–311.

Galle PC, Muss HB, McGrath KM, et al. Thrombocytopenia in two patients treated with low-dose heparin. Obstet Gynecol 1978; 52(Suppl):95–115.

Gallus A, Jackaman J, Tillet J, et al. Safety and efficacy of warfarin started early after submassive venous thrombosis or pulmonary embolism. Lancet 1986;2:1293–1296.

Gerhardt A, Scharf RE, Beckmann MW, et al. Prothrombin and factor V mutations in women with a history of thrombosis during pregnancy and the puerperium. N Engl J Med 2000;342:374–380.

Geerts WH, Jay RM, Code K, et al. A comparison of low-dose heparin with low-molecular-weight heparin as prophylaxis against venous thromboembolism after major trauma. N Engl J Med 1996;355: 701–707.

Gherman RB, Goodwin TM, Leung B, Byrne JD, Hethumumi R, Montoro M. Incidence, clinical characteristics, and timing of objectively diagnosed venous thromboembolism during pregnancy. Obstet Gynecol 1999;94:730–734.

Gillis S, Shushan A, Eldor A. Use of low molecular weight heparin for prophylaxis and treatment of thromboembolism in pregnancy. Int J Gynecol Obstet 1992;39:297–301.

Ginsberg JS. Management of venous thromboembolism. N Engl J Med 1996;334:1816–1828.

Ginsberg JS, Hirsh J. Use of antithrombotic agents during pregnancy. Chest 1992;315:1109–1114

Ginsberg JS, Hirsh J. Use of antithrombotic agents during pregnancy. Chest 1995;108:3055–3115.

Ginsberg JS, Kowalchuck G, Brill-Edwards P, et al. Heparin therapy in pregnancy: effects on the fetus. Clin Res 1988;36:A410.

Ginsberg JSA, Hirsh J, Rainbow AJ, et al. Risks to the fetus of radiologic procedures used in the diagnosis of maternal venous thromboembolic disease. Thromb Haemost 1989a;61:189–196.

Ginsberg JS, Hirsh J, Tuner C, et al. Risks to the fetus of anticoagulant therapy during pregnancy. Thromb Haemost 1989b;61:197–203.

Gold WM, McCormack KR. Pulmonary function response to radioisotope scanning of the lungs. JAMA 1966;197:146–148.

Goodwin TM, Gazit G, Gordon EM. Heterozygous protein C deficiency presenting as severe protein C deficiency and peripartum thrombosis: successful treatment with protein C concentrate. Obstet Gynecol 1995;86:662–664.

Gottlieb RH, Widjaja J, Tian L, Rubens DJ, Voci SL. Calf sonography for detecting deep vein thrombosis in symptomatic patients: experience and review of the literature. J Clin Ultrasound 1999;27(8): 415–420.

Grandone E, Margaglione M, Colaizzo D, D'Andrea G, Cappucci G, Branacaccio V, et al. Genetic susceptibility to pregnancy-related venous thromboembolism: roles of factor V Leiden, prothrombin G20210A, and methylenetetrahydrofolate reductase C677T mutations. Am J Obstet Gynecol 1998;179:1324–1328.

Griffith GC. Heparin osteoporosis. JAMA 1965;143:85–88.

Hall JG, Pauli RM, Wilson KM. Maternal and fetal sequelae of anticoagulation during pregnancy. Am J Med 1978;122–140.

Hathaway WE, Bonnar J. Perinatal coagulation. New York: Grune & Stratten, 1978.

Hellgren M, Tengborn L, Abildgaard U. Pregnancy in women with congenital antithrombin III deficiency: experience of treatment with heparin and antithrombin. Obstet Gynecol Invest 1982;14:127–130.

Henkin RE. Radionuclide detection of thromboembolic disease. In: Kwaan HC, Bowie EJQ, eds. Thrombosis. Philadelphia: WB Saunders, 1982;236–252.

Hirsch J. The treatment of venous thromboembolism. Nouv Rev Fr Hematol 1988;30:149–153.

Hirsch J. Heparin. N Engl J Med 1991;324:1565.

Hirsch J. The optimal duration of anticoagulant therapy for venous thrombosis. N Engl J Med 1995;332:1710–1711.

Hirsch J, Barrowcliffe TW. Standardization and clinical use of LMW heparin. Thromb Haemost 1988;59:333–337.

Hirsch J, Daeln JE, Deykin D, Poller L. Heparin: mechanisms of action, dosing considerations, monitoring, efficacy, and safety. Chest 1992;102:337–350.

Holm HA, Abildgaard U, Kalvenes S. Heparin assays and bleeding complications in treatment of deep venous thrombosis with particular reference to retroperitoneal bleeding. Thromb Haetmost 1985;53:278–281.

Horn JR, Danzinger LH, Davis RJ. Warfarin-induced skin necrosis: report of four cases. Am J Hosp Pharm 1981;38:1763–1768.

Howell R, Fidler J, Letsky E, deSwiet M. The risks of antenatal subcutaneous heparin prophylaxis: a controlled trial. Br J Obstet Gynecol 1983;90:1124–1128.

Huisman MV, Buller HR, ten Case JW, Vreeken JR. Seriel impedance plethysmography for suspected deep venous thrombosis in outpatients: the Amsterdam General Partitions Study. N Engl J Med 1986;314:823–882.

Hull R, Delmore T, Carter C, et al. Adjusted subcutaneous heparin versus warfarin sodium in the long-term treatment of venous thrombosis. N Engl J Med 1982;306:189–194.

Hull RD, Hirsh J, Carter CJ, et al. Pulmonary angiography, ventilation lung scanning, and venography for clinically suspected pulmonary embolism with abnormal perfusion lung scan. Ann Intern Med 1983;98:891–899.

Hux CH, Wagner R, Rattan P, et al. Surgical treatment of thromboembolic disease in pregnancy. Proceedings of the Society or Perinatal Obstetricians, January 30–February 1, 1986:62. Abstract.

Hyers TM, Hull RD, Weg JG. Antithrombotic therapy for venous thromboembolic disease. Chest 1986;89:265–355.

Jeffcoate TNA, Miller J, Roos RF, Tindall VR. Puerperal thromboembolism in relation to the inhibition of lactation by oestrogen therapy. Br Med J 1968;4:19–22.

Kakkar V. The diagnosis of deep vein thrombosis using the ^{125}I fibrinogen test. Arch Surg 1972;104:152–159.

Kakkar VV, Stamatatkis JD, Bentley PG, et al. Prophylaxis for postoperative deep-vein thrombosis: synergistic effect of heparin and dihydroergotamine. JAMA 1979;241:39–42.

Kaplan KL, Owen J. Plasma levels of B-thromboglobulin and platelet factor 4 and indices of platelet activation in vivo. Blood 1981;57:199–202.

Kaunitz AM, Hughes JM, Grimes DA, et al. Causes of maternal mortality in the United States. Obstet Gynecol 1985;65:605–612.

Kim KL, Muller NL, Mayo JR. Clinically suspected pulmonary embolism: utility of spiral CT. Radiology 1999;210:693–697.

Kipper MS, Moser KM, Kortman KE, et al. Long-term follow-up of patients with suspected pulmonary embolism and a normal lung scan. Perfusion scans in embolic subjects. Chest 1982;82:411–415.

Kohn H, Konig B, Mostbeck A. Incidence and clinical feature of pulmonary embolism in patients with deep vein thrombosis: a prospective study. Eur J Nucl Med 1987;13:S11–S13.

Koopman MMW, Prandoni P, Piovella F. Treatment of venous thrombosis with intravenous unfractionated heparin administered in the hospital as compared with subcutaneous low-molecular weight heparin administered at home. N Engl J Med 1996;334:682–687.

Kramer FL, Teitelbaum G, Merli GJ. Panvenography and pulmonary angiography in the diagnosis of deep venous thrombosis and pulmonary thromboembolism. Radiol Clin North Am 1986;24:397–418.

Lao TT, Yuen PMP, Yin JA. Protein S and Protein C levels in Chinese women during pregnancy, delivery, and puerperium. Br J Obstet Gynaecol 1989;96:167–170.

Lao TT, Yin JA, Ng WK, Yuen PMP. Relationship between maternal antithrombin III and protein C/protein S levels before, during, and after delivery. Gynecol Obstet Invest 1990;30:87–90.

Lawson HW, Atrash HK, Franks AL. Fatal pulmonary embolism during legal induced abortion in the United States from 1972 to 1985. Am J Obstet Gynecol 1990;162:986–990.

Lebsack CS, Weibert RT. "Purple toes" syndrome. Postgrad Med 1982;71:81–84.

Leclerc JR. Pulmonary embolism. In: Rakel RE, ed. Conn's current therapy—1994. Philadelphia: WB Saunders, 1994:199–205.

Leclerc JR, Geerts W, Panju A, et al. Management of antithrombin III deficiency during pregnancy without administration of antithrombin III. Thromb Res 1986;41:567–573.

Lensing AW, Prins MH, Davidson BE, et al. Treatment of deep-venous thrombosis with low molecular weight heparins: a meta-ananlysis. Arch Intern Med 1995;155:601–607.

Lepercq J, Conard J, Borel-Derlon A, et al. Venous thromboembolism during pregnancy: a retrospective study of enoxaparin safety in 624 pregnancies. Br J Obstet Gynaecol 2001;108(11):1134–1140.

Letsky EA. Coagulation problems during pregnancy. In: Lind T, ed. Current review in obstetrics and gynecology. Edinburgh: Churchill Livingstone, 1985.

Levine M, Gent M, Hirsh J, et al. A comparison of low-molecular weight heparin administered primarily at home with unfractionated heparin administered in the hospital for proximal deep-vein thrombosis. New Engl J Med 1996;334:677–681.

Lewis JF, Anderson TW, Fennel WH, et al. A clue to pulmonary embolism obtained during Swan-Ganz catheterization. Chest 1982;81:257–529.

Lindqvist P, Dahlback B, Marsal K. Thrombotic risk during pregnancy, a population study. Obstet Gynecol 1999;94:595–599.

Lipchik RJ, Goodman LR. Spiral computed tomography in the evalution of pulmonary embolism. Clin Chest Med 1999;20:731–738.

McFarlane MJ, Imperiale TF. Use of the alveolar-arterial oxygen gradient in the diagnosis of pulmonary embolism. Am J Med 1994;96:57–62.

McLean R, Mattison ET, Cochrane NE. Maternal mortality study annual report 1970–1976. NY State J Med 1979;79:39–43.

Magnani HN. Heparin induced thrombocytopenia (HIT): an overview of 230 patients treated with orgaran (Org 10172). Thromb Haemost 1993;70:554–561.

Marciniak E, Wilson HD, Marlar RA. Neonatal purpura fulminans: a genetic disorder related to the absence of protein C in blood. Blood 1985;65:15–20.

Malm J, Laurell M, Dahlbeck B. Changes in the plasma levels of vitamin K dependent protein C and S and of C4b-binding protein during pregnancy and oral contraception. Br J Haematol 1988;68:437–443.

Markisz JA. Radiologic and nuclear medicine diagnosis. In: Goldhaber SZ, ed. Pulmonary embolism and deep venous thrombosis. Philadelphia: WB Saunders, 1985:41–72.

Megha A, Finzi G, Poli T, et al. Pregnancy, antithrombin III deficiency and venous thrombosis: report of another case. Acta Heamatol 1990;83:111–114.

Middeldorp S, Henkens CM, Koopman MM, et al. The incidence of venous thromboembolism in family members of patients with factor V Leiden mutation and venous thrombosis. Ann Intern Med 1998;128:15–20.

Mills SR, Jackson DC, Older RA, et al. The incidence etiologies, and avoidance of complications of pulmonary angiography in a large series. Radiology 1980;136:295–299.

Mohr DN, Ryu JH, Litin SC, Rosenow EC III. Recent advances in the management of venous thromboembolism. Mayo Clin Proc 1988;63:281–290.

Monreal M, Salvador R, Ruiz, J. Below-knee deep venous thrombosis and pulmonary embolism. AJR 1987;149:860. Letter.

Moran KT, Jewell ER, Persson AV. The role of thrombolytic therapy in surgical practice. Br J Surg 1989;76:298–304.

Moser KM, Fedullo PE. Venous thromboembolism: threes simple decisions (part 2). Chest 1983;83:256–260.

Moser KM, LeMoine JR. Is embolic risk continued by location of deep venous thrombosis? Ann Intern Med 1981;94:439–444.

Moses DC, Silver TM, Bookstein JJ. The complementary roles of chest radiography, lung scanning and selective pulmonary angiography in the diagnosis of pulmonary embolism. Circulation 1974;44: 179–185.

National Council on Radiation Protection and Measurements. Medical Radiation Exposure of Pregnant and Potentially Pregnant Women. Bethesda, Maryland: NCRPM, 1977.

Needleman P, Minkes M, Raz A. Thromboxanes: selected biosynthesis and distinct biological properties. Science 1976;193:163–165.

Negus D, Friedgood A, Cox SJ, et al. Ultra-low dose intravenous heparin in the prevention of postoperative deep-vein thrombosis. Lancet 1980;1:891–894.

Nelson DM, Stempel LE, Fabri PJ, et al. Hickman catheter use in a pregnant patient requiring therapeutic heparin antiocoagulation. Am J Obstet Gynecol 1984;149:461–462.

Nelson DM, Stempel LE, Brandt JT. Hereditary antithrombin III deficiency and pregnancy: report of two cases and review of the literature. Obstet Gynecol 1985;65:848–853.

Nicholas GG, Lorenz RP, Botti JJ, et al. The frequent occurrence of false-positive results in phleborrheography during pregnancy. Surg Gynecol Obstet 1985;161:133–136.

Nichols AB, Beller BA, Cochari S, et al. Detection of pulmonary embolism by positron imaging of inhaled ^{15}O-labeled carbon dioxide. Semin Nucl Med 1980;10:252–258.

Park S, Schroeter AL, Park YS, Fortson J. Purple toes and livido reticularis in a patient with cardiovascular disease taking coumadin. Arch Dermatol 1993;129:775–780.

Perry PJ, Herron GR, King JC. Heparin half-life in normal and impaired renal function. Clin Pharmacol Res 1974;16:514–519.

Phillips YY, Copley JB, Stor RA. Thrombocytopenia and low dose heparin. South Med J 1983;76:526–528.

PIOPED Investigators. Value of the ventilation/perfusion scan in acute pulmonary embolism: results of the prospective investigation of pulmonary embolism diagnosis (PIOPED). JAMA 1990;263: 2753–2759.

Powrie R, Star JA, Rosene-Montella K. Deep venous thrombosis and pulmonary embolism in pregnancy. Med Health RI 1998;81(4):141–143.

Raghavendra BN, Rosen RJ, Lam S, et al. Deep venous thrombosis: detection by high-resolution real-time ultrasonography. Radiology 1984;152:789–792.

Rao AK, White GC, Sherman L, et al. Low incidence of thrombocytopenia with porcine mucosal heparin. A prospective multicenter study. Arch Intern Med 1989;149:1285–1288.

Rasmussen C, Wadt J, Jacobsen B. Thromboembolic prophylaxis with low molecular weight heparin during pregnancy. Int J Obstet Gynecol 1994;47:121–125.

Ridker PM, Miletich JP, Hennekens CH, Buring JE. Ethnic distribution of factor V Leiden in 4047 men and women. Implications for venous thromboembolism screening. JAMA 1997;277(16):1305–1307.

Robbins KC. The plasminogen-plasmin enzyme system. In: Colman RW, Hirsh J, Marder VJ, et al. eds. Hemostasis and thrombosis. Philadelphia: JB Lippincott, 1982.

Robin ED. Overdiagnosis and overtreatment of pulmonary embolism: the emperor may have no clothes. Ann Intern Med 1977;87:775–776.

Rochat RW, Koonin LM, Atrash HK, et al. Maternal mortality in the United States: report from the Maternal Mortality Collaborative. Obstet Gynecol 1988;72:91–97.

Rose PG, de Moerloose PA, Bounameaux H. Protein S deficiency in pregnancy. Am J Obstet Gynecol 1986;155:140–141.

Rosenow EC III, Osmundson PJ, Brown ML. Pulmonary embolism. Mayo Clin Proc 1981;56:161–178.

Rutherford SE, Phelan JP. Deep venous thrombosis and pulmonary embolism in pregnancy. Obstet Gynecol Clin North Am 1991;18:345–370.

Rutherford SE, Montoro M, McGehee W, et al. Thromboembolic disease associated with pregnancy: an 11-year review, SPO Abstract 139. Am J Obstet Gynecol 1991;164:286.

Sachs BP, Yeh J, Acher D, et al. Cesarean section related maternal mortality in Massachusetts, 1954–1985. Obstet Gynecol 1988;71: 385–388.

Salazar E, Zajarias A, Gutierrez N, et al. The problem of cardiac valve prostheses, anticoagulants, and pregnancy. Circulation 1984;70(Suppl I):169–177.

Salzman EW, Hirsh J. Prevention of venous thromboembolism. In: Colman RW, Hirsh J, Marder VJ, Slazman EW, eds. Hemostasis and thrombosis: basic principles and clinical practice, 2nd edn. Philadelphia: JB Lippincott, 1987:1252–1264.

Samama M. (The new heparins). Presse Med 1986;15:1631–1635.

Samson D, Stirling Y, Woolf L, et al. Management of planned pregnancy in a patient with congenital antithrombin III deficiency. Br J Haematol 1984;56:243–249.

Schiff MJ, Feinberg AW, Naidich JB. Noninvasive venous examinations as a screening test for pulmonary embolism. Arch Intern Med 1987;147:505–507.

Schulman S, Rhedin A, Lindmarker P, et al. A comparison of six weeks with six months of oral anticoagulant therapy after a first episode of venous thromboembolism. N Engl J Med 1995;332:1661–1665.

Schwartz RS, Bauer KA, Rosenberg RD, et al. Clinical experience with antithrombin III concentrate in treatment of congenital and acquired deficiency of antithrombin. Am J Med 1989;87(Suppl 3B):535–605.

Sharma GVRK, Cella, G, Parisi AF, et al. Thrombolytic therapy. N Engl J Med 1985;306:1268–1276.

Spritzer CE, Evans AC, Kay HH. Magnetic resonance imaging of deep venous thrombosis in pregnant women with lower extremity edema. Obstet Gynecol 1995;85:603–607.

Standing Advisory Committee for Haematolgoy of the Royal College of Pathologists. Drug interaction with coumarin derivative anticoagulants. Br Med J 1982;185:274–275.

Stead RB. Regulation of hemostasis. In: Goldhaber SZ, ed. Pulmonary embolism and deep venous thrombosis. Philadelphia: WB Saunders 1985:27–40.

Stevenson RE, Burton OM, Ferlauto GJ, Taylor HA. Hazards of oral anticoagulants during pregnancy. JAMA 1980;243:1549–1551.

Stringer MD, Kakkar VV. Prevention of venous thromboembolism. Herz 1989;14:135–147.

Sturridge F, Letsky E. The use of low molecular weight heparin for thrombophylaxis in pregnancy. Br J Obstet Gynecol 1994;101: 69–71.

Tenero DM, Bell HE, Deitz PA, Bertino JS Jr. Comparative dosage and toxicity of heparin sodium in the treatment of patients with pulmonary embolism versus deep-vein thrombosis. Clin Phar 1989;8:40–43.

Tengborn L, Bergqvist D, Matzsch T, et al. Recurrent thromboembolism in pregnancy and puerperium: is there a need for thromboprophylaxis? Am J Obstet Gynecol 1989;160:90–94.

Tharakan T, Baxi LV, Dinguid D. Protein S deficiency in pregnancy. A case report. Am J Obstet Gynecol 1993;168:141–142.

Thompson AR, Harker CA. Manual of thrombosis and hemostasis. Philadelphia: FA Davis, 1983.

Toglia MR, Weg JG. Venous thromboembolism during pregnancy. N Engl J Med 1996;335:108–114.

Traeger SM. Failure to wedge pulmonary hypertension during pulmonary artery catheterization: a sign of totally occlusive pulmonary embolism. Crit Care Med 1985;13:544–547.

Turrentine MA, Braems G, Ramirez MM. Use of thrombolytics for the treatment of thromboembolic disease during pregnancy. Obstet Gynecol Surv 1995;50:534–541.

Urokinase Pulmonary Embolism Trial. A national cooperative study. Circulation 1973;43(Suppl II):47.

Urokinase-Streptokinase Pulmonary Embolism Trail. Phase 2 results. A cooperative study. JAMA 1974;229:1606–1613.

Vincent WR, Goldberg SJ, Desilets D. Fatality immediately following rapid infusion a macroaggregates of ^{99m}Tc albumin (MAA) for lung scan. Radiology 1968;91:1181–1184.

Walker AM, Jick H. Predictors of bleeding during heparin therapy. JAMA 1980;244:1209–1212.

White TM, Bernene JL, Marino AM. Continuous heparin infusion requirements: diagnostic and therapeutic implications. JAMA 1979;241:2717–2720.

Woodhams BJ, Candotti G, Shaw R, et al. Changes in coagulation and fibrinolysis during pregnancy: evidence of activation of coagulation preceding spontaneous abortion. Thromb Res 1989;88:26–30.

Zimran A, Shilo S, Fisher D, et al. Histomorphometric evaluation of reversible heparin-induced osteoporosis in pregnancy. Arch Intern Med 1986;146:386–388.

Zoller B, Dahlback BD. Linkage between inherited resistance to activated protein c and factor v gene mutation in venous thrombosis. Lancet 1994;343:1536–1538.

21 Etiology and management of hemorrhage

Rosie Burton
Michael A. Belfort

In patients with major obstetric hemorrhage, measures must be taken to identify the cause, and to arrest the bleeding simultaneously with management of hypovolemic shock. Continued hemorrhage, particularly if concealed or underestimated, may result in the onset of irreversible shock.

Life-threatening hemorrhage occurs in 1 in 1,000 deliveries (Bonnar, 2000). The major obstetric causes are placental abruption, placenta previa, uterine rupture, and postpartum hemorrhage. Their specific management will be discussed in this chapter. Inherited or acquired bleeding disorders may also cause or contribute to obstetric hemorrhage. These include disorders existing prior to pregnancy (von Willebrand's disease, hemophilia)—discussed in this chapter. Conditions caused by pregnancy (HELLP syndrome, acute fatty liver of pregnancy) and disseminated intravascular coagulation are discussed in other chapters.

Massive hemorrhage may also result from surgical causes in pregnant or postpartum women. These include liver rupture in HELLP syndrome, and rupture of aortic, splenic, and renal artery aneurysms. Although rare, these should be considered in patients with hemorrhagic shock and concealed bleeding in whom an obstetric cause such as abruption, pelvic hematoma, or uterine rupture is unlikely.

Placental abruption

Placental abruption is defined as the premature separation of a normally situated placenta, and may be partial or complete. The underlying mechanism is unknown. Hemorrhage occurs into the decidua basalis, forming a hematoma which splits the decidua (Baron & Hill, 1988). As the hematoma expands, further placental separation ensues. The incidence of abruption is 0.45–1.3% of deliveries, and it may occur from the midtrimester onwards. Preeclampsia is the most common risk factor and is found in approximately 50% of women with placental abruption (Lowe & Cunningham, 1990). Other risk factors include cocaine use, smoking, multiparity, chorioamnionitis and blunt trauma; Black women are more at risk than other population groups (Pritchard et al., 1991). There is approximately a 10% recurrence rate during a subsequent pregnancy.

The classical signs of placental abruption are abdominal pain and vaginal bleeding, together with fetal distress or intrauterine death. The woman may develop uterine tenderness and uterine contractions, however these signs are not necessarily present. Vaginal bleeding may be revealed or concealed—the latter may lead to delays in seeking medical help and in diagnosis. In a major abruption blood extravasates into the myometrium, the uterus becomes "woody hard" with fetal parts no longer palpable—the Couvelaire uterus. Hemorrhagic shock and coagulopathy may be present. Blood loss may be over 50% of maternal blood volume with abruption severe enough to kill the fetus (Pritchard & Brekken, 1967). Coagulation defects appear to develop rapidly after the occurrence of a severe abruption, within a few hours, or even in minutes (Lowe & Cunningham, 1990).

Resuscitation with fluid, blood, and correction of coagulopathy must urgently be undertaken, and invasive monitoring may be necessary. Women with preeclampsia complicated by placental abruption need particular care in resuscitation. These patients tolerate hypovolemia poorly because of the contracted intravascular volume and low cardiac output, and are also highly susceptible to pulmonary edema due to volume overload (Anthony et al., 1994). If the fetus is alive and of a viable gestational age at presentation, urgent delivery by cesarean section is indicated unless vaginal delivery is imminent. Coagulopathy is uncommon with a surviving fetus; prompt delivery prevents further decompensation of both mother and fetus (Lowe & Cunningham, 1990). If severe fetal distress is diagnosed prior to cesarean, presence of fetal heart activity should be verified before anesthesia is commenced.

Major abruption sufficient to cause fetal death is life threatening for the mother. Blood loss is frequently 50% or more of blood volume (Pritchard & Brekken, 1967); up to 5 L of blood may extravasate into the myometrium, with little or no revealed bleeding (Letsky, 2001). Thromboplastin release is a powerful trigger for disseminated intravascular coagulation.

In a series of 141 cases of abruption severe enough to kill the fetus, plasma fibrinogen concentration was below 150 mg/100 mL in 38%, and below 100 mg/100 mL in 28%, and in all cases developed within 8 hours of the onset of symptoms (Pritchard & Brekken, 1967). Delivery must be expedited, with vaginal delivery the preferred route unless contraindications exist; cesarean delivery in patients with coagulopathy leads to difficulty in achieving surgical hemostasis. While the fetus is undelivered, correction of hypovolemia, blood loss, and coagulopathy must continue. If delivery does not occur within a reasonable time, recourse to cesarean may be necessary. However, the major determinant of maternal outcome is adequate replacement of fluid and blood, rather than time to delivery (Lowe & Cunningham, 1990).

Postpartum hemorrhage must be anticipated following a severe placental abruption, and prophylactic uterotonic drugs should be considered. Uterine atony may occur; myometrial contractility is impaired by fibrin degradation products rather than by the presence of extravasated blood (Letsky, 2001). Ongoing coagulopathy increases the severity of postpartum hemorrhage. Maternal deaths from abruption are frequently postpartum, when ongoing blood loss occurs in patients with inadequate correction of hemorrhagic shock and coagulopathy prior to delivery.

Uterine rupture

Uterine rupture may occur in an unscarred uterus, at the site of a previous uterine scar from a cesarean section, or a full-thickness incision secondary to gynecological surgery. The overall rate varies from 2 to 8 per 10,000 deliveries (Phelan, 1990). Asymptomatic and bloodless dehiscence of a previous cesarean section scar may occur during subsequent vaginal delivery, and may also be seen at repeat cesarean section in women who have not labored. Uterine rupture is generally considered to include only cases with complete separation of the wall of the pregnant uterus, with or without expulsion of the fetus, that may endanger the life of the mother and/or fetus (Plaunche et al., 1984).

Rupture may occur antenatally or intrapartum; however, it is commonly first suspected postpartum. The most common clinical sign in labor is the sudden onset of fetal distress, reported in 81% of cases (Phelan, 1990). Abdominal pain, cessation of contractions, and recession of the presenting part are less common. Bleeding may be intraperitoneal and into the broad ligament rather than revealed vaginally. Over 50% of cases are first diagnosed after delivery, when intractable hemorrhage follows precipitate, spontaneous, or instrumental vaginal delivery. Alternatively if bleeding is concealed, profound shock may occur before rupture is suspected. Uterine rupture should be considered in every obstetric patient with hemorrhagic shock in whom the cause is not immediately apparent.

Rupture of an unscarred uterus is frequently related to obstetric intervention. This includes use of uterotonic drugs for induction or augmentation of labor, mid-cavity forceps delivery, or breech extraction with internal podalic version (Plaunche et al., 1984). Prolonged labor in the presence of cephalopelvic disproportion or malpresentation may also cause uterine rupture; this is most common in underdeveloped countries with poor access to medical care, but also occurs due to inappropriate management of labor in industrialized nations. External trauma may cause uterine rupture at any gestation. Grand multiparity also increases the risk. Increased blood loss, transfusion rates, and fetal mortality are clinically significant with rupture of an intact uterus.

Rupture of a previously scarred uterus is more common than rupture of the intact uterus. Of 23 cases of uterine rupture reported from New Orleans between 1975 and 1983, 61.3% (14/23) involved rupture of a previous cesarean section scar, with six cases occurring prior to labor, five during labor, and the remaining three unknown (Plaunche et al., 1984). The overall risk of uterine rupture for women attempting a trial of labor following lower segment cesarean section is 1%, but higher if the trial of labor is unsuccessful (McMahon, 1998). A previous classical cesarean section has a risk of rupture of 3–6%, increased to 12% if a trial of labor takes place. Spontaneous rupture of a classical cesarean section scar has been reported as early as 15 weeks of gestation (Endres & Barnhart, 2000). Use of uterotonic drugs (prostaglandins, oxytocin, and misoprostol) in the presence of a cesarean section scar is associated with an increased risk of rupture. The risks are difficult to quantify, and their use in patients undergoing vaginal delivery after cesarean section is controversial. Recent data indicate that induction of labor and cervical ripening with prostaglandins (PGE1 and PGE2) may carry a high risk of uterine rupture (Lydon-Rochelle et al., 2001).

Management options consist of surgical repair and hysterectomy. Published case series—many spanning several decades—vary widely in reported use of each technique, with hysterectomy rates of 26–83% (Phelan, 1990). Most authors consider hysterectomy to be the procedure of choice for uterine rupture (Plaunche et al., 1984; Eden et al., 1986). Subtotal hysterectomy may be performed if the rupture is confined to the uterine corpus. Suture repair may be considered when technically feasible and there is a desire for future fertility. However, there is an increased risk of recurrence, which may be fatal. A meta-analysis from 1971 provides the most comprehensive data (Ritchie, 1971). This analysis includes 194 women, with a total of 253 pregnancies following uterine rupture; two maternal deaths occurred. Overall, repeat rupture occurred in 6% with a previous lower segment rupture, 32% with a previous upper segment rupture, and 14% where the site of previous rupture was unknown. Of note, three women in this series had repeated rupture in two or three subsequent pregnancies. Other women had an uneventful pregnancy following uterine rupture, but with a further (even fatal) rupture in a subsequent pregnancy.

If suture repair is performed, elective cesarean section has been advocated as soon as evidence of fetal lung maturity is obtained in a future pregnancy. Repair has also been advocated if successful control of hemorrhage can be attained in hemodynamically unstable patients, avoiding further blood loss and prolonged surgery during hysterectomy. Bilateral tubal ligation should be considered in these cases.

Primary postpartum hemorrhage

Primary postpartum hemorrhage is traditionally defined as blood loss of more than 500 mL within the first 24 hours of delivery (Bonnar, 2000). However, in the 1960s, studies by Pritchard involving ^{51}Cr-labeled red cells demonstrated an average blood loss of 505 mL at vaginal delivery and 930 mL at elective repeat cesarean section (Pritchard et al., 1962). Some clinicians therefore consider as clinically significant only blood loss greater than 1,000 mL, termed major obstetric hemorrhage, with a reported incidence of 1.3% (Bonnar, 2000). However, visual estimates of blood loss are commonly inaccurate, with frequent underestimation by 30–50% (ACOG, 1998). Delay in recognizing significant postpartum hemorrhage and therefore in instituting management contributes to maternal mortality from this condition; additionally the presence of concealed hemorrhage may not be appreciated. A more objective—although retrospective—definition of postpartum hemorrhage is of a 10% change in hematocrit or a need for red blood cell transfusion. On this basis, the incidence of postpartum hemorrhage is 3.9% following vaginal delivery and 6.4% following cesarean section.

Most major hemorrhage occurs within the first hour postpartum. The blood volume expansion of 1.5–2.0 L in healthy pregnant women provides a physiological reserve for blood loss at delivery (Pritchard, 1965). However, women with a below average increase in blood volume (preeclampsia, low prepregnancy body mass index) tolerate postpartum hemorrhage less readily and are therefore more at risk of hemorrhagic shock.

Etiology of primary postpartum hemorrhage

Causes of primary postpartum hemorrhage can be divided into four major categories (Table 21.1). Prolonged or severe hemorrhage is the most common cause of coagulopathy postpartum and exacerbates bleeding due to other causes (Letsky, 2001).

Uterine atony is the most common cause of primary postpartum hemorrhage, accounting for 80% of all cases. At term, the uteroplacental circulation has a blood supply of 600–800 mL per minute. Rapid cessation of blood flow at the placental site is therefore essential, occurring via myometrial contraction causing compression of uterine vasculature. If this fails to occur, life-threatening hemorrhage may rapidly ensue. Many risk factors for uterine atony have been identified. These include high parity, chorioamnionitis, uterine fibroids, overdistention of the uterus (multiple gestation, fetal macrosomia, polyhydramnios), labor-related factors (precipitate labor, prolonged labor, oxytocin use) and uterine relaxing drugs (magnesium sulfate, halogenated anesthetic agents, nitroglycerin) (ACOG, 1998). Antepartum hemorrhage due to both abruption and placenta previa carry an increased risk for postpartum hemorrhage. Previous postpartum hemorrhage confers a 10% risk of recurrence. Management of uterine atony is outlined in the next section.

Table 21.1 Causes of primary postpartum hemorrhage

Uterine atony
Retained placental tissue
Placenta accreta and other abnormal placentation
Genital tract trauma
Vaginal lacerations
Cervical lacerations
Vulval hematoma
Broad ligament hematoma
Uterine inversion
Uterine rupture—may be first diagnosed postpartum
Coagulopathy
Secondary to hemorrhage or obstetric causes
Inherited or acquired bleeding disorders
Anticoagulant drugs

Uterine atony unresponsive to medical treatment may be due to retained placental fragments. Visual examination of the placenta following removal cannot always exclude this diagnosis; a placenta appearing complete may be missing an entire or partial cotyledon, or there may be a retained succinturiate lobe. Examination under anesthesia and evacuation of retained placental tissue is necessary. Care is required with curettage since a postpartum uterus is easily perforated (Cruikshank, 1986).

Genital tract trauma is commonly associated with instrumental delivery. Other risk factors include shoulder dystocia and precipitate delivery. Lacerations may occur throughout the urogenital system, including perineum, vagina, bladder, cervix, uterus, and anorectal tissues. Hemodynamic compromise may occur if diagnosis and repair are not carried out promptly.

Genital tract hematomas may result in postpartum cardiovascular collapse due to concealed blood loss. Vulvovaginal hematomas lie below the levator ani and may contain 1.5–2.0 L of blood (Morgans et al., 1999). They probably result from contusion or avulsion of the vascular supply due to radial stretching of vaginal tissues during delivery. They may also occur in association with inadequate hemostasis during repair of episiotomy or vaginal tears. Evacuation is required, best performed by incision through the vaginal wall to minimize scarring. Bleeding vessels require ligation, but frequently vessels may retract and the source of bleeding cannot be identified. Figure-of-eight sutures may be applied; alternatively tight packing of the hematoma cavity may be necessary. If bleeding continues despite these measures, arterial ligation or angiographic embolization may be necessary (see below).

Broad ligament hematomas may result from uterine tears due to rupture or traumatic extension of a lower segment cesarean hysterotomy. Alternatively deep cervical tears during spontaneous or operative vaginal delivery may involve the uterine artery at the base of the broad ligament (Maxwell et al., 1997). Conservative management is possible if the patient is hemodynamically stable after vaginal delivery; however bleeding may be ongoing, and diagnosis may only occur following postpartum collapse. Broad ligament hematomas may be apparent clinically by the presence of a tender, boggy mass suprapubically, with a firmly contracted uterus deviated past the midline. By the time a mass is clinically apparent, it may contain several liters of blood, and continued arterial bleeding may result in broad ligament rupture. Conservative surgery may be possible, but hysterectomy may be necessary (see below).

Uterine inversion

Uterine inversion often presents with profound shock, both neurogenic (due to traction on the uterine ligaments) and hemorrhagic (if the placenta is separated) in origin. In complete inversion, clinical diagnosis may be obvious, with the uterus not palpable abdominally and the fundus visible as a mass protruding through the introitus (Kitchin et al., 1975). Partial inversion may not be apparent without vaginal examination, leading to delayed diagnosis. Risk factors relate to the management of the third stage of labor. Predisposing factors include fundal insertion of the placenta and uterine atony, together with cord traction or fundal pressure.

The placenta should not be removed prior to uterine replacement; this exacerbates blood loss (Brar et al., 1989). Manual replacement should take place without delay, by placing a hand vaginally with the fingers placed circumferentially and the fundus cupped in the palm. Replacement is such that the region of the uterus that inverted last is the first to be replaced, so avoiding multiple layers of uterine wall within the cervical ring. Uterine relaxation may be necessary, with beta-sympathomimetic agents, magnesium sulfate, or low-dose nitroglycerine (Dayan & Schwalbe, 1996). Intravaginal hydrostatic replacement is an alternative technique (O'Sullivan, 1945). The vaginal introitus is occluded and warm saline infused into the posterior fornix from a meter or more above the patient. Ensuring an adequate vaginal seal may be difficult; use of a silastic ventouse cup connected to the infusion and then inserted into the vagina has been successfully employed (Ogueh & Ayida, 1997).

Attempting initial replacement under general anesthesia may lead to delay and is associated with increased maternal morbidity; halothane may exacerbate hypotension and cause refractory atony. If these measures fail, laparotomy is required. Two procedures are described. The first involves stepwise traction on the funnel of the inverted uterus or the round ligaments, using ring or Allis forceps reapplied progressively as the fundus emerges (Huntingdon procedure). If this fails, a longitudinal incision is made posteriorly through the cervix, relieving cervical constriction and allowing stepwise replacement (Haultain procedure).

Treatment of uterine atony

Emergency procedures

Fundal massage is the simplest treatment for uterine atony, is effective and can be performed while initial resuscitation and administration of uterotonic drugs are in progress. If this fails to rapidly control hemorrhage, bimanual compression may be successful. A fist or hand is placed within the vagina such that the uterus elevated—stretching of the uterine arteries reduces blood flow. The abdominal hand continues fundal massage, whilst also compressing the uterus. A urinary catheter may be inserted; this not only aids assessment of fluid status, but a distended bladder may interfere with uterine contractility.

Aortic compression is a temporizing procedure that can be used in life-threatening hemorrhage, particularly at cesarean section. A closed fist compresses the aorta against the vertebral column just above the umbilicus (Keogh & Tsokos, 1997). Sufficient force is required to exceed systolic blood pressure—this can be assessed by absence of the femoral pulses. Intermittent release of pressure to allow peripheral perfusion then enables bleeding intra-abdominal vessels to be identified.

Following vaginal delivery, external aortic compression may be possible, due to lax abdominal musculature (Riley & Burgess, 1994). A study of the haemodynamic effects of aortic compression on healthy nonbleeding women within 4 hours of vaginal delivery found that leg blood pressure was obliterated in 55%, with a substantial reduction in a further 10%. No significant elevation in systemic blood pressure was noted, and the authors concluded that this procedure is safe, and a potentially useful maneuver for patient stabilization and transport. However there have been no studies addressing the feasibility and efficacy of external aortic compression in patients with uterine atony following vaginal delivery; a high fundus may mean that adequate compression is impossible in this situation.

Medical treatment of uterine atony

The prophylactic use of uterotonic drugs is an effective means of preventing postpartum hemorrhage from uterine atony.

Either oxytocin alone (5 IU or 10 IU intramuscularly) or syntometrine (5 IU of oxytocin plus 0.5 mg ergometrine: not available in the USA) may be used. The combination drug is more effective, but has more side effects (McDonald et al., 2000). These drugs are also first line treatment for postpartum hemorrhage due to atony.

Oxytocin

Oxytocin binds to specific uterine receptors and intravenous administration (dose 5–10 IU) has an almost immediate onset of action (Dollery, 1999). The mean plasma half-life is 3 minutes, therefore to ensure a sustained contraction a continuous intravenous infusion is necessary. The usual dose is 20–40 units per liter of crystalloid, with the dose rate adjusted according to response. Plateau concentration is reached after 30 minutes. Intramuscular injection has a time of onset of 3–7 minutes, and the clinical effect is longer lasting, at 30–60 minutes.

Oxytocin is metabolized by both the liver and kidneys. It has approximately 5% of the antidiuretic effect of vasopressin, and if given in large volumes of electrolyte-free solution can cause water overload (headache, vomiting, drowsiness, and convulsions)—symptoms that may be mistakenly attributed to other causes. Rapid administration of an intravenous bolus of oxytocin results in relaxation of vascular smooth muscle. Hypotension with a reflex tachycardia may occur, followed by a small but sustained increase in blood pressure. Oxytocin is stable at temperatures up to 25°C, but refrigeration may prolong shelf life.

Methylergonovine/ergometrine

Methylergonovine (methylergometrine) and its parent compound ergometrine result in a sustained tonic contraction of uterine smooth muscle via stimulation of α-adrenergic myometrial receptors (Dollery, 1999). The dose of methylergonovine is 0.2 mg, and of ergometrine is 0.2–0.5 mg, repeated after 2–4 hours if necessary. Time of onset of action is 2–5 minutes when given intramuscularly. These agents are extensively metabolized in the liver and the mean plasma half-life is approximately 30 minutes. However, plasma levels do not seem to correlate with uterine effect, since the clinical action of ergometrine is sustained for 3 hours or more. When oxytocin and ergometrine derivatives are used simultaneously, postpartum hemorrhage is therefore controlled by two different mechanisms, oxytocin producing an immediate response, and ergometrine a more sustained action.

Nausea and vomiting are common side effects. Vasoconstriction of vascular smooth muscle also occurs as a consequence of their α-adrenergic action. This can result in elevation of central venous pressure and systemic blood pressure and therefore pulmonary edema, stroke, and myocardial infarction. Contraindications include heart disease, autoimmune conditions associated with Raynaud's phenomenon, peripheral vascular disease, arteriovenous shunts even if surgically corrected, and hypertension. Women with preeclampsia/eclampsia are particularly at risk of severe and sustained hypertension.

Intravenous administration is associated with more severe side effects, however onset of action is almost immediate. This route may be indicated for patients in whom delayed intramuscular absorption may occur (e.g. shocked patients). The drug should be given over at least 60 seconds with careful monitoring of blood pressure and pulse. Initial reports suggested that methylergonovine resulted in hypertension less frequently than ergometrine, but no difference has since been reported in randomized controlled trials. Ergometrine and its derivatives are both heat and light sensitive, and should be stored at temperatures below 8°C and away from light.

Prostaglandins

Prostaglandin F2α results in contraction of smooth muscle cells (Dollery, 1999). Carboprost/hemabate (15-methyl prostaglandin F2α) is an established second-line treatment for postpartum hemorrhage unresponsive to oxytocic agents. It is available in single dose vials of 0.25 mg. It may be given by deep intramuscular injection or by direct injection into the myometrium—either under direct vision at cesarean section or transabdominally/transvaginally after vaginal delivery. It is not licensed for the latter route and there is concern about direct injection into a uterine sinus, although it is commonly used in this way (Bigrigg et al., 1991). Additionally it may be more efficacious in shocked patients, when tissue hypoperfusion may compromise absorption following intramuscular injection (Hayashi et al., 1984). A second dose may be given after 90 minutes, or if atony and hemorrhage continue, repeat doses may be given every 15 minutes to a maximum of 8 doses (2 mg), with ongoing bimanual compression and fundal massage.

Small case series have reported an efficacy of 85% or more in refractory postpartum hemorrhage (Toppozada et al., 1981; Hayashi et al., 1984). The largest case series to date has involved a multicenter surveillance study of 237 cases of postpartum hemorrhage refractory to oxytocics and found that it was effective in 88% (Oleen & Mariano, 1990). The majority of women received a single dose. When further oxytocics were given to treatment failures, the overall success rate was 95%. The remaining patients required surgery and many of these had a cause for postpartum hemorrhage other than atony, including laceration and retained products of conception.

Carboprost causes bronchoconstriction, venoconstriction and constriction of gastrointestinal smooth muscle. Associated side effects include nausea, vomiting, diarrhea, pyrexia, and bronchospasm. There are case reports of hypotension and intrapulmonary shunting with arterial oxygen desaturation, thus it is therefore contraindicated in patients with cardiac or pulmonary disease. Carboprost is expensive and therefore unaffordable in many developing countries. Dinoprost (prostaglandin F2α) is more readily available; intramyometrial injection of 0.5–1.0mg is effective for uterine atony. Low-dose intrauterine infusion via a Foley catheter has also been described, consisting of 20mg dinoprost in 500mL saline at 3–4mL/min for 10 minutes, then 1mL/min (Kupferminc et al., 1998). Intramuscular injection and intravenous infusion has not been shown to be effective.

Prostaglandin E2 (dinoprostone) is generally a vasodilatory prostaglandin; however, it causes contraction of smooth muscle in the pregnant uterus (Dollery, 1999). Dinoprostone is widely available on labor wards as an intravaginal pessary for cervical ripening. Rectal administration (2mg given 2 hourly) has been successful as a treatment for uterine atony—vaginal administration probably being ineffective in the presence of ongoing uterine hemorrhage. Due to its vasodilatory effect, this drug should be avoided in hypotensive and hypovolemic patients. However, it may be useful in women with heart or lung disease in whom carboprost is contraindicated (ACOG, 1998). Case reports also document the use of Gemeprost pessaries, a prostaglandin E1 analogue, but with actions resembling PGF2α rather than its parent compound. Both rectal and intrauterine administration have been reported (Barrington & Roberts, 1993; Craig et al., 1999).

Misoprostol

Misoprostol is a synthetic analogue of prostaglandin E1 and is metabolized in the liver. The tablet(s) can be given orally, vaginally, or rectally. As prophylaxis for postpartum hemorrhage, an international multicenter randomized trial reported that oral misoprostol is less successful than parenteral oxytocin administration (Gulmezoglu et al., 2001). Misoprostol may however be of benefit in treating postpartum hemorrhage.

Two small case series have reported an apparently rapid response in postpartum hemorrhage refractory to oxytocin and syntometrine, with rectal doses of 600–1,000μg. Sustained uterine contraction was reported in almost all women within 3 minutes of its administration (O'Brien et al., 1998; Abdel-Aleem et al., 2001). A single-blinded randomized trial of misoprostol 800μg rectally versus syntometrine intramuscularly plus oxytocin by intravenous infusion found that misoprostol resulted in cessation of bleeding within 20 minutes in 30/32 cases (93%) compared to 21/32 (66%) (Lokugamage et al., 2001). There was no difference in need for blood transfusion or onset of coagulopathy. Of note, misoprostol is cheap, heat and light stable, and does not require sterile needles and syringes for administration. It may therefore be of particular benefit in developing countries.

Surgical management of postpartum hemorrhage

The majority of the surgical techniques described here aim to arrest hemorrhage due to uterine atony. Many have been utilized for bleeding resulting from placenta accreta and placenta previa, or for severe genital tract trauma when simple repair is unable to control hemorrhage.

Surgical intervention for uterine atony is necessary when uterotonic agents have failed to control bleeding, and there is no evidence of retained products of conception or concurrent genital tract trauma. An examination under anesthesia is generally necessary to exclude the latter. An extensive range of surgical techniques has been advocated. Case reports and audit studies constitute the major clinical evidence. Comparison between published reports is difficult—factors such as the severity of hemorrhage, time lapse from delivery to effective surgery, hemodynamic and coagulation status, available surgical expertise, and the presence of other obstetric and medical problems all contribute to differences in outcome.

Uterine tamponade

Uterine packing is a procedure long abandoned by many units, but more recently revived with case reports detailing new techniques for tamponade of the bleeding placental bed. Historically, uterine packing was performed using sterile gauze, with up to 5m of 5–10cm gauze introduced into the uterus, either using a specific packing instrument or long forceps (Maier, 1993). Gauze is applied in layers from side to side, to give maximum pressure on the uterine wall, with the lower segment packed as tightly as possible. Indications for uterine packing include atony, placenta previa, and placenta accreta. Packs are generally left in situ for 24–36 hours, and prophylactic antibiotics given.

Uterine packing fell out of use due to concerns about concealed bleeding, infection, trauma, and problems in performing adequate packing. However there is little documented evidence to support these concerns, and it has been suggested that the risks have been overstated (Maier, 1993; Katesmark et al., 1994). Several inflatable mechanical devices have more recently been employed as alternative means of uterine tamponade. Proponents of these devices state that their advantages are that they are rapid and easy procedures to perform, and that their efficacy can readily be evaluated.

A Sengstaken–Blakemore tube has been utilized in this context (Katesmark et al., 1994; Chan et al., 1997). The first report inflated the gastric balloon with normal saline, and the second inflated only the esophageal balloon. Balloon tamponade has also been performed with a Rusch urological hydrostatic balloon catheter inflated with 400–500mL of saline. This was effective in two women with hemorrhage due to morbidly adherent placentae (Johanson et al., 2001). A continuous oxytocin infusion and prophylactic antibiotic cover are advised for these procedures.

Uterine brace suture

The B-Lynch suture is a uterine brace suture designed to vertically compress the uterine body in cases of diffuse bleeding due to uterine atony (B-Lynch et al., 1997). In order to assess whether the suture will be effective, bimanual compression is applied to the uterus. If bleeding stops, compression with a brace suture should be equally successful. The patient is placed in the Lloyd-Davies position on the operating table to enable assessment of vaginal bleeding. If delivery occurred via lower segment cesarean section, the incision is reopened; if delivery was vaginal, a similar incision is made following mobilization of the bladder. The uterus is exteriorized, and response to bimanual compression assessed. If vaginal bleeding is controlled, the "pair of braces" suture is inserted using a 70 mm round-bodied needle with number 2 chromic catgut suture (Fig. 21.1). The two ends are tied while an assistant performs bimanual compression and the lower segment incision closed as normal. The authors describe five cases in which the procedure was attempted with success in all cases. They included hemorrhage due to uterine atony, coagulopathy and placenta previa. They state that the advantages of this method are its surgical simplicity and that adequate hemostasis can be assessed immediately after its completion. Normal uterine anatomy has been demonstrated on follow-up (Ferguson et al., 2000).

A modification of the B-Lynch suture has been described (Tamizian & Arulkumaran, 2001). A less complex procedure is involved, consisting of two individual sutures, tied at the fundus. A lower segment incision is not necessary, and the authors suggest that more tension may be applied with individual sutures than with one continuous suture. They also describe tying the loose ends of the sutures together, to prevent slippage laterally. A summary of published studies is the subject of a recent review article (Dildy, 2002).

Uterine devascularization

Uterine devascularization is a long practiced technique for postpartum hemorrhage due to atony, placenta, previa, and trauma. Ligation of the uterine arteries and internal iliac

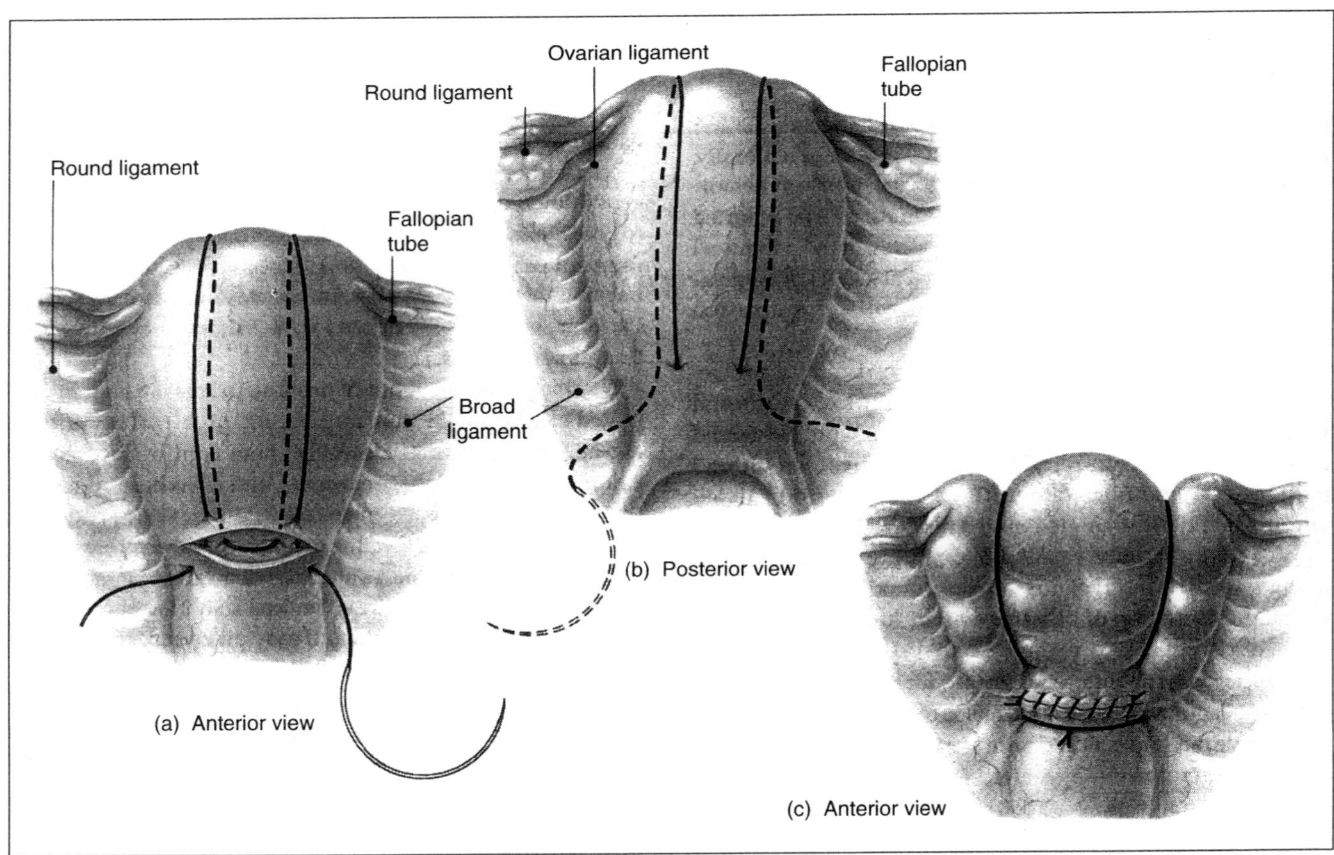

Fig. 21.1 The B-Lynch uterine brace suture. (a) Anterior and (b) posterior views are shown during insertion of the suture. (c) After successful insertion. (Reprinted from B-Lynch et al., 1997. The B-Lynch surgical technique for the control of massive postpartum haemorrhage: an alternative to hysterectomy? Five cases reported. Br J Obstet Gynaecol 104:372–375. © 1997 with permission from Elsevier Science.)

arteries are described; ovarian artery ligation may also be performed, generally as an adjunctive procedure. Evidence for the efficacy of these techniques is based on published case series. The expertise and experience of individual units are important determinants of the surgical approach to postpartum hemorrhage.

Bilateral uterine artery ligation

The pregnant uterus receives 90% of its blood supply from the uterine arteries. Bilateral ligation of the ascending branches of the uterine artery is considered by its practitioners to be a simple, safe, and efficacious alternative to hysterectomy (O'Leary & O'Leary, 1974). This procedure was originally utilized to control postpartum hemorrhage at cesarean section. Mass ligation of the uterine artery branches and veins is performed 2–3 cm below the lower segment incision. The suture is placed laterally through an avascular window in the broad ligament, and medially through almost the full thickness of the uterine wall, to include the uterine vessels and 2–3 cm of myometrium. The vessels are not divided, and inclusion of myometrium avoids vascular damage and obliterates intramyometrial ascending arterial branches. An absorbable suture such as number 1 chromic catgut on an atraumatic needle is used. Nonabsorbable and figure-of-eight sutures are avoided as they are considered to increase the risk of arteriovenous sinus formation. If vaginal delivery has occurred, the bladder may need to be adequately mobilized prior to suture insertion to avoid ureteric injury.

The largest case series was published in 1995 (O'Leary, 1995). This was a 30-year study involving 265 patients with postcesarean postpartum hemorrhage of >1,000 mL, refractory to oxytocics, methylergonovine and carboprost. Bilateral uterine artery ligation failed to control hemorrhage in only 10 women, giving a 96% success rate. An immediate effect was reported, with visible uterine blanching; myometrial contractions sometimes occurred, but even if the uterus remained atonic, hemorrhage was usually controlled (O'Leary & O'Leary, 1974). No long-term effects on menstrual patterns or fertility have been reported (AbdRabbo, 1994; O'Leary, 1995). In women who have subsequently undergone repeat caesaran section, the uterine vessels appeared to have recanalized.

Failure of this procedure is most commonly associated with placenta previa with or without accreta. More recently, low bilateral uterine artery ligation has been described for ongoing bleeding from the lower segment in these cases. A recent series of 103 patients involving stepwise uterine devascularization reported a 75% success rate with conventional uterine artery ligation (AbdRabbo, 1994). Success was highest with uterine atony and abruption. Of seven cases of placenta previa with/without accreta, hemorrhage continued in four women. A further bilateral ligation was performed 3–5 cm below the first sutures, following further mobilization of the bladder. Ligation therefore includes the ascending branches of the cervicovaginal artery and the uterine artery branches supplying the lower segment and upper cervix. This procedure was effective in all cases.

Unilateral or bilateral ligation of the ovarian artery may be performed as an adjunct to ligation of uterine arteries. The ligature is tied medial to the ovary to preserve ovarian blood supply. This was the final phase of the stepwise uterine devascularization approach described above (AbdRabbo, 1994). Following uterine artery ligation, 13/96 cases that did not involve placenta previa/accreta had ongoing bleeding. Of these, seven responded to unilateral ovarian artery and six to bilateral ovarian artery ligation. All patients in this case series therefore avoided hysterectomy.

Bilateral internal iliac artery ligation

Internal iliac artery ligation was first performed as a gynecological procedure by Kelly in 1894 (Burchell, 1968). He termed this "the boldest procedure possible for checking bleeding" and assumed that the blood supply to the pelvis would be completely arrested. From the 1950s, internal iliac ligation was increasingly performed for gynecological indications, mostly for carcinoma of the cervix. Ligation was still considered to shut off arterial flow, despite the fact that necrosis of pelvic tissues had not been observed. In the 1960s, Burchell reported cutting a uterine artery following bilateral internal iliac ligation in order to demonstrate the absence of flow. However, to the surprise of those present, blood still flowed freely.

This observation led to extensive studies of the hemodynamic effects of internal iliac ligation. These were performed on gynecological patients, but are quoted widely in the obstetric literature (Burchell, 1964; Burchell & Olson, 1966). Aortograms performed between 5 minutes and 37 months postligation demonstrated an extensive collateral circulation, with blood flow throughout the internal iliac artery and its branches. Three collateral circulations were identified: the lumbar and iliolumbar arteries; the middle sacral and lateral sacral arteries; and the superior rectal and middle rectal arteries. Ligation above the posterior division resulted in collateral and therefore reversed flow in its iliolumbar and middle sacral branches (Fig. 21.2). Ligation below the posterior division caused collateral flow only in the middle hemorrhoidal artery, again in a retrograde direction (Fig. 21.3). Flow to more distal branches of the internal iliac artery was normal.

A second study involved intra-arterial pressure recordings before and after ligation (Burchell, 1964). Following bilateral ligation, distal arterial pulse pressure decreased by 85%, with a 24% reduction in mean arterial pressure. In addition, a 48% reduction in blood flow resulted following ipsilateral ligation. The authors concluded that internal iliac ligation controls pelvic hemorrhage mainly by decreasing arterial pulse pressure. The smaller diameter of the anastomoses of the collateral circulation was proposed to explain this phenomenon. The arterial system was considered transformed into a venous-like

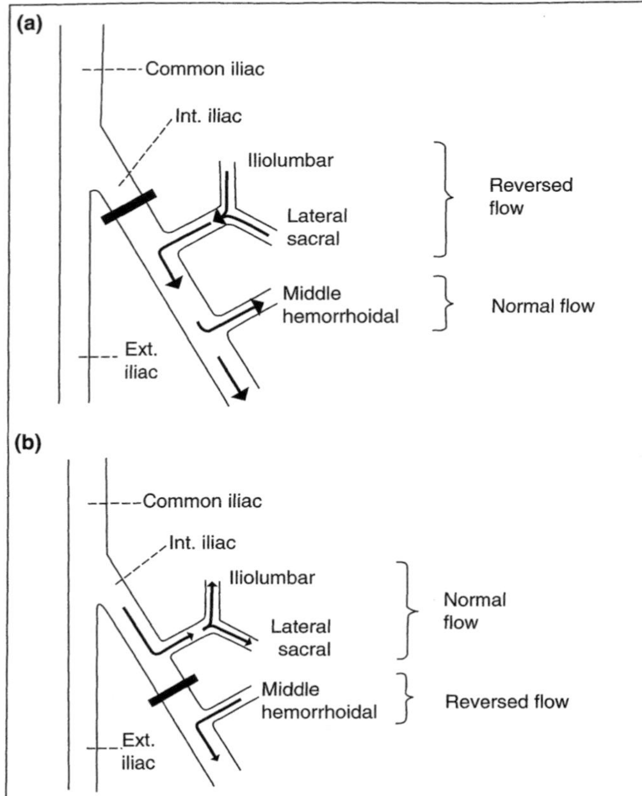

Fig. 21.2 Internal iliac artery ligation. (a) Ligation above the posterior diversion; collateral pathways result in reversed flow in the iliolumbar and lateral sacral arteries. (b) Ligation below the posterior diversion; collateral pathways result in reversed flow in the middle hemorrhoidal (middle rectal) artery. (Reprinted with permission from the American College of Obstetricians and Gynecologists. Burchell RC. Arterial physiology of the human pelvis. Obstet Gynecol 1968;31:855–860.)

circulation, with clot formation able to arrest bleeding at the site of injury. These studies have been extensively quoted, however similar studies have not been performed in postpartum women. A single case report found no change in uterine artery Doppler waveform velocity before and 2 days after bilateral internal artery ligation performed to control hemorrhage due to uterine atony (Chitrit et al., 2000).

Internal iliac artery ligation is a more complex procedure than uterine artery ligation. The bifurcation of the common iliac artery is identified at the pelvic brim, and the peritoneum opened and reflected medially along with the ureter (Tamizian & Arulkumaran, 2001). The internal iliac artery is identified, freed of areolar tissue, and a right angled clamp passed under the artery. Two ligatures are tied 1–2 cm apart. The artery is not divided. Both the uterine and vaginal arteries are branches of the anterior division, and ligation should if possible be distal to the origin of the posterior division. This is more efficacious and does not compromise blood supply to the buttocks and gluteal muscles. A retroperitoneal approach may be used when hemorrhage has followed vaginal delivery. Complications of this procedure include damage to the internal iliac vein and ureter. Tissue edema, ongoing hemorrhage, and the presence of a large atonic uterus may make identification of anatomy difficult and prolong operating time. Incorrect identification of the internal iliac artery may result in accidental ligation of the external or common iliac artery, resulting in lower limb and pelvic ischemia. Femoral pulses should therefore be checked after the procedure. Recanalization of ligated vessels may occur, and successful pregnancy has been reported whether or not recanalization has taken place.

Demonstration of the extensive collateral circulation explains why the efficacy of internal iliac ligation is less than for uterine artery ligation. Success rates are generally reported to be approximately 40% (Tamizian & Arulkumaran, 2001). A 1985 study reported a success rate of 42% in a series of 19 patients, with hysterectomy necessary in the remainder (Clark et al., 1985). Morbidity was higher than for a group of patients in whom hysterectomy was performed as a primary procedure; mean blood loss was 5,125 mL for patients with unsuccessful internal iliac artery ligation followed by hysterectomy, and 3,209 mL for those undergoing hysterectomy alone. Complications associated with unsuccessful arterial ligation in this series were associated with delay in instituting definitive treatment (hysterectomy) rather than as a consequence of arterial ligation. These authors consider that there is only a limited role for this procedure in the treatment of postpartum hemorrhage: restricted to hemodynamically stable patients of low parity in whom future fertility is of paramount concern.

Arterial embolization

Uterine devascularization by selective arterial embolization has recently gained popularity in centers with expertise in interventional radiology. Access is via the femoral artery and the site of arterial bleeding is located by injection of contrast into the aorta. The bleeding vessel is selectively catheterized, and pledgets of absorbable gelatine sponge injected (Vedantham et al., 1997). These effect only a temporary blockade and are resorbed within approximately 10 days. If the site of bleeding cannot be identified, embolization of the anterior branch of the internal iliac artery or the uterine artery is performed.

In published studies, uterine atony and pelvic trauma are the major indications for embolization, and overall success rates of 85–100% are reported (Hansch et al., 1999). Higher failure rates are associated with placenta accreta and procedures performed following failed bilateral internal iliac artery ligation (Pelage et al., 1998). Subsequent successful pregnancies have been documented.

Compared to surgical devascularization, embolization has several advantages. It is less invasive and generally results in visualization of the bleeding vessel. Occlusion of distal arteries close to the bleeding site is possible, thereby reducing the risk of ongoing bleeding from a collateral circulation (Vedentham et al., 1997). The efficacy of embolization can immediately be assessed, and repeated embolization of the same or different arteries can be performed. Disadvantages are the necessity of rapid availability of specialist equipment and personnel, and the need for transfer of a hemorrhaging patient to the radiology suite. Embolization may also be a time-consuming procedure, generally requiring between 1 and 3 hours, but with hemostasis of the major bleeding vessel frequently established in 30–60 minutes. Arterial embolization is an option in hemodynamically stable patients (Ledee et al., 2001); however, patients with life-threatening hemorrhage have also been successfully treated. A 1998 case series included 27 women with life-threatening bleeding, 12 of whom were intubated and ventilated, and four were successfully resuscitated following cardiac arrest (Pelage et al., 1998).

A variation on this theme is the prophylactic placement of inflatable balloon catheters in internal iliac arteries of patients who are expected to bleed excessively at the time of surgery, for example elective cesarean delivery in a patient with placenta percreta. In this situation the patient is taken to the interventional radiology suite prior to surgery and the balloon catheters are placed but not inflated. Following delivery of the baby the catheters can be immediately inflated. Such catheters can be deflated at the completion of surgery and left in situ during the next 24–48 hours to be re-inflated if required.

Hysterectomy

Peripartum hysterectomy is frequently considered the definitive procedure for obstetric hemorrhage, but is not without complications. In the long term, the loss of fertility may be devastating to the patient. In the emergency situation, the major concern is that peripartum hysterectomy can be a complex procedure, due to ongoing blood loss and grossly distorted pelvic anatomy due to edema, hematoma formation, and trauma. Pritchard showed an average blood loss of 1,435 mL when hysterectomy was performed at the time of elective repeat cesarean section (Pritchard et al., 1962). At emergency hysterectomy for postpartum bleeding, mean blood loss attributed to the procedure was 2,183 mL, with a mean loss of 2,125 mL by the time of decision for hysterectomy (Clark et al., 1984). Adequate hemostasis is not always achieved, and further procedures may be necessary. Uterine artery embolization has been performed for ongoing bleeding following hysterectomy, both with and without success (Pelage et al., 1998; Ledee et al., 2001). Re-look laparotomy may also be required; this has been reported in up to 13% of patients (Lau et al., 1997). The incidence of febrile morbidity is high, with rates of 5–85% in different series.

Hysterectomy is indicated if conservative procedures such as embolization or uterine devascularization fail to control bleeding. The time lapse between delivery and successful surgery is the most important prognostic factor. If the primary procedure fails, it is recommended that hysterectomy is performed promptly, without attempts at another conservative measure (Ledee et al., 2001). In severely shocked patients with life-threatening hemorrhage, hysterectomy is in most circumstances the first-line treatment (Tamizian & Arulkumaran, 2001). Hysterectomy may therefore be associated with a higher mortality than other surgical procedures (Ledee et al., 2001).

Uterine atony is the major indication for peripartum hysterectomy, although other factors such as placenta accreta and abruption are frequently present (Ledee et al., 2001). Other indications include placenta previa, uterine rupture, and other genital tract lacerations. Trauma sustained at vaginal delivery may result in concealed bleeding and is therefore associated with a worse outcome; hemorrhage at cesarean section is more readily recognized and more promptly remedied.

A subtotal hysterectomy can generally be performed if bleeding is from the uterine body. It is generally simpler than a total hysterectomy—the cervix and vaginal angles can be difficult to identify in women who have labored to full dilation. There is also less risk of injury to the ureter and bladder. One study reported the incidence of urinary tract injury to be 13% for subtotal hysterectomy, compared to 25% for total hysterectomy (Lau et al., 1997). If bleeding is from the lower segment (placenta previa, trauma) the cervical branch of the uterine artery must be ligated, and a total hysterectomy will be necessary.

Bleeding disorders

Consumptive and dilutional coagulopathies secondary to extensive blood loss and crystalloid replacement are the most common bleeding disorders associated with postpartum hemorrhage. Other obstetric causes of disseminated intravascular coagulopathy (acute fatty liver of pregnancy, abruption, anaphylactoid syndrome of pregnancy) or thrombocytopenia (HELLP syndrome, TTP) may cause or contribute to major hemorrhage. Inherited and acquired bleeding disorders unrelated to pregnancy must also be considered. These include abnormalities of the coagulation system and qualitative or quantitative platelet disorders. The most common disorders are discussed below.

Idiopathic thrombocytopenia purpura (ITP)

ITP is an autoimmune disorder resulting in increased platelet destruction. Average platelet lifespan is greatly reduced, being a tenth of the normal 7–10 days. Circulating platelets are therefore younger, larger, and functionally superior compared to normal platelets. Platelet counts are generally between 50 and 75×10^9/L, but may fall to exceedingly low levels, particularly following viral infections. Exacerbations of ITP may occur at any time during pregnancy. In nonpregnant patients, spontaneous severe bleeding is rare with platelet counts greater than 10×10^9/L, and significant bleeding following trauma unusual with platelet counts above 50×10^9/L.

Case series from the 1950s and 1960s reported no increased incidence of postpartum hemorrhage or placental abruption in patients presenting with spontaneous bleeding from other sites (Silver, 1998). Cesarean section and genital tract lacerations are associated with increased blood loss and an increased need for blood transfusion. Platelet counts should be monitored regularly. Antenatally, treatment is generally recommended with platelet counts of less than 30×10^9/L or at any level if there is clinically significant bleeding. The minimal safe platelet count for delivery is unknown. Recent US guidelines demonstrate a diversity of expert opinion (George et al., 1996); a minimum count between 10 and 50×10^9/L (mean 27×10^9/L) was recommended for vaginal delivery and 30–50 $\times 10^9$/L (mean 44×10^9/L) for cesarean section. A lower limit of 80×10^9/L is generally agreed for regional analgesia.

The most common medical treatments for ITP are corticosteroids and intravenous immunoglobulin. High-dose steroids are associated with an increased risk of hypertension in pregnancy and immunoglobulin is extremely expensive. Platelet transfusions should only be given for life-threatening bleeding or essential surgery; transfused platelets are rapidly destroyed in patients with ITP. Splenectomy remains the definitive treatment. In pregnancy this may be technically difficult, but is indicated in women who are resistant to medical treatment.

von Willebrand's disease

Von Willebrand's disease (vWD) is the most common inherited bleeding disorder (Economides et al., 1999). Pregnant women with this disorder have no increased risk of antepartum hemorrhage, however the reported incidence of primary postpartum hemorrhage is 22%, with an incidence of 20–28% for secondary postpartum hemorrhage (Kadir et al., 1998).

This disorder is characterized by quantitative or qualitative deficiency in the production of von Willebrand factor (vWF), which has a central role in hemostasis (Mannucci, 2001). First, it stabilizes the coagulation factor VIIIc, which otherwise is rapidly metabolized. Second, it mediates platelet adhesion following vascular injury. If there is a lack of functional vWF, the plasma level of factor VIIIc is low (normal range 50–150 IU/dL), and the bleeding time is prolonged. Bleeding problems are usually mild (epistaxis, menorrhagia) and the underlying problem may go undetected. However, life-threatening hemorrhage may occur postpartum.

There are three types of vWD. Types 1 and 3 are quantitative deficiencies. Type 1 is found in approximately 70% of affected individuals, and is autosomal dominant. It is a partial deficiency state of vWF, and factor VIII levels are usually in the range 5–40 IU/dL. Type 3 is rare and autosomal recessive; there is almost a complete lack of vWF leading to very low levels of factor VIII with severe bleeding problems. Type 2 consists of qualitative differences, with several different subtypes which are inherited as autosomal dominant mutations. Thrombocytopenia may occur in type 2 disease in pregnancy; increased synthesis of abnormal multimers of vWF may cause increased platelet aggregation.

In normal pregnant women and those with type 1 disease, vWF and factor VIII levels rise significantly in the second half of pregnancy. Therefore it is rare that women with mild vWD need treatment in pregnancy. However women with other types of vWD and low factor levels have an inadequate response. Factor VIII levels should be checked at the initial prenatal care visit and again in the third trimester. Following delivery, there is a rapid fall-off in factor VIII levels, resulting in a high rate of secondary postpartum hemorrhage.

Postpartum hemorrhage in women with vWD generally occurs if the factor VIII level is <50 IU/dL. Prophylactic treatment is therefore required during labor and in the early postpartum period to maintain concentrations above this threshold. The aim is to maintain higher levels for 3–4 days after vaginal delivery and 4–5 days after cesarean section. There are two options for treatment. The first is intravenous infusion of desmopressin (DDAVP; 1-deamino-8-arginine vasopressin), which acts by increasing factor VIII and vWF release into the plasma from storage sites, raising plasma concentrations by 3–5 times within 30 minutes. These levels are usually maintained for 8–10 hours and infusions therefore need to be given 1–2 times daily. Patients with type 1 disease generally respond well, but response is variable in type 3. DDAVP is contraindicated in some subtypes of type 2 because transient thrombocytopenia may result.

The second treatment option consists of factor VIII and vWF replacement. Fresh frozen plasma contains both factors, but large volumes are required to stop or prevent bleeding. Cryoprecipitate contains 5–10 times higher concentration of both factors. Factor VIII preparations for use in von Willebrand's disease must also contain some vWF, otherwise the half-life of factor VIII is 1 hour or less. Recombinant factor VIII therefore cannot be given, but commercial preparations containing both factors are available. Tranexamic acid may also be useful in women with nonlife-threatening postpartum hemorrhage.

Hemophilia

Hemophilia A (factor VIII deficiency) and hemophilia B (factor IX deficiency) are X-linked disorders, and women who are carriers may have low clotting factor levels (Kadir et al., 1997b). Some women have levels that are within the normal range (>50 IU/dL), but X-inactivation may result in inactivation of the normal chromosome and low factor levels may therefore be present (Economides et al., 1999). There is also an increased risk of primary and secondary postpartum hemorrhage in hemophilia carriers, with reported rates of 19% and 11% respectively, occurring mostly when factor levels are <50 IU/dL.

Carriers of hemophilia A generally experience a pregnancy-induced rise in factor VIII levels. However, factor IX levels are unaffected by pregnancy. Treatment is indicated for labor when factor levels are <50 IU/dL for both types of hemophilia. DDAVP may be used, or appropriate factor concentrates. Hemophilia A carriers synthesize normal amounts of vWF, and therefore recombinant factor VIII is effective in these patients.

Acquired hemophilia

Acquired hemophilia is caused by the presence of autoantibodies to factor VIII in people with previously normal factor VIII activity (Shobeiri et al., 2000). These antibodies are inhibitory, and partially or completely suppress factor VIII procoagulant activity. It is a rare disorder, and bleeding is generally severe with high morbidity and mortality. The risk of death from hemorrhage is higher in patients with this disorder than in hemophiliacs with factor VIII inhibitors.

Between 7 and 11% of cases are related to pregnancy, and most occur after the first delivery (Kadir et al., 1997a). Presentation is with major bleeding, generally within the first 3 months postpartum. Hemorrhage may be apparent at several different sites, including multiple soft-tissue hematomas, large ecchymoses, excessive vaginal loss, and postoperative bleeding. Investigations show a prolonged APTT, together with a normal prothrombin time, bleeding time, and platelet count. In the majority of patients, inhibitors spontaneously disappear and there is complete remission within a few months; however, sometimes these antibodies may persist for years. Until their disappearance, patients are at high risk for further bleeding episodes.

Hemorrhage is controlled by raising the plasma level of factor VIII, to overpower the inhibitory action. Inhibitors bind less readily to porcine factor VIII than human factor VIII, so the former is generally first-line management. DDAVP may also be used to increase endogenous factor VIII release from cellular stores. Plasmapheresis may be necessary if inhibitor levels are high. Disappearance of inhibitors can be enhanced by treatment with immunosuppressive agents such as corticosteroids, cyclophosphamide, and azathioprine. In patients with complete remission there has been no recurrence in subsequent pregnancies. However as this is a rare disorder, few cases have as yet been documented.

Secondary postpartum hemorrhage

Secondary or delayed postpartum hemorrhage is defined as blood loss of 500 mL or more from the genital tract occurring more than 24 hours after delivery and up to 6 weeks postpartum. The potential severity of this condition should not be underestimated; secondary postpartum hemorrhage may result in the rapid onset of hemorrhagic shock (Pelage et al., 1999). The peak time for presentation is the second postpartum week, with the third postpartum week the next most common. The great majority of women therefore present with this complication as outpatients.

The reported incidence is 0.5–1.3% of deliveries (Hoveyda & Mackenzie, 2001). Common causes include retained placental tissue, endometritis, and genital tract tears. Rare causes include arteriovenous fistulae and false aneurysms—possibly resulting from surgical trauma and healing at the site of cesarean section incision (Pelage et al., 1999). Scar dehiscence has also been described. Genital tract malignancy, including choriocarcinoma, may also cause excessive bleeding during the postpartum period. Bleeding disorders may also present in this way, as discussed above. Acquired hemophilia is a rare but potentially lethal cause of secondary postpartum hemorrhage.

Initial acute management of excessive bleeding from the placental bed involves medical treatment. As for primary postpartum hemorrhage, the first-line agents are intramuscular ergometrine/ergotamine and intravenous infusion of oxytocin. Prostaglandins E2, F2α, and misoprostol have been used and good responses have been reported. Antibiotics are commonly given, although positive microbial cultures are not frequently found.

Uterine curettage is commonly performed. However this is not without risk; uterine perforation is reported in 3% of women with secondary postpartum hemorrhage, and has occurred in patients up to 28 days after delivery. Histological confirmation of products of conception occurs only in about a third of cases; however, an apparent therapeutic benefit may be achieved even in its absence. Ultrasound is no more accurate in the diagnosis of retained placental tissue than clinical assessment.

If bleeding is not controlled by these means, further surgical intervention is necessary. As for primary hemorrhage, ligation of the uterine vasculature, hysterectomy, and arterial embolization have all been successfully performed, although there is little evidence to show which is the optimum procedure. Women with genital tract trauma may also undergo these procedures if primary suturing is unsuccessful or not feasible. Angiography performed prior to embolization may also result in the diagnosis of vascular causes of secondary hemorrhage where otherwise no underlying cause could be identified (Pelage et al., 1999). A case series of 14 patients revealed a false aneurysm of the uterine artery in two women and an arteriovenous fistula in one woman.

References

Abdel-Aleem H, El-Nashar I, Abdel-Aleem A. Management of severe postpartum hemorrhage with misoprostol. Int J Gynecol Obstet 2001;72:75–76.

AbdRabbo SA. Stepwise uterine devascularisation: a novel technique for management of uncontrollable postpartum hemorrhage with preservation of the uterus. Am J Obstet Gynecol 1994;171: 694–700.

ACOG Educational bulletin. Postpartum haemorrhage. Number 243,

January 1998. American College of Obstetricians and Gynecologists. Int J Gynecol Obstet 1998;61:79–86.

Anthony J, Johanson R, Dommisse J. Critical care management of severe preeclampsia. Fetal Mat Med Rev 1994;6:219–229.

Baron F, Hill WC. Placenta previa, placenta abruptio. Clin Obs Gynecol 1998;41:527–532.

Barrington JW, Roberts A. The use of gemeprost pessaries to arrest postpartum haemorrhage. Br J Obstet Gynaecol 1993;100:691–692.

Bigrigg A, Chiu D, Chissell S, Read MD. Use of intramyometrial 15-methyl prostaglandin F2α to control atonic postpartum haemorrhage following vaginal delivery and failure of conventional therapy. Br J Obstet Gynaecol 1991;98:734–736.

B-Lynch C, Coker A, Lawal AH, Abu J, Cowen MJ. The B-Lynch surgical technique for the control of massive postpartum haemorrhage: an alternative to hysterectomy? Five cases reported. Br J Obstet Gynaecol 1997;104:372–375.

Bonnar J. Massive obstetric haemorrhage. Ballière's Best Pract Res Clin Obstet Gynaecol 2000;14:1–18.

Brar HS, Greenspoon JS, Platt LD, Paul RH. Acute puerperal uterine inversion. New approaches to management. J Reprod Med 1989; 34:173–177.

Burchell RC. Internal iliac artery ligation: hemodynamics. Obstet Gynecol 1964;24:737–739.

Burchell RC. Arterial physiology of the human pelvis. Obstet Gynecol 1968;31:855–860.

Burchell RC, Olson G. Internal iliac artery ligation: aortograms. Am J Obstet Gynecol 1966;94:117–124.

Chan C, Razvi K, Tham KF, Arulkumaran S. The use of a Sengstaken-Blakemore tube to control post-partum hemorrhage. Int J Gynecol Obstet 1997;58:251–252.

Chitrit Y, Guillaumin D, Caubel P, Herrero R. Absence of flow velocity waveform changes in uterine arteries after bilateral internal iliac ligation. Am J Obstet Gynecol 2000;182:727–728.

Clark SL, Yeh S-Y, Phelan JP, Bruce S, Paul RH. Emergency hysterectomy for obstetric hemorrhage. Obstet Gynecol 1984;64:376–380.

Clark SL, Phelan JP, Yeh S-Y, Bruce SR, Paul RH. Hypogastric artery ligation for obstetric haemorrhage. Obstet Gynecol 1985;66: 353–356.

Craig S, Chau H, Cho H. Treatment of severe postpartum hemorrhage by rectally administered gemeprost pessaries. J Perinat Med 1999; 27:231–235.

Cruikshank SH. Management of postpartum and pelvic hemorrhage. Clin Obstet Gynecol 1986;29:213–219.

Dayan SS, Schwalbe SS. The use of small-dose intravenous nitroglycerin in a case of uterine inversion. Anesth Analg 1996;82:1091–1093.

Dildy GA 3rd. Postpartum hemorrhage: new management options. Clin Obstet Gynecol 2002;45(2):330–344.

Dollery C, ed. Therapeutic Drugs, 2nd edn. Edinburgh: Churchill Livingstone, 1999.

Economides DL, Kadir RA, Lee CA. Inherited bleeding disorders in obstetrics and gynaecology. Br J Obstet Gynaecol 1999;106:5–13.

Eden RD, Parker RT, Gall SA. Rupture of the pregnant uterus: a 53 year review. Obstet Gynecol 1986;68:671–674.

Endres LK, Barnhart K. Spontaneous second trimester uterine rupture after classical cesarean. Obstet Gynecol 2000;96:806–808.

Ferguson JE II, Bourgeois FJ, Underwood PB Jr. B-Lynch suture for postpartum hemorrhage. Obstet Gynecol 2000;95:1020–1022.

George JN, Woolf SH, Raskob GE, et al. Idiopathic thrombocytopenic purpura: a practice guideline developed by explicit methods for The American Society of Hematology. Blood 1996;88:3–40.

Gulmezoglu AM, Villar J, Ngoc NT, et al. WHO mulitcentre randomised trial of misoprostol in the management of the third stage of labour. Lancet 2001;358:689–695.

Hansch E, Chitkara U, McAlpine J, El-Sayed Y, Dake MD, Razavi MK. Pelvic arterial embolisation for control of obstetric hemorrhage: a five year experience. Am J Obstet Gynecol 1999;180:1454–1460.

Hayashi RH, Castillo MS, Noah ML. Management of severe postpartum hemorrhage with a prostaglandin F2α analogue. Obstet Gynecol 1984;63:806–808.

Hoveyda F, MacKenzie IZ. Secondary postpartum haemorrhage: incidence, morbidity and current management. Br J Obstet Gynaecol 2001;108:927–930.

Johanson R, Kumar M, Obhrai M, Young P. Management of massive postpartum haemorrhage: use of a hydrostatic balloon catheter to avoid laparotomy. Br J Obstet Gynaecol 2001;108:420–422.

Kadir RA, Koh MB, Lee SA, Pasi KJ. Acquired haemophilia, an unusual cause of severe postpartum haemorrhage. Br J Obstet Gynaecol 1997a;104:854–856.

Kadir RA, Economides DL, Braithewaite J, Goldman E, Lee CA. The obstetric experience of carriers of haemophilia. Br J Obstet Gynaecol 1997b;104:803–810.

Kadir RA, Lee CA, Sabin CA, Pollard D, Economides DL. Pregnancy in women with von Willebrand's disease or factor XI deficiency. Br J Obstet Gynaecol 1998;105:314–321.

Katesmark M, Brown R, Raju KS. Successful use of a Sengstaken-Blakemore tube to control massive postpartum haemorrhage. Br J Obstet Gynaecol 1994;101:259–260.

Keogh J, Tsokos N. Aortic compression in massive postpartum haemorrhage—an old but lifesaving technique. Aust NZ J Obstet Gynaecol 1997;37:237–238.

Kitchin JD III, Thiagarajah S, May HV Jr, Thornton WN Jr. Puerperal inversion of the uterus. Am J Obstet Gynecol 1975;123:51–58.

Kupferminc MJ, Gull I, Bar-Am A, et al. Intrauterine irrigation with prostaglandin F2α for management of severe postpartum haemorrhage. Acta Obstet Gynaecol Scand 1998;77:548–550.

Lau WC, Fung HYM, Rogers MS. Ten years experience of caesarean and postpartum hysterectomy in a teaching hospital in Hong Kong. Eur J Obstet Gynecol Reprod Biol 1997;74:133–137.

Ledee N, Ville Y, Musset D, Mercier F, Frydman R, Fernandez H. Management in intractable obstetric haemorrhage: an audit study on 61 cases. Eur J Obstet Gynecol Rep Biol 2001;94:189–196.

Letsky EA. Disseminated intravascular coagulation. Ballière's Best Pract Res Clin Obstet Gynaecol 2001;15:623–644.

Lokugamage AU, Sullivan KR, Niculescu I, et al. A randomized study comparing rectally administered misoprostol versus syntometrine combined with an oxytocin infusion for the cessation of primary postpartum hemorrhage. Acta Obstet Gynecol Scand 2001;80: 835–839.

Lowe TW, Cunningham FG. Placental abruption. Clin Obstet Gynecol 1990;33:406–413.

Lydon-Rochelle M, Holt VL, Easterling TR, Martin DP. Risk of uterine rupture during labor among women with a prior cesarean delivery. N Engl J Med 2001;345:3–8.

McDonald S, Prendiville WJ, Elbourne D. Prophylactic syntometrine versus oxytocin for delivery of the placenta. Cochrane Database Syst Rev 2000;(2):CD000201.

McMahon MJ. Vaginal birth after cesarean. Clin Obs Gynecol 1998; 2:369–381.

Maier RC. Control of postpartum hemorrhage with uterine packing. Am J Obstet Gynecol 1993;169:317–323.

Mannucci PM. How I treat patients with von Willebrand disease. Blood 2001;97:1915–1919.

Maxwell C, Gawler D, Green J. An unusual case of acute postpartum broad ligament haematoma. Aust NZ J Obstet Gynecol 1997; 37:239–241.

Morgans D, Chan N, Clark CA. Vulval perineal haematomas in the immediate postpartum period and their management. Aust NZ J Obstet Gynaecol 1999;39:223–227.

O'Brien P, El-Refaey H, Gordon A, Geary M, Rodeck CH. Rectally administered misoprostol for the treatment of postpartum haemorrhage unresponsive to oxytocin and ergometrine: a descriptive study. Obstet Gynecol 1998;92:212–214.

Ogueh O, Ayida G. Acute uterine inversion: a new technique of hydrostatic replacement. Br J Obstet Gynaecol 1997;104:951–952.

O'Leary JA. Uterine artery ligation in the control of postcesarean hemorrhage. J Reprod Med 1995;40:1899–1893.

O'Leary JL, O'Leary JA, Uterine artery ligation for control of postcesarean section hemorrhage. Obstet Gynecol 1974;43:849–853.

Oleen MA, Mariano JP. Controlling refractory atonic postpartum haemorrhage with Hemabate sterile solution. Am J Obstet Gynecol 1990;162:205–208.

O'Sullivan JV. A simple method of correcting puerperal uterine inversion. BMJ 1945;2:282–284.

Pelage JP, Le Dref O, Mateo J, et al. Life-threatening primary postpartum hemorrhage: treatment with emergency selective arterial embolization. Radiology 1998;208:359–362.

Pelage JP, Soyer P, Repiquet D, et al. Secondary postpartum haemorrhage: treatment with selective arterial embolisation. Radiology 1999;212:385–389.

Phelan JP. Uterine rupture. Clin Obstet Gynecol 1990;33:432–437.

Plaunche WC, von Almen W, Muller R. Catastrophic uterine rupture. Obstet Gynecol 1984;64:792–797.

Pritchard JA. Changes in the blood volume during pregnancy and delivery. Anesthesiology 1965;26:393–399.

Pritchard JA, Brekken AL. Clinical and laboratory studies on severe abruptio placentae. Am J Obstet Gynecol 1967;681–700.

Pritchard JA, Baldwin RM, Dickey JC, Wiggins KM. Blood volume changes in pregnancy and the puerperium. II. Red blood cell loss and changes in apparent blood volume during and following vaginal delivery, cesarean section, and cesarean section plus total hysterectomy. Am J Obstet Gynecol 1962;84:1271–1282.

Pritchard JA, Cunningham FG, Pritchard SA, Mason RA. On reducing the frequency of severe abruptio placentae. Am J Obstet Gynecol 1991;165:1345–1351.

Riley DP, Burgess RW. External abdominal aortic compression: a study of a resuscitation manoeuvre for postpartum haemorrhage. Anesth Intens Care 1994;22:571–575.

Ritchie EH. Pregnancy after rupture of the pregnant uterus. J Obstet Gynaecol Br Commw 1971;78:642–648.

Shobeiri SA, West EC, Kahn MJ, Nolan TE. Postpartum acquired hemophilia (factor VIII inhibitors): a case report and review of the literature. Obstet Gynecol Surv 2000;55:729–737.

Silver, RM. Management of idiopathic thrombocytopenic purpura in pregnancy. Clin Obstet Gynecol 1998;41:436–448.

Tamizian O, Arulkumaran S. The surgical management of postpartum haemorrhage. Curr Op Obstet Gynecol 2001;13:127–131.

Toppozada M, El-Bossaty M, El-Rahman HA, El-Din AH. Control of intractable atonic postpartum hemorrhage by 5-methyl prostaglandin F2α. Obstet Gynecol 1981;58:327–330.

Vedantham S, Goodwin SC, McLucas B, Mohr G. Uterine artery embolization: an underused method of controlling pelvic hemorrhage. Am J Obstet Gynecol 1997;176:938–948.

22 Severe acute asthma

William H. Barth
Theresa L. Stewart

Recent data from the National Institutes of Health (NIH) show that the prevalence of asthma is increasing, a trend which has continued over the last 20 years. The overall age-adjusted prevalence of asthma rose from 30.7 per 1,000 population in 1980 to a 2-year average of 53.8 per 1,000 in 1993–94, representing a 75% increase. This increase in prevalence has been accompanied by an increase in costs, both in terms of health care, dollars, and lives. The total cost attributable to asthma in 1998 was estimated to be 11.3 billion dollars with direct costs estimated at 7.5 billion dollars. The largest component of the direct costs is hospitalization. For those focusing on women's care this is particularly relevant since, compared to men, women are more likely to be hospitalized for asthma and when admitted, require a longer hospital stay. Asthma is among the most common chronic medical conditions in the United States, and despite the increase in health-care expenditures for asthma, the age-adjusted mortality of asthma for both men and women has continued to increase.

Currently asthma is an area of active research. New theories concerning its pathophysiology are being tested, and treatment plans have been modified to reflect this understanding. As such, there are a number of new recommendations since the last edition of this book. The National Asthma Education Program (NAEP) of the National Heart, Lung, and Blood Institute (NHLBI) established its second expert panel report for the diagnosis and management of asthma. Published in 1997, this report is readily available from the NHLBI Information Center online at http://www.nhlbi.nih.gov/nhlbi/nhlbi.htm. As with previous editions, this chapter will rely on these recommendations, the report of the Working Group on Asthma and Pregnancy of the NAEP (published in 1993), and other recent publications, as the basis for the review of current management of asthma during pregnancy. Review of the management of severe exacerbations of asthma, the main focus of this chapter, cannot be achieved optimally without understanding the management for nonacute cases. Therefore, in addition to the management of acute exacerbations of asthma, this chapter will also briefly cover long-term management of asthmatic patients as a means to prevent the recurrence of severe exacerbations.

Definitions

The traditional definition of asthma has focused on airway responsiveness and its reversibility. Although inflammation has always been considered a key component of asthma, new research is evolving supporting a more complex role for inflammation as an etiology for airway hyper-responsiveness. The new definition of asthma adopted by the NHLBI (1997) is "a chronic inflammatory disorder of the airways in which many cells and cellular elements play a role, in particular, mast cells, eosinophils, T lymphocytes, neutrophils, and epithelial cells. In susceptible individuals, this inflammation causes recurrent episodes of wheezing, breathlessness, chest tightness, and cough, particularly at night and in the early morning. These episodes are usually associated with a widespread but variable airflow obstruction that is often reversible either spontaneously or with treatment. The inflammation also causes an associated increase in the existing bronchial hyperresponsiveness to a variety of stimuli". The definition was expanded to stress the more comprehensive understanding of the pathophysiology of asthma, particularly the role of chronic inflammation, a factor that needs to be considered in the management of these patients. This NHLBI panel also recommended some changes in classification of asthma. Classification is to be based on the underlying severity of a patient's asthma, either mild intermittent, mild persistent, moderate persistent, or severe persistent. The long-term management and treatment plan is then based on this classification (Table 22.1). Patients of any severity can experience an exacerbation that may be mild, moderate, or severe (Table 22.2). This classification is based on nonpregnant asthma patients. In extending this classification to pregnant women, we need to apply our knowledge concerning the physiologic changes that occur during pregnancy, but the general concepts still apply. In the management of the pregnant asthmatic patient there will be some special considerations secondary to her pregnant state,

Table 22.1 Classification of asthma severity

	Clinical features before treatment*		
	Symptoms†	**Night-time symptoms**	**Lung function**
Step 4 Severe persistent	Continual symptoms Limited physical activity Frequent exacerbations	Frequent	FEV_1 or PEF ≤60% predicted PEF variability >30%
Step 3 Moderate persistent	Daily symptoms Daily use of inhaled short-acting β_2-agonist Exacerbations affect activity Exacerbations ≥2 times a week; may last days	>1 time a week	FEV_1 or PEF >60% but <80% predicted PEF variability >30%
Step 2 Mild persistent	Symptoms >2 times a week but <1 time a day Exacerbations may affect activity	>2 times a month	FEV_1 or PEF ≥80% predicted PEF variability 20–30%
Step 1 Mild intermittent	Symptoms ≤2 times a week Asymptomatic and normal PEFR between exacerbations Exacerbations brief (from a few hours to a few days); intensity may vary	≤2 times a month	FEV 1 or PEF ≥80% predicted PEF variability <20%

* The presence of one of the features of severity is sufficient to place a patient in that category. An individual should be assigned to the most severe grade in which any feature occurs. The characteristics noted in this table are general and may overlap because asthma is highly variable. Furthermore, an individual's classification may change over time.

† Patients at any level of severity can have mild, moderate, or severe exacerbations. Some patients with intermittent asthma experience severe and life-threatening exacerbations separated by long periods of normal lung function and no symptoms.

and although important, they are relatively few and will be stressed throughout the chapter.

Effect of pregnancy on asthma

Pregnancy may or may not affect the course of asthma in any individual patient. Turner et al. (1980), summarizing the large retrospective studies published to date, reported that 22% of patients experienced improvement in their asthma, while 40% remained unchanged and another 20% noted worsening disease. In a prospective study of 366 pregnancies complicated by asthma, Schatz and colleagues (1988) tracked both symptoms and spirometry throughout gestation and the postpartum period. Of their subjects, 28% improved, 33% remained unchanged, 35% clearly worsened, and 4% demonstrated equivocal changes. In a subsequent prospective study with 198 pregnancies reported by Stenius-Aariala et al. (1988), over 40% required additional therapy at some point during gestation.

Although predicting which gravida will experience exacerbations is generally not possible, several factors in the patient's history may be of help. Gluck and Gluck (1976) found that patients beginning pregnancy with severe disease were more likely to worsen than those beginning with mild disease. Others have shown that the natural history of asthma during one pregnancy tends to be repeated in subsequent gestations (Schatz et al., 1988). Finally, these same authors have shown that approximately 10% of pregnant women with asthma will experience exacerbations during labor and delivery.

Effect of asthma on pregnancy

Asthma, especially when severe or uncontrolled, can substantially alter pregnancy outcome. Several authors have noted significant increases in the rates of abortion, preterm labor, low birth weight, and neonatal hypoxia (Schaefer & Silverman, 1961; Bahna & Bjerkedal, 1972; Sims et al., 1976). Reporting on 277 patients with asthma in the Collaborative Study of Cerebral Palsy, Mental Retardation, and Other Allied Neurological Diseases, Gordon et al. (1970) found a perinatal mortality rate double that of controls without asthma. In 16 patients with severe asthma (repetitive attacks, persistent symptoms, or status asthmaticus), the perinatal mortality rate was 28%. Greenberger and colleagues (Fitsimons et al., 1986; Greenberger & Patterson, 1988) have shown that among women with asthma, those whose pregnancy is complicated by status asthmaticus have significantly smaller infants and a greater frequency of intrauterine growth retardation. Conversely, Schatz and coauthors (1995) reported that when asthma during pregnancy is controlled with step therapy, adverse perinatal outcomes are not increased over those in the general

Table 22.2 Classifying severity of asthma exacerbations

	Mild	Moderate	Severe	Respiratory arrest imminent
Symptoms				
Breathlessness	While walking Can lie down	While talking Prefers sitting	While at rest Sits upright	
Talks in	Sentences	Phrases	Words	
Alertness	May be agitated	Usually agitated	Usually agitated	Drowsy or confused
Signs				
Respiratory rate	Increased	Increased	Often >30/min	
Use of accessory muscles; suprasternal retractions	Usually not	Commonly	Usually	Paradoxical thoracoabdominal movement
Wheeze	Moderate, often only end expiratory	Loud; throughout exhalation	Usually loud; throughout inhalation and exhalation	Absence of wheeze
Pulse/minute	<100	100–120	>120	Bradycardia
Pulsus paradoxus	Absent <10 mmHg	May be present 10–25 mmHg	Often present >25 mmHg	Absence suggests respiratory muscle fatigue
Functional assessment				
PEFR % predicted or % personal best	>80%	Approx. 50–80% or response lasts <2 hr	<50% predicted or personal best	
$P_{a}O_2$ (on air)	Normal (test not usually necessary)	>60 mmHg (test not usually necessary)	<60 mmHg: possible cyanosis	
and/or				
PCO_2	<42 mmHg (test not usually necessary)	<42 mmHg (test not usually necessary)	≥42 mmHg: possible respiratory failure (see text)	
$S_{a}O_2$% (on air) at sea level	>95% (test not usually necessary)	91–95%	<91%	

Note:
- The presence of several parameters, but not necessarily all, indicates the general classification of the exacerbation.
- Many of these parameters have not been systematically studied, so they serve only as general guides.

population. Despite reports that aggressive management can reduce perinatal morbidity and mortality, fetal deaths secondary to maternal asthma have been described (Topilski et al., 1974; Sachs et al., 1987). Postulating a common smooth-muscle dysfunction in the vasculature and airways, Lehrer and colleagues (1993) reported an association between pregnancy-induced hypertension and maternal asthma.

In addition to its implications for fetal outcome, severe asthma during pregnancy is associated with a small but definite risk to the life of the mother. Gordon et al. (1970) reported four deaths among the 16 patients with severe disease from the Collaborative Group. Schaefer et al. (1961), Schatz et al. (1995), and Jewett (1973) have also described maternal status asthmaticus refractory to all therapy short of interrupting the pregnancy. When asthma becomes this severe, complications that directly threaten the life of the mother may include pneumothorax, pneumomediastinum, acute cor pulmonale, arrhythmias, and respiratory muscle fatigue. Levine and associates (1995) confirmed reversible severe myocardial depression with left ventricular ejection fractions between 11% and 34%. The gravity of these morbid complications is emphasized by a mortality rate over 40% when asthma has progressed to the point of requiring mechanical ventilation (Scoggin et al., 1977). Tragically, studies analyzing the causes of death in severe asthma have shown that most occur outside of a hospital and that the severity of the disease usually was not appreciated by the patient or the physician (Woolcock, 1988). Considering this, and that modern management of the severely asthmatic gravida can often avert fetal and maternal catastrophes, it is imperative that the obstetrician thoroughly evaluate and aggressively manage any pregnant woman presenting with reactive airway disease.

Pathophysiology

The pathophysiology of asthma is complex and still not fully understood. As with many diseases, we have much more information regarding clinical and pathologic findings, but only limited knowledge regarding the etiology of these changes. Components of the disease process that have been well described in the literature have been based on the pathologic lung findings from patients with fatal asthma, histologic findings from bronchial biopsies in stable asthmatic patients, and bronchoalveolar lavage specimens from patients with asthma following allergen challenge. These studies present a complex picture of an acute and chronic inflammatory process, and an underlying lung that has been altered significantly depending on the extent and duration of disease. This inflammatory process can be initiated by many factors including: infection, atopy (IgE-mediated response), exercise, cold, emotional stress, or occupational agents. In addition to the inflammatory component, asthma is characterized by an exaggerated bronchoconstrictor response, airway edema, mucus plug formation, and finally airway obstruction that leads to its clinical symptoms.

Pathologic finding include persistent hyperinflation, mucus plugging, detached bronchial epithelium, damage to extensive areas of the bronchial epithelium with exposed basal cells, inflammation with eosinophils, collagen deposition beneath the basement membrane, edema, vascular congestion, bronchial smooth muscle hyperplasia, and goblet-cell hyperplasia (Beasely et al., 1993). All of the airway cells are involved including T-lymphocytes, eosinophils, mast cells, macrophages, epithelial cells, fibroblasts, and bronchial smooth muscle cells. These cells when activated can release substances that lead to further inflammation and cellular damage. A number of known biochemical mediators of asthma are listed in Table 22.3. This cascade of events leads to a massive influx of various inflammatory cells. The extent of cellular influx is dependent on increased recruitment from the bloodstream and survival of these cells within the lung. T-cells appear to play a central role in the extent of airway inflammation.

T-cells are found in increased numbers in patients with asthma of any severity (Vignola et al., 2000). A specific subpopulation of T-lymphocytes, the Th2 phenotype, have been identified as paramount in this process. The Th2 phenotypic cells release cytokines that specifically target eosinophils, and their numbers are increased in the airways of asthmatic patients. These cells release other substances (metalloproteases and growth factors) that are important in inflammation and bronchial remodeling. Recent evidence suggests (Vignola et al., 1999) that not only are more inflammatory cells recruited to the lung, but once present, their survival appears to be prolonged. Apoptosis, or programmed cell death, tends to limit the extent of tissue injury produced by inflammatory cells. Vignola and colleagues (1999) recently described reduced numbers of apoptotic eosinophils and macrophages in the bronchial mucosa of asthmatic subjects compared to normal controls. They also noted an inverse relationship between the severity of disease and the number of apoptotic

Table 22.3 Biochemical mediators of asthma

	Source	Actions
Primary mediators		
Histamine	Mast cells, macrophages	Vasodilation, leaking venules, bronchial smooth-muscle contraction
Slow-reacting substance of anaphylaxis	Mast cells, basophils, peripheral leukocytes	Bronchial smooth-muscle contraction, increased vascular permeability
Eosinophil chemotactic factor	Basophils, mast cells	Recruitment of eosinophils, release of tissue-damaging peroxidase, cationic and major base protein
Platelet-activating factor	Mast cells, basophils	Aggregation and degranulation of platelets, increased secondary mediators
Secondary mediators		
Prostaglandins: PGF_2, PGE_2, PGD_2, PGI_2, thromboxane	Phospholipid membrane substrate	Alterations in bronchial smooth-muscle tone, alteration in pulmonary vascular resistance
Leukotrienes: LTC_4, LTD_4, LTE_4	Phospholipid membranes	Bronchoconstriction chemotaxis of neutrophils and eosinophils

eosinophils and macrophages, suggesting that reduced cell death of these cells can influence the clinical severity of the disease. The inflammatory cells with their various cellular products appear to be responsible for the thickened basement membrane that is the classic pathologic finding in many asthmatic patients.

Although the complete mechanism remains somewhat controversial, the thickened membrane appears to be a result of airway remodeling. Based on other disease processes, it would seem logical that patients with repeated clinical exacerbations of asthma would be more likely to have thickened basement membranes and therefore airway remodeling would become more prominent as the duration of disease increased. This, however, is not necessarily the case. Interestingly, Chetta et al. (1997) studied a group of asthmatic patients who were treated with inhaled β_2-agonists alone and found that the degree of subepithelial thickness was related to the clinical severity of asthma, but not related to atopy or duration of asthma. In fact, in their study the thickest subepithelial layer was obtained from a newly diagnosed subject with severe clinical grading of asthma. This would suggest that the membrane thickening is an early change in asthmatic patients, possibly occurring prior to the clinical manifestations of disease, and this may have functional and clinical significance in the treatment of the disease.

The final classic component in the pathophysiology of asthma is airway hyper-responsiveness that leads to airway obstruction. As with the other components of asthma, the airway hyper-responsiveness is not completely understood. Hyper-responsiveness is usually measured using an inhaled bronchoconstrictor stimulus such as methacholine or histamine. The individual's responsiveness is expressed as the dose required to achieve some defined degree of bronchoconstriction, usually a 20% fall in the forced expired volume in one second (FEV_1). Factors that have been shown to be associated with airway hyper-responsiveness include the degree of inflammation, the specific type of inflammatory cells involved (Foresi et al., 1990), the thickness of the basement membrane (Carroll et al., 1993), and possibly some underlying genetic predisposition of the airway to bronchoconstriction.

Clinical course

The functional result of bronchospasm is airway obstruction with a concomitant decrease in airflow. As airways constrict, the work of breathing increases and patients then present with chest tightness, wheezing, or breathlessness. Subsequent alterations in oxygenation are primarily the result of ventilation/perfusion (V/Q) mismatching, because the distribution of airway narrowing during an acute attack is uneven (Rodriguez-Roisin et al., 1989). With mild disease, initial hypoxia is well compensated, as reflected by a normal arterial oxygen tension and decreased carbon dioxide, with resultant respiratory alkalosis. As airway narrowing worsens, V/Q mismatching increases, and hypoxemia ensues. With severe obstruction, ventilation becomes impaired enough to result in early carbon dioxide retention. Superimposed on hyperventilation, carbon dioxide retention may only be manifest as an arterial carbon dioxide tension returning to the normal range. Finally, with critical obstruction, respiratory failure follows, characterized by hypoxemia, hypercarbia, and acidemia. At this extreme, oxygen consumption and cardiac work are increased, and the magnitude of pulmonary hypertension is frequently severe (Kingston & Hirshman, 1984; Rodriguez-Roisin et al., 1989). The clinical stages of asthma are presented in Table 22.4.

While such changes in pulmonary function are generally reversible and well tolerated in the healthy nonpregnant individual, even the early stages of asthma may pose grave risk to the gravida and her fetus. Maternal factors responsible for this include: (i) increased basal metabolic rate and oxygen consumption; (ii) decreased diffusing capacity; (iii) decreased available buffer; and (iv) pregnancy-induced alterations in lung volumes (Cugell et al., 1953; Fishburne, 1979; Weinberger et al., 1980; Greenberger & Patterson, 1985; Sachs et al., 1987). Most importantly, as pregnancy progresses, functional residual capacity (FRC) decreases by 10–25% and frequently falls below the critical closing volume, a phenomenon much more likely to occur during the advanced stages of pregnancy (Garrard et al., 1978; Awe et al., 1979). The smaller FRC and the increased effective shunt thus render the gravida more rapidly susceptible to the effects of hypoxia. Clinically, only 30 sec-

Table 22.4 Clinical stages of asthma

Stage	Arterial blood gases			FEV_1, peak flow % predicted	Comment
	Po_2	Pco_2	pH		
I	Normal	↓	↑	65–80	Mild respiratory alkalosis
II	↓	↓	↑	50–64	Respiratory alkalosis
III	↓	Normal	Normal	35–49	Danger zone
IV	↓	↑	↓	35–	Respiratory acidosis

Po_2, pressure of oxygen; Pco_2, pressure of carbon dioxide; FEV_1, forced expiratory volume (1 second).

onds of apnea are needed to drop maternal arterial oxygen tension to less than 60 mmHg (Levinson & Shnider, 1987). As the mother increases ventilation to maintain oxygen tension, respiratory alkalosis develops.

Data from both sheep and human studies have shown that maternal alkalosis may cause dangerous hypoxemia in the fetus before maternal oxygenation is compromised (Moya et al., 1965; Rolston et al., 1974). Mechanisms proposed to explain this include decreased uterine blood flow, decreased maternal venous return, and an alkaline-induced leftward shift of the hemoglobin–oxygen dissociation curve (Bartels et al., 1962; Wulf et al., 1972; Rolston et al., 1974). The latter mechanism, known as the Bohr effect, appears to become clinically significant when the maternal carbon dioxide tension drops to 14–17 mmHg (Bartels et al., 1962; Moya et al., 1965). Finally, when the mother can no longer maintain a normal oxygen tension, and hypoxemia develops, the fetus responds with decreased umbilical blood flow, increased systemic and pulmonary vascular resistance, and ultimately decreased cardiac output (Brinkman et al., 1970). Because the fetus may be in jeopardy before maternal disease becomes severe, it is again emphasized that the obstetrician should take an aggressive approach to the management of any pregnant women presenting with asthma.

Differential diagnosis

While over 60% of pregnant women experience a physiologic dyspnea of pregnancy, severe shortness of breath and wheezing are clearly abnormal (Cugell et al., 1953; Weinberger et al., 1980). Although a careful history and physical examination can usually assure the diagnosis, other life-threatening entities that must be excluded include severe allergic reactions, aspiration pneumonitis, pulmonary edema, pulmonary embolus, amniotic fluid embolus, left heart failure, and mitral stenosis (Cugell et al., 1953; Weinberger et al., 1980). Large airway obstruction from either a foreign body or an endobronchial tumor also should be considered. Mettam and colleagues (1992) have reported a case in which life-threatening acute respiratory distress in late pregnancy was caused by an enlarged thyroid and resultant external airway compression.

Clinical management

Although several authors have proposed the use of clinical scoring systems to predict the severity of asthma, its response to therapy, or the need for hospitalization, the prospective application of these formulas has shown them to be frequently misleading (Baker, 1988). Furthermore, their use has not been applied to or tested in a pregnant population. Recalling that fetal oxygenation may be jeopardized even with early stages of asthma, and that pregnant women are poorly tolerant of rapid ventilatory derangements, prompt and thorough evaluation and treatment of any pregnant woman with acute asthma is imperative.

The NAEP Working Group on Asthma and Pregnancy (1993) lists the essential components of effective management of asthma for pregnant women as: (i) objective measures for assessment and monitoring maternal lung function and fetal well-being in order to make appropriate therapeutic recommendations; (ii) avoiding or controlling asthma triggers in the patient's environment; (iii) pharmacologic therapy; and (iv) patient education. Importantly, the authors of the report stress that patients attempting home therapy of an acute exacerbation "should not delay in seeking medical help if therapy does not provide rapid improvement, if the improvement is not sustained, if there is further deterioration, if the asthma exacerbation is severe, or if the fetal kick count decreases." This chapter concentrates on the management of pregnant women who present with acute severe asthma or life-threatening asthma.

History and physical examination

A patient's subjective impression of the severity of her asthma frequently does not accurately reflect objective measures of airway function or ventilation. McFadden and colleagues (1973), in a classic work correlating subjective complaints with measures of lung mechanics, have shown that when patients thought their asthma had resolved, mean FEV_1 and mid-expiratory flow rates were still only 20% and 22% of predicted values, respectively. Although others have confirmed a poor correlation between dyspnea and objective assessment of airway obstruction, Rees et al. (1967) have shown that when dyspnea is so severe as to interfere with normal speech, the FEV_1 is consistently less than 0.45/1 min. Several factors in the patient's history should warn the physician of the possibility of rapid progression and potentially fatal airway obstruction. These include prior intubation for asthma, two or more hospitalizations for asthma in the past year, three or more emergency care visits for asthma in the past year, hospitalization or an emergency care visit for asthma within the past month, current use of systemic corticosteroids or recent withdrawal from systemic corticosteroids, history of syncope or hypoxic seizure due to asthma, prior admission for asthma to a hospital-base intensive care unit, and serious psychiatric disease or psychosocial problems (Miller et al., 1992; Working Group, 1993). Miller and associates (1992) have demonstrated that major psychiatric diagnoses and noncompliance are significantly related to cases of potentially fatal asthma, emphasizing the importance of increased vigilance when caring for these patients.

Physical examination of the patient with asthma, while helpful in establishing the diagnosis, is also an inaccurate predictor of the severity of airway disease. Several authors have shown that expiratory wheezing does not correlate with objective measures of airflow or derangements in arterial blood gas analysis (McFadden et al., 1973; Corre & Rothstein, 1985). Indeed, an increase in auscultated wheezing may be due to increase in airflow, while the absence of wheezing may be the result of critical airway narrowing and absence of airflow (Corre & Rothstein, 1985). Physical signs that should warn the clinician of life-threatening or severe asthma include labored breathing, tachycardia, pulsus paradoxus of greater than 10 mmHg, prolonged expiration, and use of accessory muscles of respiration. Signs that may warn of a potentially fatal attack include difficulty speaking, central cyanosis, and altered consciousness.

Pulmonary function tests

Clinical management is most appropriately guided by the use of pulmonary function tests. Measurement of either the FEV_1 or the peak expiratory flow rate (PEFR) can help to assess the severity of obstruction and monitor the response to therapy. Sims et al. (1976) have shown that pulmonary function tests in stable asthmatics, active asthmatics, and nonasthmatic controls are not altered by pregnancy. Brancazio and colleagues (1997) reported mean PEFR in normal pregnant women of 430–450 L/min, with values not changing significantly as pregnancy progresses. Unfortunately, complex bedside spirometry equipment is not commonly available. Peak flow rates, however, may now be measured with simple, hand-held peak flow meters. Predicted values based on age, height, and gender have been published in nomogram form but, in general, range between 380 and 550 L/min for women (Gregg & Nunn, 1989). Summarizing several large studies that recorded peak flow rates in acute asthma, Corre and Rothstein (1985) concluded that values less than 100 L/min correlate well with severe obstruction. Rather than relying on predicted normal values, Clark and the NAEP Working Group (1993) recommend that pregnant women should establish their own personal best PEFR after a period of monitoring when the asthma has been well controlled. Whether one uses a percent of predicted normal or personal best, pulmonary function tests should not be used to the exclusion of arterial blood gas assessment for pregnant women. Tai and Road (1967) have demonstrated a P_aO_2 less than 60 mmHg in over 16% of acute asthmatics whose FEV_1 was 1.0 L or more. Because a maternal P_aO_2 of less than 60 mmHg is associated with a rapid decline in fetal oxygenation, relying solely on reassuring pulmonary function tests may prove detrimental to an already stressed fetus. Pulmonary function test results that identify life-threatening or potentially fatal asthma for the mother include a PEFR less than 100 L/min, an FEV_1 less than 25% of predicted, or less than a 10% improvement in peak flow or FEV_1 with treatment in the emergency department (NAEP Working Group, 1993).

Arterial blood gases

While clinical signs and symptoms with acute asthma may prove misleading, arterial blood gas analysis allows direct assessment of maternal oxygenation, ventilation, and acid–base status. With this information, the clinician can correctly assess the severity of an acute attack (Table 22.4). Care must be taken, however, to interpret the results in light of normal values for pregnancy. A normal maternal P_aO_2 varies from 101 to 108 mmHg early in pregnancy and falls to 90–100 mmHg near term secondary to an increased critical closing volume, as previously discussed (Weinberger et al., 1980; Noble et al., 1988). These changes are responsible for the widened alveolar–arterial oxygen gradient [$P_{(A-a)}O_2$], which averages 20 mmHg in the third trimester (Awe et al., 1979). The normal physiologic increase in minute ventilation during pregnancy is reflected by a P_aCO_2 of 27–32 mmHg and an increase in pH from 7.40 to 7.45 (Noble et al., 1988; Hankins et al., 1996). Consequently, a P_aCO_2 greater than 35 mmHg, with a pH less than 7.35 in the presence of a falling P_aO_2, should be considered respiratory failure in a pregnant asthmatic.

As discussed, arterial blood gas assessment should be used liberally in the management of pregnant women presenting with an acute exacerbation of asthma. Guidance from the NAEP Working Group (1993) suggests that arterial blood gases must be assessed when patients present with obvious hypoventilation, cyanosis, or severe distress after initial therapy, or if the PEFR is less than 200 L/min or the FEV_1 remains less than 40% of predicted. Patients with arterial $P_aCO_2 \geq 30$ mmHg will require repeated arterial blood gas measurements to monitor their response to treatment. Finally, initiation of therapy for acute asthma in pregnancy should not be delayed while performing or awaiting the results of pulmonary function tests or arterial blood gas analysis.

Other laboratory tests

When patients without an established history of asthma present with wheezing and respiratory distress, clinicians should consider an initial ECG because these may be the signs of a more serious cardiac disease. The ECG in acute asthma may show right bundle branch block, acute enlargement of the right atrium, and ventricular ectopy (Kingston & Hirshman, 1984). Additionally, institution of a bronchodilator may precipitate or worsen such arrhythmias (Koch-Weser et al., 1977). Pulse oximetry should be employed to monitor maternal oxygenation and to ensure maintenance of an oxygen saturation greater than 95% (NAEP Working Group, 1993). If the patient is febrile or in severe distress, a chest X-ray should be obtained to rule out pneumonia or one of the severe complications of asthma, such as pneumothorax or pneumomediastinum. A Gram stain and microscopic examination of the sputum should be done to rule out a contribution from bacterial pneumonia or bronchitis (Woolcock, 1988). When the diagnosis of asthma is in question, demonstration of eosinophils on microscopic examination of the sputum may help narrow the differential (NAEP Working Group, 1993). Finally, when patients present with asthma exacerbations in the third trimester, continuous electronic fetal monitoring should be considered. As mentioned previously, significant fetal hypoxemia can occur prior to significant maternal compromise. Decreased fetal movement and fetal heart rate changes on the monitor may alert the clinician to significant fetal distress not otherwise apparent. Similarly, persistent evidence of fetal hypoxia, such as diminished variability or repetitive late decelerations, may suggest the need for increased hydration or oxygenation, even in the nominally stable mother.

Treatment

The goals of treatment of severe acute asthma in pregnancy are the prevention of maternal and fetal mortality and morbidity. Therapy should be directed toward correcting maternal hypoxia, rapid reversal of airflow obstruction, optimizing uteroplacental function, and reducing the likelihood of recurrence of the severe airflow obstruction. Recommendations on the hospital setting where the patient is best managed vary. Whether evaluated and treated in the emergency department, labor and delivery, or an observation unit, the location is not as important as the unit's capabilities. Monitoring and resuscitative equipment should be readily available (including electronic fetal heart rate monitoring if in the third trimester), and if a severe exacerbation or life-threatening asthma is suspected, provisions for intubation and ventilation should be accessible, preferably in an intensive care unit. Guidelines from both the American College of Obstetricians and Gynecologists (1996) and the NAEP Working Group on Asthma and Pregnancy (1993), suggest that in patients who respond rapidly (an FEV_1 or PEFR 70% of predicted) to bronchodilator therapy, follow-up may be continued on an outpatient basis. As discussed previously, however, clinicians caring for a pregnant woman and her fetus should have a low threshold for admission to the hospital. Clinicians should be especially liberal with admission to the hospital if the patient presents in the evening, has had the recent onset of nocturnal symptoms, has had previous episodes of severe exacerbations, or if there are concerns about social circumstances or the relatives' ability to respond if the condition should worsen (NAEP Working Group, 1993).

The first step in treatment is administration of supplemental oxygen to the mother, with a goal of maintaining a P_ao_2 greater than 65 mmHg or an oxygen saturation of at least 95% on oxygen (F_io_2) of 35–60%, and without resulting in hypercarbia. The patient should be placed in a near-sitting position, with leftward tilt, especially if in the third trimester. Awe and colleagues (1979) have shown that in the third trimester, more than 25% of normal pregnant women will develop moderate hypoxia in the supine position. In their series, simply sitting the patient up in bed changed the mean $P_{(A-a)}o_2$ from 20 to 14 mmHg.

Intravenous (IV) access should be achieved, both for administration of medications and for careful rehydration. Patients presenting in extremis are frequently volume depleted if they have been too breathless to maintain oral intake at a time when insensible losses are high (Fish & Summer, 1982). In such circumstances, rehydration may help prevent inspissation of mucus plugs and may aid in expectoration (Summer, 1985; Sawicka & Branthwaithe, 1987). The last component of the primary therapy of an acute asthma exacerbation includes the use of short-acting β_2-agonists and systemic corticosteroids (NHLBI Guidelines, 1997). The dose and the frequency with which these drugs are given are dependent on the patient's clinical findings and response to initial interventions.

Adrenergic agents

The first-line pharmacologic therapy of acute severe asthma in pregnancy should consist of an inhaled β_2-adrenergic agonist (Clark, 1993; NAEP Working Group, 1993; NHLBI Guidelines, 1997). These agents, when used alone, produce a greater degree of bronchodilation than either methylxanthines or anticholinergic drugs (Chaieb et al., 1989). Evidence now suggests that there is no clear advantage to the use of parenteral rather than inhaled β_2-agonist in patients with asthma (Leatherman, 1994). Although ingrained in clinical practice, administration of these agents via a nebulizer rarely offers advantage over the supervised use of a metered-dose inhaler (MDI) plus a holding chamber, and it is significantly more expensive (Calocone et al., 1993; Idris et al., 1993; Newhouse, 1993). In severe cases (FEV_1 30% of predicted), Idris and colleagues (1993) noted a trend toward faster improvement with an MDI plus holding chamber. In the rare situation where patients are unable to coordinate inhalation of medication from an MDI, nebulized therapy may be more effective. If, for some reason, patients cannot effectively use an MDI or nebulizer, β_2-agonists can be administered subcutaneously. The more common adrenergic agents, their dosages, and their possible routes of administration are listed in Table 22.5. The onset of action for inhaled β_2-agonists is less than 5 minutes and repetitive administration produces incremental bronchodilation.

Epidemiologic studies have demonstrated an association between the increasing use of β-agonists and an increased risk of death due to asthma (Crane et al., 1989; Spitzer et al., 1992). This association is thought to be a reflection of increasing severity of disease and not a direct effect of the medication (Burrows & Lebowitz, 1992). Spitzer et al. (1992) found that the use of more than one canister of β_2-agonist for quick relief during a 1-month period suggested an over-reliance on this drug and inadequate asthma control. Prior to 1990, short-

Table 22.5 Medications used in the treatment of acute severe asthma

	Drug	Route of administration and dosage
Inhaled β-agonists	Albuterol	Nebulizer; 2.5–5.0 mg (0.5–1.0 mL of a 5% solution, diluted with 2–3 mL normal saline) MDI with a holding chamber (90 μg/puff given as 4 puffs over 4 min)
	Metaproterenol	Nebulizer; 15 mg (0.3 mL of a 5% solution, diluted with 2–3 mL normal saline)
Subcutaneous β-agonists	Epinephrine	0.3 mg subcutaneously
	Terbutaline	0.25 mg subcutaneously
Corticosteroids	Methylprednisolone	60–80 mg IV bolus every 6–8 hr or 125 mg IV bolus followed by above or oral steroids, depending on response
	Hydrocortisone	2.0 mg/kg IV bolus every 4 hr or 2.0 mg/kg IV bolus then 0.5 mg/kg/hr continuous infusion
Anticholinergics	Ipratropium bromide	Nebulizer; 0.5 mg (one vial 0.02% solution)
	Glycopyrrolate	MDI; 18 μg/puff, 2–3 puffs Nebulizer; 0.8–2.0 mg
Magnesium sulfate		2-g IV bolus over 2 min (followed immediately by inhaled β-agonist)
Methylxanthine	Aminophylline	Loading dose of 6 mg/kg actual body weight, followed by continuous IV infusion at 0.4–0.6 mg/kg/hr (must follow serum theophylline levels with a goal of 8–12 μg/mL during pregnancy)

IV, intravenous; MDI, metered-dose inhaler.

acting β_2-agonists were prescribed as a regularly scheduled medication to improve the overall control in many asthmatic patients. In the 1990s multiple studies were published demonstrating that regularly scheduled use of β_2-agonists does not benefit asthmatic patients, and therefore prescribing short-acting β_2-agonists in this manner is no longer recommended (NHLBI guidelines, 1997).

β-agonists act in concert with specific cell-surface receptors to activate the membrane-associated enzyme, adenylate cyclase. Adenylate cyclase then promotes the conversion of adenosine triphosphate to cyclic adenosine-3′,5′-monophosphate (cAMP). Increased intracellular cAMP then mediates relaxation of bronchial smooth muscle, prevents further contraction, increases clearance of mucus, and prevents the release of mediators described earlier (Koch-Weser et al., 1977). β_2-adrenergic receptors are located primarily in the bronchia, blood vessels, pancreas, and uterus, while β_1-receptors are confined largely to the heart (Koch-Weser et al., 1977). Non-bronchodilator effects of β_2-agonists that may play a role in asthma include the following: (i) increased mucociliary clearance; (ii) inhibition of cholinergic neurotransmission; (iii) enhancement of vascular integrity; and (iv) inhibition of mediator release from mast cells, basophils, and other cells (Nelson, 1995).

One side effect of β-agonists that is observed when they are used specifically for severe asthma is a paradoxical decrease in P_ao_2 and oxygen saturation soon after initiation of therapy (Koch-Weser et al., 1977; Nelson, 1995). This is a transient phenomenon secondary to the β_1-mediated increase in cardiac output that occurs before effective bronchodilation and possible relief of compensatory hypoxic pulmonary vasoconstriction. Contraindications to β-adrenergic therapy include coronary artery disease, cardiac asthma, and cerebrovascular disease (Koch-Weser et al., 1977). While these are rare in the reproductive age group, cases of symptomatic cerebral ischemia following β-adrenergic therapy have been reported in pregnant women with a history of severe migraines (Oserne et al., 1982). Nonetheless, Schatz and colleagues (1988) have demonstrated the safety of β_2-agonists for asthma during pregnancy in a large prospective study. Comparing 259 pregnant asthmatics using β-agonists with 101 using other bronchodilators, the authors found no difference in rates of intrauterine growth retardation, congenital anomalies, or perinatal mortality.

Corticosteroids

For patients not responding immediately to bronchodilators and for those already taking regular oral corticosteroids, systemic steroids should be administered (NAEP Working Group, 1993; ACOG, 1996; NHLBI Guidelines, 1997). Corticosteroids should also be started immediately for patients with a PEFR less than 200 L/min or an FEV_1 less than or equal to 40% of predicted after an initial hour of β_2-agonist therapy (NAEP Working Group, 1993). Systemic corticosteroids should be given immediately to any patient presenting with signs or symptoms of life-threatening or potentially fatal asthma (Leatherman, 1994).

Glucocorticoids enter the cell by diffusion, bind to a specific cytoplasmic receptor, and are rapidly transported to the nucleus. There, nuclear gene expression is altered, messenger RNA is formed, and proteins subsequently produced then mediate specific pharmacologic effects (Morris, 1985a,b). Additionally, corticosteroids have a more immediate action, altering calcium entry into cells and affecting calcium-dependent enzyme systems such as the phospholipases (Morris, 1985b). Pharmacologic effects thought to play a role in acute asthma include: (i) direct bronchial smooth-muscle relaxation; (ii) constriction of the bronchial microvasculature, with reduced capillary permeability and reduced edema formation; (iii) decreased activity and number of circulating inflammatory cells; (iv) increased prostaglandin formation; and, perhaps most importantly, (v) increased responsiveness to β-adrenergic stimulation (Morris, 1985a,b; Spector, 1985; Beasely et al., 1993). This potentiation of β-adrenergic therapy is seen within 1–2 hours of steroid administration (Ellul-Micallef & Fenech, 1975). Finally, corticosteroids have been noted to improve V/Q mismatching in status asthmaticus, possibly as a result of altered prostaglandin metabolism and pulmonary perfusion (Pierson et al., 1974; Winfield et al., 1980).

Two separate studies have established the efficacy of early administration of parenteral corticosteroids in acute severe asthma. In a randomized, prospective, double-blind study using hydrocortisone for the treatment of acute asthma, Fanta and colleagues (1983) found an increase in both the rate and magnitude of improvement in FEV_1 when compared with controls. In a similar study, Littenberg and Gluck (1986) found that early administration of a 125-mg IV bolus of methylprednisolone helped to terminate the acute attack, alleviate symptoms, and decrease the need for hospitalization. Not all clinical trials have demonstrated a benefit to the early administration of corticosteroids. In a randomized, double-blind clinical trial, Rodrigo and Rodrigo (1994) did detect a difference in the duration of bronchodilator therapy, hospital admission rates, or length of stay when early administration of 500 mg of IV hydrocortisone was compared with placebo in patients receiving aggressive β_2-agonists therapy. In a similar trial, McNamarra and Rubin (1993) demonstrated that early administration decreases subsequent relapse rates in patients presenting with acute asthma exacerbations. Wendel and colleagues (1996) prospectively studied 84 pregnant women with asthma, and demonstrated a clear superiority of corticosteroids over aminophylline in the treatment of asthma exacerbation.

In the setting of acute severe asthma, corticosteroids are commonly administered parenterally. Although inhaled corticosteroids (beclomethasone dipropionate) are available, they have little systemic action and do not affect the lung parenchyma. Even though beclomethasone has been reported to be safe for severe asthma during pregnancy, it does not have a role in the acute management of women with status asthmaticus (Greenberger & Patterson, 1983). Inhaled corticosteroids or a nonsteroidal antiinflammatory drug such as nedocromil or cromolyn sodium, however, should be used regularly by patients with chronic moderate and severe asthma or by those thought to be at high risk. Recommendations for dosing systemic corticosteroids in acute severe asthma are included in Table 22.5.

Maternal side effects from corticosteroids are largely limited to long-term use. The two potential effects from short-term use are salt retention and possible suppression of the hypothalamic–pituitary–adrenal axis. If sodium retention is thought to be a concern, methylprednisolone should be used in lieu of hydrocortisone. Finally, if oral therapy is used following the initial treatment, 40 mg of prednisone per day for 10 days is sufficient, and tapering the dose is not necessary (O'Driscoll et al., 1993). The available animal and human toxicologic data regarding short-term use of systemic corticosteroids do not point to an increase in adverse fetal effects (NAEP Working Group, 1993). In fact, Fitzsimons and colleagues (1986) have noted that adverse fetal outcomes were more likely when maternal asthma was poorly controlled or complicated by status asthmaticus.

Anticholinergic agents

Although they are less potent bronchodilators than the β-agonists, anticholinergic agents may have a role in the management of acute severe asthma that is not responding to usual therapy (Leatherman, 1994; Chapman, 1996). Parasympathetic or cholinergic stimulation increases the activity of guanylate cyclase, which raises intracellular cGMP, causing mediator release and bronchial smooth-muscle contraction (Woolcock, 1988). Currently available anticholinergic agents include atropine, glycopyrrolate, and ipratropium bromide. Published experience with these agents varies. In a randomized clinical trial comparing 1.5 mg of atropine versus 15 mg of metaproterenol via nebulizer in patients not responding to standard therapy, Young and Freitas (1991) concluded that atropine was of no benefit. Two clinical trials using nebulized glycopyrrolate also failed to demonstrate significant improvement in bronchodilation when compared with β_2-agonists (Gilman et al., 1990; Cydulka & Emerman, 1994). Data on the efficacy of ipratropium bromide, a synthetic derivative of atropine, are more convincing. Rebuck and associates (1987) randomized patients with asthma to nebulized fenoterol (a β_2-agnoist), fenoterol and ipratropium, or ipratropium alone. These authors found better improvement in the FEV_1 at 45 and 90 minutes with combined therapy when compared with either therapy used alone. In a smaller study, O'Driscoll and colleagues (1989) randomized patients with asthma to salbutamol versus salbutamol plus ipratropium and found that the improvement in PEFR at 1 hour was greater with the combined therapy (31% vs 77%). Most authors now suggest that ipratropium bromide may benefit some patients and that its use should be considered when the initial response to β_2-agonists is suboptimal (Leatherman, 1994; Chapman, 1996). Dosages and routes of administration of the anticholinergic medications that may be used in acute severe asthma are listed in Table 22.5. Again, the animal and human toxicology studies suggest that anticholinergic therapy is not associated with adverse fetal effects (NAEP Working Group, 1993).

Theophylline

Theophylline is a methylxanthine that, in large concentrations, inhibits the action of phosphodiesterase and results in intracellular accumulation of cAMP (Koch-Weser et al., 1997). Although this has long been thought to be the major mechanism of action involved in bronchodilation, concentrations of theophylline that relax bronchial smooth muscle do not inhibit phosphodiesterase (Berstrand, 1980; Rossing, 1989). Other mechanisms of action established for theophylline that may play a role in the management of acute severe asthma include decreased fatigue in diaphragmatic muscles, increased mucociliary clearance, decreased microvascular leakage of plasma in airways, and a central nervous sytem effect that blocks the decrease in ventilation that occurs with sustained hypoxia (Weinberger & Hendeles, 1996). Long-term use appears to have immunomodulatory, antiinflammatory, and bronchoprotective effects (Weinberger & Hendeles, 1996).

Theophylline is available for clinical use in the form of aminophylline, an ethylenediamine salt constituting 80% theophylline by weight. For the patient not currently taking a theophylline preparation, dosing should begin with an initial 6mg/kg IV bolus over 20 minutes. Because the volume of distribution is increased in pregnancy, doses should be based on actual body weight (NAEP Working Group, 1993). The loading dose should be followed by an IV infusion of 0.5–0.7mg/kg/hr. Theophylline clearance in the third trimester falls by 20–50% (Carter et al., 1986; Gardner et al., 1987). Maternal toxic effects may include nausea and vomiting, abdominal pain, insomnia, irritability, agitation, seizures, and ventricular arrhythmias (Koch-Weser et al., 1977). Case reports of minor neonatal toxicity have been recorded when maternal levels at delivery were therapeutic (Yeh & Pildes, 1977; Arwood et al., 1979).

The efficacy of aminophylline in the modern management of status asthmaticus remains controversial. Most clinical trials have failed to show any added benefit when aminophylline was used to augment β-adrenergic therapy of acute severe asthma (Josephson et al., 1979; Fanta et al., 1982; Siegel et al., 1985; Murphy, 1993; Strauss et al., 1994). Considering its lack of proven benefit, narrow therapeutic range, and frequent side effects, as well as the availability of more effective agents, theophylline is not the first choice of therapy for status asthmaticus. To conclude that theophylline plays no role in life-threatening or potentially fatal asthma, however, would be premature. Noting that patients with respiratory failure were excluded from most of the clinical trials for ethical reasons, Weinberger and Hendeles (1996) suggest that "the addition of theophylline to drug therapy may be justified for patients with severe acute symptoms that do not respond to other measures." Although the most recent report of the Working Group on Asthma and Pregnancy (1993) continues to list theophylline in the text and flow charts for patients who have severe exacerbations requiring admission to the intensive care unit, the current guidelines from the NAEP Expert Panel Report (NHLBI, NIH) (1997) no longer list theophylline in the treatment of acute asthmatic exacerbations, noting that its benefit in patients requiring hospitalization is controversial. These newer guidelines relegated its role to that of a possible alternate, but not preferred, long-term control medication in patients with persistent asthma (NHLBI, NIH, 1997).

Magnesium sulfate

While more familiar to obstetricians as a tocolytic agent or as an effective drug for seizure prophylaxis in preeclampsia, intravenous magnesium sulfate may play a role in acute severe asthma. Several case reports and small case series suggest that intravenous magnesium sulfate is an effective bronchodilator, especially in cases not responding to more conventional therapy with β_2-agonists and corticosteroids (Noppen et al., 1990; Kuitert & Kletchko, 1991; Okayama et al., 1991; Sydow et al., 1993). Clinical trials using magnesium sulfate in acute asthma have produced mixed results. Tiffany and colleagues (1993) randomized patients with acute asthma to one of three groups: (i) a 2g IV infusion over 20 minutes followed by an infusion of 2g over 4 hours; (ii) a 2g infusion over 20 minutes plus a placebo infusion; and (iii) a placebo bolus and placebo infusion. While these authors noted no significant improvement in measures of expiratory flow with magnesium, they did note a trend toward improvement in female patients. Green and Rothrock (1992) were unable to demonstrate a difference in the required duration of treatment, need for hospitalization, or peak flows in patients with acute asthma when a 2-g infusion over 20 minutes was added to conventional therapy soon after presentation to the emergency department. Conversely, among 38 patients not responding to conventional therapy with β_2-agonists, Skobeloff and colleagues (1989) demonstrated significant improvement in PEFR and a lower hospital admission rate among patients randomized to IV magnesium sulfate when compared with placebo. One explanation for the mixed results seen in clinical trials may be the varied rates of administration of the initial magnesium bolus. Noting that a 2-g IV bolus given rapidly over 2 minutes seemed to avert the impending need for intubation in patients progressing to respiratory failure, Schiermeyer and Finkelstein (1994) suggested that the hot flushes and the slight drop in blood pressure were markers for immediate smooth-muscle relaxation associated with the rapid bolus. Noting that such rapid boluses of 4–6g are safely administered in obstetric patients for other reasons, these authors suggested that the immediate and short-lived bronchodilator effect may allow a window of opportunity to more effectively deliver nebulized β_2-agonists to the target tissues. In summary, this experience suggests that clinicians should consider the administration of a rapid bolus of magnesium sulfate for patients who are not responding to conventional therapy and who are approaching respiratory failure and the need for intubation.

Refractory status asthmaticus and respiratory failure

Pregnant women with severe asthma and impending respiratory failure (P_aCO_2 35 mmHg or measured expiratory flow less than 25% of predicted) should be managed in an intensive care unit (Clark, 1993; NAEP Working Group, 1993). Indications for intubation of the gravida with status asthmaticus include: (i) inability to maintain a P_aO_2 of greater than 60 mmHg with 90% hemoglobin saturation despite supplemental oxygen; (ii) inability to maintain a P_aCO_2 less than 40 mmHg; (iii) evidence of maternal exhaustion; (iv) worsening acidosis despite intensive bronchodilator therapy (pH 7.2–25); and (v) altered maternal consciousness (Hankins, 1987; NAEP Working Group, 1993; Leatherman, 1994). Importantly, individualization and clinical judgement must play a role in the decision to perform endotracheal intubation. Neither hypercapnia, nor respiratory acidosis without cardiorespiratory arrest, nor altered consciousness are in every case an indication for intubation before intensive bronchodilator therapy (Leatherman, 1994).

Intubation may be accomplished either orally or via a nasotracheal tube. Conventional guidance has been to use the oral route with the largest possible caliber tube to minimize airflow resistance (O'Donnell & Drazen, 1995). The clinical importance of this step, however, may have been overrated, and some authorities now recommend nasotracheal intubation for the alert, spontaneously breathing patient (Leatherman, 1994). Regardless of the route, tracheal intubation in the asthmatic patient should be preceded by 1–2 mg of nebulized atropine (or 0.5 mg subcutaneously) to prevent airway spasm and worsening airway obstruction (Leatherman, 1994).

Management of the pregnant patient with asthma-related respiratory failure requiring endotracheal intubation should be supervised by clinicians with special training and expertise in mechanical ventilation of patients with life-threatening asthma. Alterations in respiratory mechanics associated with severe asthma include increased resistance to inspiratory and expiratory flow, with resultant gas trapping or dynamic hyperinflation (DHI) (Maltais et al., 1994). Also referred to as intrinsic positive end-expiratory pressure, or auto-PEEP, the magnitude of DHI in mechanically ventilated patients is determined largely by tidal volume, expiratory time, and the degree of resistance to expiratory flow. When DHI becomes severe, the resulting cardiovascular sequelae may include decreased venous return, hypotension, decreased cardiac output, hypercapnia, and, in extreme cases, cardiac arrest and electromechanical dissociation (Leatherman, 1994; O'Donnell & Drazen, 1995). Alveolar rupture and pneumothorax are related more to the degree of DHI than to measured peak airway pressures (Leatherman, 1994). To minimize DHI, initial ventilator settings for the patient with asthma should include a tidal volume of 8–10 mL/kg, an inspiratory flow rate of 80–100 L/min, and a respiratory rate of 11–14 breaths per minute (Leatherman, 1994; O'Donnell & Drazen, 1995). This intentional hypoventilation, or permissive hypercapnia, must be balanced with other measures to minimize DHI. These include the use of a square wave of inspiratory flow, low-compliance ventilator tubing, and maneuvers that prolong the expiratory time (decreased respiratory rate, increased inspiratory flow rate) (Leatherman, 1994). The risks and benefits of permissive hypercapnia in the pregnant patient are more complex compared to the nonpregnant patient. The transfer of CO_2 across the placenta is dependent on the P_aCO_2 difference of approximately 10 mmHg between fetal and maternal circulation. This difference remains fairly constant over a wide range of CO_2 tensions (Meschia, 1999). Maternal hypercapnia could result in fetal respiratory acidosis and a shift in the fetal hemoglobin dissociation curve to the right. This would limit the ability of fetal hemoglobin to bind oxygen. These theoretical concerns warrant further research into the use of permissive hypercapnia in the pregnant patient prior to routine clinical application. Extrinsic PEEP should be avoided in patients with severe asthma, because it may contribute to hyperinflation.

Complications associated with the need for mechanical ventilation in patients with severe asthma include hypotension (25%), pneumothorax (13%), and death (13%) (Williams et al., 1992). Hypotension that develops in a ventilated asthmatic patient should be assumed to be secondary to DHI until proven otherwise. Leatherman (1994) recommends that when hypotension develops, the clinician should respond with a diagnostic trial of apnea and intravascular volume expansion. If the patient's pressure responds, the diagnosis of DHI is made, and the respiratory rate can be decreased and IV fluids increased. If there is no response, one should consider the possibility of a pneumothorax. Short-term neuromuscular blockade may be required for some patients in order to achieve an adequate level of ventilation at low peak airway pressures. Published series have documented the development of acute myopathy in patients receiving steroidal muscle relaxants and concurrent corticosteroids for severe asthma requiring mechanical ventilation (Griffin et al., 1992; Hirano et al., 1992). Although the myopathy always resolves, some patients require months of rehabilitative therapy before they could walk independently. Griffin and colleagues (1992) suggested that serum creatine phosphokinase levels should be assessed in patients treated with both corticosteroids and steroidal muscle relaxants in order to facilitate early detection. Alternatives to neuromuscular blockade include inhalational anesthesia or IV thiopental. Two series demonstrated that these alternatives may improve ventilation and respiratory mechanics in patients requiring mechanical ventilation for status asthmaticus (Grunberg et al., 1991; Maltais et al., 1994).

When traditional mechanical ventilation fails to improve maternal respiratory status, a number of additional modalities have been reported with anecdotal success. Fiberoptically directed bronchoalveolar lavage with normal saline, dilute metaproterenol, and the mucolytic, acetylcysteine, have all been successful in the critically ill asthmatic when mucus plugging was a major factor (Munakata et al., 1987; Schreier et al., 1989; Henke et al., 1994). Artificial surfactant therapy, high-frequency ventilation, extracorporeal membrane oxygenation, and controlled hypothermia have also been reported with anecdotal success (Tajimi et al., 1988; Kurashima et al., 1991; Browning & Goodrum, 1992; Raphael & Bexton, 1993; Shapiro et al., 1993).

Other therapeutic modalities

Certain medications commonly used for the management of asthma either have no role in acute therapy or are relatively contraindicated in pregnancy. Cromolyn sodium, which stabilizes mast-cell membranes, has only a preventive effect and does not reverse bronchospasm (Koch-Weser et al., 1977). Immunotherapy or desensitization therapy, although safe in pregnancy, likewise has no acute effects (Metzger et al., 1978). Antihistamines have an inconsistent action, and may actually decrease pulmonary function in asthmatics (Schuller & Turkewitz, 1986). Finally, empiric antibiotics have no proven benefit in acute asthma without evidence of infection.

Medications with adverse fetal effects include iodides and sodium bicarbonate. Long-term in utero exposure to iodides given as expectorants for asthma has clearly been associated with neonatal hypothyroidism, goiter, and critical upper airway obstruction (Hassan et al., 1968; Yaffe et al., 1976). Sodium bicarbonate therapy has been advocated by some when the maternal pH falls to less than 7.30 (Nolan et al., 1988). However, such therapy should be used with caution, because the administration of sodium bicarbonate will diminish the transfer of carbon dioxide from the fetus to the mother and may result in maternal alkalosis, with its aforementioned adverse effects (Moya et al., 1965).

Considerations for labor and delivery

Attention to the gravida with a recent history of severe asthma will avoid several pitfalls during labor, delivery, and the puerperium. Any long-term medication for the control of asthma should be continued. Women with symptoms and those whose expiratory flow is less than 80% of their personal best should be treated with inhaled β_2-agonists (NAEP Working Group, 1993). Stress-dose steroids should be administered to women who have taken systemic steroids within the past 9 months. This can be accomplished with IV hydrocortisone at a dose of 100 mg every 8 hours, continued until 24 hours postpartum. When choosing a sedative for labor, one of the nonhistamine-releasing narcotics, such as fentanyl, would be preferable to others, such as morphine and meperidine (Hermens et al., 1985; NAEP Working Group, 1993). Oxytocin is the drug of choice for induction of labor. Except for PGF_2, prostaglandin can safely be used in the patient with asthma for therapeutic abortion or labor induction with a dead fetus (Towers et al., 1991). In the second trimester, higher-dose oxytocin is equally effective for termination of pregnancy or induction for a dead fetus (Winkler et al., 1991). Because endotracheal intubation has been associated with severe bronchospasm, consideration should be given to the early placement of epidural anesthesia or access (Kingston & Hirshman, 1984). Finally, in the event of postpartum hemorrhage, PGE_2 and other uterotonics should be used in lieu of PGF_2. In two reports, PGF_2 has been associated with clinically diminished pulmonary function. Kreisman et al. (1975) documented significant bronchospasm in asthmatics receiving PGF_2 for mid-trimester abortion, while Hankins et al. (1988) noted dangerous oxygen desaturation following 15-methyl PGF_2-α given for postpartum hemorrhage.

Prevention of recurrent exacerbations

Clearly the ideal management for acute asthma exacerbations is prevention. Unfortunately, this is not always possible, but there are steps that can be taken to decrease the occurrence of such episodes. Early measures emphasized by the Working Group (NHLI, 1993) are avoidance of known exacerbating environmental factors, the development of an individual written action plan for managing exacerbations, and a stepwise pharmacotherapy approach. The NIH guidelines provide an outline for the approach to patient education in asthma management. Briefly, important components include education concerning the disease process itself, asthma medications and their appropriate uses, the use of home peak flow monitoring, an exacerbation rescue plan including stepping up the use of drugs, monitoring symptoms and responses, and when to seek medical care. Stepwise pharmacotherapy involves proper classification of the patient's asthma severity and the role of specific types of medications depending on the severity of the exacerbation. Again, these are outlined in detail in the Guidelines for the Diagnosis and Treatment of Asthma (NHLBI Guidelines, 1997).

Asthma medications are divided into long-term control medications used to achieve and maintain control of persistent asthma, and quick relief medications used to treat acute symptoms and exacerbations. Long-term medications include corticosteriods, cromolyn sodium, nedocromil (a mast cell stabilizer), long-acting β_2-agonists, methylxanthines, and leukotriene modifiers. Long-acting β_2-agonists, nedocromil, and the leukotriene modifiers are relatively new, and human data regarding their safety in pregnancy are limited. A position statement published jointly by the American College of Obstetricians and Gynecologists (ACOG) and the American College of Asthma, Allergy and Immunology (ACAAI) states that the risk–benefit considerations of nedocromil and inhaled salmeterol may favor their continuation during pregnancy in patients with moderate to severe asthma who have demonstrated a very good therapeutic response prior to becoming pregnant (2000). The leukotriene modifier drugs include zileuton, zafirlukast, and montelukast. Animal studies have demonstrated adverse effects with zileuton and therefore it is not recommended for use in pregnancy at this time. Montelukast and zafirlukast have been studied in animals with reassuring results, but no human studies have been performed in pregnancy. The joint committee recommended considering the continuation of these medications in patients with recalcitrant asthma, and who have shown a uniquely favorable response prior to becoming pregnant. The report continues to emphasize that the most effective medications for long-term therapy are those with anti inflammatory effects.

Summary

Severe acute asthma in pregnancy poses a serious threat to both maternal and fetal health. Physiologic alterations in pulmonary function render the pregnant woman rapidly susceptible to acute derangements in ventilation. Similarly, fetal health may be jeopardized, even with early stages of maternal asthma. For these reasons, the obstetrician must take an aggressive approach to the management of severe asthma complicating pregnancy.

Evaluation of the pregnant asthmatic should be objective and interpreted in light of pregnancy-induced changes. Treatment must be aggressive, with the goals of: (i) correcting maternal hypoxia; (ii) relieving bronchospasm; (iii) ensuring adequate ventilation; and (iv) optimizing uteroplacental exchange. Initial therapy should consist of supplemental oxygen and inhaled β_2-agonist. Parenteral corticosteroids should be given early in the course of therapy. Ipratropium bromide and high-dose IV magnesium sulfate should be considered for patients not responding to initial therapy and who are progressing toward respiratory failure. Finally, should maternal ventilation worsen despite pharmacologic therapy, early consideration should be given to intubation and mechanical ventilation. Appropriate long-term management of asthmatic patients has been shown to prevent exacerbations and improve pregnancy outcome (Schatz, 1999). When the acute treatment of the patient who presents with asthma exacerbation is complete, her long-term management should be appropriately addressed prior to discharge in order to avoid adverse pregnancy outcome.

References

American College of Obstetricians and Gynecologists. Pulmonary disease in pregnancy. Technical Bulletin Number 224, June 1996.

American College of Obstetricians and Gynecologists (ACOG) and The American College of Allergy, Asthma and Immunology (ACAAI). The use of newer asthma and allergy medications during pregnancy. Ann Allerg Asthma Immunol 2000;84(5):475–480.

Arrighi HM. US asthma mortality 1941–89. Ann Allerg Asthma Immunol 1995;74:321–326.

Arwood LL, Dasta JF, Friedman C. Placental transfer of theophylline: two case reports. Pediatrics 1979;63:844–846.

Awe RJ, Nicotra MB, Newsom TD, Viles R. Arterial oxygenation and alveolar-arterial gradients in term pregnancy. Obstet Gynecol 1979;53:182–186.

Bahna SL, Bjerkedal T. The course and outcome of pregnancy in women with bronchial asthma. Acta Allerg 1972;27:397–406.

Baker MD. Pitfalls in the use of clinical asthma scoring. Am J Dis Child 1988;142:183–185.

Bartels H, Moll W, Metcalfe J. Physiology of gas exchange in the human placenta. Am J Obstet Gynecol 1962;84:1714–1730.

Beasely R, Burgess C, Crane J, et al. Pathology of asthma and its clinical implications. J Allergy Clin Immunol 1993;92:148–154.

Berstrand H. Phosphodiesterase inhibition and theophylline. Eur J Respir Dis 1980;61:(suppl 109):37–44.

Brancazio LR, Laifer SA, Schwartz T. Peak expiratory flow rate in normal pregnancy. Obstet Gynecol 1997;89:383–386.

Brinkman CR, Weston P, Kirschbaum TH, Assali NS. Effects of maternal hypoxia on fetal cardiovascular hemodynamics. Am J Obstet Gynecol 1970;198:288–301.

Browning D, Goodrum DT. Treatment of acute severe asthma assisted by hypothermia. Anaesthesia 1992;47:223–225.

Burrows B, Lebowitz MD. The beta-agonist dilemma. N Engl J Med 1992;326:560–561. Editorial.

Calocone A, Afilalo M, Wolkove N, Kreisman H. A comparison of albuterol administered by metered-dose inhaler (and holding chamber) or wet nebulizer in acute asthma. Chest 1993;104:835–841.

Carter BL, Driscoll CE, Smith GD. Theophylline clearance during pregnancy. Obstet Gynecol 1986;68:555–559.

Carroll N, Elliot J, Morton A, James A. The structure of large and small airways in nonfatal and fatal asthma. Am Rev Respir Dis 1993;147:405–410.

Chaieb J, Belcher N, Rees PJ. Maximum achievable bronchodilation in asthma. Respir Med 1989;83:497–502.

Chapman KR. An international perspective on anticholinergic therapy. Am J Med 1996;100(Suppl 1A):2S–4S.

Chetta A, Foresy A, Del Donno M, et al. Airways remodeling is a distinctive feature of asthma and is related to severity of disease. Chest 1997;111:852–857.

Clark SL, and the National Asthma Education Program Working Group on Asthma and Pregnancy, National Institutes of Health, National Heart, Lung, and Blood Institute. Asthma in pregnancy. Obstet Gynecol 1993;82:1036–1040.

Corre KA, Rothstein RJ. Assess severity of adult asthma and need for hospitalization. Ann Emerg Med 1985;14:45–52.

Crane J, Pearce N, Flatt A, et al. Prescribed fenoterol and death from asthma in New Zealand, 1981–1983: case-control study. Lancet 1989;1:917–922.

Cugell DW, Frank NR, Gaensler EA, Badger TL. Pulmonary function in pregnancy. Am Rev Tuber 1953;67:568–597.

Cydulka RK, Emerman CL. The effects of combined treatment with glycopyrrolate and albuterol in acute exacerbation of asthma. Ann Emerg Med 1994;23:270–274.

Ellul-Micallef R, Fenech FF. Effect of intravenous prednisolone in asthmatics with diminished adrenergic responsiveness. Lancet 1975; 2:1269–1271.

Fanta CH, Rossing TH, McFadden ER. Emergency room treatment of asthma: relationships among therapeutic combinations, severity of obstruction and time course of response. Am J Med 1982;72:416–422.

Fanta CH, Rossing TH, McFadden ER. Glucocorticoids in acute asthma; a critical contolled trial. Am J Med 1983;74:845–851.

Fish JE, Summer WR. Acute lower airway obstruction: asthma. In: Moser KM, Spragg RG, eds. Respiratory emergencies, 2nd edn. St Louis: Mosby, 1982:144–165.

Fishburne JI. Physiology and disease of the respiratory system in pregnancy: a review. J Reprod Med 1979;22:177–189.

Fitsimons R, Greenberger PA, Patterson R. Outcome of pregnancy in women requiring corticosteroids for severe asthma. J Allergy Clin Immunol 1986;78:349–353.

Foresi A, Bertorelli G, Pesci A, Chetta A, Olivieri D. Inflammatory markers in bronchoalveolar lavage and in bronchial biopsy in asthma during remission. Chest 1990;98:528–535.

Gardner MJ, Schatz M, Coursins L, et al. Longitudinal effects of pregnancy on the pharmacokinetics of theophylline. Eur J Clin Pharmacol 1987;31:289–295.

Garrard GS, Littler WA, Redman CWG. Closing volume during normal pregnancy. Thorax 1978;33:488–492.

Gilman MJ, Meyer L, Carter J, Slovis C. Comparison of aerosolized glycopyrrolate and metaproterenol in acute asthma. Chest 1990; 98:1095–1098.

Gluck JC, Gluck PA. The effects of pregnancy on asthma: a prospective study. Ann Allergy 1976;37:164–168.

Gordon M, Niswander KR, Berendes H, Kantor AG. Fetal morbidity following potentially anoxigenic obstetric conditions: bronchial asthma. Am J Obstet Gynecol 1970;106:421–429.

Green S, Rothrock S. Intravenous magnesium sulfate for acute asthma: failure to decrease emergency treatment duration or need for hospitalization. Ann Emerg Med 1992;21:260–265.

Greenberger PA, Patterson R. Beclomethasone dipropionate for severe asthma during pregnancy. Ann Intern Med 1983;98:478–480.

Greenberger PA, Patterson R. The outcome of pregnancy complicated by severe asthma. Allergy Proc 1988;9:539–543.

Gregg I, Nunn AJ. New regression equations for predicting peak expiratory flow in adults. Br Med J 1989;298:1068–1070.

Griffin D, Fairman N, Coursin D, et al. Acute myopathy during treatment of status asthmaticus with corticosteroids and steroidal muscle relaxants. Chest 1992;102:510–514.

Grunberg G, Cohen JD, Keslin J, Gassner S. Facilitation of mechanical ventilation in status asthmaticus with continuous intravenous thiopental. Chest 1991;99:1216–1219.

Guidelines on the management of asthma. Statement by the British Thoracic Society, the British Paediatric Association, the Research Unit of the Royal College of Physicians of London, the King's Fund Centre, the National Asthma Campaign, the Royal College of General Practitioners, the General Practitioners in Asthma Group, the British Association of Accident and Emergency Medicine, and the British Paediatric Respiratory Group. Acute severe asthma in adults and children. Thorax 1993;48:S1–S24.

Hankins GDV. Acute pulmonary injury and respiratory failure during pregnancy. In: Clark SL, Phelan JP, Cotton DB, eds. Critical care obstetrics. Oradell, NJ: Medical Economics Books, 1987:290–314.

Hankins GDV, Berryman GK, Scott RT Jr, Hood D. Maternal arterial desaturation with 15-methyl prostaglandin F2 alpha for uterine atony. Obstet Gynecol 1988;72:367–370.

Hankins GDV, Clark SL, Harvey CJ, et al. Third-trimester arterial blood gas and acid base values in normal pregnancy at moderate altitude. Obstet Gynecol 1996;88:347–350.

Hassan AI, Aref GH, Kassem AS. Congenital iodide-induced goiter with hypothyroidism. Arch Dis Child 1968;43:702–704.

Henke CA, Hertz M, Gustafson P. Combined bronchoscopy and mucolytic therapy for patients with severe refractory status asthmaticus on mechanical ventilation: a case report and review of the literature. Crit Care Med 1994;22:1880–1883.

Hermens JM, Ebertz JM, Hannfin JM, et al. Comparison of histamine release in human skin mast cells induced by morphine, fentanyl, and oxymorphone. Anesthesiology 1985;62:124–129.

Hirano M, Ott BR, Raps EC, et al. Acute quadriplegic myopathy: a complication of treatment with steroids, nondepolarizing blocking agents, or both. Neurology 1992;42:2082–2087.

Idris AH, McDermott MF, Raucci JC, et al. Emergency department treatment of severe asthma: metered-dose inhaler plus holding chamber is equivalent in effectiveness to nebulizer. Chest 1993; 103:665–672.

Jewett JF. Asthma, emboli and cardiac arrest. N Engl J Med 1973; 288:265–266.

Josephson GW, Mackenzie EJ, Leitman PS, et al. Emergency treatment of asthma: a comparison of two treatment regimens. JAMA 1979; 242:639–643.

Kingston HCG, Hirshman CA. Perioperative management of the patient with asthma. Anesth Analg 1984;63:844–855.

Koch-Weser J, Webb-Johnson DC, Andrews JL. Bronchodilator therapy. Part one. N Engl J Med 1977;297:476–482. Part 2. N Engl J Med 1977;297:758–764.

Kreisman H, deWrel WV, Mitchell CA. Respiratory function during prostaglandin-induced labor. Am Rev Respir Dis 1975;111:564–566.

Kuitert LM, Kletchko SL. Intravenous magnesium sulfate in acute, life-threatening asthma. Ann Emerg Med 1991;20:1243–1245.

Kurashima K, Ogawa H, Ohka T, et al. A pilot study of surfactant inhalation in the treatment of asthma attack. Arerugi 1991;40:160–163.

Leatherman J. Life-threatening asthma. Clin Chest Med 1994;15: 453–479.

Lehrer S, Stone J, Lapinski R, et al. Association between pregnancy induced hypertension and asthma during pregnancy. Am J Obstet Gynecol 1993;168:1435–1436.

Levine GN, Posell C, Bernard SA, et al. Acute, reversible left ventricular dysfunction in status asthmaticus. Chest 1995;107:1469–1473.

Levinson G, Shnider SM. Anesthesia for surgery during pregnancy.

In: Shnider SM, Levinson G, eds. Anesthesia for obstetrics, 2nd edn. Baltimore: Williams and Wilkins, 1987:188–205.

Littenberg B, Gluck EH. A controlled trial of methylprednisolone in the emergency treatment of acute asthma. N Engl J Med 1986; 314:150–152.

McFadden ER, Kiser R, de Groot WJ. Acute bronchial asthma: relations between clinical and physiologic manifestations. N Engl J Med 1973;288:221–225.

McNamarra RM, Rubin JM. Intramuscular methylprednisolone acetate for the prevention of relapse in acute asthma. Ann Emerg Med 1993;22:1829–1835.

Maltais F, Sovilj M, Goldberg P, Gottfried SB. Respiratory mechanics in status asthmaticus: effects of inhalational anesthesia. Chest 1994;106:1401–1406.

Meschia G. Placental respiratory gas exchange and fetal oxygenation. In: Creasey RK, Resnik R, eds. Maternal-fetal Medicine. Philadelphia: W.B. Saunders; 1999:260–269.

Mettam IM, Reddy TR, Evans FE. Life-threatening acute respiratory distress in late pregnancy. Br J Anaesth 1992;69:420–421.

Metzger WJ, Turner E, Patterson R. The safety of immunotherapy during pregnancy. J Allergy Clin Immunol 1978;61:268–272.

Miller TP, Greenberger PA, Patterson R. The diagnosis of potentially fatal asthma in hospitalized adults: patient characteristics and increased severity of asthma. Chest 1992;102:516–518.

Morris HG. Mechanisms of action and therapeutic role of corticosteroids in asthma. J Allergy Clin Immunol 1985a;75:1–12.

Morris HG. Mechanisms of glucocorticoid action in pulmonary disease. Chest 1985b;88:133s–140s.

Moya F, Morishima HO, Shnider SM, James LS. Influence of maternal hyperventilation on the newborn infant. Am J Obstet Gynecol 1965;91:76–84.

Munakata M, Abe S, Fujimoto S, Kawakami Y. Bronchoalveolar lavage during third-trimester pregnancy in patients with status asthmaticus: a case report. Respiration 1987;51:252–255.

Murphy DG, McDermott MF, Rydman RJ, et al. Aminophylline in the treatment of acute asthma when beta 2-adrenergics and steroids are provided. Arch Intern Med 1993;153:1784–1788.

National Asthma Education Program Working Group. Management of asthma during pregnancy: report of the working group on asthma and pregnancy. National Asthma Education Program, National Heart, Lung, and Blood Institute, National Institutes of Health. Public Health Service, U.S. Department of Health and Human Services. NIH Publication No. 93-3279, September 1993.

National Asthma Education Program Working Group. Management of asthma during pregnancy: report of the working group on asthma and pregnancy. National Asthma Education Program, National Heart, Lung, and Blood Institute, National Institutes of Health. Public Health Service, U.S. Department of Health and Human Services. NIH Publication No. 97-4051, April 1997.

Nelson HS. Beta-adrenergic bronchodilators. N Engl J Med 1995; 333:499–506.

Newhouse MT. Emergency department management of life-threatening asthma: are nebulizers obsolete? Chest 1993;103:661–662.

Noble PW, Lavee AE, Jacobs MM. Respiratory diseases in pregnancy. Obstet Gynecol Clin North Am 1988;15:391–428.

Nolan TE, Hess LW, Hess DB, Morrison JC. Severe medical illness complicating cesarean section. Obstet Gynecol Clin North Am 1988;15:697–717.

Noppen M, Vanmaele L, Impens N, Schandevyl W. Bronchodilating effect of intravenous magnesium sulfate in acute severe bronchial asthma. Chest 1990;97:373–376.

O'Donnell WJ, Drazen JM. Life-threatening asthma. In: Ayers AM, Grenvik A, Holbrook PR, Shoemaker WC, eds. Textbook of critical care, 3rd edn. Philadelphia: WB Saunders, 1995:750–756.

O'Driscoll BR, Taylor RJ, Horsley MG. Nebulized salbutamol with and without ipratropium bromide in acute airflow obstruction. Lancet 1989;1:1418–1420.

O'Driscoll BR, Kalra S, Wilson M, et al. Double-blind trial of steroid tapering in acute asthma. Lancet 1993;341:324–327.

Okayama H, Okayama M, Aidawa T, et al. Treatment of status asthmaticus with intravenous magnesium sulfate. J Asthma 1991; 28:11–17.

Oserne KA, Featherstone JH, Benedetti TJ. Cerebral ischemia associated with parenteral terbutaline use in pregnant migraine patients. Am J Obstet Gynecol 1982;143:405–407.

Pierson WE, Bierman CW, Kelley VC. A double-blind trial of corticosteroid therapy in status asthmaticus. Pediatrics 1974;54:282–288.

Raphael JH, Bexton MD. Combined high frequency ventilation in the management of respiratory failure in late pregnancy. Anaesthesia 1993;48:596–598.

Rebuck AS, Chapman KR, Abboud R, et al. Nebulized anticholinergic and sympathomimetic treatment of asthma and chronic obstructive airways disease in the emergency room. Am J Med 1987;82:59–64.

Rees HA, Millar JS, Donald KW. A study of the clinical course and arterial blood gas tensions of patients in status asthmaticus. Q J Med 1967;37:541–561.

Rodrigo C, Rodrigo G. Early administration of hydrocortisone in the emergency room treatment of acute asthma; a controlled clinical trial. Resp Med 1994;88:755–761.

Rodriguez-Roisin R, Ballester E, Roca J, et al. Mechanisms of hypoxemia in patients with status asthmaticus requiring mechanical ventilation. Am Rev Respir Dis 1989;139:732–739.

Rolston DH, Shnider SM, de Lorimer AA. Uterine blood flow and fetal acid-base changes after bicarbonate administration to the pregnant ewe. Anesthesiology 1974;40;348–353.

Rossing TH. Methylxanthines in 1989. Ann Intern Med 1989; 110:502–504.

Sachs BP, Brown RS, Yeh J, et al. Is maternal alkalosis harmful to the fetus? Int J Gynaecol Obstet 1987;25:65–68.

Sawicka EH, Branthwaithe MA. Severe acute asthma. In: Sawicka EH, Branthwaithe MA, eds. Respiratory emergencies. London: Butterworths, 1987:23–31.

Schaefer G, Silverman F. Pregnancy complicated by asthma. Am J Obstet Gynecol 1961;82:182–191.

Schatz M. Interrelationships between asthma and pregnancy: a literature review. J Allergy Clin Immunol 1999;103(2 Pt 2):S330–336.

Schatz M, Harden K, Forsythe A, et al. The course of asthma during pregnancy, post partum, and with successive pregnancies: a prospective analysis. J Allergy Clin Immunol 1988a;81:509–517.

Schatz M, Zeiger RS, Harden KM, et al. The safety of inhaled beta-agonist bronchodilators during pregnancy. J Allergy Clin Immunol 1988b;82:686–695.

Schatz M, Zeiger RS, Hoffman CP, et al. Perinatal outcomes in the pregnancies of asthmatic women; a prospective controlled analysis. Am J Respir Crit Care Med 1995;151:1170–1174.

Schiermeyer RP, Finkelstein JA. Rapid infusion of magnesium sulfate obviates need for intubation in status asthmaticus. Am J Emerg Med 1994;12:164–166.

Schreier L, Cutler RM, Saigal V. Respiratory failure in asthma during the third trimester: report of two cases. Am J Obstet Gynecol 1989;160:80–81.

Schuller DE, Turkewitz D. Adverse effects of antihistamines. Postgrad Med 1986;79:75–86.

Scoggin CH, Sahn S, Petty TL. Status asthmaticus. A nine year experience. JAMA 1977;238:1158–1162.

Shapiro MB, Kleaveland AC, Bartlett RH. Extracorporal life support for status asthmaticus. Chest 1993;103:1651–1654.

Siegel D, Sheppard D, Gelb A, et al. Aminophylline increases the toxicity but not the efficacy of inhaled beta-adrenergic agonists in the treatment of acute exacerbations of asthma. Am Rev Respir Dis 1985;132:283–286.

Sims CD, Chamberlain GVP, De Swret M. Lung function tests in bronchial asthma during and after pregnancy. Br J Obstet Gynaecol 1976;83:434–437.

Skobeloff EM, Spivey WH, McNamara RM, Greenspon L. Intravenous magnesium sulfate for the treatment of acute asthma in the emergency department. JAMA 1989;262:1210–1213.

Spector SL. The use of corticosteroids in the treatment of asthma. Chest 1985;87:73s–79s.

Spitzer WO, Suissa S, Ernst P, et al. The use of beta-agonists and the risk of death and near death from asthma. N Engl J Med 1992; 326:501–506.

Stenius-Aarniala B, Pririla P, Teramo K. Asthma and pregnancy: a prospective study of 198 pregnancies. Thorax 1988;43:12–18.

Strauss RE, Wertheim DL, Bonagura VR, Valacer DJ. Aminophylline therapy does not improve outcome and increases adverse effects in children hospitalized with acute asthma exacerbations. Pediatrics 1994;93:205–210.

Summer WR. Status asthmaticus. Chest 1985;87:87s–94s.

Sydow M, Crozier TA, Zielman S, et al. High-dose intravenous magnesium sulfate in the management of life-threatening status asthmaticus. Intensive Care Med 1993;19:467–471.

Tai E, Road J. Blood-gas tensions in bronchial asthma. Lancet 1967; 1:644–646.

Tajimi K, Kasai T, Nakatimi T, Kobayashi K. Extracorporal lung assist for patients with hypercapnia due to status asthmaticus. Intensive Care Med 1988;14:588–589.

Tiffany BR, Berk WA, Todd IK, White SR. Magnesium bolus or infusion fails to improve expiratory flow in acute asthma exacerbations. Chest 1993;104:831–834.

Topilski M, Levo Y, Spitzer SA, et al. Status asthmaticus in pregnancy: a case report. Ann Allergy 1974;32:151–153.

Towers CV, Rojas JA, Lewis DF, et al. Usage of prostaglandin E2 (PGE_2) in patients with asthma. Am J Obstet Gynecol 1991;164:295.

Turner ES, Greenberger PA, Patterson R. Management of the pregnant asthmatic. Ann Intern Med 1980;6:905–918.

Vignola AM, Chanez P, Chiappara G, et al. Evaluation of apoptosis of eosinophils, macrophages, and T lymphocytes in mucosal biopsy specimens of patients with asthma and chronic bronchitis. J Allergy Clin Immunol 1999;103:563–573.

Vignola AM, Gagliardo R, Guerra D, et al. New evidence of inflammation in asthma. Thorax 2000;55:S59–60.

Weinberger M, Hendeles L. Theophylline in asthma. N Engl J Med 1996;334:1380–1388.

Weinberger SE, Weiss ST, Cohen WR, et al. Pregnancy and the lung. Am Rev Respir Dis 1980;121:559–581.

Weiss KB, Gergen PJ, Hodgson TA. An economic evaluation of asthma in the United States. N Engl J Med 1992;326:862–866.

Wendel PJ, Ramin SM, Barnett-Hamm C, et al. Asthma treatment in pregnancy: A randomized controlled study. Am J Obstet Gynecol 1996;175:150–154.

Williams TJ, Tuxen DV, Scheinkestel CD. Risk factors for morbidity in mechanically ventilated patients with acute severe asthma. Am Rev Respir Dis 1992;146:607–615.

Winfield CR, McAllister WA, Collins JV. Changes in effective pulmonary blood flow with prednisolone. Thorax 1980;35:238.

Winkler CL, Gray SE, Hauth JC, et al. Mid-second-trimester labor induction: concentrated oxytocin compared with prostaglandin E2 vaginal suppositories. Obstet Gynecol 1991;77:297–300.

Woolcock AJ. Asthma. In: Murray JF, Nadel JA, eds. Textbook of respiratory medicine. Philadelphia: WB Saunders, 1988:1030–1068.

Wulf KH, Kunze LW, Lehman V. Clinical aspects of placental gas exchange. In: Respiratory gas exchange and blood flow in the placenta. Bethesda, MD: National Institutes of Health, Public Health Service, 1972:505–521.

Yaffe SJ, Bierman CW, Cann HM, et al. Adverse reactions to iodide therapy of asthmas and other pulmonary diseases. Pediatrics 1976;57:272–274.

Yeh TF, Pildes RS. Transplacental aminophylline toxicity in a neonate. Lancet 1977;1:910.

Young GP, Freitas P. A randomized comparison of atropine and metaproterenol inhalational therapies for refractory status asthmaticus. Ann Emerg Med 1991;20:513–519.

23 Systemic inflammatory response syndrome and acute respiratory distress syndrome

Brian A. Mason

Systemic inflammatory response syndrome (SIRS) and acute respiratory distress syndrome (ARDS) represent two conditions causing the highest morbidity and mortality in adult critical care in general. This same pattern holds true in obstetric critical care in a subset of patients who survive initial insults such as embolic, hemorrhagic or acute infectious processes. Indeed SIRS and ARDS represent the final common pathway in the death of more long-term ICU patients than any other cause. In the United States and Europe alone up to 500,000 patients are affected annually with sepsis. Death occurs in up to 40% of patients who suffer from uncomplicated sepsis and up to a staggering 80% of those who develop multiorgan dysfunction and septic shock (Salvo et al., 1995). The annual incidence of ARDS in the United States is approximately 75 cases per 100,000 persons (Anon, 1997). Although mortality rates for ARDS have declined substantially from the 60% reported in the past, it remains as high as about 35% in recent series (Milberg et al., 1995; Abel et al., 1998).

This chapter will provide definitions and diagnostic criteria for these deadly diseases. In addition, the clinically relevant pathophysiology will be discussed, particularly as it relates to physical manifestations in the affected patient. Standard management techniques and novel approaches are discussed as well as future directions for the treatment of these conditions.

The septic inflammatory response syndrome

A great deal of progress has been made in the last decade toward understanding the unique physiology of critically ill patients. Often physiologic adaptations give way to pathophysiologic syndromes in the critically ill. One common syndrome in such patients has previously been referred to by a variety of labels, but has most commonly been called sepsis (reflecting the belief that infection was somehow universally involved as an underlying etiology in these cases). The fact that so many different labels have been applied to the condition reflects its complexity as well as our historic lack of understanding of the underlying pathophysiology. This wide variety of different terms applied to the same underlying condition led to tremendous confusion among practitioners and made research and communication among academic centers nearly impossible. In order to clarify the diagnosis and treatment of these conditions as well as to facilitate coordinated research, the American College of Chest Physicians and the American Society of Critical Care Medicine published definitions and criteria for sepsis and the systemic inflammatory response syndrome in 1991 (Table 23.1) (Bone et al., 1992).

Although the network of response to injury is extremely complex and finely balanced, the body has a fairly limited and predictable pattern of reaction to severe insult regardless of the type. Whether the body is exposed to infection, trauma, thermal or chemical burns, pancreatitis or massive blood loss, its response strategy remains, more or less, the same. This common inflammatory process response with tachycardia, tachypnea, leukocytosis or leukopenia, hyperthermia or hypothermia is referred to as the *systemic inflammatory response syndrome* (*SIRS*). Note that this definition does not require the presence of infection and that the emphasis is placed on the inflammatory process produced by the inciting conditions. By contrast, the term *sepsis* is reserved for cases of systemic inflammatory response syndrome when infection is present. If sepsis is accompanied by evidence of organ hypoperfusion it is referred to as *severe sepsis*. Likewise, if severe sepsis is complicated by hypotension (defined as systolic blood pressure less than 90 mmHg) despite adequate fluid resuscitation then the term *septic shock* is used. The term *multiple organ dysfunction syndrome* is applied if either sepsis or SIRS is accompanied by dysfunction in two or more organ systems. Note that the term septicemia has been dropped from the nomenclature entirely.

The inflammatory response

The immunoinflammatory response is a normal and desirable mechanism by which the body deals with a variety of different insults. It has often been compared to the clotting cascade in

Table 23.1 Physiologic criteria for the diagnosis of acute respiratory distress syndrome

$P\text{o}_2 < 50$ with $F_{\text{I}}\text{o}_2 > 0.6$
Pulmonary capillary wedge pressure ≤12 mmHg
Total respiratory compliance <50 mL/cm (usually 20–30 mL/cm)
Functional residual capacity reduced
Shunt (Q_S/Q_T) >30%
Dead space (V_D/V_T) >60%
Alveolar–arterial gradient on 100% oxygen ≥350 mmHg

$P\text{o}_2$, partial pressure of oxygen; $F_{\text{I}}\text{o}_2$, fraction of inspired oxygen; Q_S, blood flow to nonventilated areas; Q_T, total blood flow to both ventilated and nonventilated areas; V_D, dead space volume; V_T, tidal volume.

the sense that a stimulus precipitates a series of biological responses. Unfortunately, this analogy implies a mechanism of amplification, which may not be present in the inflammatory response, and neglects the interdependent nature of the various components of the inflammatory response. Thus, the inflammatory response is better likened to a complex interdependent network than a simple linear cascade. However, for the purposes of illustration, a simple linear pathway is presented here which will illuminate the basic mechanisms involved in this intricate biological process.

There are two basic pathways in the inflammatory response. The first is a proinflammatory mechanism, which becomes switched on in response to the initial insult. The initial insult stimulates innate immune cells (generally macrophages). These activated macrophages in turn produce the initial proinflammatory cytokines such as interleukin one (IL-1), interleukin four (IL-4), interleukin six (IL-6), interleukin eight (IL-8), interleukin 10 (IL-10), and interleukin 13 (IL-13) as well as transforming growth factor *beta* and interferon *gamma* (Koj, 1996). These cytokines cause a variety of physiologic responses including inflammation, fever and activation of the clotting system. These responses each have a role in the production of proteases and oxygen free radicals, which are key components of the cytotoxic antimicrobial system of the body (Fujishima & Aikawa, 1995). In addition to these local effects, the proinflammatory cytokines such as IL-8 have a chemoattractant effect that draws polymorphonuclear leukocytes to the area of injury. In order to facilitate the entry of the leukocyte into the tissue, the proinflammatory cytokines also tend to increase endothelial permeability.

Unfortunately, these beneficial antimicrobial strategies take a toll on the local tissues of the host as well. In order to control the proinflammatory response and prevent an uncontrolled and unrelenting inflammatory response, the body begins producing *anti*-inflammatory cytokines in response to the proinflammatory mediators. These work by a variety of mechanisms. Soluble tumor necrosis factor (TNF) receptors bind tumor necrosis factor thus preventing its action. IL-1 receptor antagonist (IL-1ra) competitively binds IL-1 receptors thus preventing IL-1 activity. The production of proinflammatory cytokines is inhibited by IL-4, IL-10, and IL-13. When the body is under appropriate balance and control, the anti-inflammatory mechanism counters the proinflammatory mechanism when the inflammatory process has accomplished its goals of eliminating or neutralizing the exogenous threat. Unfortunately, for reasons which are not entirely clear, this normal system of check and balance can become disrupted, leading either to an excessive inflammatory response (SIRS) or excessive suppression of the necessary inflammatory effect (the *compensatory anti-inflammatory response syndrome* or CARS).

The body's physiologic and pathophysiologic septic response has been conceptualized as five distinct stages, namely: *stage one*—local reaction at the site of the insult; *stage two*—initial systemic response; *stage three*—massive systemic inflammation; *stage four*—excessive immune suppression; and *stage five*—immunologic dissonance. The first stage, local reaction, is a very common occurrence. It initially involves the proinflammatory factors such as tumor necrosis factor, IL-1, IL-6, and platelet-activating factor in an initial local inflammatory response. In the ideal setting, this initial response is quickly followed by a compensatory anti-inflammatory response with factors such as IL-4, IL-10, IL-11, IL-13, and soluble tumor necrosis factor receptors. Ideally, the compensatory anti-inflammatory response is appropriately graded to switch off the proinflammatory response when the goals of inflammation have been met. This local reaction is largely compartmentalized. For example, in a case of unilobar pneumonia, bronchoscopic washings will reveal cytokine levels that are much higher on the affected side than on the unaffected one. When an insult is severe and requires a response beyond that which can be provided by the locally existing immune factors, the patient enters stage two or the initial systemic response. This systemic "spill-over" leads to the recruitment of neutrophils, T and B cells, as well as platelets to the site of injury. This response too is followed ideally by a compensatory anti-inflammatory response that is appropriate to the inflammatory response. When this normal regulation of pro- and anti-inflammatory responses is lost, there may be a massive proinflammatory systemic reaction. This excessive immune stimulation is most commonly referred to as the septic inflammatory response syndrome (SIRS). This leads to the characteristic findings of fever, hypotension, tachycardia, and endothelial dysfunction as well as disseminated intravascular coagulation (DIC) and increased microvascular permeability. Ultimately there is vasodilation and pathophysiologic shunting of the systemic circulation. If unchecked, these processes can ultimately result in end-organ compromise. When the compensatory anti-inflammatory system begins to overcompensate for a massive immune response, there may be excessive immune suppression and immune paralysis. This fourth stage is commonly referred to as the compensatory anti-inflammatory response syndrome (CARS). In the fifth and final stage, there is massive immunologic dissonance that results in multiple end-organ dysfunction (MODS). During this phase, the process of organ failure is often sequential beginning with the lung, proceeding to the liver, gastrointestinal tract, and kidneys.

One of the first organ systems to fail in a patient with sepsis or SIRS is often the respiratory system. The patient frequently presents with tachypnea, hypoxemia, and respiratory alkalosis initially. If severe and unchecked, the process may continue on to acute lung injury (ALI) and acute respiratory distress syndrome (ARDS). These pulmonic manifestations are extremely common in patients with septic shock and may complicate up to 60% of cases (Kollef & Schuster, 1995). This pathologic process is an exaggeration of the normal desirable inflammatory response in which endothelial permeability increases in response to proinflammatory cytokines in order to bring greater quantity of leukocytes to the site of injury. Unfortunately, this can be excessive, resulting in capillary endothelial dysfunction and interstitial as well as alveolar edema as proteinaceous fluid leaks from the intravascular space into the interstitium and alveolus. This may progress to destruction of the basement membrane and damage to the alveolus. Interleukin 8 is one of the principal cytokines responsible for the migration of neutrophils into the lung. Interleukin 8 concentrations from bronchoalveolar lavage specimens in patients with ARDS correlates closely with mortality (Donnelly et al., 1993).

Management of the patient with septic inflammatory response syndrome

Once established, management of SIRS is extremely difficult and often unsuccessful. Therefore, prevention or at least very early intervention should be aggressively pursued in patients who are at risk. Much of the treatment of SIRS is directed toward supportive therapies. A primary goal of these supportive therapies is to maintain organ perfusion and oxygenation. Oxygen status should be carefully monitored with pulse oximetry and blood gas evaluations and hypoxemia should be promptly treated with oxygen therapy. Often mechanical ventilation is necessary to support compromised respiratory function and noncompliant lungs. Perfusion may also require support in the form of volume expansion, vasoconstrictors, and ionotropic agents as needed. The use of such therapies is often best guided by employing a pulmonary artery catheter. Some modern pulmonary artery catheters have the advantage of oxymetric monitoring and therefore the ability to calculate oxygen delivery. As supportive care is being provided, an exhaustive evaluation of the underlying cause of the inflammatory response must be undertaken. Immediately after collecting microbiological samples such as urine, sputum, blood cultures, etc., empiric broad-spectrum antibiotic therapy should be introduced. As culture results become available, the antimicrobial therapy may then be more specifically targeted to the organisms present. Mortality has been shown to increase in cases where antibiotic therapy has not been initiated early in the course of the disease. Additionally, surgical debridement may also be required to eliminate an infectious source. Appropriate nutritional support should also be provided, preferably by the enteral route if possible to reduce mucosal atrophy of the intestine (Wheeler & Bernard, 1999).

The poor prognosis generally associated with patients suffering from the septic inflammatory response has led to a search for more effective therapies. As our understanding of the septic inflammatory response network has improved, more specifically directed therapies have been attempted to interrupt various processes in the septic inflammatory pathways. Many of these unique therapies have been directed at pathways in the immunologic pathogenesis of SIRS. Unfortunately, the search for these so-called "magic bullets" has been largely fruitless. Some of the approaches tried have included nonspecific anti-inflammatories such as corticosteroids and nonsteroidal anti-inflammatory agents. Others have sought to inhibit specific components by giving exogenous cytokine antagonists such as interleukin-1ra and soluble tumor necrosis factor receptor. Other attempts at inhibiting the progression of the systemic inflammatory response have been directed at inhibiting the initiation of the response by administering antibodies directed at endotoxin and TNF-α. Most of these specific therapies have failed to deliver any significant improvement in outcome over traditional therapies (McCloskey et al., 1994; Cohen & Carlet, 1996; Fein et al., 1997; Opal et al., 1997).

The reasons for our inability to control and manipulate the human inflammatory response are probably as many and varied as the response itself. First, our ability to detect the process is limited and many of the initial events have already come and gone before we are able to detect their presence. Second, it is becoming apparent that there is significant genetic polymorphism with respect to the cytokines and inflammatory mediators. Simply put, there are individuals who are more predisposed to excessive systemic immune responses than others (Molvig et al., 1988; Vincent, 1997). Third, the inflammatory response is a beneficial function to the host. Simply blocking the inflammatory network may be extremely detrimental to the patient. Finally, the extremely complex and redundant nature of the human inflammatory process is such that blocking a single element anywhere along the network is unlikely to produce a favorable outcome in the affected patient. Clearly, a much greater understanding of the exact nature of the signaling and function involved in the human inflammatory response system is needed before any meaningful specific therapies can be created.

Acute respiratory distress syndrome

Definitions and diagnosis

A number of different definitions for acute respiratory distress syndrome (ARDS) have been used since it was first described by Ashbaugh in 1967. The currently preferred definition is that reported by the American–European Consensus Committee. In this definition the lung injury must be of acute onset, bilateral infiltrates must be present on chest X-ray, and the patient must be without clinical evidence of left atrial hypertension and/or the pulmonary artery wedge pressure must be less than or equal to 18 mmHg. If the ratio of the measured partial pressure of oxygen (P_ao_2) divided by the fraction of inspired oxygen (F_io_2) is less than or equal to 300, then an acute lung injury (ALI) is said to be present. If the ratio of P_ao_2: F_io_2 is less than or equal to 200 then the patient is considered to have ARDS (Zimmerman et al., 1982).

Although increased vascular permeability leading to pulmonary edema is always present in the initial phases of ARDS, the clinical constellation of ARDS includes many other significant structural and functional abnormalities of the lung and has vastly different prognosis and treatment than simple pulmonary edema. In the later stages of ARDS, pulmonary vascular permeability may even return to normal as the condition progresses to its chronic stage, which is marked by significant fibrosis and a honeycomb architecture of the lungs (Tomashefski, 1990). The term, ARDS, is derived from the title of its first description in the literature by Ashbaugh et al. in which he used the term "acute respiratory distress in adults" to differentiate this condition from the respiratory distress found in premature newborns (Ashbaugh et al., 1967). It is presently accepted that ARDS may occur in patients of any age, and is not limited to adults (Faix et al., 1989). It is important to distinguish ARDS from related conditions with some similar features because of the differences in treatment and prognosis (Marinelli & Ingbar, 1994). The progression of ARDS is extremely rapid, and patients usually develop respiratory failure within 48 hours of the initial injury (Fowler et al., 1983). The radiographic appearance of ARDS is variable but it is never focal as in lobar pneumonia. ARDS is always bilateral and extensive. While cardiogenic pulmonary edema is often present in cases of severe ARDS, pulmonary capillary wedge pressures should be restored to normal (<18 mmHg in pregnant women) with no improvement in the lung infiltrates for at least 24 hours before the diagnosis of ARDS is definitively made. Lung mechanics and gas exchange are severely disrupted in ARDS (Zimmerman et al., 1982). In general, cases of ARDS require administration of oxygen concentrations exceeding a F_io_2 of 0.5 and most cases will require mechanical ventilation (Murray et al., 1988).

Pathophysiology

Regardless of the precipitating factors, ARDS tends to follow a predictable pathophysiologic course. This pathophysiologic progression is divided into three phases: the acute or exudative phase, the chronic or proliferation and fibrosis phase, and finally, the repair and recovery phase. Not every patient with ARDS proceeds through all of the phases, and patients may expire or recover at any point along the progression.

Acute or exudative phase

In this first phase of ARDS, the capillary membranes of the lungs are injured. Pulmonary edema follows due to the increased permeability of the capillary membrane and acute inflammatory changes. Microscopically, there is widespread injury to both the endothelial and epithelial cells of the lungs typically involving large cytoplasmic vacuoles, disrupted mitochondria, pyknotic nuclei, and localized swelling of the cytoplasm (Katzenstein et al., 1986). The damaged capillaries recover relatively quickly as the surviving endothelial cells spread out to close the gaps in the surface. The epithelial surface of the alveolus, on the other hand, usually shows a much more widespread and persistent level of damage. The type I epithelial cells necrose and slough away, leaving large areas of exposed basement membrane. It often takes several days for the type II epithelial cells to proliferate and close these gaps (Bachofen & Weibel, 1982). The alveolar walls become distended with edema fluid as the damaged endothelial and epithelial surfaces allow protein-rich fluid to leak into the extravascular space in the lung (Pratt et al., 1979). While some alveoli are compressed by the increased pressure in the interstitial space, others collapse due to changes in the surface tension within them, or simply fill with edema fluid. This phase is marked by the presence of hyaline membranes, which differentiates it from simple cardiogenic pulmonary edema. Alveolar macrophages begin to release cytokines, such as tumor necrosis factor, which further exacerbate the inflammation (Rinaldo & Christman, 1990). Leukocytes begin to congregate and migrate across the endothelium in response to chemoattractants released by the macrophages. The neutrophils produce oxygen free radicals as well as a variety of enzymes that cause extensive damage to the lung tissue (Weiland et al., 1986). These events occur very early in the course of the disease and neutrophils can be recovered on bronchioalveolar lavage within 48 hours of the initial lung injury (Fowler et al., 1987). Bronchoalveolar lavage studies also demonstrate significant inflammation in areas that are nondependent and not affected radiographically (Pittet et al., 1997). The similarity between these events and those of the systemic inflammatory response syndrome have led some investigators to postulate that ARDS is merely a pulmonic manifestation of a larger systemic inflammatory response. Indeed, as a group, those patients with sepsis are at the highest risk for developing ARDS, which may occur in as many as 40% of these patients (Hudson et al., 1995). Furthermore, the septic inflammatory response syndrome or its late manifestation of multiorgan dysfunction is the most common cause of death in patients with ARDS, most of whom do not die of primary respiratory causes (Doyle et al., 1995; Monchi et al., 1998; Zilberberg & Epstein, 1998). However, current thinking still maintains that ARDS is a distinct entity in which the septic inflammatory response plays a central role, but it is not a clinical subset of the septic inflammatory response syndrome.

In addition to these events within the alveolus, microthrombi begin to form in the pulmonary circulation. These occlusions further exacerbate intrapulmonic shunts and probably contribute to the thrombocytopenia that is frequently a feature of this phase of ARDS (Tomashefski et al., 1983). In some instances macrothrombi also form, and can lead to hemorrhagic infarcts in the lung (Jones et al., 1985).

Proliferation and fibrosis phase

The early proliferative changes begin in the small blood vessels of the lung as well as the alveoli. New connective tissue is deposited in the intima and media of the pulmonary arterioles by the replicating mesenchymal cells. Unfortunately, this proliferation and fibrosis tends to narrow the vessels making them susceptible to thrombosis (Marinelli et al., 1990). During this same period, which begins as early as 3 days after the initial injury, gaps in the alveolar epithelial surface are created by the death and sloughing of the type I pneumocytes. These gaps are filled in by the spread of type II pneumocytes along the alveolar wall. These migrating type II cells subsequently differentiate into type I cells and restore the surface of the alveolar wall. Fibroblasts migrate to the adjacent interstitium as well as the alveolar spaces and proliferate, forming granulation tissue (Fukuda et al., 1987). If these events are regulated, the patient may, at this point, begin to recover, and structure and function are restored. If, on the other hand, the proliferation continues unchecked, the granulation tissue in the alveoli begins to remodel and fibrosis of the alveolar and capillary membranes ensues (Kuhn, 1991).

As the pulmonary vasculature becomes thickened and distorted by progressive fibrosis, the alveoli begin to collapse or merge into larger air spaces giving rise to the classic honeycomb appearance seen on biopsy specimens. This level of fibrotic change is usually fully developed within 3 weeks from the time of injury, but it may begin to appear as early as 10 days from the onset of respiratory failure.

Those patients who have not recovered at an earlier phase of ARDS and are fortunate enough to have survived the proliferation and fibrosis phase, enter the repair and recovery phase of the disease. Obviously, few tissue specimens are taken during this time of recovery, and thus, surprisingly little is known about the actual pathophysiology of this phase (Bachofen & Weibel, 1982). What is known is that patients who survive the earlier phases will begin to recover normal function in their lungs over a period of 6–12 months despite the profound fibrosis (Eliott, 1990). Unfortunately, nearly three-quarters of the patients who recover from severe ARDS are left with a clinically detectable decrease in pulmonary function, and some suffer severe chronic debilitating lung disease (Ghio et al., 1989). The degree and nature of the residual lung injuries vary from pulmonary hypertension to new onset of reactive airway disease (Simpson et al., 1978; Hudson, 1994). In patients who fail to recover after a number of months, a correctable cause such as tracheal stenosis from an endotracheal tube site should be sought.

Radiographic manifestations

Radiographic changes in the early phase of ARDS often lag behind the pathologic changes and may even be absent when the patient first develops respiratory distress (Aberle & Brown, 1990). Initial changes may be nothing more than a minimal ground-glass infiltrate. However, most chest radiographs will show either widespread consolidation or diffuse, patchy dense infiltrates by 48 hours (Gattinoni et al., 1994). There may be a paradoxical "clearing" of these infiltrates with the initiation of positive end-expiratory pressure ventilation as some of the atelectatic air spaces are re-expanded and edema fluid is driven into the interstitial space from the alveoli (Malo et al., 1984).

As computerized tomography scans have become more available in these patients, the belief that ARDS is a homogeneous insult affecting all areas of the lung equally has been replaced with the concept that the areas of damage and consolidation can be patchy, particularly in the early phase (Maunder et al., 1986). Often the apical areas of the lung are well expanded while the more dependent portions show areas of consolidation. This pattern changes rapidly as the area of the lung that is dependent changes. These observations have led some practitioners to believe that changing the patient's position frequently from supine to prone to lateral may improve the clinical course by varying the areas of the lung which are over- or underventilated (Curley, 1999).

As the disease progresses into the chronic, or proliferation and fibrosis phase, the radiographic appearance begins to evolve. Alveolar infiltrates become less dense and are replaced by reticular infiltrates interspersed with ground glass opacities (Greene, 1987). As the lungs become more fibrotic, chest radiographs develop the "honeycomb" pattern which typifies the X-ray pattern of the disease in this late fibrotic phase. It is important to obtain chest radiographs frequently in these patients, particularly in this phase, because of the significantly increased risk of pulmonary barotrauma. In addition to the dramatic and clinically-apparent tension pneumothoraces, chest radiographs can detect more subtle findings such as pulmonary interstitial emphysema and loculated pneumothoraces.

During the repair and recovery phase, the fibrous tissue in the lungs is slowly reabsorbed and/or remodeled. This is apparent on repeated chest radiographs as a gradual but progressive clearing of the dense reticular infiltrates. Chest radiographs may return completely to normal or may show residual changes such as scattered linear densities or slightly obscured diaphragmatic and cardiac borders (Unger et al., 1989).

Clinical manifestations

Hypoxemia

One of the earliest clinical manifestations in the initial phases of ARDS is a rapidly progressive hypoxia. The hypoxemia is frequently resistant even to relatively high concentrations of inspired oxygen. This is due to the relatively large amount of blood that is shunted from right to left through the nonventilated lung segments (Dantzger, 1982). Simply increasing F_io_2 will not improve hypoxemia significantly; however, the addition of positive end-expiratory pressure in appropriate amounts can help recruit collapsed alveolar segments and decrease the shunt fraction. If a pulmonary artery catheter is in place, shunt fraction can be determined directly by measuring mixed venous and arterial partial pressures of oxygen simultaneously (Shapiro & Peters, 1977). Alternatively, shunt fraction can be estimated by measuring the alveolar–arterial gradient and dividing by 20 as the patient breathes 100% oxygen. A value of 50, for example, corresponds to a shunt fraction of approximately 50% (assuming a normal cardiac output). A shunt fraction that is greater than 50% is an ominous sign and, in such cases, central cardiac monitoring should be implemented immediately. With invasive cardiac monitoring shunt fraction can be accurately determined and corrective measures taken as soon as possible (Marini, 1990).

Decreased pulmonary compliance

Some decrease in lung compliance is present in every case of ARDS and, as a result, higher inspiratory pressures are required to inflate the stiff lungs (Shapiro & Peters, 1977). It was previously believed that this decrease in compliance was simply a function of the diffuse edema and fibrosis causing an increase in lung elasticity. It is now known that the lung injury is not homogenous and that the areas of atelectasis are intermingled with areas of normal lung. Consequently, the normal areas remain normally elastic, and the collapsed areas do not participate in ventilation. This results in an overall loss of compliance in the lung due to a decrease in total lung volume participating in ventilation, and not only because the injured lung is more inelastic (Marini, 1990). This has profound implications for the use of mechanical ventilation, and particularly positive end-expiratory pressure (PEEP) in patients with ARDS. If this theory is correct, then too much PEEP can be as deleterious as too little PEEP. Increasing PEEP (in an effort to recruit the consolidated areas) will overdistend the normally elastic segments on which the patient is relying for most of her ventilation.

Static compliance is the amount of pressure necessary to expand the entire thorax, including lungs, chest wall and diaphragm, to a given volume. Practically, serial measurements of static thoracic compliance can serve as a useful measure of clinical improvement or deterioration in ARDS as well as the effect of therapeutic interventions. The compliance of a healthy thorax, for example, is generally 100 mL of volume expansion for every centimeter of water pressure (cmH_2O) exerted on the airway at a tidal volume of 8 mL per kilogram of the patient's body weight. By contrast, in severe ARDS compliance may be as low as 10 mL/cmH_2O. If a patient is mechanically ventilated on a full-assist mode and is either deeply sedated or paralyzed such that she has no breathing effort, then static compliance can be easily estimated. One simply adjusts the ventilator to temporarily introduce a pause of approximately 0.4 seconds at the end of inspiration. This is known as a plateau airway pressure. The plateau airway pressure is measured during each breath as stepwise increases in tidal volume are delivered, usually in 200 mL increments. A pressure volume curve is then drawn by plotting these end-inspiratory plateau pressures, less PEEP, on the x-axis versus tidal volume on the y-axis. The slope of the resulting curve (i.e. tidal volume divided by [plateau pressure minus PEEP]) gives the static compliance of the thorax (Bone, 1976).

Increased airway resistance

It is generally held that airway resistance increases in ARDS because the disease process leads to *functionally* small lungs due to widespread consolidation, with overall resistance to flow increasing proportionally to the number of airways that do not participate in ventilation (Marini, 1990). This effect is compounded if there is further narrowing of the airways from secretions or bronchospasm. In patients on mechanical ventilators, it is difficult to directly assess airway resistance using standard equipment. However, expiratory airway resistance can be qualitatively assessed by noting the total time required for passive expiration. The longer the expiratory time, the greater the expiratory resistance. Total expiratory resistance of the airways can be estimated by measuring the difference between the peak airway pressure at end-inspiration and the plateau pressure. The larger this pressure difference, the greater the total inspiratory resistance of the airways. The increased airway resistance seen in ARDS has several implications for the clinical management of these patients. First, the increase in expiratory resistance necessitates a longer exhalation time and may lead to airtrapping at the end of expiration, sometimes referred to as "auto-PEEP." This becomes especially problematic in patients requiring high respiratory rates because of severe disease. Another unfortunate effect of the increased airway resistance of ARDS is that higher airway pressures are needed to overcome the airway resistance and inflate the lungs. This greatly increases the risk of barotrauma in these patients. During the recovery phase, these patients may be more difficult to wean from mechanical ventilation because of the increased work of breathing from high resistance airways.

Increased physiologic deadspace

Paradoxically, as a patient with ARDS improves and hypoxemia begins to resolve, the physiologic deadspace may actually increase (Shimada et al., 1979). This may be because ventilation is restored to poorly perfused alveoli as the injured lung begins to repair itself. Thus, the deadspace to tidal volume ratio of the lung increases. In normal individuals, the deadspace fraction is usually less than 0.35. In ARDS, on the other hand, the deadspace fraction is often greater than 0.6. The clinical effect of this is that unless minute ventilation increases dramatically, the partial pressure of carbon dioxide will begin to rise. In the past, extraordinary measures were sometimes undertaken to maintain normal $P_{a}CO_2$. Today, however, many clinicians feel that the increased morbidity from these extremely high ventilatory rates outweigh the relatively insignificant risks of elevations in the partial pressure of carbon dioxide, an approach sometimes referred to as permissive hypercapnia (Hickling et al., 1990).

Pulmonary hypertension

Mild to moderate pulmonary hypertension frequently occurs in ARDS. During the initial phase, it is believed that the perivascular edema and vasoconstriction in addition to microthrombi in the pulmonary capillaries are responsible for the pulmonary hypertension. Later in the course of the disease the increase in pulmonary vascular resistance is thought to be due to fibrosis of the pulmonary capillary vascular beds. While some patients may develop right-sided heart failure, this is relatively rare and in most cases the pulmonary hypertension resolves as the ARDS resolves (Brunet et al., 1988).

Precipitators of ARDS

Acute respiratory distress syndrome is not a single disease but a clinical syndrome. Consequently, a wide variety of disease processes may lead to the final common pathway of lung injury and pathophysiologic response. Some potential precipitators of ARDS in pregnant women include aspiration, exposure to tocolytic agents, preeclampsia/eclampsia, pyelonephritis, chorioamnionitis, endometritis, septic abortion, thromboembolism, amniotic fluid embolism, air embolism, bacterial/viral pneumonia, drug overdose and severe hemorrhage (Eriksen & Pajisi, 1990). Although large series of ARDS in pregnancy are limited, the most common causes of ARDS in pregnancy in order of frequency are infection, preeclampsia/eclampsia and hemorrhage (Smith et al., 1990). By far the most common precipitator of ARDS in pregnancy is infection, particularly infection that leads to a septic syndrome (Hudson et al., 1995). Because sepsis is the most frequent precipitator of ARDS in obstetric patients, it should be suspected in any case of ARDS in which the etiology is unknown, particularly if the patient is hypotensive and/or febrile. While Gram-negative septicemia has traditionally been associated with ARDS, any number of infectious agents can cause ARDS, including fungi and viruses (Meduri, 1993). In the gravida, infectious pneumonia is a common cause of ARDS, and may be the most common cause of nonhospital-acquired ARDS (Baumann et al., 1986). ARDS that develops in the hospital is often attributable to pneumonia as well. If a primary pulmonic source is not identified in a patient suspected of having sepsis-induced ARDS, another very common source or location of the primary infection is the abdomen, particularly in the postoperative patient (Montgomery et al., 1985). Shock, profound malnutrition, or any other severe injury or illness can interrupt the intestine–blood barrier and allow for translocation of bacteria from the intestinal lumen (Poole et al., 1992).

Pregnant women are at greatly increased risk of aspiration of gastric contents, particularly during labor-and-delivery and operative procedures. In the population at large, aspiration is a significant precipitator of ARDS, and it is estimated that up to 30% of patients who experience a documented episode of aspiration will go on to develop ARDS (Bynum & Pierce, 1976). Unfortunately, alkalization of the gastric secretions does not completely protect against this form of lung injury, as particulate matter and gastric enzymes may be sufficiently damaging to the lung to precipitate an episode of ARDS (Wynn, 1982).

Labor and delivery place the pregnant patient at greatly increased risk of severe hemorrhage and hypotension. It is now recognized that these events can lead to the systemic inflammatory response syndrome (SIRS) even when infection is not present (Demling, 1990). Aggressive treatment of blood loss with transfusions has also been implicated in precipitating acute lung injury due to rare but catastrophic leukoagglutinin reactions. These unusual reactions should be suspected in the patient who develops evidence of acute lung injury following transfusion. The diagnosis is confirmed by testing for antibodies in the transfused blood that are directed against the patient's white blood cells (Maggart & Stewart, 1987).

The high therapeutic doses of opiates used in labor can occasionally cause ARDS in susceptible individuals (Lusk & Maloley, 1988). Likewise, venous air emboli from large transected uterine veins during cesarean section, as well as neurogenic pulmonary edema following eclamptic seizures are other potential precipitators of ARDS in the gravida (Colice et al., 1984). The risk of a patient developing ARDS increases significantly if multiple predisposing factors are present (Pepe et al., 1982). In addition, underlying chronic factors such as acidosis, chronic alcohol abuse and chronic lung disease place the patient at even greater risk (Hudson et al., 1995; Moss et al., 1996). Therefore, special care should be taken to prevent possible ARDS precipitating stressors in these vulnerable patients.

Management of ARDS

General goals of management

There are three principal challenges to deal with in patients with ARDS. First is the immediate problem of achieving appropriate pulmonary gas exchange. The second is the careful weaning of the patient from mechanical ventilation. The plan of management must incorporate a wide variety of clinical details including identifying and treating the underlying cause of injury when possible, treatment of secondary infections and other developing complications, keeping the patient adequately nourished and hydrated, and limiting iatrogenic injuries. A third major challenge in dealing with the ARDS patient is the ability to provide realistic evaluation of the patient's condition and to accurately determine prognosis. Given the present mortality rates for this disease, a number of patients will come to a point in therapy where assisted life-prolonging measures are futile.

To overcome these challenges, care is best individualized and delivered with a multidisciplinary approach (Surratt & Troiano, 1994). However, certain basic elements are common to most patients with ARDS, and an appropriate treatment plan should include the following elements. First, an effort should be made to identify and eliminate any precipitators of the syndrome. Second, one should use the minimal F_iO_2 necessary to support the partial pressure of oxygen at between 60 and 80 mmHg, which corresponds to an oxygen saturation of approximately 90%. Oxygen may be toxic in any patient, but there is a suggestion that there is enhanced oxygen toxicity in ARDS. Furthermore, every effort should be made to optimize the delivery of oxygen (DO_2) by maintaining an optimal cardiac output and a hemoglobin concentration of approximately 10 g/dL. In most cases, mechanical ventilation will become necessary and supraphysiologic levels of PEEP may be necessary to maintain adequate oxygenation. One must constantly keep in mind that the desired endpoint is not a given partial pressure of oxygen in the arterial blood (PO_2), but rather an optimal oxygen delivery (DO_2). To this end, invasive monitoring with a pulmonary artery (PA) catheter may assist in not only excluding cardiogenic pulmonary edema, but also in optimizing PEEP and pre-load. The optimal level of PEEP is not necessarily that which provides the highest P_aO_2, but is that level which is associated with the optimum oxygen delivery. Third, sources of sepsis should be actively sought out and aggressively treated. Fourth, it is best to keep the patient at a volume status that provides the lowest pulmonary capillary wedge pressure compatible with adequate cardiac output. In this way, optimal cardiac output and thus, optimal DO_2 is achieved, but the risk of increasing the hydrostatic pressure (which may lead to pulmonary edema) is minimized. There are few effective direct and specific therapies for ARDS. Consequently, the emphasis is on minimizing further injury and providing adequate supportive care until the lungs can repair themselves.

Specific approaches to management

Exudative phase

Oxygen

In the initial phase of ARDS, the first line of therapy is supplemental oxygen to prevent pulmonary morbidity and mortality due to extreme hypoxemia. In pregnant women, ample oxygen therapy should be given to keep the P_aO_2 above at least 60 mmHg, which corresponds roughly to an oxygen saturation of 90%. Increasing levels of oxygen must be provided as ARDS begins to worsen. In some cases, patients' symptoms will resolve and endotracheal intubation might be avoided simply by providing adequate oxygen with a facemask. Some authors advocate using positive pressure "aviator type" masks, which can deliver higher F_iO_2 and positive end-expiratory pressure (Venus et al., 1979). This method to avoid intubation is less desirable in the gravida (particularly in the late third trimester and during labor and delivery) because of the increased risk for aspiration. Unfortunately, the hypoxemia of ARDS tends to be resistant to supplemental oxygen alone; a function of the increased right-to-left shunt past collapsed or flooded alveoli. Oxygen toxicity may become problematic at higher F_iO_2 concentrations. It is currently held that any level of inspired oxygen greater than 21% has some level of toxicity and that this toxicity is enhanced in the ARDS patient. At least one study suggests that exposing a patient with ARDS to an F_iO_2 level greater than 0.6 for more than 24 hours may cause permanent lung damage (Elliot et al., 1987). Oxygen delivery is of greater biologic significance than P_aO_2 or oxygen saturation. Oxygen delivery is a function of oxygen content and cardiac output. Oxygen content is in turn a function of hemoglobin concentration. Given the nature of these relationships, much greater increases in oxygen delivery can be obtained by raising hemoglobin concentrations and cardiac output to appropriate levels than can be achieved by simply increasing F_iO_2. Furthermore, these increases in oxygen delivery can be made without the potentially toxic effects to the lung of increasing oxygen concentration (Clark, 1974).

PEEP

To avoid the problems of oxygen toxicity and to more directly address the underlying pathophysiology of the right-to-left shunt, positive end-expiratory pressure is frequently used in the treatment of ARDS. As a general rule, when a patient requires more than 48 hours of high dose oxygen therapy at F_iO_2

levels approaching 0.9, strong consideration should be given to endotracheal intubation and initiation of mechanical ventilation with PEEP. Positive end-expiratory pressure helps to reduce the right-to-left shunt across the lungs by helping to restore the lung's functional residual capacity (FRC) (Ranieri et al., 1991). PEEP may also favorably affect the compliance of the lung (Suter et al., 1975). There is no doubt that PEEP can increase P_ao_2 in ARDS. As a result, patients with ARDS may survive longer with the addition of PEEP, but an increase in overall survival had never been rigorously demonstrated until recently (Amato et al., 1998). However, the recent prospective controlled randomized clinical trial that demonstrated an increase in overall survival with the use of PEEP is small and needs to be independently confirmed. PEEP is not without risks and may be associated with significant side effects, such as barotrauma, overdistension of alveoli and decreased cardiac output with subsequent decrease in oxygen delivery. Moreover, most deaths due to ARDS are not directly due to hypoxemia (Montgomery et al., 1985).

In addition to the more dramatic and obvious potential deleterious effects of PEEP, such as barotrauma, there are a number of other significant side effects of PEEP. PEEP can decrease venous return to the thorax due to an increase in the pleural pressure. This increased pressure compresses the walls of the great veins and the right side of the heart, both of which are quite compliant. As a result, stroke volume is decreased, leading to a decrease in cardiac output, and ultimately, hypotension. At pressures of greater than 15 cmH_2O, PEEP may actually have a direct negative inotropic effect on the left ventricle (Jardin et al., 1981). PEEP also decreases cardiac output by increasing right ventricular afterload. Despite these drawbacks, PEEP has several positive effects on lungs affected with ARDS. Among these is prevention of small airway collapse during expiration thereby improving the ventilation/perfusion ratio, a decrease in right-to-left shunt fraction, a redistribution of water into the interstitial space from the intra-alveolar space, and the recruitment of some alveoli that may otherwise not be ventilated. Care must be taken not to use excessive PEEP, which has been shown to overdistend lung regions with normal alveoli and cause acute lung injury (Dreyfuss et al., 1988). In determining the appropriate level of PEEP to apply to a given patient, one must keep in mind the therapeutic goals of PEEP. Initially, the desired endpoint is the effective restoration of an acceptable P_ao_2 at a nontoxic F_io_2 level. Once this has been established, there is time to determine the patient's optimal or "best-PEEP." Until noninvasive methods are available, this is best accomplished using a pulmonary artery catheter (Belfort & Saade, 1994). If a pulmonary artery catheter is not in place, one approach is to increase PEEP until P_ao_2 is acceptable or there is a clinically significant fall in blood pressure. If F_io_2 is still at a toxic level and hypoxemia remains a problem, then decreased cardiac output and blood pressure may be dealt with by using inotropes and vasopressors such as dobutamine and norepinephrine. Once the cardiac performance is restored, PEEP may be increased until nontoxic levels of oxygen and acceptable oxygenation are achieved. If a pulmonary artery catheter is available, then a PEEP trial may be undertaken. In a PEEP trial, PEEP is incrementally increased while the inspired oxygen concentration is held constant at less than 60%. The optimal PEEP is determined by that level of PEEP that provides the *appropriate* oxygen delivery (DO). Do_2 is a product of oxygen concentration and cardiac output and thus takes into account the amount of oxygen in a given volume of blood as well as the perfusion of the peripheral tissues with that blood. Therefore, it is the best single index of tissue oxygenation (Suter et al., 1975). Alternatively, a higher initial F_io_2 may be chosen, the optimal level of PEEP determined by a PEEP trial, and then PEEP held constant while tapering the patient's inspired oxygen concentration down to less toxic levels. Once a less toxic range is achieved ($F_io_2 < 0.6$), an effort is made to lower PEEP as the patient's P_ao_2 allows. This is frequently a slow process and must be done carefully as an overly aggressive withdrawal of PEEP may cause adverse effects on oxygenation that may take many hours to fully correct, even when the previous level of PEEP is reinstituted (Lamy et al., 1976). One must not be overly committed to any one principle of management; if higher levels of oxygen are required to avoid potentially damaging levels of airway pressure then current thinking suggests that excessive pressure may be more damaging than high F_io_2 (Dreyfuss et al., 1988).

New approaches to mechanical ventilation

Several important principles should be taken into account when patients with ARDS require mechanical ventilation. First, in contrast to previous thinking, large tidal volumes should not be used. Second, one should avoid the overdistension of the alveoli (Cole & Shouse, 1995). The simplest clinical measure of the pressure needed to hold open the alveolar units is mean airway pressure. In the gravida with ARDS, increasing P_ao_2 generally requires increasing mean airway pressure regardless of the method used to increase that pressure (i.e. PEEP, tidal volume, etc.) (Marini & Ravenscraft, 1992). The adverse effects of mechanical ventilation correlate closely with mean airway pressures (Cournand et al., 1948). Thus, the higher the mean airway pressure, the more likely the patient will suffer from increased lung water, barotrauma, and decreased cardiac performance. Mean airway pressure may be altered by increasing minute ventilation, extending the inspiratory time, changing the inspiratory peak pressure, altering the pressure wave form, and of course, increasing PEEP. Because of its correlation with respiratory complications, the minimal amount of mean airway pressure needed to maintain appropriate oxygen delivery should be used.

Because of potential complications of volutrauma, high tidal volumes are rarely the method of choice for increasing mean airway pressure, and thus arterial oxygenation. Likewise, increasing inspiratory frequency excessively can lead to complications of air trapping within the bronchioles (auto-

PEEP). Thus, at higher minute ventilations, increases in mean airway pressure, for the purpose of increasing oxygenation, are usually accomplished by either increasing end-expiration (PEEP) or by extending the inspiratory time (increase I:E ratio). Small increases in inspiratory time (in contrast to PEEP) do not tend to adversely affect the driving pressure needed for ventilation, provided that the patient does not require extremely high minute ventilations and that the I:E ratio does not exceed 2:1 (Pesenti et al., 1985). Historically, volume-cycled ventilators replaced negative pressure units such as the iron lung, principally because of their ability to guarantee a defined minute ventilation, which can be controlled by the operator. Unfortunately, in disease processes such as ARDS, as the resistance to flow increases, these modes allow airway pressures to increase to overcome the resistance. Because we now know these increased pressures can lead to lung damage, there is an increase in the use of pressure-controlled, time-cycled ventilators (Morris, 1994; Shapiro & Peruzzi, 1995). Pressure-controlled ventilation allows the operator to select and control mean airway pressure as well as peak airway pressure while tidal volumes remain variable. When the operator presets the maximal airway pressure, the tidal volume that is ultimately delivered depends upon the compliance of the respiratory system, the time available for inspiration, and the resistance to air flow. If the operator elects to add PEEP (or if there is auto-PEEP present) this is subtracted from the total pressure, and it is the difference between total pressure and end-expiratory pressures which determines the pressure difference available to ventilate the lung. This mode of ventilation has a theoretical advantage over volume-cycled modes for avoiding lung trauma, namely mean, peak, and end-expiratory alveolar pressure can be controlled and specifically limited (Marini, 1994). This may be useful in restrictive lung diseases such as ARDS, where low compliance can lead to dangerously high airway pressures (Benito & Lemaire, 1990). Pressure-cycled ventilation has not been proven to be superior in clinical practice, but rigorous data are lacking (Lessard et al., 1994).

Inverse inspiratory to expiratory ratio ventilation is another modality that can be used particularly in refractory cases of low P_ao_2. Although some authors feel that inverse ratio ventilation adds little benefit and can be dangerous, others are using this method and reporting significant success (Kacmarek & Hess, 1990). Unfortunately, there is a paucity of randomized controlled trials in the literature specifically addressing pregnant women (Tharratt et al., 1988). Although details of the mechanism have not been fully investigated, there is experimental evidence in both animal and human lung injury models of small, but significant improvements in ventilatory efficiency and P_ao_2, an effect that is most likely due to increased average lung volume through the respiratory cycle (Marini & Ravenscraft, 1992). One of the principal risks of inverse ratio ventilation is barotrauma if inappropriate peak alveolar pressures are chosen. Much of the negative experience with this complication stems from studies in which larger tidal volumes were used, producing peak airway pressures greater than pressures that are currently considered safe (Tharratt et al., 1988). To avoid these possibly catastrophic complications, smaller tidal volumes and higher partial pressures of carbon dioxide may be allowed. Furthermore, peak airway pressure should be kept below 33 mmHg and I:E ratios of greater than 3:1 should be avoided until more experience is gained with this technique (even though considerably higher ratios have been successfully employed) (Marcy & Marini, 1991). As noted above, one of the most important factors in reducing the risk of exacerbating lung injury is to reduce mean airway pressure and minute ventilation. At minute ventilations that may allow for an adequate P_ao_2, P_aco_2 may be significantly elevated. Increased arterial carbon dioxide, itself, is relatively benign. The ill effects of an elevated P_aco_2 are primarily due to the rate and degree of change in intracellular pH. If these pH changes are attenuated by buffering with bicarbonate or by allowing a very gradual increase in P_aco_2, the potential ill effects of decreased intracellular pH (such as muscular weakness, increased pulmonary vascular resistance and central nervous system dysfunction) can usually be limited. This strategy of reducing minute ventilation and slowly allowing P_aco_2 to reach relatively high levels is referred to as *permissive hypercapnia*. There is clinical evidence to suggest that mortality rates can be favorably affected using low tidal volume permissive hypercapnia in patients with ARDS (Lewandowski et al., 1992). Other, somewhat extreme, methods for reducing airway pressures and minute ventilation involve the extrapulmonic removal of CO_2 from the blood. Although successful in some cases, these methods suffer from being expensive, invasive, and relatively experimental (Mortensen, 1991). For these reasons, the simple, inexpensive and relatively safe permissive hypercapnia approach has enjoyed considerably more popularity.

High frequency ventilation is another strategy for minimizing barotrauma, and for keeping peak airway pressures and tidal volumes small without sacrificing oxygenation. A conventional volume control ventilator can be used at rates of over 50 breaths per minute and low tidal volumes of approximately 5 mL/kg of body weight, resulting in lower airway pressures. The term high frequency ventilation, however, usually refers to extremely high ventilation rates, often exceeding 100 breaths per minute with even smaller tidal volumes (Slusky, 1988). This mode of ventilation has been shown to provide adequate oxygenation while keeping tidal volumes and peak airway pressures low, but carbon dioxide removal may be limited and an alternative form of CO_2 removal may be needed. The usual indication for this type of ventilation has been in cases of bronchopleural fistula. High frequency or "jet" ventilation seems to work well in patients without underlying lung disease (Carlon et al., 1982). Unfortunately, in patients with ARDS who develop fistulae, the results are poor and, in many cases, air-leak actually increases with high frequency ventilation (Bishop et al., 1987). Consequently, this form of ventilation should be employed with extreme caution, if at all, in these patients (Carlon et al., 1983).

Nosocomial infection

A new, persistent, or recurring fever in the patient with ARDS provides a significant diagnostic dilemma for the practitioner. If the fever is coupled with an infiltrate on chest radiographs, the chance that it is in response to pneumonia is greatly increased. However, there are a variety of other clinical conditions in these patients which can lead to the presence of a fever with an infiltrate, such as fibroproliferation in the late phase of ARDS, chemical aspirations, atelectases or pulmonary embolism. To further complicate this issue, two separate coexisting causes of fever and infiltrate may be present, for example an extrapulmonary infection with a pleural effusion, or drug reaction in the presence of congestive heart failure, or a blood transfusion reaction coexisting with pulmonary hemorrhage. In addition, the full spectrum of the traditional clinical findings for pneumonia such as new pulmonary infiltrate, fever, sputum production, cough, and leukocytosis may not be present in the severely compromised patient with a nosocomial pneumonia. The results of clinical studies testing the utility of clinical parameters in predicting nosocomial pneumonia have been extremely disappointing. Using purely clinical assessments, one study showed a 10% false-positive rate and a 62% false-negative rate for the detection of pneumonia when compared to histologic evaluation (Johanson et al., 1972). Another study comparing 16 clinical variables such as leukocytosis, hypoxia, and fever among others, found no combinations that were useful in determining which patient had bacterial pneumonia (Chastre et al., 1988). In the chronically ventilated patient, the addition of microscopic evaluation of tracheal secretions often adds little to the diagnostic accuracy given the high rate of colonization with potential pulmonary pathogens in these patients (Hill et al., 1976). The unfortunate result of this reliance on clinical signs and symptoms for the diagnosis of nosocomial pneumonia are several. First, some patients with nosocomial pneumonias may not be recognized clinically due to an atypical presentation. Second (and probably more commonly) a great many patients are treated with antibiotics for "pneumonia" in which no bacterial infection is present. As a result, there is a delay in the diagnosis of the actual etiology of the infiltrate and fever, and exposure to unnecessary drugs for both mother and fetus, as well as the risk of superinfection with highly resistant strains of hospital-acquired microorganisms. Furthermore, even if the diagnosis of a nosocomial bacterial pneumonia is accurately made, a reliance on blind, broad-spectrum coverage, or treating culture results from tracheal aspirates (which may not reflect the actual pathogens) does not constitute optimum therapy.

Several techniques have been proposed to deal with this dilemma. The most promising of these methods centers on the use of flexible fiberoptic bronchoscopy to direct sampling of the lower pulmonic tract. One of the best of these is a modified bronchioalveolar lavage method that utilizes a protected transbronchoscopic balloon-tipped catheter, which avoids exposing the instilled and aspirated bronchioalveolar lavage solution to upper airway contaminants. Results with this technique have been extremely favorable giving diagnostic sensitivities of up to 97% and specificities of up to 92% (George et al., 1992). Other advantages of this technique are that it allows sampling of a sizable area of the lower respiratory tract, allows for the collection of suitable material for culture, and provides an immediate provisional result based on microscopic analysis and Gram stain (Trouillet et al., 1990).

Potential concerns about this strategy for rapidly and accurately diagnosing nosocomial infections include cost, the need for appropriate equipment and expertise, and potential risks of the procedure in critically ill patients. Although the procedure does require some expertise and incurs some additional cost, these facts are probably far outweighed by the ability to make precise and timely diagnosis of potentially devastating illnesses. Furthermore, the relative risk of bronchoscopy is extremely small using current techniques.

Proliferative/fibrosis phase

Pathologic features that differentiate the exudative and proliferative phases of ARDS have been previously discussed. These pathologic characteristics give rise to differences in clinical features that necessitate some differences in therapeutic approach. Much of the supportive care in the early and late phases of ARDS is identical. Two areas, however, which differ somewhat between the two phases, are the approach to the evaluation and treatment of fever, and the use of PEEP. Unlike the exudative phase, the proliferative and fibrosis phase is characterized by complete obliteration of a large number of alveoli by the fibroproliferative changes. Consequently, increasing PEEP does little or nothing to improve gas exchange because it is impossible to recruit these obliterated alveoli. Indeed, increasing PEEP often not only fails to improve oxygenation, it may actually reduce oxygen delivery by decreasing preload, and thus reducing cardiac output (Kiiski et al., 1992).

Fever is an extremely important physical finding in late ARDS. Fibroproliferation itself can cause fever in late ARDS, even in the absence of infection. This is probably mediated by the elaboration of inflammatory cytokines within the pulmonic tissue (Meduri et al., 1991). Fibroproliferative fever without any other source of infection may account for up to 25% of the febrile morbidity seen in the proliferative phase of ARDS (Belenchia et al., 1991). Unfortunately, sepsis is such a serious complication of ARDS that fever cannot be simply attributed to fibroproliferation without an exhaustive search for a site of potential infection.

Although there are many potential sources of infection, ventilator-associated pneumonia is the most commonly identified primary source in advanced ARDS. It is believed that pulmonary superinfection and ensuing sepsis is the leading cause of death in patients who survive the initial phase of ARDS (Seidenfeld et al., 1986). Pulmonic infections are not the only source of sepsis in ARDS patients. Other sites which have been regularly identified include catheter-related infections, sinusitis, urinary tract infections, intra-abdominal infections, wound infections, empyema, and primary candidemia. This wide range of infections underscores the importance of accurately identifying and precisely treating the source of fever in the patient with ARDS. If at all possible, empiric therapy should be avoided if more precise identification of the infectious agent can be made (Meduri, 1993).

New techniques for maintaining gas exchange

A concept that has been proposed by several authors is that of "lung rest." Theoretically, an alternate method of gas exchange is temporarily employed to free the lung from its ventilatory duties so that it can heal itself without further injury while the body maintains adequate oxygenation and perfusion. Several methods of accomplishing this have been used with varying degrees of success.

One such method is extracorporeal membrane oxygenation, or ECMO, which has been used successfully in pregnancy (Plotkin et al., 1994). This method has been employed in patients who have severe life-threatening hypoxemia despite 100% F_iO_2 levels and maximal mechanical ventilation. In these cases, the lung injury is so severe that the intrinsic ability of the lung to oxygenate the blood is impaired to a point that is incompatible with life. In these extreme circumstances, an artificial "auxiliary lung" may be placed in a vascular circuit and allowed to supplant or supplement pulmonary oxygenation. Some investigators have even suggested that this might become a first line therapy (once the technique is improved) because it allows the lung to repair itself under a situation of complete rest while supporting the gas exchange requirements of the body. The "lung rest" hypothesis has not been proven in fact, but it is known that, in some cases, hyaline membrane formation may be prevented, and renal and hemodynamic functions improved when the stresses on the lung are minimized (Pesenti et al., 1982). Despite its theoretic appeal, the technique has been plagued by technical problems such as hemolysis, bleeding, and infection. ECMO has been compared to conventional ventilation in a controlled prospective multicenter trial in patients with ARDS (Zapol et al., 1979). The results of this study have been questioned for a variety of reasons. The incidence of viral pneumonia in this study was much higher than in other series, nonvalidated entry criteria were used, and an overall much higher mortality rate in both the control and ECMO groups was reported as compared to other series. In this series, mortality was nearly 90% as compared to an average 60% mortality in most clinical experiences. Nonetheless, this study failed to show any advantage in the use of ECMO over conventional techniques when applied to this population of patients with ARDS. In an attempt to overcome some of the drawbacks of ECMO, the emphasis in extracorporeal gas exchange shifted from oxygenation to the removal of carbon dioxide using a technique sometimes known as extracorporeal CO_2 removal (ECCO2R) or extracorporeal lung assist (ECLA) (Cottingham & Habashi, 1995). In this technique, some oxygenation is provided across the artificial membrane thus avoiding oxygen toxicity to the lungs, but the primary goal is the removal of carbon dioxide and thus allowing reduction of the minute ventilation and prevention of alveolar damage. Unlike ECMO, ECLA utilizes a lower pressure, lower flow venous-to-venous system (Gattinoni et al., 1986). Although the results are preliminary, ECCO2R seems to have greater success and fewer complications than ECMO, but early results in controlled trials have not shown a significant advantage over conventional therapy. Nonetheless, several institutions have begun to use this method for severe ARDS in patients who fail to respond to PEEP. With increasing experience in this method, clinicians will develop a better understanding of when to apply this expensive technology (Gattinoni et al., 1980). Until the safety and utility of this technique is better defined, its use remains investigational.

Specific therapy in ARDS

By it's very nature, specific therapy requires an accurate understanding of the precise pathophysiology of a disease process in order to appropriately target correctable problems. The historic failure of some specific therapies may, in part, be due to an incomplete understanding of the precise mechanisms involved in the respiratory distress syndrome as well as the closely related, multisystem organ dysfunction (MODS) (Bernard et al., 1994). Recent thinking on the cause of ARDS centers on a lung injury either precipitating, or arising secondary to, sepsis-induced organ dysfunction that is mediated by endotoxin or similar substances stimulating the release of the host's own cytokines and lipid mediators. These lipid mediators may directly damage the lung but may also act through increasing the production of oxygen free radicals (Vercellotti et al., 1988). New approaches to specific therapy in the adult respiratory distress syndrome are being directed toward the modification or interruption of these events.

Corticosteroids

The clinical application of corticosteroids to both ARDS and multisystem organ failure has generally been disappointing. This is somewhat surprising because corticosteroids have significant theoretical benefits such as the ability to decrease the production of arachidonic acid metabolites, inhibit neutrophil aggregation and decrease the production of tumor necrosis factor. In addition, a few animal studies (as well as anecdotal clinical reports) have suggested some benefit from the use of corticosteroids in the disease process. Unfortunately, current clinical trials are not nearly as encouraging.

High-dose corticosteroids have been shown to be relatively ineffective in improving the outcome of patients with ARDS when examined in a rigorous, randomized, double-blind clinical trial (Bernard et al., 1987). In another study, corticosteroids did not prevent the development of ARDS or change overall outcome in patients with septic shock when administered prophylactically prior to the development of clinical symptoms of ARDS (Luce et al., 1988). Such findings tend to suggest that corticosteroids should not be used except in a very limited subset of patients in the fibrosing-alveolitis phase of the disease (Menduri et al., 1991, 1994). Clearly, more effective agents that have fewer side effects are needed, but until these are available, steroids may have some minimal indication in a highly defined subset of patients with late ARDS (Menduri et al., 1998).

Surfactant

Acute respiratory distress syndrome was often referred to as adult respiratory distress syndrome because of its clinical similarity to the neonatal respiratory distress syndrome, which has been shown to be the result of a lack of surfactant in the immature neonatal lung. It is now known that the principal pathogenesis of ARDS is due to increased capillary-alveolar permeability. There is, however, a decrease in functional surfactant in ARDS. This could contribute to alveolar instability and worsening hypoxemia. Theoretically, by restoring normal levels of surfactant activity within the damaged alveoli, some improvement in oxygenation and lung compliance might be realized. This could help reduce the need for more aggressive mechanical ventilation that leads to alveolar over-distension and damage. Unfortunately, studies of artificial surfactant instillation failed to show any sustained clinical improvement (Haslam et al., 1994; Anzueto et al., 1996). Clearly additional studies are needed before any benefit of surfactant replacement can be determined accurately.

Nitric oxide

Nitric oxide is an endothelial-derived relaxing agent that can selectively dilate pulmonary vasculature when the gas is inhaled. As previously noted, the lung in ARDS is often associated with some degree of pulmonary hypertension. As a result, there is an element of intrapulmonic shunt as blood passes by damaged and poorly ventilated lung segments. When nitric oxide is inhaled, it would theoretically travel only to the well-ventilated lung units and cause local vasodilation. Nitric oxide would not travel to the unventilated regions and, therefore, they would not experience the same degree of vasodilation and increased perfusion as the well-ventilated units. This would lead to a redistribution of blood flow from the poorly-ventilated to the well-ventilated lung units, and thus could reduce intrapulmonic shunting and improve systemic oxygenation. Because of its extremely short half-life, nitric oxide could accomplish this without decreasing systemic arterial pressure (Rossaint et al., 1994). Several clinical reports have demonstrated that P_aO_2 can be favorably influenced by the inhalation of very low concentrations of nitric oxide (Grover et al., 1993). Interestingly, the degree of vasodilation appears to correlate directly with the degree of vasoconstriction present in a given vascular bed; the greater the degree of pulmonary hypertension, the better the response to nitric oxide inhalation (Zapol et al., 1993). This may add some level of safety in the clinical application of this agent, as normally perfused lung segments may not become overdilated. Furthermore, tachyphylaxis has not been seen even with extended periods of exposure to nitric oxide (Rossaint et al., 1993). Unfortunately, the beneficial effects of nitric oxide disappear very quickly after the agent is discontinued and can lead to rebound pulmonary vasoconstriction (Bigatello et al., 1993). Enthusiasm for these beneficial effects of nitric oxide must be tempered with concern over its potential toxicity; both short-term exposure at high levels and long-term exposure at low levels of nitric oxide have demonstrated toxicity. Nitric oxide has failed to improve outcome overall in phase 2 and phase 3 trials, and therefore should not be used except in rare instances as a rescue therapy in patients with hypoxia unresponsive to other measures (Dellinger et al., 1998; Payen, 1999).

Immunotherapy

Current thinking suggests that a neutrophil response may be part of the common pathway of both ARDS and multiple organ dysfunction. The initiating insult may either be exogenous, such as the presence of bacterial endotoxin, or some other failure of endogenous mediation of neutrophil response. Consequently, a therapy that can counteract the effect of endotoxin or mediate the over-reaction of endogenous host defenses may prove effective therapy, not only for ARDS, but for the multiple-system organ failure syndrome as well.

Monoclonal-antibody therapy directed against endotoxin has enjoyed some limited success in decreasing mortality in certain subsets of patients with Gram-negative sepsis. Unfortunately, the improved survival in these select patients was not associated with a decrease in the occurrence of ARDS. Because one of the major factors affecting mortality from ARDS is concomitant sepsis and multisystem organ failure, these therapies may nonetheless still prove to be beneficial in improving overall survival. Additionally, research is progressing rapidly toward the development of agents that may successfully block other steps in the pathway of neutrophil expression. One of the initiating steps in neutrophil-mediated organ injury is the binding of neutrophils to the endothelial cells themselves, a process that involves linking molecules such as CD11b. By blocking CD11b with anti-CD11b antibodies, it may be possible to temporarily inhibit this element of the host defenses and thus limit tissue injury (Wortel & Doerschuk, 1993). These investigations need to be confirmed by appropriate clinical trials, but are very appealing on theoretic grounds.

Lipid mediator antagonists

The inflammatory response relies on a number of lipid mediators including various metabolites of arachidonic acid and platelet-activating factors. Some of these mediators appear to be associated with the initial inflammatory phase in ARDS. It has been demonstrated that there are large quantities of both prostacyclin and thromboxane in patients who are septic (Bernard et al., 1991). The effect of the prostaglandin inhibitor, ibuprofen, was studied in patients with sepsis in a prospective, double-blind, randomized clinical trial. There was a significant reduction in prostaglandins as well as a significant improvement in clinical factors such as blood pressure, arterial blood gases, body temperature, peak airway pressure, and minute ventilation (Bernard et al., 1991).

Many of the pathologic stigmata of ARDS can be produced when platelet-activating factors are administered to experimental animals (Christman et al., 1988). The effects of an antiplatelet activating factor agent in ARDS were investigated in a prospective, double-blind randomized clinical trial. While there was no significant difference in overall mortality between the treatment and control groups, there was a significant decrease in the mortality of the subset of patients who had documented Gram-negative sepsis and received the antiplatelet activating factor (Tenaillon et al., 1993). While these results are encouraging, they remain very preliminary.

Antioxidants

One mechanism of injury due to neutrophil and macrophage activation is mediated by oxygen free radicals and hydrogen peroxide. The release of these highly cytotoxic agents has been associated with diffuse capillary injury of the type seen in ARDS. These findings led to the suspicion that providing antioxidants to patients with ARDS might limit the severity of the injury. In one randomized, double-blind controlled clinical trial, patients with ARDS were given either the antioxidant *N*-acetylcysteine or placebo. The treatment group showed significant improvement in chest radiograph appearance, cardiac output, and a transient improvement in thoracic compliance (Bernard, 1991). While not definitive, such findings suggest that antioxidants may have some role in the treatment of ARDS in the future.

Conclusions

As our understanding of the complex pathophysiology of the adult respiratory distress syndrome improves, so does our ability to effectively and selectively influence the factors that contribute to this devastating condition. In addition to improved specific therapies, our supportive management has seen significant advances over the past decade (Demling, 1993; Temmesfeld-Wollbruck & Walmrath, 1995). There is some evidence that overall survival has somewhat increased in recent years (Kollef & Schuster, 1995). In order to continue this trend, it is essential to carefully and objectively evaluate new therapies for ARDS. Their use should be incorporated only after careful evaluation and outcomes-based research. This rigor and caution will help to minimize unnecessary costs and excessive risks that are often incurred with the overzealous clinical application of unproven therapies.

References

Abel SJC, Finney SJ, Brett SJ, Keogh BF, Morgan CJ, Evans TW. Reduced mortality in association with the acute respiratory distress syndrome (ARDS). Thorax 1998;53:292–294.

Aberle DR, Brown K. Radiologic considerations in the adult respiratory distress syndrome. Clin Chest Med 1990;11:737–754.

Amato MBP, Barbas CSV, Medeiros DM, et al. Effect of a protective-ventilation strategy on mortality in the acute respiratory distress syndrome. N Engl J Med 1998;338:347–354.

Anon. Mechanisms of acute respiratory failure. Am Rev Respir Dis 1977;115:1071–1078.

Anzueto A, Baughman RP, Guntupalli KK, et al. Aerosolized surfactant in adults with sepsis-induced acute respiratory distress syndrome. N Engl J Med 1996;334:1417–1421.

Ashbaugh DG, Bigelow DB, Petty TL, et al. Acute respiratory distress in adults. Lancet 1967;2:319–323.

Bachofen M, Weibel ER. Structural alterations of lung parenchyma in the adult respiratory distress syndrome. Clin Chest Med 1982; 3:35–36.

Baumann WR, Jung RC, Koss M, et al. Incidence and mortality of adult respiratory distress syndrome: A prospective analysis from a large metropolitan hospital. Crit Care Med 1986;14:1–4.

Belenchia JM, Meduri GI, Massey JD, et al. Sources of fever in the ventilated patient: Diagnostic value of gallium-67 citrate scan. Chest 1991;100:145S.

Belfort MA, Saade GR. Oxygen delivery and consumption in critically ill pregnant patients: association with ophthalmic artery diastolic velocity. Am J Obstet Gynec 1994;171:211–217.

Benito S, Lemaire F. Pulmonary pressure-volume relationship in acute respiratory distress syndrome in adults: role of positive end-expiratory pressure. J Crit Care 1990;5:27.

Bernard GR. N-acetylcysteine in experimental and clinical acute lung injury. Am J Med 1991;91:54.

Bernard GR, Luce JM, Sprung CL, et al. High-dose corticosteroids in patients with the adult respiratory distress syndrome. N Engl J Med 1987;317:1565–1570.

Bernard GR, Reines HD, Halushka PV, et al. Prostacyclin and thromboxane A2 formation is increased in human sepsis syndrome: effects of cyclooxygenase inhibition. Am Rev Respir Dis 1991;144: 1095–1101.

Bernard GR, Artigas A, Brigham KL, et al. The American–European Consensus Conference on ARDS. Definitions, mechanisms, relevant outcomes, and clinical trial coordinations. Am J Respir Crit Care Med 1994;149:818–824.

Bigatello LM, Hurford WE, Kacmarek RM, et al. The hemodynamic and respiratory response of ARDS patients to prolonged nitric oxide inhalation. Am Rev Respir Dis 1993;147:A720.

Bishop MJ, Benson MS, Sato P, et al. Comparison of high-frequency jet ventilation with conventional mechanical ventilation for bronchopleural fistula. Anesth Analg 1987;66:833–838.

Bone RC. Diagnosis of causes for acute respiratory distress by pressure-volume curves. Chest 1976;70:740–746.

Bone RC, Balk RA, Cerra FB, et al. ACCP/SCCM consensus conference: definitions for sepsis and organ failure and guidelines for the use of innovative therapies in sepsis. Chest 1992;101:1644–1655.

Brunet I, Dhainaut JF, Devaux JY, et al. Right ventricular performance in patients with acute respiratory failure. Intensive Care Med 1988; 14(Suppl 2):474–477.

Bynum LJ, Pierce AK. Pulmonary aspiration of gastric contents. Am Rev Respir Dis 1976;114:1129–1136.

Carlon GC, Ray C, Pierri NK, et al. High frequency jet ventilation: Theoretical considerations and clinical observations. Chest 1982; 81:350–354.

Carlon GC, Howland WS, Ray C, Miodownik S, Griffin JP, Groeger JS. High-frequency jet ventilation: a prospective randomized evaluation. Chest 1983;84:551–559.

Chastre J, Fagon JY, Soler P, et al. Diagnosis of nosocomial bacterial pneumonia in intubated patients undergoing ventilation: Comparison of the usefulness of bronchoalveolar lavage and the protected specimen brush. Am J Med 1988;85:499–506.

Christman BW, Lefferts PL, King GA, et al. Role of circulating platelets and granulocytes in PAF-induced pulmonary dysfunction in awake sheep. J Appl Physiol 1988;64:2033–2041.

Clark JM. The toxicity of oxygen. Am Rev Respir Dis 1974;110:40–50.

Cohen J, Carlet J. Intersept: An international, multicenter, placebo-controlled trial of monoclonal antibody to human tumor necrosis factor—in patients with sepsis. International Sepsis Trial Study Group. Crit Care Med 1996;24:1431–1440.

Cole FJ Jr, Shouse BA. Alternative modalities of ventilation in acute respiratory failure. Surg Annu 1995;27:55–69.

Colice GL, Matthay MA, Bass E, et al. Neurogenic pulmonary edema. Am Rev Respir Dis 1984;130:941–948.

Cottingham CA, Habashi NM. Extracorporeal lung assist in the adult trauma patient. AACN Clin Issues 1995;6:229–241.

Cournand A, Motley HL, Werko L, et al. Physiologic studies of the effects of intermittent positive pressure breathing on cardiac output in man. Am J Physiol 1948;152:162.

Curley MA. Prone positioning of patients with acute respiratory distress syndrome: a systematic review. Am J Crit Care 1999;8(6): 397–405.

Dantzger DR. Gas exchange in the adult respiratory distress syndrome. Clin Chest Med 1982;3:57.

Dellinger RP, Zimmerman JL, Taylor RW, et al. Effects of inhaled nitric oxide in patients with acute respiratory distress syndrome: results of a randomized phase II trial. Crit Care Med 1998;26:15–23.

Demling RH. Current concepts on the adult respiratory distress syndrome. Circ Shock 1990;30:297–309.

Demling RH. Adult respiratory distress syndrome: current concepts. New Horiz 1993;1:388–401.

Donnelly SC, Strieter RM, Kunkel SL. Interleukin-8 and development of adult respiratory distress syndrome in at risk patient groups. Lancet 1993;341:643–647.

Doyle RL, Szaflarski N, Modin GW, Wiener-Kronish JP, Matthay MA. Identification of patients with acute lung injury: predictors of mortality. Am J Respir Crit Care Med 1995;152:1818–1824.

Dreyfuss D, Soler P, Basset G, Saumon G. High inflation pressure pulmonary edema: respective effects of high airway pressure, high tidal volume, and positive end-expiratory pressure. Am Rev Respir Dis 1988;137:1159–1164.

Eliott CG. Pulmonary sequelae in survivors of ARDS. Clin Chest Med 1990;11:789.

Elliot CG, Rasmusson BY, Crapo RO, et al. Prediction of pulmonary function abnormalities after adult respiratory distress syndrome (ARDS). Am Rev Respir Dis 1987;135:634–638.

Eriksen NL, Pajisi VM. Adult respiratory distress syndrome and pregnancy. Semin Perinatal 1990;14:68–78.

Faix R, Viscardi RM, DiPietro MA, et al. Adult respiratory distress syndrome in full-term newborns. Pediatrics 1989;83:971–976.

Fein AM, Bernard GR, Criner GJ, et al. Treatment of severe systemic inflammatory response syndromes and sepsis with a novel bradykinin antagonist, deltibant (CP-0127): Results of a randomized, double-blind, placebo-controlled trial. CP-1027 SIRS and Sepsis Study Group. JAMA 1997;277:482–487.

Fowler AA, Hamman RF, Good JT, et al. Adult respiratory distress syndrome: Risk with common predispositions. Ann Intern Med 1983;98:593–597.

Fowler AA, Hyers TM, Fisher BJ, et al. The adult respiratory distress syndrome: cell populations and soluble mediators in the airspaces of patients at high risk. Am Rev Respir Dis 1987;136: 1225–1231.

Fujishima S, Aikawa N. Neutrophil-mediated tissue injury and its modulation. Intensive Care Med 1995;21:277–285.

Fukuda Y, Ishizaki M, Masuda Y, et al. The role of intra-alveolar fibrosis in the process of pulmonary structural remodeling in patients with diffuse alveolar damage. Am J Pathol 1987;126:171–182.

Gattinoni L, Agostoni A, Pesenti A, et al. Treatment of acute respiratory failure with low frequency positive pressure ventilation and extracorporeal removal of CO_2. Lancet 1980;ii:292–294.

Gattinoni L, Pesenti A, Mascheroni D, et al. Low frequency positive-pressure ventilation with extracorporeal CO_2 removal in severe acute respiratory failure. JAMA 1986;256:881.

Gattinoni L, Bombino M, Pelosi P, et al. Lung structure and function in different stages of severe adult respiratory distress syndrome. JAMA 1994;271:1772–1779.

George DL, Falk PS, Meduri GU, et al. The epidemiology of nosocomial pneumonia in medical intensive care unit (MICU) patients: A prospective study based on bronchoscopic sampling. Infect Control Hosp Epidemiol 1992;21:496.

Ghio AJ, Elliott CG, Crapo RO, et al. Impairment after adult respiratory distress syndrome. Am Rev Respir Dis 1989;139:1158–1162.

Greene R. Adult respiratory distress syndrome: Acute alveolar damage. Radiology 1987;163:57–66.

Grover R, Smithies M, Bihari D. A dose profile of the physiological effects of inhaled nitric oxide in acute lung injury. Am Rev Respir Dis 1993;147:A350.

Haslam PL, Hughes DA, MacNaughton PD, et al. Surfactant replacement therapy in late stage adult respiratory distress syndrome. Lancet 1994;343:1009–1011.

Hickling KG, Henderson SJ, Jackson R. Low mortality associated with permissive hypercapnia in severe adult respiratory distress syndrome. Intensive Care Med 1990;16:372–377.

Hill JD, Ratliff JL, Parrott JCW, et al. Pulmonary pathology in acute respiratory insufficiency: Lung biopsy as a diagnostic tool. J Thorac Cardiovasc Surg 1976;71:64–71.

Hudson LD. What happens to survivors of the adult respiratory distress syndrome? Chest 1994;105:S123–126.

Hudson LD, Milberg JA, Anardi D, Maunder RJ. Clinical risks for development of the acute respiratory distress syndrome. Am J Respir Crit Care Med 1995;151:293–301.

Jardin F, Farcot JC, Boisante L, et al. Influence of positive end-expiratory pressure on left ventricular performance. N Engl J Med 1981;304:387–392.

Johanson WG Jr, Pierce AK, Sanford JP, et al. Nosocomial respiratory infections with gram negative bacilli: The significance of colonization of the respiratory tract. Ann Intern Med 1972;77:701–706.

Jones B, Reid LK, Zapol WK, et al. Pulmonary vascular pathology: human and experimental studies. In: Zapol WM, Falke KJ, eds. Acute Respiratory Failure. New York: Marcel Dekker, 1985:23.

Kacmarek RM, Hess D. Panacea or auto-PEEP? Respir Care 3 1990; 5:945.

Katzenstein AA, Myers JL, Mazur MT. Acute interstitial pneumonia: A clinicopathologic, ultrastructural, and cell kinetic study. Am J Surg Pathol 1986;10:256–257.

Kiiski R, Takala J, Kari A, et al. Effect of tidal volume on gas exchange and oxygen transport in the adult respiratory distress syndrome. Am Rev Respir Dis 1992;146:1131–1135.

Koj A. Initiation of acute phase response and synthesis of cytokines. Biochim Biophy Acta 1996;1317:84–94.

Kollef ME, Schuster DP. The acute respiratory distress syndrome. N Engl J Med 1995;332:27–37.

Kuhn C. Patterns of lung repair: A morphologist's view. Chest 1991; 99:11S.

Lamy K, Fallat RJ, Koeniger E, et al. Pathologic features and mechanisms of hypoxemia in adult respiratory distress syndrome. Am Rev Respir Dis 1976;114:267–284.

Lessard MR, Guerot E, Lorino H, Lemaire F, Brochard L. Effects of pressure-controlled with different I:E ratios versus volume-controlled ventilation on respiratory mechanics, gas exchange, and hemodynamics in patients with adult respiratory distress syndrome. Anesthesiology 1994;80:983–991.

Lewandowski K, Slama K, Falke KJ. Approaches to improve survival in severe ARDS: In: Vincent JL, ed. Update in Intensive Care and Emergency Medicine. Berlin: Springer-Verlag, 1992:372–377.

Luce JM, Montgomery AB, Marks JD, et al. Ineffectiveness of high-dose methylprednisolone in preventing parenchymal lung injury and improving mortality in patients with septic shock. Am Rev Respir Dis 1988;138:62–68.

Lusk JA, Maloley PA. Morphine-induced pulmonary edema. Am J Med 1988;84:367–368.

McCloskey RV, Straue RC, Sanders C, et al. Treatment of septic shock with human monoclonal antibody HA-1A: A randomized, double-blind, placebo-controlled trial. CHESS Trial Study Group. Ann Intern Med 1994;121:1–5.

Maggart M, Stewart S. The mechanisms and management of non-cardiogenic pulmonary edema following cardiopulmonary bypass. Ann Thorac Surg 1987;43:231–236.

Malo J, Ali J, Wood LD. How does positive end-expiratory pressure reduce intrapulmonary shunt in canine pulmonary edema? J Appl Physiol 1984;57:1002–1010.

Marcy TW, Marini JJ. Inverse ratio ventilation in ARDS: rationale and implementation. Chest 1991;100:494–504.

Marini JJ. Monitoring during mechanical ventilation. Clin Chest Med 1988;9:73–100.

Marini JJ. Lung mechanics in ARDS. Clin Chest Med 1990;11:673–690.

Marini JJ. Pressure-targeted, lung-protective ventilatory support in acute lung injury. Chest 1994;105:S109–115.

Marinelli WA, Henke CA, Harmon KR, et al. Mechanisms of alveolar fibrosis after acute lung injury. Clin Chest Med 1990;11:657–672.

Marini JJ, Ravenscraft SA. Mean airway pressure: physiologic determinants and clinical importance: Part 1 and 2. Crit Care Med 1992; 20:1461–1472, 1604–1616.

Marinelli WA, Ingbar DH. Diagnosis and management of acute lung injury. Clin Chest Med 1994;15:517–546.

Maunder RJ, Shuman WP, McHugh JW, et al. Preservation of normal lung regions in the adult respiratory distress syndrome: analysis by computed tomography. JAMA 1986;255:2463–2465.

Meduri GU. Diagnosis of ventilator-associated pneumonia. Infect Dis Clin North Am 1993;7:295–329.

Meduri GU, Belenchia JM, Estes RJ, et al. Fibroproliferative phase ARDS: Clinical findings and effects of corticosteroids. Chest 1991; 100:943–952.

Meduri GU, Chinn AJ, Leeper KV, et al. Corticosteroid rescue treatment of progressive fibroproliferation in late ARDS: patterns of response and predictors of outcome. Chest 1994;105:1516–1527.

Meduri GU, Headley AS, Golden E, et al. Effect of prolonged methylprednisolone therapy in unresolving acute respiratory distress syndrome: a randomized controlled trial. JAMA 1998;280:159–165.

Milberg JA, Davis DR, Steinber KP, Hudson LD. Improved survival of patients with acute respiratory distress syndrome (ARDS):1983–1993. JAMA 1995;273:306–309.

Molvig J, Baek L, Christensen P, et al. Endotoxin-stimulated human monocyte secretion of interleukin 1, tumor necrosis factor, and prostaglandin E2 shows stable interindividual differences. Scand J Immunol 1988;27:705–716.

Monchi M, Bellenfant F, Cariou A, et al. Early predictive factors of survival in the acute respiratory distress syndrome: a multivariate analysis. Am J Respir Crit Care Med 1998;158:1076–1081.

Montgomery AB, Stager MA, Carrico J, et al. Causes of mortality in patients with the adult respiratory distress syndrome. Am Rev Respir Dis 1985;132:485–489.

Morris AH. Adult respiratory distress syndrome and new modes of mechanical ventilation: reducing the complications of high volume and high pressure. New Horiz 1994;2:19–33.

Mortensen JD. Augmentation of blood gas transfer by means of an intravascular blood gas exchanger (IVOX). In: Marini JJ, Roussos C, eds. Ventilatory Failure. New York: Springer-Verlag, 1991: 318–346.

Moss M, Bucher B, Moore FA, Moore EE, Parsons PE. The role of chronic alcohol abuse in the development of acute respiratory distress syndrome in adults. JAMA 1996;275:50–54.

Murray JF, Mathay MA, Luce J, et al. An expanded definition of the adult respiratory distress syndrome. Am Rev Respir Dis 1988; 138:720–723.

Opal SM, Fisher CJ Jr, Dhainaut JF, et al. Confirming interleukin-1 receptor antagonist trial in severe sepsis: A phase III, randomized, double-blind, placebo-controlled, multicenter trial. The Interleukin-1 Receptor Antagonist Sepsis Investigation Group. Crit Care Med 1997;25:1115–1124.

Payen D, Vallet B, Genoa Group. Results of the French prospective multicentric randomized double-blind placebo-controlled trial on inhaled nitric oxide in ARDS. Intensive Care Med 1999;25(Suppl): S166 (abstract).

Pepe PE, Potkin RT, Reus DH, Hudson LD, Carrico CJ. Clinical predictors of the adult respiratory distress syndrome. Am J Surg 1982;144: 124–130.

Pesenti A, Kolobow T, Buckhold DK, et al. Prevention of hyaline membrane disease in premature lambs by apneic oxygenation and extracorporeal carbon dioxide removal. Intensive Care Med 1982;8: 11–17.

Pesenti A, Marcolin R, Prato P, et al. Mean airway pressure vs. positive end-expiratory pressure during mechanical ventilation. Crit Care Med 1985;13:34–37.

Pittet JP, MacKersie RC, Martin TR, Matthay MA. Biological markers of acute lung injury: prognostic and pathogenetic significance. Am J Respir Crit Care Med 1997;155:1187–1205.

Plotkin JS, Shah JB, Lofland GK, et al. Extracorporeal membrane oxygenation in the successful treatment of traumatic adult respiratory distress syndrome: case report and review. J Trauma 1994;37: 127–130.

Poole GV, Muakkassa IF, Griswold JA. Pneumonia, selective decontamination and multiple organ failure. Surgery 1992;11:1–3.

Pratt PC, Vollmer RT, Shelburne JD, et al. Pulmonary morphology in a multihospital collaborative extracorporeal membrane oxygenation project: I. Light microscopy. Am J Pathol 1979;95:191–214.

Ranieri VM, Eissa NT, Corbeil C, et al. Effects of positive end-expiratory pressure on alveolar recruitment and gas exchange in patients with the adult respiratory distress syndrome. Am Rev Respir Dis 1991;144:544–551.

Rinaldo JE, Christman JW. Mechanisms and mediators of ARDS. Clin Chest Med 1990;11:621–632.

Rossaint R, Falke KF, Lopez F, et al. Inhaled nitric oxide for the adult respiratory distress syndrome. N Engl J Med 1993;328:399–405.

Rossaint R, Gerlach H, Falke KJ, Inhalation of nitric oxide—a new approach in severe ARDS. Eur J Anaesthesiol 1994;11:43–51.

Salvo I, de Cian W, Mussico M, et al. The Italian SEPSIS study: preliminary results on the incidence and evolution of SIRS, sepsis, severe sepsis and septic shock. Intensive Care Med 1995; 21:S244–249.

Seidenfeld JJ, Pohl DF, Bell RC, et al. Incidence, site and outcome of infections in patients with the adult respiratory distress syndrome. Am Rev Respir Dis 1986;134:12–16.

Shapiro AR, Peters RM. A nomogram for planning respiratory therapy. Chest 1977;72:197–200.

Shapiro VA, Peruzzi WT. Changing practices in ventilator management: a review of the literature and suggested clinical correlations. Surgery 1995;117:121–133.

Shimada Y, Yoshiya I, Tanaka K, et al. Evaluation of the progress and prognosis in the adult respiratory distress syndrome. Chest 1979; 76:180–186.

Simpson DL, Goodman M, Spector SL, et al. Long-term follow-up and bronchial reactivity testing in survivors of the adult respiratory distress syndrome. Am Rev Respir Dis 1978;117:449–454.

Slusky AS. Non-conventional methods of ventilation. Am Rev Respir Dis 1988;138:175.

Smith JL, Thomas F, Orme JF, et al. Adult respiratory syndrome during pregnancy and immediately postpartum. West J Med 1990;153:508–510.

Surratt N, Troiano NH. Adult respiratory distress in pregnancy: critical care issues. J Obstet Gynecol Neonatal Nurs 1994;23:773–780.

Suter PM, Fairley BB, Isenberg MD. Optimum end-expiratory airway pressure in patients with acute pulmonary failure. N Engl J Med 1975;292:284–289.

Temmesfeld-Wollbruck B, Walmrath D, Grimminger F, et al. Prevention and therapy of the adult respiratory distress syndrome. Lung 1995;173:139–164.

Tenaillon A, Dhainaut JF, Letulzo Y, et al. Efficacy of P.A.F. antagonist (BN 520210) in reducing mortality of patients with severe gram-negative sepsis. Am Rev Respir Dis 1993;147;A196.

Tharratt RS, Allen RP, Albertson TE. Pressure controlled inverse ratio ventilation in severe adult respiratory failure. Chest 1988;94:755.

Tomashefski JF. Pulmonary pathology of the adult respiratory distress syndrome. Clin Chest Med 1990;11:593–619.

Tomashefski JF, Davies P, Boggis L, et al. The pulmonary vascular lesions of the adult respiratory distress syndrome. Am J Pathol 1983;112:112–126.

Trouillet JL, Guiguet M, Gilbert C, et al. Fiberoptic bronchoscopy in ventilated patients: Evaluation of cardiopulmonary risk under midazolam sedation. Chest 1990;97:927–933.

Unger JM, England DM, Bogust GA. Interstitial emphysema in adults: Recognition and prognostic implications. J Thorac Imaging 1989;4: 86–94.

Venus B, Jacobs HK, Lim L. Treatment of the adult respiratory distress syndrome with continuous positive airway pressure. Chest 1979;76: 257–261.

Vercellotti GM, Yin HQ, Gustafson KS, et al. Platelet-activating factor primes neutrophil responses to agonists: role in promoting neutrophil endothelial damage. Blood 1988;71:1100–1107.

Vincent J. New therapies in sepsis. Chest 1997;112:330S–338S.

Weiland JE, Davis WB, Holter JF, et al. Lung neutrophils in the adult respiratory distress syndrome: Clinical and pathophysiological significance. Am Rev Respir Dis 1986;133:218–225.

Wheeler AP, Bernard GR. Treating patients with severe sepsis. New Engl J Med 1999;340:207–214.

Wortel CH, Doerschuk CM. Neutrophils and neutrophil-endothelia cell adhesion is adult respiratory distress syndrome. New Horiz 1993;1:631–637.

Wynne JW. Aspiration pneumonitis: Correlation of experimental models with clinical disease. Clin Chest Med 1982;3:25–34.

Zapol WK, Snider MT, Hill JD, et al. Extracorporeal membrane oxygenation in severe acute respiratory failure: A randomized prospective study. JAMA 1979;242:2193–2196.

Zapol WM, Falke KJ, Rossaint R. Inhaled nitric oxide for the adult respiratory distress syndrome. N Engl J Med 1993;329:207.

Zilberberg MD, Epstein SK. Acute lung injury in the medical ICU: comorbid conditions, age, etiology, and hospital outcome. Am J Respir Crit Care Med 1998;157:1159–1164.

Zimmerman GA, Morris AH, Cengiz M. Cardiovascular alterations in acute respiratory distress syndrome. Am J Med 1982;73:25–34.

24 Pulmonary edema

William C. Mabie

The lung is divided into alveoli, interstitium, and vessels. Fluid enters the lung interstitium and is pumped out by the lymphatics to the thoracic duct at about 20 mL/hr at rest. With strenuous exercise, interstitial edema may be cleared at a rate up to 200 mL/hr. In patients with mitral stenosis or chronic congestive heart failure, compensatory hypertrophy of the pulmonary lymphatics and vasculature prevents alveolar flooding even with elevated hydrostatic pressure (e.g. pulmonary artery wedge pressure [PAWP] >18 mmHg) and interstitial edema formation rates.

If the fluid clearance mechanisms are exceeded and alveolar edema results, type I and type II alveolar epithelial cells actively transport fluid back into the interstitium. Fluid enters the cells via the apical sodium channel and is extruded at the base of the cells via the Na,K-ATPase pump with water following isosmotically (Fig. 24.1).

There are also water channels called aquaporins within cells and between cells. Aquaporins presumably have a role in water homeostasis as evidenced by their increased expression in the perinatal period during rapid fluid absorption following the initiation of alveolar respiration (Dematte & Sznajder, 2000).

Pathophysiology

Hydrostatic pulmonary edema

While it is easy to think of pulmonary edema as being either cardiogenic or noncardiogenic in origin, the subject is more complicated. Pulmonary edema is best thought of in terms of the four mechanisms outlined in Table 24.1 (Ingram & Baunwald, 2001). The first is hydrostatic pulmonary edema. Hydrostatic pulmonary edema includes cardiogenic causes, colloid osmotic pressure (COP) problems, and rare states resulting in negative interstitial pressure such as rapid reexpansion of a pneumothorax or acute airway obstruction (e.g. blocked endotracheal tube). Excessive intravenous infusions of saline, plasma, or blood can lead to a rise in PAWP and pulmonary edema.

Cardiogenic pulmonary edema can be further divided into disease resulting from systolic dysfunction (decreased myocardial squeeze, ejection fraction <45%), diastolic dysfunction (impaired ventricular muscle relaxation resulting in high filling pressures), or valvular disease (either stenosis or insufficiency). Systolic dysfunction is one of the major causes of pulmonary edema in pregnancy (e.g. peripartum cardiomyopathy) and is the classic pathophysiologic mechanism of congestive heart failure (Heider et al., 1999; Pearson et al., 2000). Congestive heart failure may be thought of from different points of view—backward failure versus forward failure, or left heart failure versus right heart failure. Discussing these viewpoints illustrates pathophysiologic mechanisms for the development of the signs and symptoms of heart failure.

With backward failure there is accumulation of excess fluid behind the failing ventricle. In backward failure of the left heart, the ventricle does not empty normally. Left ventricular end-diastolic pressure, wedge pressure, and pulmonary artery pressure increase. There is a redistribution of intravascular volume from the systemic circulation to the pulmonary circulation resulting in alveolar flooding. With backward failure of the right heart, there is decreased emptying of the right ventricle and elevated central venous pressure (CVP) resulting in peripheral edema, neck vein distension, hepatojugular reflux, hepatic congestion, and jaundice.

Clinical manifestations of forward failure result from an inadequate discharge of blood into the arterial system. If left ventricular forward output is decreased, blood pressure falls. The kidneys sense decreased effective blood volume and increase renin, angiotensin, and aldosterone production resulting in salt and water retention and increased systemic vascular resistance (SVR). With forward failure of the right heart, there is an interventricular septal shift to the left compromising the left ventricular cavity and decreasing stroke volume. This results in increased left ventricular filling pressure, decreased blood flow through the lungs returning to the left atrium, and decreased left ventricular output and systemic blood pressure (Ingram & Baunwald, 2001).

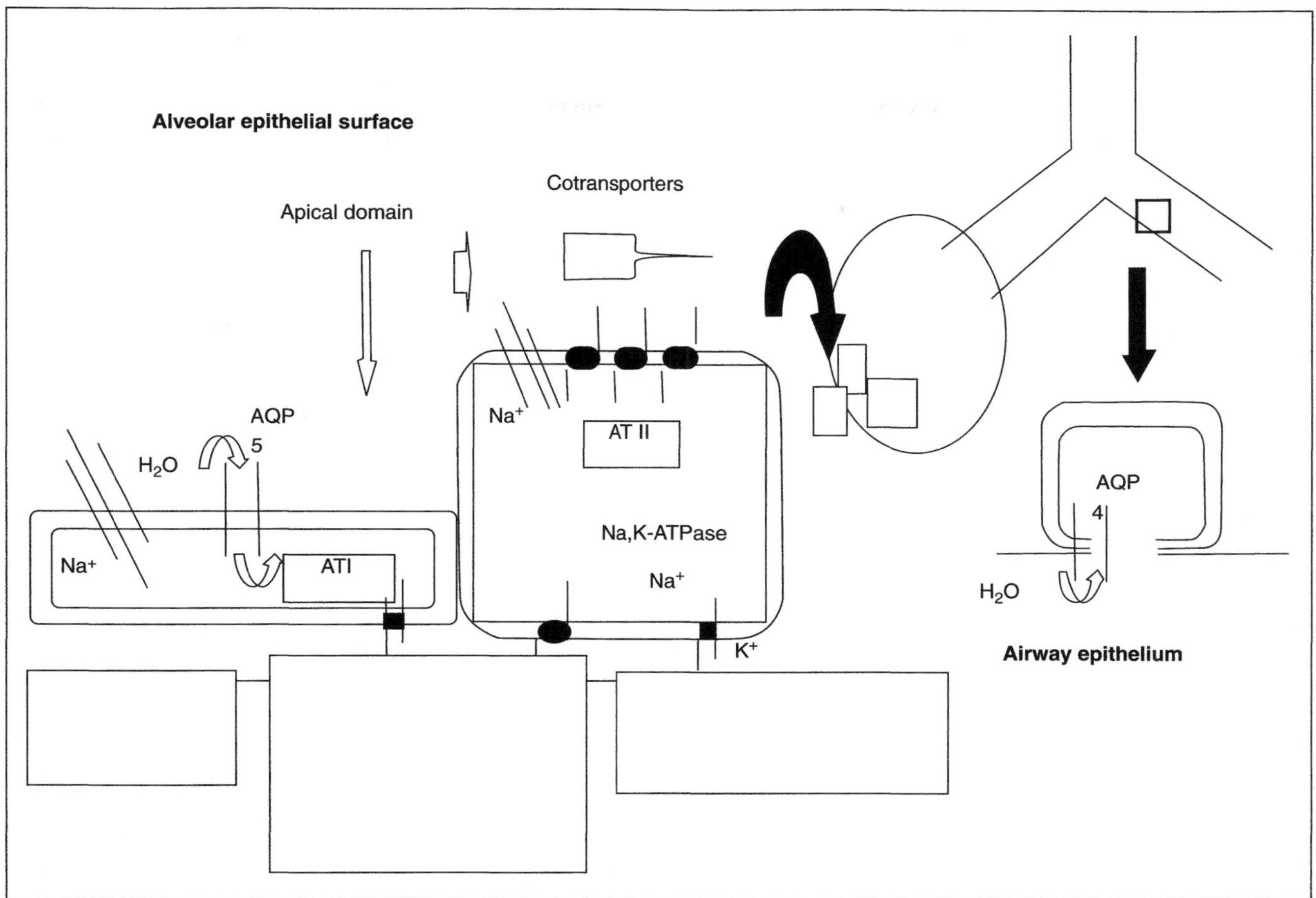

Fig. 24.1 Schematic representation of alveolar epithelial cells, types I and II, depicting the apical Na^+ channels, the basolaterally located Na,K-ATPase, the aquaporins (AQPs) and some of the co-transporters. Sodium enters through the apical membrane via NA^+ channels and is extruded by the Na,K-ATPase with water following isosmotically. Also shown is an airway epithelial cell with associated basolateral aquaporins. (Reproduced by permission of the publisher, Springer-Verlag, from Dematte JE, Sznajder JI. Mechanisms of pulmonary edema clearance: from basic research to clinical implication. Intensive Care Med 2000;26:477–480.)

Despite the usefulness of these concepts, the ventricular muscles are interdependent. If one ventricle fails, the other will fail.

One of the most interesting developments in cardiology during the last 20 years has been the discovery of congestive heart failure in the absence of systolic dysfunction. Largely based on echocardiographic findings, it is now recognized that, depending on the population studied, about half of patients with heart failure have normal systolic function and presumed diastolic dysfunction (Gandhi et al., 2001). This is particularly common in patients with chronic hypertension and left ventricular hypertrophy. Diastolic relaxation is an active energy-requiring process. The echocardiographic diagnosis of diastolic dysfunction is complex, still evolving, and beyond the scope of this discussion. Some of the parameters measured echocardiographically are the E wave to A wave peak velocity ratio of transmitral filling and the rate of left ventricular posterior wall thinning. Many pregnant patients have been found to have diastolic dysfunction as a cause of pulmonary edema, particularly those with both exogenous obesity and chronic hypertension in which the heart has undergone dimorphic adaptation. Obesity results in chamber dilation while hypertension results in concentric hypertrophy (Mabie et al., 1988; Desai et al., 1996).

During pregnancy, the valvular heart disease which commonly results in pulmonary edema is rheumatic mitral stenosis. Pregnancy complicates mitral stenosis in two ways: (i) an increase in blood volume; and (ii) an increase in heart rate, shortening diastolic filling time. The pregnant patient with mitral stenosis has a shorter time interval to get an increased amount of blood across a stenotic valve than a nonpregnant patient with mitral stenosis. This results in increased left atrial pressure and, since there are no valves in the pulmonary circulation, increased pressure in the entire pulmonary circuit

Table 24.1 Mechanisms of pulmonary edema

Hydrostatic
Cardiogenic
Systolic dysfunction (e.g. peripartum cardiomyopathy)
Diastolic dysfunction (e.g. chronic hypertension)
Valvular disease (e.g. mitral stenosis)
Decreased COP
Hypoalbuminemia secondary to preeclampsia, renal, liver, intestinal disease, or malnutrition
Increased negative interstitial pressure
Rapid expansion of pneumothorax
Acute airway obstruction
Permeability (ARDS)
Pneumonia (bacterial or viral)
Septic shock
Aspiration
Inhaled toxins (e.g. "crack" cocaine, smoke, chlorine gas)
Pancreatitis
Lymphatic insufficiency
Lymphangitic carcinomatosus
Fibrosing lymphangitis (e.g. silicosis)
Post lung transplant
Unknown or incompletely understood
Tocolytic-induced
Preeclampsia
Narcotic overdose (e.g. intravenous heroin)
Neurogenic (e.g. head trauma)
High altitude

manifested by elevated pulmonary artery pressure and right ventricular afterload. Thus, the pregnant patient with mitral stenosis is closer to being in pulmonary edema when she is pregnant than when she is not pregnant. These women are apt to go into pulmonary edema postpartum after autotransfusion from the contracting uterus. This autotransfusion is associated with an approximately 10 mmHg increase in the PAWP. Heart rate control with beta-blockers and judicious diuresis using Swan–Ganz catheter measurements for guidance has been discussed in an original paper by Clark et al. in 1985.

Colloid osmotic pressure (COP) refers to the pressure resulting from the effect of albumin and globulins that hold water in the vascular space. Intravascular COP opposes hydrostatic pressure and interstitial COP which tend to pull water from the vasculature into the interstitium. The normal intravascular COP in the nonpregnant state is 25 mmHg. Normal PAWP is 6–12 mmHg. Therefore, the normal COP-wedge gradient is about 12 mmHg. Low albumin can occur with liver disease, renal losses, and malnutrition. In normal pregnancy at term, because of increased plasma volume and dilution of albumin, COP falls to 22 mmHg. With blood loss and crystalloid replacement postpartum, COP falls to 15 mmHg (Cotton et al., 1984). In patients with preeclampsia and hypoalbuminemia, COP may fall from 18 antepartum to 13 mmHg postpartum (Benedetti & Carlson, 1979). Pulmonary edema has been shown to occur when the COP-wedge gradient is less than 4 mmHg. This narrowing of the COP-wedge gradient reflects predisposition to pulmonary edema. The situation is not so simple, however. When COP falls, the intravascular and interstitial COP decrease in parallel, so that the next flux across the membrane should be zero. In addition, patients with nephrotic syndrome and low COP are not more prone to pulmonary edema. Decreased COP is rarely responsible for pulmonary edema on its own, but it can exaggerate the edema that occurs when some other precipitating factor is present (West, 1998).

Permeability edema

In permeability pulmonary edema (the second mechanism outlined in Table 24.1), the tight junctions between the endothelial cells open up allowing water, proteins, and cells into the interstitial and alveolar space. The spectrum of severity for permeability edema ranges from acute lung injury to the acute respiratory distress syndrome (ARDS) (Bernard et al., 1994). The mechanisms for this edema formation are numerous. Bacterial or viral pneumonia cause release of prostaglandins, cytokines, and complement components. Septic shock acts similarly by releasing a myriad of mediators including myocardial depressant factor. Aspiration causes a chemical acid injury to the lung as well as bacterial and obstructive components of injury. Inhaled toxins cause direct injury to the alveoli and vasculature (e.g. chlorine gas, smoke). Finally, pancreatitis acts by systemic transport of a locally-initiated cytokine cascade. Permeability edema can be substantiated by obtaining edema fluid (e.g. suctioned from an endotracheal tube) and measuring the edema fluid to plasma protein ratio. In hydrostatic pulmonary edema, there should be a low protein content in the edema fluid; whereas, in permeability pulmonary edema, there should be a high protein content. Thus, the edema fluid protein to plasma protein ratio is ≥0.6 in permeability pulmonary edema.

Another way to look at the difference between hydrostatic pulmonary edema and permeability edema is to consider the histologic picture of the lung. In hydrostatic pulmonary edema, one sees nice, lacy alveoli filled with salt water. In permeability edema (particularly in ARDS), one sees "chopped chicken liver." Distorted alveoli are filled with inflammatory cells, protein, blood, hyaline membranes due to fibrin deposition, and collagen.

Hydrostatic pulmonary edema clears in a few hours with aggressive diuresis, whereas permeability edema takes days or weeks to clear, because polymorphonuclear leukocytes have to ingest and eliminate the protein and debris in the lung.

One may also use a Swan–Ganz catheter to differentiate hydrostatic from permeability edema. Hydrostatic pulmonary edema is accompanied by a PAWP >18 mmHg (usually >24–30 mmHg). Noncardiogenic edema is thus associated with a normal PAWP or at least a PAWP <18 mmHg. There are problems with trying to document an elevated wedge pressure. There may be "flash" pulmonary edema where the wedge pressure goes to 35 mmHg and then falls because of decompression of the pulmonary vasculature with alveolar flooding, delay in inserting the Swan–Ganz catheter, or partial treatment with diuretics.

Lymphatic insufficiency

The third mechanism of pulmonary edema in Table 24.1 is lymphatic insufficiency. This is rarely seen in pregnancy and will not be discussed further.

Unknown or poorly understood mechanisms of pulmonary edema

The fourth category (Table 24.1) includes diseases in which the mechanisms of pulmonary edema are incompletely understood. Tocolytic-induced pulmonary edema, which was one of the main causes of pulmonary edema in obstetrics two decades ago, is now infrequently seen except in aggressive treatment of preterm labor following fetal surgery. Tocolytic-induced pulmonary edema is associated with twin gestation, maternal anemia, low maternal weight, use of intravenous ritodrine or terbutaline for more than 24 hours, simultaneous use of two or three tocolytic agents, and corticosteroid therapy to accelerate fetal lung maturity. Several mechanisms have been proposed for the development of tocolytic-induced pulmonary edema. These include underlying heart disease, fluid overload, occult chorioamnionitis, hypokalemia, myocardial ischemia, mineralocorticoid effect of corticosteroids, catecholamine injury to the myocardium, and permeability edema. The most plausible explanation is that catecholamine tocolytics increase antidiuretic hormone release from the posterior pituitary causing oliguria. This has been confirmed clinically by finding a hematocrit fall of 6–8 points after a 24-hour infusion of beta-agonist tocolytics. Many times occult abruption has been suspected because of this hematocrit fall. The mineralocorticoid effect of steroid therapy is now thought to be too small to be contributing to pulmonary edema. With the switch from catecholamine tocolytics to magnesium sulfate as the first agent of choice for tocolysis and the limitation of intravenous therapy to 24 hours, the incidence of tocolytic-induced pulmonary edema has waned (Pisani & Rosenow, 1989; Lampert et al., 1993; Leduc et al., 1996).

Preeclampsia should also be considered in the unknown or incompletely understood category. Preeclamptic patients frequently have multiple abnormalities including increased capillary permeability due to endothelial cell injury, hypoalbuminemia, and afterload-induced left ventricular dysfunction (Strauss et al., 1980; Keefer et al., 1981; Benedetti et al., 1985).

Narcotic overdose pulmonary edema has been thought to be due to contaminants. Neurogenic pulmonary edema, as seen in head trauma, has been thought to be due to a massive sympathetic discharge with an acute rise in PAWP. High altitude pulmonary edema is thought to be caused by hypoxic pulmonary vasoconstriction. The wedge pressure is normal, but PA pressures are high. The pulmonary edema fluid has a high protein content, however, suggesting capillary leak (West, 1998).

Several physiologic changes of pregnancy may predispose to the development of pulmonary edema. These include increased cardiac output, increased blood volume, decreased plasma colloid osmotic pressure, increased heart rate, and decreased functional residual capacity in the lung (Zlatnik, 1997).

A chronological review of some of the advancements in our knowledge of pulmonary edema in pregnancy is found in Table 24.2 (Berkowitz & Rafferty, 1980; Strauss et al., 1980; Keefer et al., 1981; Hankins et al., 1984; Benedetti et al., 1985; Cotton et al., 1986; Sibai et al., 1987; Mabie et al., 1988, 1993).

Lung mechanics and gas exchange

Pulmonary edema reduces the distensibility of the lung and edematous alveoli shrink in size. Ventilation of fluid-filled alveoli cannot occur and perfusion of unventilated alveoli results in shunting and hypoxemia. Hypoxic pulmonary vasoconstriction reduces the shunt, but pulmonary vascular resistance rises thereby increasing the right ventricular work load. Airway resistance is increased, especially if the large airways are filled with fluid. Rapid, shallow breathing occurs early in the course of pulmonary edema because of stimulation of J receptors in the alveolar walls. This breathing pattern minimizes the high elastic work of breathing. Arterial hypoxemia is an additional stimulus to breathing (West, 1998).

Diagnosis

The diagnosis of pulmonary edema is based on the history, physical examination, laboratory data, and chest radiograph. In the history, one seeks the onset and duration of symptoms, precipitating factors, comorbidity (e.g. anemia, underlying heart, lung, kidney, or liver disease), and any medication the patient is taking. Symptoms of pulmonary edema include dyspnea, orthopnea, paroxysmal nocturnal dyspnea, Cheyne–Stokes or periodic respiration, and decreased exercise tolerance. Signs include tachypnea, upright posture, air hunger, sweating, rales, use of accessory muscles of respiration, resting tachycardia, displaced point of maximal impulse, third heart sound, neck vein distension, hepatojugular reflux, hepatomegaly, jaundice, and peripheral edema. The chest X-ray usually shows bilateral air space disease more prominent in the bases. There may be perihilar infiltrates in a "bat-wing"

Table 24.2 Selective literature review of pulmonary edema in obstetrics

Year	Authors	Cardiac monitoring	Significant findings
1980	Berkowitz, Rafferty	Swan–Ganz	Used in 20 obstetric patients over 3 years. Differentiated cardiogenic from noncardiogenic pulmonary edema. Followed patients with multiple organ system failure. Early detection of loss of cardiac reserve and effectiveness of therapeutic manipulations
1980	Strauss et al.	Swan–Ganz	Three cases of preeclampsia with pulmonary edema. Elevated PAWP (22–33 mmHg). Simultaneous CVP normal. Isolated left ventricular dysfunction was primarily the result of increased afterload and responded to vasodilators (sodium nitroprusside, hydralazine). Cardiac output nearly doubled without a significant change in heart rate or blood pressure. Limit nitroprusside therapy to 30 minutes if fetus still in utero
1981	Keefer et al.	Swan–Ganz	Four cases of noncardiogenic pulmonary edema treated with supportive care with mechanical ventilation and positive end-expiratory pressure. Pulmonary artery catheter allowed documentation of normal wedge pressure
1984	Hankins et al.	Swan–Ganz	Eight primigravid women with eclampsia. Initial hemodynamic findings: low CVP and PAWP, high cardiac output, and elevated SVR. Postpartum, women without spontaneous diuresis had elevated PAWP and cardiac output. Proposed concept of delayed mobilization of extravascular fluid occurring 24–72 hours postpartum
1985	Benedetti et al.	Swan–Ganz	Ten preeclamptic patients with pulmonary edema. Eight of 10 developed pulmonary edema postpartum. Five patients had COP-wedge gradient $\leq$4. Three had findings consistent with pulmonary capillary leak. Two had left ventricular failure. CVP did not correlate with PAWP. Eight of 10 received colloidal fluid before onset of pulmonary edema raising the possibility that colloid was contributory
1986	Cotton et al.	Swan–Ganz	Used intravenous nitroglycerin to drop mean arterial pressure by 20% in three preeclamptic women with pulmonary edema. Mean PAWP decreased from 27 ± 4 to 14 ± 6 mmHg resulting in a COP-wedge gradient change from −10 to 2 mmHg. There was no change in heart rate, CVP, or cardiac output
1987	Sibai et al.	None	Retrospective chart review of 37 patients. Incidence of pulmonary edema 2.9% among 1,290 severe preeclampsia/eclampsia patients. Incidence was higher in older, multiparas with chronic hypertension. Seventy percent of cases occurred postpartum. Four maternal deaths. Perinatal mortality 530/1,000. Sick patients with much comorbidity: 18 had disseminated intravascular coagulation, 17 sepsis, 12 abruptio placenta, 10 acute renal failure, 6 hypertensive crisis, 5 cardiopulmonary arrest, 2 liver rupture, and 2 ischemic cerebral damage
1988	Mabie et al.	Echocardiography	Used the concept of diastolic dysfunction to explain pulmonary edema in four obese, chronically hypertensive pregnant women
1993	Mabie et al.	Echocardiography	Prospective study of 45 obstetric patients with pulmonary edema. Three therapeutically and prognostically distinct groups were identified: (i) systolic dysfunction ($n = 19$); (ii) diastolic dysfunction ($n = 17$); and (iii) normal heart ($n = 9$). Two patients with systolic dysfunction died and one underwent cardiac transplantation. Patients with systolic dysfunction required short- and long-term treatment with digoxin, diuretics, and angiotensin-converting enzyme inhibitors. Those with diastolic dysfunction received diuretics and long-term antihypertensive therapy. Women with normal hearts required acute therapy only. Because clinical and roentgenographic findings do not accurately differentiate patients with respect to the presence and type of cardiac dysfunction, echocardiography was recommended to evaluate all pregnant women with pulmonary edema

distribution, redistribution of blood flow with prominence of the upper lobe veins, or pleural effusions. Interstitial edema causes short, linear, horizontal markings originating near the pleural surface, so-called B lines of Kerley. Cardiomegaly may be present; although with a portable anterior–posterior projection, it is difficult to interpret heart size. Chest radiography cannot reliably distinguish hydrostatic from permeability edema, although claims to the contrary have been made.

Arterial blood gases are measured less frequently now, because noninvasive pulse oximetry allows continuous oxygen saturation measurement. If the patient is critically ill or has comorbid conditions such as renal disease, chronic obstructive pulmonary disease, or sepsis, an arterial blood gas measurement may be needed to check for acidosis or carbon dioxide retention. Typical blood gases in pulmonary edema reveal hypoxemia with low or normal $P_a\text{CO}_2$. With florid pulmonary edema, carbon dioxide retention and respiratory acidosis may develop.

A twelve-lead electrocardiogram should be performed to detect chamber hypertrophy, ischemia, conduction defects, or arrhythmias.

An extremely useful diagnostic test in pulmonary edema is the echocardiogram. This allows noninvasive evaluation of cardiac structure and function. In a prospective study of pregnant women with pulmonary edema, Mabie et al. used echocardiography to differentiate between cardiogenic and noncardiogenic forms of pulmonary edema, determine the type of cardiac dysfunction (systolic, diastolic, or valvular), and plan long-term therapy (Mabie et al., 1993). It is important to recognize that the echocardiogram does not have to be done acutely while the patient is in pulmonary edema. The underlying cardiac abnormalities do not change rapidly despite therapy. With the development of new, lightweight, portable echocardiography machines, it may be possible to initiate "point of care" echocardiography, but there are still several questions: (i) the portable machines are not as good as the $250,000 state-of-the-art platforms; (ii) echocardiography technicians require years of experience to obtain the data and the average cardiologist cannot perform the study as well as an experienced technician; (iii) the setting in an ICU (lighting, bandages, uncooperative patient, ventilator) may decrease the sensitivity of the portable exam; and (iv) reimbursement may change if the echo lab is dismantled and bedside echocardiograms are performed by the cardiology consultants (Schiller, 2001).

A Swan–Ganz catheter may be needed for diagnosis and/or management of patients with pulmonary edema. The Swan–Ganz catheter can be used to diagnose hypovolemia; hydrostatic pulmonary edema (PAWP >18 mmHg); severe mitral regurgitation (V wave); pulmonary hypertension; low, normal, or high cardiac output state; cardiac tamponade (equalization of pressures PAWP, CVP, pulmonary artery diastolic), and ventricular septal rupture (step-up in oxygenation). Many of these diagnostic uses have been replaced by echocardiography. The Swan–Ganz catheter is primarily useful for management to obtain CVP, PAWP, intermittent or continuous cardiac output, mixed venous oxygen saturation, and right ventricular ejection fraction—depending on the type of catheter used. The author has found the Swan–Ganz catheter most useful in treating pregnant patients with tight mitral stenosis (valve area <1 cm^2), severe systolic dysfunction (e.g. ejection fraction <30%), a "white out" on chest X-ray, and those patients who do not respond after 2 hours of aggressive diuresis with furosemide.

The Swan–Ganz catheter provides information that one could not obtain by history, physical examination, and chest X-ray (Connors et al., 1996). Nevertheless, it has become highly controversial with calls for a moratorium on its use (Dahlen & Bone, 1996). Problems are lack of prospective, randomized studies showing benefit in any clinically significant outcome, lack of physician ability to interpret hemodynamic waveforms, and nonrandomized trials showing increased length of stay with increased cost and mortality in patients undergoing Swan–Ganz monitoring (Iberti et al., 1990; Dahlen, 2001). It has been suggested that use of the right heart catheter is a marker for a more aggressive and morbid style of care (Connors et al., 1996). On the other hand, the Swan–Ganz catheter generates data that provoke questions, to which the search for the answers produces better understanding of the disease process.

The differential diagnosis of pulmonary edema includes pneumonia, asthma, and pulmonary embolism. These can usually be differentiated by the history, physical, and chest X-ray. The evaluation and treatment of pulmonary edema must begin simultaneously. While a pulmonary embolism can occur in association with pulmonary edema, it is rare. Transporting a patient with pulmonary edema for a lung scan or computed tomographic scan to rule out pulmonary embolism wastes valuable time.

Treatment

The range of treatments for pulmonary edema is listed in Table 24.3. Treatment includes sitting the patient upright and administering oxygen, furosemide, and morphine. Oxygen may be given be nasal cannula at rates of up to 4 L/min. Flow rates above this do not increase the inhaled oxygen fraction and cause nasal irritation. Face mask oxygen can be given with a nonrebreathing mask using flow rates up to 15 L/min. Continuous positive airway pressure (CPAP) may be given noninvasively with a tight-fitting face mask or nasal mask. This increases intra-alveolar pressure, reduces transudation of fluid from alveolar capillaries, and impedes venous return to the thorax. It is most useful as a temporizing measure to maintain oxygenation until furosemide-induced diuresis clears the lungs. Intubation and mechanical ventilation may be required for patient exhaustion or refractory hypoxemia. Mechanical

Table 24.3 Treatment of pulmonary edema

Sit patient upright
Oxygen
Furosemide
Morphine
Antihypertensives (hydralazine, labetalol, nicardipine)
Nitroglycerin
Nitroprusside
Aminophylline
Digoxin
Dobutamine
Dopamine
Norepinephrine
Epinephrine
Phosphodiesterase inhibitors (amrinone, milrinone)
Mechanical ventilation
Intra-aortic balloon counterpulsation
Biventricular assist device
Heart transplant

ventilation decreases the work of breathing, allows delivery of increased inhaled oxygen fractions, and permits the use of positive end-expiratory pressure to recruit atelectatic alveoli or to maintain partially expanded alveoli. The route of oxygen administration depends on the severity of the pulmonary edema and the response to initial therapy. The goal is to maintain the arterial partial pressure of oxygen >60 mmHg and the oxygen saturation >90%.

Furosemide may be given in a dose of 40–80 mg intravenously. This causes venodilation, decreasing preload, and blockage of chloride and sodium reabsorption in the ascending limb of the loop of Henle. The aim should be to obtain roughly a 2,000 mL diuresis over a few hours. This is often associated with radiographic clearing of the pulmonary edema.

Morphine (2–5 mg intravenously) is also a venodilator and will decrease the patient's anxiety. Frequently in obstetrics, these mainstays of therapy are all that are needed. In fact, oxygen and furosemide are frequently all that is required.

When pulmonary edema is associated with severe hypertension, antihypertensive therapy with intravenous hydralazine, labetalol, or nicardipine will reduce afterload and improve cardiac performance. Sodium nitroprusside, a balanced arterial and venular vasodilator, can be used for minute-to-minute titration of blood pressure; however, it is rarely used in pregnancy because of the risk of fetal cyanide and thiocyanate toxicity. Nitroglycerin is primarily a venular vasodilator that has arterial vasodilator effects when given in higher intravenous doses. Although it crosses the placenta, nitroglycerin is safe for the fetus. It is the drug of choice in hypertension associated with acute coronary syndromes such as myocardial infarction or unstable angina; however, symptomatic coronary artery disease is uncommon in pregnancy.

In patients with systolic dysfunction and pulmonary edema, there are a number of supportive agents that can be used. In pregnancy, systolic dysfunction would most commonly be seen in a patient with peripartum, familial, or idiopathic dilated cardiomyopathy. Current therapy for systolic dysfunction centers around afterload reduction rather than inotropic therapy. If the systolic blood pressure exceeds 70 mmHg, dobutamine, an inotropic vasodilator, may be given to increase cardiac output and lower SVR. Digoxin is not recommended acutely, except for rate control, because of its proarrhythmia potential. If hypotension is present, dopamine, an inotropic vasoconstrictor, may be used. A combination of dopamine and dobutamine may be used, or norepinephrine, a more powerful inotropic vasoconstrictor, may be tried. Noncatecholamine inotropes, which do not increase oxygen consumption as much, include amrinone and milrinone (phosphodiesterase inhibitors). The rest of the armamentarium includes intra-aortic balloon counterpulsation, biventricular assist device, and heart transplant.

Long-term therapy of patients with pulmonary edema can be based on echocardiographic findings. In pregnancy, treatment of systolic dysfunction consists of an inotrope, a diuretic, and an afterload reducer (i.e. digoxin, furosemide, and hydralazine). Isosorbide dinitrate, a long-acting oral nitroglycerin preparation, may be combined with hydralazine for preload and afterload reduction. Therapeutic anticoagulation with heparin may be needed with severe cardiomyopathy (ejection fraction <15%), atrial fibrillation, previous mural thrombus, or a previous pulmonary embolism. Following delivery, afterload reduction with an angiotensin-converting enzyme inhibitor can replace hydralazine and isosorbide dinitrate. Aldosterone antagonists (e.g. spironolactone) and beta-blockers (e.g. carvedilol, metoprolol) have both been shown to prolong life in congestive heart failure.

Patients with diastolic dysfunction require treatment to control blood pressure. No lusitropic drug is available. Beta-blockers to control heart rate and allow time for diastolic filling are most useful.

Patients with normal hearts require no long-term treatment once pulmonary edema has cleared (Mabie et al., 1993).

Prevention

Tocolytic-induced pulmonary edema is the etiology most amenable to prevention by the obstetrician. A strategy for prevention includes: (i) attention to contraindications to tocolytic therapy (e.g. preeclampsia, infection); (ii) careful intake and output with total fluid administration limited to 2,500 mL/day; (iii) recognition of predisposing factors (e.g. twins, anemia, low maternal weight); and (iv) use of magnesium sulfate as the tocolytic agent of first choice.

Other strategies to prevent pulmonary edema include: (i) invasive hemodynamic monitoring in patients with New York Heart Association Class III or IV cardiac disease, particularly mitral stenosis with a valve area less than 1.0 cm^2; and (ii) close monitoring of the patient undergoing "conservative" management of severe preeclampsia.

References

Benedetti TJ, Carlson RW. Studies of colloid osmotic pressure in pregnancy-induced hypertension. Am J Obstet Gynecol 1979; 135(3):308–311.

Benedetti TJ, Kates R, Williams V. Hemodynamic observations in severe preeclampsia complicated by pulmonary edema. Am J Obstet Gynecol 1985;152(3):330–334.

Berkowitz RL, Rafferty TD. Invasive hemodynamic monitoring in critically ill pregnant patients: Role of Swan–Ganz catheterization. Am J Obstet Gynecol 1980;137(1):127–134.

Bernard GR, Artigas A, Brigham KL, et al. and the Consensus Committee. The American-European Concensus Conference on ARDS: Definitions, mechanisms, relevant outcomes, and clinical trial coordination. Am J Respir Crit Care Med 1994;149:818–824.

Clark SL, Phelan JP, Greenspoon J, Aldahl D, Horenstein J. Labor and delivery in the presence of mitral stenosis: Central hemodynamic observations. Am J Obstet Gynecol 1985;152(8):984–988.

Connors AF, Speroff T, Dawson NV, et al. for the SUPPORT (Study to Understand Prognoses and Preferences for Outcomes and Risks of Treatments) Investigators. The effectiveness of right heart catheterization in the initial care of critically ill patients. JAMA 1996;276(11): 889–897.

Cotton DB, Gonik B, Spillman T, Dorman KF. Intrapartum to postpartum changes in colloid osmotic pressure. Am J Obstet Gynecol 1984;149(2):174–177.

Cotton DB, Jones MM, Longmire S, Dorman KF, Tessem J, Joyce TH 3rd. Role of intravenous nitroglycerin in the treatment of severe pregnancy-induced hypertension complicated by pulmonary edema. Am J Obstet Gynecol 1986;154(1):91–93.

Dahlen JE. The pulmonary artery catheter—friend, foe, or accomplice? JAMA 2001;286(3):348–350.

Dahlen JE, Bone RC. Is it time to pull the pulmonary artery catheter? JAMA 1996;276(11):916–918.

Dematte JE, Sznajder JI. Mechanisms of pulmonary edema clearance: From basic research to clinical implication. Intensive Care Med 2000;26(4):477–480.

Desai DK, Moodley J, Naidoo DP, Bhorat I. Cardiac abnormalities in pulmonary edema associated with hypertensive crises in pregnancy. Br J Obstet Gynaecol 1996;103(6):523–528.

Gandhi SK, Powers JC, Nomeir AM, et al. The pathogenesis of acute pulmonary edema associated with hypertension. N Engl J Med 2001;344(1):17–22.

Hankins GDV, Wendel GD, Cunningham FG, Leveno KJ. Longitudinal evaluation of hemodynamic changes in eclampsia. Am J Obstet Gynecol 1984;150(5pt1):506–512.

Heider AL, Kuller JA, Strauss RA, Wells SR. Peripartum cardiomyopathy: A review of the literature. Obstet Gynecol Surv 1999;54(1): 526–531.

Iberti TJ, Fischer EP, Leibowitz AB, Panacek EA, Silverstein JH, Albertson TE, and the Pulmonary Artery Catheter Study Group. A multicenter study of physicians' knowledge of the pulmonary artery catheter. JAMA 1990;264(22):2928–2932.

Ingram RH Jr, Baunwald E. Dyspnea and pulmonary edema. In: Braunwald E, Fauci AS, Kasper DL, Hauser SL, Longo DL, Jameson JL, eds. Harrison's Principles of Internal Medicine, 15th edn. New York: McGraw-Hill, 2001:199–203.

Keefer JR, Strauss RG, Civetta JM, Burke T. Noncardiogenic pulmonary edema and invasive cardiovascular monitoring. Obstet Gynecol 1981;58(1):46–51.

Lampert MB, Hibbard J, Weinert L, Briller J, Lindheimer M, Lang RM. Peripartum heart failure associated with prolonged tocolytic therapy. Am J Obstet Gynecol 1993;168(2):493–495.

Leduc D, Naeije K, Leeman M, Homans C, Kahn RJ. Severe pulmonary edema associated with tocolytic therapy: Case report with hemodynamic study. Intensive Care Med 1996;22(11):1280–1281.

Mabie WC, Ratts TE, Ramanathan KB, Sibai BM. Circulatory congestion in obese hypertensive women: A subset of pulmonary edema in pregnancy. Obstet Gynecol 1988;72(4):553–558.

Mabie WC, Hackman BB, Sibai BM. Pulmonary edema associated with pregnancy: Echocardiographic insights and implications for treatment. Obstet Gynecol 1993;81(2):227–234.

Pearson GD, Veille JC, Rahimtoola S, et al. Peripartum cardiomyopathy: National Heart, Lung, and Blood Institute and Office of Rare Diseases (National Institute of Health) workshop recommendations and review. JAMA 2000;283(9):1183–1188.

Pisani RJ, Rosenow EC 3rd. Pulmonary edema associated with tocolytic therapy. Ann Intern Med 1989;110(9):814–818.

Schiller NB. Hand-held echocardiography: Revolution or hassle? J Am Coll Cardiol 2001;37(8):2023–2024.

Sibai BM, Mabie BC, Harvey CJ, Gonzales AR. Pulmonary edema in severe preeclampsia-eclampsia: Analysis of 37 consecutive cases. Am J Obstet Gynecol 1987;156(4):1174–1179.

Strauss RG, Keefer JR, Burke T, Civetta JM. Hemodynamic monitoring of cardiogenic pulmonary edema complicating toxemia of pregnancy. Obstet Gynecol 1980;55(2):170–174.

West JB. Vascular diseases. In: Pulmonary Pathophysiology: The essentials, 5th edn. Philadelphia, PA: Lippincott, Williams and Wilkins, 1998:95–112.

Zlatnik MG. Pulmonary edema: Etiology and treatment. Semin Perinatol 1997;21(4):298–306.

25 The acute abdomen

Howard T. Sharp

There is often a tendency to treat the pregnant patient with a nonobstetric problem as the "Faberge Egg," particularly when performing exploratory surgery, or ordering diagnostic testing involving exposure to ionizing radiation. The fact that there are two patients involved, both with unique vulnerabilities, should not cause delay or indecision but rather a heightened sense of awareness. For it is often treatment delay which can ultimately be the greatest danger in terms of morbidity and mortality. As a general rule, the acute abdomen during pregnancy should be treated as it would in the nonpregnant state, with an emphasis on making a timely diagnosis and performing appropriate surgery. It is also important for physicians caring for obstetric patients with acute surgical issues to be aware of the unique circumstances associated with each trimester of pregnancy. In particular, organogenesis is ongoing in the first trimester, and preterm labor issues may arise with surgery during the later part of the second and the third trimester. Lastly, with the popularization of laparoscopy, surgical approaches are continually evolving, the limits of which are currently being investigated for safety and efficacy.

This chapter will review the contemporary diagnostic and surgical modalities available for patients with the acute abdomen in pregnancy. The morbidity and mortality associated with these surgical conditions will also be reviewed. The vast majority of data regarding the acute abdomen in pregnancy are based upon experience, case reports and case series, and are therefore considered level III data as outlined by the US Preventive Services Task Force.

Laparoscopy during pregnancy

The popularization of operative laparoscopy has caused a significant shift in the way many surgeries are performed during pregnancy. Questions have arisen regarding the potential for decreased uterine blood flow due to increased intra-abdominal pressures from insufflation, and possible fetal carbon dioxide absorption. Some data from animal models suggest that fetal acidosis may be higher than expected (Amos et al., 1997). Other possible drawbacks of laparoscopic surgery during pregnancy include injury of the pregnant uterus, and the technical difficulty of laparoscopic surgery due to the growing mass of the gravid uterus.

In reviewing the literature for case series and surveys, data can be obtained from a total of 518 laparoscopic surgeries during pregnancy (Lachman et al., 1999). The most commonly performed laparoscopic surgery during pregnancy is cholecystectomy. This procedure is routinely performed during the second trimester at many hospitals, and is becoming more common during the first and third trimesters at selected centers. Appendectomy, adnexal surgery, and miscellaneous rare surgeries (liver biopsy, exploratory surgery) are performed less often during pregnancy.

Due to the small number of reported cases and the lack of prospective studies, data on laparoscopic surgery during pregnancy are insufficient to allow firm conclusions regarding safety and complication rates to be drawn (Fatum & Rojansky, 2001). Most reports come from surgeons with significant interest and skill in laparoscopy. Therefore, their results may not accurately reflect complication rates at other centers. However, the trend of the cumulative experience over the past 10 years suggests that laparoscopic surgery may be performed safely during pregnancy, although more studies are needed to establish its exact complication rate.

If laparoscopic surgery is to be performed after the first trimester, open laparoscopy is recommended to best avoid trocar or Veress needle injury to the gravid uterus. The use of a uterine manipulator is contraindicated in pregnancy.

Diagnostic imaging during pregnancy

There is often undue concern over the use of diagnostic imaging during pregnancy. According to the American College of Radiology, no single diagnostic X-ray procedure results in enough radiation exposure to threaten the well-being of the developing preembryo, embryo, or fetus. Radiation exposure of less than 5 rads is not associated with an increased fetal risk.

However, ultrasound should be considered a first-line diagnostic procedure if appropriate for the suspected condition.

All diagnostic X-ray procedures result in fetal exposure of less than 5 rads (Table 25.1). These range from approximately 100 mrad for a single view abdominal film to 2–4 rads for a barium enema or small bowel series. The amount of radiation exposure is largely dependent upon the number of exposures. Consultation with a radiologist can assist in estimating the amount of ionizing radiation to the fetus before tests are performed.

Magnetic resonance imaging (MRI) uses magnets that alter the energy state of hydrogen protons instead of using ionizing radiation. Though there have been no reported adverse fetal effects from its use, the National Radiological Protection Board has arbitrarily advised against its use in the first trimester.

Appendicitis during pregnancy

The most common cause of the acute abdomen in pregnancy is appendicitis, which occurs with a rate of approximately 1 in 1,500 deliveries (Black, 1960; Babaknia et al., 1977). The diagnosis of appendicitis in pregnancy can be difficult because pregnancy may alter classic signs and symptoms of appendicitis. In addition, appendiceal location changes as pregnancy advances. When appendicitis is suspected during pregnancy, the physician must balance the risks associated with delaying surgery with the effects of surgery on the mother and fetus. Ultimately, the decision to operate should be made on clinical grounds, as in the nonpregnant state, accepting that there is a necessary inherent negative exploration rate. Most larger series of appendectomy during pregnancy quote a negative exploration rate of approximately 20–35%. If the appendix appears normal at surgery, it is important to look for both other nonobstetric causes (Table 25.2) as well as obstetric causes (Table 25.3).

Presentation of appendicitis during pregnancy

It is important to realize the changes that the uterus undergoes throughout the nine months of gestation. In 1932, Baer et al. demonstrated the migration of the appendix based on serial radiographs in pregnant women (Baer et al., 1932). They described a progressive upward displacement of the appendix after the third month, reaching the level of the iliac crest at the end of the sixth month. The appendix was noted to return to its normal position by the 10th postpartum day.

The most typical presentation of appendicitis is colicky epigastric or periumbilical pain (referred from the appendiceal viscera), which eventually localizes to the right side of the abdomen. The location of the pain often reflects the changing location of the appendix. Anorexia and vomiting, though common in pregnant women with appendicitis, are not necessarily specific or sensitive indicators; likewise, fever is often not present. The single most reliable symptom in pregnant patients with appendicitis is right lower quadrant pain (Mourad et al., 2000), yet rebound tenderness and guarding are not particularly specific.

Due to the natural physiology of pregnancy, laboratory values are not reliably predictive of appendicitis during pregnancy. In the first and second trimesters, the white blood cell count may normally range from 6,000 to 16,000 cells/mm^3. During

Table 25.1 Estimated fetal exposure from radiologic procedures

Procedure	Fetal exposure
Abdominal film	100 mrad
Intravenous pyelogram	>1 rad
Barium enema	2–4 rad
Small bowel series	2–4 rad
CT of abdomen	3.5 rad
Helical CT of abdomen	300 mrad

Table 25.2 Nonobstetric conditions mimicking appendicitis

Pyelonephritis
Urinary calculi
Cholecystitis/cholelithiasis
Bowel obstruction
Pancreatitis
Gastroenteritis
Acute mesenteric adenitis
Carcinoma of large bowel
Rectus hematoma
External hernia
Ischemic mesentaric necrosis
Acute intermittent porphyria
Perforated duodenal ulcer

Table 25.3 Obstetric conditions mimicking appendicitis

Preterm labor
Abruptio placenta
Chorioamnionitis
Adnexal torsion
Ectopic/heterotopic pregnancy
Pelvic inflammatory disease
Round ligament pain
Utero-ovarian vein rupture
Rupture of uterine arteriovenous malformation
Myomatous red degeneration
Uterine rupture
(placenta percreta)
(rudimentary uterine horn)

labor, it may rise to 20,000–30,000 cells/mm^3. Therefore, leukocytosis may not be helpful in diagnosing appendicitis in pregnancy; however, a persistent white blood cell count less than 10,000/mm^3 gives reassurance. Recent larger series have questioned the usefulness of relying on laboratory data to confirm or dismiss a diagnosis of appendicitis in pregnancy (Baer et al., 1932; Andersen & Nielsen, 1999).

Diagnostic imaging for appendicitis during pregnancy

In the nonpregnant state, graded compression ultrasound (GCU) has been used to diagnose acute appendicitis with a sensitivity of 86%, and because of its favorable safety profile, it should be considered as the initial diagnostic imaging test of choice for evaluating pregnant women. In pregnancy, GCU has been shown to be accurate in the first and second trimesters, but technically difficult in the third. In a series of 42 women with suspected appendicitis during pregnancy, GCU was found to be 100% sensitive, 96% specific, and 98% accurate in diagnosing appendicitis (Lim et al., 1992). Three patients were unable to be adequately evaluated due to the technical difficulties associated with gestational ages over 35 weeks.

Helical computed tomography is a newer technology which is currently being evaluated for its efficacy during pregnancy. The initial results are promising; however, to date only one case series has been reported which includes seven patients (Castro et al., 2001). The potential advantages of this modality are the rapidity with which it can be performed and the safety that it offers compared to standard computed tomography. Helical computed tomography of the pregnant abdomen can be accomplished in 15 minutes with an exposure of approximately 300 mrads to the fetus. Larger studies are needed to validate the initial favorable results of this case series.

Mortality and morbidity associated with appendicitis during pregnancy

Babler wrote in 1908, "The mortality of appendicitis complicating pregnancy and the puerperium is the mortality of delay" (Babler, 1908). Though the fetal mortality rate associated with appendicitis has improved over the past 50 years, when appendiceal perforation occurs, the fetal loss rate may be as high as 36% (Babaknia et al., 1977). In contrast, in the absence of appendiceal perforation, the incidence of fetal loss is 1.5% or less (Babaknia et al., 1977). This is of particular concern in the third trimester, when the likelihood of intact fetal viability is high. Appendiceal rupture has been reported to occur twice as often in the third trimester (69%) as in the first and second trimesters (31%) (Weingold, 1983). This is probably secondary to delayed diagnosis in advanced gestation.

Preterm labor is a concern due to peritoneal irritation and its inflammatory response. Though preterm contractions are common after appendectomy in pregnancy (83%), they rarely result in preterm labor and delivery (5–14%) (Baer et al., 1932; Andersen & Nielsen, 1999). Therefore tocolytic agents are not routinely recommended in the absence of cervical change.

Over the past 30 years, maternal mortality rates associated with appendicitis have dropped sharply. This is likely due to the development of improved antibiotics and surgical techniques. Maternal death from appendicitis, which was not uncommon in the early 20th century (25% mortality rate), is now a rarity and is usually associated with significant surgical delay.

Prompt surgical intervention has been shown to decrease the morbidity and mortality associated with appendicitis during pregnancy in several case series. Horowitz reported on a series of 12 patients with a preoperative diagnosis of appendicitis, 10 of which were documented to have appendicitis (Horowitz et al., 1995). Surgery was delayed more than 24 hours in seven of the 12 patients. Six of the seven patients had appendiceal perforation resulting in two fetal deaths, one preterm delivery, and one maternal death. A larger series by Tamir reported appendiceal perforation in 66% of patients when surgical delay occurred for greater than 24 hours ($n=35$), yet no cases of perforation in patients taken to surgery within 24 hours of presentation (Tamir et al., 1990). The old adage "if you cannot rule it out, take it out," probably still applies to the diagnosis of appendicitis in pregnancy.

Preparing for surgery

When preparing for surgery in the pregnant patient, it is useful for care to be coordinated between consulting services in a timely fashion. Obstetrics, General Surgery, Anesthesia, and Neonatology Services each may have important details to convey to optimize the team approach.

If laparotomy is to be performed, the patient should be placed in the supine position with a right hip roll, rotating the patient 30° to the left to optimize blood flow to the fetus. Uterine manipulation should be avoided as much as possible to decrease the risk of uterine irritability and preterm labor. Intraoperative external fetal monitoring is rarely indicated unless the mother is hemodynamically unstable. There is nothing intrinsic to the process of exploratory laparotomy or appendectomy which predisposes to fetal asphyxia or death. If perforation has occurred, an important part of therapy is the use of copious irrigation and broad-spectrum antibiotics, including anaerobic coverage. The use of an intraperitoneal drain has been advocated in such cases.

Various incisions have been recommended. The most popular is a muscle-splitting incision over the point of maximum tenderness, which is particularly useful in the second and third trimesters. The paramedian and midline vertical incisions should be used if there is significant doubt about the diagnosis, for improved access to the left adnexa if necessary.

In a case–control study of 22 laparoscopic appendectomies, compared to 18 open appendectomies, all were performed without birth defects, fetal loss or uterine injury. Preterm delivery rates in both groups were similar. Neither birth weights nor Apgar scores were significantly different between groups (Affleck et al., 1999).

In a recent prospective series, outcomes in pregnant women undergoing laparoscopic appendectomy were compared with a control group of pregnant women who underwent open appendectomy (Lyass et al., 2001). There was no significant difference in the length of procedure (60 vs 46 min) or complications rate. There was no conversion to laparotomy in the laparoscopic group, and the length of postoperative stay was shorter in the laparoscopic group (3.6 vs 5.2 days; $P = 0.05$). There was no fetal loss or other adverse outcome of pregnancy in either group, and all the women in both groups had normal full-term delivery. The infants' development was normal in both groups for a mean follow-up period of 30 months.

Cholecystitis during pregnancy

Cholecystitis is the second most common surgical condition in pregnancy, occurring in between 1 in 1,600 and 1 in 10,000 pregnancies. During pregnancy, there is an increase in cholesterol synthesis with an increased concentration of cholesterol in the gallbladder, and stasis of bile in the gallbladder. Cholelithiasis is the cause of cholecystitis in pregnancy in over 90% of cases. The incidence of cholelithiasis in pregnant women undergoing routine obstetric ultrasound examinations is 3.5%; however, it is unclear whether pregnancy predisposes women to cholecystitis, as statistically fewer cholecystectomies are performed on pregnant women than on nonpregnant women (Stauffer et al., 1982). This lower rate may be due to physicians' reluctance to perform surgery on pregnant patients.

Presentation of cholecystitis during pregnancy

The presentation of cholecystitis in pregnancy is essentially the same as in the nonpregnant state. Nausea, vomiting, and an acute onset of a colicky or stabbing pain that begins over the midepigastrium or right upper abdominal quadrant with radiation to the back is common. Biliary colic, usually sudden in onset, may persist for approximately 3 hours after a meal. Symptoms also may be localized to the flank, right scapula, or shoulder. Murphy's sign (tenderness under the right costal margin upon deep inspiration) is less common in pregnant women with cholecystitis. Fever, tachycardia, and tachypnea may be present. When upper abdominal pain presents during pregnancy, the differential diagnosis should include potentially life-threatening processes such as myocardial infarction, acute fatty liver in pregnancy, and HELLP syndrome. Other less serious but significant conditions should also be considered in the differential diagnosis (Table 25.4).

Table 25.4 Differential diagnosis of cholecystitis during pregnancy

Appendicitis
Acute hepatitis
Herpes zoster
Myocardial infarction
Pancreatitis
Peptic ulcer disease
Pneumonia
Severe preeclampsia
Pyelonephritis

Diagnosing cholecystitis during pregnancy

Leukocytosis and hyperamylasemia are common, the latter usually resolving upon hydration. Serum transaminases and direct bilirubin levels may also be elevated. Jaundice is rare, but if present, may be associated with common bile duct stones. Alkaline phosphatase is less helpful in diagnosing cholecystitis in pregnancy because estrogen causes the level of this enzyme to be elevated.

Ultrasound of the gallbladder is indicated when there is significant right upper-quadrant pain in pregnancy. It is the diagnostic test of choice in pregnancy because it is noninvasive, readily available, and accurate. The diagnostic accuracy of ultrasound for detecting gallstones is approximately 95% (Stauffer et al., 1982). Good views of the gallbladder can usually be obtained during pregnancy without fasting.

Clinical management of cholecystitis during pregnancy

The initial treatment for cholecystitis in pregnancy has typically been medical, especially in the third trimester. Surgery has generally been reserved for those women in whom medical treatment has failed after several days, or in patients who experienced repeated attacks of biliary colic. Surgery is performed as initial therapy in patients with suspected perforation, sepsis, or peritonitis. This traditional approach is now being challenged by some investigators in favor of a more aggressive surgical approach, managed by laparoscopy or laparotomy regardless of trimester.

Medical management

The medical treatment of cholecystitis in pregnancy consists of supportive intravenous hydration, enteric rest with nasogastric suction, and judicious use of narcotics. Morphine is avoided because it can exacerbate biliary colic. The routine use of broad-spectrum antibiotics is controversial, but is clearly indicated in patients with signs of sepsis.

Active surgical management

In 1987, Dixon made an argument for a more aggressive approach during the second trimester. He reported a retrospective study of 44 pregnant women with biliary colic, 26 who received conservative medical management and 18 who underwent primary open cholecystectomy in the second trimester (Dixon et al., 1987). In the group receiving medical management, 58% suffered recurrent episodes. Total parenteral nutrition was necessary in 8% of patients for an average of 29 days, and one patient developed pancreatitis. The mean hospital stay was 14 days which did not include hospital days for subsequent cholecystectomy. Spontaneous abortion occurred in 12% of patients, whereas 15% of the patients underwent elective abortion. In the group of women treated primarily by surgery, two were lost to follow-up, 12 delivered healthy infants at term, three underwent elective abortion, and one had a premature delivery at 8 months, secondary to severe preeclampsia. The mean hospital stay was 6 days. Recently, this study was corroborated in a report of 35 patients which demonstrated improved pregnancy outcomes in women who underwent surgical management (Lee et al., 2000).

The laparoscopic cholecystectomy experience in pregnancy was reviewed in 1998 (Graham et al., 1998). The authors concluded that this procedure compared favorably with open cholecystectomy. There was a decreased risk both of spontaneous abortion in the first trimester and of preterm labor in the third trimester in women undergoing laparoscopic cholecystectomy. In a review of 16 women who underwent laparoscopic cholecystectomy during pregnancy, 9 of 11 women who underwent cholecystectomy more than 5 weeks after onset of symptoms experienced recurrent attacks necessitating 15 hospital admissions and four emergency room visits (Muench et al., 2001). Moreover four women who developed symptoms in the first and second trimesters with surgery delayed to the third trimester had 11 hospital admissions and four emergency room visits. Three of those four women developed premature contractions necessitating tocolytics. Cholecystectomy was completed laparoscopically in 14 women. There was no hospital infant or maternal mortality or morbidity. As a result, the authors recommend that prompt laparoscopic cholecystectomy in pregnant women with symptomatic biliary disease be considered as a means of reducing hospital admissions and frequency of premature labor.

Bowel obstruction during pregnancy

Bowel obstruction occurs in approximately 1 in 3,000 pregnancies. Adhesions are the cause of obstruction in many cases. The frequency of adhesions as the cause of intestinal obstruction during pregnancy was found to be 6% in the first trimester, 27% in the second trimester, 44% in the third trimester, and 21% postpartum (Connolly et al., 1995). In the first trimester this is probably caused by the uterus becoming a suprapubic organ, and later due to rapid uterine size changes that take place during delivery and the puerperium. Volvulus is the second most common cause of bowel obstruction in pregnancy, occurring in approximately 25% of cases (Wenetick et al., 1973). Other causes such as intussusception, hernia, and cancer are rare. The incidence of bowel obstruction has been climbing since the 1940s, largely because of an increase in the number of surgeries performed in the population in general. As with appendicitis, the morbidity and mortality of bowel obstruction is related to diagnostic and therapeutic delay. Beware of the diagnosis of hyperemesis gravidarum in the second and third trimesters in patients who have had abdominal surgery, as this is a common misdignosis.

Bowel obstruction can result in significant maternal and fetal morbidity and mortality. Perdue et al. (1992) reviewed the literature written between 1966 and 1991 and found four maternal deaths in 66 reported cases of bowel obstruction in pregnancy. The fetal mortality rate was 26%. Bowel strangulation requiring resection occurred in 23% of cases. The mean length of time from admission to surgery in these cases was 48 hours.

Presentation of bowel obstruction during pregnancy

The symptoms associated with bowel obstruction in pregnancy are crampy abdominal pain, obstipation, and vomiting. In the case of a high obstruction, the period between attacks is usually short, 4 or 5 minutes, and is frequently characterized by diffuse, poorly localized upper-abdominal pain. Colonic obstruction may manifest itself as low abdominal or perineal pain with a longer interval between pain attacks, 15–20 minutes. The abdomen is frequently distended and tender. Fever, leukocytosis, and electrolyte abnormalities increase the likelihood of finding intestinal strangulation.

Diagnosing bowel obstruction during pregnancy

Upright and flat-plate abdominal films should be obtained if intestinal obstruction is suspected. It is often helpful to compare serial radiographic findings at 4–6 hour intervals to identify the presence of air-fluid levels or progressive bowel dilation, in order to assess whether conservative management is effective. In one series, flat and upright radiographs showed typical patterns of obstruction in 75% of cases (Wenetick et al., 1973). Additional radiologic studies following the administration of oral contrast media should be performed if bowel obstruction still is suspected in the absence of typical findings on flat and upright abdominal images.

Clinical management of bowel obstruction during pregnancy

The clinical management of bowel obstruction during pregnancy is essentially no different from treatment in the nonpregnant state. Initial treatment consists of fluid and electrolyte replacement, and bowel decompression via a nasogastric tube. Surgery is generally reserved for failed medical management. Fluid is lost by way of vomiting, nasogastric suctioning, intralumenal losses, bowel wall edema, and free peritoneal fluid. A Foley catheter should be placed to monitor urine output. The amount of fluid loss is often underestimated and may result in renal insufficiency, hypovolemia, shock, and death.

If the decision is made to take the patient to surgery, a midline vertical incision is recommended. Exposure is often a challenge, and depending on the gestational age in the third trimester, cesarean delivery may be necessary before the bowel can be adequately explored. The entire bowel should be examined, as there may be more than one area of obstruction. Bowel viability should be assessed carefully by a surgeon experienced in the management of necrotic bowel. Segmental resection with or without anastomosis may be needed.

Adnexal torsion during pregnancy

Adnexal torsion is one of the few causes of the acute abdomen that is more common in pregnancy than in the nonpregnant state (28% vs 7%). The typical presentation is lateralized lower quadrant pain, often sudden in onset. Though nausea, vomiting, fever, and leukocytosis may be present, none of these are reliable findings during pregnancy. On physical examination, the abdomen is tender, often with peritoneal signs. If torsion occurs in the first trimester, the adnexum is usually enlarged and exquisitely tender on bimanual exam.

Ultrasonography is the diagnostic modality of choice, as the presence of an adnexal mass is usually detectable. Doppler studies may assist to document the presence or absence of ovarian blood flow. However, the diagnosis of ovarian and adnexal torsion cannot be based solely on the absence or presence of flow on color Doppler sonography, because the presence of arterial or venous flow does not exclude the diagnosis of adnexal torsion. Doppler studies of the ovarian vessels in pregnancy have not been investigated at the time of this writing.

If adnexal torsion is suspected, surgery should not be delayed, as the viability of the ovary may be compromised. If a laparotomy is to be performed, a midline vertical incision is recommended. This gives the surgeon excellent access to the adnexa and allows for enough room to properly explore the upper abdomen as is standard for the presence of an adnexal mass. Recently, the laparoscopic approach to adnexal torsion in pregnancy has been reported with favorable outcomes (Morice et al., 1997; Abu-Musa et al., 2001).

There has been a common misconception that the untwisting of an ovary that has undergone torsion may cause venous embolism. A review of the literature failed to document any cases of venous embolic phenomena associated with this practice. A total of 133 cases (nonpregnant) have been successfully documented as being treated with detorsion (Cohen et al., 1999). In a series of 54 women with ovarian torsion resulting in black–bluish ovaries, all underwent detorsion with sparing of the affected ovary. On follow-up, 93% were documented to have normal ovarian size with follicular development. The authors conclude that ovaries that have undergone torsion should be untwisted regardless of color and that cystectomy should be performed instead of oophorectomy.

References

Abu-Musa A, Nassar A, Usta I, Khalil A, Hussein M. Laparoscopic unwinding and cystectomy of twisted dermoid cyst during second trimester of pregnancy. J Am Assoc Gynecol Laparosc 2001; 8:456–460.

Affleck DG, Handrahan DL, Egger MJ, Price RR. The laparoscopic management of appendicitis and cholelithiasis during pregnancy. Am J Surg 1999;178:523–529.

Amos JD, Schorr SJ, Norman PF, et al. Laparoscopic surgery during pregnancy. Am J Surg 1997;174:222.

Andersen B, Nielsen TF. Appendicitis in pregnancy: diagnosis, management and complications. Acta Obstet Gynecol Scand 1999; 78:758–762.

Babaknia A, Parsa H, Woodruff JD. Appendicitis during pregnancy. Obstet Gynecol 1977;50:40–44.

Babler EA. Perforative appendicitis complicating pregnancy. JAMA 1908;51:1313.

Baer JL, Reis RA, Arens RA. Appendicitis in pregnancy with changes in position and axis of the normal appendix in pregnancy. JAMA 1932;52:1359–1364.

Black WP. Acute appendicitis in pregnancy. BMJ 1960;1:1938–1941.

Castro MA, Shipp TD, Castro EE, Ouzounian J, Rao P. The use of helical computed tomography in pregnancy for the diagnosis of acute appendicitis. Am J Obstet Gynecol 2001;184:954–957.

Cohen SB, Oelsner G, Seidman DS, Admon D, Mashiach S, Goldenberg M. Laparoscopic detorsion allows sparing of the twisted ischemic adnexa. J Am Assoc Gynecol Lapaorsc 1999;6:139–143.

Connolly MM, Unit JA, Nora PF. Bowel obstruction in pregnancy. Surg Clin North Am 1995;75:101–113.

Dixon NP, Faddis DM, Silberman H. Aggressive management of cholecystitis during pregnancy. Am J Surg 1987;154:292–294.

Fatum M, Rojansky N. Laparoscopic surgery during pregnancy. Obstet Gynecol Surv 2001;56:50–59.

Graham G, Baxi L, Tharakan T. Laparoscopic cholecystectomy during pregnancy: a case series and review of the literature. Obstet Gynecol Surv 1998;53:566–574.

Horowitz MD, Gomez GA, Santiesteban R, Burkett G. Acute appendicitis during pregnancy. Arch Surg 1995;120:1362–1367.

Lachman E, Schienfield A, Voss E, et al. Pregnancy and laparoscopic surgery. J Am Assoc Gynecol Laparosc 1999;6:347–351.

Lee S, Bradley JP, Mele MM, Sehdev HM, Ludmir J. Cholelithiasis in pregnancy: Surgical versus medical management. Obstet Gynecol 2000;95:S70–S71.

Lim HK, Bae SH, Seo GS. Diagnosis of acute appendicitis in pregnant women: value of sonography. Am J Roentgenol 1992;159:539–542.

Lyass S, Pikarsky A, Eisenberg VH, Elchalal U, Schenker JG, Reissman P. Is laparoscopic appendectomy safe in pregnant women? Surg Endosc 2001;15:377–379.

Morice P, Louis-Sylvestre C, Chapron C, Dubuisson JB. Laparoscopy for adnexal torsion in pregnant women. J Reprod Med 1997; 42:435–439.

Mourad J, Elliott JP, Erickson L, Lisboa L. Appendicitis in pregnancy: new information that contradicts long-held clinical beliefs. Am J Obstet Gynecol 2000;182:1027–1029.

Muench J, Albrink M, Serafini F, Rosemurgy A, Carey L, Murr MM. Delay in treatment of biliary disease during pregnancy increases morbidity and can be avoided with safe laparoscopic cholecystectomy. Am Surg 2001;67:539–542.

Perdue PW, Johnson HW, Stafford PW. Intestinal obstruction complicating pregnancy. Am J Surg 1992;164:384–388.

Stauffer RA, Adams A, Wygal J, Lavery PJ. Gallbladder disease in pregnancy. Am J Obstet Gynecol 1982;6:661–664.

Tamir IL, Bongard FS, Klein SR. Acute appendicitis in the pregnant patient. Am J Surg 1990;160:571–576.

Weingold AB. Appendicitis in pregnancy. Clin Obstet Gynecol 1983;26:801–809.

Wenetick LH, Roschen FP, Dunn JM. Volvulus of the small bowel complicating pregnancy. J Reprod Med 1973;14:82–83.

26 Acute pancreatitis

Karen A. Zempolich

Pancreatitis occurring during pregnancy is a potential threat to maternal and fetal well-being, with an associated increase in morbidity and mortality frequently cited. A clearer understanding of the natural history of this disease as it exists in the gravid woman has evolved over the past two decades. As with all abdominal processes, the diagnosis of pancreatitis during pregnancy may be challenging; maternal outcome, however, does not appear to be altered by the concurrent state of pregnancy. Indeed, reports of maternal mortality range from 0% to 3.4%, comparing favorably with an overall mortality of 9% in the general population (Klein, 1986; Block & Kelly, 1989; Steinberg & Tenner, 1994; Swisher et al., 1994; Ramin et al., 1995; Gullo et al., 2002). Fetal and neonatal outcomes, however, are often adversely affected by this disease, with prematurity accounting for a substantial portion of morbidity (Ramin et al., 1995). However, earlier reports of mortality as high as 35% have been tempered by studies demonstrating fetal loss directly attributable to pancreatitis of 0% to 11% (Corlett & Mishell, 1972; Wilkinson, 1973; Jouppila et al., 1974; Block & Kelly, 1989; Swisher et al., 1994; Ramin et al., 1995).

Pancreatitis spans the clinical spectrum from mild disease to multisystem organ failure. This chapter focuses on the epidemiology, clinical course, diagnosis, prognostic indicators, and management of pancreatitis occurring in pregnancy.

Epidemiology

The reported incidence of pancreatitis complicating pregnancy varies widely, with studies demonstrating rates as frequent as 1 in 459 and as uncommon as 1 in 4,350 (Langmade & Edmondson, 1951; Herfort et al., 1981). Many retrospective studies have been generated from tertiary care hospitals evaluating the frequency of pancreatitis within individual institutions. Compiling data from seven such reports shows the estimated incidence of pancreatitis is approximately one case per 2,000 deliveries (Langmade & Edmondson, 1951; Corlett & Mishell, 1972; Wilkinson, 1973; Jouppila et al., 1974; Herfort et al., 1981; Swisher et al., 1994; Ramin et al., 1995). In a review of cholecystectomies performed for gallstone pancreatitis, Block and Kelly (1989) found that among 152 female patients, 21 (13.8%) were either pregnant at the time of surgery or within 6 weeks postpartum.

Many studies have shown an increasing incidence of pancreatitis with advancing gestational age, although first trimester pancreatitis is well described (Legro & Laifer, 1995). While pancreatitis may occur throughout pregnancy and the puerperium, as many as 35–50% of cases occur during the third trimester. Approximately 70–80% of patients are multigravidas, correlating with the overall distribution within the general obstetric population. Parity, therefore, does not appear to influence the development of pancreatitis. Increased risk among ethnic groups has not been demonstrated within the obstetric population. Incidence rates, however, do correlate with the prevalence of etiologic factors such as cholelithiasis (Opie, 1901) and alcohol abuse, which are known to vary among populations.

Early reports of phenomenally high maternal mortality led to a long-held belief that pancreatitis in pregnancy gravely endangered maternal well-being. It is now accepted that previous maternal mortality figures approaching 35–50% considerably overestimated the lethality of the disease (Langmade & Edmondson, 1951; Wilkinson, 1973). Klein collected data from five single institution series and found only three maternal deaths among 87 cases of pancreatitis, a mortality rate of 3.4%. Other studies also have corroborated this finding, with no deaths occurring among 94 cumulative cases (Block & Kelly, 1989; Swisher et al., 1994; Ramin et al., 1995). Biased reporting of more severe cases, as well as confounding concurrent disease, such as fatty liver of pregnancy, may have contributed to the higher mortality reported in earlier studies. Commonly used pharmacologic agents, including methyldopa, may produce unpredictable idiosyncratic or hypersensitivity reactions, including hepatitis and pancreatitis (Rominger et al., 1978; Scarpelli, 1989; Underwood & Frye, 1993; Webster & Koch, 1996; Eland et al., 1999). Additionally, two drugs previously used more liberally in pregnancy, thiazide diuretics and tetracycline, have been linked to pancreatitis (Greenberger et al., 1991; Steinberg & Tenner 1994; Gorelick, 1995). The course of pancreatitis associated with these drugs may have incited a more frequently fulminant disease process. Conversely, improvements in laboratory assays and radiologic modalities may now enable detection of a greater number of mild cases. Regardless of the underlying cause of this discrepancy, current maternal mortality from pancreatitis is only a tenth of previously reported rates.

Etiology

Acute pancreatitis is caused by many different factors. While the list of etiologies is extensive (Table 26.1), approximately 80% of cases are attributable to either biliary tract disease or alcohol abuse in the general population (Steinberg & Tenner, 1994; Steer, 1995). Gallstones are the most common cause of pancreatitis in the United States, Western Europe, and Asia, accounting for 45% of cases (Steinberg & Tenner, 1994). Alcoholism accounts for another 35%, roughly 10% are idiopathic, and the remainder are divided among miscellaneous causes.

Among pregnant patients, causes of pancreatitis parallel those of the general population. Physiologic changes in biliary function, however, appear to influence the incidence of cholelithiasis, although not necessarily gallstone pancreatitis, during pregnancy. Behavioral changes secondary to teratogenic concerns also may decrease the relative proportion of alcohol-induced pancreatitis. This section focuses on those causes most commonly seen in pregnancy: gallstones, hypertriglyceridemia, and drug-associated pancreatitis.

Biliary disease in pregnancy

Cholelithiasis is the most common etiology of pancreatitis in pregnancy, representing a larger percentage of cases than in the nonpregnant population. Biliary disease has been identified in 68–100% of pregnant patients with pancreatitis (Block & Kelly, 1989; Swisher et al., 1994; Ramin et al., 1995). The increased proportion of gallstone-induced pancreatitis may be attributable to the direct effects of pregnancy on gallstone formation, rather than a decreased incidence of other etiologies, and remains an area of active investigation.

Table 26.1 Causes of acute pancreatitis in pregnancy

Obstruction (cholelithiasis)
Drugs (ethanol, thiazides, azathioprine, valproic acid)
Hyperlipidemia
Abdominal trauma
Hypercalcemia
Infection (viral, parasitic)
Vascular disease (systemic lupus erythematosus)
Miscellaneous (Crohn's disease, perforating ulcer, cystic fibrosis)

Physiology of the biliary system during gestation appears to promote the incidence of gallstone formation through changes in both gallbladder function and bile composition. Using direct observation, intravenous contrast, and, most recently, serial ultrasound evaluation, residual gallbladder volume has been shown to increase throughout pregnancy (Potter, 1936; Gerdes & Boyden, 1938; Braverman et al., 1980). Braverman et al. also demonstrated a slower rate of gallbladder emptying in the latter part of pregnancy. It is felt that these functional changes result in bile stasis, thereby facilitating gallstone formation. Furthermore, studies of bile composition have demonstrated an increase in the lithogenic index of bile, as well as increased bile acid pool size, increased cholesterol secretion, and decreased enterohepatic circulation (Kern et al., 1981; Scott, 1992). The functional changes that contribute to bile stasis act in concert with physiologic changes that increase the lithogenicity of bile constituents, leading to gallstone formation during pregnancy. In a study of gallstones in Chilean women, Valdivieso et al. (1993) demonstrated the effect of pregnancy on the incidence of gallstone formation, noting gallstones in 12.2% of puerperal women, compared with 1.3% in age-matched controls.

The mechanism by which gallstones initiate pancreatitis remains poorly understood. In 1901, Opie proposed the "common channel theory," by which stone impaction at the ampulla of Vater occludes the biliopancreatic duct, creating a channel that allows bile to reflux into the pancreatic duct. Another theory suggests that the pancreatic duct itself becomes blocked, obstructing the outflow of pancreatic secretions, which, in turn, damage the pancreatic acini. While further investigations have challenged these theories, the actual sequence of events remains elusive. Regardless of the mechanism by which stone passage initiates pancreatitis, it is clear that passage is temporally related to the onset of symptoms. Recovery of stones from stool collections has been reported to be as high as 85% (Gorelick, 1995).

Hypertriglyceridemia

Elevation of plasma triglycerides is a well-established cause of pancreatitis. The physiologic changes of pregnancy can exacerbate and unmask an underlying familial disorder and can compound the effects of other secondary causes of hypertriglyceridemia. The mechanism by which hyperlipidemia causes pancreatitis is not fully understood. Local injury to the pancreatic acini, however, is felt to occur through the release of free fatty acids by the action of lipases on the excessive triglycerides (Klein, 1986; DeChalain, 1988). Patients with triglyceride levels exceeding 1000 mg/dL are at greatest risk for pancreatitis, especially those with type V hyperlipidemia (Klein, 1986).

Pregnancy alters lipid metabolism by several mechanisms. An increase in triglyceride production and very low density lipoprotein (VLDL) secretion, as well as a decrease in lipolysis, result in a 50% increase in cholesterol and a threefold increase in triglycerides, with the peak effect seen in the third trimester (Montes, 1984; Klein, 1986; DeChalain, 1988). Superimposed on a familial hyperlipidemia, the metabolic changes of pregnancy can lead to markedly elevated serum levels and greatly increase the risk of pancreatitis. Postpartum total cholesterol and VLDL fall to baseline by 6 weeks (Montes, 1984).

Several features of a patient's medical and family history may suggest an underlying lipid disorder. A history of pancreatitis, recurrent (unexplained) abdominal pain, and known familial disorders can suggest the presence of inherited hyperlipidemia. Chronic renal failure, poorly controlled diabetes mellitus, hypothyroidism, alcohol use, and drugs such as glucocorticoids and beta-blockers can lead to elevated lipid levels (Stone, 1994). In the presence of such conditions in a patient with a familial lipid disorder, the superimposition of pregnancy may result in fulminant pancreatitis (Stone, 1994). Intravenous fat emulsions administered to patients receiving parenteral nutrition are also a rare cause of pancreatitis.

Drugs

Numerous drugs may occasionally cause pancreatitis. One review classified the following drugs as toxic to the pancreas: azathioprine, estrogens, furosemide, methyldopa, pentamidine, procainamide, sulfonamides, and thiazide diuretics (Scarpelli, 1989). The immunosuppressants 6-mercaptopurine and azathioprine and the common AIDS therapies pentamidine and 2′,3′-dideoxyinosine have been strongly associated with this condition (Gorelick, 1995). Antibiotics, including erythromycin and sulfonamides, also have been implicated.

More pertinent to the pregnant population, thiazide diuretics and tetracycline historically accounted for a significant portion of pancreatitis during pregnancy. When these agents were used more commonly in the treatment of preeclampsia, thiazides were associated with 8% of cases of pancreatitis in pregnancy (Wilkinson, 1973). In the same review, tetracycline accounted for nearly 28% of cases and was also commonly associated with acute fatty liver of pregnancy. With subsequent elucidation of the teratogenic effects of tetracycline, this agent should no longer cause pancreatitis in pregnancy. Similarly, use of thiazide diuretics has little or no role in the modern management of preeclampsia.

Pathology and pathophysiology

The pancreas secretes approximately 20 enzymes in 2,000–3,000 mL of alkaline fluid each day. The fluid is rich in bicarbonate, which serves to neutralize gastric acid and provide the correct pH within the interstinal tract for activation of the pancreatic enzymes. Under hormonal and neural control, amylolytic, lipolytic, and proteolytic enzymes are released into the duodenum. The pancreas is normally protected from autodigestion by the presence of protease inhibitors and storage of proteases as precursors (zymogens).

Pancreatitis can be classified based on its chronicity and severity. Acute pancreatitis implies return of normal pancreatic function, while chronic disease represents residual damage to the gland. The acute form can be further classified as either mild (interstitial or edematous) or severe (necrotizing or hemorrhagic) pancreatitis. Edematous pancreatitis represents roughly 75–90% of cases and is typically self-limiting in its course (Reynaert et al., 1990; Steinberg & Tenner, 1994). Morphologically, pancreatic interstitial edema and fat necrosis are present, but pancreatic necrosis is absent. In severe cases, the parenchyma of the gland undergoes necrosis and can lead to parenchymal and extrapancreatic hemorrhage.

Multiple diverse etiologies appear to trigger a sequence of events that ultimately leads to parenchymal inflammation and premature activation of pancreatic enzymes. Zymogen activation results in local damage by direct action on the acinar cells and pancreatic blood vessels. Systemic effects occur when complement and kallikrein activation induce disseminated intravascular coagulation and cardiovascular compromise. Degradation of surfactant by activated phospholipase A2 has been implicated as a possible mechanism of pulmonary injury in acute pancreatitis (Buchler, 1989).

Clinical manifestations

Symptoms of acute pancreatitis may develop abruptly or intensify over several hours. Present in nearly 100% of patients, epigastric or umbilical pain is constant and noncolicky in nature and often radiates to the back (Swisher et al., 1994). The pain is variable in severity, often peaking in a matter of hours but frequently continuing for many days. In some patients, the pain is worse in the supine position and relieved partially by sitting and leaning forward. Nausea and vomiting affect 80% of patients, but vomiting does not usually relieve the pain (Swisher et al., 1994; Gorelick, 1995).

Physical examination generally reveals anxious and restless behavior as the patient strives to attain a comfortable position. Fever is present in as many as 60% of patients. Tachycardia and hypotension may result from hemorrhage, vasodilation, increased vascular permeability, or sequestration of fluids in the retroperitoneum or peritoneal cavity (ascites). Pulmonary findings are present in a minority of patients, ranging from decreased breath sounds secondary to effusions (more often left-sided) to severe respiratory distress. Evaluation of the abdomen reveals areas of tenderness, both epigastric and generalized. Voluntary and involuntary guarding is frequently present. Pancreatic pseudocysts may be palpable. The abdomen is commonly distended, and bowel sounds are diminished or absent. Bluish discoloration around the umbilicus (Cullen's sign) or at the flanks (Grey Turner's sign) occurs in less than 1% of patients but represents the ominous development of hemorrhagic pancreatitis with retroperitoneal dissection.

Complications

Severe cases of pancreatitis can lead to both local and systemic complications (Table 26.2). Locally, pancreatic necrosis and infection may occur early in the course of disease, often within the first 2 weeks. Necrosis of greater than 50% of the pancreas is associated with high rates of infection. Increased abdominal tenderness, fever, and leukocytosis signal the onset of infection. Late complications include pseudocyst and abscess formation. Pseudocysts are collections of pancreatic secretions that lack epithelial linings and develop in 1–8% of cases of acute pancreatitis (Steinberg et al., 1994; Gorelick, 1995). They usually occur 2–3 weeks after the onset of illness. Patients frequently complain of upper abdominal pain and may develop symptoms related to growth and pressure on adjacent structures. Abscesses differ from pseudocysts by the presence of a capsule surrounding a purulent fluid collection. Abscesses complicate 1–4% of cases and are most often diagnosed 3–4 weeks after the onset of pancreatitis (Steinberg et al., 1994).

Systemic complications arising in severe cases of pancreatitis are often manifest within the first week of illness and are potentially life-threatening. Multisystem organ failure may involve the pulmonary, cardiovascular, and renal systems, contributing to a mortality rate of nearly 9% (Steinberg et al., 1994; Gullo et al., 2002). Pulmonary involvement ranges from pleural effusions and pneumonia to acute respiratory distress syndrome (ARDS). The frequency of ARDS as a cause of death has previously been underestimated. In a review of 405 autopsy cases, 60% of deaths occurred in the first week of illness; among these patients, pulmonary failure was the most common cause of death (Renner et al., 1985). The exact mechanism of pulmonary injury has not been elucidated. As mentioned earlier, however, patients with pancreatitis-associated pulmonary complications have been noted to have higher phospholipase A and phospholipase A2 catalytic activity (Buchler et al., 1989).

Various other organ systems are at risk in severe pancreatitis. Cardiovascular compromise may occur secondary to several mechanisms. Hemorrhage (intra- or retroperitoneal), fluid sequestration, and activation of vasoactive substances can lead to profound, refractory hypotension. Renal failure may develop following hypotensive episodes and acute tubular necrosis. Overwhelming sepsis is the most common cause of death after the first week of illness (Buchler et al., 1989).

Uncommon complications also may occur during severe cases of pancreatitis. Stress ulcers leading to gastrointestinal hemorrhage, pancreatic pseudoaneurysms, or colonic obstruction or fistulas may develop. Sudden blindness rarely has been reported (Purtscher's angiopathic retinopathy), with funduscopy revealing cotton-wool spots and flame-shaped hemorrhages found solely at the optic disk and macula.

Table 26.2 Complications of acute pancreatitis in pregnancy

Hypovolemic shock (third-space sequestration)
Disseminated intravascular coagulation
Acute respiratory distress syndrome
Acute tubular necrosis
Hypocalcemia, hyperglycemia
Pseudocyst formation
Pancreatic abscess
Upper gastrointestinal hemorrhage
Premature labor and delivery

Diagnosis

Laboratory evaluation

While serum amylase has been the cornerstone of diagnosis for many decades, a variety of biochemical indicators have been identified as markers of pancreatitis. Amylase isoenzymes, serum lipase, and more recently, trypsinogen-2 may increase the diagnostic accuracy of more standard serum assays. Several factors influence the accuracy of these tests. For example, amylase levels may be falsely elevated by nonpancreatic production, impaired renal clearance, or acidemia, as in diabetic ketoacidosis. Furthermore, concurrent conditions, such as hypertriglyceridemia, can falsely lower measured values.

Serum amylase is a rapidly performed, readily available serum marker of pancreatic enzyme levels. Many organs contribute to total amylase values. The pancreas contributes roughly 40%, while salivary glands contribute 60%, as measured by the P-isoenzyme and S-isoenzyme levels, respectively. Other tissues, such as the lung and fallopian tubes, also produce S-isoamylase. Isoenzyme measurement can improve the sensitivity of amylase testing. However, it is not as widely available. Amylase rises in the first few hours of disease onset and falls rapidly, returning to normal in 24–72 hours. It is, therefore, not an accurate test for patients presenting more than several days after the onset of symptoms. Overall, serum amylase has a sensitivity of 95–100% and a specificity of 70% (Agarwal et al., 1990).

In contrast, serum lipase rises in a fashion parallel to amylase but remains elevated for a longer period (as many as 7–14 days). Serum lipase, therefore, has greater sensitivity in the subset of patients with late presentation. It is also unaffected by diabetic ketoacidosis. Lipase is produced mainly by the pancreas but is produced by other gastrointestinal sources as well, namely, liver, intestine, biliary tract, and salivary glands. The effect of nonpancreatic production on serum lipase levels, however, is unclear. It is generally regarded that lipase is more specific (99%) and as sensitive (99–100%) as serum amylase and merits wider use in the evaluation of pancreatitis (Agarwal et al., 1990).

The effect of pregnancy on amylase and lipase levels has been investigated. Strickland et al. (1984) studied 413 asymptomatic women of varying gestational ages. In contrast to earlier studies reporting higher levels in pregnancy that vary through gestation, they concluded that mean amylase activities did not significantly differ among gestational age groups, nor compared with women 6 weeks' postpartum (Kaiser et al., 1975; Strickland et al., 1984). Amylase levels measured as high as 150 IU/L. Ordorica et al. (1991) and Karsenti et al. (2001) corroborated these findings, noting no difference in amylase activity related to pregnancy. Lipase levels were also studied, and no significant difference was found between the second and third trimesters or compared with nonpregnant controls, although one study noted a lower lipase level in the first trimester (Karsenti et al., 2001). Mean values of lipase in 175 women were approximately 12 IU/L, with none exceeding 30 IU/L.

As a screening tool for acute pancreatitis, urinary trypsinogen-2 has also been evaluated in the general population. Using a dipstick test for urinary trypsinogen-2, Kemppainen et al. (1997) evaluated 500 consecutive patients presenting to the emergency room with abdominal pain. The authors found a 94% sensitivity and 95% specificity in detecting acute pancreatitis. While requiring further study, the 99% negative predictive value achieved with this urinary dipstick test may prove a useful adjunctive test to standard serum evaluation of amylase and lipase.

Radiologic evaluation

Radiologic tests aid in the diagnosis of acute pancreatitis and can be used to monitor the development and progression of complications. A plain film of the abdomen may show dilation of an isolated loop of intestine (sentinel loop) adjacent to the pancreas. Pleural effusions may be detected on chest X-ray. While overlying bowel gas patterns may obscure imaging, ultrasound is very useful in evaluating the biliary tree and for ruling out other differential diagnoses. Free peritoneal fluid, abscess or pseudocyst formation, and morphologic changes of the pancreas can be visualized ultrasonographically. Computed tomography (CT) is superior in evaluating the severity of pancreatitis. Unhindered by bowel gas patterns, CT scans can demonstrate pancreatic necrosis and pseudocysts and provide guidance for directed sampling of abscess cavities (Figs 26.1, 26.2).

Differential diagnosis

Abdominal complaints in pregnancy present unique diagnostic challenges (Table 26.3). Nonobstetric conditions include cholecystitis, duodenal ulcer, appendicitis, splenic rupture, perinephric abscess, mesenteric vascular occlusion, pneumonia, and diabetic ketoacidosis. In the pregnant patient, preeclampsia, hyperemesis gravidarum, and ruptured ectopic pregnancy must be added to the differential diagnosis.

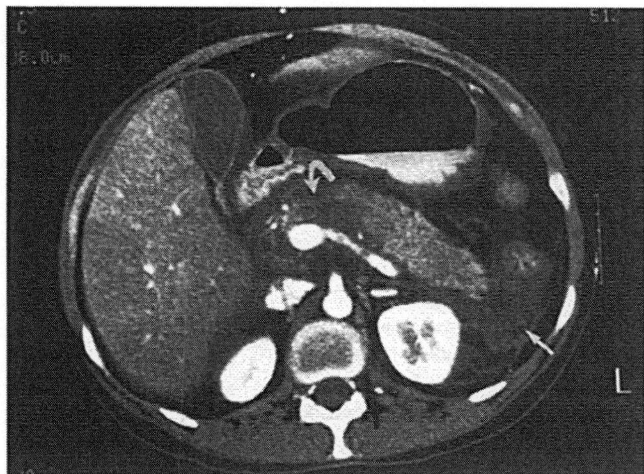

Fig. 26.1 Computed tomography scan demonstrating necrosis in the head of the pancreas (curved arrow) and free fluid in the anterior pararenal space (straight arrow). (Courtesy of Dr Paula Woodward.)

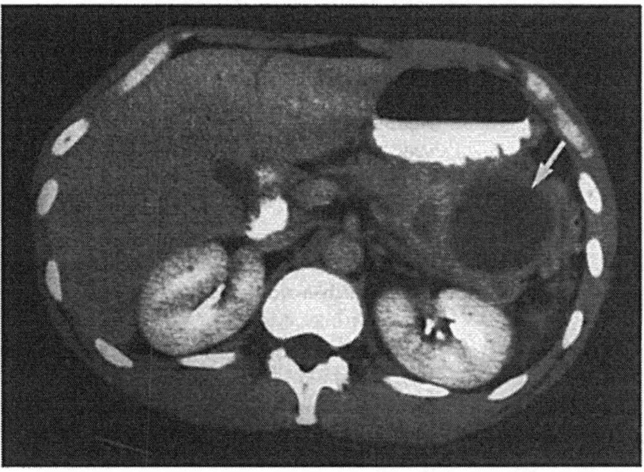

Fig. 26.2 Computed tomography scan demonstrating pseudocyst in the tail of the pancreas (arrow). (Courtesy of Dr Paula Woodward.)

Preeclampsia may mimic pancreatitis with upper abdominal pain, nausea, and vomiting. Concomitant hypertension, proteinuria, and edema, however, will usually be present. Hyperemesis gravidarum most often affects patients in the first trimester, without a significant component of pain. Ruptured ectopic pregnancy may produce symptoms similar to those seen in acute pancreatitis. Hemoperitoneum can occur with either and will often require laparotomy for diagnosis.

Prognostic indicators

Several methods utilizing clinical and laboratory data have been developed to indicate the severity of acute pancreatitis

Table 26.3 Differential diagnosis of acute pancreatitis

Nonobstetric conditions
Acute cholecystitis
Appendicitis
Duodenal ulcer
Splenic rupture
Mesenteric vascular occlusion
Perinephric abscess
Pneumonia
Pulmonary embolus
Myocardial infarction
Diabetic ketoacidosis
Obstetric conditions
Preeclampsia
Ruptured ectopic pregnancy
Hyperemesis gravidarum

Table 26.4 Clinical indicators of poor prognosis: Ranson's criteria

Nongallstone pancreatitis
On admission
Age >55 yr
WBC >16,000/mm^3
Glucose >200 mg/dL
LDH >350 IU/L
AST >250 IU/L
Within 48 hr
Decrease in hematocrit >10%
Increase in BUN >5 mg/dL
Calcium <8 mg/dL
Pa_{O_2} <60 mmHg
Base deficit >4 mmol/L
Fluid deficit >6 L
Gallstone pancreatitis
On admission
Age >70 yr
WBC >18,000/mm^3
Glucose >220 mg/dL
LDH >400 IU/L
AST >250 IU/L
Within 48 hr
Decrease in hematocrit >10%
Increase in BUN >2 mg/dL
Calcium <8 mg/dL
Base deficit >5 mmol/L
Fluid deficit >4 L

AST, aspartate amino transferase; LDH, lactic dehydrogenase.

and allow refinement of prognosis (Ranson et al., 1974; Imrie et al., 1978; Ranson, 1979). The most widely used criteria were developed by Ranson for gallstone pancreatitis (Table 26.4). The number of criteria met correlates with the mortality risk

Table 26.5 Acute Physiology and Chronic Health Evaluation (APACHE) III prognostic system for critically ill adults

Temperature	Serum sodium
Mean BP	Serum glucose
Heart rate	Serum creatinine
Respiratory rate	BUN
Pa_{O_2}	Bilirubin
$P_{(A-a)}O_2$	Albumin
Arterial pH	Hematocrit
Urine output	Leukocyte count

Age, comorbidities, and neurologic state also are scored. A numerical value is assigned to each category (total score 0–299) and weighted by its deviation from the normal range. (Reproduced by permission from Gorelick FS. Acute pancreatitis. In: Yamada T, Alpers DH, Power DW, et al., eds. Textbook of Gastroenterology, 2nd edn. Philadelphia: JB Lippincott, 1995:2064–2091.)

for the individual. For nongallstone pancreatitis, patients with fewer than three signs have rates of mortality less than 3% and morbidity less than 5%. Patients with three or more positive signs carry a 62% mortality rate and a 90% morbidity rate. Utilizing a modified set of criteria for gallstone pancreatitis, individuals with fewer than three signs have a 1.5% mortality rate, while those with three or more signs demonstrate a 29% mortality rate. Critics of this system cite poor specificity, delayed assessment (due to the labs required at 48 hours), and inability to perform repeated assessments as major deterrents to its usefulness.

Another method of clinically evaluating the severity of several types of critical illnesses, including pancreatitis, is the Acute Physiology and Chronic Health Evaluation (APACHE) III criteria (Table 26.5) (Knaus et al., 1991). Unlike Ranson's criteria, the APACHE assessment can be updated and the patient's course monitored on a continuing basis. This system evaluates several variables, both biochemical and physiologic, and calculates scores based on deviation from normal values. A 5-point increase in score is independently associated with a statistically significant increase in the relative risk of hospital death within a specific disease category. Within 24 hours of admission, 95% of patients admitted to the intensive care unit could be given a risk estimate for death within 3% of that actually observed (Knaus et al., 1991). Although more complex and computer-dependent, the APACHE scoring system appears more accurate than Ranson's criteria in predicting morbidity (Larvin & McMahon, 1989).

Several single prognostic indicators have been investigated in order to achieve early identification of pancreatic necrosis. Paracentesis can be performed; return of dark, prune-colored fluid is characteristic of necrotizing pancreatitis. Utilizing color charts, Mayer and McMahon (1985) identified 90% of the patients who subsequently died and 72% of patients with severe morbidity.

Biochemical indicators that have been evaluated as predictors of severity of disease include C-reactive protein (Buchler et al., 1986; Mantke et al., 2002; Mayer et al., 2002), trypsinogen activation peptide (Tenner et al., 1997; Neoptolemos et al., 2000; Lempinen et al., 2001), procalcitonin (Kylanpaa-Back, 2001a,b), thrombomodulin (Mantke et al., 2002), and serum amyloid A (Mayer et al., 2002). Only C-reactive protein is currently used clinically, but is limited in that it is predictive only after 48–72 hours following onset of symptoms. Serum amyloid A, thrombomodulin, trypsinogen activation peptide and procalcitonin all show promise in identifying, on admission, patients destined for a severe clinical course. All await confirmatory trials and acceptance into routine clinical use.

Compared with scoring systems and laboratory markers, contrast-enhanced CT scans offer broader information regarding intra-abdominal anatomy. Location and extent of necrosis are identified and can be serially evaluated (see Fig. 26.1). Infection within pseudocysts is suggested by evidence of gas production. This test, however, may be limited in its availability and is difficult to obtain in severely ill patients.

Management

The initial treatment of acute pancreatitis is supportive medical management. Because most cases are mild and self-limiting, this approach is largely successful. Avoidance or cessation of exacerbating factors, such as alcohol or drugs, is a basic principle to be observed. Assessment of prognostic indicators, as discussed earlier, permits appropriate surveillance. Patients with more severe disease should be transferred to an intensive care unit for continuous monitoring, because shock and pulmonary failure often present early in the course of disease and require prompt recognition and management.

Medical therapy is comprised of fluid and electrolyte management, adequate analgesia, and elimination of oral intake. Intravenous fluid resuscitation is a vital component of treatment in both mild and severe cases. Restoration of intravascular volume and avoidance of hypotension is important for cardiovascular stability and renal perfusion. Electrolyte abnormalities are common, including hypokalemia and metabolic alkalosis from severe vomiting and hypocalcemia from fat saponification. Serial assessment of electrolytes and appropriate replacement are essential. Parenteral analgesia is frequently necessary; morphine compounds, however, should be avoided secondary to their actions on the sphincter of Oddi. Oral intake is withheld for the duration of illness. Parenteral nutrition should be implemented early in the hospital course.

Nasogastric suction may be appropriate in a subset of patients with acute pancreatitis. Nasogastric suction, however, does not appear to influence duration of disease or its symptoms. Several studies have investigated the role of nasogastric suction in mild-to-moderate pancreatitis and found no difference in duration of abdominal pain, tenderness, nausea, and elevated pancreatic enzymes or time to resumption of oral feeding (Levant et al., 1974; Naeije et al., 1978; Loiudice et al., 1984). Therefore, nasogastric suction should be utilized on an elective basis for symptomatic relief for those patients with severe emesis or ileus.

Prophylactic antibiotics also have been advocated in an effort to prevent the development of infectious complications. Mild cases of pancreatitis do not appear to benefit from antibiotic prophylaxis, although studies are few (Howes et al., 1975; Finch et al., 1976). In contrast, severe cases with pancreatic necrosis have a high rate (40%) of bacterial contamination and represent a subset of patients that might benefit from antibiotic administration (Berger et al., 1986). A study of 74 patients with acute necrotizing pancreatitis treated with prophylactic imipenem demonstrated a significantly decreased incidence of pancreatic sepsis (12% vs 30%) (Pederzoli et al., 1993). Similar results were observed by Sainio and colleagues (1995). While further studies are needed to better define both patient and antibiotic selection, antibiotic prophylaxis appears to be indicated in patients at high risk for septic complications.

Antienzyme and hormonal therapies have been designed to reduce the severity of disease by halting the production of pancreatic enzymes and the subsequent cascade activation of the complement, kallikrein–kinin, fibrinolytic, and coagulation systems. Studies evaluating atropine, calcitonin, glucagon, somatostatin, and the enzyme inhibitors, aprotinin and gabexate, however, have not shown improved morbidity or mortality in severe acute pancreatitis (Reynaert et al., 1990; Steinberg & Tenner, 1994). Octreotide, a somatostatin analogue, has received considerable attention as a means to improve the course of acute pancreatitis. Five randomized trials have been performed (Beechey-Newman, 1993; Paran et al., 1995; McKay et al., 1997; Karakoyunlar et al., 1999; Uhl et al., 1999) which failed to demonstrate a clinical benefit.

Surgical therapy

Although supportive measures are the mainstay of therapy, surgical intervention also has a place in the management of acute pancreatitis. The exact role, timing, and form of surgery remain a matter of debate. The one clear indication for surgery is for diagnosis of an acute abdomen. An uncertain diagnosis mandates exploration for possible surgically correctable conditions. Two other situations also may require surgery: gallstone pancreatitis and select anatomic or infectious complications.

The goals of biliary surgery in cases of gallstone pancreatitis are to prevent recurrence and to decrease morbidity and mortality by removing the instigating agent. Cholecystectomy and bile duct exploration are not performed, however, during the acute episode. Because nearly 95% of stones pass during the first week of illness, the utility of surgery early in the illness does not weigh heavily against the high mortality rates that have been reported for early biliary surgery (Osborne et al., 1981). While not indicated in the acute phase of illness, biliary surgery should be performed after the acute pancreatitis subsides, prior to discharge from the hospital.

An alternative to open surgical removal of bile duct stones has been developed utilizing endoscopic retrograde cholangiopancreatography (ERCP). Combined with endoscopic sphincterotomy, ERCP offers both diagnostic and therapeutic advantages in the critically ill patient (Venu et al., 2002). If performed within the first 72 hours of illness, this procedure has been shown to decrease morbidity and length of hospital stay in patients with severe pancreatitis (Neoptolemos, 1988). It has been applied in a small number of pregnant patients without complications and avoids the potential risks of major surgery during pregnancy (Buchner et al., 1988; Baillie et al., 1990; Uomo et al., 1994; Nesbitt et al., 1996).

Surgery for early and late complications of pancreatitis has also been the subject of controversy. A few situations appear to be clear indications for surgical intervention, such as acute, life-threatening hemorrhage. However, the timing and type of surgical procedures for later complications, such as sterile necrosis, pseudocyst, and abscess, are less straightforward. Using the development or persistence of organ failure despite 72 hours of intensive medical therapy as indications for surgery, Gotzinger and colleagues (2002) reported on 340 patients who underwent surgical exploration for acute pancreatitis. Control of pancreatic necrosis (total removal of necrotic tissue) was accomplished in 73% of patients, requiring an average of 2.1 operations. Mortality was 100% in patients in whom surgical control of necrosis could not be accomplished versus 19% in those patients who did achieve surgical control of necrosis.

Arterial hemorrhage occurs in 2% of patients with severe pancreatitis. Necrosis and erosion into surrounding arteries of the gastrointestinal tract result in massive intra-abdominal or retroperitoneal hemorrhage. Arteriographic embolization followed by surgical debridement and artery ligation improved survival from 0% to 40% (Waltman et al., 1986). In contrast, the development of sterile pancreatic necrosis is not an automatic indication for surgery, because up to 70% of cases will resolve spontaneously. While few studies have been performed, no benefit for early debridement has been demonstrated (Bradley & Allen, 1991; Karimigani et al., 1992).

The formation of pseudocysts may mandate surgical debridement based on clinical characteristics. Occurring in as many as 10–20% of patients with severe acute pancreatitis, pseudocysts resolve in approximately 50% of cases (Reynaert et al., 1990). Surgery is performed if symptoms of hemorrhage, infection, or compression develop or if the pseudocyst exceeds 5–6 cm or persists longer than 6 weeks. Internal drainage represents the superior surgical approach, although percutaneous drainage may temporize a critically ill patient. Fluid should be collected for culture to rule out infection.

Finally, pancreatic abscess formation occurs in 2–4% of patients with severe pancreatitis and is 100% lethal if left undrained. Although percutaneous drainage may be temporizing, the catheter often becomes occluded secondary to the thick purulent effluent. With early and aggressive surgical debridement, mortality is reduced to 5% (Warshaw & Gongliang, 1985). Either transperitoneal or retroperitoneal approaches may be appropriate. Postoperatively, 20% will require reoperation for incomplete drainage, ongoing infection, fistulas, or hemorrhage (Warshaw & Gongliang, 1985).

Considerations in pregnancy

Treatment of pancreatitis does not differ in the pregnant patient. Supportive measures are identical to those of the nonpregnant patient, and severe complications are managed aggressively. Two situations, however, merit special consideration in pregnancy: the treatment of biliary disease and hypertriglyceridemia.

The management of biliary disease in pregnancy raises the issue of timing of surgery. On resolution of acute pancreatitis, cholecystectomy is typically performed in a nonpregnant patient prior to discharge from the hospital. Some advocate continued conservative management in pregnancy to avoid operative complications and fetal morbidity. A high relapse rate (72%), however, is often encountered (Swisher et al., 1994). For patients presenting in the first trimester, this may be as high as 88%. Surgical intervention decreases the incidence of relapse and the risk of systemic complications.

Several studies support the use of second-trimester cholecystectomy for cholecystitis or pancreatitis (Block & Kelly, 1989; Swisher et al., 1994; Ramin et al., 1995; Martin et al., 1996; Cosenza et al., 1999). The second trimester appears optimal in order to avoid medication effect on organogenesis and a possible increased rate of spontaneous abortion in the first trimester (vida infra). Third-trimester patients are best managed conservatively because they are close to the postpartum period when operative risks are reduced. Cholecystectomy may be performed by laparotomy or open laparoscopy. The open technique for the laparoscopic approach is often best, in order to avoid puncture of the gravid uterus with blind trocar insertion.

Fetal loss following cholecystectomy was once reported to be as high as 15% (Green et al., 1963). Many earlier reports, however, included patients undergoing surgery in the first trimester suffering spontaneous abortion many weeks postoperatively. Because at least 15% of all pregnancies are now known to end in spontaneous abortion, and preterm labor is seen in up to 10% of all continuing pregnancies, it would appear that the actual rate of complications related to surgery probably approaches nil, a figure confirmed by several recent studies (McKellar et al., 1992; Kort et al., 1993; Swisher et al., 1994). A review of studies from 1963 to 1987, evaluating fetal loss in patients undergoing cholecystectomy, revealed an 8% spontaneous abortion rate and an 8% rate of premature labor (McKellar et al., 1992). In a similar manner, laparoscopic cholecystectomy in the second trimester has been reported in a small number of patients, with no increase in fetal or maternal morbidity or mortality (Morrell et al., 1992; Elerding, 1993).

Treatment of hypertriglyceridemia in pregnancy is aimed primarily at prevention of pancreatitis. Fats should be limited to fewer than 20 g/day. This restrictive diet, however, is not palatable and is difficult for patients to maintain. Sanderson et al. (1991) reported successful management of hypertrigliceridemia during an episode of pancreatitis and the remainder of gestation by utilizing intravenous fluid therapy to provide calories in the form of 5% dextrose and restricting oral intake to clear liquids. Total parenteral nutrition offers another therapeutic approach when dietary adjustments are inadequate to prevent excessive triglyceride elevations. Plasma exchange and immunospecific apheresis also have been investigated and have suggested that long-term extracorporeal elimination of lipoproteins may offer a safe and effective method of prevention and treatment of hypertriglyceridemic pancreatitis in pregnancy (Swoboda et al., 1993).

References

Agarwal N, Pitchumoni CS, Sivaprasad AV. Evaluating tests for acute pancreatitis. Am J Gastroenterol 1990;85:356–366.

Baillie J, Cairns SR, Putnam WS, Cotton PB. Endoscopic management of choledocholithiasis during pregnancy. Surg Gynecol Obstet 1990;171:1–4.

Beechey-Newman N. Controlled trial of high-dose octreotide in treatment of acute pancreatitis. Dig Dis Sci 1993;38:644–647.

Berger HG, Bittner R, Block S, Buchler M. Bacterial contamination of pancreatic necrosis: a prospective clinical study. Gastroenterology 1986;91:433–438.

Block P, Kelly TR. Management of gallstone pancreatitis. Surg Gynecol Obstet 1989;168:426–428.

Bradley EL, Allen K. A prospective longitudinal study of observation versus surgical intervention in the management of necrotizing pancreatitis. Am J Surg 1991;16:19–25.

Braverman DZ, Johnson ML, Kern F Jr. Effects of pregnancy and contraceptive steroids on gallbladder function. N Engl J Med 1980;302:362–364.

Buchler M, Malfertheiner P, Schoetensack C, Uhl W, Beger HG. Sensitivity of antiproteases, complement factors and C-reactive protein in detecting pancreatic necrosis. Results of a prospective clinical study. Int J Pancreatol 1986;1(3–4):227–235.

Buchler M, Malfertheiner P, Schadlich H, et al. Role of phospholipase A2 in human acute pancreatitis. Gastroenterology 1989;97:1521–1526.

Buchner WF, Stoltenberg PH, Kirtley DW. Endoscopic management of severe gallstone pancreatitis during pregnancy. Am J Gastroenterol 1988;83:1073.

Corlett RC, Mishell DR. Pancreatitis in pregnancy. Am J Obstet Gynecol 1972;113:281–290.

Cosenza CA, Saffari B, Jabbour N, et al. Surgical management of biliary gallstone disease during pregnancy. Am J Surg 1990;178(6):545–548.

DeChalain TMB, Michell WL, Berger GMB. Hyperlipidemia, pregnancy and pancreatitis. Surg Gynecol Obstet 1988;167:469–473.

Eland IA, van Puijenbroek EP, Sturkenboom MJ, Wilson JH, Stricker BH. Drug-associated acute pancreatitis: twenty-one years of spontaneous reporting in The Netherlands. Am J Gastroenterol 1999;94(9):2417–2422.

Elerding SC. Laparoscopic cholecystectomy in pregnancy. Am J Surg 1993;165:625–627.

Finch WT, Sawyers JL, Schenker S. A prospective study to determine the efficacy of antibiotics in acute pancreatitis. Ann Surg 1976;183:667–671.

Gerdes M, Boyden EA. The rate of emptying of the human gallbladder in pregnancy. Surg Gynecol Obstet 1938;66:145.

Gorelick FS. Acute pancreatitis. In: Yamada T, et al., eds. Textbook of gastroenterology, 2nd edn. Philadelphia: JB Lippincott, 1995: 2064–2091.

Gotzinger P, Sautner T, Kriwanek S, et al. Surgical treatment for severe acute pancreatitis: extent and surgical control of necrosis determine outcome. World J Surg 2002;26(4):474–478.

Green J, Rogers A, Rubin L. Fetal loss after cholecystectomy during pregnancy. Canad Med Assoc J 1963;88:576–577.

Greenberger NJ, Toskes PP, Isselbacher KJ. Acute and chronic pancreatitis. In: Wilson JD, et al., eds. Harrison's principles of internal medicine, 12th edn. New York: McGraw-Hill, 1991;1372–1378.

Gullo L, Migliori M, Olah A, et al. Acute pancreatitis in five European countries: etiology and mortality. Pancreas 2002;24(3):223–227.

Herfort K, Fialova V, Srp B. Acute pancreatitis in pregnancy. Mater Med Pol 1981;13:15–17.

Howes R, Zuidema GD, Cameron JL. Evaluation of prophylactic antibiotics in acute pancreatitis. J Surg Res 1975;18:197–200.

Imrie CW, Benjamin IS, Ferguson JC. A single-centre double-blind trial of Trasylol therapy in primary acute pancreatitis. Br J Surg 1978;65:337–341.

Jouppila P, Mokka R, Larmi TK. Acute pancreatitis in pregnancy. Surg Gynecol Obstet 1974;139:879–882.

Kaiser R, Berk JE, Fridhandler L. Serum amylase changes during pregnancy. Am J Obstet Gynecol 1975;122:283–286.

Karakoyunlar O, Sivrel E, Tani N, Denecli AG. High-dose octreotide in the management of acute pancreatitis. Hepatogastroenterology 1999;46:1968–1972.

Karimigani I, Porter KA, Langevin RE, Banks P. Prognostic factors in sterile pancreatic necrosis. Gastroenterology 1992;103:1636–1640.

Karsenti D, Bacq Y, Brechot JF, Mariotte N, Vol S, Tichet J. Serum amylase and lipase activities in normal pregnancy: a prospective case-control study. Am J Gastroenterol 2001;96(3):697–699.

Kemppainen EA, Hedstrom JI, Puolakkainen PA, et al. Rapid measurement of urinary trypsinogen-2 as a screening test for acute pancreatitis. N Engl J Med 1997;336(25):1788–1793.

Kern F Jr, Everson FT, Demark B, et al. Biliary lipids, bile acids, and gallbladder function in the human female. Effects of pregnancy and the ovulatory cycle. J Clin Invest 1981;68:1229–1242.

Klein KB. Pancreatitis in pregnancy. In: Rustgi VK, Cooper JN, eds. Gastrointestinal and hepatic complications in pregnancy. New York: Wiley, 1986.

Knaus WA, Wagner DP, Draper EA, et al. The APACHE III prognostic system. Risk prediction of hospital mortality for critically ill hospitalized adults. Chest 1991;100:1619–1636.

Kort B, Katz VL, Watson WJ. The effect of nonobstetric operation during pregnancy. Surg Gynecol Obstet 1993;177:371–376.

Kylanpaa-Back ML, Takala A, Kemppainen EA, et al. Procalcitonin, soluble interleukin-2 receptor, and soluble E-selectin in predicting the severity of acute pancreatitis. Crit Care Med 2001a;29(1): 63–69.

Kylanpaa-Back ML, Takala A, Kemppainen EA, et al. Procalcitonin strip test in the early detection of severe acute pancreatitis. Br J Surg 2001b;88(2):222–227.

Langmade CF, Edmondson HA. Acute pancreatitis during pregnancy and the postpartum period: a report of nine cases. Surg Gynecol Obstet 1951;92:43–46.

Larvin M, McMahon MJ. APACHE-II score for assessment and monitoring of acute pancreatitis. Lancet 1989;2:201–205.

Legro RS, Laifer SA. First trimester pancreatitis: Maternal and neonatal outcome. J Reprod Med 1995;40:689.

Lempinen M, Kylanpaa-Back ML, Stenman UH, et al. Predicting the severity of acute pancreatitis by rapid measurement of trypsinogen-2 in urine. Clin Chem 2001;47(12):2103–2107.

Levant JA, Secrist DM, Resin HR, et al. Nasogastric suction in the treatment of alcoholic pancreatitis. JAMA 1974;229:51–52.

Loiudice TA, Lang J, Mehta H, Banta L. Treatment of acute alcoholic pancreatitis: the roles of cimetidine and nasogastric suction. Am J Gastroenterol 1984;79:553–558.

McKay C, Baxter J, Imrie C. A randomized, controlled trial of octreotide in the management of patients with acute pancreatitis. Int J Pancreatol 1997;21:13–19.

McKellar DP, Anderson CT, Boynton CJ. Cholecystectomy during pregnancy without fetal loss. Surg Gynecol Obstet 1992;174: 465–468.

Mantke R, Pross M, Kunz D, et al. Soluble thrombomodulin plasma levels are an early indication of a lethal course in human acute pancreatitis. Surgery 2002;131(4):424–432.

Martin IG, Dexter SP, McMahon MJ. Laparoscopic cholecystectomy in pregnancy. A safe option during the second trimester? Surg Endosc 1996;10(5):508–510.

Mayer DA, McMahon MJ. The diagnostic and prognostic value of peritoneal lavage in patients with acute pancreatitis. Surg Gynecol Obstet 1985;160:507–512.

Mayer JM, Raraty M, Slavin J, et al. Serum amyloid A is a better early predictor of severity than C-reactive protein in acute pancreatitis. Br J Surg 2002;89(2):163–171.

Montes A, Walden CE, Knopp RH, et al. Physiologic and supraphysiologic increases in lipoprotein lipids and apoproteins in late pregnancy and postpartum. Arteriosclerosis 1984;4:407–417.

Morrell DG, Mullins JR, Harrison PB. Laparoscopic cholecystectomy during pregnancy in symptomatic patients. Surgery 1992;112:856–859.

Naeije R, Salingret E, Clumeck N, et al. Is nasogastric suction necessary in acute pancreatitis? Br Med J 1978;2:659–660.

Neoptolemos JP, Carr-Locke DL, London NJ, et al. Controlled trial of urgent endoscopic retrograde cholangiopancreatography and endoscopic sphincterotomy versus conservative treatment for acute pancreatitis due to gallstones. Lancet 1988;2:979–983.

Neoptolemos JP, Kemppainen EA, Mayer JM, et al. Early prediction of severity in acute pancreatitis by urinary trypsinogen activation peptide: a multicentre study. Lancet 2000;355(9219): 1955–1960.

Nesbitt TH, Kay HH, McCoy MC, Herbert WN. Endoscopic management of biliary disease during pregnancy. Obstet Gynecol 1996;87(5 Pt 2):806–809.

Opie EL. The relation of cholelithiasis to disease of the pancreas and to fat necrosis. Am J Med Surg 1901;12:27–43.

Ordorica SA, Frieden FJ, Marks F, et al. Pancreatic enzyme activity in pregnancy. J Reprod Med 1991;36:359–362.

Osborne DH, Imrie CW, Carter DC. Biliary surgery in the same admission for gallstone-associated acute pancreatitis. Br J Surg 1981;68:758–761.

Paran H, Neufeld D, May A, et al. Preliminary report of a prospective randomized study of octreotide in the treatment of severe acute pancreatitis. J Am Coll Surg 1995;181:121–124.

Pederzoli P, Bassi C, Vesentini S, Campedelli A. A randomized multicenter clinical trial of antibiotic prophylaxis of septic complications in acute necrotizing pancreatitis with imipenem. Surg Gynecol Obstet 1993;176:480–483.

Potter MG. Observations of the gallbladder and bile during pregnancy at term. JAMA 1936;106:1070.

Ramin KD, Ramin SM, Richey SD, Cunningham FG. Acute pancreatitis in pregnancy. Am J Obstet Gynecol 1995;173:187–191.

Ranson JC. The timing of biliary surgery in acute pancreatitis. Ann Surg 1979;189:654–663.

Ranson JHC, Rifkind KM, Roses DF, et al. Prognostic signs and the role of operative management in acute pancreatitis. Surg Gynecol Obstet 1974;139:69–81.

Renner IG, Savage WT, Pantoja JL, Renner VJ. Death due to acute pancreatitis. Dig Dis Sci 1985;30:1005–1018.

Reynaert MS, Dugernier T, Kestens PJ. Current therapeutic strategies in severe acute pancreatitis. Intensive Care Med 1990;16:352–362.

Rominger JM, Gutierrez JG, Curtis D, Chey WY. Methyldopa-induced pancreatitis. Am J Dig Dis 1978;23(8):756–758.

Sainio V, Kemppainen E, Puolakkainen P, et al. Early antibiotic treatment in acute necrotizing pancreatitis. Lancet 1995;346:663.

Sanderson SL, Iverius P, Wilson DE. Successful hyperlipemic pregnancy. JAMA 1991;265:1858–1860.

Scarpelli DG. Toxicology of the pancreas. Toxicol Appl Pharmacol 1989;101(3):543–554.

Scott LD. Gallstone disease and pancreatitis in pregnancy. Gastroenterol Clin North Am 1992;21:803–815.

Steer ML. Acute pancreatitis. In: Ayres SM, Gronvik A, Holbrook PR, Shoemaker WC, eds. Textbook of critical care, 3rd edn. Philadelphia: WB Saunders, 1995.

Steinberg W, Tenner S. Acute pancreatitis. N Engl J Med 1994;330:1198–1210.

Stone NJ. Secondary causes of hyperlipidemia. Med Clin North Am 1994;78:117–141.

Strickland DM, Hauth JC, Widish J, et al. Amylase and isoamylase activities in serum of pregnant women. Obstet Gynecol 1984;64:389–391.

Swisher SG, Hunt KK, Schmit PJ, et al. Management of pancreatitis complicating pregnancy. Am Surg 1994;60:759–762.

Swoboda K, Derfler K, Koppensteiner R, et al. Extracorporeal lipid elimination for treatment of gestational hyperlipidemic pancreatitis. Gastroenterology 1993;104:1527–1531.

Tenner S, Fernandez-del Castillo C, Warshaw A, et al. Urinary trypsinogen activation peptide (TAP) predicts severity in patients with acute pancreatitis. Int J Pancreatol 1997;21(2):105–110.

Uhl W, Buchler MW, Malfertheiner P, et al. A randomized, double-blind, multicentre trial of octreotide in moderate to severe acute pancreatitis. Gut 1999;45:97–104.

Underwood TW, Frye CB. Drug-induced pancreatitis. Clin Pharm 1993;12(6):440–448.

Uomo G, Manes G, Picciotto FO, Rabitti PG. Endoscopic treatment of

acute biliary pancreatitis in pregnancy. J Clin Gastroenterol 1994;18:250–252.
Valdivieso V, Covarrubias C, Siegel F, Cruz F. Pregnancy and cholelithiasis: pathogenesis and natural course of gallstones diagnosed in early puerperium. Hepatology 1993;17:1–4.
Venu RP, Brown RD, Halline AG. The role of endoscopic retrograde cholangiopancreatography in acute and chronic pancreatitis. J Clin Gastroenterol 2002;34(5):560–568.
Waltman AC, Luers PR, Athanasoulis CA, Warshaw AL. Massive arterial hemorrhage in patients with pancreatitis. Arch Surg 1986;121:439–443.
Warshaw AL, Gongliang J. Improved survival in 45 patients with pancreatic abscess. Ann Surg 1985;202:408–417.
Webster J, Koch HF. Aspects of tolerability of centrally acting antihypertensive drugs. J Cardiovasc Pharmacol 1996;27(Suppl 3):S49–54.
Wilkinson EJ. Acute pancreatitis in pregnancy: a review of 98 cases and a report of 8 new cases. Obstet Gynecol Surv 1973;28:281–303.

27 Acute renal failure

Shad H. Deering
Gail L. Seiken

Renal failure is now an uncommon complication of pregnancy, occurring in less than 1% of all pregnancies in developing countries (Pertuiset et al., 1984). In fact, the incidence of acute renal failure (ARF) requiring dialysis is not significantly different in pregnant women in Western countries compared with the worldwide population. In one large analysis, the incidence of ARF in pregnancy fell from 1/3,000 to 1/18,000 between the years 1958 and 1994 (Stratta et al., 1996). In previous decades, rates of ARF as high as 20–40% were reported in pregnancy, largely attributed to the high incidence of septic abortion (Lindheimer et al., 1988; Stratta et al., 1989; Turney et al., 1989). In underdeveloped parts of the world, when ARF does present, it is often secondary to limited prenatal care and illegal abortion.

As the incidence of pregnancy-related ARF in developed countries has sharply declined and treatment has improved, so have maternal mortality rates. This improvement is related both to earlier recognition and intervention, as well as availability of dialytic support. Stratta et al. reported no deaths over the last 7 years of their experience, as compared with previously reported rates as high as 31% (Stratta et al., 1996). This is in sharp contrast, however, to another study at an inner-city hospital in Georgia from 1986 to 1996 which documented 15% maternal and 43% perinatal mortality rates, respectively (Nzerue et al., 1998). Acute renal failure does, however, remain a potentially devastating complication, with a substantial number of those affected requiring chronic therapy.

Etiologies of acute renal failure

The approach to the pregnant patient with ARF is similar to that of the nonpregnant patient, although diseases unique to pregnancy (Table 27.1) must be considered in the differential diagnosis (Thadhani et al., 1996). Disorders causing ARF in pregnancy include prerenal azotemia, intrinsic renal disease, urinary obstruction, as well as preeclampsia, HELLP syndrome (*h*emolysis, *e*levated *l*iver enzymes, *l*ow *p*latelets), acute fatty liver of pregnancy (AFLP), and postpartum renal failure, also known as postpartum hemolytic uremic syndrome (HUS). Bilateral renal cortical necrosis (BRCN) is another consideration in the evaluation of the pregnant women with ARF, which, though not unique to the pregnant state, is seen overwhelmingly in pregnancy.

In the past, a bimodal incidence of ARF was seen in pregnancy, with a peak in the first trimester corresponding to the high incidence of septic abortion, and a second peak in the third trimester corresponding to a number of other disorders seen uniquely in pregnancy. Currently, the majority of ARF is seen in the latter part of gestation. Additionally, accelerated loss of renal function, along with more difficult to control hypertension and increased proteinuria, is seen in 10% of women entering pregnancy with underlying moderate to severe renal insufficiency due to a variety of causes (Jones & Hayslett, 1996). Although less common, significant deterioration in renal function may also occur during pregnancy in women with underlying diabetic nephropathy (Gordon et al., 1996).

Renal biopsy is infrequently performed during pregnancy as the clinical presentation and timing of renal failure is usually adequate to establish a diagnosis. A renal biopsy may be indicated in pregnancy if there is a sudden deterioration of renal function without a definite cause before 32 weeks of gestation, especially if a diagnosis of preeclampsia is in doubt and a premature delivery may be avoided by the information obtained. A large retrospective study of over 1,000 percutaneous renal biopsies performed during pregnancy between 1970 and 1996 reported a complication rate of only 2.4% (Gonzalez et al., 2000). Another recent but smaller study of 18 renal biopsies performed in pregnancy and the early postpartum period reported a 38% incidence of renal hematoma, with nearly one-third of those affected requiring a blood transfusion (Kuller et al., 2001). Because of advances in neonatal intensive care and the favorable long-term prognosis for infants born after 32 weeks of gestation, renal biopsy is generally not performed after this gestational age as prolongation of pregnancy is less of a concern.

Table 27.1 Differential diagnosis of acute renal failure in pregnancy

Prerenal azotemia
Acute tubular necrosis
Acute interstitial nephritis
Acute glomerulonephritis
Obstruction
Preeclampsia
HELLP syndrome
Acute fatty liver of pregnancy
Postpartum renal failure
Pyelonephritis
Bilateral renal cortical necrosis

Table 27.2 Laboratory evaluation of acute renal failure

	Prerenal azotemia	Acute tubular necrosis
BUN : creatinine ratio	>20 : 1	10 : 1
Urine Na^+ (mEq/L)	<20	>40
Fractional excretion of Na^+ ($FENa^+$)	<1%	>2%
Urine osmolality (mosm/kg H_2O)	>500	<350
Urine sp gr	>1.020	1.010
Urine sediment	Bland	Granular casts, renal tubular epithelial cells

Prerenal azotemia

Prerenal azotemia is the result of decreased renal perfusion, either due to true intravascular volume depletion, decreased cardiac output, or altered renal perfusion. The latter can be seen with cirrhosis, the nephrotic syndrome, renal artery stenosis, or the use of nonsteroidal anti-inflammatory agents. By definition, prerenal azotemia is readily reversible with restoration of renal perfusion.

Early in pregnancy, hyperemesis gravidarum is one of the more common causes of ARF secondary to profound volume depletion resulting from poor oral intake and vomiting. Similarly, any gastrointestinal illness with vomiting or diarrhea, excessive use of cathartics or laxatives, or bulimia may result in prerenal azotemia. Generally, these disorders are readily apparent on the basis of history and laboratory findings. However, eating disorders, which occur in up to 1% of pregnancies, are often difficult to diagnose and require a high index of suspicion (Turton et al., 1999). To prevent the development of fixed renal tubular injury, prerenal azotemia, due to hemorrhage or other causes, must be treated aggressively with blood product support and fluid resuscitation.

Laboratory studies that may be of benefit in establishing the diagnosis of prerenal azotemia include urinary electrolytes and osmolality (Table 27.2). The urine sodium is typically low, as is the fractional excretion of sodium [(urine Na^+/serum Na^+)/(urine creatinine/serum creatinine) × 100%], reflecting a sodium avid state, and urine osmolality is high, indicating intact urinary concentrating ability. A low urine chloride may also provide a clue to surreptitious vomiting.

Uterine hemorrhage is an important cause of hypovolemia and subsequent prerenal azotemia late in pregnancy. Hemorrhage may be concealed in patients with placental abruption or may occur in the postpartum period secondary to lacerations, uterine atony, or retained products of conception. Hemorrhage with resultant hypotension was a major cause of pregnancy-associated ARF in 7% of patients studied at the Necker Hospital, and was a contributing factor in as many as 79% of cases in other studies (Pertuiset et al., 1984). A more recent study implicated postpartum hemorrhage in nearly 10% of ARF cases, and placental abruption in another 4% (Nzerue et al., 1998).

Patients with preeclampsia may be particularly susceptible to ARF associated with hemorrhage, due to preexisting alterations in maternal physiology, including decreased intravascular volume, heightened vascular responsiveness to catecholamines and angiotensin II, and altered prostaglandin synthesis (Grunfeld et al., 1980). In a study of 31 patients with preeclampsia and acute renal failure, Sibai and colleagues reported that 90% had experienced some form of significant hemorrhage (Sibai et al., 1990).

Intrinsic renal disease

Acute renal failure may result from a variety of intrinsic renal diseases similar to those in the nonpregnant patient. Involvement of the glomeruli may predominate in one of the many primary or secondary glomerulonephritides. The renal tubules and interstitium are the primary areas of injury in acute tubular necrosis (ATN) and acute interstitial nephritis (AIN). Both clinical presentation and examination of the urinary sediment can provide valuable clues to the diagnosis, although renal biopsy may eventually be required to distinguish among the many glomerular disease and to predict prognosis (Table 27.3).

Acute glomerulonephritis

The numerous causes of acute glomerulonephritis (GN) include primary glomerular disease such as poststreptococcal GN, membranoproliferative GN, idiopathic rapidly progressive (or crescentic) GN (RPGN), as well as secondary glomerular diseases such as lupus nephritis, systemic vasculitis, and bacterial endocarditis (Table 27.4).

The classic presentation of acute GN is that of hypertension, edema and volume overload, nephrotic range proteinuria, and an active urinary sediment with red blood cell casts (Table 27.3). In those women with preexisting renal disease, these features are often noted in the first two trimesters of gestation, although systemic lupus erythematosus (SLE) may manifest at

Table 27.3 Acute renal failure: evaluation of intrinsic renal disease

	Acute tubular necrosis	Acute interstitial nephritis	Acute glomerulonephritis
Urine sediment	Brown granular casts, renal tubular cells	Hematuria, pyuria, eosinophils, WBC casts	Hematuria, RBC casts, oval fat bodies
Proteinuria	<2 g/day	<2 g/day	>2 g/day, possible nephrotic syndrome
FENa+	>2%	>2%	<1%
Hypertension	Uncommon	Uncommon	Common
Systemic manifestations	Hypotension, sepsis, hemorrhage	Fever, skin rash, new medication	Collagen-vascular disease, infection

Table 27.4 Causes of glomerulonephritis

Primary
Minimal change disease
Focal segmental glomerulosclerosis
IgA nephropathy
Membranoproliferative GN
Membranous nephropathy
Poststreptococcal GN
Secondary
SLE
Henoch–Schönlein purpura
Cryoglobulinemia
Polyarteritis nodosa
Wegener's granulomatosis
Hypersensitivity vasculitis
Goodpasture's syndrome
Infection-related (i.e. shunt nephritis, endocarditis)

Table 27.5 Causes of acute interstitial nephritis

Drug-induced
Infection
Viral: CMV, infectious mononucleosis, hemorrhagic fever
Bacterial: streptococcal infections, diphtheria, Legionnaires' disease
Parasitic: malaria, leptospirosis, toxoplasmosis
Systemic disease
Sarcoidosis
SLE
Sjögren's syndrome
Transplant rejection
Leukemic or lymphomatous infiltration
Idiopathic

CMV, cytomegalovirus.

any time during pregnancy. Laboratory analysis including serum complement levels, antinuclear antibodies, antistreptolysin-O titers, antineutrophil cytoplasmic antibodies, and other autoantibodies may be helpful in establishing a diagnosis, although in most cases renal biopsy is eventually necessary. Preeclampsia may mimic acute glomerulonephritis in presentation, although serologic evaluation should be negative. Treatment of acute GN is largely supportive, including diuretics, antihypertensive agents, and occasionally dialysis. Depending on the underlying disease, corticosteroids or cytotoxic agents may be employed as well.

Acute interstitial nephritis

The most common cause of AIN is drug exposure; an extensive list of agents have been implicated. Among those more commonly noted are the beta-lactam antibiotics such as the semisynthetic penicillins, sulfa-based drugs, histamine H-2 blockers, and nonsteroidal anti-inflammatory agents. Acute interstitial nephritis may also occur in association with viral infections, including cytomegalovirus and infectious mononucleosis, direct bacterial invasion, parasitic infections such as malaria and leptospirosis, and systemic diseases such as SLE and sarcoidosis (Table 27.5). Unlike acute GN, interstitial nephritis typically presents with modest proteinuria (<2 g/day), pyuria, eosinophiluria, hematuria, and white blood cell casts on urinalysis. Systemic manifestations may include fever, rash, arthralgias, and other signs of a hypersensitivity reaction in those patients with drug-induced interstitial nephritis. Hypertension and edema are infrequently seen with AIN, except in those cases of severe renal failure. Withdrawal of the offending agent or treatment of the underlying infection or disease usually results in improvement of renal function. In some cases of drug-induced or idiopathic AIN, steroids have been used with varying degrees of success. When history, physical examination, and laboratory evaluation are inadequate to establish a diagnosis, renal biopsy may be necessary.

Acute tubular necrosis

Acute tubular necrosis may result from a variety of toxic exposures, including aminoglycosides, radiographic contrast, heavy metals, and several chemotherapeutic agents. Pigment-induced ATN may occur in cases of rhabdomyolysis or massive hemolysis. More commonly in pregnancy, however, ATN is ischemic in nature, as a result of a hemodynamic insult with hypotension and impaired renal perfusion. In those patients with preeclampsia who develop renal failure, ATN appears to be the underlying renal lesion. Clinically, it may be difficult to distinguish between severe prerenal azotemia and ATN, although urinary indices and urinalysis may be helpful (Table 27.2). Urinalysis typically reveals muddy brown granular casts and renal tubular epithelial cells. In light of impaired renal tubular function, laboratory evaluation reveals a high urinary sodium excretion as well as urine that is neither concentrated nor dilute. Acute tubular necrosis may be either oliguric (urine output <400 mL/day) or nonoliguric (>400 mL/day), depending on the mechanism of injury and the severity. Treatment of ATN is supportive and necessitates optimization of hemodynamics, avoidance of potential nephrotoxin exposure, nutritional support with careful monitoring of fluids and electrolytes, and, occasionally, dialysis. Renal function typically recovers in 7–14 days with appropriate treatment.

Urinary obstruction

Although urinary obstruction is a relatively uncommon cause of ARF in pregnancy, it is readily reversible and, therefore, must be considered in the differential. Obstruction may occur at any level of the urinary tract due to a wide variety of causes, the majority of which are not unique to pregnancy (Table 27.6). Additionally, gravidas with an abnormally configured or overdistended uterus, such as those with uterine leiomyomata, polyhydramnios, or multiple gestations, may be particularly susceptible. Ureteral compression by the gravid uterus, with resultant ARF and hypertension, has been reported (Satin, 1993) and large leiomyomata have even been reported to cause ureteral obstruction in the first trimester (Courban et al., 1997). Other risk factors for urinary obstruction in pregnancy include pyelonephritis, renal calculi, ureteral narrowing, and low abdominal wall compliance (Brandes & Fritsche, 1991). Renal ultrasound is the first step in the evaluation of possible urinary tract obstruction, although results may be inconclusive due to the physiologic dilation of the collecting system often seen in pregnancy due to both the effects of progesterone and the mechanical pressure of the gravid uterus. Thus, anterograde or retrograde pyelography may be necessary for definitive diagnosis. Relief of the obstruction may be accomplished by ureteral stent placement, percutaneous nephrostomy, or amniocentesis in the case of polyhydramnios. If the fetus is significantly premature, this may allow for a substantial delay in delivery as well as recovery of renal function. If the patient is near term, however, delivery may be indicated to remove both the mechanical and hormonal causes of the obstruction. It should be noted that the fetal mortality rate for reversible obstructive uropathy with associated renal failure has been reported to be as high as 33% (Khanna & Nguyen, 2001).

Table 27.6 Causes of urinary obstruction

Upper tract	Lower tract
Stones	Stones
Blood clots	Blood clots
Tumor	Tumor
Sloughed papillae	Neuropathic bladder
Ureteral stricture or ligation	Urethral stricture
Retroperitoneal fibrosis	
Extrinsic compression by tumor, gravid uterus	

Pyelonephritis

Pyelonephritis is an important cause of ARF during pregnancy. As a result of the normal physiologic changes that accompany pregnancy, the urinary collecting system is prone to dilation and urinary stasis. This results in an increased incidence in both upper and lower tract infections. The incidence of pyelonephritis in pregnancy is approximately 2% (Cunningham & Lucas, 1994). Presenting symptoms generally include fever, flank pain, nausea, vomiting, and possibly urinary frequency, dysuria, and urgency. The most common causative organism is *E. coli*, which accounts for nearly 75% of cases (Davison & Lindheimer, 1999). Prompt and appropriate antibiotic treatment is generally very effective in treating pyelonephritis during pregnancy, with improvement generally seen in the first 24–48 hours. After resolution of the initial infection, suppressive antibiotic treatment throughout pregnancy should be considered as the recurrence rate is as high as 20%.

Although pyelonephritis rarely results in a significant decline in renal function in nonpregnant patients, Gilstrap and colleagues demonstrated a substantial decrease in creatinine clearance among gravidas with pyelonephritis, with a return to normal or near-normal renal function in the majority of women re-evaluated following antibiotic therapy (Whalley et al., 1975; Gilstrap et al., 1981). It has been postulated that this decline in renal function is related to an increased vascular sensitivity to bacterial endotoxins and vasoactive mediator release in pregnancy (Pertuiset et al., 1984). It is this sensitivity to endotoxin that may account for the greater incidence of septic shock and adult respiratory distress syndrome from pyelonephritis during pregnancy.

Preeclampsia

Among those causes of ARF unique to pregnancy, preeclampsia-eclampsia accounts for the majority. One study of ARF in pregnancy performed in Uruguay, which included patients from 1976 to 1994, reported that preeclampsia was the cause of ARF in approximately 47% of cases (Ventura et al., 1997). Another retrospective study conducted at an inner-city hospital in Georgia described preeclampsia in more than one-third of 21 cases of ARF diagnosed at their institution from 1986 to 1996 (Nzerue et al., 1998).

Classically, preeclampsia is defined as the development of hypertension, proteinuria, and edema after the 20th week of gestation. Elevated liver enzymes, coagulation abnormalities, and microangiopathic hemolytic anemia may be seen in severe preeclampsia as well. The diagnosis is established clinically and rarely confirmed by renal biopsy. Pathologically, preeclampsia is characterized by swollen glomerular capillary endothelial cells or glomerular endotheliosis, with resultant capillary obstruction and glomerular ischemia (Antonovych & Mostofi, 1981). Importantly, the extent of the morphologic lesion does not necessarily correspond to the degree of renal functional impairment (Lindheimer et al., 1988). In addition, the presence of subtle volume depletion and enhanced sensitivity of the renal vasculature to vasoconstriction may contribute to superimposed ATN, which many believe to be the lesion associated with significant ARF in preeclampsia.

Treatment of severe preeclampsia and the associated renal failure ultimately depends on termination of the pregnancy with delivery of the infant. Recovery of renal function is usually seen within days to weeks with isolated preeclampsia, although 20% may have some degree of residual impairment (Suzuki et al., 1997). In contrast, when patients with chronic hypertension and underlying renal disease experience ARF in pregnancy, approximately 80% will require long-term renal replacement therapy (Sibai et al., 1990). Histologic evaluation in those patients with persistent renal impairment, proteinuria, or hypertension postpartum has revealed evidence of underlying chronic renal disease, presumably unmasked by pregnancy and/or preeclampsia (Stratta et al., 1989).

HELLP syndrome

HELLP is an acronym used to describe a constellation of findings, including *h*emolysis, *e*levated *l*iver enzymes, and *l*ow *p*latelets. Nausea, epigastric or right upper quadrant pain, and tenderness are common at presentation, as are proteinuria and renal dysfunction. Coagulation studies including fibrinogen, prothrombin time, and partial thromboplastin time may be useful in distinguishing this disorder from others associated with disseminated intravascular coagulation (DIC), in that they are often normal in patients with HELLP syndrome in the absence of placental abruption.

HELLP syndrome has been described in 4–12% of patients with severe preeclampsia (Martin et al., 1991) and is considered to represent a variant of severe preeclampsia. However, in a small study by Krane, in which patients with HELLP syndrome underwent renal biopsy, less than half had the glomerular endotheliosis classic for preeclampsia (Krane, 1988). Sibai et al. observed acute renal failure in 7.4% of 32 patients with HELLP syndrome, and approximately one-third of these patients required hemodialysis (Sibai & Ramadan, 1993). Evidence of disseminated intravascular coagulation was present in 84% of these patients, and 44% had abruptio placentae. HELLP syndrome associated with acute renal failure in this study carried a maternal mortality rate of 18% and perinatal mortality rate of 34%. The poor prognoses described by Sibai likely reflect the severity of disease seen in his patient population.

Generally, treatment of the HELLP syndrome consists of expeditious delivery once the diagnosis is established, with rapid recovery of renal function. In a group of 23 patients with HELLP syndrome who were normotensive prior to pregnancy, no residual renal impairment was observed following delivery. However, 40% of patients with chronic hypertension and subsequent HELLP syndrome eventually required chronic dialysis (Sibai & Ramadan, 1993; Nakabayashi et al., 1999).

Acute fatty liver of pregnancy

Acute fatty liver of pregnancy is another uncommon cause of ARF in pregnancy, with an incidence reported between one in 6,700 and one in 13,000 deliveries (Kaplan, 1985; Castro et al., 1999). The disease exhibits a slight predominance in nulliparas; it has been diagnosed as early as 24 weeks of gestation and as late at 7 days' postpartum (Lindheimer et al., 1988; Castro et al., 1999), but usually occurs in the last few weeks of gestation. Initial manifestations are nonspecific, including nausea, vomiting, headache, malaise, and abdominal pain. Laboratory evaluation reveals mild elevation of serum transaminase levels, hyperbilirubinemia, and leukocytosis. Renal failure develops in the majority of cases. Left untreated, patients may progress to fulminant hepatic failure with jaundice, encephalopathy, disseminated intravascular coagulopathy, gastrointestinal hemorrhage, and death. Maternal and fetal mortality rates as high as 85% were seen in the past, although with earlier diagnosis and treatment a recent analysis of 28 consecutive cases reported no maternal deaths (Castro et al., 1999).

Diagnosis of fatty liver may be established by liver biopsy revealing microvesicular fatty infiltration. Computed tomography (CT) may reveal decreased hepatic attenuation. A report by Usta and colleagues described their experience with 13 patients (14 cases) of AFLP over an 8-year period, all of whom had ARF on presentation (Usta et al., 1994). They reported 100% maternal survival, with 13% perinatal mortality. Although nine of 14 cases were initially diagnosed as preeclampsia, the diagnosis of AFLP was subsequently confirmed either by liver biopsy (10/14), CT of the liver (2/14), or clinically. One patient experienced a recurrence of AFLP in a subsequent pregnancy. Although CT revealing hepatic density below the normal range of 50–70 Hounsfield units has been reported as suggestive of AFLP, Usta's study demonstrated a high false-negative rate with only two of 10 abnormal scans, including nine biopsy-proven cases (Usta et al., 1994). Contributing to the diagnostic dilemma in these women is the frequent occurrence of hypertension, edema, and proteinuria suggestive of preeclampsia, although renal pathology has failed to reveal evidence of glomerular endotheliosis. As is the case with severe preeclampsia, expeditious delivery is warranted, with prompt improvement in both hepatic and renal failure noted in nearly all cases (Kaplan, 1985; Castro et al., 1999).

Postpartum renal failure

Idiopathic postpartum renal failure, also referred to as postpartum HUS, is a unique cause of pregnancy-associated ARF that typically develops in the puerperium following an uncomplicated pregnancy and delivery. Women may present up to several months following delivery with severe hypertension, microangiopathic hemolytic anemia, and oliguric renal failure, often with congestive heart failure and CNS manifestations. A prodromal flu-like illness or initiation of oral contraceptives may be associated with postpartum renal failure as well as with idiopathic HUS, suggesting a toxic or hormonal influence.

Pathologically, the disease is often indistinguishable from the thrombotic microangiopathies, idiopathic HUS and thrombotic thrombocytopenic purpura (TTP), with arteriolar injury, fibrin deposition, and microvascular (arteriolar and glomerular capillary) thrombosis. The major pathologic involvement is renal, as opposed to CNS involvement seen in TTP. The pathogenesis of the thrombotic microangiopathies remains unclear, although intravascular coagulation, disordered platelet aggregation, endothelial damage, and alterations in prostaglandins have been suggested (Hayslett, 1985). Therapies have been chosen in an attempt to intervene in one or more of these processes, including plasma exchange, plasma infusion, antiplatelet agents, and anticoagulation. In addition, acute and long-term dialytic support is often necessary, with approximately 12–15% of patients developing end-stage renal disease. The maternal mortality rate was estimated to between 46% and 55% in the 1980s (Weiner, 1987; Li et al., 1988) but appears to be improving with the use of plasma exchange and other treatments.

Although treatment guidelines are not well established, plasma exchange is recommended due to an apparent benefit in survival in a small number of patients. Due to the continuum of disease, both HUS and TTP have been considered together in most clinical trials. The Canadian Apheresis Study Group and a group at Johns Hopkins University examined therapeutic outcomes in TTP and HUS-TTP, respectively (Bell et al., 1991; Rock et al., 1991). Both reported the superiority of plasma exchange therapy in terms of clinical response and survival, with mortality rates of 22% and 9% respectively, in those receiving such treatment. Additional therapeutic interventions varied, including aspirin, dipyridamole, and corticosteroids. Greater than 50% of all patients had evidence of renal dysfunction, although those with severe ARF or anuria were excluded from the Canadian multicenter trial.

Nine of the 76 women seen at Johns Hopkins presented in their third trimester of pregnancy, although there was no comment as to the degree of renal impairment in this subset of patients. A recent report of three patients with postpartum HUS at the Rhode Island hospital who were treated with frequent plasma exchange and prednisone reported survival in all three patients (Shemin & Dworkin, 1998). Additionally, Hayward and colleagues described nine pregnant women presenting between the first trimester of gestation and one month postpartum with TTP-HUS (Hayward et al., 1994). Of these 21 women from three institutions, all but one survived, and none required renal replacement therapy.

Bilateral renal cortical necrosis

Acute, bilateral renal cortical necrosis is a pathologic entity consisting of partial or complete destruction of the renal cortex, with sparing of the medulla. While not unique to pregnancy, this rare and catastrophic form of ARF occurs most commonly in pregnancy, with obstetric causes accounting for 50–70% of cases (Donohoe, 1983). Although BRCN represents less than 2% of cases of ARF in the nonpregnant population, it has been reported to account for 10–38% of obstetric cases of renal failure, perhaps secondary to the hypercoagulable state and altered vascular sensitivity of pregnancy (Krane, 1988; Prakash et al., 1996). Patients typically present between 30 and 35 weeks of gestation in association with profound shock and renal hypoperfusion, such as that seen with abruptio placentae, placenta previa, and other causes of obstetric hemorrhage. Acute BRCN has also been observed early in pregnancy associated with septic abortion. Abruption placentae, with either overt or concealed hemorrhage, appears to be the most common antecedent event (Donohoe, 1983).

Patients with BRCN present with severe and prolonged oliguria or anuria (urine output <50 mL/day), flank pain, gross hematuria, and urinalysis demonstrating RBC and granular casts. Diagnosis is established by renal arteriogram demonstrating virtual absence of cortical blood flow (interlobular arteries), despite patency of the renal arteries. Diagnosis may be established by ultrasonography, contrast-enhanced CT demonstrating areas of cortical lucency, and MRI (Francois et al., 2000). The prognosis for patients with BRCN is extremely poor, again likely related to the severity of illness, with one study of 15 cases during pregnancy reporting a mortality rate of 93% (Prakash et al., 1996).

Management of acute renal failure

Management of ARF in pregnancy is similar to that in the nonpregnant patient, including supportive therapy as well as dialysis. Close attention to fluid balance is critical because

Table 27.7 Classification of pregnancy-associated acute renal failure

Preeclampsia	HELLP syndrome	Acute fatty liver of pregnancy	Postpartum (HUS) renal failure	Pyelonephritis	Bilateral renal cortical necrosis
Proteinuria	RUQ pain	Elevated LFTs	Occurring postpartum	Positive urine culture	Hemorrhage
Hypertension	Proteinuria	Hyperbilirubinemia	MAHA	Fever	Hypotension/shock
Edema	Hemolysis	Coagulopathy	Oliguria		Oliguria/anuria
	Elevated LFTs	Oliguria	Severe HTN		Flank pain
	Thrombocytopenia	Nausea	Prodromal illness		Gross hematuria
	Normal coags	Abdominal pain	Thrombocytopenia		
		Leukocytosis	CNS involvement		

HTN, hypertension; LFTs, liver function tests; MAHA, microangiopathic hemolytic anemia; RUQ, right upper quadrant.

superimposed volume depletion or fluid overload may exacerbate ARF or necessitate earlier dialytic intervention. Correction of the metabolic acidosis seen with ARF may require bicarbonate therapy or dialysis, if it remains refractory to medical therapy or occurs in the setting of congestive heart failure. Prevention of hyperphosphatemia includes dietary phosphate restriction and nonabsorbable or calcium-containing phosphate binders given with meals. Dietary potassium restriction also is imperative to avoid potentially life-threatening hyperkalemia. A cation-exchange resin, such as kayexalate, can be used for mild hyperkalemia or until dialysis is available. For hyperkalemia with associated electrocardiographic changes, acute therapy includes intravenous calcium gluconate to stabilize the cardiac membrane, infusion of glucose and insulin or inhaled beta-agonists to transiently shift potassium intracellularly, and acute dialysis. Additional conservative measures include avoiding further nephrotoxic exposure and hypotension, control of hypertension, and medication dose adjustment according to the degree of renal impairment.

In patients with severe metabolic abnormalities that are unresponsive to conservative medical management, volume overload and pulmonary congestion that cannot be corrected with diuretics, or signs and symptoms of uremia, including pericarditis and encephalopathy, dialysis is indicated.

Summary

Evaluation of the pregnant patient with ARF encompasses a broad range of disorders, some of which are unique to pregnancy. Prerenal azotemia, intrinsic renal disease, including ATN, GN, and interstitial nephritis, and urinary obstruction should be considered based on clinical presentation. Evaluation of ARF during pregnancy is similar to that in the nonpregnant patient, including urinalysis and urinary diagnostic indices, and in some cases, renal biopsy. In addition, diseases unique to pregnancy and those more common during pregnancy must be considered, including preeclampsia, HELLP syndrome, AFLP, postpartum renal failure, and BRCN (Table 27.7). Treatment often necessitates prompt termination of pregnancy and delivery of the infant, even at early gestational ages when issues of prematurity may exist.

References

Antonovych TT, Mostofi FK. Atlas of kidney biopsies. Washington, DC: Armed Forces Institute of Pathology 1981:266–275.

Bell WR, Braine HG, Ness PM, Kickler TS. Improved survival in thrombotic thrombocytopenic purpura-hemolytic uremic syndrome. N Engl J Med 1991;325:398–403.

Brandes JC, Fritsche C. Obstructive acute renal failure by a gravid uterus: a case report and review. Am J Kidney Dis 1991;18:398–401.

Castro MA, Fassett MJ, Reynolds TB, Shaw KJ, Goodwin TM. Reversible peripartum liver failure: A new perspective on the diagnosis, treatment, and cause of acute fatty liver of pregnancy, based on 28 consecutive cases. Am J Obstet Gynecol 1999; 181(2):389–395.

Courban D, Blank S, Harris MA, Bracy J, August P. Acute renal failure in the first trimester resulting from uterine leiomyomas. Am J Obstet Gynecol 1997;177(2):472–473.

Cunningham FG, Lucas MJ. Urinary tract infections complicating pregnancy. Baillieres Clin Obstet Gynaecol 1994;8:353–373.

Davison JM, Lindheimer MD. Renal disorders. In: Creasy RK, Resnick R, eds. Maternal Fetal Medicine, 4th edn. Philadelphia: WB Saunders 1999:873–894.

Donohoe JF. Acute bilateral cortical necrosis. In: Brenner BM, Lazarus JM, eds. Acute Renal Failure, 1st edn. Philadelphia: WB Saunders 1983:252–269.

Francois M, Tostivint I, Mercadal L, Bellin M, Izzedine H, Deray G. MR imaging features of acute bilateral renal cortical necrosis. Am J Kidney Dis 2000;35(4):745–748.

Gilstrap LC, Cunningham FG, Whalley PJ. Acute pyelonephritis during pregnancy: an anterospective study. Obstet Gynecol 1981;57:409–413.

Gonzalez M, Chew W, Soltero L, Gamba G, Correa R. Percutaneous kidney biopsy, analysis of 26 years: complication rate and risk factors. Rev Invest Clin 2000;52:125–131.

Gordon M, Landon MB, Samuels P, et al. Perinatal outcome and long-term follow-up associated with modern management of diabetic nephropathy. Obstet Gynecol 1996;87:401–409.

Grunfeld JP, Ganeval D, Bournerias F. Acute renal failure in pregnancy. Kidney Int 1980;18:179–191.

Hayslett JP. Postpartum renal failure. N Engl J Med 1985;312: 1556–1559.

Hayward CPM, Sutton DMC, Carter WH, et al. Treatment outcomes in patients with adult thrombotic thrombocytopenic purpura-hemolytic uremic syndrome. Arch Intern Med 1994;154:982–987.

Jones DC, Hayslett JP. Outcome of pregnancy in women with moderate or severe renal insufficiency. N Engl J Med 1996;335:226–232.

Kaplan MM. Acute fatty liver of pregnancy. N Engl J Med 1985;313:367–370.

Khanna N, Nguyen H. Reversible acute renal failure in association with bilateral ureteral obstruction and hydronephrosis in pregnancy. Am J Obstet Gynecol 2001;184(2):239–240.

Krane NK. Acute renal failure in pregnancy. Arch Intern Med 1988;148:2347–2357.

Kuller JA, D'Andrea NM, McMahon MJ. Renal biopsy and pregnancy. Am J Obstet Gynecol 2001;184(6):1093–1096.

Li PK, Lai FM, Tam JS, Lai KN. Acute renal failure due to postpartum hemolytic uremic syndrome. Aust N Z J Obstet Gynaecol 1988;28(3):228–230.

Lindheimer MD, Katz AI, Ganeval D, et al. Acute renal failure in pregnancy. In: Brenner BN, Lazarus JM, eds. Acute Renal Failure. New York: Churchill Livingstone, 1988:597–620.

Martin JN, Blake PG, Perry KG, et al. The natural history of HELLP syndrome: patterns of disease progression and regression. Am J Obstet Gynecol 1991;164:1500–1513.

Nakabayashi M, Adachi T, Itoh S, Kobayashi M, Mishina J, Nishida H. Perinatal and infant outcome of pregnant patients undergoing chronic hemodialysis. Nephron 1999;82:27–31.

Nzerue CM, Hewan-Lowe K, Nwawka C. Acute renal failure in pregnancy: A review of clinical outcomes at an inner-city hospital from 1986–1996. J Natl Med Assoc 1998;90:486–490.

Pertuiset N, Ganeval D, Grunfeld JP. Acute renal failure in pregnancy: an update. Semin Nephrol 1984;3:232–239.

Prakash J, Tripathi K, Pandey LK, Gadela SR. Renal cortical necrosis in pregnancy-related acute renal failure. J Indian Med Assoc 1996;94(6):227–229.

Rock GH, Shumak KH, Buskard NA, et al. Comparison of plasma exchange with plasma infusion in the treatment of thrombotic thrombocytopenic purpura. N Engl J Med 1991;325:393–397.

Satin AJ, Seiken GL, Cunningham FG. Reversible hypertension in pregnancy caused by obstructive obstetric uropathy. Obstet Gynecol 1993;81:823–825.

Shemin D, Dworkin LD. Clinical outcome in three patients with postpartum hemolytic uremic syndrome treated with frequent plasma exchange. Ther Apher 1998;2(1):43–48.

Sibai BM, Ramadan MK. Acute renal failure in pregnancies complicated by hemolysis, elevated liver enzymes, and low platelets. Am J Obstet Gynecol 1993;168:1682–1690.

Sibai BM, Villar MA, Mabie BC. Acute renal failure in hypertensive disorders of pregnancy. Pregnancy outcome and remote prognosis in thirty-one consecutive cases. Am J Obstet Gynecol 1990;162(3): 777–783.

Stratta P, Canavese C, Dogliani M, et al. Pregnancy-related renal failure. Clin Nephrol 1989;32:14–20.

Stratta P, Besso L, Canavese C, et al. Is pregnancy-related acute renal failure a disappearing clinical entity? Ren Fail 1996;18(4):575–584.

Suzuki S, Gejyo F, Ogino S. Post-partum renal lesions in women with pre-eclampsia. Nephrol Dial Transplant 1997;12:2488–2493.

Thadhani R, Pascual M, Bonventre JV. Acute renal failure. N Engl J Med 1996;334:1448–1460.

Turney JH, Ellis CM, Parsons FM. Obstetric acute renal failure 1956–1987. Br J Obstet Gynaecol 1989;96:679–687.

Turton P, Hughes P, Bolton H, Sedgwick P. Incidence and demographic correlates of eating disorder symptoms in a pregnant population. Int J Eat Disord 1999;26:448–452.

Usta IM, Barton JR, Amon EA, et al. Acute fatty liver of pregnancy: an experience in the diagnosis and management of fourteen cases. Am J Obstet Gynecol 1994;171(5):1342–1347.

Ventura JE, Villa M, Mizraji R, Ferreiros R. Acute renal failure in pregnancy. Ren Fail 1997;19(2):217–220.

Weiner CP. Thrombotic microangiopathy in pregnancy and the postpartum period. Semin Hematol 1987;24:119–129.

Whalley PJ, Cunningham FG, Martin FG. Transient renal dysfunction associated with acute pyelonephritis of pregnancy. Obstet Gynecol 1975;46:174–177.

28 Acute fatty liver of pregnancy

T. Flint Porter

Acute fatty liver of pregnancy (AFLP) is a rare, yet potentially fatal complication of late pregnancy. Also known as acute fatty metamorphoisis or acute yellow atrophy, the incidence ranges between 1 in 7,000 and 1 in 15,000 depending on the population studied (Reyes et al., 1994; Castro et al., 1999). Older published series reported maternal and perinatal mortality rates as high as 75 and 85%, respectively (Kaplan, 1985). However, since the early 1980s, experience suggests that both morbidity and mortality can be reduced by early recognition and prompt treatment (Usta et al., 1994; Castro et al., 1999).

Pathophysiology

The yellow appearance of the liver and fulminant hepatic failure which are characteristic of AFLP are the result of progressive accumulation of hepatocellular lipid. The cause remains a mystery, but similar diffuse microvesicular fatty infiltration of the liver occurs in other conditions as well. Both tetracycline and valproic acid toxicity result in fatty infiltration (Peters et al., 1967); however, their infrequent use during pregnancy makes them unlikely causative agents in most cases of AFLP. The hepatocellular changes of Reye's syndrome also resemble those of AFLP and both have similar abnormalities in mitrochondrial enzymatic function and structure (Weber et al., 1979). However, the histologic appearance of the liver is noticeably different in children with Reye's syndrome.

Inherited defects in intramitochondrial β-oxidation of fatty acids have been reported in pregnancies affected by AFLP by several investigators (Treem et al., 1994; Sims et al., 1995; Ibdah, et al., 1999; Matern et al., 2001). In one case series of 12 affected pregnancies, several of the offspring delivered of mothers with AFLP were subsequently diagnosed with a homozygous form of long-chain hydroxyacyl coenzyme A dehydrogenase deficiency while some mothers and even fathers were found to be heterozygous carriers (Treem et al., 1994). In another study of 24 infants with confirmed fatty acid oxidation defects, Ibdah and colleagues (1999) reported that 80% of mothers were afflicted with AFLP or HELLP during pregnancy. In the same study, three of ten multiparous mothers had AFLP in a previous pregnancy. Other investigators have reported similar findings (Schoeman et al., 1991).

Preeclampsia syndromes such as HELLP and AFLP may represent two points along a spectrum of disease. In addition to their shared relationship to fatty acid oxidation defects, both exhibit similar histologic hepatic changes (Minakami et al., 1988). At least 40% of women with AFLP also exhibit clinical findings consistent with preeclampsia (Minakami et al., 1988; Barton et al., 1990; Castro et al., 1999) and like preeclampsia, AFLP typically resolves 2–3 days after delivery.

Clinical presentation

Acute fatty liver of pregnancy most often presents during the third trimester of pregnancy (Pockros et al., 1984; Usta et al., 1994; Castro et al., 1999), though mid-trimester cases have also been reported (Monga & Katz, 1999). AFLP never has its onset postpartum but may be diagnosed after delivery (Bacq, 1998). Women with AFLP are more likely to be in their first pregnancy (Bacq, 1998), carrying male fetuses (Burroughs et al., 1982), and have multiple gestation (Bacq, 1998; Davidson et al., 1998). The most common presenting symptoms are nausea, vomiting, anorexia, abdominal pain, and jaundice (Reyes et al., 1994; Usta et al., 1994; Bacq, 1998; Castro et al., 1999) (Table 28.1). These may be acute or go on for several days. Fever, headache, and pruritis are not uncommon (Reyes et al., 1994; Castro et al., 1999). For some women, the presentation may also include obstetric complaints such as contractions, decreased fetal movement, and vaginal bleeding (Castro et al., 1999).

At least 50% of women are jaundiced and ill-appearing at the time of presentation (Usta et al., 1994; Castro et al., 1999). Liver size is usually normal or small. Around 50% of affected patients have symptoms of preeclampsia including hypertension, proteinuria, and edema (Bacq, 1998) and tachycardia is common, especially during the acute phase of illness.

The systemic effects of hepatic failure are many and may contribute most to the morbidity and mortality associated

Table 28.1 Signs and symptoms of acute fatty liver of pregnancy

Symptoms	
Nausea, vomiting	Almost always
Malaise	Always
Abdominal pain	Almost always, may be variable in position, severity
Physical signs	
Hypertension	Almost always
Edema	Almost always
Proteinuria	Variable
Jaundice	Always
Elevated liver transaminases	Always
Hypoglycemia	Always, may be masked by administration of intravenous fluids
Coagulopathy	Common
Diabetes insipidus	Common
Encephalopathy	Common, may correlate with ammonia levels

with AFLP. The neurological consequences may be seen early in the disease process and include restlessness, confusion, disorientation, asterixis, seizures, psychosis, and ultimately coma (Reyes et al., 1994; Usta et al., 1994; Castro et al., 1999). Some form of renal insufficiency occurs in all women with AFLP (Castro et al., 1999). Initially, kidney damage is due to fatty infiltration. The hepatorenal syndrome eventually leads to oliguria and acute tubular necrosis (Castro et al., 1999). Damage to the proximal renal tubules also results in decreased sensitivity to endogenous vasopressin leading to the development of transient diabetes insipidus (Tucker et al., 1993; Kennedy et al., 1994).

Virtually all women with AFLP have laboratory evidence of DIC and at least 50% have bleeding complications requiring replacement of blood components (Usta et al., 1994; Castro et al., 1996, 1999). Specific coagulation abnormalities include profound antithrombin III deficiency, hypofibrinogenemia, and prolonged prothrombin time (PT) and activated partial thromboplastin time (aPTT). Coagulopathy may worsen in the postpartum period, probably secondary to low antithrombin III levels (Liebman, 1983).

Likewise, all women with AFLP have at least mild hypoglycemia though routine administration of dextrose solutions at the time of admission may mask all but the most severe cases. Other systemic effects include respiratory failure, sometimes requiring assisted ventilation (Usta et al., 1994), ascites (Bacq, 1998), and gastrointestinal bleeding from gastric ulceration and Mallory Weiss syndrome (Bacq, 1998).

Laboratory abnormalities

Serum transaminase concentrations are typically mildly increased, usually between 100 and 1,000 U/L. Bilirubin levels are variable but generally exceed 5 mg/dL. Alkaline phosphatase is elevated but is not helpful in making the diagnosis because of placental production. Serum albumin is usually low. Ammonia levels are elevated, due to decreased utilization by urea cycle liver enzymes, and may predict the degree of altered sensorium. Elevated amylase and lipase should raise suspicions of concomitant pancreatitis (Lauersen et al., 1983). Liver function tests usually return to normal 4–8 weeks after delivery (Kaplan, 1985).

Impaired hepatic synthesis of coagulation factors leads to prolongation of prothrombin time (PT) and hypofibrinogenemia. Thrombocytopenia is common. Factor VIII levels most accurately reflect the extent of coagulopathy and while not predictive of ultimate clinical outcome, their return toward normal signals recovery.

Laboratory evidence of renal dysfunction is evident early in the disease with increased serum creatinine levels. Serum concentration of uric acid and blood urea nitrogen are also elevated, and with the onset of jaundice, urobilinogen appears in the urine. Serum electrolytes may reflect metabolic acidosis and plasma glucose is often below 60 mg/dL suggesting reduced hepatic glycogenolysis (Purdie & Waters, 1988).

The gold standard used for confirmation of AFLP remains the liver biopsy. However, it is rarely necessary when other clinical and laboratory parameters are consistent with the diagnosis. Microscopic examination of fresh specimens stained with special fat stains, most commonly oil red, demonstrate hepatocellular cytoplasm distended by numerous fine vacuoles giving the cells a distinct foamy appearance (Fig. 28.1). The myriad of tiny vacuoles are separated from each other by thin eosinophilic cytoplasmic strands and do not coalesce to form a single large vacuole. In contrast to the cytoplasm, the cell nucleus is located centrally and is normal in size and appearance.

Histologic changes are most prominent in the central portion of the lobule with a thin rim of normal hepatocytes at the periphery. The lobular architecture is usually preserved and, with rare exceptions, necrosis and inflammation are absent (Duma et al., 1965). This is distinct from the periportal fibrin deposition and hemorrhagic necrosis reported in preeclampsia (Fig. 28.2). Characteristic histologic changes may be present up to 3 weeks after the onset of jaundice.

Imaging studies

Ultrasonography, computerized tomography (CT), and magnetic resonance imaging (MRI) are often performed as part of the diagnostic work-up for jaundice during pregnancy. Ultrasound demonstrates echogenicities within the liver of women with AFLP (Bacq, 1998). While very nonspecific, ultrasound may also identify subcapsular hematoma, cholecystitis, and/or cholangitis. Both CT and MRI may suggest AFLP

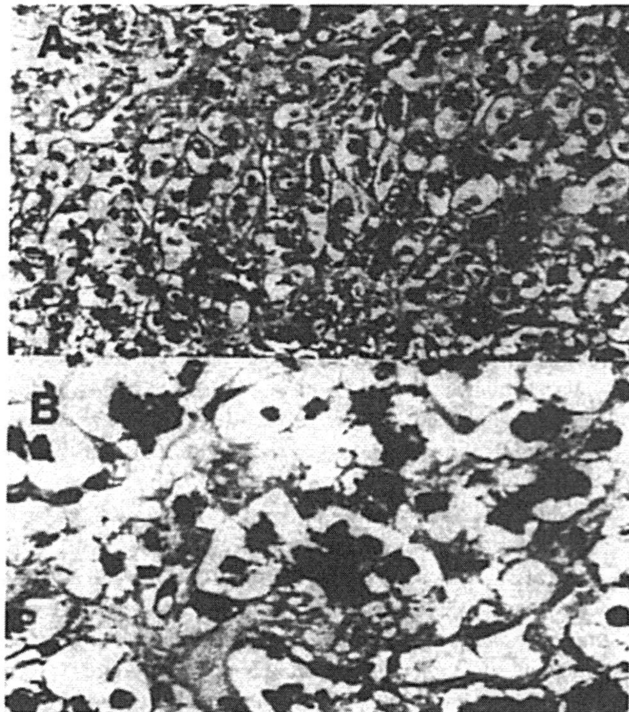

Fig. 28.1 (A) Acute fatty liver of pregnancy (H&E stain). Note diffuse fatty infiltration and absence of necrosis and inflammation. (Magnification, 200×.) (B) Higher magnification demonstrates the fine cytoplasmic vacuoles and centrally placed nuclei (H&E stain). (Magnification, 1,000×.) (Courtesy of Dr Patricia Latham, University of Maryland Hospital.)

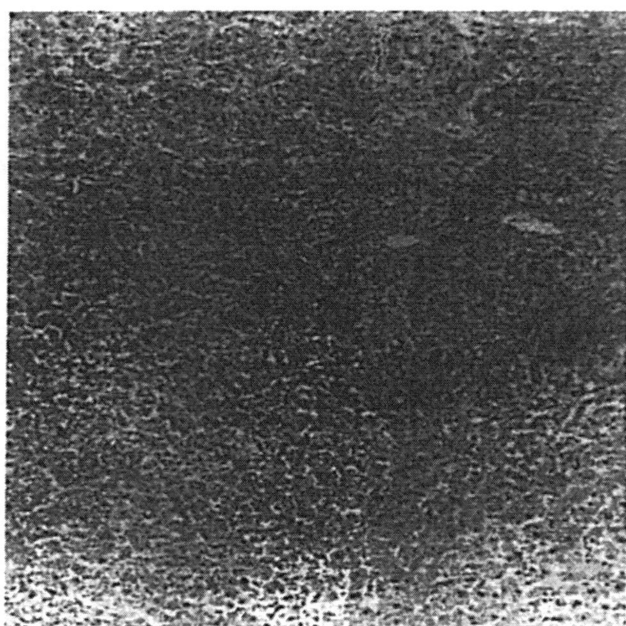

Fig. 28.2 Liver section from a patient who died of complications of preeclampsia (H&E stain). Note extensive hepatocellular inflammation and necrosis. (Magnification 40×.) (Courtesy of Dr James Kelley, Madigan AMC.)

based on lower density that occurs with fatty infiltration of the liver (Clements et al., 1990; Farine et al., 1990). However, both have high false negative rates that limit their usefulness (Castro et al., 1999). In clinical practice, complementary imaging studies are not necessary to make the diagnosis of AFLP and their performance should not delay appropriate treatment. On the other hand, they may be useful in detecting other liver and biliary tract abnormalities.

Diagnosis

The correct interpretations of laboratory tests correlated with clinical manifestations are usually sufficient to make the diagnosis of AFLP (Bacq, 1998; Castro et al., 1999). Liver biopsy, while confirmatory, is usually not necessary and may be relatively contraindicated because of coagulopathy. Most common among the differential diagnoses are preeclampsia, viral hepatitis, and cholestasis (Table 28.2). Women with either AFLP or preeclampsia may have elevated serum transaminases, thrombocytopenia or coagulation defects. However, clinically apparent liver failure and jaundice rarely occur in preeclampsia. Notwithstanding, both AFLP and preeclampsia may occur concomitantly (Castro et al., 1999). The diagnosis of viral hepatitis can be established quickly and with reasonable certainty via specific serologic testing. In addition, serum transaminase levels in women with AFLP are usually elevated well beyond those normally seen in AFLP. Women with cholestasis of pregnancy are usually not nearly so ill-appearing as those with either AFLP, preeclampsia, or viral hepatitis. While liver function tests are abnormal in cholestasis of pregnancy, concentrations of bilirubin and transaminases are usually much lower compared to those of AFLP or viral hepatitis. In addition, the signs and symptoms of preeclampsia are rarely present.

Treatment

Women suspected of having AFLP should be hospitalized in an intensive care setting where comprehensive support can be given and preparations for delivery can be made. All series have reported improved maternal and perinatal outcome when prompt delivery is accomplished (Kaplan, 1985; Reyes et al., 1994; Usta et al., 1994; Bacq, 1998; Castro et al., 1999). Patients begin to show clinical improvement and resolution of laboratory abnormalities by the second postpartum day (Usta et al., 1994). There are no reported cases in which patients have recovered prior to delivery, making expectant management absolutely contraindicated.

While delivery should be accomplished as expeditiously as

Table 28.2 Differential diagnosis of acute fatty liver of pregnancy

	Acute fatty liver of pregnancy	Acute hepatitis	Cholestasis of pregnancy	Severe preeclampsia
Trimester	Third	Variable	Third	Third
Clinical manifestations	Nausea, vomiting, malaise, encephalopathy, abdominal pain, coagulopathy	Malaise, nausea, vomiting, jaundice, anorexia, encephalopathy	Pruritus, jaundice	Hypertension, edema, proteinuria, oliguria, CNS hyperexcitability
Bilirubin	Elevated	Elevated	Elevated	Normal or elevated
Transaminases	Minimally elevated	Markedly elevated	Minimally elevated	Normal or minimal to moderate increase
Alkaline phosphatase	Usually normal for pregnancy	Minimally elevated	Moderately elevated	Normal for pregnancy
Histology	Fatty infiltration, no inflammation or necrosis	Marked inflammation and necrosis	Biliary stasis, no inflammation	Inflammation, necrosis, fibrin deposition
Recurrence	Reported	No	Yes	Yes

possible, immediate cesarean has no clear advantage over induction and vaginal delivery as long as adequate maternal supportive care and fetal surveillance are possible. Most hemorrhagic complications in women with AFLP occur as a result of surgical trauma (Castro et al., 1999). On the other hand, protracted inductions in critical circumstances are potentially dangerous to the mother and the fetus. In the end, fetal compromise during labor is common and abdominal delivery is often necessary (Castro et al., 1999). The decision should be individualized based on maternal and fetal condition as well as the favorability of the cervical exam.

Anesthetic options in patients with AFLP are limited. General anesthesia can further damage an already compromised liver and regional anesthesia poses a risk of local hemorrhage when coagulopathy is present. If general anesthesia must be used, inhalation agents with potential hepatotoxicity (e.g. halothane) should be avoided. Isoflurane is a logical choice since it has little or no hepatotoxicity and may preserve liver blood flow (Goldfarb et al., 1990; Holzman et al., 2001). Epidural anesthesia is the optimal choice because it preserves liver blood flow with no hepatotoxic effects (Antognini & Andrews, 1991; Holzman et al., 2001). However, recognition and correction of thrombocytopenia and coagulopathy is essential prior to administration.

Supportive care

Supportive care of patients with AFLP should include diligent monitoring for evidence of progressive hepatic failure, hypoglycemia, and coagulopathy. Prevention of worsening hypoglycemia and reduction of endogenous production of nitrogenous wastes can be accomplished by providing approximately 2,000–2,500 calories per day, primarily in the form of glucose. Most patients require solutions containing more than 5% dextrose, sometimes as high as 25%, administered intravenously or through a nasogastric tube. Nitrogenous waste production can be reduced further by exclusion of protein intake during the acute phase of the illness. Once clinical improvement is evident, protein intake should gradually be restored. With rare exceptions, any drug that requires hepatic metabolism should be withheld from the patient. Colonic emptying should be facilitated through the use of enemas and/or magnesium citrate. Ammonia production by intestinal bacteria may be diminished by the administration of neomycin, 6–12 g orally per day. Finally, exchange transfusion, hemodialysis, plasmapheresis, extracorporeal perfusion, and corticosteroids have all been used to treat fulminant hepatic failure (Katelaris & Jones, 1989) and should be considered in cases unresponsive to traditional management.

Mild coagulation abnormalities need not be corrected if delivery can be accomplished atraumatically. However, in the presence of hemorrhagic complications or if surgery is contemplated, the coagulation abnormalities should be corrected with platelets, fresh frozen plasma, or cryoprecipitate, as indicated by laboratory parameters. The administration of antithrombin preparations has also been reported (Castro et al., 1999).

Morbidity from other potential complications may be prevented by prophylactic treatment and careful surveillance. The liberal use of broad-spectrum antibiotics has been shown to decrease the incidence of concomitant infection (Castro et al., 1999). Prophylactic administration of antacid solutions and H_2 blocking agents may decrease the risk of gastrointestinal bleeding.

Successful liver transplantation has been reported in women with AFLP who continue to deteriorate in spite of delivery and appropriate supportive care (Ockner et al., 1990;

Amon et al., 1991; Franco et al., 2000). However, the pathophysiologic changes associated with AFLP are considered reversible making transplantation inappropriate in all but the most extreme cases (Doepel et al., 1996; Castro et al., 1999). Successful temporary auxiliary liver transplant has also been reported (Franco et al., 2000).

Summary

Acute fatty liver of pregnancy is uncommon but is always associated with significant morbidity and potential for mortality in the worst cases. Early diagnosis and prompt treatment remain the best defense against AFLP. Defects in long-chain fatty acid oxidation appear to place women at risk for both AFLP and HELLP syndrome. Like HELLP, delivery is the treatment of choice and supportive care and treatment of systemic manifestations of AFLP improve both maternal and perinatal survival.

References

Amon E, Allen SR, Petrie RH, Belew JE. Acute fatty liver of pregnancy associated with preeclampsia: Management of hepatic failure with postpartum live transplantation. Am J Perinat 1991;8:278–279.

Antognini JF, Andrews S. Anaesthesia for caesarean section in a patient with acute fatty liver of pregnancy. Can J Anaesth 1991;38: 904–907.

Bacq Y. Acute fatty liver of pregnancy. Semin Perinatol 1998;22(2):134–140.

Burroughs AK, Seong NG J, Dojcinov DM, et al. Idiopathic acute fatty liver of pregnancy in twelve patients. Q J Med 1982;204: 481–497.

Castro MA, Ouzounian JG, Colletti PM, Shaw KJ, Stein SM, Goodwin TM. Radiologic studies in acute fatty liver of pregnancy. A review of the literature and 19 new cases. J Reprod Med 1996;41(11):839–843.

Castro MA, Fassett MJ, Reynolds TB, Shaw KJ, Goodwin TM. Reversible peripartum liver failure: a new perspective on the diagnosis, treatment, and cause of acute fatty liver of pregnancy, based on 28 consecutive cases. Am J Obstet Gynecol 1999;181(2): 389–395.

Clements D, Young WT, Thornton JG, Rhodes J, Howard C, Hibbard B. Imaging in acute fatty liver of pregnancy. Case report. Br J Obstet Gynaecol 1990;97:631–633.

Davidson KM, Simpson LL, Knox TA, D'Alton ME. Acute fatty liver of pregnancy in triplet gestation. Obstet Gynecol 1998;91(5 Pt 2): 806–808.

Doepel M, Backas HN, Taskinen EI, et al. Spontaneous recovery of postpartus liver necrosis in a patient listed for transplantation. Hepato Gastroenterol 1996;43:1084–1087.

Duma RJ, Dowling EA, Alexander HC, et al. Acute fatty liver of pregnancy: Report of a surviving patient with serial liver biopsies. Ann Intern Med 1965;63:851–858.

Farine D, Newhouse J, Owen J, Fox HE. Magnetic resonance imaging and computed tomography scan for the diagnosis of acute fatty liver of pregnancy. Am J Perinatol 1990;7:316–318.

Franco J, Newcomer J, Adams M, Saeian K. Auxiliary liver transplant in acute fatty liver of pregnancy. Obstet Gynecol 2000;95: 1042.

Goldfarb G, Debaene B, Ang ET, Roulot D, Jolis P, Lebrec D. Hepatic blood flow in humans during isoflurane N_2O and halothane-N_2O anesthesia. Anesth Analg 1990;71:349–353.

Holzman RS, Riley LE, Aron E, Fetherston J. Perioperative care of a patient with acute fatty liver of pregnancy. Anesth Analg 2001; 92(5):1268–1270.

Ibdah JA, Bennett MJ, Rinaldo P, et al. A fetal fatty-acid oxidation disorder as a cause of liver disease in pregnant women. N Engl J Med 1999;340(22):1723–1731.

Kaplan MM. Acute fatty liver of pregnancy. N Engl J Med 1985; 313:367–370.

Katelaris PH, Jones DB. Fulminant hepatic failure. Med Clin N Am 1989;73:955–970.

Kennedy SK, Hall PM, Seymore AE, Hague WM. Transient diabetes insipidus and acute fatty liver of pregnancy. Br J Obstet Gynecol 1994;101:387–391.

Laursen L, Frost L, Mortensen JZ, et al. Acute fatty liver of pregnancy with complicating disseminated intravascular coagulation. Acta Obstet Gynecol Scand 1983;62:403–407.

Liebman HA, McGhee WG, Patch MJ, Feinstein DI. Severe depression of antithrombin III associated with disseminated intravascular coagulation in women with fatty liver of pregnancy. Ann Intern Med 1983;98:330–333.

Matern D, Hart P, Murtha AP, et al. Acute fatty liver of pregnancy associated with short-chain acyl-coenzyme A dehydrogenase deficiency. J Pediatr 2001;138(4):585–588.

Minakami H, Oka N, Sato T, Tamada T, Yasuda Y, Hirota N. Preeclampsia: A microvesicular fat disease of the liver? Am J Obstet Gynecol 1988;159:1043–1047.

Monga M, Katz AR. Acute fatty liver in the second trimester. Obstet Gynecol 1999;93(5 Pt 2):811–813.

Ockner SA, Brunt E, Cohn SM, Krul ES, Hanto DW, Peters MG. Fulminant hepatic failure caused by acute fatty liver of pregnancy by orthotopic liver transplantation. Hepatology 1990;11: 59–64.

Peters RL, Edmondson HA, Mikkelsen WP, et al. Tetracycline-induced fatty liver in nonpregnant patients. A report of six cases. Am J Surg 1967;113:622–632.

Pockros PJ, Peters RL, Reynolds TB. Idiopathic fatty liver of pregnancy: Findings in ten cases. Medicine 1984;63:1–11.

Purdie JM, Waters BNJ. Acute fatty liver of pregnancy. Clinical features and diagnosis. Aust N Z J Obstet Gynaecol 1988;28:62–67.

Reyes H, Sandoval L, Wainstein A, et al. Acute fatty liver of pregnancy: a clinical study of 12 episodes in 11 patients. Gut 1994;35:101–106.

Schoeman MN, Batey RG, Wilcken B. Recurrent acute fatty liver of pregnancy associated with a fatty-acid oxidation defect in the offspring. Gastroenterology 1991;100:544–548.

Sims HF, Brackett JC, Powell CK, et al. The molecular basis of pediatric long chain 3-hydroxyacyl-CoA dehydrogenase deficiency associated with maternal acute fatty liver of pregnancy. Proc Natl Acad Sci 1995;92:841–845.

Treem WR, Rinaldo P, Hale DE, et al. Acute fatty liver of pregnancy and long-chain 3-hydroxyacyl-coenzyme A dehydrogenase deficiency. Hepatology 1994;19:339–345.

Tucker ED, Calhoun BC, Thorneycroft IH, Edwards MS. Diabetes insipidus and acute fatty liver: A case report. J Reprod Med 1993; 38:835–838.

Usta IM, Barton JR, Amon EA, Gonzalez A, Sibai BM. Acute fatty live of pregnancy: An experience in the diagnosis and management of fourteen cases. Am J Obstet Gynecol 1994;171:1342–1347.

Weber FL, Snodgrass PJ, Powell DE, et al. Abnormalities of hepatic mitochondrial urea-cycle enzyme activities and hepatic ultrastructure in acute fatty liver of pregnancy. J Lab Clin Med 1979;94:27–41.

29 Sickle-cell crisis

Lisa E. Moore
James N. Martin, Jr

The sickle-cell diseases are heritable disorders of hemoglobin structure and synthesis that include sickle-cell anemia ($\beta^S\beta^S$), sickle-cell trait ($\beta\beta^S$), SC disease ($\beta^S\beta^C$), and sickle β-thalassemia ($\beta^S\beta^{Thal}$). With the exception of sickle-cell trait, these disorders are characterized by chronic hemolytic anemia and episodic vaso-occlusive crises that can cause heightened susceptibility to infection and organ failure. SC disease is associated with an increased incidence of preeclampsia, preterm labor, spontaneous abortion, and stillbirth compared to unaffected pregnancies (Seoud et al., 1994; Sun et al., 2001).

Epidemiology

The sickle-cell mutation arose independently in five different geographic locations worldwide (Bain, 2001). The mutations are identified by their association with different β-globin gene haplotypes. Four occurred in Africa (Senegal-type, Bantu-type, Benin-type, and Cameroon-type) and one originated in southern India (Indian/Saudi Arabian-type). The high prevalence of such a deleterious gene among some ethnic groups has been attributed to selective pressure from falciparum malaria. Heterozygotes (sickle trait) are usually asymptomatic and have partial protection against the malarial parasite.

Approximately, 1 in 12 Americans of African descent in the United States have sickle-cell trait. The incidence of sickle-cell disease in African-Americans is 1 in 500–600. Hemoglobin-SC disease has an approximate frequency of 1 in 1,250 and the sickle β-thalassemias occur in approximately 1 in 24,000 African-Americans (Whitten & Whitten-Shurney, 2001). Because American society is made up of immigrants from many countries, it is useful to be aware that the sickle hemoglobin gene has a prevalence of 25% in some parts of Saudi Arabia and 30% among some Indian populations. The gene has also been identified in parts of the former Soviet Union, in Arabs living in Israel, in Central and South America, and in the Mediterranean countries of Greece, Italy, and Spain (Bain, 2001; Sergeant & Sergeant, 2001). Similarly, the β-thalassemia mutations are common in Africa, some parts of India and around the Mediterranean, and in Southeast Asia.

Fertility is not impaired in women with sickle-cell disease. Although no statistics are available on the number of births to affected women, the high prevalence of the disease makes it very likely that a clinician will at some time be responsible for the care of a pregnant sickle-cell patient.

Molecular basis of the sickle hemoglobinopathies

The sickle hemoglobinopathies are inherited as autosomal recessive traits (Table 29.1). Hemoglobin-S is caused by a missense mutation in the gene coding for β-globin that causes valine to be substituted for glutamic acid at the sixth position in the hemoglobin chain. Hemoglobin-C is the result of a missense mutation causing lysine to be inserted rather than glutamic acid at the sixth position.

A second mutation sometimes occurs resulting in a hemoglobin with two amino acid substitutions. These variants retain the tendency to sickle, but migrate differently when electrophoresed. Six double mutations are known (Table 29.2). These amino acid substitutions result in abnormalities of the tertiary structure of the resulting globin chain (Bain, 2001). Low oxygen tension causes bonds to form between sickle hemoglobin chains resulting in strands of deoxyhemoglobin tetramers within the erythrocyte. These structures deform the red blood cell causing the classic sickle shape.

While the sickle gene causes production of a defective globin chain, the thalassemia gene results in an abnormality in the amount of globin produced. The β-thalassemia mutations are divided into two categories, β^0 and β^+. In β^+ there is reduced production of β-chains. Multiple mutations causing this effect have been identified. In β^0 there is a gene deletion or an abnormal gene that results in total failure to produce β-chains.

Table 29.1 Mutations that cause sickle-cell disease

$\beta^{6glu\to val}\,\beta^{6glu\to val}$	Sickle-cell anemia
$\beta^{6glu\to val}\,\beta^{6glu\to lys}$	SC disease
$\beta^{6glu\to val}\,\beta^{0}$ or β^{+}	Sickle β-thalassemia
$\beta^{6glu\to val}\,\beta^{A}$	Sickle trait

Table 29.2 Known double mutations

$\beta^{6glu\to val\ 121glu\to lys}$
$\beta^{6glu\to val\ 73asp\to asn}$
$\beta^{6glu\to val\ 142ala\to val}$
$\beta^{6glu\to val\ 23val\to ile}$
$\beta^{6glu\to val\ 82lys\to asn}$
$\beta^{6glu\to val\ 58pro\to arg}$

Pathophysiology

Under conditions of normal oxygenation, sickle hemoglobin has normal form and function. Under conditions that cause reduced oxygen concentrations, the deoxyhemoglobin molecules form hydrophobic bonds between adjacent amino acids. This is facilitated by the neutrally charged valine that substitutes for glutamic acid. Tetramers of deoxyhemoglobin polymerize to form deoxyhemoglobin strands within the erythrocyte (Rust & Perry, 1995; Bunn, 1997). Fully oxygenated sickle hemoglobin is sterically prevented from polymerization. Most importantly, there is a delay between the deoxygenation and the formation of the hemoglobin polymer that is inversely dependent upon the concentration of sickle hemoglobin (Steinberg, 2001). This explains why the persistence of fetal hemoglobin decreases the severity of sickle-cell anemia. Fetal hemoglobin has a higher affinity for oxygen and does not polymerize. Patients with 20–30% hemoglobin-F rarely experience crises because the speed of sickling is reduced and the presence of the alternate globin chain inhibits the polymerization process (Mentzer & Wang, 1980; Noguchi et al., 1988; Bunn, 1997; Sergeant & Sergeant, 2001).

Sickling can be precipitated by extremes of temperature (cold or hot), acidosis, increased concentration of 2,3-diphosphoglycerate, dehydration, hypoxia, and infection. Initially, oxygen can restore the erythrocyte to normal, but with repeated episodes of deoxygenation the red blood cell membrane becomes rigid and irreversibly sickled (Mentzer & Wang, 1980; Bunn, 1997).

Because of their molecular alterations, sickled erythrocytes have a lifespan of 10–20 days compared to approximately 120 days for a normal red blood cell. These permanently damaged erythrocytes are cleared by the reticuloendothelial system, where the majority of hemolysis occurs. About one-third of hemolysis of these cells occurs intravascularly. This accounts for the depression of serum haptoglobin and the loss of iron in the urine, the elevation in the serum level of indirect unconjugated bilirubin, and the appearance of icterus in the affected patient. A chronic compensated anemia is achieved by bone marrow and extramedullary erythropoiesis.

During vaso-occlusive crises, obstruction to blood flow first occurs in the microcapillary beds. These capillaries have diameters smaller than the diameter of red blood cells. Normal cells change shape to move through these vessels, but sickled cells have a rigid membrane and are unable to change shape. They become stuck in the capillary. Sickled cells also have increased adhesiveness to vascular endothelium (Bunn, 1997). The vessel becomes occluded and the area becomes deoxygenated, which causes more cells to sickle and the cycle perpetuates. Infection is postulated to disrupt the vascular endothelium causing enhanced sickle-cell adhesion.

Secondary organ system effects

Chronic anemia and episodic vaso-occlusion affects multiple organ systems. Almost all patients with sickle-cell anemia have cardiac abnormalities. Cardiac output is increased to compensate for the reduced oxygen-carrying capacity of the blood caused by the anemia. This increase in output occurs without an elevation of heart rate, and thus must be accomplished by increasing stroke volume. Cardiomegaly is found in 80–100% of adult sicklers. The right and left ventricle and left atrium are usually enlarged and the interventricular septum is thickened (Lindsay et al., 1974). On an EKG, 10% of sicklers have prolongation of the PR interval and 50% have evidence of left ventricular hypertrophy (Mentzer & Wang, 1980). These physiologic adaptations to chronic anemia combined with the volume changes of pregnancy place the pregnant sickler at an increased risk of heart failure should volume overload occur.

Sickle-cell anemia is also associated with alterations in renal morphology and function. Light microscopy has demonstrated sickled blood cells in glomerular capillaries and afferent arterioles. Capillary engorgement and dilation are found in both the medulla and the cortex (Buckalew & Someren, 1974). The hypertonic milieu of the medulla dehydrates sickle red cells, inducing sickling and causing vaso-occlusion with destruction of the vasa recta. As a consequence, sickle patients have a defect in the mechanism for concentrating urine that causes a tendency toward dehydration and sickling.

Sickle crisis (Fig. 29.1)

Sickle crisis is a potentially life-threatening complication of sickle-cell disease. Crises can be divided into two major categories: hematologic and vaso-occlusive. Hematologic crises are most common in the pediatric population and are rare in pregnancy. They are characterized by a sudden worsening of

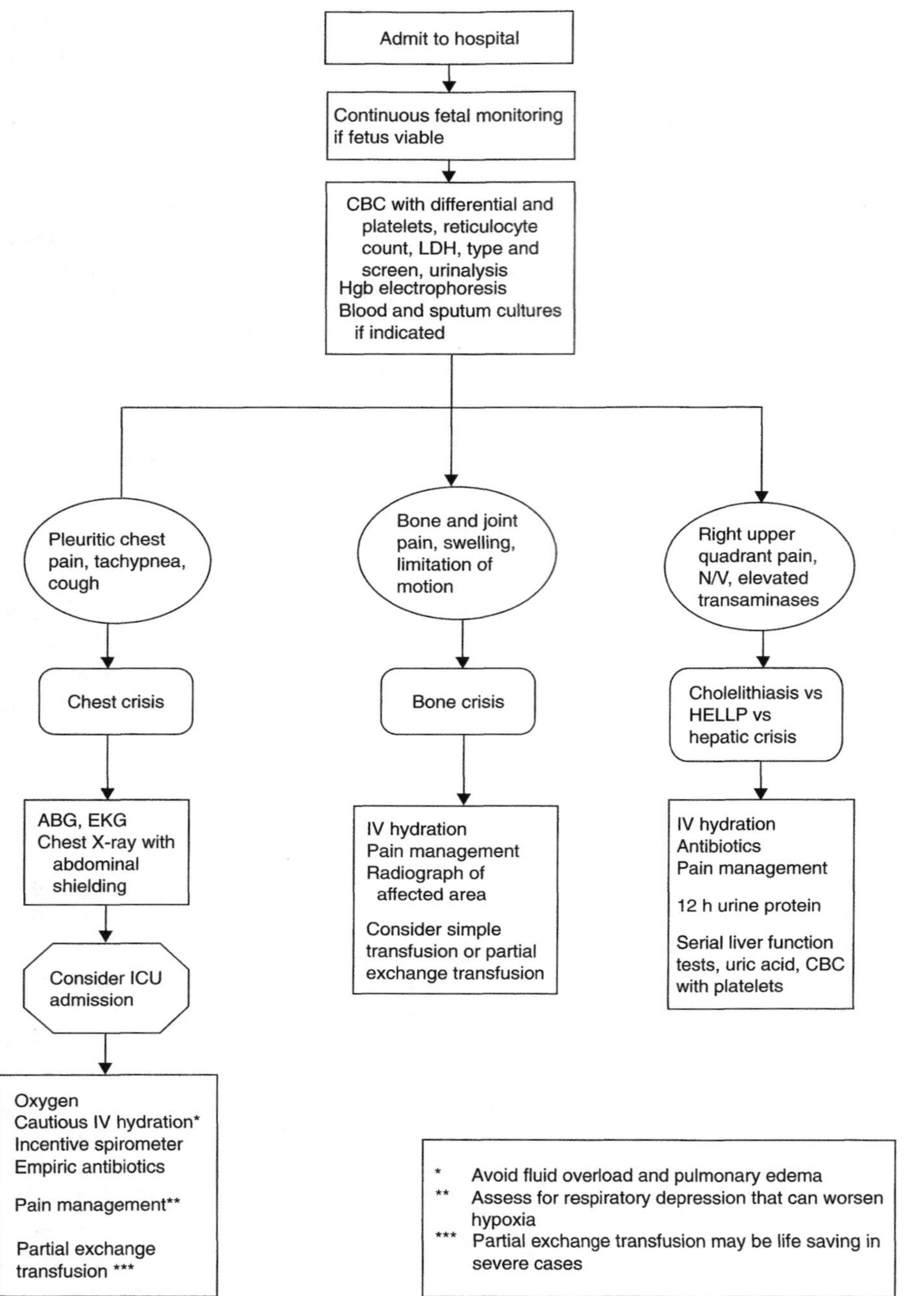

Fig. 29.1 Algorithm for management of sickle-cell crisis. ABG, arterial blood gas; CBC, complete blood count; ICU, intensive care unit; N/V, nausea/vomiting.

anemia. Patients present with weakness and exertional dyspnea and may show signs of high-output cardiac failure.

The most common type of hematologic crisis is the aplastic crisis characterized by decreased red blood cell production in the bone marrow. This is typically precipitated by a bacterial or viral infection. The most common causative agent is parvovirus B-19 infection (Rao et al., 1992). Human parvovirus attacks erythrocyte precursors in the marrow. Failure of red blood cell production combined with increased destruction of sickled cells produces a severe anemia. The finding of giant pronormoblasts during examination of a bone marrow aspirate is diagnostic. The infection is self-limiting and marrow aplasia usually resolves within 2 weeks of the onset of infection. During the period of severe anemia, patients are at risk for cerebrovascular accidents. Transfusion of packed red blood cells is indicated for symptomatic patients with a hematocrit of less than 25% and evidence of decreased reticulocytosis. Infection with parvovirus during pregnancy has been associated with fetal death, nonimmune hydrops, and congenital anomalies.

Other types of hematologic crises include splenic sequestration due to trapping of sickled cells in the spleen, hepatic sequestration, and hyperhemolytic crises in which hemolysis is elevated to a level that cannot be compensated by reticulocytosis. As stated previously, these are more common in children and so are not discussed in detail here.

Vaso-occlusive acute pain crises are by far the most common type of sickle-cell crisis experienced during pregnancy (Koshy et al., 1987). These crises are painful, can involve any part of the body at multiple sites, and can lead to single or multiple organ dysfunction.

Uncomplicated acute pain crisis

Pain crises without major organ involvement are the most common types of crises during pregnancy. Clinical features of acute pain crises vary with age and sex and frequently recur in a pattern, which is stereotypical for each individual. Pregnancy and the puerperium are associated with an increased frequency of painful episodes.

Musculoskeletal pain, limited motion and swollen tender joints with effusions may be present. Dark urine is a common complaint, reflecting excretion of urinary porphyrin. The diagnosis of pain crisis is a diagnosis of exclusion because objective laboratory and physical findings are lacking. Approximately 50% of patients with pain crises have alterations in vital signs, including mild to moderate fever (37.8°C or higher), elevations of blood pressure, tachycardia, and tachypnea. Fever can occur in the absence of infection due to release of endogenous pyogens by ischemic tissue. Nonetheless, when fever is encountered, an infectious cause should be sought. Moderate leukocytosis ($12–17 \times 10^3/mm^3$) usually occurs even in the absence of infection and is most likely a reaction to tissue ischemia. In the presence of infection the white blood cell count can exceed $20 \times 10^3/mm^3$ with an associated bandemia. Serum lactate dehydrogenase (LDH) values, especially isoenzymes 1 and 2, are elevated in sickle pain crises most likely due to marrow infarction (Mentzer & Wang, 1980). Levels of LDH rise in proportion to the severity of systemic vaso-occlusion. C-reactive protein is elevated within 1–2 days of onset of the crises and the erythrocyte sedimentation rate is decreased. Approximately one-third of pain crises are associated with infection. The most common infections during pregnancy are pneumonia, urinary tract infections, endomyometritis, and osteomyelitis.

Standard management of sickle pain crises is supportive: rest, hydration, oxygenation, and pain control. The majority of patients will be dehydrated due to an inability to concentrate urine. Fluid resuscitation should be initiated with normal saline. Fluid therapy probably has no effect on irreversibly sickled cells but euvolemia will decrease blood viscosity and thereby decrease the predisposition to ongoing vaso-occlusion. Input and output should be followed closely to limit the occurrence of pulmonary edema, though urinary catheterization should be avoided, if possible, to decrease the risk of infection. If infection is suspected, blood and urine cultures and a chest radiograph should be taken and broad-spectrum antibiotic coverage should be started empirically.

Fetal assessment

During and immediately after a vaso-occlusive crisis, there is significant risk for fetal distress, premature labor, and fetal loss. Continuous electronic fetal monitoring should be initiated for fetuses at the age of viability, and continued until the patient is stable. A nonreactive fetal heart tracing is common during vaso-occlusive crises. One-third of fetuses will have a biophysical profile score of 6 or less (Anyaegbunum et al., 1991). Fetal assessments typically improve as the sickle crisis resolves. The maternal condition should be stabilized and intrauterine resuscitation initiated before emergency operative delivery is considered. Once the patient is well hydrated, her vital signs are stable, there is no evidence of major organ involvement or severe infection, and her pain is well controlled, continuous fetal monitoring can be replaced by intermittent fetal assessment, such as a daily nonstress test. As in most pregnancy complications, obstetric care should be individualized to the patient and her presentation.

Chest syndrome

Acute chest syndrome or pulmonary crisis is a potentially fatal complication of sickle-cell disease characterized by fever, pleuritic chest pain, tachypnea, and pulmonary infiltrates (Kirkpatrick & Bass, 1989; Stuart & Yamaha, 1999). If a cough is present it is usually nonproductive.

The syndrome results from infarction of the pulmonary vasculature or pulmonary infection or a combination of these. The differential diagnosis of chest syndrome includes pulmonary embolus, fat embolus from bone marrow infarction, and amniotic fluid embolus (Vichinsky et al., 2000). The ventilation–perfusion scan may be abnormal due to recurrent episodes of pulmonary infarction.

Treatment is supportive. The goals of therapy are adequate oxygenation, hydration, treatment of infection, and pain relief. An arterial blood gas should be obtained and oxygen provided to keep arterial oxygen tension above 70 mmHg. Hypoventilation due to pleuritic chest pain can worsen hypoxia. Likewise, narcotics should be used cautiously to prevent respiratory depression. Use of an incentive spirometer may minimize atelectasis and infiltrates (Bellet et al., 1995). Empiric antibiotic coverage for community-acquired pneumonia should be started. In a multicenter trial with 538 patients, the most frequent organisms identified in sputum were *Chlamydia pneumoniae*, *Mycoplasma pneumoniae*, and respiratory syncytial virus (Vichinsky et al., 2000). Transfusion to increase the level of hemoglobin-A to 30–50% without exceeding a hematocrit of 30% has been shown to reverse acute respiratory distress during pulmonary crisis (Mallouh & Asha, 1988; Vichinsky et al., 2000).

Davies et al. (1984) recommended exchange transfusion for worsening hypoxia, continuing fever, and tachycardia or worsening chest radiograph. Atz and Wessel (1997) reported the successful use of inhaled nitric oxide in two patients with chest syndrome. Inhaled nitric oxide selectively dilates the pulmonary vasculature and increases oxygenation and potentially alleviates the vaso-occlusive process.

Hepatic crisis

Hepatic crisis due to disseminated vaso-occlusion of the hepatic microvasculature with sickled red cells simulates acute cholecystitis, with fever, right upper quadrant pain, leukocytosis, and elevations in transaminases and bilirubin. Differentiating this syndrome from cholecystitis or the syndrome of hemolysis, elevated liver enzymes and low platelets (HELLP) can be a diagnostic challenge. It is reasonable to manage such patients with parenteral hydration, broad-spectrum antibiotics, pain control, and serial laboratory assessments of liver function, uric acid, and complete blood count with platelets.

Pain management (Fig. 29.2)

The management of pain in the sickle-cell population presents difficulties to the clinician for multiple reasons. Sickle-cell patients are often economically disadvantaged and sometimes noncompliant. There are no objective criteria for identifying a pain crisis or for quantifying the pain. The patient's self-report of her level of pain is the only assessment tool available. Factitious disorder and Munchausen syndrome are well documented among sickle patients. On the other hand, patients who require large doses of narcotics to control their pain may be incorrectly labeled as drug seeking.

The initial dose of pain medicine should be individualized

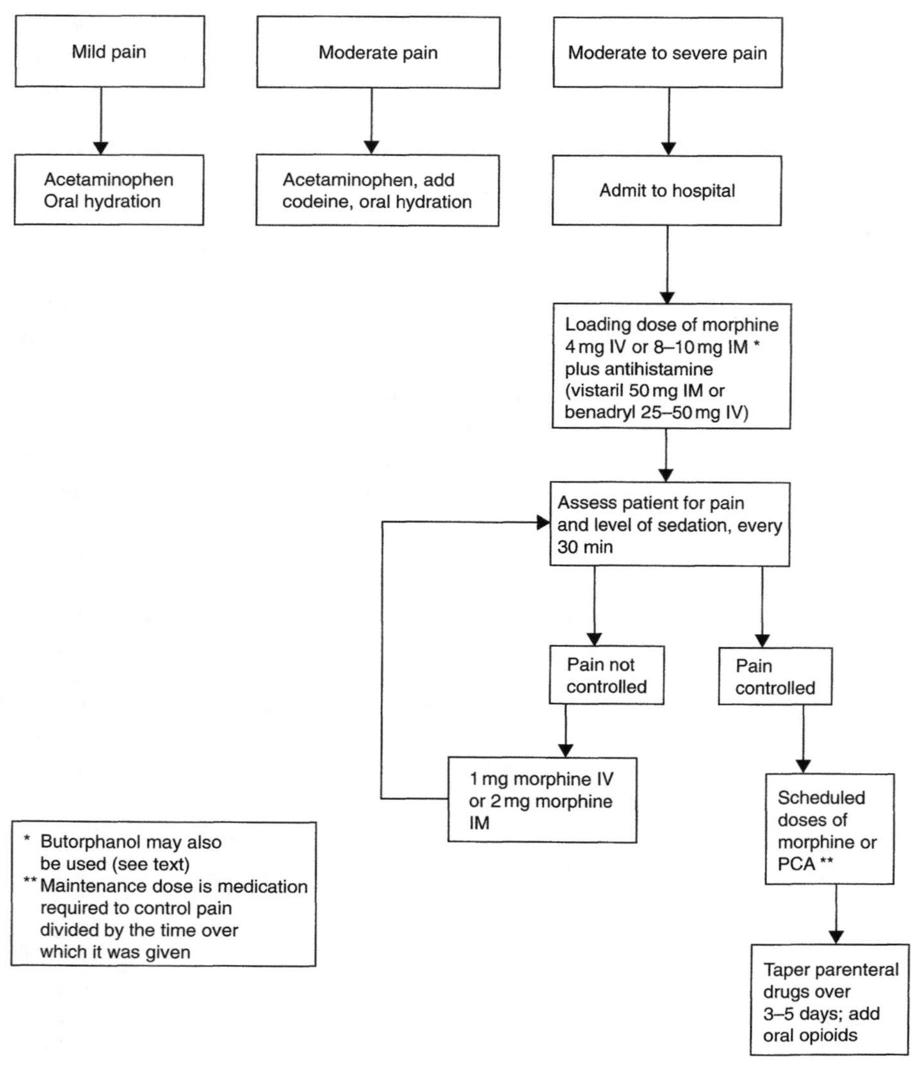

Fig. 29.2 Algorithm for management of pain crisis.

based on the patient's prior use of analgesia, including the type, route and frequency of dosage. Traditional therapy includes nonopioid and opioid analgesics with analgesic adjuvants.

For mild pain, peripherally acting oral analgesia, such as acetaminophen, may be sufficient, combined with aggressive oral hydration. Acetaminophen is an analgesic and antipyretic; the recommended adult dosage should not exceed 6 g in a 24-hour period. Mild to moderate pain can be managed by the addition of codeine.

Hospitalization is recommended for greater than mild to moderate pain. Opioids combined with nonopioids and adjuvant analgesics are the mainstay of treatment. Morphine is the preferred opioid. Demerol should be avoided, if possible, because of the increased potential for dependency and abuse.

Morphine should be given in a loading dose to provide pain relief. The loading dose should be based on the patient's previous use of narcotics. A possible starting dose is 4 mg of morphine sulfate IV or 8–10 mg IM. After the loading dose, subsequent doses are titrated with the goal of providing quick and sustained relief of pain. The patient should be reassessed every 30 minutes for amount of pain and sedation. One-fourth of the initial loading dose should be given at each reassessment until the pain is relieved or there is concern about sedation. Once relief of pain is achieved, maintenance dosing should be started either at scheduled intervals or by patient-controlled pump. Sickle-cell patients with pain crises who are provided with patient-controlled analgesia (PCA) use less medication, develop less respiratory depression, and report better pain control than those receiving bolus injections on demand (Shapiro et al., 1993). The maintenance dose can be calculated as the medication required during the titration phase divided by the number of hours over which it was given.

An alternative to morphine, for those patients who report morphine allergies, is butorphanol. An intramuscular injection of 2 mg of butorphanol has equivalent analgesic effect to 10 mg morphine IM or 80 mg meperidine IM. It is a mixed agonist/antagonist and can precipitate withdrawal in addicted patients. In a study comparing butorphanol to morphine for the control of pain due to sickle-cell crisis, no difference was found in pain relief or level of alertness (Gonzalez et al., 1988). Butorphanol can be given as 2 mg IM or 1 mg IV with assessment of the patient in 30 minutes and repeated doses until pain is relieved. Maintenance dosing should be the initial dose given at schedule times every 2–4 hours.

Adjuvant analgesics are often added to improve the effect of the opioids and minimize side effects. The most commonly used adjuvants are antihistamines (Steinberg & Rodgers, 2001). They counteract the opioid-induced release of histamines that cause pruritis, reduce nausea, and have a mild sedative effect. Once consistent pain control has been achieved, the parenteral opioids should be tapered over several days while maintaining pain control with oral opioids. We have had good success with OxyContin; however this drug has tremendous potential for abuse.

Therapeutic options

Oxygen therapy

The benefit of oxygen therapy in nonhypoxic patients is uncertain. Although oxygen has been shown to reduce the number of reversibly sickled cells in vitro, clinical trials of such therapy have not produced a reduction in the duration of pain, analgesic administration, or length of hospitalization (Zippursky et al., 1992). The therapeutic goal is to maintain a normal P_aO_2.

If oxygen therapy is needed, 3 L supplied by nasal canula is usually sufficient. In severe oxygenation failure refractory to supplemental oxygen, continuous positive airway pressure or positive end-expiratory pressure may be necessary.

Exchange transfusion

Prophylactic partial exchange transfusion during pregnancy, prior to the onset of a vaso-occlusive crisis, is controversial (Morrison & Morrison, 1989). It has been shown to improve both maternal and fetal outcomes in one study (Morrison & Wiser, 1976). In contrast, no improvement in pregnancy outcome was found in a retrospective review of matched patients who received prophylactic exchange during pregnancy compared to those who did not (Miller et al., 1981). The major disadvantage is the potential for isosensitization. Patients can become so severely sensitized that cross-matching becomes nearly impossible. During an emergency requiring transfusion, inability to find compatible blood can be fatal. During pain crises, exchange transfusion has been shown to provide symptomatic relief within 1 hour of initiation of the procedure (Martin et al., 1986). This procedure rapidly decreases the amount of hemoglobin-S and increases hemoglobin-A, thereby improving oxygenation and decreasing the risk of sickling and associated complications. The goal is to achieve a hemoglobin-A concentration of at least 60–70% with a hematocrit of 30–35%.

Tables are available to calculate the required volume of transfusion given a target percentage of hemoglobin-A, the hematocrit of the transfused blood, and the patient's weight in kilograms. Patients usually require placement of a double-lumen central catheter prior to the procedure. They should also be premedicated as with any blood transfusion. We have found that a standard exchange of 6 units of washed packed red blood cells results in a hemoglobin-A concentration of approximately 70%.

Simple transfusion

Simple transfusion of packed red cells is indicated for a hematocrit of less than 15% or hemoglobin less than 6 g/dL. A hematocrit of 30–35% is considered optimal and should not be exceeded due to the increased viscosity of sickled cells, which can precipitate a crisis when the hematocrit is elevated.

Hydroxyurea

Hydroxyurea is an antineoplastic agent that has been shown to induce production of hemoglobin-F (Bunn, 1999). It is commonly used in nonpregnant sicklers and has been shown to decrease the frequency of pain crises, acute chest syndrome, and the necessity of transfusions (Charache et al., 1995; Steinberg, 1999). Hydroxyurea works by selectively killing cells in the bone marrow, thus increasing the number of erythroblasts producing hemoglobin-F (Steinberg, 1999). Because it is cytotoxic, the risk of teratogenesis when used during the first trimester, its long-term effect, and the risk of carcinogenesis is a concern. No randomized studies exist on its use in pregnancy. There are case reports indicating favorable outcomes even when administered in the first trimester of pregnancy.

Diav-Citrin et al. (1999) reported a case of hydroxyurea use during the first 9 weeks of pregnancy and additionally reviewed case reports of 15 other exposures to the drug during pregnancy. Nine cases had first-trimester exposure. All of these pregnancies had phenotypically normal children. However, there is no long-term follow up on these children. At this time, use of hydroxyurea in pregnancy cannot be advocated. However, for patients with unplanned exposure to the drug during pregnancy, the prognosis may not be as grim as expected.

Erythropoietin

Erythropoietin is a hormone that stimulates red blood cell production. It has been shown to increase the number of reticulocytes containing fetal hemoglobin in humans (Rodgers et al., 1993). It has been used alone and in alternating doses with hydroxyurea to increase the amount of hemoglobin-F (Rodgers et al., 1993; Steinberg, 1999). Studies have produced conflicting results about its efficacy in either augmenting the effect of hydroxyurea or of enhancing production of fetal hemoglobin (Goldberg et al., 1990; Rodgers et al., 1993). Erythropoietin is currently not used for induction of fetal hemoglobin in sickle-cell patients, but may be useful in sickle patients with renal insufficiency.

References

Anyaegbunum A, Morel M, Merkatz IR. Antepartum fetal surveillance tests during sickle cell crisis. Am J Obstet Gynecol 1991;165: 1081–1083.

Atz AM, Wessel DL. Inhaled nitric oxide in sickle cell disease with acute chest syndrome. Anesthesiology 1997;87:988–990.

Bain BJ. Haemoglobinopathy Diagnosis. Oxford: Blackwell Science, 2001:113–117.

Bellet PS, Kalinyak KA, Shukla R, Gelfand JM, Rucknagel DL. Incentive spirometry to prevent acute pulmonary complications in sickle cell disease. N Engl J Med 1995;333:699–703.

Buckalew VM Jr, Someren A. Renal manifestations of sickle cell disease. Arch Intern Med 1974;133:660–669.

Bunn HF. Pathogenesis and treatment of sickle cell disease. N Engl J Med 1997;337:762–769.

Bunn HF. Induction of fetal hemoglobin in sickle cell disease. Blood 1999;93:1787–1789.

Charache TS, Moore RD, Dover GJ, Barton FB, Eckert SV, McMahon RP, Bonds DR. Effect of hydroxyurea on the frequency of painful crisis in sickle cell anemia. N Engl J Med 1995;332:1317–1322.

Davies SC, Win AA, Luce PJ, Riordan JF. Acute chest syndrome in sickle cell disease. Lancet 1984;8367:36–38.

Diav-Citrin O, Hunnisett L, Sher GD, Koren G. Hydroxyurea use during pregnancy: a case report in sickle cell disease and review of the literature. Am J Hematol 1999;60:148–150.

Goldberg MA, Brugnara C, Dover GJ, Schapira L, Charache S, Bunn HF. Treatment of sickle cell anemia with hydroxyurea and erythropoietin. N Engl J Med 1990;323:366–372.

Gonzalez ER, Ornato JP, Ware D, Bull D, Evens RP. Comparison of intramuscular analgesic activity of butorphanol and morphine in patients with sickle cell disease. Ann Emerg Med 1988;17:788–791.

Kirkpatrick MB, Bass JB. Pulmonary complications in adults with sickle cell disease. Pulmonary Perspective 1989;6:6.

Koshy M, Burd L, Hoff G. Frequency of pain crisis during pregnancy. Prog Clin Biol Res 1987;240:305–311.

Lindsay J Jr, Meshel JC, Patterson RH. The cardiovascular manifestations of sickle cell disease. Arch Intern Med 1974;133:643–650.

Mallouh AA, Asha MA. Beneficial effect of blood transfusion in children with sickle cell chest syndrome. Am J Dis Child 1988;142: 178–182.

Martin JN Jr, Martin RW, Morrison JC. Acute management of sickle cell crisis in pregnancy. Clin Perinatol 1986;13:853–869.

Mentzer WC Jr, Wang WC. Sickle-cell disease: pathophysiology and diagnosis. Pediatr Ann 1980;9:287–296.

Miller JM, Horger EO, Key TC, Walker EM. Management of sickle hemoglobinopathies in pregnant patients. Am J Obstet Gynecol 1981;141:237–241.

Morrison JC, Morrison FS. Prophylactic transfusions in pregnant patients with sickle cell disease. N Engl J Med 1989;320:1286–1287.

Morrison JC, Wiser WL. The use of prophylactic partial exchange transfusions in pregnancies associated with sickle cell hemoglobinopathies. Obstet Gynecol 1976;48:516–520.

Noguchi CT, Rodgers GP, Serjeant RG, Schechter AN. Levels of fetal hemoglobin necessary for treatment of sickle cell disease. N Engl J Med 1988;318:96–99.

Rao SP, Miller ST, Cohen BJ. Transient aplastic crisis in patients with sickle cell disease: B19 parvovirus studies during a 7 year period. Am J Dis Child 1992;146:1328–1330.

Rodgers GP, Dover GJ, Uyesaka N, Noguchi CT, Schecter AN, Nienhuis AW. Augmentation by erythropoietin of the fetal-hemoglobin response to hydroxyurea in sickle cell disease. N Engl J Med 1993;328:73–80.

Rust OA, Perry KG Jr. Pregnancy complicated by sickle hemoglobinopathy. Clin Obstet Gynecol 1995;38:472–484.

Seoud MA, Cantwell C, Nobles G, Lerry DL. Outcome of pregnancies complicated by sickle cell and sickle-C hemoglobinopathies. Am J Perinatol 1994;11:187–191.

Sergeant GR, Sergeant BE. Sickle Cell Disease, 3rd edn. Oxford: Oxford University Press, 2001.

Shapiro BS, Cohen DE, Howe CJ. Patient-controlled analgesia for sickle-cell-related pain. J Pain Symptom Manage 1993;8:22–28.

Steinberg MH. Management of sickle cell disease. N Engl J Med 1999;340:1021–1030.

Steinberg MH, Rodgers GP. Pathophysiology of sickle cell disease: role of cellular and genetic modifiers. Semin Hematol 2001;38: 299–306.

Stuart MJ, Yamaha S. Sickle cell acute chest syndrome: pathogenesis and rationale for treatment. Blood 1999;94:1555–1560.

Sun PM, Wilburn W, Raynor D, Jamieson D. Sickle cell disease in pregnancy: twenty years of experience at Grady Memorial Hospital, Atlanta, Georgia. Am J Obstet Gynecol 2001;184:1127–1130.

Vichinsky EP, Neumayr LD, Earles AN, et al. Causes and outcomes of the acute chest syndrome in sickle cell disease. N Engl J Med 2000;342:1855–1865.

Whitten CF, Whitten-Shurney W. Sickle cell. Clin Perinatol 2001;28: 435–448.

Zipursky A, Robieux I, Brown EJ, et al. Oxygen therapy in sickle cell disease. Am J Pediatr Hematol Oncol 1992;14:222–228.

30 Disseminated intravascular coagulopathy

Luis Diego Pacheco*
James W. Van Hook
Alfredo F. Gei

Disseminated intravascular coagulopathy (DIC) occurs in all areas of medicine and can have a number of varied clinical presentations. Consumption of hemostatic factors and systemic fibrin deposition characteristically lead to both bleeding and thrombosis, with tissue or organ system damage in those organs affected by DIC. DIC is a hemostatic and systemic feature of many pathophysiologic disorders (Bick, 1994, 2000; ten Cate, 2001). In obstetrics, the leading causes of direct maternal mortality in the perinatal period include thromboembolic events, pregnancy-induced hypertension, surgical hemorrhage, and infection; and DIC is a common complication of each. Therefore, understanding DIC is essential for obstetricians.

DIC is a thrombohemorrhagic disorder with concurrent activation of the coagulation and fibrinolytic pathways, resulting in simultaneous fibrin clot formation and lysis (Marder, 1990). The occlusion of small vessels by fibrin deposition leads to tissue ischemia and organ dysfunction, such as acute renal failure, hepatic damage, acute respiratory distress syndrome, and cerebral infarction. This effect is exacerbated by concomitant bleeding due to thrombocytopenia and consumption of clotting factors, leading to hypovolemia and hypoperfusion. The disorder is always the result of an underlying disease process. Several conditions where DIC can occur are unique to pregnancy: placental abruption, septic abortion, intrauterine fetal demise, amniotic fluid embolism, acute fatty liver of pregnancy, induced abortion, gestational trophoblastic disease, and dilutional coagulopathy often due to washout of clotting factors from uncorrected hemorrhage. In this chapter we discuss the pathophysiology, diagnosis, etiology, and treatment of DIC associated with pregnancy.

Normal coagulation

In the traditional model of coagulation, the coagulation pathway is divided into extrinsic, intrinsic, and common pathways (Fig. 30.1). The pathways function as a cascade with near-sequential serial activation of factors. The end result of coagulation is the formation of fibrin through the cleavage of fibrinogen by the serine protease thrombin.

Hemostasis is thought to occur in four major phases. The first phase is the vascular phase, which is characterized by local vasospasm. After vasospasm, platelet migration and activation produces a platelet plug at the site of hemorrhage. At this point, the coagulation mechanism forms a fibrin-rich clot. Finally, as the tissue injury that initiated the hemorrhage is repaired, the fibrinolytic system lyses the hemostatic clot. Overall, a very complex system of processes must all function correctly to properly stop bleeding, form a clot, and restore circulation.

Although hemostasis is multifaceted and complex, an understanding of coagulation is necessary for insight into DIC. Under normal circumstances, platelet activation or tissue disruption causes activation of the clotting cascade. The end result of coagulation activation is the formation of fibrin through activation of fibrinogen by thrombin. Thrombin is a serine protease, cleaving the inactive fibrinogen into hemostatically active fibrin. Thrombin itself is the active form of prothrombin. Thrombin is formed from protease cleavage of prothrombin by factor Xa (activated). This process is potentiated by the presence of cofactor Va (activated) (Wessler & Gitel, 1984; Aird, 2001).

Using traditional nomenclature, fibrin clot formation as initiated by factor Xa and thrombin is referred to as the common pathway. Activation of factor X to Xa (activated) is promulgated via the extrinsic and intrinsic pathways. The intrinsic pathway is activated after contact of blood with artificial surfaces having a negative charge. Factor XIIa transforms factor XI to XIa, thereby initiating the conversion of factor IX to IXa. Factor IXa activates factor Xa of the common pathway. The extrinsic pathway is initiated after exposure to membrane-bound glycoprotein tissue factor. Factor VII is converted to factor VIIa, which in turn induces activation of cofactor VIIIa. Cofactor VIIIa significantly propagates factor IXa-mediated activation of factor X (Rosenberg & Aird, 1999; Aird, 2001).

*This chapter is dedicated to my father, mother and lovely wife.

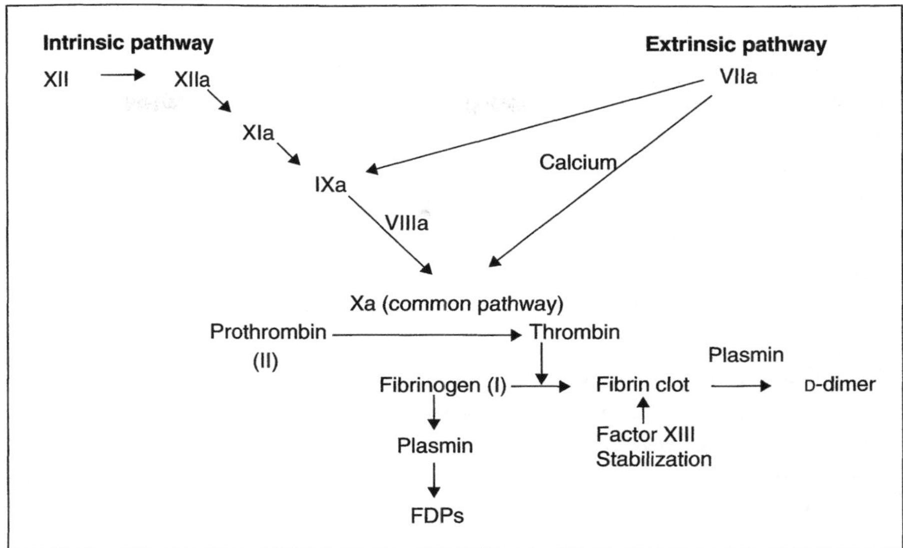

Fig. 30.1 Normal hemostasis. Fibrin degradation products (FDPs) come from plasmin action on both fibrinogen and fibrin.

In order to achieve coagulation, relatively low concentrations of the different clotting factors are needed (Table 30.1). Normal plasma contains an excess of clotting factors, allowing a patient to receive up to a full volume replacement of packed red blood cells and crystalloid/colloid solutions without requiring fresh frozen plasma (American Association of Blood Banks, 1999a). This may not be applicable to the patient with hepatic disease (HELLP syndrome, acute fatty liver of pregnancy, etc.), since the clotting factor reserve in such patients may be less than normal.

For normal hemostasis to occur, the fibrinogen level should be greater than 100 mg/dL. It is important to remember that obstetric patients will have a significant elevation of fibrinogen and factors VII, VIII, IX and X, while factors V and II remain nearly constant. In contrast, factors XI and XIII decrease during pregnancy to approximately 70% of their normal value (Hobisch-Hagen et al., 1997).

The activation of coagulation is balanced by the activity of the anticlotting system, and both systems exist harmoniously in the normal patient. The regulation of coagulation is mediated by the supply of factors, the presence or absence of events which incite anticoagulation, and the naturally present anticoagulant mechanisms that serve to dampen the procoagulant response. Natural anticoagulation occurs via specific serine protease inhibitors and the fibrinolytic system. Antithrombin III (AT III) is a circulating serine protease inhibitor that neutralizes thrombin and to a lesser degree factors IXa, Xa, XI, XIIa, and plasmin (Savelieva et al., 1995). Approximately 75% of the thrombin formed is inactivated by AT III, while the remaining 25% is inactivated by other minor inhibitors. Thrombin itself initiates another important serine protease inhibitor system by activation of protein C. Thrombomodulin and protein S serve as cofactors for protein C. Proteins C and S are vitamin K dependent. Stimulation of protein C inactivates factors V and VIII (Aird, 2001). The natural fibrinolytic system is headed by plasmin. Tissue plasminogen activator converts plasminogen into plasmin, which degrades fibrin and factors V, VIII, IX, and XII (Bick, 1994; Rosenberg & Aird, 1999).

Table 30.1 Clotting factors: percent of normal needed for hemostasis

Factor	Name (common synonym)	Percent needed
I	Fibrinogen	12–50
II	Prothrombin	10–25
V	Proaccelerin (labile)	10–30
VII	Proconvertin (stable)	>10
VIII	Antihemophilic factor	30–40
IX	Plasma thromboplastin component (Christmas)	15–40
X	Stuart factor (Stuart–Prower)	10–40
XI	Plasma thromboplastin antecedent	20–30
XIII	Fibrin stabilizing factor	<5

(Adapted with permission from the American Association of Blood Banks.)

Some differences may be present in the thrombolytic and coagulation regulatory systems during pregnancy when compared to nonpregnant controls. Most evidence suggests that fibrinolytic system activity is reduced in normal pregnancy (Ostlund et al., 1998; Baker & Cunningham, 1999). Conflicting results regarding plasminogen activator inhibitors have been noted by other investigators (Koh et al., 1993). One conclusion regarding the conflicting data is that the concomitant evidence of both increased and decreased fibrinolysis during pregnancy underscores the difficulty in interpreting measures of fibrinolysis (Cunningham et al., 2001). Available data suggest that neither antigenic nor functional levels of protein C appreciably change during pregnancy (Faught et al., 1995). Free protein S has been shown to decrease during normal pregnancy and during use of oral contraceptives by nonpregnant women. Total protein S antigenic levels are generally decreased as well (Faught et al., 1995; Lefkowitz et al., 1996).

Pathophysiology

The pathophysiology of DIC is extremely complex. It involves activation of the clotting cascade and the fibrinolytic system and these two interact in a circular self-perpetuating fashion until the underlying disease is treated.

DIC is characterized by systemic activation of the clotting cascade with resultant increase in the circulating levels of both thrombin and plasmin (Bick, 2000). Clotting factors are consumed and degraded both by plasmin and by monocyte enzymes. The factors more profoundly depleted are fibrinogen, prothrombin, factor V, and factor VIII. Once this activation has taken place, the pathophysiology of the coagulation disorder is similar regardless of the etiology of the DIC.

As thrombin circulates, fibrinopeptides A and B are cleaved from fibrinogen, leaving the fibrin monomer. This monomer polymerizes into fibrin (clot), which leads to microvascular and macrovascular thrombosis. The deposition of fibrin initiates platelet adhesion and consumption, with resultant thrombocytopenia. The development of these thrombi compromises the perfusion to multiple organs such as the liver, kidneys, and central nervous system.

Concomitant with the activation of coagulation, DIC is characterized by systemic activation of the fibrinolytic system. Plasminogen is converted into plasmin, which cleaves fibrinogen into fibrin(ogen) degradation products: fragments X, Y, D, and E (Bick, 2000). These fragments may combine with the fibrin monomer before polymerization takes place, leading to solubilized fibrin monomers and impaired hemostasis. Fragments D and E have high affinity for the platelet membrane, inducing platelet dysfunction and impaired hemostasis. Particularly in obstetrics, these products have a significant pathophysiologic effect; they inhibit adequate myometrial contraction, worsening postpartum hemorrhage secondary to uterine atony. This is believed to be due to weak myometrial contractility in association with placental abruption and intrauterine fetal demise.

Fibrinogen degradation products are known to induce macrophage liberation of interleukins 1 and 6, which produce further endothelial damage. Macrophages also secrete plasminogen activator inhibitor 1, a substance that inhibits fibrinolysis with concomitant thrombus formation (Robson et al., 1994).

Thrombin alone induces liberation by monocytes of interleukins 1 and 6 and tumor necrosis factor (TNF), contributing to the endothelial damage and exposing more subendothelial collagen to favor the formation of thrombi.

Another significant action of thrombin is the stimulation of endothelial cells to liberate proteins such as soluble thrombomodulin, endothelin-1, and selectin (Okajima et al., 1997). Endothelin induces severe vasospasm, leading to end-organ damage. Selectin binds to granulocytes, lymphocytes, monocytes, and macrophages to produce further cytokine release and a concomitant increase in endothelial damage. The inflammatory cells also liberate platelet activating factor, favoring more thrombi formation and leading to end-organ damage due to hypoperfusion. Ischemic tissues release tissue factor, thereby activating the extrinsic pathway of the clotting cascade with an increase in thrombin formation. Finally, granulocytes bind to the endothelium and liberate cathepsins and elastases, enzymes that contribute to tissue damage and the degradation of procoagulant and profibrinolytic factors.

As the coagulation system is activated, there is concomitant activation of the fibrinolytic system. High concentrations of plasmin will lead to degradation of fibrinogen and factors V, III:C, IX, and XI. As plasmin degrades cross-linked fibrin, specific fibrin degradation products such as D-dimer appear. Plasmin also is responsible for the activation of C1 and C3, leading to activation of C8 and C9 with subsequent red cell and platelet lysis.

Complement is also activated by TNF that is liberated by monocytes under the stimulation of thrombin, as described previously. The lysis of red cells liberate ADP and red cell membrane phospholipids, which are strong procoagulant materials. The systemic deposition of fibrin leads to microangiopathic hemolysis, with subsequent development of schistocytes and helmet cells increasing the liberation of ADP and red cell membrane phospholipids. Complement activation also induces increased vascular permeability, leading to hypotension and potential shock.

The diffuse endothelial lesion seen in DIC activates factor XII and induces the conversion of prekallikrein to kallikrein; subsequently the transformation of kininogens to kinins occurs, thereby increasing vascular permeability. Once the cycle of thrombin-induced microvascular thrombosis and plasmin-induced hemorrhage is established, it can become self-perpetuating. The pathophysiology of DIC is summarized in Fig. 30.2.

Diagnosis

Clinical

Hemorrhage and/or thrombosis associated with one of the clinical conditions listed in Table 30.2 are strongly suggestive of DIC. Laboratory confirmation of DIC is recommended; however, this should not delay the institution of treatment if clinical suspicion is strong.

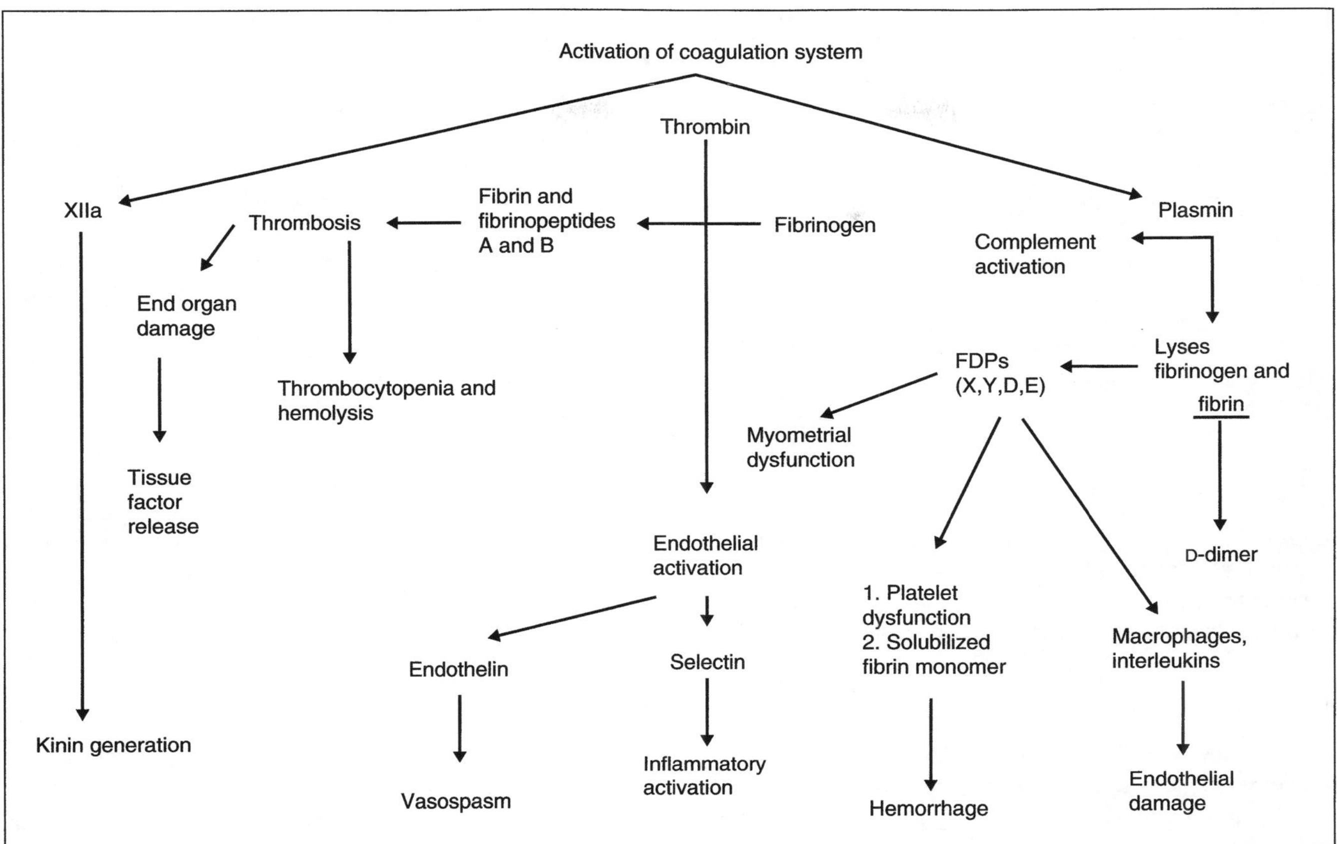

Fig. 30.2 Pathophysiology of DIC. FDPs, fibrin degradation products.

Table 30.2 Conditions associated with DIC in obstetrics

Abruptio placenta (most frequent etiology)
Preeclampsia/eclampsia
Intrauterine fetal demise
Induced abortion
Acute fatty liver of pregnancy
Amniotic fluid embolism
Sepsis (bacterial, viral, protozoan, fungal, mycobacterial)
Trauma
Hemolytic transfusion reactions
Dilutional or washout coagulopathy

The onset of acute DIC is characterized by multiple hemostatic defects that may result in venipuncture oozing, epistaxis, hematuria, gingival/mucosal bleeding, and purpura or petechiae, particularly over pressure sites (blood pressure cuffs, external monitors, splints, etc.). On the other hand, chronic compensated DIC (due to malignancy or intrauterine fetal demise) rarely leads to dramatic bleeding, and thus laboratory confirmation may be more important in these cases. Chronic compensated DIC has a predominance of thrombosis over bleeding; however, these patients often develop minor mucosal bleeding, hematuria, epistaxis, or easy bruising (Bick, 1978).

In the case of low-grade DIC, coagulation tests are frequently normal or nearly normal, although the chronic turnover and ongoing consumption results in an increase in fibrin(ogen) degradation products (Bick, 2000). The clot assay may be a useful bedside test. A sample of blood is placed in a red-topped tube. If a clot does not form in 6 minutes or forms and lyses in less than 30 minutes, there is a high chance that there is a coagulation defect and the fibrinogen level will be less than 150 mg/dL (Gabbe et al., 2002).

Although the morbidity associated with the hemorrhagic consequences of DIC is generally recognized, thrombosis actually accounts for a large degree of the serious complications from DIC. These can include renal cortical necrosis, peripheral gangrene, central nervous system thrombosis, and acute ulceration with gastrointestinal bleeding. Evidence suggests that microvascular thrombosis with inconsistent reperfusion injury is the major mechanism for thrombotic damage in DIC (Aird, 2001). Attenuation of microvascular thrombosis may be instituted in successful treatment of DIC.

Table 30.3 Abnormal laboratory tests seen in DIC

Elevated D-dimer
Prolonged PT and aPTT
Low platelet count
Decreased fibrinogen
Elevated fibrin degradation products
Prolonged thrombin time
Decreased antithrombin III
Elevated fibrinopeptide A
Elevated platelet factor 4
Elevated prothrombin fragments 1 and 2

aPTT, activated partial thromboplastin time; PT, prothrombin time.

Laboratory analysis

Appropriate laboratory tests provide objective criteria for diagnosis and treatment of DIC. The laboratory abnormalities seen in DIC are listed in Table 30.3. In this section we discuss the most relevant laboratory tests for the diagnosis of DIC.

Prothrombin time

Prothrombin time (PT) reflects the integrity of the extrinsic and common pathways. It measures the activity of factors VII, X, V, II, and fibrinogen. Commercially prepared rabbit brain and/or lung tissue thromboplastin and calcium are added to citrate-anticoagulated plasma from the patient, making the clotting time observable by a variety of manual or automated techniques.

Prolongation of the PT generally occurs when the factor levels are less than 50% of normal or the fibrinogen level is less than 100 mg/dL (Cunningham et al., 2001). Overall, the PT may be normal in up to 50% of patients with DIC. This is due to the presence of circulating activated clotting factors such as thrombin and factor X, thus accelerating the formation of fibrin in vitro (Bick et al., 1999).

Another reason for a normal PT in patients with DIC is that early degradation products may be rapidly clotted by thrombin, causing the test system to register a normal or even fast PT. The PT can be evaluated by using the international normalized ratio (INR), which shows the relationship between the normal PT value and that of the patient. The normal INR value is 1.2.

Activated partial thromboplastin time

Activated partial thromboplastin time (aPTT) reflects the integrity of the intrinsic and common pathways and measures the activity of factors XII, XI, IX, VIII, X, V, II, and fibrinogen (Reiss, 2000). The partial thromboplastin reagent is essentially a platelet factor 3 or a phospholipid substitute with one of a variety of activators added to speed up the glass contact activation of factors XII and XI. Plasma is then added and preincubated, and the clotting time is observed by manual or automated technique.

The aPTT test is as reliable as the PT. Similar to the PT, the aPTT is prolonged when the clotting factors are less than 50% of normal or fibrinogen is less than 100 mg/dL. This test is prolonged only in 50% of the patients. The same reasons for a normal or fast PT as detailed earlier also apply to the aPTT.

While important for the evaluation of the clotting cascade itself, the aPTT (like the PT) may not be reflective of microvascular thrombosis and hemorrhage. Also, DIC can exist with relatively normal PT and aPTT assays.

Thrombin time

The thrombin time (TT) measures the time required to convert fibrinogen to fibrin and is frequently prolonged in DIC. It is an indication of completion of the final step of the common pathway of the clotting cascade. The prolongation of this test is associated with a decreased level of fibrinogen. However, the same limitations that apply to the use of PT and aPTT for the diagnosis of DIC apply to the use of TT as well.

Fibrin(ogen) degradation products

Fibrin(ogen) degradation products (FDPs) are elevated in 85–100% of patients with DIC (Bick et al., 1999). They are indicative of the enzymatic degradation of fibrinogen and fibrin by plasmin. FDPs may be elevated in other medical conditions such as myocardial infarction, renal disease, chronic hepatic disease, arterial or venous thrombosis, and pulmonary embolism. Of patients with acute DIC, 15% have normal FDP levels (Myers et al., 1970). This may be secondary to incomplete or excessive degradation of FDPs that results in levels undetectable by commercially available kits.

D-dimer

The most specific and reliable test for the diagnosis of DIC is the monoclonal assay for D-dimer, a breakdown product of the cross-linked fibrin polymer (Carr et al., 1989). It is a rapid (1 hour) widely available test and should be used, if possible, instead of relying on FDP levels. The D-dimer indicates the presence of circulating plasmin and thrombin. This text is abnormal in more than 90% of patients with DIC. The D-dimer level increases as pregnancy progresses, with the highest values seen during delivery. This test must be interpreted in association with other clinical and laboratory findings during gestation (Ghirardini et al., 1999).

Platelets and fibrinogen

During normal pregnancy fibrinogen levels range between 400 and 700 mg/dL, representing a 74% increase in concentration. Therefore, a "normal" fibrinogen level could represent a relative hypofibrinogenemia (Gerbasi et al., 1990). The platelet count is usually significantly decreased, but the range is quite variable. Most tests of platelet function, such as bleeding time and platelet aggregation, are abnormal and add little to the diagnosis.

Other diagnostic tests

Free thrombin and plasmin cannot be detected by routine biochemical assays because of their extremely short half-life and rapid binding to antagonists. The measurement of free thrombin and plasmin is demonstrated indirectly by other laboratory tests that reflect the biochemistry of their generation, inactivation, and action (Schuster, 1998).

The AT III level is decreased in 89% of patients with DIC (Bick, 1994). This is secondary to the rapid binding of this molecule to free thrombin, resulting in the generation of thrombin–antithrombin (TAT) complexes. AT III levels are a highly sensitive test, because abnormal consumption of this coagulation inhibitor must occur if DIC is present. TAT complexes can be measured and are also very sensitive for the diagnosis of DIC (Teitel et al., 1982).

The formation of thrombin from prothrombin results in the liberation of prothrombin fragment 1 + 2 (PF 1 + 2). Subsequently, the cleavage of fibrinogen produces fibrinopeptide A, which is elevated in 88% of patients with DIC. PF 1 + 2 is a reliable marker for factor Xa generation, and fibrinopetide A is a reliable marker for thrombin generation (Sorensen et al., 1992).

Platelet factor 4 and β-thromboglobulin are markers of platelet reactivity and are usually elevated in DIC.

Plasmin is also elevated in DIC. Once generated, plasmin will bind to α_2-antiplasmin. The levels of this inhibitor will be decreased in DIC, and the level of plasmin–antiplasmin complexes will rise (Takahashi et al., 1986). Many of these molecular markers are now available in the USA for the evaluation of DIC; however, their availability in other countries may still be limited.

Obstetric causes

Pregnancy is a well-documented hypercoaguable state (Weiner et al., 1984; Eby, 1993). Less established is the association between pregnancy and an increased risk of DIC (Gerbasi et al., 1990). The purpose of this section is not to discuss treatment of each of the obstetric conditions, but rather to understand how each of these conditions is associated with DIC in pregnancy. Parturients may be at greater risk for this syndrome than nonpregnant women because of the complications unique to pregnancy (placental abruption, amniotic fluid embolism and fetal death) associated with DIC. The different etiologies of DIC in obstetrics are summarized in Table 30.4.

Table 30.4 Mechanisms of DIC in obstetrics

Cause	Mechanism
Placental abruption Intrauterine fetal demise Amniotic fluid embolism Traumatic delivery	Thromboplastin material liberation and activation of extrinsic pathway (factor VII)
Massive transfusion	Dilutional coagulopathy
Preeclampsia	Diffuse endothelial lesion
Sepsis	Cytokines, endotoxins
Fatty liver of pregnancy	Hepatic dysfunction

Placental abruption

Abruption is the most common cause of DIC in pregnancy (Gilabert et al., 1985). The incidence of these disorders varies according to the population studied and the diagnostic criteria used, but it ranges from 0.45 to 1.3% (Richey et al., 1995). Clinically significant DIC is present in only 10% of cases of abruption, being more common in severe cases associated with fetal death and severe hemorrhage (grade III abruptios). Grade III placental abruption involves fetal death and a fibrinogen level of less than 150 mg/dL (Gabbe et al., 2002). In severe cases of placental abruption, the development of DIC is expected in up to 35% of cases (Rath et al., 2000).

The development of a large extravascular clot that consumes clotting factors does not explain all the coagulation anomalies seen in severe cases of abruption. In fact, activation of the fibrinolytic system and systemic consumption of soluble components frequently occurs out of proportion to blood loss, due to systemic activation of the extrinsic pathway of the clotting cascade. The degree of thrombocytopenia, AT III consumption, hypofibrinogenemia, and D-dimer elevation is correlated with the clinical severity of the abruption and with the time interval between the placental separation and delivery. If this interval is longer than 4 hours, the severity of DIC and acute renal failure is substantially higher (Kobayashi et al., 2001).

Placental abruption in the second trimester of pregnancy carries a significant risk of DIC that can be life-threatening and out of proportion to the degree of placental separation (Olah et al., 1988). In these second-trimester cases, even small areas of disruption can liberate significant amounts of thromboplastin material, greater than that seen in the third trimester (Olah et al., 1988). The inciting event is the liberation of thromboplastins from the site of placental injury. These substances are capable of activating the clotting cascade mainly through the extrinsic pathway by binding factor VII (see Fig. 30.1).

Plasma fibrinolytic activity is similar in the uterine artery and vein during normal pregnancy. Following normal delivery, there is an increase in FDPs in the uterine vein; a similar increase occurs after an episode of abruption. Thus, it appears that the process of placental separation contributes to the increase in FDPs. The elevation of these products is associated with an increased risk of postpartum bleeding, since they inhibit myometrial contraction (Basu, 1971). This situation is seen when FDP levels are higher than 330 mg/mL. Further, the concentration of FDPs in the lochia of women who have experienced placental abruption is significantly higher than concentrations in normal controls. There are enough data to support a direct pathophysiologic relationship between elevated FDPs and postpartum hemorrhage in cases of placental abruption (Zaitsev et al., 1997).

Management of acute placental abruption thus includes emptying the uterus so that the source of thromboplastin material is removed as fast as possible. Euvolemia should be maintained by use of crystalloid solutions and the oxygen-carrying capacity improved by transfusion of packed red blood cells. The coagulation deficit may require blood component therapy according to the guidelines below.

Preeclampsia–eclampsia syndrome

DIC is considered a manifestation of the severity of preeclampsia (Pritchard et al., 1976). While the causal relationship between preeclampsia–eclampsia and overt DIC is unclear, there is substantial clinical evidence that the majority of women with preeclampsia have a subclinical consumptive coagulopathy. Both fibrin and fibrin-like substances have been identified as variable constituents of the typical renal lesion seen in preeclampsia, namely glomerular endotheliosis. The activation of coagulation may cause fibrin deposition in both the kidney and the lung (Birmingham Eclampsia Study Group, 1971). Also, fibrin deposition is consistently seen in liver biopsies obtained from women with preeclampsia (Anas & Mancilla-Jimenez, 1976). There is an increased incidence of fibrin deposition in placental microvessels and in the perivillous spaces. Levels of D-dimer are elevated in women with preeclampsia (Trofatter et al., 1989). Kanfer et al. (1996) demonstrated increased fibrin deposition and increased antifibrinolytic activity in preeclamptic placentas.

The liberation of blood-borne products from the diseased placenta may induce endothelial cell damage and dysfunction, with increased liberation of vasoconstrictive substances such as endothelin and decreased activity of prostacyclin. The exposure of subendothelial collagen may activate the clotting cascade through the intrinsic pathway. The activation of the clotting cascade is reflected by an increase in plasma TAT complexes and a significant decrease in plasma levels of AT III (Terao et al., 1991; Halim et al., 1995; Savelieva et al., 1995). A characteristic fall in the platelet count occurs (Redman et al., 1978), coupled with platelet damage and dysfunction (Halim et al., 1996). Additionally, the levels of fibrinopeptide A are significantly higher in the preeclamptic pregnancy (Douglas et al., 1982). The elevation of fibrinopeptide A reflects fibrinogen transformation into fibrin.

Although a subclinical consumptive state may be demonstrated in preeclampsia by using sophisticated laboratory tests, frank DIC or alterations in clinically measured clotting parameters (other than thrombocytopenia) are virtually never seen in severe preeclampsia or eclampsia in the absence of placental abruption or HELLP syndrome.

DIC has been reported in 4–38% of cases of HELLP syndrome (Reubinoff & Schenker, 1991). The frequency of DIC in HELLP syndrome is probably associated with the incidence of coexistent placental abruption. DIC is neither an initial nor a principal symptom of HELLP syndrome; it actually reflects a secondary pathophysiologic process of the primary disease. In patients with preeclampsia where DIC is proven by laboratory means, immediate delivery is recommended before clinical manifestations occur (Rath et al., 2000).

Treatment of DIC in the pregnant preeclamptic patient is generally supportive in nature. Specific treatment of DIC is often not necessary, provided delivery is effected.

Hemostatic defects in massive transfusion

Massive transfusion is defined as the transfusion, within 24 hours, of a volume of whole blood, or its equivalent in red cells and crystalloid or colloid, that is greater than the total blood volume of the patient receiving the transfusion (Reiss, 2000). Most healthy pregnant women can tolerate this situation without developing dilutional coagulopathy. Complications are usually seen when blood is lost and replaced at a greater rate.

Severe bleeding diatheses in a patient undergoing massive transfusion are manifested by microvascular bleeding in the operative field and oozing from venipuncture sites. The practice of prophylactic transfusions of platelets and fresh frozen plasma (FFP) to prevent coagulopathy in massive transfusion is not indicated. This practice does not decrease the bleeding or the transfusion requirements (Reed et al., 1986).

The most common alterations in hemostasis observed after massive transfusion are dilutional thrombocytopenia and dilutional coagulopathy. Patients who receive large amounts of blood products should be screened periodically with a platelet count, aPTT, PT, and fibrinogen level. The PT and aPTT become progressively and simultaneously prolonged in simple hemodilution (no other hemostatic anomalies present). Usually the PT is more prolonged than the aPTT since it exceeds the upper reference limit faster than the aPTT (because the PT normal interval is narrower than the aPTT normal interval). The PT becomes prolonged earlier than the aPTT because of the extremely short half-life of factor VII. The fibrinogen level decreases in direct proportion to the level of hemodilution since most of the fibrinogen is intravascular and has a prolonged half-life (Reiss, 2000).

Normal hemostasis requires no more than 30% of normal values of the clotting factors; consequently, bleeding after massive transfusion would not be expected until the PT and aPTT have exceeded 1.5 times their reference values (Reiss, 2000).

Transfusion of platelets is recommended when the platelet count falls below 50,000/mm^3. If bleeding continues after platelet transfusion, and prolongation of the PT and aPTT is such that the concentration of clotting factors may be less than 30% of normal (PT of 21 seconds and aPTT of 74 seconds), then FFP is indicated (College of American Pathologists, 1994). The clinician treating a patient for bleeding after massive transfusion should always consider coexisting hemostatic defects and treat them accordingly.

Intrauterine fetal demise

The association between prolonged retention of a dead fetus in utero and a coagulation disorder was first reported by Weiner et al. in 1950. Thanks to aggressive management, the prolonged retention of a dead fetus is rarely the cause of coagulopathy in modern obstetrics.

Coagulopathy can occur following the death of either a singleton or one or more fetuses in a multiple gestation. The development of hemostatic anomalies usually occurs about 5 weeks after the demise (Pritchard & Ratnoff, 1959). The onset of the coagulopathy is gradual, and consists of varying degrees of hypofibrinogenemia, decreased plasminogen, decreased AT III, thrombocytopenia, and elevation of FDPs. The proposed mechanism in the development of DIC in the fetal death syndrome is the release of tissue thromboplastin from the fetoplacental unit activating the clotting cascade through the extrinsic pathway (Bick, 1994).

The main cause of the low fibrinogen in these patients is the increased activity of thrombin, indicating a consumptive process (Romero et al., 1985). One-third of patients will have fibrinogen concentrations below 150 mg/dL when more than 5 weeks have elapsed. Patients presenting with a fetal demise usually should be screened with coagulation studies because initial clinical manifestations of hemostatic dysfunction often are minimal; the first sign may be severe postpartum bleeding. The recommended laboratory tests include a complete blood cell count, fibrinogen, PT, aPTT, fibrin(ogen) split products, and D-dimer. The two earliest abnormalities include the elevation in fibrin(ogen) split products and the fall in fibrinogen (Romero et al., 1985).

Heparin is the treatment of choice for the chronic DIC associated with intrauterine fetal demise. Low-dose subcutaneous heparin (5,000–10,000 units twice daily) is adequate for most patients. Treatment should be continued until there is correction of the hypofibrinogenemia, after which time delivery may be carried out. A reasonable goal is to achieve a fibrinogen level of 200–300 mg/dL and a platelet count above 50,000/mm^3.

If labor is in progress at the time of the diagnosis, potential areas of vascular disruption and injury are likely to develop (i.e. at the placental implantation site or in lacerations). In these situations heparin administration may exaggerate the bleeding tendency and is not recommended (Romero et al., 1985). Fibrinogen replacement may be accomplished with cryoprecipitate in these cases.

After the demise of one fetus in a multiple pregnancy, there is a 12% risk of neurologic compromise in the surviving fetus. This is thought to be the result of profound hypotension in the surviving twin in the presence of a monochorionic placenta. The risk of DIC in the mother in this situation has been overestimated. A baseline set of coagulation indices after the diagnosis of a demise of one fetus is probably the only test needed. Subsequent laboratory surveillance with coagulation profile studies is probably unnecessary (Creasy & Resnik, 1999).

Acute fatty liver

Acute fatty liver is a rare, potentially fatal disorder of the third trimester of pregnancy. DIC and profound depression of AT III are hallmarks of this condition, but rarely do they have an impact on the clinical outcome. Holzbach (1974) proposed that the coagulopathy associated with this condition was the result of DIC initiated by severe hepatic dysfunction. Acute fatty liver of pregnancy is characterized by profound liver failure, as indicated by hypoglycemia and a severe reduction in clotting factors. Castro et al. (1996) found laboratory evidence of DIC in all of the cases of acute fatty liver in their series. Typically, there is a profound decrease in levels of AT III, to levels significantly lower than those seen in severe preeclampsia and HELLP syndrome (Vigil De Gracia, 2001). This difference may aid in the diagnosis of acute fatty liver of pregnancy earlier in the course of the disease or when the overlap with HELLP syndrome obscures the diagnosis.

Treatment consists of delivery, aggressive fluid resuscitation, and replacement of blood products as needed. The use of AT III concentrates may be useful in the patient who presents with active bleeding (Castro et al., 1996).

Sepsis

Severe infections such as septic abortion, pyelonephritis, chorioamnionitis, or endomyometritis may be associated with shock and DIC. Most of these cases are associated with Gram-negative microorganisms, although Gram-positive organisms and viral, fungal, protozoan and mycobacterial etiologies must be considered.

The bacterial endotoxin (lipopolysaccharide) or exotoxin provides the initiating insult. Endotoxins activate factor XII, induce platelet release, cause endothelial sloughing, release of granulocyte procoagulants, and ultimately liberate histamine, kinins, and serotonin. Any of these events might trigger DIC.

Activation of the intrinsic pathway (via factor XII) does not play a significant role in DIC associated with sepsis; however, it provides a powerful stimulus for the production of kinins that will induce profound hypotension. The most important mechanism of DIC in sepsis is the activation of the extrinsic pathway via tissue factor and TNF-α (Levi et al., 1993). Tissue factor is released by TNF-α stimulation of monocytes and by exposure of subendothelially located tissue factor following diffuse endothelial damage. The quantity of kinin and kallikrein production correlates directly with the severity of the shock (Mason et al., 1970). Heparin is contraindicated in these patients, since there is significant disruption of the vascular tree. The coagulopathy generally resolves rapidly after removal of the septic focus and antibiotic therapy. Unless the patient is actively bleeding or a surgical procedure is anticipated, no attempt to treat DIC through transfusion should be made. If the platelet count falls to 5,000–10,000/mm^3, even in the asymptomatic patient, platelet transfusion may be indicated to prevent spontaneous hemorrhage. The best treatment for DIC associated with sepsis is to treat the underlying condition.

Abortion

In this setting, coagulopathy may occur as a result of septic abortion, massive hemorrhage with shock, or after intrauterine instillation of hypertonic saline. With the development of safer newer alternatives for pregnancy termination, saline abortion has been relegated largely to historic status. The pathophysiology of DIC in saline-induced abortion is unclear (Laros & Penner, 1976). Some have proposed that hypertonic saline produces cellular disruption in the products of conception and this may lead to the passage of thromboplastic substances into the maternal circulation. If DIC does occur, the management includes evacuation of the uterus, restoration of volume status with crystalloid solutions, and blood component therapy as needed. (More detail is provided in the therapy section.)

Amniotic fluid embolism

Amniotic fluid embolism is rare, but is associated with a maternal mortality of up to 80% (Locksmith, 1999). If the initial cardiovascular insult is not fatal, DIC can follow in 45% or more of cases. The mechanism that leads to DIC in this condition is similar to that of massive placental abruption, with activation of the clotting cascade following exposure of the maternal circulation to a variety of fetal antigens with varying thromboplastin-like effects (Clark, 1995). Amniotic fluid has the capability in vitro to activate factor X and induce platelet aggregation. The hemorrhage of amniotic fluid embolism is treated by volume and component replacement, often in massive quantities. The clinician is advised to continue replacement therapy until normalization of laboratory parameters. Amniotic fluid embolism can present clinically with isolated DIC in the absence of significant cardiopulmonary findings (Davies, 1999). Chapter 34 provides a detailed review on amniotic fluid embolism.

Therapy

The morbidity and mortality of DIC result from both the coagulopathy and the precipitating illness. The primary therapeutic goal is to treat the underlying disorder, accompanied by aggressive support of blood volume, blood pressure, and tissue oxygenation (Lurie et al., 2000). Insufficient volume expansion and fluid resuscitation are the most common therapeutic errors. An approach applicable to most patients with pregnancy-associated DIC is outlined in Table 30.5.

Volume replacement, blood pressure maintenance, and evacuation of the uterus (thus terminating the source of the DIC) constitute adequate therapy in the vast majority of obstetric-related DIC syndromes (Marinoff et al., 1999). Volume replacement generally should be accomplished with the use of crystalloid solutions accompanied by packed red blood cells in order to increase the oxygen-carrying capacity. Colloid solutions such as dextran 40, dextran 70, albumin, and starches provide no benefit over isotonic crystalloid solutions. Colloids have also been associated with a transient decrease in platelet count, prolongation of PT and aPTT, and accelerated fibrinoly-

Table 30.5 Treatment outline for DIC in pregnancy

Goals of therapy
Treat/remove underlying etiology (most critical step)
Maintain blood volume and oxygenation
Stop intravascular clotting and inhibit fibrinolysis
Management protocol
Maintenance of blood volume (crystalloids, albumin, plasma expanders); ideally, use crystalloid solutions and maintain oxygen-carrying capacity with packed red blood cells
Maintenance of blood pressure (pressors if necessary)
Maintenance of oxygenation (oxygen administration or mechanical ventilation)
Additional supportive therapy as required
Treatment of underlying etiology of DIC
Evacuation of the uterus, if indicated
Broad-spectrum antibiotics for sepsis
Component therapy (aggressive replacement with packed red blood cells; and choice of coagulation components based on deficiencies)
Consideration of specific therapies (heparin therapy or possible other advanced therapies)
Critical laboratory tests
CBC with platelet count, PT, aPTT, fibrinogen, FDPs, D-dimer, thrombin time, and antithrombin III levels
Consultation
Hematology

aPTT, activated partial thromboplastin time; CBC, complete blood cell count; FDPs, fibrin degradation products; PT, prothrombin time.

sis. In obstetrics, elimination of the cause of DIC can sometimes be easily achieved by cesarean section, forceps delivery, or dilation and curettage (Yaw & Wan, 1998). Vaginal delivery is recommended when feasible, since it is less demanding for the hemostatic system than a cesarean section (Brandjes et al., 1991). In infection-mediated DIC, appropriate antibiotic therapy is added to the plan of care. The next defense is replacement therapy of the deficient clotting factors. The argument that this "adds fuel to the fire" and worsens DIC is unfounded; it may instead be life-saving. The following information pertains to the use of blood products for the treatment of DIC in obstetrics.

Replacement therapies

Fresh frozen plasma

FFP has an added anticoagulant preservative and must be stored at −18°C or colder. It contains both the labile (factors V and VIII) and nonlabile factors at a concentration of 1 IU/mL. Although FFP has a shelf-life of 12 months after the date of total blood collection, once the product is thawed it should be transfused immediately or stored for no more than 24 hours at 1–6°C.

The use of FFP is indicated in patients with bleeding due to clotting factor deficiency. Clinically, these patients usually have significant prolongations of the aPTT and PT, defined as an aPTT > 54 seconds, a PT > 18 seconds and an INR > 1.6 (American Association of Blood Banks, 1999a).

In DIC, circulating thrombin induces widespread fibrin deposition in the microcirculation, leading to depletion of platelets and clotting factors such as fibrinogen, factor V, and factor VIII. When the fibrinogen level falls below 100 mg/dL, FFP is usually indicated. FFP increases the fibrinogen level by 10 mg/dL per unit transfused (Naef & Morrison, 1995; Gabbe et al., 2002). Each unit has a volume of 200–250 mL, and the usual dose is 10–20 mL/kg (4–6 units). This dose will increase the level of clotting factors by 20% immediately after infusion. Only ABO-compatible plasma is appropriate. This product should never be used for volume expansion purposes only.

Cryoprecipitate

Cryoprecipitate is the cold, insoluble portion of plasma that precipitates at the time that FFP is thawed. It is suspended in less than 15 mL of plasma. Each unit contains at least 150 mg of fibrinogen as required by the American Association of Blood Banks (usually 250 mg per bag) and more than 80 units of factor VIII (both VIII:C and von Willebrand factor), as well as factor XIII and fibronectin.

This blood derivative is stored at −18°C or colder. Once thawed, it should be transfused immediately or stored at 20–24°C for no more than 6 hours if intended as a source for factor VIII (American Association of Blood Banks, 1999b).

Since it contains high concentrations of fibrinogen, each unit of cryoprecipitate will elevate the fibrinogen level by 5–15 mg/dL. Fibrinogen levels less than 100 mg/dL signify an indication for cryoprecipitate. The initial transfusion dose is 1 unit for every 10 kg of weight. After transfusion, only 75% of the fibrinogen remains in the intravascular space (Gabbe et al., 2002). Cryoprecipitate is particularly useful in patients with severe depletion of clotting factors and high risk of volume overload, and in cases where FFP might be relatively contraindicated.

Since cryoprecipitate does not contain all of the clotting factors, it is not indicated as the sole treatment for DIC. Each unit contains only small amounts of plasma, so ABO compatibility is not required; however, special care should be taken in pediatric cases where even small volumes may be significant.

Platelets

The normal lifespan of a platelet is 9.5 days, although this decreases as the severity of thrombocytopenia increases. Platelet concentrates have small amounts of red blood cells, which is particularly important in obstetrics. If Rh-positive platelets are given to a patient who is Rh negative, RhoGAM prophylaxis should be instituted. In situations like DIC where active bleeding is present, the RhoGAM should not be administered intramuscularly due to the risk of hematoma formation. A recent form of intravenous RhoGAM has been approved by the FDA. Whenever possible, ABO-compatible platelets should be used; urgent transfusions should however not be delayed if they are not available.

Platelets transfused to patients usually have a shorter lifespan. The platelet count can be assessed anywhere from 10 to 60 minutes after completion of the transfusion. Adequate response to allogeneic platelet transfusion can be evaluated by the corrected count increment (CCI):

$$\text{CCI of platelets at 1 hr} = \frac{\left[\begin{pmatrix}\text{Platelet}\\ \text{count (post)}\end{pmatrix} - \begin{pmatrix}\text{Platelet}\\ \text{count (pre)}\end{pmatrix}\right] \times \text{BSA}(\text{m}^2)}{\text{Number of units transfused}}$$

(A CCI above 4,000–5,000/mL suggests an adequate response to allogeneic platelet transfusion; adapted with permission from the American Association of Blood Banks.)

The usual dose for transfusion of platelets is 1 unit per 10 kg of weight with each unit usually containing 50–70 mL of plasma. Platelet transfusion is usually indicated in patients with active bleeding and a platelet count less than 50,000/mm^3 or before surgery or any other invasive procedure when the platelet count is less than 50,000/mm^3. The risk of spontaneous bleeding in the nonsurgical patient with a platelet count about 5,000–10,000/mm^3 is low. The role of prophylactic transfusions of platelets in patients without active bleeding, and the traditional threshold of 20,000/mm^3 or fewer platelets as an indication for transfusion, have both been questioned. Studies have failed to demonstrate the benefit of such transfusions in nonbleeding patients. In patients not actively bleeding or in those presenting with only petechiae and ecchymoses the transfusion of platelets should be avoided unless the platelet count is less than 5,000–10,000/mm^3. However, conditions such as fever and sepsis increase the risk of bleeding secondary to thrombocytopenia; and in these situations a threshold of 20,000/mm^3 may be considered for platelet transfusion.

Extensive mucous membrane bleeding dictates platelet transfusion irrespective of platelet count, in order to avoid significant hemorrhage.

If spontaneous vaginal delivery is anticipated, classically a platelet count of 20,000/mm^3 has been the threshold for platelet transfusion.

Platelets should be transfused in DIC only when the patient is actively bleeding. The typical dose for a bleeding thrombocytopenic patient is 1 unit per 10 kg of weight (usually 6 units for an adult). In a 70-kg adult, each unit of platelets will increase the platelet count by 5,000/mm^3.

Occasionally the response to platelet transfusion may be poor, usually due to the presence of antibodies to human leukocyte antigens (HLA). Clinically, the antibodies should be suspected in DIC cases with poor clinical response after transfusion and a poor post-transfusion platelet count increment (calculated by the CCI method previously described). This situation is treated by administering either cross-matched or HLA-matched platelets.

Red blood cells

Red blood cells are capable of increasing oxygen-carrying capacity; however they should not be used as plasma expanders. The infusion of excessive amounts of packed red blood cells may result in hypervolemia.

One unit of red blood cells has a volume of 250 mL. The components of red blood cells have hematocrits ranging from 52 to 80% depending on the storage method used in the blood bank. Each unit increases the hemoglobin by about 1 g/dL and the hematocrit by approximately 3%.

Heparin

In many conditions, heparin therapy may be the next line of treatment for intravascular thrombosis (Rubin & Colman, 1992; Gilbert & Scalzi, 1993; Bick, 1994), although heparin is rarely indicated in the obstetric patient because of the presence of vascular disruption and active bleeding. The only time heparin therapy may be indicated in obstetric patients is for the treatment of hypofibrinogenemia associated with intrauterine fetal death with no active bleeding. Low-dose subcutaneous heparin appears to be effective and safer than larger doses of intravenous heparin (Sakurawaga et al., 1993). In this case, AT III levels should be determined when possible, because low levels of AT III (frequently seen in cases of DIC) are associated with a lack of response to heparin therapy (Nishiyama et al., 2000).

New treatment strategies

New therapeutic options have been described for the treatment of DIC in the last decade. These include antithrombin concentrates, synthetic serine protease inhibitors, and activated protein C concentrates. Their use should neither be considered first-line therapy nor standard care until further research data are available.

Antithrombin concentrates

Antithrombin is a serine protease inhibitor that inhibits activity of thrombin, factors Xa, XIa, VIIa, IX, XIIa, plasmin, and kallikrein (Bucur et al., 1998). Infusion of this product might therefore stop the pathologic activation of both the clotting system and the fibrinolytic system. Intravenous infusions of 1,500–3,000 units a day are used.

In obstetrics, the use of antithrombin has resulted in decreased levels of FDPS and increased fibrinogen and platelet levels. The prophylactic use of antithrombin concentrates prior to surgery or delivery can be recommended, since delivery or surgical procedures in patients with DIC and low levels of AT III can result in severe bleeding. Antithrombin monotherapy is preferably employed (Kobayashi et al., 2001).

Synthetic serine protease inhibitors

Synthetic serine protease inhibitors such as gabexate mesilate and nafamostat mesilate are used for the treatment of DIC in obstetrics in other countries, but their use in the USA has been limited. Theses substances inhibit the clotting activity of thrombin, and they competitively inhibit the enzymatic reactions needed for the activation of factor X, plasmin, and kallikrein. Gabexate mesilate has been used in doses of 20–39 mg/kg IV per day (Kobayashi et al., 2001). The protease inhibitors are capable of inhibiting the clotting cascade through a mechanism independent of AT III (Yokota et al., 2001). Nafamostat is 10 to 100 times more potent than gabexate (Keck et al., 2001). The use of synthetic protease inhibitors in DIC may block the generation of thrombin as well as the resultant increase in fibrinolysis.

Activated protein C

Protein C is a naturally occurring anticoagulant protein. It can inhibit factors V and VIII and also activate the fibrinolytic system. Once again, Kobayashi et al. (1999) have used intravenous infusions of activated protein C in patients with obstetric DIC. Patients with placental abruption and DIC received infusions of 5,000–10,000 units for as long as 48 hours, resulting in significant increases in fibrinogen levels 48 hours after the administration. The investigators concluded that protein C concentrates are a safe and effective option for the treatment of DIC in obstetrics. Protein C concentrates may hold hope for future treatment of DIC.

Conclusions

DIC continues to be an important contributor to maternal morbidity and mortality in the obstetric setting. This syndrome is generally associated with well-defined clinical disorders, some of which are seen exclusively in pregnancy. The practicing obstetrician should be familiar with the pathophysiology, clinical presentation, and treatment of DIC in order to institute early treatment so that both short-term and long-term sequelae can be minimized. Further understanding of the clotting mechanisms has yielded new therapeutic options that may soon be available for clinical practice.

References

Aird WC. Vascular bed-specific hemostasis: role of endothelium in sepsis pathogenesis. Crit Care Med 2001;29:S28–34.

American Association of Blood Banks. Technical Manual, 13th edn. Bethesada, MD: American Association of Blood Banks, 1999a.

American Association of Blood Banks. Blood Transfusion Therapy, 6th edn. Bethesda, MD: American Association of Blood Banks, 1999b.

Anas F, Mancilla-Jimenez R. Hepatic fibrinogen deposits in preeclampsia: immunofluorescent evidence. N Engl J Med 1976;295:578.

Baker PN, Cunningham FG. Platelet and coagulation abnormalities. In: Lindheimer MD, Roberts JM, Cunningham FG, eds. Chesley's Hypertensive Disorders in Pregnancy, 2nd edn. Stamford, CT: Appleton & Lange, 1999:349.

Basu HK. Fibrinolysis and abruptio placenta. Br J Obstet Gynaecol 1971;109:604.

Bick RL. Disseminated intravascular coagulation and related syndromes: etiology, pathophysiology, diagnosis, and management. Am J Hematol 1978;5:265–282.

Bick RL. Disseminated intravascular coagulation: objective criteria for diagnosis and management. Med Clin North Am 1994;78: 511–543.

Bick RL. Syndromes of disseminated intravascular coagulation in obstetrics, pregnancy and gynecology. Objective criteria for diagnosis and management. Hematol Oncol Clin North Am 2000;14:999–1044.

Bick RL, Arun B, Frenkel EP. Disseminated intravascular coagulation: clinical and pathophysiological mechanisms and manifestations. Hemostasis 1999;29:111–134.

Birmingham Eclampsia Study Group. Intravascular coagulation and abnormal lung-scans in preeclampsia and eclampsia. Lancet 1971;ii:889–891.

Brandjes DP, Schenk BE, Buller HR, et al. Management of disseminated intravascular coagulation in obstetrics. Eur J Obstet Gynecol Reprod Biol 1991;42:S87–89.

Bucur SZ, Levy GJ, Despotis GJ, et al. Uses of antithrombin III concentrate in congenital and acquired deficiency states. Transfusion 1998;38:481–498.

Carr JN, McKinney M, McDonagh J. Diagnosis of disseminated intravascular coagulation role of D-dimer. Am J Clin Pathol 1989;91:280–287.

Castro MA, Goodwin TM, Shaw KJ, et al. Disseminated intravascular coagulation and antithrombin III depression in acute fatty liver of pregnancy. Am J Obstet Gynecol 1996;174:211–216.

Clark SL, Hankins GD, Dudley DA, et al. Amniotic fluid embolism: an analysis of a national registry. Am J Obstet Gynecol 1995;172: 1158–1169.

College of American Pathologists. Practice parameter for the use of fresh frozen plasma, cryoprecipitate, and platelets. Fresh Frozen Plasma, Cryoprecipitate and Platelets Administration Practice Guidelines, Development Task Force of the College of American Pathologists. JAMA 1994;271:777.

Creasy R, Resnik R, eds. Maternal Fetal Medicine, 4th edn. Philadelphia: WB Saunders, 1999.

Cunningham FG, Gant NF, Leveno KJ, Gilstrap LC, Hauth JC, Wenstrom KD. Williams Obstetrics, 21st edn. New York: McGraw-Hill, 2001.

Davies S. Amniotic fluid embolism and isolated disseminated intravascular coagulation. Can J Anaesth 1999;46:456.

Douglas JT, Shah M, Lowe GD, et al. Plasma fibrinopeptide A and beta thromboglobulin levels in preeclampsia and hypertensive pregnancy. Thromb Haemost 1982;47:54–55.

Eby CS. A review of the hypercoagulable state. Hematol Oncol Clin North Am 1993;7:1121–1142.

Faught W, Garner P, Johnes G, Ivey B. Changes in protein C and protein S levels in normal pregnancy. Am J Obstet Gynecol 1995;172:147–150.

Gabbe S, Niebyl J, Simpson JL. Obstetrics, Normal and Problem Pregnancies, 4th edn. New York: Churchill Livingstone, 2002.

Gerbasi FP, Bottoms S, Farag A, Mammen E. Increased intravascular coagulation associated with pregnancy. Obstet Gynecol 1990; 75:385–389.

Ghirardini G, Battioni M, Bertellini C, et al. D-dimer after delivery in uncomplicated pregnancies. Clin Exp Obstet Gynecol 1999;26: 211–212.

Gilabert J, Estelles A, Aznar J, Galbis M. Abruptio placentae and disseminated intravascular coagulation. Acta Obstet Gynecol Scand 1985;64:35–39.

Gilbert JA, Scalzi RP. Disseminated intravascular coagulation. Emerg Med Clin North Am 1993;11:465–480.

Halim A, Bhuiyan AB, Azim FA, et al. Blood coagulation and fibrinolysis in eclamptic patients and their correlation with the clinical signs. Gynecol Obstet Invest 1995;39:97–102.

Halim A, Kanayama N, el Maradny E, et al. Plasma P selectin (GMP-140) and glycocalicin are elevated in preeclampsia and eclampsia: their significance. Am J Obstet Gynecol 1996;174:272–277.

Hobisch-Hagen P, Mortl M, Schobersberger W. Hemostatic disorders in pregnancy and the peripartum period. Acta Anesthesiol Scand 1997;111:216–217.

Holzbach RT. Acute fatty liver of pregnancy with disseminated intravascular coagulation. Obstet Gynecol 1974;43:740–744.

Kanfer A, Bruch JF, Nguyen G, et al. Increased placental antifibrinolytic potential and fibrin deposits in pregnancy-induced hypertension and preeclampsia. Lab Invest 1996;74:253–258.

Keck T, Balcom M, Antoniu BA, et al. Regional effects of nafamostat, a novel potent protease and complement inhibitor, on severe necrotizing pancreatitis. Surgery 2001;130:175–181.

Kobayashi T, Terao T, Maki M, et al. Activated protein C is effective for disseminated intravascular coagulation associated with placental abruption. Thromb Haemost 1999;82:1363.

Kobayashi T, Terao T, Maki M, et al. Diagnosis and management of acute obstetrical DIC. Semin Thromb Hemost 2001;27:161–167.

Koh SCL, Anandakumar C, Montan S, Ratnam SS. Plasminogen activators, plasminogen activator inhibitors and markers of intravascular coagulation in pre-eclampsia. Gynecol Obstet Invest 1993; 35:214–221.

Laros RK Jr, Penner AJ. Pathophysiology of disseminated intravascular coagulation in saline-induced abortion. Obstet Gynecol 1976;48:353–356.

Lefkowitz JB, Clarke SH, Barbour LA. Comparison of protein S functional antigenic assays in normal pregnancy. Am J Obstet Gynecol 1996;175:657–660.

Levi M, ten Cate H, van der Poll T, et al. Pathogenesis of disseminated intravascular coagulation in sepsis. JAMA 1993;270:975–979.

Locksmith GJ. Amniotic fluid embolism. Obstet Gynecol Clin North Am 1999;26:435–444.

Lurie S, Feinstein M, Mamet Y. Disseminated intravascular coagulopathy in pregnancy: thorough comprehension of etiology and management reduces obstetrician's stress. Arch Gynecol Obstet 2000;263:126–130.

Marder VJ. Consumptive thrombohemorrhagic disorders. In: Williams WJ, Beutler E, Ersleu AJ, et al., eds. Hematology, 4th edn. New York: McGraw-Hill, 1990:1522.

Marinoff DN, Honegger MM, Girard JB. Spontaneous resolution of disseminated intravascular coagulopathy in the second trimester. Am J Obstet Gynecol 1999;181:759–760.

Mason JW, Kleeberg U, Dolan P, et al. Plasma kallikrein and Hageman factor in gram negative bacteremia. Ann Intern Med 1970;1973: 545–551.

Myers AR, Bloch KJ, Coleman RW. A comparative study of four methods for detecting fibrinogen degradation products in patients with various diseases. N Engl J Med 1970;283:663–668.

Naef RW, Morrison JC. Transfusion therapy in pregnancy. Clin Obstet Gynecol 1995;38:547–557.

Nishiyama T, Matsukawa T, Hanaoka K. Is protease inhibitor a choice for the treatment of pre- or mild disseminated intravascular coagulation? Crit Care Med 2000;28:1419–1422.

Okajima K, Uchiba M, Murakami K, et al. Plasma levels of soluble E-selectin in patients with disseminated intravascular coagulation. Am J Hematol 1997;54:219–224.

Olah KS, Gee H, Needham PG. The management of severe disseminated intravascular coagulopathy complicating placental abruption in the second trimester of pregnancy. Br J Obstet Gynaecol 1988;95:419–420.

Ostlund E, Bremme K, Wiman B. Soluble fibrin in plasma as a sign of activated coagulation in patients with pregnancy complications. Acta Obstet Gynecol Scand 1998;77:165–169.

Pritchard JA, Ratnoff OD. Studies of fibrinogen and other hemostatic factors in women with intrauterine death and delayed delivery. Surg Gynecol Obstet 1959;101:467.

Pritchard JA, Cunningham FG, Mason RA. Coagulation changes in eclampsia: their frequency and pathogenesis. Am J Obstet Gynecol 1976;124:855–864.

Rath W, Faridi A, Dudenhausen JW. HELLP syndrome. J Perinat Med 2000;28:249–260.

Redman CWG, Bonnar J, Berlin L. Early platelet consumption in preeclampsia. Br Med J 1978;1:467–469.

Reed RL, Ciavarella D, Heimbach DM, et al. Prophylactic platelet administration during massive transfusion: a prospective randomized double-blind clinical study. Ann Surg 1986;203:40–48.

Reiss RF. Hemostatic defects in massive transfusion: rapid diagnosis and management. Am J Crit Care 2000;9:158–165.

Reubinoff BE, Schenker JG. HELLP syndrome—a syndrome of hemolysis, elevated liver enzymes and low platelet count—complicating preeclampsia-eclampsia. Int J Gynecol Obstet 1991;36:95–102.

Richey ME, Gilstrap LC, Ramin SM. Management of disseminated intravascular coagulopathy. Clin Obstet Gynecol 1995;38:514–520.

Robson S, Shephard E, Kirsch R. Fibrin degradation product D-dimer induces the synthesis and release of biologically active IL-1 beta, IL-6 and plasminogen activator inhibitors from monocytes in vitro. Br J Haematol 1994;86:322–326.

Romero R, Copel JA, Hobbins JC. Intrauterine fetal demise and hemostatic failure: the fetal death syndrome. Clin Obstet Gynecol 1985;28:24–31.

Rosenberg RD, Aird WC. Vascular bed specific hemostasis and hypercoagulable states. N Engl J Med 1999;340:1555–1564.

Rubin RN, Colman RW. Disseminated intravascular coagulation: approach to treatment. Drugs 1992;44:963–971.

Sakuragawa N, Hasegawa H, Maki M, et al. Clinical evaluation of low-molecular-weight-heparin (FR-860) on disseminated intravascular coagulation (DIC): a multicentric cooperative double-blind trial in comparison with heparin. Thromb Res 1993;72:475–500.

Savelieva GM, Efimov VS, Grishin VL, Shalina RI, Kashezheva AZ. Blood coagulation changes in pregnant women at risk of developing preeclampsia. Int J Gynaecol Obstet 1995;48:3–8.

Schuster H. Epilogue: Disseminated intravascular coagulation and antithrombin III in intensive care medicine: pathophysiological insights and therapeutic hopes. Semin Thromb Hemost 1998;24:81–83.

Sorensen JV, Jensen HP, Rahr HR, et al. F 1 + 2 and FPA in urine from patients with multiple trauma and healthy individuals: a pilot study. Thromb Res 1992;67:429–434.

Takahashi H, Koike T, Yoshida N, et al. Excessive fibrinolysis in suspected amyloidosis: demonstration of plasmin–alpha-2 plasmin inhibitor complex and von Willebrand factor fragment in plasma. Am J Hematol 1986;23:153–166.

ten Cate H, Schoenmakers S, Franco R, et al. Microvascular coagulopathy and disseminated intravascular coagulation. Crit Care Med 2001;29;S95–97.

Teitel JM, Bauer KA, Lau HK, et al. Studies of the prothrombin activation pathway utilizing radioimmunoassays for the F_2/F_{1+2} fragment and thrombin–antithrombin complex. Blood 1982;59: 1086–1097.

Terao T, Maki M, Ikenoue T, et al. The relationship between clinical signs and hypercoagulable state in toxemia of pregnancy. Gynecol Obstet Invest 1991;31:74–85.

Trofatter KF, Howell MD, Greenberg CS, Hage ML. Use of the fibrin D-dimer in screening for coagulation abnormalities in preeclampsia. Obstet Gynecol 1989;73:435–440.

Vigil De Gracia P. Acute fatty liver and HELLP syndrome: two distinct pregnancy disorders. Int J Gynaecol Obstet 2001;73:215–220.

Weiner AE, Reid DE, Roby CC, et al. Coagulation defects with intrauterine death from Rh isosensitization. Am J Obstet Gynecol 1950;60:1015.

Weiner C, Kwaan H, Hauck WW, et al. Fibrin generation in normal pregnancy. Obstet Gynecol 1984;64:46–48.

Wessler S, Gitel SN. Warfarin: from bedside to bench. N Engl J Med 1984;311:645–652.

Yaw RH, Wan YL. Successful management of intractable puerperal hematoma and severe post partum hemorrhage with DIC through transcatheter arterial embolization: two cases. Acta Obstet Gynecol Scand 1998;77:129.

Yokata T, Yamada Y, Takahashi M, et al. Successful treatment of DIC with a serine proteinase inhibitor. Am J Emerg Med 2001;19:334.

31 Thrombotic microangiopathies

Christopher A. Sullivan
James N. Martin, Jr

The term "thrombotic microangiopathy" (TMA) defines a fairly uncommon and severe group of syndromes that are pathologically distinguished by (i) vessel wall thickening (mainly arterioles and capillaries), (ii) swelling or detachment of the endothelial cell from the basement membrane, (iii) accumulation of fluffy material in the subendothelial space, (iv) intraluminal platelet thrombosis, and (v) obstruction of the vessel lumina (Ruggenenti et al., 2001). These syndromes can have numerous associated clinical features, depending on the particular organ system(s) affected. In the future, as the etiologies of these syndromes become more clear, differentiation between the disorders may be distinguished by clinical and laboratory investigation. However, at this time, no specific testing to distinguish a particular disease state is available.

The inclusive term "thrombotic microangiopathy" was first introduced by Symmers (1952). Terminology in this area is often confusing, as is the relationship of pregnancy to these conditions, such as hemolytic–uremic syndrome (HUS), more commonly seen in nonpregnant individuals. TMA is perhaps best conceptualized by considering the terms "hemolytic–uremic syndrome" and "thrombotic thrombocytopenic purpura" (TTP) to refer to different points in the spectrum of presentation of these diseases in a particular patient. TMA can be initiated by a number of seemingly different antecedent events, such as infection, autoimmune disease, and pregnancy. However, this spectrum can also include the HELLP (hemolysis, elevated liver enzymes, and low platelets) syndrome variant of severe preeclampsia or, as with other disorders involving renal compromise, can predispose the patient to develop this condition (Isler et al., 2001).

Various forms of TMA can be associated with pregnancy. Some of these are pregnancy-specific. Others are uncommon in the nonpregnant adult woman but are noted to occur with greater frequency during gestation, such as TTP and HUS. A few TMAs are considered only rarely in pregnancy and have distinguishable clinical or laboratory features that can facilitate diagnosis (Evans' syndrome, acute allograft rejection, complications of certain medications, or TMA associated with autoimmune disease) (Martin et al., 1991).

Except for the spectrum of severe preeclampsia–eclampsia, few obstetricians or their maternal–fetal medicine or internal medicine consultants have much experience with these pregnancy-associated syndromes. Thus, the management of affected patients can be a bewildering exercise. Consequently, the aim of this chapter is to describe the differential diagnosis of pregnancy-associated TMAs, elaborate the pathophysiologic mechanisms that may underlie the more common forms seen during pregnancy (TTP/HUS), and develop a rational approach to management of the pregnant patient with a TMA, focusing in particular on TTP/HUS.

Historic considerations

The first recorded case of TTP was described by Moschcowitz (1925), who noted a previously undescribed symptom complex of hemolytic anemia, hemorrhage, neurologic abnormalities, and renal failure, resulting in the death of a 16-year-old girl. Although thrombocytopenia was never documented, autopsy findings were consistent with widespread microvascular thromboses, which Moschcowitz attributed to a powerful toxin with hemolytic and agglutinative properties. Numerous case reports followed until the 1950s, when the clinical and pathologic features of the disease were established (Gore, 1950; Barondess, 1952).

A similar constellation of signs and symptoms, including hemolytic anemia and thrombocytopenia but associated primarily with acute renal failure, was first described by Gasser et al. (1955). The disturbance was believed to be a distinct entity confined to the kidney and it was therefore named "hemolytic–uremic syndrome." Further investigation has not confirmed Gasser's suspicions (Amorosi & Ultman, 1966; Eknoyan & Riggs, 1986), because both TTP and HUS have been associated with multiorgan involvement, including cerebral disturbances (originally thought to be specific to TTP) and acute renal failure. Until very recently, the prevailing opinion was that these disorders represented a spectrum of disease of common etiology, with similar pathologic features of TMA

(Byrnes & Moake, 1986). Subsequent investigation has helped elucidate the biochemical mechanism by which TTP develops, a process which could be different from HUS (see below).

An explosion of various therapies designed to alleviate the devastating effects of these syndromes has occurred during the past 20 years. The list includes corticosteroids, immunosuppressive agents, antiplatelet drugs, plasma exchange (PEX), plasma infusion (PI), and whole blood exchange transfusion. Utilization of a combination of these various modalities has contributed to a dramatic improvement in survival and much speculation concerning the etiology of these disorders (Ruggenenti & Remuzzi, 1990; Moake, 1991; Egerman et al., 1996).

Thrombotic thrombocytopenic purpura/hemolytic–uremic syndrome

Disease profile

TTP/HUS is more common in females (10:1, female–male ratio), with no apparent racial predilection. A genetic basis for disease susceptibility has not been demonstrated to date, but is likely. It usually appears in the third decade of life, although certain forms of the syndrome can appear from infancy through the geriatric period. Because TTP/HUS is rare, the true incidence of the disease is difficult to determine. One report from a major teaching institution noted an average of six cases per 50,000 yearly admissions (Bell, 1991). The incidence in pregnancy has been estimated to be 1 in 25,000 live births (Dashe et al., 1998).

There is no seasonal variation in the incidence of this syndrome. Although it can occur at any time during pregnancy, the disease appears more commonly in the peripartum period (late third trimester, early puerperium) (Bell, 1991; Egerman et al., 1996).

Associated agents or conditions

In a significant number of patients with TTP/HUS, it is likely that infectious agents or certain pharmaceuticals can trigger the development of the syndrome. A prodromal illness similar to a viral infection occurs in 40% of patients. Associated agents include coxsackievirus A and B, *Mycoplasma* pneumonia, or recent vaccinations (Neumann & Urizar, 1994). A significant relationship between bacterial endotoxins and HUS has been described in numerous reports and is discussed in detail in the section dealing with pathogenesis (Moake, 1994). A TTP/HUS-like syndrome has been noted in certain patients infected with the human immunodeficiency virus (HIV) (Ucar et al., 1994).

There is also a strong association between TTP/HUS and antineoplastic and immunosuppressive agents. Triggering chemotherapeutic agents include mitomycin C, bleomycin, mithramycin, cytosine arabinoside, and daunorubicin, while the immunosuppressants cyclosporin A and FK-506 have been associated with a TTP/HUS-like arteriopathy leading to renal allograft loss. More recently, drug reactions to ticlopidine and clopidogrel have been seen in association with a TTP/HUS-like syndrome (Allford & Machin, 2000). Certain neoplastic conditions also can coexist with the syndrome, including non-Hodgkin's lymphoma, certain forms of leukemia, and particular adenocarcinomas (Kwaan, 1987; Holman et al., 1993). Oral contraceptives and levonorgestrel implants have also been linked to TMA-type syndromes (Fraser et al., 1996).

There are familial forms of TTP/HUS. One report described five families with multiple members who contracted TTP, including two sisters who developed the condition during and immediately after pregnancy (Wiznitzer et al., 1992). The condition is most likely inherited in an autosomal recessive pattern. In these patients, TTP/HUS is associated with a high mortality rate (70%) and a significant risk of recurrence (Berns et al., 1992). Since the last edition of this book, the genetic mechanism of disease in inheritable cases has been elucidated (Levy et al., 2001; Ruggenenti et al., 2001).

There appears to be a significant relationship between the microangiopathic syndromes and underlying connective tissue disease. TTP/HUS has been described in patients with systemic lupus erythematosus (SLE) (especially in patients with the associated antiphospholipid antibody syndrome; Huang et al., 1998), Sjogren's syndrome, rheumatoid arthritis, and polyarteritis. The most frequent association appears to be between SLE and TTP/HUS, although the incidence varies widely. The postulated mechanism in this situation involves immune-mediated vasculopathy, immune complex deposition, or both (Byrnes & Moake, 1986; Meyrier et al., 1991; Stricker et al., 1992).

Finally, there is a strong association between TTP/HUS and pregnancy, with most cases occurring in the latter part of gestation and/or the puerperium. The etiologic basis between the two conditions is speculative at present but could include an immune mechanism, vascular endothelial damage, or prostanoid imbalance (Pinette et al., 1989).

Clinical features

Neuologic symptoms often predominate in TTP and can include headache, aphasia, altered consciousness (stupor, confusion, coma), parasthesia, paresis, syncope, cranial nerve palsies, seizures, or stroke (Egerman et al., 1996). Characteristically, the neurologic symptoms are transient and fluctuating, probably secondary to microvascular platelet aggregation and occlusion of susceptible cerebral arterioles. Patients with HUS can present with neurologic manifestations, but renal involvement is more dramatic. With HUS, the majority of patients require dialysis, a feature which helps to distinguish between the two syndromes. Other findings elicited during the history and physical examination are listed in Table 31.1.

Table 31.1 The spectrum of clinical features in adult TTP/HUS

Presenting symptoms	Frequency	Presenting signs
Neurologic (60%) (often intermittent)	Very common	Fever (98%)
Confusion		Hemorrhage (96%)
Mental status changes		Petechiae ecchymoses
Dizziness		
Headache		Neurologic (92%)
Focal/central losses		Tremor
Bleeding (44%)		Hemiparesis
		Seizures
Gastrointestianl (30%)		Coma
Abdominal pain (11%)		
Nausea/vomiting (24%)		Pallor (96%)
Diarrhea		Jaundice (42%)
Nonspecific		Abdominal tenderness (13%)
Fatigue (25%)		
Viral prodrome (40%)		
Arthralgia (7%)	Least common	

(Adapted from Bell W. Thrombotic thrombocytopenic purpura. JAMA 1991;265:91.)

Although fever is not often a notable clinical symptom, it is commonly found on physical examination, as are pallor and hemorrhage.

TTP/HUS continues to be a diagnosis of exclusion. Although there is no single laboratory test that can be used to reliably differentiate it from other disorders, there is a certain group of laboratory findings that should guide the clinician to consider the diagnosis (Table 31.2). The test that provides the most immediate clue to TTP/HUS is examination of the peripheral blood smear. Evidence of a fulminant hemolytic process (microangiopathic hemolytic anemia), including red-cell fragmentation (burr cells, helmet cells, and schistocytes) and severe thrombocytopenia (platelet count 50,000/mm^3), strongly suggests TTP/HUS. Intravascular hemolysis is reflected by a high serum lactic dehydrogenase (LDH), elevated indirect bilirubin, reduced haptoglobin, hemoglobinemia, and occasionally hemoglobinuria. Direct Coombs' testing should be negative.

Both TTP and HUS are commonly associated with renal dysfunction, including proteinuria, hematuria, and azotemia. Histologic confirmation by bone marrow core biopsy (megakaryocytic hyperplasia), skin biopsy of a petechial spot, or renal biopsy (Droz et al., 2000) can sometimes substantiate the diagnosis in confusing cases. The classic clinical pentad associated with TTP/HUS thus consists of fever, thrombocytopenia, microangiopathic hemolytic anemia, neurologic abnormalities, and renal disease (Amorosi & Ultman, 1966; Ridolfi & Bell, 1981; Bartholomew & Bell, 1986).

Table 31.2 Laboratory features of TTP

Laboratory features
Microangiopathic hemolytic anemia (100%)
Anemia: often severe (96%)
Reticulocytosis
Red-cell fragmentation (100%)
Nucleated red cells, spherocytes, myelocytes, schistocytes, helmet cells
High LDH
Negative direct Coombs' test
Indirect hyperbilirubinemia (60%)
Hemoglobinemia (occasional)
Leukocytosis
Absent serum haptoglobin
Thrombocytopenia: usually severe (100%)
Azotemia: usually mild to moderate (88%)
Normal coagulation parameters: PT, PTT, fibrinogen, AT III, fibronectin
Abnormal urinary sediment
Microscopic hematuria
Proteinuria
Hemoglobinuria
Bone marrow aspirate: marked megakaryocytic hyperplasia
Gingival/skin biopsy of petechial spot: platelet microthrombi

AT III, antithrombin III; LDH, lactate dehydrogenase; PT, prothrombin time; PTT, partial thromboplastin time.
(Adapted from Bell W. Thrombotic thrombocytopenic purpura. JAMA 1991;265:91.)

Differential diagnosis

Given the wide range of clinical symptomatology and laboratory findings observed in patients with a TMA, the differential diagnosis for TTP/HUS is considerable (Table 31.3). For the obstetrician encountering a pregnant patient with a TMA syndrome, the most important disease process to exclude is any form of severe preeclampsia. When adult TTP/HUS is present

Table 31.3 Differential diagnoses of adult TTP/HUS

Disseminated intravascular coagulopathy
Evans' syndrome (immune-mediated thrombocytopenic purpura + immune-mediated hemolytic anemia)
Vasculitis
  Systemic lupus erythematosus
  Severe glomerulonephritis
Other causes of microangiopathic hemolytic anemia
  Vascular malformation
  Prosthetic valves
  Metastatic adenocarcinoma
  Malignant hypertension
Adult TTP/HUS-like syndromes
  Acute fatty liver of pregnancy
  Postpartum acute renal failure
  Severe preeclampsia–eclampsia/HELLP

Table 31.4 Distinguishing TTP/HUS from preeclampsia

Feature	TTP/HUS	Preeclampsia
Microangiopathic hemolytic anemia	Frequent	Only with HELLP
Thrombocytopenia	Frequent	Occasional/HELLP
Neurologic dysfunction	Frequent/variable	Occasional
Fever	Variable	Absent
Renal dysfunction	Variable/frequent	Frequent
Hypertension	Variable/frequent	Frequent
Purpuric skin lesions	Variable	Rare
Low fibrinogen	Rare	Variable
Elevated fibrin split products	Infrequent	Variable
Antithrombin III	Usually normal	Often decreased
24-hour calcium excretion	Variable	Usually decreased
Elevated transaminases	Rare	Frequent/HELLP

during the first trimester of pregnancy, the diagnosis is relatively easy to make, and some successful pregnancies after therapy have been reported. Later in gestation, the differential diagnostic problem is more difficult because of striking similarities between the HELLP syndrome and adult TTP/HUS (Vandekerckhove et al., 1984; Thorp et al., 1991). Both diseases can present with thrombocytopenia and microangiopathic hemolytic anemia, as well as with neurologic and renal dysfunction. Parturients with severe preeclampsia–eclampsia often manifest elevation of liver function tests (AST/ALT), and may have hypofibrinogenemia and depressed antithrombin III level (Weiner, 1987). These findings are infrequent in patients with TTP/HUS, who are also more often febrile and do not initially manifest the acute elevations in blood pressure commonly seen in preeclampsia–eclampsia.

It is important to differentiate between the two syndromes, because patients with HELLP/severe preeclampsia or eclampsia usually respond dramatically to delivery, while patients with TTP/HUS require other therapy. Because preeclampsia–eclampsia is the more common condition, it should generally be assumed to be present if clinical and pathologic data are not helpful in differentiating these disorders. Generally, it is not in the best interest of the mother or fetus to prolong a gestation beyond 34 weeks in patients with microangiopathic hemolytic anemia, thrombocytopenia, or elevated liver enzyme levels on the premise that the disease may not actually be severe preeclampsia. If the disease is considered initially to represent severe preeclampsia–eclampsia, yet delivery does not ameliorate the disease process within 48–72 hours, the patient can be considered to have the less likely diagnosis of adult TTP/HUS and alternate therapy can be undertaken (Martin et al., 1991).

It is not unusual for TTP/HUS and preeclampsia to be present concomitantly, making it impossible to distinguish between syndromes and forcing the clinician to direct therapy to alleviate both disorders (Weiner, 1987). A complete listing of the findings common to these disorders and their frequencies is found in Table 31.4. Table 31.5 lists other associated diseases that also may be considered, such as acute fatty liver of pregnancy or autoimmune thrombocytopenic purpura, and their associated differential features (Pinette et al., 1989; Volcy et al., 2000).

Table 31.5 Comparison between TTP/HUS and autoimmune thrombocytopenic purpura (ITP), atypical preeclampsia–eclampsia as HELLP syndrome, and acute fatty liver of pregnancy (AFLP)

	TTP	ITP	HELLP	HUS	AFLP
CNS	+	–	+	–	–
Hypertension	–	–	±	–	±
Fever	+	–	–	–	±
Petechiae	+	+	+	–	–
MHA	+	–	+	+	–
DIC	–	–	±	–	+
Antibodies	–	+	–	–	–
Protein	+	–	+	+	±
LDH	I	N	I	I	I
AST/ALT	N	N	I	N	I
Cr/BUN	I	N	I	I	N/I

Cr/BUN, creatinine/blood urea nitrogen; DIC, disseminated intravascular coagulopathy; I, increased; LDH, lactate dehydrogenase; MHA, microangiopathic hemolytic anemia; N, no change.

Disseminated intravascular coagulation is not commonly seen in microangiopathic disorders. It is a thrombin-driven disorder characterized by increased turnover of both platelets and fibrinogen, accompanied by a secondary fibrinolytic response. In contrast, TMA disorders are platelet-driven processes in which there is increased platelet consumption, normal fibrinogen turnover, absent local fibrinolysis, and no coagulopathy, although fibrin split products may be increased in some patients with adult HUS (secondary to platelet–fibrinogen degradation).

Evans' syndrome describes the coexistence of immune-mediated idiopathic thrombocytopenic purpura and hemolytic anemia and could be confused with adult TTP. In the immune-mediated disorders, platelet or red-cell antibodies should be present and red-cell fragmentation should be absent. As stated before, in patients with TTP, the Coombs' test should be negative. The distinction between adult TTP and vasculitic disorders is best made on the basis of the composite clinical picture, although biopsy of involved vessels may be useful in making the diagnosis. Other causes of microangiopathy also should be considered and include a connective tissue disorder, vascular malformations, prosthetic heart valves, metastatic adenocarcinoma, and malignant hypertension, all of which are usually easy to distinguish clinically (Bell, 1991; Martin et al., 1991).

Etiology and pathogenesis

Although HUS and TTP are considered together as TMAs, certain etiologic agents can be specifically associated with one form of the syndrome.

About 90% of HUS cases are pediatric and occur in late infancy and early childhood. They are preceded by the onset of bloody diarrhea (known as D-positive HUS). *Shigella dysenteriae* serotype I and various *Escherichia coli* serotypes have been identified as etiologic agents, and various other organisms have also been implicated, including *Salmonella typhi*, *Campylobacter jejuni*, *Streptococcus*, and viruses of the coxsackie, echo, influenza, and Epstein–Barr varieties (Karmali et al., 1985). These organisms produce a powerful protein exotoxin that is detectable in feces.

The prototype of the 70-kDa exotoxin is shiga toxin (ST), encoded in *S. dysenteriae* DNA. The structurally related exotoxins SLT-1 and SLT-2 (SLT, shiga-like toxin) are encoded in bacteriophage DNA that is incorporated in the genome of specific *E. coli* serotypes. Of these serotypes, the one most frequently associated with HUS is *E. coli* 0157:H7 (50% of the cases) (Karmali, 1992; Ashkenazi, 1993). These bacteria may be ingested in contaminated food (beef or poultry) that is insufficiently cooked; they then colonize the large intestine and adhere, invade, and destroy colonic mucosal epithelial cells, finally entering the maternal circulation.

ST, SLT-1, and SLT-2 are internalized by endocytosis, preferentially in the renal glomerular endothelial cell. Byproducts of this toxin inhibit protein elongation and lead to overall suppression of protein synthesis (van de Kar et al., 1992). Light and electron microscopy studies demonstrate that toxin invasion leads to swelling and detachment of the endothelial cells in capillaries and small arterioles and to eventual necrosis. Exposure of the subendothelial space allows for enhancement of platelet thrombi formation in these areas. In addition, glomerular endothelial cell injury leads to release of various substances, including von Willebrand factor (vWF or factor VIII). Levels of this substance correlate with the degree of microvascular injury associated with HUS. The development of this syndrome following an episode of bloody diarrhea has been termed the classic or postinfectious form of HUS (Habib, 1992).

HUS can develop weeks to months after exposure to various other previously described triggering agents (D-negative HUS), such as oral contraceptive or immunosuppressive medications, or it can develop spontaneously during or after an uncomplicated pregnancy. Exactly why HUS occurs remains a mystery, although substantial progress regarding the etiology of the disease has occurred in recent years (see below). In general, HUS that is not associated with diarrhea carries a substantially worse prognosis than the D-positive form (Moake, 1994).

TTP is thought to involve an extreme form of microvascular platelet clumping, a process that can be activated by various substances. These include a 37-kDa (Siddiqui & Lian, 1985) or 59-kDa (Chen & Lian, 1989) protein, a calcium-rich enzyme that cleaves vWF multimers into fragments with increased platelet-binding capacity (Moore et al., 1990), or unusually large vWF (ULvWF) multimeric forms (Moake et al., 1982; Moake & McPherson, 1989).

The vWF monomers are naturally linked by disulfide bonds to form large aggregates or multimers (ULvWF) of varying sizes that range into the millions of daltons. Multimers are stored inside both endothelial cells and platelets (although the main source of plasma vWF appears to be the endothelial cell) to be degraded by a specific plasma reductase prior to their entrance into the vascular lumen (Frangos et al., 1989; Moake et al., 2001).

Patients who develop TTP are found to have large amounts of circulating plasma ULvWF during the acute episode. This occurs presumably because of endothelial cell injury or intense stimulation of ULvWF release that overwhelms the degradation capability inherent in plasma. Patients who survive the initial episode and have no relapse almost always have absent plasma ULvWF multimer levels. In contrast, those who have persistent plasma ULvWF multimers will most likely have recurrent episodes of TTP secondary to continued endothelial cell pertubation (chronic relapsing TTP). ULvWF will then stimulate platelet aggregation to the subendothelial collagen, thus triggering microthrombi formation. Those patients with the chronic relapsing form of TTP may have a congenital defect of the endothelial cell that permits augmented release of ULvWF multimers at frequent and regular intervals (Moake et al., 1982; Moake & McPherson, 1989).

Recently, two groups of investigators have helped to link the evidence described earlier into a common pathogenic mechanism for TMA. Landmark studies of Furlan et al. (1998) and Tsai and Lian (1998), published concomitantly, found that deficiencies or antibodies directed against the vWF-cleaving protease play a critical role in the pathogenesis of TTP.

The vWF-cleaving protease cleaves the peptide bond

between tyrosine at position 842 and methionine at position 843 in monomeric units of vWF, degrading the large multimeter released by endothelial cells. Both groups of investigators noted that all patients with TTP had little, if any, vWF-cleaving protease activity during the acute episode of the disease. Most patients who made a full recovery restored protease activity to normal levels during recovery. An IgG autoantibody directed against the enzyme probably accounted for the lack of protease activity during the acute phase of the disease. What triggers release of the autoantibody is still not known.

In patients who carried the familiar form of the disease, no protease activity was noted either in the acute phase or in remission. These patients have chronic-relapsing TTP, and always have ULvWF multimers in their plasma between episodes. What happens between disease exacerbations still remains a mystery. However it is clear that lack of the protease itself is responsible, at least in part, for the manifestations which ultimately result during a clinical exacerbation of TTP.

The clinical penalty for failing to eliminate the large multimers of vWF secreted by the endothelial cells in the microcirculation is the development of platelet aggregation and subsequent thrombocytopenia. The vWF multimers bind to the platelet glycoprotein receptors, leading to large protein thrombi that ultimately obstruct the microcirculation and lead to the clinical manifestations of TTP. Immunohistochemical examination of specimens obtained during these episodes shows that the platelet thrombi occluding microvessels contain vWF but not fibrinogen (Asada et al., 1985). Taking into account all of the above findings, it seems clear that the unprocessed forms of vWF are the deadly aggregating agents of TTP (Moake, 1998). The clinical relevance of these findings explains why plasma therapy is a significant component of disease treatment.

Clinical overlap between the syndromes of TTP and HUS as noted above has now come into question. Certainly, patients with TTP can have renal involvement and patients with HUS not infrequently exhibit extrarenal manifestations of their disease. However, Furlan et al. (1998) have shown that patients with HUS exhibit normal plasma activity of the enzyme, a feature which may lead to clear definition between the two syndromes. This could in the future make it possible for clinicians to order a single laboratory test to differentiate between the two diseases. However, some investigators (Te Loo et al., 2000) feel that this theory is too simplistic (Warwicker et al., 1999), since patients with HUS as well as other disorders have also been found to have no evidence of vWF protease activity. It may be that similar mechanisms are localized to the renal glomerular endothelial cell, or that an alternative pathway exists which results in manifestations that mimic certain findings that overlap between the two disease states (Noris et al., 1999).

A molecular mechanism for deficiency of vWF-cleaving protease has been discovered recently by Levy and colleagues, at least in patients who possessed the familial form of TTP. Mutations in the *ADAMTS13* gene on chromosome 9 led to a decrease in the production of active protease that cleaves vWF (Levy et al., 2001).

Whether this same mechanism could explain both the high risk of TTP/HUS in pregnancy and the strong association with preeclampsia remains to be elucidated. In the studies referenced above, only a small number of patients were pregnant at the time of the investigation, and any association with preeclampsia or the HELLP syndrome was not noted.

Pregnancy

There have been numerous case reports and literature summaries concerning TTP/HUS associated with pregnancy (Ambrose et al., 1985; Kwaan, 1985; Permezel et al., 1992; Helou et al., 1994; Egerman et al., 1996; Dashe et al., 1998). The largest summary of cases in the English language noted 40 cases of well-documented TTP in 65 women and 40 cases of HUS in 62 women over a 19-year period (Weiner, 1987). Cases that appear clinically consistent with preeclampsia were rejected, with the author nothing a bias toward rejecting mild cases of the syndrome.

The majority of cases (40/45) of TTP developed during the antepartum period at a mean gestational age of 23.5 ± 10.4 weeks; 58% of the cases presented prior to the twenty-fourth week of pregnancy. The mean maternal age at the time of onset was 23 years. Symptoms and signs consistent with preeclampsia were identified in 9 of 24 (38%) patients, although only three of these patients were thought to have TTP and preeclampsia simultaneously. Only 25% (10/40) of maternal–fetal pairs survived when TTP was diagnosed during the antepartum period, and the fetal mortality rate was 80% (32/40). Maternal mortality was 44% overall in his series but was highly dependent on the treatment modality utilized. For example, if plasma therapy as infusion or exchange was employed, the mortality rate was 0% (0/17). If this form of therapy was not used, however, the mortality rate substantially increased to 68% (19/28).

HUS is first recognized in the postpartum period in most patients (58/62, 94%), although symptoms generally precede delivery when viewed retrospectively. In cases presenting during the postpartum period, there is an average symptom-free interval of 26.6 ± 35.0 days (range 0–180 days). In most cases, the distinction between HUS and severe preeclampsia is clear, and in only 15% do both syndromes occur in combination. Maternal mortality was high (55%) and was considered to be an underestimate, because almost half of the survivors were on or nearing dialysis at the time of publication. The overall outcome for patients with HUS was thought to be worse than that in patients with TTP, even though only a small number of women received plasma therapy in one series (3/62), all of whom survived (Weiner, 1987).

In a more recent series (Egerman et al., 1996), which included long-term follow-up of patients averaging 9 years, a survival rate of 80–90% was noted. However, 9 of 11 women developed multiple recurrences of TMA, chronic renal insufficiency, including end-stage renal disease requiring dialysis and/or transplantation, severe hypertension, and blood-borne infectious diseases. Two women died, one of AIDS contracted as a consequence of plasma therapy and the other from complications of dialysis. It is clear from this study and others that the development of TMA during pregnancy has significant long-term complications and/or morbidity.

Treatment

A considerable improvement in survival has been recorded in those patients affected with TTP/HUS. In 1964, overall survival was only 10% (Amorosi & Ultman, 1966). In a series of cases reported from 1964 to 1980, survival had increased to 46% (Ridolfi & Bell, 1981). By 1991, the largest reported series of patients treated for TTP/HUS noted a survival rate of 91% (Bell et al., 1991). Undoubtedly, this increase in survival can be attributed to increased availability of improved supportive therapies, including dialysis and antihypertensive regimens and treatment for life-threatening neurologic involement. In addition, earlier diagnosis has allowed detection and rapid intervention in patients with less fulminant disease. Most authors, however, credit the improved survival of patients with TTP/HUS to the therapeutic effect of PI or PEX therapies, which have become a mainstay of treatment for this disorder (Table 31.6) (Caggiano et al., 1983; Shepard & Bukowski, 1987; Roberts et al., 1991; Egerman et al., 1996).

The goals of therapy in TTP/HUS are threefold: (i) to improve the patient's renal and/or neurologic status, (ii) to control episodes of hypertension, and (iii) to reverse the TMA.

Primary therapy

Plasma manipulations

Bukowski et al. (1977) suggested the use of plasmapheresis and replacement with fresh-frozen plasma (FFP) as primary treatment of TTP/HUS. Subsequent reports followed of disease remission following the simple infusion of FFP (PI) (Byrnes & Khurana, 1977; Shepard & Bukowski, 1987). The beneficial effects of PI were thought to be due to a combination of factors, including increased PGI_2 availability, replacement of a deficient PGI_2-stimulating factor, or normalization of vWF metabolism (Goodman et al., 1982). It is now postulated that this is probably not the mechanism that leads to recovery from the disease, and that FFP provides the vWF-cleaving protease needed in those with a deficiency of the enzyme. Plasma exchange (PEX) is thought to derive its benefit, at least in part, from the removal of possibly deleterious circulating substances such as immune complexes, antiendothelial antibodies, abnormal vWF multimers, and products of damaged red cells, platelets, and white blood cells. PEX could also supply via FFP putative lacking factors involved in the pathogenesis of disease (Ruggenenti & Remuzzi, 1990).

Due to current advances in understanding the etiology and pathogenesis of the syndrome, patients who have an antibody directed against the vWF-cleaving protease benefit from PEX, while those with the familial form derive the same benefit by the addition of plasma containing high levels of the vWF-cleaving protease. At this time, differentiation between the two groups of patients is purely investigational and PEX continues to be the recommended treatment of choice. A benefit of PEX over PI is the avoidance or lessening of risk to develop fluid overload.

The fundamental principle of PEX is separation of the blood into its components. This is accomplished by a cell separator, which uses centrifugal force to separate the blood components. Essentially, there are two types of device: continuous flow and intermittent flow. The continuous-flow type is usually favored because it allows simultaneous withdrawal and infusion of blood components and minimizes the amount of blood that is extracorporeal at any given time. Two intravenous lines of at least 17–18 gauge are required in both arms, one to withdraw blood and the other to reinfuse the separated red cells and donor FFP. Complications of PEX include arrhythmia, cardiac arrest, hypovolemia or volume overload (probably accentuated during pregnancy), complications related to vascular access, anaphylaxis, citrate toxicity, metabolic alkalosis (Marques & Huang, 2001), or transmission of infectious organisms (Watson et al., 1990). The estimated risk of posttransfusion hepatitis is 1% per unit of infused FFP, while the risk of HIV is estimated to be between 1 in 40,000 to 1 in 250,000 (Food and Drug Administration, 1989). This is especially important, because a typical adult patient with TTP/HUS who requires multiple PEXs will receive on average more than 200 units of FFP during a disease exacerbation (Bell et al., 1991).

In contrast to PI, PEX minimizes volume fluctuations and is thus the treatment of choice for patients with marginal renal function and severe oliguria (Mokrzycki & Kaplan, 1994). During PEX in the undelivered patient with a viable pregnan-

Table 31.6 Therapeutic approaches to adult TTP/HUS

Primary therapy	*Tertiary therapy*
Fresh-frozen plasma infusion	Splenectomy
Plasma exchange (PEX)	Immunosuppressants
Hemodialysis (HUS)	Azathioprine
	Chemotherapeutic agents
Secondary therapy	Vincristine
Glucocorticoids	Cyclophosphamide
Antiplatelet agents	High-dose immune globulin
Aspirin	
Dipyridamole	
Dextran 70	
Prostacyclin	

cy, we recommend continuous electronic fetal monitoring and vigilant monitoring of maternal pulmonary status. Although each patient's therapy is individualized, the usual policy is to exchange 2–4 L of plasma on a daily basis until a platelet count of more than 150,000/mm^3 is established and then convert to an alternate-day or every-third-day cycle (Martin et al., 1991). A general approach to management is shown by the algorithm in Fig. 31.1.

The goal of PI is to administer the equivalent of one plasma volume (30 mL/kg) over 24 hours, followed by half to one plasma volume per day until improvement is noted. Risks involved are similar to those of PEX, except that PI is more commonly associated with volume overload.

There is evidence that PEX may be more beneficial than PI for the treatment of TTP/HUS. Rock et al. (1991) reported the results of a 7-year multicenter, prospective, randomized trial of PI versus PEX in 102 nonpregnant patients with TTP. Patients in the PEX group received FFP and PEX for a minimum of seven procedures over the first 9 hospital days, with 1.5 times the predicted plasma volume exchanged over the first 3 days, followed 1.0 times the predicted volume thereafter. The other group received PI daily in a cycle of 30 mL/kg over the first 24 hours, followed by 15 mL/kg each day thereafter. In addition to this therapy, all patients received dipyridamole (400 mg/day) and aspirin (325 mg/day) by mouth for at least 2 weeks following entry into the trial.

PEX proved superior to PI for all clinical endpoints. Overall, more patients on PEX (24/51, 47%) had an increase in the platelet count compared with those on PI (13/51, 25%). Only 2 of 51 (4%) patients in the PEX group died during the first treatment cycle, compared with 8 of 51 (16%) of those randomized to PI. More importantly, after 6 months, patients who received PEX demonstrated a lower rate of relapse and a significantly lower mortality rate. The overall mortality in both groups was 29%. These results are conservative, because a large number of patients in the PI group were classified as treatment failures (31/51) and received PEX as a salvage treatment during the study protocol.

Bell et al. (1991) reported a 91% survival in 108 patients with TTP/HUS who were treated with a combination of corticosteroids and PEX. Of the patients in this study, 9% were pregnant at the time of the initial episode. The largest series of TTP reported from one institution during pregnancy detailed eight episodes in 16 pregnancies of five patients (Ezra et al., 1996), with successful disease process reversal in 8 of 12 patients treated initially with PEX. In addition to PEX, patients also received corticosteroids (300 mg of hydrocortisone or its equivalent per day), aspirin (100–500 mg/day), and dipyridamole

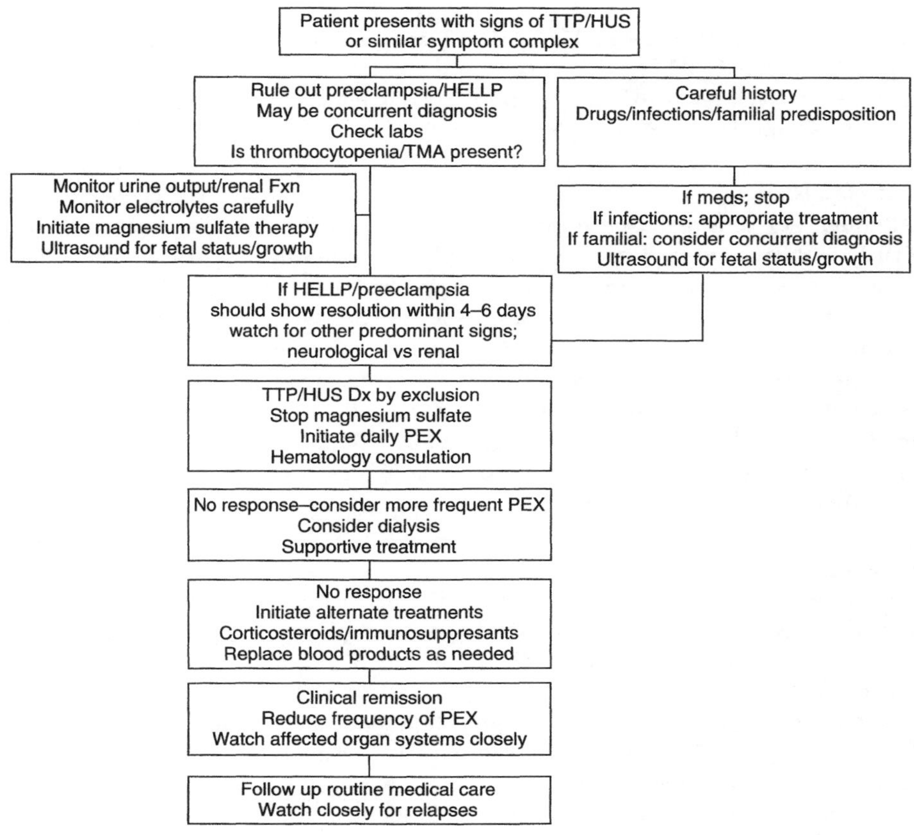

Fig. 31.1 An algorithm for the management of TTP/HUS.

(225 mg/day). In agreement with previous case reports, these authors noted that termination of pregnancy did not affect the course of the disease, although there was a higher incidence of relapse if the patient survived the initial episode and became pregnant again. If therapy were immediate and intensive, the maternal–infant pair could survive.

Based on these reports, we recommend a course of PEX as the initial therapeutic modality in those affected with TTP/HUS during pregnancy. Other therapies (aspirin, steroids, etc.) can be utilized during the primary event or to prevent relapse in accordance with the consulting hematologist's preference.

Secondary treatments

While the therapeutic benefits of plasma for TTP/HUS appear to be well established, the value of a number of adjunctive therapeutic agents is less certain.

Corticosteroids

Corticosteroids were the earliest treatment advocated for TTP/HUS. The rationale for their use was the response seen in occasional patients and the knowledge that platelet survival time is improved with steroid use. Although the efficacy of steroid regimens is debated, nevertheless most patients affected with the syndrome have been treated with steroids in combination with other drugs, making it difficult to evaluate recommendations for their use in the treatment of TTP (Ridolfi & Bell, 1981; Bell et al., 1991). Dosages are variable, but an equivalent of 100–400 mg of hydrocortisone administered daily for 1 week and tapered thereafter until hematologic parameters improve is a reasonable regimen.

Antiplatelet agents

Although not considered beneficial for those affected primarily with HUS, therapy inclusive of antiplatelet agents in noncontrolled studies has proven successful in obtaining remissions in patients with TTP (Amorosi & Karpatkin, 1977; Bukowski et al., 1981). As with corticosteroids, the common use of antiplatelet agents in combination with other therapies makes it difficult to evaluate their actual efficacy. Possible modalities include aspirin (325–1,500 mg/day), dipyridamole (400–600 mg/day), sulfinpyrazone (400 mg/day), and dextran 70 (500 mL IV every 12 hours).

Prostacyclin

The use of prostacyclin infusion in TTP/HUS is consistent with the hypothesis that affected patients may lack a plasma factor required to stimulate prostacyclin production. Given the current theory of the genesis of the disease, prostacyclin infusion may help to prevent platelet aggregation that results from the presence of vWF mulitmers. Unfortunately, experience with this mode of therapy is limited. Some investigators have noted dramatic remissions after failure to respond to PEX as well as PGI_2 infusion failures. The authors of a review of this subject noted that most treatment failures were associated with insufficient dosing or duration of therapy (Tardy et al., 1991). They recommended an initial intravenous infusion of 4–9 ng/kg/min for the first 120 hours of infusion, followed by 48 hours at 9 ng/kg/min. One side effect of prostacyclin infusion is hypotension, which may limit its potential usefulness in pregnancy.

Tertiary treatments

The value of these approaches is even less well established and should be considered investigational.

Splenectomy

Patients with relapsing disease, especially after PEX, occasionally benefit from splenectomy (Wells et al., 1991; Onundarson et al., 1992). This may be due to the removal of the source of the autoantibodies directed against the cleaving protease. Most investigators, however, consider this operation to be ineffective (Ruggenenti & Remuzzi, 1990). In the investigation of Bell et al. (1991), six patients underwent splenectomy as a salvage procedure. All of them experienced a rapid deterioration in clinical status, four patients became comatose, and one died abruptly. Thus, splenectomy for TTP/HUS may be ill advised if not contraindicated.

Immunosuppressive and chemotherapeutic agents

These agents include vincristine, azathioprine, and cyclophosphamide. Vincristine may be efficacious because its depolymerizing effect on platelet microtubules produces secondary alterations in the exposure of cell-surface receptors. This therapy, however, may be teratogenic and should not be employed in the presence of a live fetus. It is administered intravenously at an initial dose of 2 mg, followed by 1 mg every 4 days for a period of 4–6 weeks (Levin & Grunwald, 1991).

The use of azathioprine (Moake et al., 1985) and cyclophosphamide (Wallach et al., 1979) has been associated with the disappearance of ULvWF forms and complete recovery in patients with frequently relapsing TTP. These observations suggest that autoantibodies directed against the protease may be suppressed by this therapeutic approach.

The effectiveness of all these drugs is unproven at present, although vincristine has been shown to produce remission as a single drug treatment.

High-dose immunoglobulins

Intravenous immunoglobulins in large doses for extended periods (0.5 mg/kg daily for 5 consecutive days) have been advocated as a means to neutralize platelet aggregating factors in patients with TTP. The effectiveness of this therapy needs to be established by controlled trials (Raniele et al., 1991; Finazzi et al., 1992).

Table 31.7 Treatment of major electrolyte abnormalities seen in HUS

Abnormality	Preferred treatment	Doses	Comment
Hyponatremia (<130 mEq/L)	Fluid restriction		If hypervolemic
	Diuretics		
	Furosemide	1–2 mg/kg	
	Bumetanide	0.1–0.2 mg/kg	
	Dialysis		
Hypernatremia (>150 mEq/L)	Provide free (H_2O) (D_5W)		If normal glomerular filtration rate
	Dialysis		
Hyperkalemia (>6.5 mEq/L)	IV Ca gluconate (10%)*	1 g/kg	If no hypertension or hypervolemia
	IV $NaHCO_3$*	1–3 mEq/kg over 3–5 min	If no hypertension or hypervolemia
	IV glucose (D_5W)	500 mg/kg over 2 hours	
	IV insulin	0.1 units/kg	
	Cation-exchange resin	1 g/kg	
	Dialysis		If no hypertension or colitis. Removes approximately 10 mEq K^+/hour
Metabolic acidosis (pH < 7.35) (HCO_3 < 15 mEq/L)	$NaHCO_3$	1 mEq/kg	If no hypertension or hypervolemia
	Dialysis		

* Calcium gluconate and $NaHCO_3$ should be given in separate IV lines to avoid calcium carbonate formation and precipitation. Lines must be well flushed between infusions when these substances are given sequentially through the same IV access.

Supportive therapy

In gravidas with adult HUS syndrome, it is critically important to initiate comprehensive supportive therapy to correct fluid and electrolyte imbalance, including, when necessary, dialysis for the control of renal failure. Meticulous attention to salt and water management and correction of hyperkalemia is imperative (Table 31.7). Thereafter, or in concert, PEX is begun as previously described.

Although a significant number of patients with TTP/HUS will be severely thrombocytopenic, with spontaneous bleeding and purpura, the infusion of platelet concentrates should be restricted to circumstances of life-threatening hemorrhage or immediately prior to surgery or any invasive procedure in the patient with a platelet count less than 50,000/mm^3. Administration of platelet concentrates has been associated with worsening of intravascular thrombus formation. Their purported acceleration of the disease process is consistent with the view that intravascular platelet aggregation is probably the initiating event in this disorder (Gordon et al., 1987).

Patients with TTP/HUS are best monitored with sequential blood counts, platelet count, serum creatinine, LDH, and indirect bilirubin determinations. Frequent neurologic examinations are indicated. The two most sensitive laboratory indicators of patient recovery are a rising trend in the platelet count and a decreasing serum concentration of LDH (Patton et al., 1994).

References

Allford SL, Machin SJ. Current understanding of the pathophysiology of thrombotic thrombocytopenic purpura. J Clin Pathol 2000;53: 497–501.

Ambrose A, Welham RG, Cefalo RC. Thrombotic thrombocytopenic purpura in early pregnancy. Obstet Gynecol 1985;66:267–272.

Amorosi EL, Karpatkin S. Antiplatelet treatment of thrombotic thrombocytopenis purpura. Ann Intern Med 1977;86:102–106.

Amorosi EL, Ultman JE. Thrombotic thrombocytopenic purpura: report of 16 cases and review of the literature. Medicine (Baltimore) 1966;45:139.

Asada Y, Sumiyoshi A, Hayashi T, Suzumiva J, Kaketani K. Immunohistochemistry of vascular lesions in thrombotic thrombocytopenic purpura, with special reference to factor VIII related antigen. Thromb Res 1985;38:469–479.

Ashkenazi S. Role of bacterial cytotoxins in hemolytic uremic syndrome and thrombotic thrombocytopenic purpura. Annu Rev Med 1993;44:11–18.

Barondess JA. Thrombotic thrombocytopenic purpura: review of the literature and report of three cases. Am J Med 1952;13:294.

Bartholomew JR, Bell WR. Thrombotic thrombocytopenic purpura. J Intensive Care Med 1986;1:341.

Bell W. Thrombotic thrombocytopenic purpura. JAMA 1991;265:91.

Bell WR, Braine HG, Ness PM, Kickler TS. Improved survival in thrombotic thrombocytopenic purpura–hemolytic uremic syndrome. N Engl J Med 1991;325:398–403.

Berns JS, Kaplan BS, Mackow RC, Hefter LG. Inherited hemolytic uremic syndrome in adults. Am J Kidney Dis 1992;19:331–334.

Bukowski RM, King JW, Hewlett JS. Plasmapheresis in the treatment of thrombotic thrombocytopenic purpura. Blood 1977;50:413–417.

Bukowski RM, Hewlett JS, Reimer RR, et al. Therapy of thrombotic thrombocytopenic purpura: an overview. Semin Thromb Hemost 1981;7:1–8.

Byrnes JJ, Khurana M. Treatment of thrombotic thrombocytopenic purpura with plasma. N Engl J Med 1977;297:1386–1389.

Byrnes JJ, Moake JL. Thrombotic thrombocytopenic purpura and the haemolytic–uraemic syndrome: evolving concepts of pathogenesis and therapy. Clin Haematol 1986;15:413–442.

Caggiano V, Fernando LP, Schneider JM, et al. Thrombotic thrombocytopenic purpura: report of 14 cases—occurrence during pregnancy and response to plasma exchange. J Clin Apheresis 1983;1:71–85.

Chen SH, Lian EC-Y. Purification and some properties of a 59 kDa platelet-aggregating protein from the plasma of a patient with thrombotic thrombocytopenic purpura. Thromb Haemost 1989; 62:568.

Dashe JS, Ramin SM, Cunningham FG. The long-term consequences of thrombotic microangiopahy (thrombotic thrombocytopenic purpura and hemolytic uremic syndrome) in pregnancy. Obstet Gynecol 1998;91:662–668.

Droz D, Nochy D, Noël LH, Heudes D, Nabarra B, Hill GS. Thrombotic microangiopathies: renal and extrarenal lesions. Adv Nephrol Necker Hosp 2000;30:235–259.

Egerman RS, Witlin AG, Friedman SA, Sibai BM. Thrombotic thrombocytopenic purpura and hemolytic uremic syndrome in pregnancy: review of 11 cases. Am J Obstet Gynecol 1996;175:950–956.

Eknoyan G, Riggs SA. Renal involvement in patients with thrombotic thrombocytopenic purpura. Am J Nephrol 1986;6:117–131.

Ezra Y, Rose M, Eldor A. Therapy and prevention of thrombotic thrombocytopenic purpura during pregnancy: a clinical study of 16 pregnancies. Am J Hematol 1996;51:1–6.

Finazzi G, Bellavita P, Falanga A, et al. Inefficacy of intravenous immunoglobulin in patients with low-risk thrombotic thrombocytopenic purpura/hemolytic–uremic syndrome. Am J Hematol 1992;41:165–169.

Food and Drug Administration. Use of blood components. FDA Drug Bull 1989;19:14.

Frangos JA, Moake JL, Nolasco L, et al. Cryosupernatant regulates accumulation of unusually large vWF multimers from endothelial cells. Am J Physiol 1989;256:H1635–1644.

Fraser JL, Millenson M, Malynn ER, Uhl L, Kruskall MS. Possible association between the Norplant contraceptive system and thrombotic thrombocytopenic purpura. Obstet Gynecol 1996;87:860–863.

Furlan M, Robles R, Galbusera M, et al. von Willebrand factor-cleaving protease in thrombotic thrombocytopenic purpura and the hemolytic–uremic syndrome. N Engl J Med 1998;339:1578–1584.

Gasser C, Gautier E, Steck A, et al. Haemolytisch–uramische syndromes bilaterale nierenrin-dennkrosen bei akuten erworbencheuschr hamolytischen anamien. Schweiz Med Wochenschr 1955;85:905.

Goodman RP, Killam AP, Brash AR, Branch RA. Prostacyclin production during pregnancy: comparison of production during normal pregnancy and pregnancy and pregnancy complicated by hypertension. Am J Obstet Gynecol 1982;142:817–822.

Gordon LI, Kwaan HC, Rossi EC. Deleterious effects of platelet transfusions and recovery thrombocytosis in patients with thrombotic microangiopathy. Semin Hematol 1987;24:194–201.

Gore I. Disseminated arteriolar and capillary platelet thrombosis: a morphologic study of its histogenesis. Am J Pathol 1950;26:155.

Habib R. Pathology of the hemolytic uremic syndrome. In: Kaplan BS, Trompeter RS, Moake JL, eds. Hemolytic–Uremic Syndrome and Thrombotic Thrombocytopenic Purpura. New York: Marcel Dekker, 1992:315.

Helou J, Nakhle S, Shoenfeld S, et al. Postpartum thrombotic thrombocytopenic purpura: report of a case and review of the literature. Obstet Gynecol Surv 1994;49:785–789.

Holman MJ, Gonwa TA, Cooper B, et al. FK506-associated thrombotic thrombocytopenic purpura. Transplantation 1993;55:205–206.

Huang JJ, Chen MW, Sung JM, Lan RR, Wang MC, Chen FF. Postpartum haemolytic uraemic syndrome associated with antiphospholipid antibody. Nephrol Dial Transplant 1998;13:182–186.

Isler CM, Barrilleaux PS, Magann EF, Bass JD, Martin JN Jr. A prospective, randomized trial comparing the efficacy of dexamethasone and betamethasone for the treatment of antepartum HELLP syndrome. Am J Obstet Gynecol 2001;184:1332–1337.

Karmali MA. The association of verotoxins and the classical hemolytic uremic syndrome. In: Kaplan BS, Trompeter RS, Moake JL, eds. Hemolytic–Uremic Syndrome and Thrombotic Thrombocytopenic Purpura. New York: Marcel Dekker, 1992:199.

Karmali MA, Petric M, Lim C, et al. The association between idiopathic hemolytic uremic syndrome and infection by verotoxin-producing Escherichia coli. J Infect Dis 1985;151:775–782.

Kwaan HC. Thrombotic thrombocytopenic purpura and hemolytic uremic syndrome in pregnancy. Clin Obstet Gynecol 1985;28:101.

Kwaan HC. Miscellaneous secondary thrombotic microangipathy. Semin Hematol 1987;24:141–147.

Levin M, Grunwald HW. Use of vincristine in refractory thrombotic thrombocytopenic purpura. Acta Haematol 1991;85:37–40.

Levy GG, Nichols WC, Lian EC, et al. Mutations in a member of the ADAMTS gene family cause thrombotic thrombocytopenic purpura. Nature 2001;413:488–494.

Marques MB, Huang ST. Patients with thrombotic thrombocytopenic purpura commonly develop metabolic alkalosis during therapeutic plasma exchange. J Clin Apheresis 2001;16:120–124.

Martin JN Jr, Files JC, Morrison JC. Peripartal adult thrombotic thrombocytopenic purpura and hemolytic–uremic syndrome. In: Clark SL, Cotton DB, Hankins GDV, Phelan JP, eds. Critical Care Obstetrics, 2nd edn. Oxford: Blackwell Scientific Publications, 1991;464.

Meyrier A, Becquemont L, Weill B, et al. Hemolytic–uremic syndrome with anticardiolipin antibodies revealing paraneoplastic systemic scleroderma. Nephron 1991;59:493–496.

Moake JL. TTP: desperation, empiricism, progress. N Engl J Med 1991;325:426–428.

Moake JL. Haemolytic–uraemic syndrome: basic science. Lancet 1994;343:393–397.

Moake JL. Moschcowitz, multimers, and metalloprotease. N Engl J Med 1998;339:1629–1631.

Moake JL, McPherson PD. Abnormalities of von Willebrand factor multimers in thrombotic thrombocytopenic purpura and the hemolytic–uremic syndrome. Am J Med 1989;87:N9–15.

Moake JL, Rudy CK, Troll JH, et al. Unusually large plasma factor VIII: von Willebrand factor multimers in chronic relapsing thrombotic thrombocytopenic purpura. N Engl J Med 1982;307:1432–1435.

Moake JL, Rudy CK, Troll JH, et al. Therapy of chronic relapsing thrombotic thrombocytopenic purpura with prednisone and azathioprine. Am J Hematol 1985;20:73–79.

Moake JL, Sadler JE, Mannucci P, Ganguly P. Report on the workshop: von Willebrand factor and thrombotic thrombocytopenic purpura. Am J Hematol 2001;68:122–126.

Mokrzycki MH, Kaplan AA. Therapeutic plasma exchange: complications and management. Am J Kidney Dis 1994;23:817–827.

Moore JC, Murphy WG, Kelton JG. Calpain proteolysis of von Willebrand factor enhances its binding to platelet membrane glycoprotein IIb/IIIa: an explanation for platelet aggregation in thrombotic thrombocytopenic purpura. Br J Haematol 1990;74:457–464.

Moschcowitz E. Acute febrile pleiochromic anemia with hyaline thrombosis of the terminal arterioles and capillaries. An undescribed disease. Arch Intern Med 1925;36:89.

Neumann M, Urizar R. Hemolytic uremic syndrome: current pathophysiology and management. ANNA J 1994;21:137.

Noris M, Ruggenenti P, Perna A, et al. Hypocomplementemia discloses genetic predisposition to hemolytic uremic syndrome and thrombotic thrombocytopenic purpura: role of factor H abnormalities. Italian Registry of Familial and Recurrent Hemolytic Uremic Syndrome/Thrombotic Thrombocytopenic Purpura. J Am Soc Nephrol 1999;10:281–293.

Onundarson PT, Rowe JM, Heal JM, Francis CW. Response to plasma exchange and splenectomy in thrombotic thrombocytopenic purpura. A 10-year experience at a single institution. Arch Intern Med 1992;152:791–796.

Patton JF, Manning KR, Case D, Owen J. Serum lactate dehydrogenase and platelet count predict survival in thrombotic thrombocytopenic purpura. Am J Hematol 1994;47:94–99.

Permezel M, Lee N, Corry J. Thrombotic thrombocytopenic purpura in pregnancy. Aust N Z J Obstet Gynaecol 1992;32:278–280.

Pinette MG, Vintzileos AM, Ingardia CJ. Thrombotic thrombocytopenic purpura as a cause of thrombocytopenia in pregnancy: literature review. Am J Perinatol 1989;6:55–57.

Raniele DP, Opsahl JA, Kjellstrand CM. Should intravenous immunoglobulin G be first-line treatment for acute thrombotic thrombocytopenic purpura? Case report and review of the literature. Am J Kidney Dis 1991;28:264–268.

Ridolfi RL, Bell WR. Thrombotic thrombocytopenic purpura: report of 25 cases and review of the literature. Medicine (Baltimore) 1981;60:413–428.

Roberts AW, Gillett EA, Fleming SJ. Hemolytic uremic syndrome/thrombotic thrombocytopenic purpura: outcome with plasma exchange. J Clin Apheresis 1991;6:150–154.

Rock GA, Shumak KH, Buskard NA, et al. Comparison of plasma exchange with plasma infusion in the treatment of thrombotic thrombocytopenic purpura. Canadian Apheresis Study Group. N Engl J Med 1991;325:393–397.

Ruggenenti P, Remuzzi G. Thrombotic thrombocytopenic purpura and related disorders. Hematol Oncol Clin North Am 1990;4: 219–241.

Ruggenenti P, Noris M, Remuzzi G. Thrombotic microangiopathy, hemolytic uremic syndrome, and thrombotic thrombocytopenic purpura. Kidney Int 2001;60:831–846.

Shepard KV, Bukowski RM. The treatment of thrombotic thrombocytopenic purpura with exchange transfusions, plasma infusions, and plasma exchange. Semin Hematol 1987;24:178–193.

Siddiqui FA, Lian EC. Novel platelet-agglutinating protein from a thrombotic thrombocytopenic purpura plasma. J Clin Invest 1985;76:1330–1337.

Stricker RB, Davis JA, Gershow J, et al. Thrombotic thrombocytopenic purpura complicating systemic lupus erythematosus. Case report of literature review from the plasmapheresis era. J Rheumatol 1992;19:1469–1473.

Sugio Y, Okamura T, Shimoda K, et al. Ticlopidine-associated thrombotic thrombocytopenic purpura with an IgG-type inhibitor to von Willebrand factor-cleaving protease activity. Int J Hematol 2001;74:347–351.

Symmers VStC. Thrombotic microangiopathic haemolytic anaemia (thrombotic microangiopathy). Br Med J 1952;2:897.

Tardy B, Page Y, Comtet C, et al. Intravenous prostacyclin in thrombotic thrombocytopenic purpura: case report and review of the literature. J Intern Med 1991;230:279–282.

Te Loo DM, Levtchenko E, Furlan M, et al. Autosomal recessive inheritance of von Willebrand factor-cleaving protease deficiency. Pediatr Nephrol 2000;14:762–765.

Thorp JM Jr, Wells SR, Bowes WA Jr. The obfuscation continues. Severe preeclampsia versus thrombotic thrombocytopenic purpura. N C Med J 1991;52:126–128.

Tsai HM, Lian EC. Antibodies to von Willebrand factor-cleaving protease in acute thrombotic thrombocytopenic purpura. N Engl J Med 1998;339:1585–1594.

Ucar A, Fernandez HF, Byrnes JJ, et al. Thrombotic microangiopathy and retroviral infections: a 13-year experience. Am J Hematol 1994;45:304–309.

van de Kar NC, Monnens LA, Karmali MA, van Hinsbergh VW. Tumor necrosis factor and interleukin-1 induce expression of the verocytotoxin receptor globotriaosylceramide on human endothelial cells: implication for the pathogenesis of the hemolytic uremic syndrome. Blood 1992;80:2755–2764.

Vandekerckhove F, Noens L, Colardyn F, et al. Thrombotic thrombocytopenic purpura of seven pregnancies mimicking toxemia of pregnancy. Am J Obstet Gynecol 1984;150:320–322.

Volcy J, Nzerue CM, Oderinde A, Hewman-Iowe K. Cocaine-induced acute renal failure, hemolysis, and thrombocytopenia mimicking thrombotic thrombocytopenic purpura. Am J Kidney Dis 2000;35:E3.

Wallach HW, Oren ME, Herskowitz A. Treatment of thrombotic thrombocytopenic purpura with plasma infusion and cyclophosphamide. South Med J 1979;72:1346–1347.

Warwicker P, Goodship JA, Goodship TH. Van Willebrand factor-cleaving protease in thrombotic thrombocytopenic purpura and the hemolytic-uremic syndrome. N Engl J Med 1999;340:1368–1369.

Watson WJ, Katz VL, Bowes WA Jr. Plasmapheresis during pregnancy. Obstet Gynecol 1990;76:451–457.

Weiner CP. Thrombotic microangiopathy in pregnancy and the postpartum period. Semin Hematol 1987;24:119–129.

Wells AD, Majumdar G, Slater NG, Young AE. Role of splenectomy as a salvage procedure in thrombotic thrombocytopenic purpura. Br J Surg 1991;78:1389–1390.

Wiznitzer A, Mazor M, Leigerman JR, et al. Familial occurrence of thrombotic thrombocytopenic purpura in two sisters during pregnancy. Am J Obstet Gynecol 1992;166:20–21.

32 Endocrine emergencies

Carey L. Winkler
Lowell E. Davis

This chapter reviews the management of diabetic ketoacidosis, thyroid disorders, pheochromocytoma, adrenal crisis, and altered parathyroid states during pregnancy.

Diabetic ketoacidosis

In recent years, diabetes has accounted for approximately 3–5% of all maternal mortality. Approximately 15% of these deaths were secondary to diabetic ketoacidosis (DKA) (Gabbe et al., 1976). However, with prompt recognition and treatment, the risk of maternal death from an episode of DKA is now 1% or less (Drury & Greene, 1977). Unfortunately, the fetus has not fared as well. Despite aggressive treatment of the mother and improvements in neonatal care, studies suggest a 10–25% fetal loss rate for a single episode of DKA (Kilvert et al., 1993; Montoro et al., 1993).

Factors that predispose pregnant women to DKA include accelerated starvation, dehydration, and/or decreased caloric intake secondary to nausea, decreased buffering capacity (respiratory alkalosis of pregnancy), stress, and increased insulin antagonists such as human placental lactogen, prolactin and cortisol (Chauhan & Perry, 1995). Precipitating events in DKA include viral or bacterial infections in 30% of cases, inadequate insulin treatment or noncompliance in approximately 30%, insulin pump failure, and medications (glucocorticoids and/or β-adrenergic agents) for preterm labor (Bedalov & Balasubramanyam, 1997; Bouhanick et al., 2000; Kitabchi et al., 2001). In one series, 7 of 11 patients decreased their insulin dosage because of decreased food intake and lower glucose levels (Cullen et al., 1996). In addition, Montoro et al. (1993) noted that 6 of 20 patients (30%) who presented with DKA were newly diagnosed as diabetic. Finally, it is important to note that DKA may develop in pregnant women at plasma glucose levels less than usually expected. In four patients reported by Cullen et al. (1996), the initial plasma glucose levels were less than 200 mg/dL.

The underlying cause of DKA is an absolute, or more commonly in pregnancy a relative, deficiency in circulating insulin levels in relation to an excess of insulin counter-regulatory hormones, specifically catecholamines, glucagon, cortisol, and growth hormone. The sequence of events has recently been reviewed by Kitabchi et al. (2001). The levels of catecholamines (700–800%), glucagon (400–500%), cortisol (400–500%), and growth hormone (200–300%) are all increased during DKA when compared to baseline. An increase in glucagon leads to inhibition of phosphofructokinase, the rate-limiting step in the glycolytic pathway, decreasing glycolysis. The decrease in insulin reduces glycogen synthase, and glucagons, in combination with cortisol, additionally increase gluconeogenesis through stimulation of several enzymes including glucose-6-phosphatase and phosphoenolpyruvate kinase. The net result is an increase in glucose levels and hyperglycemia. In addition, the decrease in insulin results in proteolysis and increased glucose production from alanine in the liver and from glutamine in the kidney. Epinephrine results in increased tissue lipase and glucagon increases production of hepatic ketone bodies from fatty acids. Because insulin is also needed for the effective degradation of ketone bodies, the excessive degree of ketonemia is due to both overproduction as well as continued under-metabolization.

The main ketone bodies are β-hydroxybutyric acid, acetic acid, and acetone. These moderately strong acids, when released into the maternal circulation, exceed the maternal buffering capability of serum bicarbonate resulting in the metabolic acidosis component of DKA. As hydrogen ions move into the intracellular space from the extracellular compartment, potassium ions shift in the opposite direction. As a result, there is a depletion of intracellular potassium stores that may be greater than indicated by plasma levels. Maternal respiratory changes to excrete carbon dioxide include an increase in the rate and depth of inspiration, also known as Kussmaul respirations. This results in a compensatory respiratory alkalosis. As the degree of hyperglycemia and ketonemia increases, there is a rise in serum osmolarity. In addition, the hyperglycemia and ketonuria result in a profound osmotic diuresis and severe dehydration. Hypovolemia and hypotension soon follow resulting in decreased peripheral perfusion, increased production of lactic acid, and a further decrease in serum pH. This sequence of events sets up a vicious cycle of worsening dehydration, increasing serum osmolarity, increasing release of insulin counter-regulatory hormones from stress and cellular dysfunction, and worsening acidosis.

The loss of free water from osmotic diuresis can be extensive, up to 150 mL/kg body weight. In a typical pregnant patient, this equates to 7–10 L of free water. Along with the loss of urinary water, there is the depletion of many electrolytes, specifically sodium, potassium, and phosphorus. The hypovolemia and hypotension may result in emesis, which can exacerbate dehydration and electrolyte losses. Finally, the increased respiratory rate can cause additional water loss and dehydration.

Usually the diagnosis is quite obvious from a clinical perspective. The patient will present with feelings of malaise, emesis, weakness/lethargy, polyuria, polydipsia, tachypnea, and signs of dehydration (decreased skin turgor, dry mucous membranes, tachycardia, hypotension). The patient may complain of fever, suggesting infection as a precipitating event. Because of the decreased peripheral perfusion and resultant ischemia, patients may have abdominal pain of such severity that it may mimic an intra-abdominal process such as appendicitis. Acetone is highly volatile and is excreted in the patient's breath, causing a classic fruity smell.

Laboratory evaluation should include serum electrolytes, osmolality, creatinine, blood urea nitrogen, urine leukocyte esterase, and arterial blood gases. Classically, the serum glucose will be elevated to 300 mg/dL or more. An arterial blood gas will confirm an acidotic pH (<7.30) along with a decreased serum bicarbonate level. The anion gap will be increased (>12) suggesting the presence of nonvolatile acids. Finally, the serum will test strongly for acetone (1:2 dilution or greater). The predominant ketone produced in DKA is β-hydroxybutyric acid. A commonly used test for evaluating the presence of ketones is the nitroprusside reaction. Neither β-hydroxybutyric acid nor acetone reacts as strongly with nitroprusside as acetoacetate. Therefore, the severity of the ketonemia may be severely underestimated by this test. If possible, direct measurement of plasma β-hydroxybutyric acid should be performed. In addition, as insulin therapy is begun, there is a preferential fall in the level of β-hydroxybutyric acid and increased conversion to acetoacetate. Paradoxically, the nitroprusside reaction may worsen as the condition of the patient improves. However, there should be an improvement in the patient's pH, a decrease in the anion gap, and an overall improvement in the patient's clinical condition. Of note, creatinine may be falsely elevated because acetoacetate interferes with colorimetric methods and elevations of amylase from extrapancreatic secretion do not necessarily correlate with pancreatitis (Kitabchi et al., 2001).

In order to optimize maternal–fetal outcome, the diagnosis needs to be made quickly with immediate initiation of treatment (Montoro et al., 1993). Therapy should consist of rapidly correcting the volume deficits, initiation of insulin, treatment of infection if present, and careful monitoring to aid in correction of the metabolic and electrolyte abnormalities. A transurethral catheter should be placed and urine sent for culture and sensitivity. The initial intravenous solution replacement consists of isotonic saline (0.9% NaCl) at 1,000 mL/hr for at least 2 hours. Using a hypotonic intravenous solution such as half-normal saline (0.45% NaCl) solution can lead to a rapid decline in serum osmolarity. If this occurs too quickly for intracellular equilibrium to take place, rarely cellular swelling can occur, leading to cerebral edema (Van der Meulen et al., 1987). After 2 L of an isotonic solution over 2 hours, the solution should be changed to one more similar to electrolyte losses during osmotic diuresis (0.45% NaCl), given at 250 mL/hr until serum glucose is between 200 and 250 mg/dL. Continuing the use of an isotonic saline solution can result in excessive chloride and metabolic acidosis during the resolution phase. Once glucose reaches 250 mg/dL, intravenous fluids should be changed to 0.45% NaCl with 5% dextrose to prevent an excessively rapid drop in serum glucose. Approximately 75% of the total fluid replacement should occur during the first 24 hours and the remaining 25% over the next 24–48 hours. Unless there are signs of severe dehydration and cardiovascular collapse, a good estimate of the total fluid loss is 100 mL/kg actual body weight.

Since DKA is precipitated by an absolute or relative deficiency in insulin, it is critical that insulin therapy is started in order to correct the many metabolic abnormalities that have occurred. Treatment should be an initial intravenous bolus followed by continuous infusion. Intramuscular or subcutaneous therapy should be avoided as decreased perfusion may result in inadequate absorption (Kitabchi et al., 2001). The initial bolus should be in the neighborhood of 10 units of regular insulin (0.1 units/kg) followed by a continuous infusion of 0.1 units/kg/hr. Serum glucose levels should be determined every hour. The decrease in serum glucose levels should be gradual to prevent excessive movement of water into the cells from a rapid drop in serum osmolarity. A reasonable target is a decrease of 50–70 mg/dL every hour. If serum glucose levels fail to decrease by at least 50 mg/dL in the first 2 hours, the rate of infusion should be doubled (Kitabchi et al., 2001). The insulin infusion should be maintained until most of the metabolic abnormalities have corrected and the patient is feeling well enough to eat. At that time, subcutaneous insulin can be initiated and the insulin infusion discontinued. A thorough search and treatment of the precipitating cause and continuation of insulin is necessary to limit recurrence (Fig. 32.1).

In DKA, there is a significant loss in total body sodium and potassium. The total body loss of potassium can approach over 300 mEq. As the acidosis is corrected, potassium ions shift intracellularly. The intracellular movement of potassium is accelerated in the presence of insulin and can lead to a precipitous decrease in the serum potassium level. As the patient's volume status improves, potassium levels must be followed

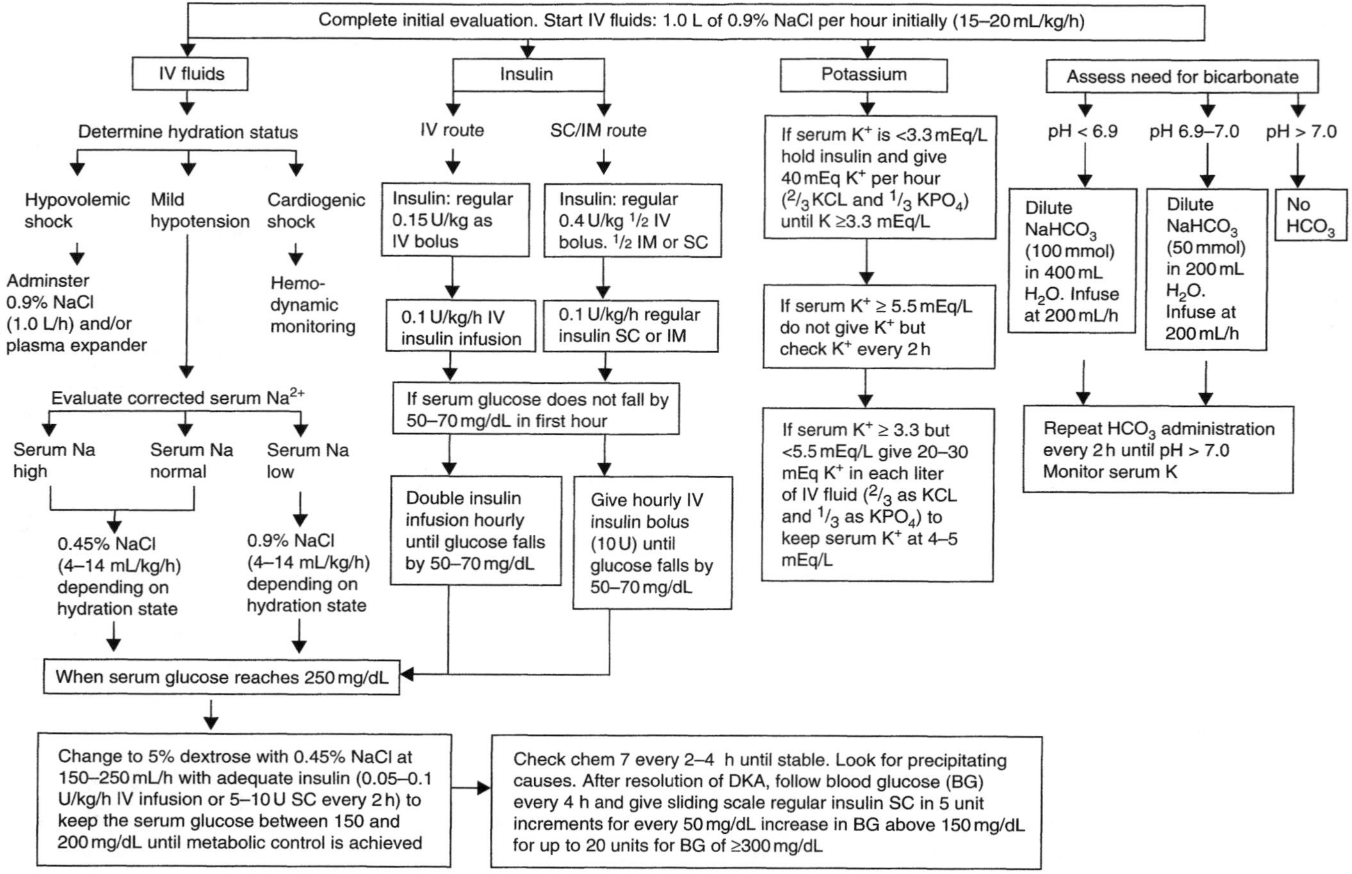

Fig. 32.1 Management of diabetic ketoacidosis. DKA diagnostic criteria: blood glucose >250 mg/dL; arterial pH <7.3; bicarbonate <15. (From Kitabchi A, Umpierrez G, Murphy M, Barrett E. Diabetes Care 2001;24:131.)

closely and immediately corrected when low. It is important to replace potassium slowly and not cause hyperkalemia. Serum potassium levels should be determined every 2–4 hours depending on the levels. Two ways to replace potassium are as follows.

1 Add KCl (40 mEq/L) to each liter of replacement fluids and run at the usual 150–250 mL/hr. This will give approximately 5–10 mEq/hr replacement.
2 Intermittent intravenous infusion boluses: in an additional intravenous port, give 10 mEq/hr infusion for 4–6 hours, check the serum potassium level, and continue the "piggy-back" infusion as necessary.

Because of concerns for toxicity/cardiac arrhythmias, potassium supplements should not be given more quickly than 20 mEq/hr. After the patient is stable and eating a regular diet, oral supplementation can be given for 1–2 days.

The use of intravenous bicarbonate to increase pH and improve organ function is controversial. Sodium bicarbonate treatment has failed to show a difference in outcome in DKA with a pH in the range 6.8–7.1 (Viallon et al., 1999; Kitabchi et al., 2001). However, due to the paucity of patients with pH 6.9–7.0 studied, if the patient has a pH less than 7.0 or the serum bicarbonate level is <5 mEq/L, administration of one ampule (44 mEq) is prudent. Rapid administration of sodium bicarbonate has the potential to cause paradoxical central nervous system acidosis as the blood–brain barrier is freely permeable to carbon dioxide but not bicarbonate.

One final point is evaluation and care of the fetus. Fetal distress may occur due to several mechanisms. Uterine blood flow may decrease due to catecholamine-induced vasoconstriction or dehydration. Secondly, fetal β-hydroxybutyric acid and glucose concentrations parallel maternal levels (Miodovnik et al., 1982) and fetal hyperglycemia may in itself lead to an osmotic diuresis, fetal intravascular volume depletion, and decreased placental perfusion. Finally, a leftward shift of the oxygen dissociation curve with decreased 2,3-diphosphoglycerate increases hemoglobin affinity for oxygen and reduces tissue oxygen delivery. In any case, uterine blood flow is reduced in poorly controlled diabetics (Nylund et al., 1982). A significant reduction in the maternal pH thus will result in a corresponding decrease in the fetal pH. This will often be reflected in abnormal fetal heart rate tracings. Unless there are other overriding reasons for prompt delivery, it is usually prudent to correct the underlying DKA, as the abnormal fetal heart rate tracings and Doppler studies seen in maternal ketoacidosis improve with diabetic control (Hughes, 1987; Takahashi et al., 2000). In the majority of cases, improving the maternal condition allows prolongation of the pregnancy.

Thyroid dysfunction

Multiple changes occur in the maternal and fetal thyroid gland during pregnancy. These physiologic changes have been extensively detailed (Burrow et al., 1994; Glinoer & Delange, 2000). A brief review of changes that affect the interpretation of thyroid tests or thyroid hormone metabolism in relationship to clinical management follows.

Maternal iodide blood levels fall during gestation in part due to an increase in glomerular filtration rate, as well as transplacental iodide transport. When iodide intake is mildly decreased, maternal thyroid volume increased by 30%, there is a marked increase in serum thyroglobulin, and 16% of women develop a goiter (Glinoer et al., 1995). In severely iodide-deficient areas, 50% of individuals have a visible goiter and neonatal hypothyroidism ranges from 2 to 9% (Xue-Yi et al., 1994). In contrast, dietary iodide supplementation in the United States is usually sufficient to maintain normal thyroid function and neonatal hypothyroidism is rare, occurring in 1 of 4,500 infants (Larsen, 1989). A recent survey has suggested however that iodide intake in the United States has decreased in the last 15 years and 7% of pregnant women may have evidence of moderate dietary deficiency (Hollowell et al., 1998). Although some investigators have found that in iodide-replete areas thyroid volume, as measured by ultrasound, is unchanged during pregnancy (Berghout et al., 1994), a mild increase in thyroid volume of 10–20% may be seen (Burrow et al., 1994). Therefore goiter should be investigated and not ascribed to pregnancy changes. Thyroid nodules, particularly solid nodules greater than 2 cm, cystic nodules larger than 4 cm, or enlarging nodules while on thyroid suppression, can be evaluated by ultrasound and fine-needle aspiration (Doherty et al., 1995).

Changes in thyroid hormone levels during pregnancy occur both in the maternal circulation and in the developing fetus. Thyroid-binding globulin (TBG) and total thyroxine (T_4) blood levels increase in the maternal circulation (Fig. 32.2). Sensitive thyroid-stimulating hormone (TSH) and free T_4 assays have largely replaced the free T_4 index and have improved the diagnosis of thyroid disorders during pregnancy. Maternal free T_4 and free triiodothyronine (T_3) blood levels remain within the range of normal values but are minimally decreased in the second and third trimester (Berghout et al., 1994; Burrow et al., 1994). One exception to the interpretation of free T_4 and TSH during pregnancy (Figs 32.3 & 32.4) is the increase in maternal free T_4 and decrease in TSH at 8–12 weeks of gestation when human chorionic gonadotropin (hCG) levels peak (Glinoer et al., 1990). This is thought in part to reflect the weak

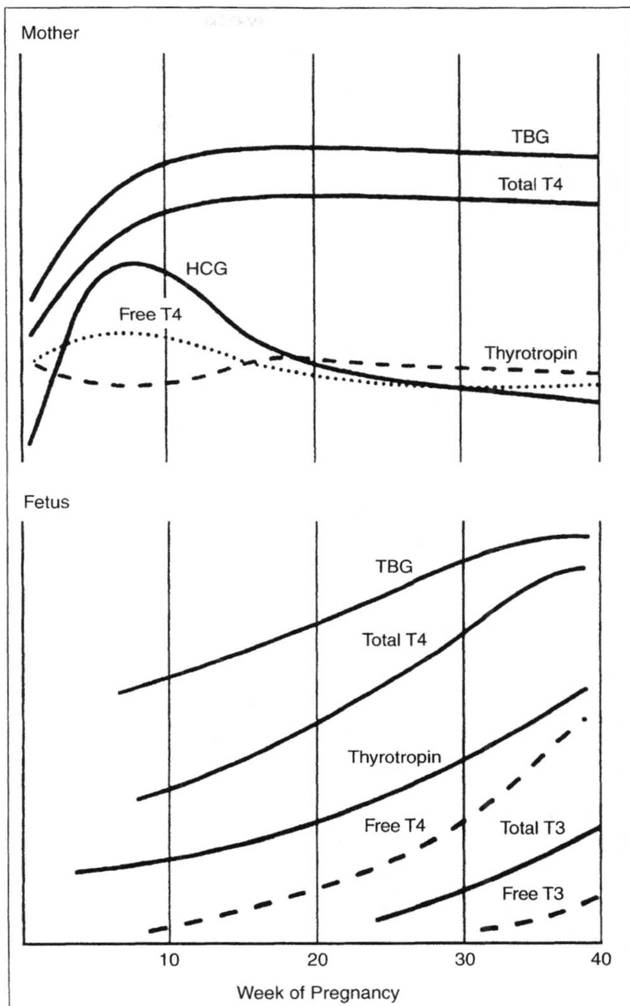

Fig. 32.2 Relative changes in maternal and fetal thyroid function during pregnancy. (Reproduced by permission from Burrow GN, Fisher DA, Larsen PR. Maternal and fetal thyroid function. N Engl J Med 1994;331:1072.)

thyrotropic activity of hCG. Thus, a mild elevation of free T_4 and suppressed TSH level in the first trimester, in the absence of clinical signs of thyrotoxicosis, is likely to be physiologic and does not suggest hyperthyroidism. In some circumstances, it may be reasonable to confirm increased free T_4 levels by equilibrium dialysis as high free T_4 levels may be falsely elevated in some assays due to changes in binding proteins (Mandel & Cooper, 2001; Stockigt, 2001). TSH assays also differ in their sensitivity: third-generation assays have detection limits that approximate 0.005 mIU/L compared to second-generation assays with detection limits of 0.05 mIU/L (Woeber, 2000).

Much remains to be known of the metabolism of thyroid hormones in pregnancy. The daily production of thyroid hormones as measured in nonpregnant individuals is roughly 90 µg of T_4 and 32 µg of T_3 (Degroot et al., 1984). Virtually 80%

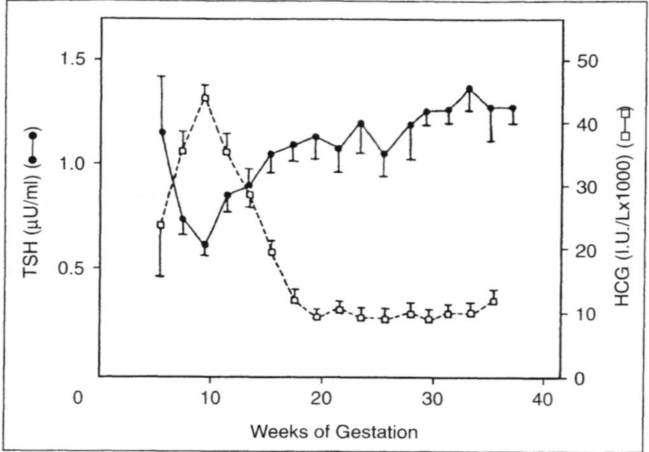

Fig 32.3 Serum TSH and hCG as a function of gestational age. (Reproduced by permission from Glinoer D, De Nayer P, Bourdoux P, et al. Regulation of maternal thyroid during pregnancy. J Clin Endocrinol Metab 1990;71:276.)

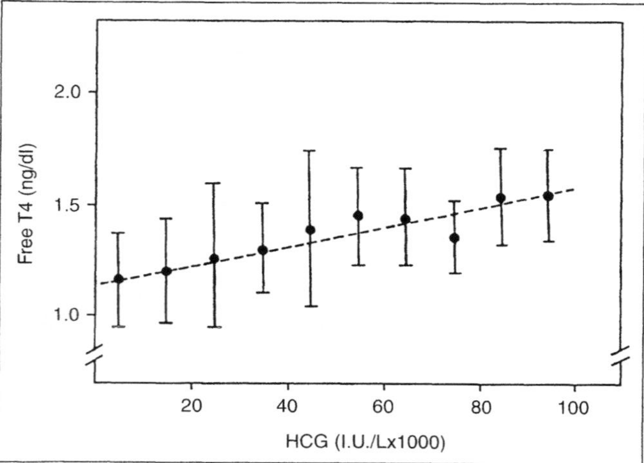

Fig 32.4 Free T_4 in relation to hCG concentrations. (Reproduced by permission from Glinoer D, De Nayer P, Bourdoux P, et al. Regulation of maternal thyroid during pregnancy. J Clin Endocrinol Metab 1990;71:276.)

of T_3 is produced by peripheral conversion of T_4 by 5′-deiodination. Only 0.02% of T_4 is unbound and in free form as compared to 0.3% of T_3. In addition, the half-life of T_4 is 8 days (Hermann et al., 1994) and that of T_3 1 day. Taken together, these data suggest that the relative metabolic potency of T_3 is three times that of T_4.

The clinical consequences of T_4 metabolism are threefold. The first is that thyroid replacement in hypothyroid patients is usually initiated at 100 µg/day (Mandel et al., 1990; Toft, 1994) and often increases during pregnancy. Mandel et al. (1990) found that to normalize TSH levels in pregnant women, the mean T_4 dose increased from 102 to 147 µg/day, an increase of 45%. Similarly, estrogen replacement in nonpregnant women who are hypothyroid is accompanied by an increase in TSH

Table 32.1 Causes of hyperthyroidism

Autoimmune
Graves' disease
Hashimoto's disease
Autonomous
Toxic multinodular goiter
Solitary toxic adenoma
Thyroiditis (transient)
Postpartum thyroiditis
Subacute thyroiditis
Painless thyroiditis
Drug induced
Iodide-induced (Jod–Basedow)
Radiocontrast agents
Thyroxine (factitous or dietary supplements containing thyroid hormones)
Secondary
TSH-secreting tumor
hCG dependent (hyperemesis gravidarum, hydatidiform mole)
Thyroid hormone resistance
Ectopic struma ovarii
Metastatic follicular carcinoma

and decrease in free T_4 levels (Arafah, 2001). Second, in the acute setting of thyroid storm, it is logical to use propylthiouracil instead of methimazole as the former inhibits peripheral conversion of T_4 to T_3, while the latter does not. Finally, clinical symptomatic improvement in patients with acute hyperthyroidism treated with propylthiouracil (measured in days) precedes normalization of thyroid function tests (which may take 6–8 weeks).

Hyperthyroidism during pregnancy is rare, complicating less than 0.2% of all births (Davis et al., 1989; Wing et al., 1994). Early treatment and normalization of maternal thyroid function is important because poor metabolic control increases the risk of preterm delivery, fetal wastage, and thyroid crisis (Davis et al., 1989; Kriplani et al., 1994). By far the most common cause of thyrotoxicosis during pregnancy is Graves' disease, accounting for 60–90% of cases. Less common causes are listed in Table 32.1 and include thyroid adenomas, thyroiditis, or secondary hCG-dependent disorders.

It is generally accepted that Graves' disease is an autoimmune disorder (Weetman, 2000). Prior to the use of thionamides, it was recognized that some 25% of patients undergo long-term remission without therapy (Volpe, 1991). During pregnancy, the course is variable. As in other autoimmune disorders, some patients appear to improve during pregnancy and relapse post partum. Amino et al. (1982) noted in women with Graves' disease near remission at the onset of pregnancy that the free T_4 index was increased in the first trimester, fell in the second and third trimester, and was again increased post partum. A fall in antimicrosomal antibodies during pregnancy and an increase post partum was also measured in patients with Graves' disease or postpartum thyroiditis (Amino et al., 1978). For further information, the reader is referred to a recent review of postpartum thyroiditis, which occurs in 5–7% of patients (Muller et al., 2001).

The diagnosis of Graves' disease is suggested by the presence of thyrotoxicosis, ophthalmopathy, a diffuse goiter, dermopathy, and thyroid receptor antibodies. The diagnosis is clinical and is supported by thyroid function tests; thyroid receptor antibody tests are often not necessary. However, pretibial dermopathy is rarely present in pregnant women, and active clinical ophthalmopathy is evident in only half of patients with Graves' disease (Epstein, 1993; Weetman, 2000). The ocular signs of sympathetic overactivity (lid retraction, widening of the palpebral fissure, lid lag, and staring) generally regress with treatment of hyperthyroidism. Exophthalmos, weakness of the extraocular muscles, chemosis, and impairment of convergence are signs of infiltrative ophthalmopathy and may remain despite normalization of thyroid hormone levels.

In pregnancy, the signs and symptoms of hyperthyroidism are slightly more difficult to interpret due to the normal changes that occur during gestation. Heart rate and cardiac output increase, and heat intolerance, nausea, and weight loss are common. Thyrotoxicosis is suggested by clinical findings, which include a pulse rate persistently greater than 100 that fails to decrease with Valsalva in the presence of a tremor, previously mentioned signs, thyroid bruit, thyromegaly, and mild systolic hypertension. The cardiac effects of hyperthyroidism are summarized in Table 32.2. An elevated free T_4 and low serum TSH by a sensitive assay confirms the diagnosis. Clinical signs of thyrotoxicosis without elevated total or free T_4 should suggest free T_3 thyrotoxicosis or deficient TBG states (Bitton & Wexler, 1990).

"Thyroid receptor antibodies" is a generalized term that may be used to include both thyroid-stimulating immunoglobulins (TSI) as well as thyrotropin-binding inhibitor immunoglobulins (TBII) and may be useful predictors of neonatal thyroid dysfunction (Peleg et al., 2002). The more common receptor assay measures the inhibition of TSH binding to its receptor by displacement of labeled TSH. As such, the assay does not directly measure receptor activation or thyroid activity; therefore TSI or TBII antibodies may be measured (Mortimer et al., 1990; Weetman, 2000). Tests for TSI specifically measure the production of cyclic AMP following stimulation of TSH receptors, but are expensive and not often used. Although antimicrosomal antibodies do not cross the placenta, thyroid receptor antibodies do. Consequently, neonatal thyroid effects may occur years after the diagnosis of Graves' disease, when the mother is either euthyroid or hypothyroid after radioactive thyroid ablation (Volpe et al., 1984).

Table 32.2 Cardiovascular changes in hyperthyroid and hypothyroid states

	Hyperthyroid	Hypothyroid
Cardiac output	↑	↓
Heart rate	↑	↓
Stroke volume	↑	↓
Cardiac contractility	↑	↓
Systemic vascular resistance	↓	↑
Mean arterial pressure	↑	↑
Blood volume	↑	↓
Other	Atrial fibrillation ↓QT ↑PR interval ST elevation	Ascites Pleural effusion ↑QT interval ↑Conduction abnormalities

(Sources: Dillman, 1989;Easterling et al., 1991; Woeber, 1992; Klein & Ojamaa, 2001.)

Neonatal thyroid status may be affected transiently by either thionamide therapy or thyroid receptor antibodies. The incidence of neonatal hyperthyroidism or hypothyroidism due to maternal passive transmission of thyroid receptor antibodies appears to be 1–3%. Mitsuda et al. (1992) reported overt thyrotoxicosis in six neonates of 230 women with Graves' disease. In four of the mothers, TBII levels were elevated. In addition, transient hypothyroidism was found in five neonates with normal TBII levels and thionamide treatment. Mortimer et al. (1990) reported a higher incidence of neonatal thyrotoxicosis in four infants of 44 mothers with Graves' disease; in all four cases the mothers had TBII levels >70%. These investigators observed that the neonatal free T_4 index correlated inversely with maternal thionamide dose. In addition, women who had a free T_4 index in the lower half of the reference range on thionamides were more likely to deliver a child with an elevated TSH than women with a free T_4 index in the upper half of the reference range. Similarly, Momotani et al. (1986) studied 43 women maintained on thionamide therapy until delivery and 27 women in whom thionamide therapy was discontinued due to normalization of thyroid function tests prior to delivery. They found in women who took thionamides until delivery a greater number had fetuses with increased TSH levels, lower T_4 levels, and higher maternal TBII levels. It is important to note that in both of these studies there was only evidence of mild chemical, not clinical, hypothyroidism. However, taken together these data suggest that the minimal dose of thionamide therapy should be used to keep maternal thyroid function at the upper limits of normal. Because TBII antibodies are positive although at lower levels in 50–80% of women with Graves' disease (Momotani et al., 1986; Mortimer et al., 1990; Weetman, 2000), their utility remains to be further demonstrated. The fetal heart rate is an indicator of fetal thyroid function and should be evaluated at each prenatal visit.

Wing et al. (1994) found that only one infant of 185 women treated with propylthiouracil or methimazole had transient hypothyroidism at birth. Similarly, Davis et al. (1989) found one neonate had transient hypothyroidism and a second was euthyroid with an asymptomatic goiter among 43 mothers receiving propylthiouracil. Both were on high doses of propylthiouracil at the time of delivery. This is consistent with a review of the literature by Mandel et al. (1994) in which the incidence of neonatal goiter in women exposed to antithyroid medications was 4%. If necessary, when fetal goiter is detected on ultrasound, umbilical cord blood sampling can be used to differentiate between maternal passive transmission of thyroid receptor antibodies or thionamide treatment (Davidson et al., 1991; Nicolini et al., 1996). Intra-amniotic injection of T_4 is effective in treating fetal hypothyroidism. Indications for umbilical cord sampling have recently been reviewed by Kilpatrick (2003).

In thyroid crisis or storm, an acute increase in the signs and symptoms of thyrotoxicosis may be life-threatening. The overall incidence of thyroid crisis in women who receive thionamide treatment during pregnancy, some of whom remain thyrotoxic, is about 2% (Davis et al., 1989). A clinical diagnosis must be established and treatment initiated well before confirmatory thyroid function tests are available. The classic signs of thyroid storm (altered mental status, temperature >41°C, hypertension, and diarrhea) are not necessarily present. Postpartum congestive heart failure, tachycardia, and severe hypertension should suggest the diagnosis and prompt an evaluation for other signs of thyrotoxicosis. Rarely, loss of consciousness following cesarean section (Pugh et al., 1994) or seizures mimicking eclampsia (Mayer et al., 1995) may complicate the presentation of thyrotoxicosis.

The risks appear to be related to metabolic status and to the precipitating cause. Perkonen et al. (1978) reported that two of seven untreated thyrotoxic women in labor developed thyroid crisis. Similar results were described in eight untreated women in labor, of whom five developed heart failure, and four had stillbirths (Davis et al., 1989). In that series, among 16 other women who had received thionamides but were still thyrotoxic at the time of delivery, two had stillbirths and one developed heart failure, whereas there were no complications in 36 women who were euthyroid. In an expanded review Sheffield and Cunningham (2003) found that nearly 10% of thyrotoxic women developed reversible congestive heart failure. Kriplani et al. (1994) also reported three patients who developed thyroid storm, including one maternal death, among 32 patients who were hyperthyroid during pregnancy. Although thyroid functions were not specifically detailed, thyroid storm was associated with either emergent operative delivery or infection. Thionamide therapy, even of short duration, is generally effective in preventing storm. Therefore, congestive heart failure that occurs after administration of propylthiouracil should suggest other precipitating events: underlying infection, hypertension, or anemia.

The treatment of thyroid storm is somewhat empiric and consists of thionamides, iodide, and β-blockers (Table 32.3). Therapy differs from the usual management of hyperthyroidism in the dose and choice of thionamide. Although propylthiouracil and methimazole are equally effective in the treatment of hyperthyroidism in pregnancy (Wing et al., 1994),

Table 32.3 Treatment of thyroid storm

Propylthiouracil 800 mg administered orally, then 150–200 mg every 4–6 hr
Starting 1–2 hours after propylthiouracil administration
Saturated solution of potassium iodide 2–5 drops orally every 8 hours, *or*
Sodium iodide 0.5–1.0 g IV every 8 hours
Dexamethasone 2 mg IV every 6 hours for four doses
Propranolol 1–2 mg IV repeated every 5 min, up to a total of 6 mg for extreme tachycardia
Phenobarbital 30–60 mg every 8 hours as needed for extreme restlessness
Search for precipitating event, in particular infection
Control temperature if hyperthermic
Critical tests
Free T_4, TSH, urine culture
Evaluate for other autoimmune disorders
Chest X-ray if indicated
EKG (atrial fibrillation)

in the setting of thyroid storm, propylthiouracil is administered by mouth and if necessary by nasogastric tube to inhibit peripheral conversion of T_4 to T_3. Despite inhibition of T_4 synthesis, it may take 7–8 weeks of therapy to deplete thyroid colloid stores and normalize thyroid function tests (Davis et al., 1989; Wing et al., 1994). Clinical improvement commonly precedes resolution of the tachycardia due to the long half-life of T_4. Iodide inhibits thyroid release rapidly (Wartofsky et al., 1970; Tan et al., 1989). Iodide should be given only after propylthiouracil is administered and should be discontinued when there is clinical improvement to avoid the risk of congenital goiter if the pregnancy continues. Propranolol (1 mg IV every 5 minutes and repeated as necessary) may be used to control autonomic symptoms. Although β-adrenergic blockade may inhibit peripheral conversion of T_4 to T_3, this does not alter thyroid release and does not prevent thyroid storm (Eriksson et al., 1997; Ashikaga, 2000). Because large increases in pulmonary diastolic pressure may be precipitated (Ikram, 1985) and because congestive heart failure may be a common presentation of thyroid crisis in pregnant women, propranolol should be used with caution.

Corticosteroids have been advocated for inhibiting peripheral conversion of T_4 and to prevent adrenal insufficiency, but there are few data to support their use. Fever should be treated with cooling blackets or acetaminophen to decrease cardiovascular demands. Salicylate use is best avoided as T_4 and T_3 may be displaced from TBG (Larsen, 1972). A thorough search for underlying infection is necessary because pyelonephritis, endometritis, or sepsis are common precipitating factors. Because of the increased incidence of atrial arrhythmia and central nervous system emboli, thromoembolic disease should be considered in patients with altered mental status that does not respond to the above therapy (Woeber, 1992). Complications of propylthiouracil and methimazole include chemical hepatitis, rash or other drug reactions (5%) and rarely agranulocytosis (0.3%) (Cooper et al., 1983). Because of the seriousness of the latter, patients with fever or sore throat should be instructed to discontinue medication until a white blood cell count is checked. Agranulocytosis, as defined by a total leukocyte count of <1,000/mm^3 or granulocyte count of less than 250/mm^3, is generally seen in older patients and within 2 months of the onset of therapy (Cooper et al., 1983). Finally lactation may be continued if total doses of propylthiouracil do not exceed 450 mg/day and if methimazole dosage does not exceed 20 mg/day (Azizi et al., 2000; Mandel & Cooper, 2001).

Thyroid hormones are known to affect both the myocardium and systemic vasculature; however, the cause of thyrotoxic heart failure is still controversial. Despite parallels to catecholamine excess, catecholamine levels and secretion rates of norepinephrine are not altered in thyrotoxicosis (Levey, 1990) and when thyroid hormone concentrations have been measured in thyroid storm, they do not differ from thyrotoxic patients (Jacobs et al., 1973). Exogenous T_3 administration in the pig as well as other species produces eccentric cardiac hypertrophy and an increase in β-adrenergic receptors that are reversible when therapy is discontinued (Hammond et al., 1987). However, the increase in β-adrenergic receptors does not necessarily produce an increase in sensitivity of the heart to catecholamines as adenylyl cyclase is downregulated in cardiac myocytes (Woeber, 1992; Klein & Ojamaa, 2001).

Thyroid hormones increase myocardial myosin isozyme ATPase activity, sarcoplasmic reticulum calcium-ATPase, and several voltage-gated potassium channels, increasing cardiac contractility and heat production (Dillmann, 1989; Kinugawa et al., 2001; Klein & Ojamaa, 2001). Thus, as cardiac work increases due to increases in stroke volume, afterload, and heat production, contractile reserve may be limited (Woeber, 1992). This would help explain the observation that left ventricular ejection fraction is increased at rest in thyrotoxicosis, but decreases with exercise (Forfar et al., 1982). This effect is reversible, as after thionamide therapy left ventricular ejection fraction again increases in response to exercise (Forfar et al., 1982). It is important to note that responses of the left ventricule are not normalized with propranolol alone and require normalization of thyroid hormone levels.

The similarities of thyrotoxicosis and pregnancy are striking. Both demonstrate increased blood volume, cardiac output, stroke volume, heart rate, and decreased systemic vascular resistance (Woeber, 1992; Klein & Ojamaa, 2001). T_3 is known to directly promote smooth muscle dilation of arteriole resistance vessels (Ojamaa et al., 1996) and in part this accounts for the decrease in systemic vascular resistance. The subnormal response to exercise is thought in part to result from an inability to lower vascular resistance further (Klein & Ojamaa, 2001). Consequently, labor (exercise) as well as the volume shifts that occur with delivery may explain the increased incidence of heart failure seen in pregnant women. Despite this, congestive heart failure when it presents as thyroid storm is rapidly reversible when treated with propylthiouracil, iodide, and diretics (Davis et al., 1989).

Overt hypothyroidism during pregnancy is uncommon as many women are anovulatory. The most common etiologies are prior surgical thyroidectomy, radioiodine ablation, and autoimmune thyroiditis. Clinical signs and symptoms include delayed deep tendon reflexes, fatigue, weight gain, cold intolerance, hair loss, dry skin, brawny edema, thickened tongue, hoarse voice, hypertension, and bradycardia, some of which are more difficult to ascertain during pregnancy. The hemodynamic changes of hypothyroidism are summarized in Table 32.2. Hyponatremia, ascites, pericardial effusions, or psychosis are not commonly present but may herald myxedema coma. Laboratory confirmation of hypothyroidism can be established by a low free T_4 in the presence of an elevated TSH. However, TSH levels may be supressed in the first trimester with less sensitive tests and undetectable in as many as 13% of women (Glinoer et al., 1990). More sensitive third-generation TSH assays are unlikely to return undetectable.

Although earlier studies of hypothyroidism suggested an increase in congenital anomalies, perinatal mortality, and infant neurologic dysfunction, more recent studies report better outcomes with adequate replacement (Abalovich et al., 2002). Leung et al. (1993) studied 23 women with overt hypothyroidism and 45 women with subclinical hypothyroidism (elevated TSH level with a normal T_4 index). One stillbirth occurred in an untreated overtly hypothyroid patient who was also eclamptic. Other than one infant with clubfeet, neonatal outcomes were satisfactory. Preeclampsia, pregnancy-induced hypertension, and eclampsia were common in women who were not yet euthyroid at delivery (9/30 subjects). In another study of 16 pregnancies in overtly hypothyroid women and 12 cases of subclinical hypothyroidism, complications were more common in overtly hypothyroid women including postpartum hemorrhage, anemia, preeclampsia, and placental abruption (Davis et al., 1988). Two women also had evidence of cardiac dysfunction, one of whom developed congestive heart failure. It is likely that the etiology of the increase in abruption was secondary to the higher incidence of chronic hypertension in hypothyroid patients (Bing et al., 1980). Rarely, hypothyroid patients may have prolonged bleeding times that normalize with T_4 replacement (Myrup et al., 1995).

Cardiac dysfunction, although rare, is of particular importance in an acute setting. As discussed earlier, the relationship of thyroid hormones to cardiac function is complex. Indices of cardiac contractility, left ventricular developed pressure, and the maximal rate of left ventricular developed pressure, as well as cardiac Na^+, K^+-ATPase activity are lower in a thyroidectomized rat model (Galinanes et al., 1994). These effects, along with the increase in systemic vascular resistance and afterload in hypothyroidism as well as volume changes at delivery, may lead to temporary cardiac dysfunction. Finally, it should be noted that in nonpregnant patients with subclinical hypothyroidism, echocardiographic indices of contractility improve after replacement therapy (Monzani et al., 2001).

As previously mentioned, thyroid replacement requirements may increase during pregnancy (Abalovich et al., 2002; Chopra & Baber, 2003). Mandel et al. (1990) found it necessary to increase the mean T_4 dose from 102 to 147 μg/day in 9 of 12 patients in order to normalize TSH levels. Another group of investigators studied 35 pregnancies and noted that only 20% of women required an increase in T_4 dosage (Girling & de Swiet, 1992). TSH measurements should be used to guide replacement because of the advantages of treating subclinical thyroid disease (Toft, 1994; Monzani et al., 2001). Caution should be taken in overtly hypothyroid patients with a history of heart disease; replacement is started at 50 μg/day initially and increased progressively to avoid angina.

Of recent concern is the effect of prolonged hypothyroidism upon the fetus and newborn. One of the great successes in clinical medicine is the prevention of the neurologic sequelae of congenital hypothyroidism by neonatal thyroid screening programs (Burrow et al., 1994). Two factors that appear to be important in the prevention of the neurologic sequelae of congenital hypothyroidism are maternal–fetal transfer of T_4 and pituitary increases in type II deiodinase, which regulates conversion of T_4 to T_3 in hypothyroid states (Burrow et al., 1994). A study of infants unable to iodinate thyroid proteins and therefore unable to make T_4 found that maternal–fetal transfer of T_4 could account for T_4 levels in newborns that approximated 30–50% of normal values (Vulsma et al., 1989). Secondly, in rat models of fetal hypothyroidism induced by maternal administration of methimazole, fetal brain T_3 levels can be maintained by maternal T_4 supplementation. Thus, increases in type II deiodinase activity may serve to normalize brain T_3 concentrations despite peripheral manifestations of hypothyroidism (Ruiz De Ona et al., 1988). Recently a study using 25,216 second-trimester maternal serum α-fetoprotein samples (Haddow et al., 1999) selected 62 women with TSH levels greater than the 98th percentile. At 8 years of age, the children of women with elevated TSH levels had a mean IQ 4 points less than matched controls ($P = 0.06$). In 48 of the women who did not receive thyroid replacement during pregnancy, the IQ was 7 points less than matched controls ($P = 0.05$) and these children scored lower on 8 of 15 neuropsychological tests. Within 11 years, 64% of the untreated women and 4% of the matched control women had confirmed hypothyroidism. Similar differences have been found by Pop et al. (2003). Although universal thyroid screening is not currently recommended (ACOG Bulletin, 2001), screening of women with a history of thyroid disorders and normalization of TSH levels would be prudent.

Myxedema coma is an extremely rare life-threatening disorder with a mortality of 15–20%. It deserves mention as an acute manifestation of hypothyroidism. The clinical presentation as reviewed by Jordan (1995) includes coma, respiratory hypoventilation with carbon dioxide retention, hypothermia, bradycardia, hyponatremia, hypoglycemia, and often the presence of an associated infection, most commonly urosepsis. Therapy includes mechanical ventilation to correct hypoxia or hypercarbia, T_4 replacement in larger doses (400 μg IV followed by 50 μg daily), steroids, passive rewarming to slowly increase body temperature, and correction of hypotension if present. Correction of hyponatremia by fluid restriction or cautious use of hypertonic saline may be necessary. As in thyroid storm, a thorough search for an infectious precipitating event is necessary. Laboratory tests are the same as in hypothyroidism, with the exception that TSH levels may be suppressed (euthyroid sick syndrome). Obtundation in the presence of hypothyroidism suggests the diagnosis.

Pheochromocytoma

Pheochromocytoma is a rare tumor of catecholamine-secreting chromaffin cells. Recent reviews have noted some 43 cases associated with pregnancy between 1988 and 1997 (Ahlawat et al., 1999; Hermayer & Szpiech, 1999; Almog et al., 2000). Compared to the period 1980–87, maternal mortality fell from 16 to 2%, fetal loss decreased from 26 to 11%, and cases diagnosed antenatally increased from 52 to 83%.

The most common signs are hypertension (90%), headache, excessive truncal sweating, and paroxysmal attacks in 40–50% of patients. Pallor, flushing, anxiety, chest pain, nausea, and vomiting are less common. The diagnosis should be considered in the differential with hyperthyroidism and preeclampsia as higher maternal mortality is increased with hypertensive crisis when the diagnosis is not established prior to delivery (Ahlawat et al., 1999). Most (90%) pheochromocytomas occur sporadically and some 10% are associated with familial disorders including multiple endocrine neoplasia (MEN) II syndromes, von Recklinghausen's disease, or von Hippel–Lindau syndrome (Prys-Roberts, 2000). Hypertension in the setting of café-au-lait spots and neurofibromas should raise the suspicion of pheochromocytoma. Genetic screening may be warranted not only in familial syndromes (Pacak, 2001) but also in sporadic cases (Neumann et al., 2002). MEN 2A is an autosomal dominant syndrome in which medullary thyroid carcinoma is associated with pheochromocytoma and hyperparathyroidism. The reader is referred to a recent review of pheochromocytoma for futher details (Prys-Roberts, 2000).

Advances in biochemical testing have improved the diagnosis. Table 32.4 summarizes the sensitivity and specificity of plasma and urine tests (Pacak et al., 2001).

In borderline circumstances, the clonidine suppression test may be helpful in distinguishing between elevated blood levels of norepinephrine due to increased sympathetic nerve stimulation from that due to pheochromocytoma. Clonidine inhibits neurally mediated catecholamine release (Ahlawat et al., 1999). After an overnight fast, a heparin lock is placed at least 30 minutes prior to baseline levels being drawn. Plasma catecholamine levels are sampled at baseline and hourly for 3 hours after the patient is given clonidine (0.3 mg per 70 kg

Table 32.4 Biochemical tests for pheochromocytoma

Biochemical test	Sensitivity (%)	Specificity (%)
Plasma metanephrine	99	89
Plasma catecholamine	85	80
Urinary catecholamine	88	64
Urinary metanephrine	94	53
Urinary vanillylmandelic acid	63	94

body weight). A normal response is a decrease of more than 50% in plasma norepinephrine levels or minimal norepinephrine of 500 pg/mL or less. False-positive results can occur in patients taking diuretics and particularly tricyclic antidepressants. Finally, MRI can be safely performed in pregnancy to confirm the presence of an adrenal mass, as 90% of pheochromocytomas arise in the adrenal glands. After delivery, radioactive iodine-labeled metiodobenzylguanidine scintigraphy offers greater than 95% specificity in detection (Pacak et al., 2001).

The most frequently used treatment consists of nonspecific α-adrenergic blockade with phenoxybenzamine given by mouth 10 mg daily, increased to 0.5–1.0 mg/kg/daily (Hermayer & Szpiech, 1999; Prys-Roberts, 2000). Alternatively, the shorter-acting selective α_1-blocker prazosin is less likely to cause tachycardia. The initial dosage is 1 mg three times a day increased to 2–5 mg three times a day. β-Blockers should be used in conjunction only after adrenergic blockade is initiated as unopposed α-adrenegic activity may lead to vasoconstriction and a marked increase in blood pressure. Commonly, labetalol is used as it has both α- and β-adrenergic antagonist properties. As hypertension is the most common presenting feature, preeclampsia will often be included in the differential diagnosis. Interestingly, magnesium sulfate given as a bolus followed by 2 g infusion has been used in nonpregnant patients for operative control during surgical removal of pheochromocytoma (James, 1989, 2001). The use of magnesium sulfate may therefore be advantageous.

Hyperparathyroidism

Primary hyperparathyroidism is more common in women than men (3 : 1 ratio). Since the average age of diagnosis is 55 years, the combination of hyperparathyroidism and pregnancy is uncommon. Approximately 145 cases of primary hyperparathyroidism have been reported during pregnancy, which is proportionately less than the expected incidence of eight new cases per 100,000 per year in women of child-bearing age (Carella & Gossain, 1992; Schnatz & Curry, 2002). The discrepancy is in part due to the asymptomatic nature of most cases of hyperparathyroidism. Combining the results of two series (Gelister et al., 1989; Kort et al., 1999), the majority of patients were diagnosed post partum following the presentation of neonatal tetany. A recent review summarizes parathyroid disorders (Marx, 2000).

Whether pregnant or not, the diagnosis of hyperparathyroidism is suggested by elevated levels of ionized calcium in the presence of inappropriately elevated parathyroid hormone (PTH). The majority of calcium is bound to albumin. The reduced serum albumin levels in pregnancy, acquisition by the fetus of 25–30 g of calcium, increase in glomerular filtration rate, and the expanded extracellular fluid volume result in an overall decrease in total serum calcium levels of 0.5 mg/dL (Pitkin, 1985). However, ionized calcium levels are not affected. Pregnant women with primary hyperparathyroidism have biochemical parameters similar to those who are not pregnant (Ammann et al., 1993). In normal gestation, PTH levels, when measured by new two-site immunoradiometric assays, are stable or slightly lower in the second trimester, refuting earlier studies of elevated PTH levels (Seki et al., 1991; Kohlmeier & Marcus, 1995; Seely et al., 1997). Thus, repeatedly elevated PTH levels in the presence of increased ionized calcium, or total calcium adjusted for albumin, must be considered significant.

When hyperparathyroidism is diagnosed, a search for MEN is indicated (Marx, 2001). Most nonparathyroid causes of hypercalcemia are associated with suppression of PTH and urinary cAMP levels. Nonparathyroid causes of hypercalcemia include malignancy (breast, myeloma, lymphoma), hypocalcuric hypercalcemia (familial, thiazides, lithium), granulomatous disease (sarcoidosis, tuberculosis), thyrotoxicosis, drug-induced causes (hypervitaminosis D or A, calcium, milk-alkali syndrome), adrenal insufficiency, and immobilization. Hypercalcemia secondary to PTH-related protein produced by breast tissue during pregnancy and lactation with normal PTH levels has also been reported (Lepre et al., 1993). A history should include the use of over-the-counter vitamin preparations and other medications.

Primary hyperparathyroidism may be due to parathyroid adenomas (89% of cases), parathyroid hyperplasia (9%), or parathyroid cancer (2%) (Kelly, 1991). The majority of patients with primary hyperparathyroidism are thought to be asymptomatic and are found to have elevated serum calcium levels on routine screening. However, on closer questioning, nearly half of these patients may complain of weakness or fatigue (Bilezikian et al., 2001). Approximately 20% of patients with hyperparathyroidism will have nephrolithiasis. Other common signs and symptoms include nausea or vomiting, mental disturbances, pancreatitis, and bone pain (Kristoffersson et al., 1985; Carella & Gossain, 1992; Murray et al., 1999). Hypercalcemic crisis is characterized by progressive hypercalcemia with hypovolemia, renal insufficiency, altered mentation, and pancreatitis in the most severe cases. Rarely, seizures from hypercalcemia may mimic eclampsia (Whalley, 1963).

The only definitive treatment is surgical removal of the glands. Since only 25% of asymptomatic patients will have progressive disease, which is usually in the form of a decrease in bone mass, the management of asymptomatic hyperparathyroidism is somewhat controversial. In nonpregnant patients with mild to moderate hyperparathyroidism that were left untreated, no increase in mortality was seen. The only increase in mortality occurred in those patients with serum calcium levels in the uppermost quartile (Silverberg et al., 1999). Treatment during pregnancy, however, may be warranted in view of the risk of neonatal tetany as well as the increase in perinatal complications including miscarriage and stillbirth seen in maternal hypercalcemia (Shangold et al., 1982).

There is no satisfactory medical treatment for primary hyperparathyroidism in the pregnant or nonpregnant state. Mithramycin and bisphosphonates are contraindicated during pregnancy. Asymptomatic patients with mild hypercalcemia can be followed closely through pregnancy, with surgery deferred until after delivery (Croom & Thomas, 1984; Gelister et al., 1989; Hill et al., 1989). Occasionally, patients with significant symptoms due to hypercalcemia but who are not surgical candidates have been controlled safely and effectively with oral phosphate therapy (1.5 g/day in divided doses) throughout gestation (Montoro et al., 1980). This therapy is only indicated in patients in whom the initial serum phosphorus level is less than 3 mg/dL; phosphate administration should be adjusted to maintain serum phosphate below 4 mg/dL. Furosemide increases the excretion of calcium in the urine and can be given orally to help lower the serum calcium levels on a chronic basis. In contrast, patients with progressive symptoms, significant hypercalcemia (>12 mg/dL), or deterioration of renal function should be treated surgically by an experienced parathyroid surgeon (Kelly, 1991; Carella & Gossain, 1992). Neck exploration should not be deferred in the symptomatic woman because of pregnancy, unless delivery is imminent (Carella & Gossain, 1992).

Medical management for stabilization in hypercalcemic crisis includes hydration with normal saline (2–3 L over 3–6 hours); correction of electrolyte abnormalities; furosemide, which decreases distal tubular calcium reabsorption (10–40 mg IV every 2–4 hours) to maintain urine output at 200 mL/hr; and calcium restriction. Hypercalcemia resistant to this regimen may be alleviated with more potent agents, such as calcitonin (100–400 units/day). Although effective initially, tachyphylaxis to calcitonin generally occurs in 4–6 days. Glucocorticoids can be used to decrease gastrointestinal calcium absorption. The reader is referred to a recent review (Schnatz & Curry, 2002) for greater detail.

In hyperparathyroid mothers, neonatal hypocalcemia is predictable and can be prevented. Transient neonatal tetany should not be associated with long-term sequelae. Management of maternal hyperparathyroidism diagnosed during pregnancy should be individualized, taking into consideration the patient's symptoms, the gestational age of the fetus, and the severity of the disease.

Hypoparathyroidism

Hypocalcemia caused by hypoparathyroidism is an extremely rare disorder in pregnancy. The most common cause of hypoparathyroidism is nonproduction of PTH because of excision of the parathyroid gland, usually following thyroidectomy. Anywhere from 0.5 to 3.5% of thyroid surgeries result in hypoparathyroidism. As mentioned earlier, although total calcium concentration decreases in pregnancy, ionized calcium does not (Pitkin, 1985; Seki et al., 1991). In response to hypocalcemia, PTH normally increases, which in turn augments renal tubular calcium reabsorption and phosphate excretion. PTH also increases 25-hydroxyvitamin D transformation to the active hormone 1,25-dihydroxyvitamin D, which stimulates intestinal calcium and phosphate absorption as well as osteoclastic bone reabsorption (Marx, 2000). Ineffective PTH syndromes may be caused by failure to respond to increased PTH (pseudohypoparathyroidism), deficient vitamin D from malabsorption, or increased vitamin D metabolism seen with phenytoin or other anticonvulsants (Zalonga & Eil, 1989; Potts, 2001).

Other causes of hypocalcemia include massive citrated blood transfusions (generally transient); alkalosis, with increased ionized calcium binding to albumin; increased phosphate in renal failure; pancreatitis; sepsis; and hypomagnesemia or hypermagnesemia (Reber & Heath, 1995). The hypocalcemia of respiratory alkalosis is rarely clinically important, although metabolic alkalosis secondary to bicarbonate administration can be significant. Seriously ill patients often may have depressed total calcium levels; however, the frequency of hypocalcemia when corrected for hypoalbuminemia or when ionized calcium is evaluated is approximately 10% (Potts, 2001).

Chronic candidiasis, alopecia, vitiligo, and multiple endocrinopathies should suggest the autoimmune polyendocrinopathy–candidiasis–ectodermal dystrophy syndrome (Ahonen et al., 1990; Marx, 2000). Perioral paresthesias, psychiatric disturbances, and Chvostek's or Trousseau's sign may be present. Trousseau's sign, also known as the "obstetrician's hand," or carpal spasm due to ulnar and median nerve ischemia, is elicited by inflating a sphygmomanometer cuff around the arm to 20 mmHg above systolic pressures (Cain, 1973). The thumb adducts and the fingers are extended, except at the metacarpophalangeal joints, within minutes, indicating latent tetany. Cardiac changes of hypocalcemia are nonspecific but include electrocardiogram Q–T prolongation, hypotension, and reversible congestive cardiomyopathy (Zalonga & Eil, 1989; Csanady et al., 1990). Hypopharyngeal tetany may present as stridor and seizures and may be life-threatening. Magnesium sulfate rarely has been implicated in hypocalcemia and should be used cautiously when preeclampsia is superimposed on hypoparathyroidism (Eisenbud & LoBue, 1976). Dilantin may increase vitamin D metabolism. In one case, decreased fetal heart rate variability was reported, although there was no evidence of acidosis (Hagay et al., 1986). Secondary fetal or neonatal hyperparathyroidism, bone demineralization, skeletal and skull fractures have been reported.

Medical treatment of hypocalcemia can be divided into long-term and acute management. Vitamin D (50,000–100,000 units/day) or 1,25-dihydroxyvitamin D (calcitriol 0.5–3.0 μg/day) and 1–2 g/day of elemental calcium have been used successfully in pregnancy (Pitkin, 1985). Vitamin D_2 is the least expensive form of vitamin D, but several weeks may be needed for its full effect. Calcitriol has a faster onset of action (1–2 days) but requires more frequent monitoring to prevent hypercalcemia. Requirements during pregnancy may increase in the latter half of pregnancy, presumably due to increased vitamin D-binding protein. It is often necessary to reduce replacement doses in the postpartum period to avoid hypercalcemia, even in women who are breastfeeding (Caplan & Beguin, 1990). The latter require closer monitoring of calcium levels, because it may be difficult to predict calcium needs during lactation. Of interest, in some species (cattle in particular) the onset of lactation can result in hypocalcemia and parturient paresis (Goff et al., 1989).

Acute hypocalcemia or impending signs of tetany are treated by 10% calcium gluconate (10 mL diluted in 150 mL of D_5W given over 10 minutes), followed by continuous infusions of calcium (0.5–2.0 mg/kg/hr). Serial calcium measurements should be measured initially every 2–4 hours to assess the adequacy of the administered dose and adjust the infusion rate accordingly (Reber & Heath, 1995). Laboratory evaluation in addition to ionized calcium should include magnesium, phosphorus, and PTH levels. Hypoparathyroidism is diagnosed by normal serum magnesium concentration, low or inappropriately normal PTH level, and low ionized calcium. High PTH and low phosphorus levels suggest vitamin D deficiency, whereas high PTH and high phosphorus levels are consistent with the diagnosis of pseudohypoparathyroidism or renal insufficiency.

Adrenal crisis

Adrenal insufficiency may be primary or secondary. The most common cause of primary adrenal insufficiency (Addison's disease) is idiopathic or autoimmune adenitis. Less frequently, tuberculosis, sarcoidosis, AIDS, or bilateral hemorrhage (antiphospholipid syndrome or anticoagulation) may be the cause. Autoimmune adenitis may be associated with gonadal failure, hypothyroidism, hyperthyroidism, Hashimoto's thyroiditis, vitiligo, hypoparathyroidism, and pernicious anemia (polyglandular failure type I or II). For further details, the reader is referred to the review of Williams and Dluhy (2001). Except for those patients on corticosteroid therapy for other medical reasons, secondary adrenal insufficiency is rare in pregnancy. In 1962 Osler reported that the birth weights of children of mothers with adrenal insufficiency average 500 g below normal. More recent case reports do not confirm growth retardation or adverse outcomes other than related to maternal diagnosis and treatment (Seaward et al., 1989; Perlitz et al., 1999).

Adrenal insufficiency is more commonly diagnosed during the puerperium than earlier in pregnancy, in part due to the similar symptoms of pregnancy, including nausea, fatigue, anorexia, and hyperpigmentation. The latter may be seen as a diffuse tan or bronze darkening of the elbows or creases of the hands, and bluish-black patches may appear on the mucous membranes. Axillary and pubic hair may be reduced as adrenal androgens are diminished. The diagnosis may not be suspected until adrenal crisis develops, with potentially serious sequelae. Pregnancy may be well tolerated until stresses such as infection, trauma, surgery, labor, or dehydration from vomiting or diarrhea precipitate adrenal crisis. The clinical features of acute primary adrenocortical insufficiency include hypotension and shock (cardiovascular collapse), weakness, apathy, nausea, vomiting, anorexia, abdominal or flank pain, and hyperthermia. Electrolyte abnormalities include hyponatremia, hyperkalemia, mild azotemia, and metabolic acidosis. Hypoglycemia and mild hypercalcemia may also be seen. Importantly, secondary adrenal insufficiency may present similarly, but without electrolyte changes (normal renin–aldosterone response) and should be considered in patients previously on corticosteroids.

The diagnosis of adrenal insufficiency rests on the lack of cortisol response to adrenocorticotropic hormone (ACTH) stimulation, or on unstimulated subnormal cortisol levels during stress. The rapid ACTH test can be performed at any time of the day (Williams & Dluhy, 2001). Normally, the plasma cortisol should rise more than 18 μg/dL above baseline 30–60 minutes after the intravenous administration of 250 μg of ACTH (Cosyntropin). If the response is abnormal, then primary and secondary adrenal insufficiency can be distinguished by measuring aldosterone levels from the same blood samples. In secondary, but not primary, adrenal insufficiency the aldosterone increment will be normal (5 ng/dL). Additionally, a plasma ACTH level may also be used to differentiate primary from secondary adrenal insufficiency. In Addison's disease, early-morning ACTH levels are more than 250 pg/mL but in secondary adrenal insufficiency are less than 50 pg/mL. It is important to note that some patients with a partial ACTH deficit and absence of adrenal atrophy will have a normal cortisol response; in pregnancy, increased corticosteroid-binding globulin may increase levels. In these circumstances, the low-dose (1 μg) ACTH test may be used to further differentiate adrenal insufficiency (Helal et al., 2000).

Treatment for acute adrenal insufficiency includes hydrocortisone 100 mg IV every 6 hours for 24 hours. This dose can be reduced to 50 mg every 6 hours if the patient is improving, and tapered to an oral maintenance dose in 4–5 days. Doses of hydrocortisone in the range 100–200 mg maximize mineralocorticoid effects and therefore supplementary mineralocorticoid is not necessary (Williams & Dluhy, 2001). Additional therapy includes intravenous saline and glucose and correction of precipitating factors (infection) and electrolyte abnormalities. Volume replacement is critical in improving cardiovascular status. Patients with cardiovascular collapse may not respond well to pressor agents until hydrocortisone is given. This decrease in pressor responsiveness and hypotension in adrenalectomized animals is thought in part to be due to excessive production of nitric oxide (Orbach et al., 2001).

Patients on chronic corticosteroid therapy should receive stress doses for infections, surgery, labor, and delivery. Adrenal suppression is unlikely to occur when corticosteroids are used for less than 3 weeks (Jabbour, 2001). Following withdrawal of prolonged corticosteroids, approximately 70% of patients will have normal function within a month, but in some individuals up to 9 months may be necessary for restoration of normal function (Graber et al., 1965; Aceto et al., 1966). However, abnormal ACTH testing measures physiologic reserve and does not necessarily predict whether adrenal crisis will develop following stress. The risk of clinically apparent adrenal insufficiency developing in unsupplemented patients undergoing surgery is well recognized (Kehlet & Binder, 1973). In obstetric patients, chemical adrenal suppression has been noted in women receiving two courses of betamethasone for fetal lung maturation, yet none of these patients had clinical signs of adrenal insufficiency during pregnancy (Helal et al., 2000). One suggested regimen is to use hydrocortisone 100 mg every 8 hours for 24 hours if the patient has received more than 20 mg of prednisone daily for more than 3 weeks within the previous year (Jabbour, 2001).

For chronic replacement in patients with primary adrenocortical insufficiency, doses are similar to those in the nonpregnant patient: hydrocortisone 20 mg each morning and 10 mg each evening. Since this dosage of hydrocortisone does not replace the adrenal mineralocorticoid component, mineralocorticoid supplementation is usually needed. This is accomplished by the administration of 0.05–0.2 mg/day fluorocortisone by mouth. Patients should also be instructed to maintain an ample intake of sodium (3–4 g/day). During conditions of increased sweating, exercise, nausea and vomiting, these doses may need to be increased.

References

Abalovich M, Gutierrez S, Alcaraz G, et al. Overt and subclinical hypothyroidism complicating pregnancy. Thyroid 2002;12:63–68.

Aceto T, Beckhorn G, Jorgensen J, et al. Iatrogenic ACTH–cortisol insufficiency. Pediatr Clin North Am 1966;13:543.

ACOG Practice Bulletin 32. Thyroid Disease in Pregnancy. November 2001.

Ahlawat S, Jain S, Kumari S, et al. Pheochromocytoma associated with pregnancy: case report and review of the literature. Obstet Gynecol Surv 1999;54:728–737.

Ahonen P, Myllarniemi S, Sipila I, et al. Clinical variation of autoimmune polyendocrinopathy–candidiasis–ectodermal dystrophy (APECED) in a series of 68 patients. N Engl J Med 1990;322:1829–1836.

Almog B, Kupferminc M, Many A, Lessing J. Pheochromocytoma in pregnancy: a case report and review of the literature. Acta Obstet Gynecol Scand 2000;79:709–711.

Amino N, Kuro R, Tanizawa O, et al. Changes of serum anti-thyroid antibodies during and after pregnancy in autoimmune thyroid diseases. Clin Exp Immunol 1978;31:30–37.

Amino N, Tanizawa O, Mori H, et al. Aggravation of thyrotoxicosis in early pregnancy and after delivery in Graves' disease. J Clin Endocrinol Metab 1982;55:108–112.

Ammann P, Irion O, Gast J, et al. Alterations of calcium and phosphate metabolism in primary hyperparathyroidism during pregnancy. Acta Obstet Gynecol Scand 1993;72:488–492.

Arafah BM. Increased need for thyroxine in women with hypothyroidism during estrogen therapy. N Engl J Med 2001;344: 1743.

Ashikaga H. Propranolol administration in a patient with thyroid storm. Ann Intern Med 2000;132:681–682.

Azizi F, Khoshniat M, Bahrainian M, et al. Thyroid function and intellectual development of infants nursed by mothers taking methimazole. J Clin Endocrinol Metab 2000;85:3233–3238.

Bedalov A, Balasubramanyam A. Glucocorticoid induced ketoacidosis in gestational diabetes. Diabetes Care 1997;20:922–924.

Berghout A, Endert E, Ross A, et al. Thyroid function and thyroid size in normal pregnant women living in an iodine replete area. Clin Endocrinol (Oxf) 1994;41:375–379.

Bilezikian JP, Silverberg SJ, Gartenberg F, et al. Clinical presentation of primary hyperparathyroidism. In: Bilezikian JP, Levine MA, Marcus R, eds. The Parathyroids: Basic and Clinical Concepts, 2nd edn. San Diego, CA: Academic Press, 2001.

Bing RF, Briggs RSJ, Burden AC, et al. Reversible hypertension and hypothyroidism. Clin Endocrinol (Oxf) 1980;13:339–342.

Bitton RN, Wexler C. Free triiodothyronine toxicosis: a distinct entity. Am J Med 1990;88:531–533.

Bouhanick B, Biquard F, Hadjadj S, et al. Does treatment with antenatal glucocorticoids for the risk of premature delivery contribute to ketoacidosis in pregnant women with diabetes who receive CSII? Arch Intern Med 2000;160:242–243.

Burrow GN, Fisher DA, Larsen PR. Maternal and fetal thyroid function. N Engl J Med 1994;331:1072–1078.

Cain A. The thyroid gland. In: Clain A, ed. Hamilton Bailey's Demonstrations of Physical Signs in Clinical Surgery, 15th edn. Bristol: John Wright & Sons, 1973:164.

Caplan RH, Beguin EA. Hypercalcemia in a calcitriol-treated hypoparathyroid woman during lactation. Obstet Gynecol 1990; 76:485–489.

Carella MJ, Gossain V. Hyperparathyroidism and pregnancy. J Gen Intern Med 1992;7:448–453.

Chauhan SP, Perry KG. Management of diabetic ketoacidosis in the obstetric patient. Obstet Gynecol Clin North Am 1995;22:143–155.

Chopra I, Baber K. Treatment of primary hypothyroidism during pregnancy: is there an increase in thyroxine dose requirement in pregnancy? Metabolism 2003;52:122–128.

Cooper DS, Goldminz D, Levin A, et al. Agranulocytosis associated with antithyroid drugs. Ann Intern Med 1983;98:26–29.

Croom RD, Thomas CG. Primary hyperparathyroidism during pregnancy. Surgery 1984;96:1109–1118.

Csanady M, Forster T, Julesz J. Reversible impairment of myocardial function in hypoparathyroidism causing hypocalcaemia. Br Heart J 1990;63:58–60.

Cullen MT, Reece EA, Homko CJ, Sivan E. The changing presentations of diabetic ketoacidosis during pregnancy. Am J Perinatol 1996;13:449–451.

Davidson KM, Richards DS, Schatz DA, et al. Successful in utero treatment of fetal goiter and hypothyroidism. N Engl J Med 1991;324:543–546.

Davis LE, Leveno KJ, Cunningham FG. Hypothyroidism complicating pregnancy. Obstet Gynecol 1988;72:108–112.

Davis LE, Lucas MJ, Hankins GD, et al. Thyrotoxicosis complicating pregnancy. Am J Obstet Gynecol 1989;160:63–70.

DeGroot L, Larsen PR, Refetoff S, Stanbury JB, eds. Hormone synthesis, secretion and action. In: The Thyroid and its Diseases. New York: John Wiley & Sons, 1984:76.

Dillmann WH. Diabetes and thyroid hormone induced changes in cardiac function and their molecular basis. Annu Rev Med 1989;40:373.

Doherty CM, Shindo ML, Rice DH, et al. Management of thyroid nodules during pregnancy. Laryngoscope 1995;105:251–255.

Drury MI, Greene AT, Stronge JM. Pregnancy complicated by clinical diabetes mellitus: a study of 600 pregnancies. Obstet Gynecol 1977;49:519–522.

Easterling TR, Schmucker BC, Carlson KL, et al. Maternal hemodynamics in pregnancies complicated by hyperthyroidism. Obstet Gynecol 1991;78:348–352.

Eisenbud E, LoBue C. Hypocalcemia after therapeutic use of magnesium sulfate. Arch Intern Med 1976;136:688–691.

Epstein RH. Pathogenesis of Graves' ophthalmopathy. N Engl J Med 1993;329:1468.

Eriksson M, Rubenfeld S, Garber AJ, et al. Propranolol does not prevent thyroid storm. N Engl J Med 1977;296:263–264.

Forfar JC, Muir AL, Sawers SA, et al. Abnormal left ventricular function in hyperthyroidism. N Engl J Med 1982;307:1165–1170.

Gabbe SG, Mestman JH, Hibbard LT. Maternal mortality in diabetes mellitus: an 18 year survey. Obstet Gynecol 1976;48:549–551.

Galinanes M, Smolenski R, Haddock P, et al. Early effects of hypothyroidism on the contractile function of the rat heart and its tolerance to hypothermic ischemia. J Thorac Cardiovasc Surg 1994;107:829–837.

Gelister JS, Sanderson JD, Chapple CR, et al. Management of hyperparathyroidism in pregnancy. Br J Surg 1989;76:1207–1208.

Girling JC, de Swiet M. Thyroxine dosage during pregnancy in women with primary hypothyroidism. Br J Obstet Gynaecol 1992;99:368–370.

Glinoer D, Delange F. The potential repercussions of maternal, fetal and neonatal hypothyroxinemia on the progeny. Thyroid 2000;10:871–887.

Glinoer D, de Nayer P, Bourdoux P, et al. Regulation of maternal thyroid during pregnancy. J Clin Endocrinol Metab 1990;71:276–278.

Glinoer D, De Nayer P, Delange F, et al. A randomized trial for the treatmeant of mild iodine deficiency during pregnancy: maternal and neonatal effects. J Clin Endocrinol Metab 1995;80:258–269.

Goff JP, Reinhardt TA, Horst RL. Recurring hypocalcemia of bovine parturient paresis is associated with failure to produced 1,25-dihydroxyvitamin D. Endocrinology 1989;125:49–53.

Graber A, Ney R, Nicholson W, et al. Natural history of pituitary–adrenal function recovery after long-term suppression with corticosteroids. J Clin Endocrinol 1965;25:11.

Haddow J, Palomaki G, Allan W, et al. Maternal thyroid deficiency during pregnancy and subsequent neurophyschological development of the child. N Engl J Med 1999;341:549–555.

Hagay S, Mazor M, Leiberman J, et al. The effect of maternal hypocalcemia on fetal heart rate baseline variability. Acta Obstet Gynecol Scand 1986;65:513–515.

Hammond HK, White FC, Buxton IL, et al. Increased myocardial B-receptors and adrenergic responses in hyperthyroid pigs. Am J Physiol 1987;252:H283–290.

Helal K, Gordon MC, Lightner CR, et al. Adrenal supresssion induced by betamethasone in women at risk for premature delivery. Obstet Gynecol 2000;96:287–290.

Hermann M, Richter B, Roka R, et al. Thyroid surgery in untreated severe hyperthyroidism: perioperative kinetics of free thyroid hormones in the glandular venous effluent and peripheral blood. Surgery 1994;115:240–245.

Hermayer K, Szpiech M. Diagnosis and management of pheochromocytoma during pregnancy: a case report. Am J Med Sci 1999; 318:186–189.

Hill NC, Lloyd-Davies SV, Bishop A, et al. Primary hyperparathyroidism and pregnancy. Int J Gynaecol Obstet 1989;29:253–255.

Hollowell JG, Staehling NW, Hannon WH, et al. Iodine nutrition in the United States. Trends and public health implications: iodine excretion data from National Health and Nutrition Examination Surveys I and III (1971–1974 and 1988–1994). J Clin Endocrinol Metab 1998;83:3401–3408.

Hughes AB. Fetal heart rate changes during diabetic ketosis. Acta Obstet Gynecol Scand 1987;66:71–73.

Ikram H. The nature and prognosis of thyrotoxic heart disease. Q J Med 1985;54:19–28.

Jabbour S. Steroids and the surgical patient. Med Clin North Am 2001;85:1311–1317.

Jacobs HS, Mackie DB, Eastman CJ, et al. Total and free triiodothyronine and thyroxine levels in thyroid storm and recurrent hyperthyroidism. Lancet 1973;ii:236–238.

James MF. Use of magnesium sulphate in the anaesthetic management of phaeochromocytoma: a review of 17 anaesthetics. Br J Anaesth 1989;62:616–623.

James M. Phaeochromocytoma: recent progress in its management. Br J Anaesth 2001;86:594–595.

Jordan RM. Myxedema coma. Pathophysiology, therapy, and factors affecting prognosis. Med Clin North Am 1995;79:185–194.

Kehlet J, Binder C. Adrenocortical function and clinical course during and after surgery in unsuplemented glucocorticoid-treated patients. Br J Anaesth 1973;45:1043–1048.

Kelly TR. Primary hyperparathyroidism during pregnancy. Surgery 1991;110:1028–1033.

Kilpatrick S. Umbilical blood sampling in women with thyroid disease in pregnancy: is it necessary? Am J Obstet Gynecol 2003;189:1.

Kilvert JA, Nicholson HO, Wright AD. Ketoacidosis in diabetic pregnancy. Diabet Med 1993;10:278–281.

Kinugawa K, Yonekura K, Ribeiro R, et al. Regulation of thyroid hormone receptor isoforms in physiological and pathological cardiac hypertrophy. Circ Res 2001;89:591–598.

Kitabchi A, Umpierrez G, Murphy M, Barrett E. Management of hyperglycaemic crises in patients with diabetes. Diabetes Care 2001;24:131–153.

Klein I, Ojamaa K. Thyroid hormone and the cardiovascular system. N Engl J Med 2001;344:501–509.

Kohlmeier L, Marcus R. Calcium disorders of pregnancy. Endocrinol Metab Clin North Am 1995;24:15–39.

Kort KC, Schiller HJ, Numann PJ. Hyperparathyroidism and pregnancy. Am J Surg 1999;177:66–68.

Kriplani A, Buckshee K, Bhargava VL, et al. Maternal and perinatal outcome in thyrotoxicosis complicating pregnancy. Eur J Obstet Gynecol Reprod Biol 1994;54:159–163.

Kristoffersson A, Dahlgren S, Lithner F, et al. Primary hyperparathyroidism in pregnancy. Surgery 1985;97:326–330.

Larsen P. Salicylate-induced increases in free triiodothyronine in human serum. Evidence of inhibition of triiodothyronine binding to thyroxine-binding globulin and thyroxine-binding prealbumin. J Clin Invest 1972;51:1125–1134.

Larsen PR. Maternal thyroxine and congenital hypothyroidism. N Engl J Med 1989;321:13–16.

Lepre F, Grill V, Ho PW, et al. Hypercalcemia in pregnancy and lactation associated with parathyroid hormone-related protein. N Engl J Med 1993;328:666–667.

Leung AS, Millar LK, Koonings PP, et al. Perinatal outcome in hypothyroid pregnancies. Obstet Gynecol 1993;81:349–353.

Levey GS. Catecholamine-thyroid hormone interactions and the cardiovascular manifestations of hyperthyroidism. Am J Med 1990;88:642–646.

Mandel SJ, Cooper DS. The use of antithyroid druges in pregnancy and lactation. J Clin Endocrinol Metab 2001;86:2354–2359.

Mandel SJ, Larsen RP, Seely EW, et al. Increased need for thyroxine during pregnancy in women with primary hypothyroidism. N Engl J Med 1990;323:91–96.

Mandel SJ, Brent GA, Larsen PR. Review of antithyroid drug use during pregnancy and a report of aplasia cutis. Thyroid 1994;4:129–133.

Marx SJ. Hyperparathyroid and hypoparathyroid disorders. N Engl J Med 2000;343:1863–1875.

Mayer DC, Thorp J, Baucom D, et al. Hyperthyroidism and seizures during pregnancy. Am J Perinatol 1995;12:192–194.

Miodovnik M, Lavin J, Harrington D, et al. Effect of maternal ketoacidemia on the pregnant ewe and the fetus. Am J Obstet Gynecol 1982;144:585–593.

Mitsuda N, Tamaki H, Amino N, et al. Risk factors for developmental disorders in infants born to women with Graves disease. Obstet Gynecol 1992;80:359–364.

Momotani N, Noh J, Oyanagi, Ishikawa N, Ito K. Antithyroid drug therapy for Grave's disease during pregnancy. Optimal regimen for fetal thyroid status. N Engl J Med 1986;315:24–28.

Montoro MN, Collear JV, Mestman JH. Management of hyperparathyroidism in pregnancy with oral phosphate therapy. Obstet Gynecol 1980;55:431–434.

Montoro MN, Myers VP, Mestman JH, et al. Outcome of pregnancy in diabetic ketoacidosis. Am J Perinatol 1993;10:17–20.

Monzani F, Di Bello V, Caraccio N, et al. Effect of levothyroxine on cardiac function and structure in subclinical hypothyroidism: a double blind, placebo-controlled study. J Clin Endocrinol Metab 2001;86:1110–1115.

Mortimer RH, Tyuack SA, Galligan JP, et al. Graves' disease in pregnancy: TSH receptor binding inhibiting immunoglobulins and maternal and neonatal thyroid function. Clin Endocrinol 1990;32: 141–152.

Muller A, Drexhage H, Berghout A. Postpartum thyroiditis and autoimmune thyroiditis in women of childbearing age: recent insights and consequences for antenatal and postnatal care. Endocrine Rev 2001;22:605–630.

Murray J, Newman W, Dacus J. Hyperparathyroidism in pregnancy: diagnostic dilemma? Obstet Gynecol Surv 1999;541:183.

Myrup B, Bregengard C, Faber J. Primary haemostasis in thyroid disease. J Intern Med 1995;238:59–63.

Neumann H, Bausch B, McWhinney SR, et al. Germ-line mutations in nonsyndromic pheochromocytoma. N Engl J Med 2002;346:1459–1466.

Nicolini U, Venbegoni E, Acaia B, et al. Prenatal treatment of fetal hypothyroidism: is there more than one option? Prenat Diagn 1996;16:443–448.

Nylund L, Lunell N, Lewander R, et al. Uteroplacental blood flow in diabetic pregnancy: measurements with indium 113m and a computer-linked gamma camera. Am J Obstet Gynecol 1982;144:298–302.

Ojamaa K, Klemperer J, Klein I. Acute effects of thyroid hormone on vascular smooth muscle. Thyroid 1996;6:505–512.

Orbach P, Wood C, Keller-Wood M. Nitric oxide reduces pressor responsiveness during ovine hypoadrenocorticism. Clin Exp Pharmacol Physiol 2001;28:459–462.

Osler M. Addison's disease and pregnancy. Acta Endocrinol 1962;41:67.

Pacak K, Linehan WM, Eisenhofer G, et al. Recent advances in genetics, diagnosis, localization and treatment of pheochromcytoma. Ann Intern Med 2001;134:315–329.

Pekonen F, Lamberg BA, Ikonen E. Thyrotoxicosis and pregnancy. An analysis of 43 pregnancies in 42 thyrotoxic mothers. Ann Chir Gynaecol 1978;67:1–7.

Peleg D, Cada S, Peleg A, Ben-Ami M. The relationship between maternal serum thyroid stimulating immunoglobulin and fetal and neonatal thyrotoxicosis. Obstet Gynecol 2002;99:1040–1043.

Perlitz Y, Varkel J, Markovitz J, et al. Acute adrenal insufficiency during pregnancy and puerperium: case report and literature review. Obstet Gynecol Surv 1999;54:717–722.

Pitkin RM. Calcium metabolism in pregnancy and the perinatal period. A review. Am J Obstet Gynecol 1985;151:99–109.

Pop VJ, Brouwers EP, Vader HL, et al. Maternal hypothroxinaemia during early pregnancy and subsequent child development: a 3 year follow up study. Clin Endocrinol 2003;59:282–288.

Potts JT. Diseases of the parathyroid gland and other hyper and hypocalcemic disorders. In: Braunwald E, Fauci AS, Isselbacher KJ, et al., eds. Harrison's Principles of Internal Medicine, 15th edn. New York: McGraw-Hill, 2001:Chapter 341.

Prys-Roberts C. Phaeochromocytoma: recent progress in its management. Br J Anaesth 2000;85:44–57.

Pugh S, Lalwani K, Awal A. Thyroid storm as a cause of loss of consciousness following anaesthesia for emergency caesarean section. Anaesthesia 1994;49:35–37.

Reber PM, Heath H. Hypocalcemic emergencies. Med Clin North Am 1995;79:93.

Ruiz De Ona C, Obregon MJ, Escobar Del Rey F, et al. Developmental changes in rat brain 5′-deiodinase and thyroid hormones during the fetal period: the effects of fetal hypothyroidism and maternal thyroid hormones. Pediatr Res 1988;24:588–594.

Schnatz P, Curry S. Primary hyperparathyroidism in pregnancy: evidence based management. Obstet Gynecol Surv 2002;57:365–376.

Seaward P, Guidozzi F, Sonnendecker E. Addisonian crisis in pregnancy. Case report. Br J Obstet Gynaecol 1989;96:1348–1350.

Seely EW, Brown EM, DeMaggio DM, et al. A prospective study of calciotropic hormones in pregnancy and post partum: reciprocal changes in serum intact parathyroid hormone and 1,25-dihydroxyvitamin D. Am J Obstet Gynecol 1997;176:214–217.

Seki K, Makimura N, Mitsui C, et al. Calcium-regulating hormones and osteocalcin levels during pregnancy: a longitudinal study. Am J Obstet Gynecol 1991;164:1248–1252.

Shangold MN, Dor N, Welt S, et al. Hyperparathyroidism and pregnancy: a review. Obstet Gynecol Surv 1982;37:217–228.

Sheffield J, Cunningham FG. Thyrotoxicosis and heart failure complicating pregnancy. Am J Obstet Gynecol 2003 (in press).

Silverberg SJ, Shane E, Jacobs TP, Siris E, Bilezikian JP. A 10 year prospective study of primary hyperparathyroidism with or without parathyroid surgery. N Engl J Med 1999;341:1249–1255.

Stockigt J. Free thyroid hormone measurement. A critical appraisal. Endocrinol Metab Clin North Am 2001;30:265–289.

Takahashi Y, Kawabata I, Shinohara A, Tamaya T. Transient fetal blood flow redistribution induced by maternal diabetic ketoacidosis diagnosed by Doppler ultrasonography. Prenat Diagn 2000;20:524–525.

Tan TT, Morat P, Ng ML, et al. Effects of Lugol's solution on thyroid function in normals and patients with untreated thyrotoxicosis. Clin Endocrinol 1989;30:645–649.

Toft AD. Thyroxine therapy. N Engl J Med 1994;331:174–180.

Van der Meulen JA, Klip A, Grinstein S. Possible mechanisms for cerebral oedema in diabetic ketoacidosis. Lancet 1987;ii:306–308.

Viallon A, Zeni F, Lafond P, et al. Does bicarbonate therapy improve the management of severe diabetic ketoacidosis? Crit Care Med 1999;27:2690–2693.

Volpe R. Graves' disease. In: Braverman LE, Utiger RD, eds. Werner and Ingbars' The Thyroid, 6th edn. Philadelphia: JB Lippincott, 1991:648.

Volpe R, Ehrlich R, Steiner G, et al. Graves' disease in pregnancy years after hypothyroidism with recurrent passive-transfer neonatal Graves' disease in offspring. Therapeutic considerations. Am J Med 1984;77:572–578.

Vulsma T, Gons MH, de Vijlder JM. Maternal–fetal transfer of thyroxine in congenital hypothyroidism due to a total organification defect or thyroid agenesis. N Engl J Med 1989;321:13–16.

Wartofsky L, Ransil B, Ingbar S. Inhibition by iodine of the release of thyroxine from the thyroid gland of patients with thyrotoxicosis. J Clin Invest 1970;49:78–86.

Weetman AP. Graves' disease. N Engl J Med 2000;343:1236–1248.

Whalley PJ. Hyperparathyroidissm and pregnancy. Am J Obstet Gynecol 1963;86:517.

Williams G, Dluhy R. Primary adrenocortical deficiency (Addison's disease). In: Braunwald E, Fauci AS, Isselbacher KJ, et al., eds. Harrison's Principles of Internal Medicine, 15th edn. New York: McGraw Hill: 2001:Chapter 331.

Wing DA, Millar LK, Koonings PP, et al. A comparison of propylthiouracil versus methimazole in the treatment of hyperthyroidism in pregnancy. Am J Obstet Gynecol 1994;170:90–95.

Woeber K. Thyrotoxicosis and the heart. N Engl J Med 1992;327:94–98.

Woeber K. Update on the management of hyperthyroidism and hypothyroidism. Arch Intern Med 2000;160:1067–1071.

Xue-Yi C, Xin-Min J, Zhi-Hong D, et al. Timing of vulnerability of the brain to iodine deficiency in endemic cretinism. N Engl J Med 1994;331:1739–1744.

Zalonga GP, Eil C. Diseases of the parathyroid glands and nephrolithiasis during pregnancy. In: Brody SA, Ueland K, Kase N, eds. Endocrine Disorders in Pregnancy. Norwalk, CT: Appleton & Lange, 1989:231.

33 Complications of preeclampsia

Gary A. Dildy III

Hypertensive disorders complicate 6–8% of pregnancies and remain significant contributors to maternal and perinatal morbidity and mortality (Report of the National High Blood Pressure Education Program Working Group, 2000). Classification systems of hypertensive diseases during pregnancy tend to be confusing. Recently an NIH sponsored working group proposed a modified classification system (Table 33.1) for the purpose of providing clinical guidance in managing hypertensive patients during pregnancy. Chronic hypertension is defined as hypertension that is present before pregnancy or diagnosed before the 20th week of gestation. Preeclampsia is defined as the appearance of hypertension plus proteinuria, usually occurring after 20 weeks of gestation. Chronic hypertension may be complicated by superimposed preeclampsia or eclampsia. In this classification system, gestational hypertension is reassigned retrospectively following the puerperium as transient hypertension of pregnancy or chronic hypertension.

In the United States, preeclampsia is one of the top three causes of maternal mortality in advanced gestations (Kaunitz et al., 1985; Pritchard et al., 1985; Grimes, 1994; Berg et al., 1996). Pathologic changes commonly affect the maternal cardiovascular, renal, hematologic, neurologic, and hepatic systems (Table 33.2). Equally important are the adverse effects on the uteroplacental unit, resulting in fetal and neonatal complications (Lin et al., 1982; Sibai & Ramadan, 1993; Sibai et al., 1993). Our goal is to help guide the clinician in managing potentially severe complications of preeclampsia. Therapy for pregnant women with chronic hypertension will not be addressed in this chapter (Sibai, 1996).

Etiology of preeclampsia

Preeclampsia has been a recognized pathologic entity since the time of the ancient Greeks (Chesley, 1974, 1984). The inciting factor remains unknown, however, and an empty shield located on a portico at the Chicago Lying-In Hospital awaits inscription of the name of the person who discovers the etiology of the disease (Zuspan, 1978). A significant amount of investigation has been undertaken during recent decades to elucidate the cause and improve the treatment of this disease. During the past 40 years of medical research, the number of published articles has grown in geometric manner.

Numerous risk factors are associated with the development of preeclampsia (Table 33.3), allowing for antenatal recognition of potential problems in some cases. Multiple interrelated pathophysiologic processes have been proposed as etiologic in the development of this disease (Worley, 1984; Conde-Agudelo et al., 1994; Stone et al., 1994), including prostaglandin imbalance (Lewis et al., 1981; Dadek et al., 1982; Downing et al., 1982; Friedman, 1988; Sorensen et al., 1993), immunologic mechanisms (Balasch et al., 1981; Redman, 1981; Rote & Caudle, 1983; Massobrio et al., 1985; Robillard et al., 1994), hyperdynamic increase in cardiac output (Easterling & Benedetti, 1989), and subclinical blood coagulation changes (Savelieva et al., 1995). Endothelial involvement and the role of tumor necrosis factor, β-carotene, and reduced antithrombin III have also been investigated, but remain incompletely understood (Weenink et al., 1984; Weiner et al., 1985; Rodgers et al., 1988; Friedman et al., 1994; Kupferminc et al., 1994; Mikhail et al., 1994).

Increased vascular reactivity to vasoactive agents was demonstrated by Dieckmann and Michel in 1937. In 1961, Abdul-Karim and Assali found that normal pregnant women were less responsive to angiotensin II than nonpregnant women. Gant et al. (1973) published data that demonstrated an early loss of refractoriness to angiotensin II in those patients who later were to develop preeclampsia. Although clinical improvement may follow hospitalization and bed rest, vascular sensitivity to angiotensin II does not decrease until after delivery of the fetus (Whalley et al., 1983).

A molecular variant of the angiotensinogen gene (T235), found to be associated with essential hypertension, also has been associated with preeclampsia (Ward et al., 1993). It is postulated that increased concentrations of plasma or tissue angiotensinogen could lead to increased baseline or reactive production of angiotensin II, chronically stimulating autoregulatory mechanisms, thus increasing vascular tone and pro-

Table 33.1 Classification of hypertensive diseases during pregnancy

Chronic hypertension
Hypertension that is present before pregnancy or diagnosed before 20 weeks of gestation

Preeclampsia—eclampsia
Hypertension plus proteinuria usually occurring after 20 weeks of gestation or earlier with trophoblastic diseases

Preeclampsia superimposed upon chronic hypertension
Chronic hypertension with signs and symptoms of preeclampsia such as:
- Blood pressure ≥ 160/110 mmHg
- Proteinuria ≥ 2.0 g/24 hr
- Serum creatinine > 1.2 mg/dL unless previously elevated
- Thrombocytopenia
- Persistent epigastric pain
- Elevated hepatic transaminases
- Persistent neurologic disturbances

Gestational hypertension
These are retrospective diagnoses. If preeclampsia is not present at the time of delivery and elevated blood pressure:
- Transient hypertension of pregnancy: returns to normal by 12 weeks post partum
- Chronic hypertension: persists beyond 12 weeks

(Modified from the Working Group Report on High Blood Pressure in Pregnancy. National Heart, Lung, and Blood Institute. NIH Publication No. 00-3029, July 2000.)

Table 33.2 Complications of severe pregnancy-induced hypertension

Cardiovascular
Severe hypertension
Pulmonary edema

Renal
Oliguria
Renal failure

Hematologic
Hemolysis
Thrombocytopenia
Disseminated intravascular coagulopathy

Neurologic
Eclampsia
Cerebral edema
Cerebral hemorrhage
Amaurosis

Hepatic
Hepatocellular dysfunction
Hepatic rupture

Uteroplacental
Abruption
Intrauterine growth retardation
Fetal distress
Fetal death

ducing vascular hypertrophy. These changes then may impede pregnancy-induced plasma volume expansion, which occurs in normal pregnancies, and result in general circulatory maladaptation.

One of the more striking clinical risk factors for the development of preeclampsia is the antiphospholipid syndrome. At the University of Utah, Branch et al. (1989) studied 43 women who presented with severe preeclampsia prior to 34 weeks of gestation and found 16% to have significant levels of antiphospholipid antibodies. They recommended that women with early-onset severe preeclampsia be screened for antiphospholipid antibodies and, if detected, be considered for prophylactic therapy in subsequent pregnancies. The same group (Branch et al., 1992) found a high incidence of preeclampsia (51%) and severe preeclampsia (27%) in 70 women with antiphospholipid syndrome whose pregnancies progressed beyond 15 weeks of gestation, despite various medical treatment protocols.

An integrated model of preeclampsia pathophysiology has been proposed by Romero et al. (1988a). Abnormal placentation is thought to be the first step in the development of the disease, possibly related to immune mechanisms. Trophoblastic prostacyclin, which may be important with respect to trophoblast invasion and prevention of blood clotting in the intervillous space, becomes deficient. A relative decrease in the prostacyclin–thromboxane ratio allows platelet aggregation,

Table 33.3 Risk factors for the development of pregnancy-induced hypertension

Risk factor	Risk ratio
Nulliparity	3
Age > 40 years	3
African-American race	1.5
Family history of pregnancy-induced hypertension	5
Chronic hypertension	10
Chronic renal disease	20
Antiphospholipid syndrome	10
Diabetes mellitus	2
Twin gestation	4
Angiotensinogen gene T235 mutation	
Homozygous	20
Heterozygous	4

(Revised from ACOG. Hypertension in pregnancy. ACOG Technical Bulletin 219. Washington, DC: American College of Obstetricians and Gynecologists, 1996.)

thrombin activation, and fibrin deposition in systemic vascular beds. Thrombosis and vasospasm develop and lead to multiorgan involvement, including renal, hepatic, neurologic, hematologic, and uteroplacental dysfunction.

All of the preceding theories still do not allow accurate prediction of which gravidas will develop preeclampsia, and an ideal screening test is currently not available (Masse et al., 1993; Conde-Agudelo et al., 1994). Furthermore, it is still not clear which process or processes separate mild disease from the development of critical illness and multiorgan dysfunction.

Diagnosis of preeclampsia

The diagnosis of preeclampsia is often clinically confusing and erroneous (Goodlin, 1976; Fisher et al., 1981; Chesley, 1985; Sibai, 1988). Blood pressure (BP) criteria include a systolic BP of at least 140 mmHg or a diastolic BP of at least 90 mmHg. The relative rise from baseline values in systolic pressure of 30 mmHg or diastolic pressure of 15 mmHg appears to be of questionable value (Villar & Sibai, 1989; Conde-Agudelo et al., 1993). Significant proteinuria is defined as at least 300 mg in a 24-hour period. Semiquantitative dipstick analysis of urinary protein is poorly predictive of the actual degree of proteinuria measured by 24-hour urinary collections; thus, classification of preeclampsia based on proteinuria should be confirmed with a 24-hour quantitative collection (Meyer et al., 1994). Edema and weight gain historically have been included in the diagnostic triad (hypertension, proteinuria, edema) of preeclampsia, but have been deemphasized recently due to the ubiquitous nature of edema during pregnancy (Report of the National High Blood Pressure Education Program Working Group, 2000). These changes usually occur after 20 weeks of gestation, except when there exists hydatidiform changes of the chorionic villi, such as seen with hydatidiform mole or hydrops fetalis.

The signs and symptoms of severe preeclampsia are summarized in Table 33.4. The development of these manifestations necessitates careful evaluation, management in a tertiary care facility, and consideration for delivery (Pritchard et al., 1985).

Table 33.4 Diagnostic criteria for severe preeclampsia

Blood pressure > 160–180 mmHg systolic or > 110 mmHg diastolic
Proteinuria > 5 g/24 hr
Oliguria defined as < 500 mL/24 hr
Cerebral or visual disturbances
Pulmonary edema
Epigastric or right upper quadrant pain
Impaired liver function of unclear etiology
Thrombocytopenia
Fetal intrauterine growth retardation or oligohydramnios
Elevated serum creatinine
Grand mal seizures (eclampsia)

(Revised from ACOG. Hypertension in pregnancy. ACOG Technical Bulletin 219. Washington, DC: American College of Obstetricians and Gynecologists, 1996.)

General management principles for preeclampsia

On suspecting the diagnosis of preeclampsia, several steps are initiated simultaneously to treat and further evaluate the mother and her fetus. A peripheral intravenous line is placed and fluid therapy initiated. These patients are often volume-depleted and benefit from intravenous hydration, but are also susceptible to volume overload, so meticulous monitoring of intake and output is recommended.

Routine laboratory evaluation for preeclampsia (Table 33.5) includes complete blood count, platelet count, serum creatinine, and liver enzyme analyses (Pritchard et al., 1976; Weinstein, 1985; Romero et al., 1988a,b, 1989). If delivery is not felt to be imminent, a 24-hour collection of urine should be started for volume, creatinine clearance, and total protein excretion. The patient should be placed in a lateral recumbent position and fetal assessment (ultrasound, nonstress test, or biophysical profile) performed as indicated (Dildy, 2003). Amniocentesis for fetal lung maturity should be considered in those cases in which fetal maturity is in question and the disease process is not severe enough to mandate delivery.

When severe preeclampsia is diagnosed, immediate delivery, regardless of gestational age, has generally been recommended (National High Blood Pressure Education Program Working Group, 1990). Conservative management has been proposed in select cases (MacKenna et al., 1983; Thiagarajah et al., 1984; Van Dam et al., 1989). Sibai and colleagues retrospectively reviewed 60 cases of conservatively managed severe preeclampsia during the second trimester (18–27 weeks' gestation). They found a high maternal morbidity rate, with complications such as abruptio placentae, eclampsia, coagulopathy, renal failure, hypertensive encephalopathy, intracerebral hemorrhage, and ruptured hepatic hematoma. Additionally, an 87% perinatal morality rate was noted (Sibai et al., 1985a). In subsequent prospective studies, Sibai and colleagues reported improved perinatal outcomes with no increased rate of maternal complications in a select group of women with severe preeclampsia between 24–27 weeks of gestation and 28–32 weeks of gestation (Sibai et al., 1994) who were managed with intensive fetal and maternal monitoring under strict protocols in a tertiary care center. In another randomized controlled trial, expectant management in selected

Table 33.5 Laboratory evaluation for preeclampsia

Complete blood count
Platelet count
Liver function tests (ALT and AST)
Renal function tests (creatinine, blood urea nitrogen, uric acid)
Urinalysis and microscopy
24-hour urine collection for protein and creatinine clearance
Blood type and antibody screen

severe preeclamptics between 28 and 34 weeks of gestation was not associated with an increase in maternal complications, but did result in a significant prolongation of the pregnancy, reduction of neonates requiring ventilation, and a reduction in the number of neonatal complications (Odendaal et al., 1990).

The presence of preeclampsia does not guarantee accelerated lung maturation, and a high incidence of neonatal respiratory complications has been associated with premature delivery for preeclampsia (Weinstein, 1982; Pritchard et al., 1984). In a stable maternal–fetal environment, steroid therapy may be considered if amniocentesis reveals fetal lung immaturity or the clinical situation is consistent with prematurity. Although delivery is generally indicated for severe preeclampsia regardless of gestational age, we feel that conservative therapy in a tertiary care center is appropriate in select premature patients with proteinuria exceeding 5 g/per 24 hr, mild elevations of serum transaminase levels, or borderline decreases in platelet count and blood pressure that is controllable.

Fluid therapy for preeclampsia

Fluid management in severe preeclampsia consists of crystalloid infusions of normal saline or lactated Ringer's solution at 100–125 mL/hr. Additional fluid volumes, in the order of 1,000–1,500 mL, may be required prior to use of epidural anesthesia or vasodilator therapy to prevent maternal hypotension and fetal distress (Wasserstrum & Cotton, 1986).

Epidural anesthesia appears to be safe and is the anesthetic method of choice in severe preeclampsia, if preceded by volume preloading to avoid maternal hypotension (Joyce et al., 1979; Graham & Goldstein, 1980; Jouppila et al., 1982; Gutsche, 1986; Newsome et al., 1986). Likewise, severely hypertensive patients receiving vasodilator therapy may require careful volume preloading to prevent an excessive hypotensive response to vasodilators. Abrupt and profound drops in blood pressure lading to fetal bradycardia and distress may occur in severe preeclampsia when vasodilator therapy is not accompanied by volume expansion (Cotton et al., 1986a; Kirshon et al., 1988b; Wasserstrum et al., 1989).

Intravenous fluids are known to cause a decrease in colloid oncotic pressure (COP) in laboring patients (Gonik & Cotton, 1984). In addition, baseline COP is decreased in patients with preeclampsia and may decrease further post partum as a result of mobilization of interstitial fluids. This may be clinically relevant with respect to the development of pulmonary edema in preeclamptic patients (Cotton et al., 1984a). Therefore, close monitoring of fluid intake and output, hemodynamic parameters, and clinical signs must be undertaken to prevent an imbalance of hydrostatic and oncotic forces that potentiate the occurrence of pulmonary edema.

Kirshon et al. (1988b) placed systemic and pulmonary artery catheters in 15 primigravid patients with severe preeclampsia during labor. A hemodynamic protocol requiring strict control of COP, pulmonary capillary wedge pressure (PCWP), and mean arterial pressure (MAP) throughout labor, delivery, and the postpartum period was followed. Low COP and PCWP were corrected with the administration of albumin. Severe hypertension was treated as needed with intravenous nitroglycerin, nitroprusside, or hydralazine. Furosemide was administered for elevated PCWP. These investigators found that the only benefit of such management was avoidance of sudden profound drops in systemic blood pressure and fetal distress during antihypertensive therapy. The overall incidence of fetal distress in labor was not affected, however. Because of a significant requirement for pharmacologic diuresis to prevent pulmonary edema in the study group, these authors recommended that COP not be corrected with colloid unless markedly decreased (12 mmHg) or a prolonged negative COP–PCWP gradient was identified. While the infusion of colloids has been shown to result in less of a decrease in COP when compared with crystalloids, there is no evidence of any clinical benefit of colloids over crystalloids for the pregnant patient (Jones et al., 1986). Thus, in the absence of a firm clinical indication for colloid infusion, carefully controlled crystalloid infusions appear to be the safest mode of fluid therapy in severe preeclampsia.

Seizure prophylaxis for preeclampsia

Magnesium sulfate ($MgSO_4 \cdot 7H_2O$ USP) has been used for the prevention of eclamptic seizures since the early twentieth century (Dorsett, 1926; Lazard, 1933; Eastman & Steptoe, 1945) and has long been the standard treatment of preeclampsia –eclampsia in the United States (Pritchard, 1955; Pritchard & Pritchard, 1975). The mechanism of action of magnesium sulfate remains controversial (Shelley & Gutsche, 1980). Some investigators feel that magnesium acts primarily via neuromuscular blockade, while others believe that magnesium acts centrally (Borges & Gucer, 1978; Pritchard, 1979). Two separate investigations evaluating the effect of parenteral magnesium sulfate on penicillin-induced seizure foci in cats report conflicting data (Borges & Gucer, 1978; Koontz & Reid, 1985). Koontz and Reid (1985) postulate that magnesium may be effective as an anticonvulsant only when the blood–brain barrier is disrupted. Human data reveal that abnormal EEG findings are common in preeclampsia–eclampsia, and they are not altered by levels of magnesium considered to be therapeutic (Sibai et al., 1984a). In the rat model, Hallak et al. (1994) and Hallak (1998) proposed that magnesium's anticonvulsant mechanism of action was central, mediated through excitatory amino acid (*N*-methyl-D-aspartate) receptors. In a randomized placebo-controlled study, Belfort et al. (1992) evaluated the effect of magnesium sulfate on maternal retinal blood flow in preeclamptics by way of Doppler blood flow measurements of central retinal and posterior ciliary arteries. Their findings suggested that magnesium sulfate vasodilates small vessels in the retina and proposed that this may reflect similar changes occurring in the cerebral circulation.

Magnesium sulfate regimens are illustrated in Table 33.6. Because a regimen of a 4-g IV loading dose followed by a 1–2-g/hr IV maintenance dose failed to prevent eclampsia in a significant number of preeclamptic women, Sibai et al. (1984b) modified this regimen to a 4-g IV loading dose followed by a 2–3-g/hr IV maintenance dose. Sibai compared Pritchard's regimen of a 4-g IV and 10-g IM loading dose followed by a 5-g IM maintenance dose every 4 hours, with a 4-g IV loading dose followed by a 1–2-g/hr continuous IV maintenance infusion. The IV loading dose with maintenance dose of 1 g/hr did not produce adequate serum levels of magnesium (4–7 mEq/L); thus, they recommended a 2–3-g/hr maintenance dose (Sibai et al., 1984b). We employ a regimen of a 4–6-g IV loading dose over 20 minutes, followed by a 2–3-g/hr continuous IV infusion. The maintenance infusion may be adjusted according to clinical parameters and serum magnesium levels. Pruett et al. (1988) found no significant effects on neonatal Apgar scores at these doses.

Until relatively recently there remained considerable controversy regarding the best agent for eclampsia prophylaxis. In the United States, magnesium sulfate has been the agent of choice (Pritchard et al., 1984; National High Blood Pressure Education Program Working Group, 1990; Atkinson et al., 1991), whereas in the United Kingdom and in a few US centers, conventional antiepileptic agents have been advocated (Donaldson, 1992; Hutton et al., 1992; Repke et al., 1992; Duley & Johanson, 1994). Recently, several important randomized clinical trials of magnesium sulfate for prevention or control of eclamptic seizures have been published (Table 33.7).

Table 33.6 Magnesium sulfate protocols

	Loading dose	Maintenance dose
Pritchard (1955),		
Eclampsia	4 g IV and 10 g IM	5 g IM every 4 hr
Zuspan (1966)		
Severe preeclampsia	None	1 g/hr IV
Eclampsia	4–6 g IV over 5–10 min	1 g/hr IV
Sibai et al. (1984b)		
Preeclampsia–eclampsia	6 g IV over 15 min	2 g/hr

In a randomized trial comparing magnesium sulfate with phenytoin for the prevention of eclampsia, Lucas et al. (1995) found a statistically significant difference ($P = 0.004$) in the development of seizures between the magnesium sulfate group (0/1,049) and the phenytoin group (10/1,089), with no significant differences in eclampsia risk factors between the two study groups.

The Eclampsia Trial Collaborative Group (1995) enrolled 1,687 women with eclampsia in an international multicenter randomized trial comparing standard anticonvulsant regimens of magnesium sulfate, phenytoin, and diazepam. Women allocated magnesium sulfate had a 52% lower risk of recurrent convulsions than those allocated diazepam, and a 67% lower risk of recurrent convulsions than those allocated phenytoin. Women allocated magnesium sulfate were less likely to require mechanical ventilation, to develop pneumonia, and to be admitted to intensive care than those allocated phenytoin. Furthermore, the babies of mothers allocated magnesium sulfate were less likely to be intubated at delivery and less likely to be admitted to the newborn intensive care nursery when compared with babies of mothers treated with phenytoin. The Eclampsia Trial Collaborative Group concluded that magnesium sulfate is the drug of choice for routine anticonvusant management of women with eclampsia, rather than diazepam or phenytoin, and recommended that other anticonvulsants be used only in the context of randomized trials.

Coetzee et al. (1998) conducted a blinded, randomized, controlled trial ($n = 822$) of intravenous magnesium sulfate versus placebo in the management of women with severe preeclampsia. They found that use of intravenous magnesium sulfate significantly reduced the development of eclampsia (0.3%

Table 33.7 Randomized trials comparing magnesium sulfate ($MgSO_4$) with other agents in prophylaxis (preventing eclampsia in preeclamptics) and treatment (preventing recurrent seizures) of eclampsia

Reference	Study population	*n*	$MgSO_4$	Placebo	Phenytoin	Diazepam	Lytic cocktail	Nimodipine
Bhalla (1994)	Eclamptics	91	2.2%	—	—	—	24.4%	—
Lucas et al. (1995)	Mixed preeclamptics	2,138	0%	—	0.9%	—	—	—
Eclampsia Trial Collaborative	Eclamptics	905	13.2%	—	—	27.9%	—	—
Group (1995)	Eclamptics	775	5.7%	—	17.1%	—	—	—
Coetzee et al. (1998)	Severe preeclamptics	685	0.3%	3.2%	—	—	—	—
Magpie Trial Collaborative Group (2002)	Mixed preeclamptics	10,141	0.8%	1.9%	—	—	—	—
Belfort et al. (2003)	Severe preeclamptics	1,650	0.8%	—	—	—	—	2.6%

vs 3.2%, relative risk 0.09; 95% confidence interval 0.01–0.69; $P = 0.003$) compared to placebo.

Thus at present, magnesium sulfate is strongly endorsed as the agent of choice for eclampsia prophylaxis and treatment (Chien et al., 1996; Rey et al., 1997; Report of the National High Blood Pressure Education Program Working Group, 2000; Hypertensive, 2001; ACOG, 2002). The Cochrane Review of randomized clinical trials found magnesium superior to lytic cocktail (chlorpromazine, promethazine, pethidine), diazepam, and phenytoin for prevention and/or treatment of eclampsia (Duley & Gulmezoglu, 2002; Duley & Henderson-Smart, 2002a,b; Duley et al., 2002). The role of magnesium sulfate seizure prophylaxis for mild preeclamptics is still subject to debate.

Plasma magnesium levels maintained at 4–7 mEq/L are felt to be therapeutic in preventing eclamptic seizures (Pritchard et al., 1985). Patellar reflexes usually are lost at 8–10 mEq/L, and respiratory arrest may occur at 13 mEq/L (Pritchard, 1955; Chesley, 1979). Urine output, patellar reflexes, and respiratory rates should be monitored closely during magnesium sulfate administration. In those patients who have renal dysfunction, serum magnesium levels should be monitored as well. Calcium gluconate, oxygen therapy, and the ability to perform endotracheal intubation should be available in the event of magnesium toxicity (Chesley, 1979). Calcium will reverse the adverse effects of magnesium toxicity. Calcium gluconate is administered as a 1-g dose (10 mL of a 10% solution) IV over a period of 2 minutes (ACOG, 1996).

Bohman and Cotton (1990) reported a case of supralethal magnesemia (38.7 mg/dL) with patient survival and no adverse sequelae. The essential elements in the resuscitation and prevention of toxic magnesemia are (i) respiratory support as determined by clinical indicators; (ii) use of continuous cardiac monitoring; (iii) infusion of calcium salts to prevent hypocalcemia and the enhanced cardiotoxicity associated with concurrent hypocalcemia and hypermagnesemia; (iv) use of loop or osmotic diuretics to excrete the magnesium ion more rapidly, as well as careful attention to fluid and electrolyte balances; (v) a consideration that toxic magnesium is neither anesthetic nor amnestic to the patient; and (vi) assurance that all magnesium infusions be administered in a buretrol-type system or by intramuscular injection to prevent toxic magnesemia.

Magnesium sulfate is not an antihypertensive agent (Pritchard, 1955). Administration produces a transient decrease in BP in hypertensive, but not normotensive, nonpregnant subjects (Mroczek et al., 1977). Young and Weinstein (1977) noted significant respiratory effects and a transient fall in maternal BP in patients who received a 10-g IM loading dose of magnesium sulfate followed by maintenance push doses of 2 g every 1–2 hours, but not in patients who received the 10-g loading dose followed by a 1-g/hr continuous infusion (Young & Weinstein, 1977). Cotton et al. (1984b) observed a transient hypotensive effect related to bolus infusion, but not with continuous infusion in severe preeclampsia.

Antihypertensive therapy for severe preeclampsia

Preeclampsia is sometimes manifested by severe systemic hypertension. Careful control of hypertension must be achieved to prevent complications such as maternal cerebral vascular accidents and placental abruption. Medical intervention is usually recommended when the diastolic BP exceeds 110 mmHg (Naden & Redman, 1985; Lubbe, 1987; ACOG, 1996). The degree of systolic hypertension requiring therapy is less certain, but most would treat for a level exceeding 160–180 mmHg, depending on the associated diastolic pressure. In the previously normotensive patient, cerebral autoregulation is lost and the risk of intracranial bleeding increases when MAP exceeds 140–150 mm Hg, as illustrated in Fig. 33.1 (Zimmerman, 1995). Although many different antihypertensive agents are available, we confine our discussion to those agents most commonly used for acute hypertensive crises in pregnancy (Table 33.8).

Hydralazine hydrochloride

Hydralazine hydrochloride (Apresoline) has long been the gold standard of antihypertensive therapy for use by obstetricians in the United States. Hydralazine reduces vascular resistance via direct relaxation of arteriolar smooth muscle, affecting precapillary resistance vessels more than postcapillary capacitance vessels (Koch-Weser, 1976). Assali et al. (1953) noted the hypotensive effect to be marked and prolonged in preeclamptic patients, moderate in patients with essential hypertension, and slight in normotensive subjects. Using M-mode echocardiography, Kuzniar et al. (1985) found an attenuated response to a 12.5-mg IV dose of hydralazine in

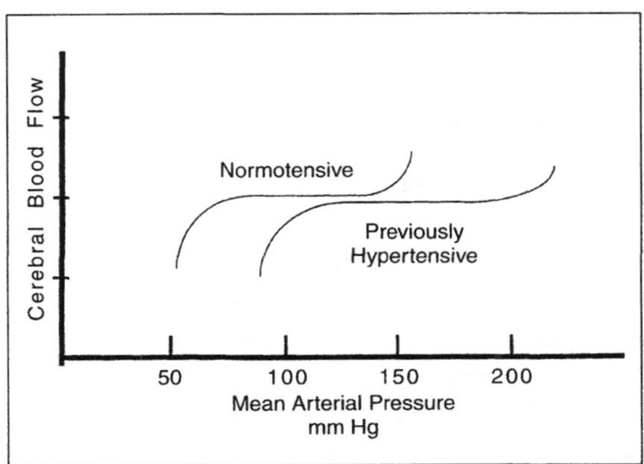

Fig. 33.1 Cerebral blood flow remains constant over a wide range of pressures in normotensive individuals. This range is shifted to the right in individuals with chronic hypertension. (Modified from Zimmerman JL. Hypertensive crisis: emergencies and urgencies. In: Ayers SM, ed. Textbook of Critical Care. Philadelphia: WB Saunders, 1995.)

Table 33.8 Pharmacologic agents for antihypertensive therapy in preeclampsia–eclampsia

Generic name	Trade name	Mechanism of action	Dosage	Comment
Hydralazine	Apresoline	Arterial vasodilator	5 mg IV, then 5–10 mg IV/20 min up to total dose of 40 mg; titrated IV infusion 5–10 mg/hr	Must wait 20 min for response between IV doses; possible maternal hypotension
Labetalol	Normodyne Trandate	Selective α- and nonselective β-antagonist	20 mg IV, then 40–80 mg IV/10 min to 300 mg total dose; titrated IV infusion 1–2 mg/min	Less reflex tachycardia and hypotension than with hydralazine
Nifedipine	Procardia Adalat	Calcium channel blocker	10 mg PO, may repeat after 30 min	Oral route only; possible exaggerated effect if used with $MgSO_4$
Nitroglycerin	Nitrostat IV Tridil Nitro-Bid IV	Relaxation of venous (and arterial) vascular smooth muscle	5 μg/min infusion; double every 5 min	Requires arterial line for continuous blood pressure monitoring; potential methemoglobinemia
Nitroprusside	Nipride Nitropress	Vasodilator	0.25 μg/kg/min infusion; increase by 0.25 μg/kg/min every 5 min	Requires arterial line for continuous blood pressure monitoring; potential cyanide toxicity

(Modified from Dildy GA, Cotton DB. Hemodynamic changes in pregnancy and pregnancy complicated by hypertension. Acute Care 1988–89;14–15:26–46.)

patients with preexisting hypertension, compared with those with severe preeclampsia. Cotton et al. (1985) studied the cardiovascular alterations in six severe preeclamptics following intravenous administration of a 10-mg bolus of hydralazine. They observed a significant increase in maternal heart rate and cardiac index (CI), with a decrease in MAP and systemic vascular resistance (SVR) index. There was a wide range of individual response with respect to peak and duration. Jouppila et al. (1985) measured maternal–fetal effects with Doppler in severe preeclamptics receiving dihydralazine and demonstrated a fall in maternal BP with no change in intervillous blood flow and an increase in umbilical vein blood flow. Dihydralazine also has been shown to cross the placenta to the fetus (Liedholm et al., 1982). The administration of hydralazine may result in maternal hypotension and fetal distress (Spinnato et al., 1986). For this reason, we recommend an initial dose of 2.5–5.0 mg IV, followed by observation of hemodynamic effects. If appropriate change in BP is not achieved, 5–10 mg IV may be administered at 20-minute intervals to a total acute dose of 30–40 mg. Hypertension refractory to the preceding approach warrants the use of alternative antihypertensive agents (Cotton et al., 1986b; Clark & Cotton, 1988).

Diazoxide

Diazoxide (Hyperstat) is a benzothiadiazine derivative that exerts its antihypertensive effect by reducing peripheral vascular resistance through direct relaxation of arterioles (Rubin et al., 1962). The commonly used 300-mg bolus injection to treat severe hypertension may induce significant hypotension with resultant morbidity. Minibolus diazoxide titration is clinically effective and relatively free of side effects in nonpregnant, severely hypertensive adults; a suggested dose would be 30–60 mg IV in 5-minute intervals, titrating to desired clinical response. Thien et al. (1980) recommended that diazoxide for the treatment of severe preeclampsia–eclampsia be administered by the infusion method (15 mg/min; total amount, 5 mg/kg body weight) rather than by bolus injection (300 mg within 10 sec), because the infusion method results in a more gradual decline in BP and can be interrupted in cases of exaggerated drop in BP.

Calcium channel blockers

Calcium channel blockers such as nifedipine (Procardia, Adalat) lower BP primarily by relaxing arterial smooth muscle. An initial oral dose of 10 mg is administered, which may be repeated after 30 minutes, if necessary, for the acute management of severe hypertension; 10–20 mg may then be administered orally every 3–6 hours as needed (Naden & Redman, 1985). Principal side effects in severe preeclamptics include headache and cutaneous flushing. Care must be given when nifedipine is administered to patients receiving concomitant magnesium sulfate because of the possibility of an exaggerated hypotensive response (Waisman et al., 1988). In a randomized clinical trial, 49 women with severe preeclampsia and severe hypertension between 26 and 36 weeks of gestation were primarily treated with sublingual (then oral) nifedipine or intravenous (then oral) hydralazine (Fenakel et al., 1991). Effective control of BP (values consistently below 160/110 mmHg) was achieved in 96% of the nifedipine group and 68% of the hydralazine group ($P < 0.05$), with acute fetal distress occurring more commonly in the hydralazine group. A beneficial effect may also be seen on urine output in women with severe preeclampsia treated with nifedipine (Vermillion et al., 1999; Aali & Nejad, 2001). Other calcium channel blockers (nimodipine) have been studied in the management of preeclampsia (Belfort et al., 1993, 1994, 1999a,b) and are the subject of ongoing investigation.

Labetalol

Labetalol (Normodyne, Trandate) is a combined α- and β-adrenoceptor antagonist that may be used to induce a controlled rapid decrease in BP via decreased SVR in patients with severe hypertension (Lund-Johnson, 1983b). Reports on the efficacy and safety of labetalol in the treatment of hypertension during pregnancy have been favorable (Lamming & Symonds, 1979; Michael, 1979; Coevoet et al., 1980; Lunell et al., 1981; Riley, 1981; Mabie et al., 1987; Pickles et al., 1989). Mabie et al. (1987) compared bolus intravenous labetalol with intravenous hydralazine in the acute treatment of severe hypertension. They found that labetalol had a quicker onset of action and did not result in reflex tachycardia. Labetalol also may exert a positive effect on early fetal lung maturation in patients with severe hypertension who are remote from term (Michael, 1979, 1982). An initial dose of 10 mg is given and is followed by progressively increasing doses (20, 40, 80 mg) every 10 minutes, to a total dose of 300 mg. Alternately, constant intravenous infusion may be started at 1–2 mg/min until therapeutic goals are achieved, then decreased to 0.5 mg/min or completely stopped (Naden & Redman, 1985). Lunell et al. (1984) studied the effects of labetalol on uteroplacental perfusion in hypertensive pregnant women and noted increased uteroplacental perfusion and decreased uterine vascular resistance. Morgan et al. (1993) evaluated the effects of labetalol on uterine blood flow in the hypertensive gravid baboon and found that low doses (0.5 mg/kg) significantly reduced MAP without adversely affecting uterine blood flow.

Nitroglycerin

Nitroglycerin (Nitrostat IV, Nitro-Bid IV, Tridil) relaxes predominantly venous but also arterial vascular smooth muscle, decreasing preload at low doses and afterload at high doses (Herling, 1984). It is a rapidly acting potent antihypertensive agent with a very short hemodynamic half-life. Using invasive hemodynamic monitoring, Cotton et al. (1986a,b) noted that the ability to control BP precisely was dependent on volume status. Although larger doses of nitroglycerin were required following volume expansion, the ability to effect a smoother and more controlled drop in BP required prevasodilator hydration (Cotton et al., 1986a). Nitroglycerin is administered via an infusion pump at an initial rate of 5 μg/min and may be doubled every 5 minutes. Methemoglobinemia may result from high-dose (7 μg/kg/min) intravenous infusion. Patients with normal arterial oxygen saturation who appear cyanotic should be evaluated for toxicity, defined as a methemoglobin level greater than 3% (Herling, 1984).

Sodium nitroprusside

Sodium nitroprusside (Nipride, Nitropress) is another potent antihypertensive agent that may be used to control severe hypertension associated with preeclampsia. A dilute solution may be started at 0.25 μg/kg/min and titrated to the desired effect through an infusion pump by increasing the dose by 0.25 μg/kg/min every 5 minutes. The solution is light sensitive and should be covered in foil and changed every 24 hours (Pasch et al., 1983). Arterial blood gases should be monitored for developing metabolic acidosis, which may be an early sign of cyanide toxicity. In nonpregnant subjects, sodium nitroprusside infusion rates in excess of 4 μg/kg/min led to red blood cell cyanide levels that after 2–3 hours of administration extended into the toxic range (>40 nmol/mL); infusion rates of less than 2 μg/kg/min for several hours remained nontoxic (Pasch et al., 1983). Treatment time should be limited because of the potential for fetal cyanide toxicity (Strauss et al., 1980). Correction of hypovolemia prior to initiation of nitroprusside infusion is essential in order to avoid abrupt and often profound drops in BP.

Angiotensin-converting enzyme inhibitors

Angiotensin-converting enzyme (ACE) inhibitors (captopril, enalapril) interrupt the renin–angiotensin–aldosterone system, resulting in a lowering of BP (Oates & Wood, 1988). The risk of inducing neonatal renal failure and other serious complications would contraindicate the use of ACE inhibitors during pregnancy (Hurault de Ligny et al., 1987; Schubiger et al., 1988; Barr & Cohen, 1991; Hanssens et al., 1991). Fetal abortion has been reported in pregnant rabbits (Ferris & Weir, 1983). Additionally, the ACE inhibitors as a class do not appear to be useful in acute treatment of severe hypertension because of a 1–4-hour delay in achievement of peak serum levels after ingestion (Oates & Wood, 1988).

Severe hypertension

We recommend hydralazine for initial management of severe

hypertension (BP 180–160/110 mmHg). Hydralazine will be effective in restoring BP to a desired range (160–130/110–80 mmHg) in the majority of cases. When maximum doses of hydralazine (40 mg) have not corrected severe hypertension, we then proceed to nifedipine or labetalol. In rare cases, these agents are ineffective, and we resort to intravenous infusion of nitroglycerin or nitroprusside, which requires an intensive care setting.

Analgesia–anesthesia for preeclampsia

The use of conduction anesthesia in preeclampsia was, at one time, controversial. Concerns have been voiced by some authors that the sympathetic blockade and peripheral vasodilation resulting from epidural anesthesia may lead to hypotension and fetal distress in patients who are already volume-contracted (Pritchard & Pritchard, 1975; Lindheimer & Katz, 1985; Pritchard et al., 1985). However, induction of general endotracheal anesthesia is not without its own inherent risks. General anesthesia has been shown to result in significant rises in systemic arterial pressure in patients with severe preeclampsia. An average increase in systolic arterial BP of 56 mmHg during endotracheal intubation of 20 patients with hypertension was reported by Connell et al. (1987).

Hodgkinson et al. (1980) evaluated 10 severe preeclampticeclamptic patients undergoing general anesthesia using the pulmonary artery catheter. They noted severe systemic and pulmonary hypertension during endotracheal intubation and extubation. Ten patients undergoing epidural anesthesia with 0.75% bupivacaine for cesarean section maintained stable systemic and pulmonary arterial pressures, with the exception of one patient who developed systemic hypotension that responded promptly to ephedrine.

Newsome et al. (1986) demonstrated a drop in MAP and a slight but insignificant decrease in SVR without change in CI, peripheral vascular resistance (PVR), central venous pressure (CVP), or PCWP in 11 patients with severe preeclampsia undergoing lumbar epidural anesthesia. Jouppila et al. (1982) measured intervillous blood flow in nine patients with severe preeclampsia during labor with lumbar epidural block and found a significant increase in uterine blood flow. Ramos-Santos et al. (1991) studied the effects of epidural anesthesia on uterine and umbilical artery blood flow by way of Doppler velocimetry in mild preeclamptics, chronic hypertensives, and normal controls during active term labor. In the preeclamptic group, the uterine artery systolic/diastolic ratios decreased to levels similar to those of the control group, suggesting a possible beneficial effect in reducing uterine artery vasospasm.

Deleterious hypotension may be avoided by lateral maternal tilt, thus preventing aortocaval occlusion, and preloading with crystalloid solution to compensate for peripheral vasodilation (Jouppila et al., 1982). Contraindications to epidural anesthesia include patient refusal, fetal distress requiring immediate delivery, local infection, septicemia, severe spinal deformities, and coagulopathy (Gutsche, 1986). If preceded by volume loading, epidural anesthesia appears beneficial and safe in severe preeclampsia (Joyce et al., 1979; Graham & Goldstein, 1980; Jouppila et al., 1982; Gutsche, 1986; Newsome et al., 1986; Wasserstrum & Cotton, 1986; Clark & Cotton, 1988). Clark and Cotton (1988) state, "In skilled hands, a cautiously administered epidural anesthetic is, in our opinion, not only justified, but the method of choice for anesthesia in cesarean section or for control of the pain of labor in the patient with severe preeclampsia." The safety and efficacy of neuraxial analgesia for severe preeclamptics appears to be well supported by recent studies (Hogg et al., 1999; Head et al., 2002). When general anesthesia is necessary, careful control of maternal BP, especially around the time of induction and awakening, is essential. Small doses of nitroglycerin or other similar agents are often useful in this regard.

Hemodynamic monitoring for preeclampsia

The pulmonary artery catheter, introduced over 30 years ago, has been very useful in the management of critically ill patients (Swan et al., 1970). In cases of severe preeclampsia, most clinicians have obtained excellent results without invasive monitoring (Pritchard et al., 1984). Protocols developed to study the central hemodynamic parameters of severe preeclampsia have revealed interesting data, which are sometimes confounded by differences in clinical patient management prior to and at the time of catheterization (Wasserstrum & Cotton, 1986). Hemodynamic changes observed in normal pregnancies and pregnancies complicated by hypertension are summarized by Dildy and Cotton (1988, 1991). Central hemodynamic findings in severe preeclampsia are summarized by Clark and Cotton (1988) in Table 33.9. Hemodynamic findings in nonpregnant women, normal third-trimester pregnancy, and severe preeclamptics are provided in Table 33.10.

Current indications for the use of a pulmonary artery catheter in preeclampsia are listed in Table 33.11 (Clark et al., 1985a,b; Clark & Cotton, 1988; Cotton et al., 1988). Routine use of the pulmonary artery catheter in uncomplicated severe preeclampsia is not recommended. In these cases, the potential morbidity of pulmonary artery catheterization does not appear to be justified. Known complications of invasive monitoring at the time of insertion include cardiac arrhythmias, pneumothorax, hemothorax, injury to vascular and neurologic structures, pulmonary infarction, and pulmonary hemorrhage. Later complications include balloon rupture, thromboembolism, catheter knotting, pulmonary valve rupture, and catheter migration into the pericardial and pleural spaces, with subsequent cardiac tamponade and hydrothorax (Mitchell & Clark, 1979; Cotton & Benedetti, 1980; Kirshon & Cotton, 1987). It should be noted, however, that Clark et al.

(1985a) observed no significant complications from pulmonary artery catheterization in a series of 90 patients who underwent the procedure on an obstetrics–gynecology service. A retrospective study of 115 pregnant women with severe preeclampsia and eclampsia managed by pulmonary artery catheterization concluded that catheterization was subjectively beneficial in 93% of cases with an acceptable complication rate of 4% (Gilbert et al., 2000).

Table 33.9 Hemodynamic findings in severe pregnancy-induced hypertension

Cardiac output is variable
Mean arterial pressure is elevated; systemic vascular resistance is normal (early) or elevated (late)
Central venous pressure is usually low to normal and does not correlate with pulmonary capillary wedge pressure
Pulmonary hypertension and pulmonary vascular resistance are not present, but low pulmonary artery pressure may occur in the presence of hypovolemia
Pulmonary capillary wedge pressure may be low, normal, or high
Oliguria may not reflect volume depletion
Ventricular function is usually hyperdynamic, but may be depressed in the presence of marked elevation in systemic vascular resistance
Colloid oncotic pressure is usually low

(Reproduced with permission from Clark SL, Cotton DB. Clinical indications for pulmonary artery catheterization in the patient with severe preeclampsia. Am J Obstet Gynecol 1988;158:453–458.)

Cardiopulmonary complications of preeclampsia

During normal pregnancy, plasma volume increases approximately 42% while red blood cell volume increases approximately 24% (Chesley, 1972). Earlier studies of cardiovascular changes in preeclampsia revealed increased vascular resistance, decreased circulatory volume, and decreased perfusion of various organ systems, most notably the renal and uteroplacental circulations, when compared with normal nonpregnant subjects (Zuspan, 1978; Hays et al., 1985), In pregnancies complicated by preeclampsia, a reduction in plasma volume with hemoconcentration occurs in proportion to the severity of the disease (Chesley, 1972). Significant plasma volume depletion and reduction in circulating plasma protein may occur prior to the clinical manifestations of preeclampsia (Bletka et al., 1970; Gallery et al., 1979; Hays et al., 1985). In subjects who developed hypertension during pregnancy, various degrees of

Table 33.10 Hemodynamic profiles of nonpregnant women, normal women during the late third trimester, and severe preeclamptics

	Normal nonpregnant ($n = 10$)* (mean ± SD)	Normal late third trimester ($n = 10$)* (mean ± SD)	Severe preeclampsia ($n = 45$)† (mean ± SEM)	Severe preeclampsia ($n = 41$)‡ (mean ± SEM)
Heart rate (beats/min)	71 ± 10	83 ± 10	95 ± 2	94 ± 2
Systolic blood pressure (mmHg)	N/A	N/A	193 ± 3	175 ± 3
Diastolic blood pressure (mmHg)	N/A	N/A	110 ± 2	106 ± 2
Mean arterial blood pressure (mmHg)	86.4 ± 7.5	90.3 ± 5.8	138 ± 3	130 ± 2
Pulse pressure (mmHg)	N/A	N/A	84 ± 2	70 ± 2
Central venous pressure (mmHg)	3.7 ± 2.6	3.6 ± 2.5	4 ± 1	4.8 ± 0.4
Pulmonary capillary wedge pressure (mmHg)	6.3 ± 2.1	7.5 ± 1.8	10 ± 1	8.3 ± 0.3
Pulmonary artery pressure (mmHg)	11.9 ± 2.0§	12.5 ± 2.0§	17 ± 1	15 ± 0.5
Cardiac output (L/min)	4.3 ± 0.9	6.2 ± 1.0	7.5 ± 0.2	8.4 ± 0.2
Stroke volume (mL)	N/A	N/A	79 ± 2	90 ± 2
Systemic vascular resistance (dynes · sec · cm^{-5})	1,530 ± 520	1,210 ± 266	1,496 ± 64	1,226 ± 37
Pulmonary vascular resistance (dynes · sec · cm^{-5})	119 ± 47	78 ± 22	70 ± 5	65 ± 3
Serum colloid osmotic pressure (mmHg)	20.8 ± 1.0	18.0 ± 1.5	19.0 ± 0.5	N/A
Body surface area (m^2)	N/A	N/A	N/A	N/A
Systemic vascular resistance index (dynes · sec · cm^{-5} · m^2)	N/A	N/A	2,726 ± 120	2,293 ± 65
Pulmonary vascular resistance index (dynes · sec · cm^{-5} · m^2)	N/A	N/A	127 ± 9	121 ± 7
Right ventricular stroke work index (g · m · M^{-2})	N/A	N/A	8 ± 1	10 ± 0.5
Left ventricular stroke work index (g · m · M^{-2})	41 ± 8	48 ± 6	81 ± 2	84 ± 2
Cardiac index (L · min^{-1} · m^2)	N/A	N/A	4.1 ± 0.1	4.4 ± 0.1
Stroke volume index (mL · beat · m^2)	N/A	N/A	44 ± 1	48 ± 1
COP–PCWP (mmHg)	14.5 ± 2.5	10.5 ± 2.7	N/A	N/A

Data from * Cotton et al. (1988); † Clark et al. (1989); ‡ Mabie et al. (1989); § Clark et al., unpublished data.
N/A, not available; SD, standard deviation; SEM, standard error of the mean.

Table 33.11 Indications for use of pulmonary artery catheter in pregnancy-induced hypertension

Complications related to central volume status
Pulmonary edema of uncertain etiology
Pulmonary edema unresponsive to conventional therapy
Persistent oliguria despite aggressive volume expansion
Induction of conduction anesthesia in hemodynamically unstable patients
Medical complication that would otherwise required invasive monitoring

increased cardiac output (CO) and/or SVR were noted (Lees, 1979).

Although the precise cause of these changes remains unknown, further insight into the exact cardiovascular parameters associated with pregnancy-related disease states evolved around 1980, when obstetric and gynecologic indications for use of the pulmonary artery catheter were described, and measurements of CVP, pulmonary artery pressure (PAP), PCWP, CO, and mixed venous oxygen became available (Cotton & Benedetti, 1980).

Rafferty and Berkowitz (1980) studied three preeclamptic patients with a pulmonary artery catheter and noted an increased left ventricular stroke index (LVSWI) and normal pulmonary artery resistance. At delivery, the CI and PCWP increased in these patients, probably secondary to increased venous return. These investigators noted an increased PCWP post partum, which also was felt to be secondary to increased circulatory volume. These findings suggest that the pulmonary vasculature is not involved in the vasospastic process and that pulmonary hypertension is not present in severe preeclampsia.

Observations made from pulmonary artery catheterization in 10 patients with severe preeclampsia during labor showed an increased LVSWI (suggesting hyperdynamic ventricular function), normal PAP, and poor correlation between CVP and PCWP (Benedetti et al., 1980). The poor correlation of PCWP and CVP has been verified by subsequent investigations (Strauss et al., 1980; Cotton et al., 1985).

Hemodynamic studies have consistently demonstrated hyperdynamic left ventricular function in preeclamptic patients (Phelan & Yurth, 1982; Cotton et al., 1984b; Henderson et al., 1984). Phelan and Yurth (1982) studied 10 severe preeclamptics and noted hyperdynamic cardiac function with elevated CO and variable elevation of SVR. Immediately post partum, a transient fall in left ventricular function with a rise in CVP and PCWP was noted in 6 of 10 patients, possibly secondary to an autotransfusion effect. Hyperdynamic ventricular function returned 1 hour post partum. One criticism of this study as it related to CO is the fact that several of these patients received intrapartum hydralazine, which could account for the elevated CO.

Groenendijk et al. (1984) noted a low CI, low PCWP, and high SVR in preeclamptics prior to volume expansion. Volume expansion resulted in an elevation of PCWP and CI to normal pregnant values, a drop in SVR, and no change in BP. Vasodilation using hydralazine then resulted in a further drop in SVR and BP, with a rise in CI, and no change in PCWP.

Eclamptics studied by Hankins et al. (1984) initially demonstrated hyperdynamic left ventricular function and elevated SVR, as well as low right and left ventricular filling pressures. Following labor management, consisting of fluid restriction, magnesium sulfate, and hydralazine, the authors observed a postpartum rise in PCWP in patients who did not have an early spontaneous diuresis. This rise in PCWP was thought to be secondary to mobilization of extravascular fluids before the diuresis phase. They concluded that the hemodynamic status was influenced by the severity and duration of the disease, other underlying disease states, and therapeutic interventions such as epidural anesthesia.

Cotton et al. (1988) summarized the hemodynamic profile in 45 patients with severe preeclampsia or eclampsia. They observed a wide variety of hemodynamic measurements in these patients; however, the majority were found to have an elevated BP, variably elevated SVR, hyperdynamic left ventricular function, normal to increased PCWP, and low CVP. They hypothesized that the elevated PCWP with decreased CVP was secondary to elevated left ventricular afterload, combined with a hypovolemic state. These findings are summarized in Table 33.9.

Clark et al. (1989) documented for the first time central hemodynamic parameters in normotensive late third-trimester pregnant patients (see Table 33.10). They demonstrated that most reported patients with severe preeclampsia have SVR in the normal range for pregnancy, and that left ventricular function in normal pregnancy as assessed by LVSWI is not hyperdynamic. This supports the model of an initially hyperdynamic hypertension without vasospasm in preeclampsia. This may be followed by the development of elevated SVR associated with vasospasm and a secondary decline in CO and LVSWI. Such a phenomenon has been documented in untreated nonpregnant patients with essential hypertension (Lund-Johansen, 1983a).

Pulmonary edema

Sibai et al. (1987) reported a 2.9% incidence of pulmonary edema in severe preeclampsia–eclampsia; 70% of these 37 cases developed post partum. In 90% of the cases that developed antepartum, chronic hypertension was identified as an underlying factor. A higher incidence of pulmonary edema was noted in older patients, multigravidas, and patients with underlying chronic hypertension. The development of pulmonary edema was also associated with the administration of excess infusions, either colloids or crystalloids.

Reduction of COP, alteration of capillary membrane permeability, and elevated pulmonary vascular hydrostatic pressures may lead to extravasation of fluids into the interstitial and alveolar spaces, resulting in pulmonary edema (Henderson et al.,

1984). Cotton et al. (1985) observed a negative COP–PCWP gradient in five preeclamptic patients who developed pulmonary edema. Interestingly, Clark et al. (1985b) compared the hemodynamic alterations in severe preeclamptics and eclamptics and suggested that the occurrence of eclamptic seizures may have also been associated with decreased COP rather than with the intensity of peripheral vasospasm.

The etiology of pulmonary edema in preeclamptic patients appears to be multifactorial, as illustrated by Benedetti's work involving 10 preeclamptic women with pulmonary edema (Benedetti et al., 1985). Of these patients eight developed pulmonary edema in the postpartum period. Five patients had an abnormal COP–PCWP gradient, three demonstrated increased pulmonary capillary permeability, and two suffered left ventricular failure. Pulmonary edema secondary to capillary leak versus that due to increased hydrostatic pressure was distinguished by evaluating the ratio of edema fluid protein to plasma protein (Fein et al., 1979). The diagnosis of capillary leak was made in Benedetti's study when the ratio of protein in pulmonary edema fluid to serum protein was greater than 0.4 (Benedetti et al., 1985). Again, CVP was found not to correlate with PCWP. A decreased COP–PCWP gradient has long been correlated with the development of pulmonary edema in nonpregnant patients (Fein et al., 1979). Pregnancy is known to lower COP, and COP is lower in preeclamptic patients than in normal pregnant patients. COP decreases further post partum, secondary to supine positioning, bleeding at the time of delivery, and intrapartum infusion of crystalloid solutions (Weil et al., 1979). In 50% of Benedetti's preeclamptic patients, a lowered COP–PCWP gradient may have contributed to pulmonary edema (Benedetti & Carlson, 1979).

From the foregoing discussion, it is clear that nonhydrostatic factors (pulmonary capillary leak and deceased COP) may cause or contribute to pulmonary edema in patients with preeclampsia. In other patients, highly elevated SVR may lead to decreased CO and LVSWI and secondary cardiogenic pulmonary edema. A similar hydrostatic pulmonary edema may have been seen with normal left ventricular function following iatrogenic fluid overload.

The diagnosis of pulmonary edema is made on clinical grounds. Symptoms of dyspnea and chest discomfort are usually elicited. Tachypnea, tachycardia, and pulmonary rales are noted on examination. Chest X-ray and arterial blood gas analysis confirm the diagnosis. Other life-threatening conditions, such as thromboembolism, should be considered and ruled out as quickly as possible.

Initial management of pulmonary edema includes oxygen administration and fluid restriction. A pulse oximeter should be placed so that oxygen saturation may be monitored continuously. A pulmonary artery catheter may be considered for severe preeclamptic patients who develop pulmonary edema antepartum, in order to distinguish between fluid overload, left ventricular dysfunction, and nonhydrostatic pulmonary edema, each of which may require different approaches to therapy.

Furosemide (Lasix) 10–40 mg IV over 1–2 minutes represents the first line of conventional therapy for patients with pulmonary edema associated with fluid overload. If adequate diuresis does not commence within 1 hour, an 80-mg dose may be slowly administered to achieve diuresis. In severe cases of pulmonary edema, a diuresis of 2–3 L needs to be achieved before oxygenation begins to improve. Again, the degree of diuresis appropriate for these hemodynamically complex patients may be clarified by complete hemodynamic evaluation, using parameters derived by a pulmonary artery catheter. An alternative approach in patients without evidence of fluid overload, but with congestive failure secondary to intense peripheral vasospasm (Strauss et al., 1980), involves the administration of intravenous nitroprusside. While hydrostatic derangements may be corrected quickly, rapid improvement in arterial oxygenation may not be seen (Herling, 1984; Cotton, et al., 1986a). Continuous arterial BP monitoring is often helpful in this setting because of the potent activity of some arteriodilating agents.

When hypoxemia persists despite initial treatment, mechanical ventilation may be required for respiratory support, pending correction of the underlying problem. In all cases, close monitoring of the patient's respiratory status with arterial blood gas analysis should be performed. Fluid balance is maintained by careful monitoring of intake and output. An indwelling catheter with urometer should be placed to follow hourly urine output. Serum electrolytes should also be closely monitored, especially in patients receiving diuretics.

Renal complications of preeclampsia

Renal plasma flow and glomerular filtration rate are diminished significantly in preeclamptic women (Chesley & Duffus, 1971). Renal biopsy of preeclamptic patients often demonstrates a distinctive glomerular capillary endothelial cell change, termed "glomerular endotheliosis." Damage to the glomerular membrane results in renal dysfunction (Morris et al., 1964; Sheehan, 1980). Urinary sediment changes (granular, hyaline, red-cell, and tubular cell casts) are common in severe preeclampsia; they reflect renal parenchymal damage but do not correlate with or predict the clinical course of disease (Leduc et al., 1991; Gallery et al., 1993).

Acute renal failure in preeclamptic pregnancies is uncommon (Krane, 1988). In 245 cases of eclampsia reported by Pritchard et al. (1984), none required dialysis for renal failure. Among a group of 435 women with HELLP syndrome, however, 7% developed acute renal failure. Maternal and perinatal complications were extremely high, although subsequent pregnancy outcome and long-term prognosis were usually favorable in the absence of preexisting chronic hypertension (Sibai & Ramadan, 1993). Acute renal failure secondary to preeclampsia is usually the result of acute tubular necrosis but may be secondary to bilateral cortical necrosis (Sibai & Ramadan, 1993; Sibai et al., 1993). Precipitating factors include abruption, coagulopathy, hemorrhage, and severe hypotension (Grunfeld & Pertuiset, 1987). The urine sediment may show granular casts and renal tubular cells (Krane, 1988; Gallery et al., 1993). Renal cortical necrosis may be associated with preeclampsia and may present as anuria or oliguria. Renal failure presenting in association with preeclampsia may be secondary to other underlying medical disorders, especially in the older multiparous patient (Fisher et al., 1981). Should acute renal failure occur, hemodialysis or peritoneal dialysis may be required, pending return of renal function (Krane, 1988).

Oliguria

Severe renal dysfunction in preeclampsia is most commonly manifested as oliguria, defined as urinary output less than 25–30 mL/hr over two consecutive hours. This often parallels a rise in serum creatinine and blood urea nitrogen (BUN) and a fall in creatinine clearance. Reversible hyperuricemia is a common feature of preeclampsia and usually precedes the development of uremia and proteinuria (Redman et al., 1976). Significant alterations in albumin/creatinine ratio have also been described (Baker & Hacket, 1994).

Clark et al. (1986a) have described three different hemodynamic subsets of preeclamptic–eclamptic patients with persistent oliguria, based on invasive monitoring parameters. The first group was found to have a low PCWP, hyperdynamic left ventricular function, and mild to moderately increased SVR. These patients responded to further volume replacement. This is the most common clinical scenario, and it is felt to be secondary to intravascular volume depletion.

The second group is characterized by normal or increased PCWP, normal CO, and normal SVR, accompanied by intense uroconcentration. The pathophysiologic basis of oliguria in this group is thought to be secondary to intrinsic renal arterial spasm out of proportion to the degree of generalized systemic vasospasm. Low-dose dopamine (1–5 µg/kg/min) has been shown to produce a significant rise in urine output in severe preeclamptic patients in this hemodynamic subgroup (Kirshon et al., 1988a). Alternatively, afterload reduction may also improve urine output in this setting.

The third group of oliguric patients has markedly elevated PCWP and SVR, with depressed ventricular function. These patients respond to volume restriction and aggressive afterload reduction. In many cases, a forced oliguria in this subgroup may often be accompanied by incipient pulmonary edema, with fluid accumulation in the pulmonary interstitial space. Such patients would certainly not benefit from further volume infusion, yet they may be clinically indistinguishable from patients in the first group, who do respond to additional fluid infusion. Central hemodynamic assessment will allow the clinician to distinguish the preceding subgroups and tailor therapy accordingly.

Lee et al. (1987) studied seven preeclamptic women with oliguria, utilizing the pulmonary artery catheter, and also found that oliguria was not a good index of volume status. They determined that urinary diagnostic indices such as urine–plasma ratios of creatinine, urea nitrogen, and osmolality were clinically misleading if applied to fluid management. Five of seven patients were found to have urinary diagnostic indices consistent with prerenal dehydration, but PCWP consistent with euvolemia. Normal PCWPs in preeclamptics with oliguria support the hypothesis that oliguria is often secondary to severe regional vasospasm (Pritchard et al., 1984; Lee et al., 1987).

Close monitoring of fluid intake and output is of paramount importance in all patients diagnosed with preeclampsia. If urine output falls below 25–30 mL/hr over two consecutive hours, oliguria is said to be present, and a management plan should be instituted. Given the fact that plasma volume is diminished in preeclamptics, the cause of oliguria may be considered prerenal in most instances (Chesley, 1972; Gallery et al., 1979; Clark et al., 1986a). A fluid challenge of 500–1,000 mL of normal saline or lactated Ringer's solution may be administered over 30 minutes. If urine output does not respond to an initial fluid challenge, additional challenges should be withheld pending delivery or the institution of pulmonary artery catheterization for a more precise definition of hemodynamic status (Clark et al., 1986a). If at any time oxygen saturation drops during a volume challenge, pulmonary artery catheterization is indicated if further fluid is contemplated in an effort to resolve the oliguria (Clark et al., 1985a, 1986a; Clark & Cotton, 1988; Cotton et al., 1988). Repetitive fluid challenges are to be avoided in the absence of close monitoring of oxygenation status. In the presence of oliguria, delivery is of course indicated.

HELLP syndrome

The HELLP syndrome is a variant of severe preeclampsia, affecting up to 12% of patients with preeclampsia–eclampsia. In one study, the incidence of HELLP syndrome (442 cases) was 20% among women with severe preeclampsia (Sibai et al., 1993). HELLP syndrome is characterized by hemolysis, elevated liver enzymes, and low platelets (Weinstein, 1982). The acronym, HELLP syndrome, was coined by Weinstein in 1982, but the hematologic and hepatic abnormalities of three cases were described by Pritchard et al. in 1954. Pritchard credited association of thrombocytopenia with severe preeclampsia to Stahnke in 1922, and hepatic changes to Sheehan in 1950. Despite the high maternal and perinatal mortality rates associated with the HELLP syndrome, considerable controversy exists as to the proper management of these patients, who constitute a heterogeneous group with a wide array of clinical and laboratory manifestations. In addition, HELLP syndrome may be the imitator of a variety of nonobstetric medical entities (Killam et al., 1975; Goodlin, 1976) and serious medical–surgical pathology may be misdiagnosed as HELLP syndrome (Goodlin, 1991).

Unlike most forms of preeclampsia, HELLP syndrome is not primarily a disease of primigravidas. For example, several studies have found that nearly half of HELLP syndrome patients were multigravidas, the incidence among multigravidas being almost twice that seen in primigravid patients (MacKenna et al., 1983; Weinstein, 1985; Sibai et al., 1986a, 1991).

Clinically, many HELLP syndrome patients do not meet the standard BP criteria for severe preeclampsia. In one series of 112 women with severe preeclampsia–eclampsia complicated by HELLP syndrome, diastolic BP was less than 110 mmHg in 31% of cases and less than 90 mmHg in 15% at admission (Sibai et al., 1986b).

The multisystem nature of preeclampsia is often manifested by hepatic dysfunction. Hepatic artery resistance is increased in patients with HELLP syndrome (Oosterhof et al., 1994). Liver dysfunction, as defined by an elevated SGOT, was retrospectively identified in 21% of 355 patients with preeclampsia (Romero et al., 1988b). Liver dysfunction has been associated with intrauterine growth retardation (IUGR), prematurity, increased cesarean section rates, and lower Apgar scores (Romero et al., 1988b). Using immunofluorescent staining, Arias and Mancilla-Jimenez (1976) found fibrin deposition in hepatic sinusoids of preeclamptic women, thought to be the result of ischemia secondary to vasospasm. Continued prolonged vasospasm may lead to hepatocellular necrosis (Arias & Mancilla-Jimenez, 1976; Shukla et al., 1978).

The clinical signs and symptoms of patients with HELLP syndrome are classically related to the impact of vasospasm on the maternal liver. Thus, the majority of patients present with signs or symptoms of liver compromise. These include malaise, nausea (with or without vomiting), and epigastric pain. In most series, hepatic or right-upper-quadrant tenderness to palpation is seen consistently in HELLP syndrome patients (Weinstein, 1982, 1985; MacKenna et al., 1983; Sibai et al., 1986b).

Laboratory studies often create the illusion of medical conditions unrelated to pregnancy or preeclampsia. Peripheral smears demonstrate burr cells and/or schistocytes with polychromasia, consistent with microangiopathic hemolytic anemia. Hemolysis can also be demonstrated by abnormal haptoglobin or bilirubin levels (Vardi & Fields, 1974; Cunningham & Pritchard, 1978; Gibson et al., 1982; Cunningham et al., 1985). Scanning electron microscopy demonstrates evidence of microangiopathic hemolysis in patients with HELLP syndrome (Cunningham et al., 1985). The microangiopathic hemolytic anemia is felt to occur secondary to passage of the red cells through thrombosed, damaged vessels (Cunningham & Pritchard, 1978; Gibson et al., 1982; Burrows et al., 1987; Entman et al., 1987; Romero et al., 1988b). Increased red-cell turnover has also been evidenced by increased levels of carboxyhemoglobin and serum iron (Entman et al., 1987). Although some degree of hemolysis is noted, anemia is uncommon.

Table 33.12 Differential diagnoses of HELLP syndrome

Autoimmune thrombocytopenic purpura
Chronic renal disease
Pyelonephritis
Cholecystitis
Gastroenteritis
Hepatitis
Pancreatitis
Thrombotic thrombocytopenic purpura
Hemolytic–uremic syndrome
Acute fatty liver of pregnancy

Thrombocytopenia is defined as a platelet count of less than 100,000–150,000/μL. This process is not usually encountered in pregnant patients with essential hypertension (Pritchard et al., 1954). Thrombocytopenia in preeclampsia occurs secondary to increased peripheral platelet destruction, as manifested by increased bone marrow megakaryocytes, the presence of circulating megathrombocytes, evidence of reduced platelet lifespan, and platelet adherence to exposed vascular collagen (Gibson et al., 1982; Burrows et al., 1987; Entman et al., 1987; Hutt et al., 1994). Thrombocytopenia has been found in as many as 50% of preeclamptic patients studied prospectively for hemostatic and platelet function (Burrows et al., 1987). Evidence for platelet destruction, impaired platelet function, and elevated platelet-associated IgG has been found in thrombocytopenic preeclamptic patients.

In a retrospective review of 353 patients with preeclampsia, Romero et al. (1989) reported an 11.6% incidence of thrombocytopenia, defined as a platelet count less than 100,000/μL. Patients with thrombocytopenia had an increased risk for cesarean section, blood transfusion, preterm delivery, IUGR, and low Apgar scores. Thrombocytopenia has also been reported to occur in the neonates of preeclamptic women (Klechner et al., 1977; Weinstein, 1982, 1985), although others have disputed these findings (Pritchard et al., 1987).

Clotting parameters, such as the prothrombin time, partial thromboplastin time, fibrinogen, and bleeding time, in the patient with HELLP syndrome are generally normal in the absence of abruptio placentae or fetal demise (Sibai et al., 1986b). Platelet or fresh frozen plasma transfusion is necessary in 8–10% of patients with HELLP syndrome (Pritchard et al., 1954; Sibai et al., 1986b).

Significant elevation of alkaline phosphatase is seen in normal pregnancy; the elevation of SGOT and/or SGPT, however, indicates hepatic pathology. In HELLP syndrome, SGOT and SGPT are rarely in excess of 1,000 IU/L; values in excess of this level suggest other hepatic disorders, such as hepatitis. However, HELLP syndrome progressing to liver rupture may be associated with markedly elevated hepatic transaminases.

Laboratory abnormalities usually return to normal within a short time after delivery; it is not unusual, however, to see transient worsening of both thrombocytopenia and hepatic function in the first 24–48 hours post partum (Neiger et al., 1991). An upward trend in platelet count and a downward trend in lactate dehydrogenase concentration should occur in patients without complications by the fourth postpartum day (Martin et al., 1991). Martin et al. (1991) evaluated postpartum recovery in 158 women with HELLP syndrome at the University of Mississippi Medical Center. A return to a normal platelet count (100,000/μL) occurred in all women whose platelet nadir was below 50,000/μL by the 11th postpartum day, and in all women whose platelet nadir was 50,000–100,000/μL by the sixth postpartum day.

HELLP syndrome can be a "great masquerader," and both clinical presentation and laboratory findings associated with this syndrome may suggest an array of clinical diagnoses (Table 33.12). Because of the numerous misdiagnoses associated with this syndrome, and because a delay in diagnosis may be life-threatening, a pregnant woman with thrombocytopenia, elevated serum transaminase levels, or epigastric pain should be considered as having HELLP syndrome until proven otherwise.

Complications associated with HELLP syndrome include placental abruption, acute renal failure and hepatic hematoma with rupture, and ascites. Placental abruption in HELLP syndrome occurs at a rate 20 times that seen in the general obstetric population; the reported incidence ranges from 7 to 20% (Pritchard et al., 1954; Cunningham et al., 1985; Sibai et al., 1986b; Messer, 1987). Abruption in the presence of HELLP syndrome is frequently associated with fetal death and/or consumptive coagulopathy.

A review of the literature discloses significantly elevated maternal (Table 33.13) and perinatal (Table 33.14) mortality rates associated with HELLP syndrome. As with other severe preeclampsia variants, delivery is ultimately the treatment of choice. The timing of delivery, however, remains controversial. Several investigators recommend immediate delivery, while others reasonably suggest that under certain conditions with marked fetal immaturity, delivery may safely be delayed for a short time (Killam et al., 1975; Weinstein, 1982; MacKenna et al., 1983; Thiagarajah et al., 1984; Goodlin & Mostello, 1987; Heyborne et al., 1990). In support of this latter approach, Clark et al. (1986b) have demonstrated transient improvement in patients with HELLP syndrome following bed rest and/or corticosteroid administration. Following an initial improvement, however, each patient's clinical condition worsened. Similar observations were seen in 3 of 17 (18%) patients in Sibai's series following steroid administration to enhance fetal pulmonary maturity (Sibai et al., 1986b). Thus, it appears that in the mother with a very premature fetus and

Table 33.13 Maternal outcomes in HELLP syndrome

Reference	Location	Years	Cases (*n*)	Incidence (%)	Maternal mortality (%)	Cesarean rate (%)
MacKenna et al. (1983)	Greenville, NC	1978–82	27	12*	0	N/A
Weinstein (1985)	Tucson, AZ	1980–84	57	0.67†	3.5	58
Sibai et al. (1986b)	Memphis, TN	1977–85	112	9.7‡	1.8	63
Romero et al. (1988b)	New Haven, CT	1981–84	58	21*	N/A	57
Sibai et al. (1993)	Memphis, TN	1977–92	442	20§	0.9	42

* Among all preeclamptic–eclamptic patients.
† Among all live births.
‡ Among severe preeclamptic–eclamptic pregnancies.
§ Among severe preeclamptic women.
N/A, not available.

Table 33.14 Perinatal outcomes in HELLP syndrome

Reference	Location	Years	Cases (*n*)	Perinatal mortality (%)	Small for gestational age (%)	Respiratory distress syndrome (%)
MacKenna et al. (1983)	Greenville, NC	1978–82	27	11	N/A	8
Weinstein (1985)	Tucson, AZ	1980–84	57	8	N/A	16
Sibai et al. (1986b)	Memphis, TN	1977–85	112	33	32	N/A
Romero et al. (1988b)	New Haven, CT	1981–84	58	7	41	31

N/A, not available.

borderline disturbances in platelet count or serum transaminase values, and in the absence of other absolute indications for delivery, careful in-hospital observation may at times be appropriate. Certainly, uncontrollable BP or significantly changing liver enzymes or platelet count would mandate delivery irrespective of gestational age.

The mode of delivery should depend on the state of the cervix and other obstetric indications for cesarean birth. HELLP syndrome, by itself, is not an indication for cesarean delivery. At least half of patients with HELLP syndrome, however, will undergo operative delivery (see Table 33.13). A commonly encountered situation involves a mother with a premature fetus, an unfavorable cervix, and a platelet count less than 100,000/μL. In such patients, cesarean delivery is often preferred in order to avoid the necessity of later operative delivery for failed induction in the face of more significant thrombocytopenia.

Sullivan et al. (1994) evaluated 481 women who developed HELLP syndrome at the University of Mississippi Medical Center; 195 subsequent pregnancies occurred in 122 patients. The incidence of recurrent HELLP syndrome was 19–27%, and the recurrence of any form of preeclampsia–eclampsia was 42–43%. Sibai et al. (1995) reviewed 442 pregnancies complicated by HELLP syndrome at the University of Tennessee in Memphis; follow-up data were available in 341 cases. In 192 subsequent pregnancies, obstetric complications were common, including preeclampsia (19%), although only 3% experienced recurrent HELLP syndrome. They attributed the discrepancy in recurrence risk between their study and that of Sullivan et al. (1994) to differences in definitions of the syndrome and patient populations.

Schwartz and Brenner (1985) reported the use of exchange plasmapheresis with fresh frozen plasma to treat hemolysis and thrombocytopenia that did not resolve following delivery and standard medical treatment.

Liver rupture

Hepatic infarction may lead to intrahepatic hemorrhage and development of a subcapsular hematoma, which may rupture into the peritoneal space and result in shock and death (Rademaker, 1943; Arias & Mancilla-Jimenez, 1976). Subcapsular hematomas usually develop on the anterior and superior aspects of the liver (Herbert & Brenner, 1982). The diagnosis of a liver hematoma may be aided by use of ultrasonography, radionuclide scanning, computed tomography (CT), magnetic resonance imaging (MRI), and selective angiography (Herbert & Brenner, 1982; Henny et al., 1983).

Henny et al. (1983) described a biphasic chronologic sequence of events during rupture of the subcapsular hematoma. The initial presenting symptoms are constant, progressively worsening pain in the epigastrium or right upper quadrant of the abdomen, with or without nausea and vomiting. The second phase is manifested by the development of vascular collapse, shock, and fetal death. The maternal and fetal prognoses of liver rupture are poor. Bis and Waxman (1976) reported a 59% maternal and 62% fetal mortality rate.

Significant or persistent elevations of serum transaminase levels in conjunction with preeclampsia and right-upper-quadrant or epigastric tenderness indicate delivery regardless of gestational age. Especially when such dysfunction occurs in the presence of thrombocytopenia, careful clinical observation during the postpartum period is essential. When the diagnosis of liver hematoma is suspected in severe preeclampsia prior to delivery of the fetus, immediate exploratory laparotomy and cesarean section should be performed in order to prevent rupture of the hematoma secondary to increased abdominal pressure in the second stage of labor, with vomiting, or during eclamptic convulsions (Henny et al., 1983). When the diagnosis of liver hematoma is made in the postpartum period, conservative management with blood transfusion and serial ultrasonography may be reasonable (Henny et al., 1983; Goodlin et al., 1985).

Smith et al. (1991) reviewed the medical literature for the period 1976–90 (28 cases) and reported their experience at Baylor College of Medicine for the period 1978–90 (seven new cases) of spontaneous rupture of the liver during pregnancy. The incidence was 1 per 45,145 live births in the Baylor series. A significant improvement in maternal outcome ($P = 0.006$) was seen among patients who were managed by packing and drainage (82% survival) compared with those managed by hepatic lobectomy (25% survival). This conservative approach is supported by the trauma literature. At Baylor College of Medicine, 1,000 consecutive cases of liver injury were evaluated; extensive resection of the liver or lobectomy with selective vascular ligation resulted in a 34% mortality rate, whereas conservative surgery (packing and drainage and/or use of topical hemostatic agents) resulted in a 7% mortality (Feliciano et al., 1986). Smith et al. (1991) proposed an algorithm for antepartum and postpartum management of hepatic hemorrhage in their review.

Liver rupture with intraperitoneal hemorrhage, when suspected, requires laparotomy. Hemostasis may be achieved by compression, simple suture, topical coagulant agents, arterial embolization, omental pedicles, ligation of the hepatic artery, or lobectomy, depending on the extent of the hepatic damage (Lucas & Ledgerwood, 1976). Temporary control of bleeding may be achieved by packing the rupture site or by application of a gravity suit (Gardner & Storer, 1966; Lucas & Ledgerwood, 1976). Management by liver transplant has been reported (Hunter et al., 1995; Reck et al., 2001).

Few cases of pregnancy following hepatic rupture have been reported. There have been several reported cases of non-recurrence in subsequent pregnancies (Sakala & Moore, 1986) and one case of recurrence with survival in a subsequent pregnancy (Greenstein et al., 1994). Spontaneous splenic rupture associated with preeclampsia has been reported (Barrilleaux et al., 1999).

Neurologic complications of preeclampsia

Cerebral hemorrhage, cerebral edema, temporary blindness (amaurosis), and eclamptic seizures are separate but related neurologic conditions that may occur in preeclampsia. Cerebral hemorrhage and cerebral edema are two major causes of maternal mortality in preeclampsia (Hibbard, 1973). Intracranial hemorrhage may result from the combination of severe hypertension and hemostatic compromise (Romero et al., 1988a).

Cerebral edema

Cerebral edema is defined as increased water content of one or more of the intracranial fluid compartments of the brain (Bell, 1983). Signs of diffuse cerebral edema may be found in eclamptic women on CT scan (Kirby & Jaindl, 1984) and may develop when the forces affecting the Starling equilibrium are disturbed. The three most important etiologic factors include increased intravascular pressure, damage to the vascular endothelium, and reduced plasma COP (Miller, 1979). Miller's classification of cerebral edema includes (i) vasogenic edema with breakdown of the blood–brain barrier, secondary to vascular damage; (ii) cytotoxic edema, secondary to damage to the cellular sodium pump; (iii) hydrostatic edema from increased intravascular pressure; (iv) interstitial edema related to acute obstructive hydrocephalus; and (v) hypoosmotic edema, in which intravascular free water decreases plasma osmolality (Miller, 1979). In the general population, vasogenic edema, which predominantly occurs in the cerebral white matter, is the most common type of cerebral edema (Weiss, 1985).

In preeclampsia, cerebral edema is thought to occur secondary to anoxia associated with eclamptic seizures or secondary to loss of cerebral autoregulation as a result of severe hypertension (Benedetti & Quilligan, 1980). Cerebral edema is diagnosed on CT scan by the appearance of areas with low density or a low radiographic absorption coefficient (Beeson & Duda, 1982; Kirby & Jaindl, 1984; Weiss, 1985). MRI has also been useful in providing an index of water content in select areas of the brain (Weiss, 1985).

General therapeutic principles in the treatment of cerebral edema include correction of hypoxemia and hypercarbia, avoidance of volatile anesthetic agents, control of body temperature, and control of hypertension (Miller, 1979; Weiss, 1985). Assisted hyperventilation reduces intracranial hypertension and the formation of cerebral edema. The partial pressure of carbon dioxide is maintained between 25 and 30 mmHg (Miller, 1979).

The administration of hypertonic solutions such as mannitol increases serum osmolality and draws water from the brain into the vascular compartment, thus reducing brain tissue water and volume. A 20% solution of mannitol is given as a dose of 0.5–1.0 g/kg over 10 minutes or as a continuous infusion of 5 g/hr. The serum osmolality is maintained in a range between 305 and 315 mosmol (Miller, 1979; Weiss, 1985). Steroid therapy (dexamethasone, betamethasone, methylprednisolone) is thought to be most effective in the treatment of focal chronic cerebral edema, which may occur in association with a tumor or abscess. Steroid therapy is less beneficial in cases of diffuse or acute cerebral edema (Miller, 1979). Other pharmacologic agents that have been used to reduce intracranial pressure and cerebral edema include acetazolamide (Diamox), furosemide (Lasix), spironolactone (Aldactone), and ethacrynic acid (Edecrin).

In preeclamptic–eclamptic patients diagnosed with cerebral edema, therapy should be directed at correcting hypoxemia, hypercarbia, hyperthermia, and/or hypertension or hypotension. If assisted ventilation is employed, hyperventilation with controlled hypocapnia should be used. Mannitol may be administered with careful observation of pulmonary, cardiovascular, and renal function. The inciting factor of cerebral edema in preeclampsia and eclampsia, albeit unknown, is eliminated by delivery of the products of conception and thus the condition is ultimately treatable in this patient population.

Temporary blindness

Temporary blindness may complicate 1–3% of cases of preeclampsia–eclampsia (Beal & Chapman, 1980; Beck et al., 1980; Beeson & Duda, 1982; Hill et al., 1985; Seidman et al., 1991) and was recently reported in 15% of women with eclampsia at Parkland Hospital (Cunningham et al., 1995). Pregnancy-related blindness has been associated with eclampsia, cavernous sinus thrombosis, and hypertensive encephalopathy (Beal & Chapman, 1980; Beck et al., 1980; Beeson & Duda, 1982; Hill et al., 1985). Beeson and Duda (1982) reported one case associated with eclampsia and occipital lobe edema. Hill et al. (1985) noted that recovery of vision correlated with the return of a normal PCWP in severe preeclamptics with amaurosis. The injury is usually the result of severe damage to the retinal vasculature or occipital lobe ischemia (Beal & Chapman, 1980). Cunningham et al. (1995) evaluated the clinical courses of 15 women with severe preeclampsia or eclampsia who developed cortical blindness over a 14-year period. Blindness persisted from 4 hours to 8 days but resolved completely in all cases. Based on data from CT imaging and MRI, the Parkland group concluded that cortical blindness resulted from petechial hemorrhages and focal edema in the occipital cortex. Hinchey et al. (1996) described a syndrome of reversible posterior leukoencephalopathy, with neuroimaging findings characteristic of subcortical edema without infarction in patients who presented with headache, altered mental functioning, seizures, and loss of vision.

Transient blindness usually resolves spontaneously after delivery of the fetus (Beck et al., 1980; Beeson & Duda, 1982; Hill et al., 1985). Nevertheless, focal neurologic deficits such as this require ophthalmologic and neurologic consultation and CT or MRI of the brain. Generally, management guidelines are the same as for preeclamptics without this complication (Cunningham et al., 1995). Associated conditions, such as cerebral edema, should be treated as indicated. Paralysis of the sixth cranial nerve has been reported as a complication of eclampsia (Kinsella et al., 1994).

Eclampsia

The precise cause of seizures in preeclampsia remains unknown. Hypertensive encephalopathy, as well as vasospasm, hemorrhage, ischemia, and edema of the cerebral hemispheres, have been proposed as etiologic factors. Thrombotic and hemorrhagic lesions have been identified on autopsy of preeclamptic women (Sheehan, 1950; Govan, 1961). Clark et al. (1985b) noted lower COP associated with eclamptic patients, as opposed to matched severe preeclamptic patients. The importance of low COP in the development of pulmonary dysfunction has been described previously (Benedetti et al., 1985).

Douglas and Redman (1994) reported that the incidence of eclampsia in the United Kingdom during 1992 was 4.9 per 10,000 maternities. During the period 1979–86, the incidence of eclampsia in the United States was 5.6 per 10,000 births (Saftlas et al., 1990). The eclampsia rate decreased by 36% from 6.8 per 10,000 births during the first half of the series to 4.3 per 10,000 births during the latter half of the series.

Eclamptic seizures usually occur without a preceding aura, although many patients will manifest some form of apprehension, excitability, or hyperreflexia prior to the onset of a seizure. Eclampsia unheralded by hypertension and proteinuria occurred in 38% of cases reported in the United Kingdom (Douglas & Redman, 1994). Douglas and Redman conclude that "the term pre-eclampsia is misleading because eclampsia can precede pre-eclampsia." In a study of 179 cases of eclampsia, approximately one-third of patients received obstetric care that met standards for delivery of obstetric services and were thus classified as "unavoidable" cases of eclampsia (Sibai et al., 1986c). Sibai and colleagues have recommended magnesium prophylaxis in all preeclamptics, regardless of degree, because a significant percentage of eclamptics demonstrated only mild signs and symptoms of preeclampsia prior to the onset of seizures (Sibai et al., 1986c). Once a seizure occurs, it is usually a forerunner of more convulsions unless anticonvulsant therapy is initiated.

Eclamptic seizures occur prior to delivery in roughly 80% of patients (Table 33.15). In the remainder, convulsions occur post partum, and have been reported up to 23 days following delivery (Sibai et al., 1980; Brown et al., 1987). Douglas and Redman (1994) observed that most antepartum convulsions (76%) occurred prior to term, while most intrapartum or postpartum convulsions (75%) occurred at term. Late postpartum eclampsia (convulsions more than 48 hours but less than 4 weeks after delivery) constituted 56% of total postpartum eclampsia and 16% of all cases of eclampsia in a series collected at the University of Tennessee, Memphis, between 1977 and 1992 (Lubarsky et al., 1994). Severe headache or visual disturbances were noted in 83% of patients before the onset of convulsions. When seizures occur more than 24 hours post partum, however, a thorough search for other potential causes is mandatory.

A maternal seizure typically results in fetal bradycardia,

Table 33.15 Eclampsia: maternal–fetal complications

Reference	Location	Years	Cases (*n*)	Antepartum eclampsia (%)	Cesarean rate (%)	Maternal mortality (%)	Perinatal mortality (%)
Bryant & Fleming (1940)	Cincinnati, OH	1930–40	120	62	0	1.7	29*
Zuspan (1966)	Augusta, GA	1956–65	69	88	1.4†	2.9	32*
Harbert et al. (1968)	Charlottesville, VA	1939–63	168	78	6†	4.8	22*
Pritchard & Pritchard (1975)	Dallas, TX	1955–75	154	82	23	0	15†
Lopez-Llera (1982)	Mexico City, Mexico	1963–79	704	83	57†	14	27
Pritchard et al. (1984)	Dallas, TX	1975–83	91	91	33†	1.1	16†
Adetoro (1989)	Ilorin, Nigeria	1972–87	651	N/A	N/A	14	N/A
Sibai (1990)	Memphis, TN	1977–89	254	71	49†	0.4	12*
Douglas & Redman (1994)	United Kingdom	1992	383	56	54†	1.8	7*
Majoko & Mujaji (2001)	Harare, Zimbabwe	1997–98	151	68	63	26.5	N/A
Onwuhafua et al. (2001)	Kaduna Stage, Nigeria	1990–97	45	60	53	42	44

* All cases.
† Antepartum and intrapartum cases only.
N/A, not available.

and the fetal heart rate pattern usually returns to normal upon resolution the seizure. Appropriate steps should be taken to enhance maternal–fetal well-being, including maintenance of the maternal airway, oxygen administration, and maternal lateral repositioning. Complete maternal recovery following eclampsia usually is expected.

The standard therapy for the management of eclampsia includes magnesium sulfate and delivery of the fetus. We administer magnesium sulfate 4–6 g IV over 20 minutes, and initiate an intravenous infusion at 2–3 g/hr. If control of seizures is not successful after the initial intravenous bolus, a second 2-g bolus of magnesium sulfate may be cautiously administered. No more than a total of 8 g of magnesium sulfate is recommended at the outset of treatment.

Seizures may recur despite apparently appropriate magnesium therapy. The incidence of recurrent seizures ranges from 8 to 13% (Sibai et al., 1986c). Both intramuscular and intravenous magnesium sulfate regimens may be associated with recurrent seizures. Of such patients, half may have subtherapeutic magnesium levels (Sibai et al., 1986c). This underscores the importance of individualized therapy in order to achieve adequate serum magnesium levels and minimize the risk of recurrent seizures. Seizures refractory to standard magnesium sulfate regimens may be treated with a slow 100-mg IV dose of thiopental sodium (Pentothal) or 1–10 mg of diazepam (Valium). Alternatively, sodium amobarbital (up to 250 mg IV) may be administered. In a clinical study, Lucas et al. (1994) described a simplified regimen of phenytoin for the treatment of preeclampsia. An intravenous infusion rate of 16.7 mg/min over 1 hour provided an initial dose of 1,000 mg; an additional 500 mg of phenytoin administered orally 10 hours after treatment initiation maintained therapeutic levels for an additional 14 hours.

Eclamptic patients with repetitive seizures despite therapeutic magnesium levels may warrant CT evaluation of the brain. Dunn et al. (1986) found five of seven such patients to have abnormalities including cerebral edema and cerebral venous thrombosis. However, Sibai et al. (1985b) reported 20 cases of eclampsia with neurologic signs or repetitive seizures who all had normal CT findings. Their recommendation regarding CT scan was restricted to patients with late-onset postpartum preeclampsia or those patients with focal neurologic deficits.

Eclamptic patients require delivery without respect to gestational age (Cunningham & Gant, 1994). Cesarean delivery should be reserved for obstetric indications or deteriorating maternal condition. As demonstrated in Table 33.15, vaginal delivery may be achieved in at least half of eclamptic patients. Pritchard et al. (1984) reported successful vaginal delivery in 82% of oxytocin-induced patients.

Maternal mortality rates are increased in eclamptics, although the rates have declined dramatically in recent years (Pritchard et al., 1984). According to Chesley (1984), the average maternal mortality rate of eclampsia during the mid-nineteenth century (1837–67) was approximately 30%. In the latter half of the nineteenth century, the average maternal mortality rate was around 24%. During the early twentieth century (1911–25), the maternal mortality rate was 11% and 22% among women managed conservatively and delivered operatively, respectively. Lazard (1933) reported a 13% gross mortality rate among 225 eclamptics treated in Los Angeles between 1924 and 1932. Eastman and Steptoe (1945) reported a 7.6% maternal mortality and 21.7% fetal mortality rate of eclampsia in Baltimore between 1924 and 1943.

Contemporary maternal mortality rates of eclampsia are under 2% in developed countries but are significantly higher in developing nations (see Table 33.15). In Pritchard's series of 245 eclamptics, one maternal death occurred, which was attributed to magnesium intoxication (Pritchard et al., 1984). In Sibai's series of 254 eclamptic women, there was one maternal death in a woman who suffered seizures prior to arrival at the hospital and who arrived in a moribund state (Sibai et al., 1992). In the United Kingdom during 1992, a 1.8% maternal case mortality rate was reported for eclampsia (Douglas & Redman, 1994).

At a referral hospital in Mexico City, 704 eclamptic women were managed during a 15-year period (Lopez-Llera, 1982). The maternal mortality rate was 14%, a relatively high rate likely secondary to a high proportion of advanced cases of disease. According to Lopez-Llera (1982), maternal mortality rates are higher in those women with seizures prior to (15%) than after (10%) delivery. The most common cause of death in the Mexico City series among 86 fatal cases of antepartum and intrapartum eclampsia was cerebrovascular damage (72%), followed by severe respiratory insufficiency (12%), postpartum hemorrhage (6%), and disseminated intravascular coagulation (4%). Autopsy findings have mirrored these observations (Sheehan, 1950).

Overall, the contemporary perinatal mortality rate among eclamptics ranges from 7 to 16% in the United States and the United Kingdom (see Table 33.15) and is most commonly secondary to placental abruption, prematurity, and perinatal asphyxia. Antenatal deaths accounted for a significant proportion of the overall perinatal mortality. Depending on the gestational age and the clinical circumstances, it may be prudent to have a person capable of neonatal resuscitation immediately available at delivery.

Eclamptic patients are at increased risk for developing preeclampsia–eclampsia in a subsequent pregnancy (Sibai et al., 1986a, 1992). Remote mortality is not greater for White primiparous eclamptics but is increased from two to five times the expected rate for White multiparous eclamptics and all Black eclamptics (Chesley et al., 1976). Moreover, these women appear to be at a greater risk of developing chronic hypertension and diabetes mellitus (Chesley et al., 1976; Chesley, 1978; Sibai et al., 1986a). However, long-term neurologic deficits are rare and long-term anticonvulsant therapy is usually not necessary in the eclamptic woman (Sibai et al., 1985b).

Uteroplacental–fetal complications of preeclampsia

Uteroplacental blood flow is significantly decreased in preeclamptic patients (Browne & Veall, 1953; Dixon et al., 1963; Lunell et al., 1982, 1984; Friedman, 1988) and may lead to IUGR, fetal distress, or fetal death. Hypertensive patients are also at higher risk for abruption. The pathophysiology of placental abruption in preeclamptic patients has been proposed to result from thrombotic lesions in the placental vasculature, leading to decidual necrosis, separation, and hemorrhage. A vicious cycle then continues as the decidual hemorrhage results in further separation. This cycle may be aggravated by coexisting hemostatic compromise. Abdella et al. (1984) evaluated 265 cases of abruption and estimated an incidence of approximately 1% in the total obstetric population; 27% were complicated by a hypertensive disorder. Preeclamptics, chronic hypertensives, and eclamptics were found to have a 2, 10, and 24% incidence of abruption, respectively (Hurd et al., 1983; Abdella et al. 1984). Severe preeclamptic patients with chronic hypertension have a significantly increased perinatal mortality rate, abruption rate, and frequency of growth-retarded infants compared with severe preeclamptics without preexisting hypertension (Sibai et al., 1984a). Fetal growth retardation appears to occur frequently in multiparous women with preeclampsia compared with nulliparous women with preeclampsia; the cause of this difference, however, is uncertain (Eskenazi et al., 1993). Oxygen transport and extraction may be negatively affected by preeclampsia. Wheeler et al. (1996) demonstrated a strong negative linear correlation between base deficit and oxygen delivery index and suggested that a base deficit exceeding –8.0 mEq/L consistently predicted fetal acidosis, death, and maternal end-organ ischemic injury (Belfort et al., 1995). The reader is referred to a recent review of antenatal fetal surveillance techniques for hypertensive women (Dildy, 2003).

Conclusions

Preeclampsia and eclampsia have the potential to produce significant maternal and fetal complications. Advances in clinical medicine have provided for improved outcomes for our patients. While the critically ill preeclamptic today is much better off than her predecessors, continued evolution of medical services and technology are needed to reduce these complications to an acceptable level.

References

Aali BS, Nejad SS. Nifedipine or hydralazine as a first-line agent to control hypertension in severe preeclampsia. Acta Obstet Gynecol Scand 2002;81:25–30.

Abdella TN, Sibai BM, Hays JM Jr, Anderson GD. Relationship of hypertensive disease to abruptio placentae. Obstet Gynecol 1984;63:365–370.

Abdul-Karim R, Assali NS. Pressor response to angiotensin in pregnant and nonpregnant women. Am J Obstet Gynecol 1961;82: 246–251.

ACOG. Hypertension in pregnancy. ACOG Technical Bulletin 219. Washington, DC: American College of Obstetricians and Gynecologists, 1996.

ACOG. Diagnosis and management of preeclampsia and eclampsia. ACOG Committee on Practice Bulletins. Obstet Gynecol 2002; 99(Suppl):159–167.

Adetero OO. A sixteen year survey of maternal mortality associated with eclampsia in Ilorin, Nigeria. Int J Gynecol Obstet 1989;30: 117–121.

Arias F, Mancilla-Jimenez R. Hepatic fibrinogen deposits in preeclampsia. N Engl J Med 1976;295:578–582.

Assali NS, Kaplan S, Oighenstein S, Suyemoto R. Hemodynamic effects of 1-hydrazinophthalazine (Apresoline) in human pregnancy: results of intravenous administration. J Clin Invest 1953;32:922–930.

Atkinson MW, Belfort MA, Saade GR, Moise K. The relation between magnesium sulfate therapy and fetal heart rate variability. Obstet Gynecol 1991;83:967–970.

Atkinson MW, Maher JE, Owen J, et al. The predictive value of umbilical artery Doppler studies for preeclampsia or fetal growth retardation in a preeclampsia prevention trial. Obstet Gynecol 1994;83:609–612.

Baker PN, Hacket GA. The use of urinary albumin–creatinine ratios and calcium–creatinine ratios as screening tests for pregnancy-induced hypertension. Obstet Gynecol 1994;83:745–749.

Balasch J, Mirapeix E, Borche L, et al. Further evidence against preeclampsia as an immune complex disease. Obstet Gynecol 1981;58:435.

Barr M, Cohen M. ACE inhibitor fetopathy and hypocalvaria: the kidney–skull connection. Teratology 1991;44:485–495.

Barrilleaux PS, Adair D, Johnson G, Lewis DF. Splenic rupture associated with severe preeclampsia. A case report. J Reprod Med 1999;44:899–901.

Beal MF, Chapman PH. Cortical blindness and homonymous hemianopia in the postpartum period. JAMA 1980;244:2085–2087.

Beck RW, Gamel JW, Willcourt RJ, Berman G. Acute ischemic optic neuropathy in severe preeclampsia. Am J Ophthalmol 1980; 90:342–346.

Beeson JH, Duda EE. Computed axial tomography scan demonstration of cerebral edema in eclampsia preceded by blindness. Obstet Gynecol 1982;60:529–532.

Belfort MA, Saade GR, Moise KJ. The effect of magnesium sulfate on maternal retinal blood flow in preeclampsia: A randomized placebo-controlled study. Am J Obstet Gynecol 1992;167:1548–1553.

Belfort MA, Carpenter RJ Jr, Kirshon B, Saade GR, Moise KJ Jr. The use of nimodipine in a patient with eclampsia: color flow Doppler demonstration of retinal artery relaxation. Am J Obstet Gynecol 1993;169:204–206.

Belfort MA, Saade GR, Moise KJ Jr, et al. Nimodipine in the management of preeclampsia: maternal and fetal effects. Am J Obstet Gynecol 1994;171:417–424.

Belfort MA, Saade GR, Wasserstrum N, et al. Acute volume expansion with colloid increases oxygen delivery and consumption but does not improve the oxygen extraction in severe preeclampsia. J Maternal-Fetal Med 1995;4:57–64.

Belfort MA, Anthony J, Saade GR, Prevention of eclampsia. Semin Perinatol 1999a;23:65–78.

Belfort MA, Saade GR, Yared M, et al. Change in estimated cerebral perfusion pressure after treatment with nimodipine or magnesium sulfate in patients with preeclampsia. Am J Obstet Gynecol 1999b;181:402–407.

Belfort MA, Anthony J, Saade GR, Allen JC Jr, Nimodipine Study Group. A comparison of magnesium sulfate and nimodipine for the prevention of eclampsia. N Engl J Med 2003;348:304–311.

Bell BA. A history of the study of cerebral edema. Neurosurgery 1983;13:724–728.

Benedetti TJ, Carlson RW. Studies of colloid osmotic pressure in pregnancy-induced hypertension. Am J Obstet Gynecol 1979;135: 308–317.

Benedetti TJ, Quilligan EJ. Cerebral edema in severe pregnancy-induced hypertension. Am J Obstet Gynecol 1980;137:860–862.

Benedetti TJ, Cotton DB, Read JC, Miller FC. Hemodynamic observations in severe preeclampsia with a flow-directed pulmonary artery. Am J Obstet Gynecol 1980;136:465–470.

Benedetti TJ, Kates R, Williams V. Hemodynamic observations in severe preeclampsia complicated by pulmonary edema. Am J Obstet Gynecol 1985;152:330–334.

Berg CJ, Atrash HK, Koonin LM, Tucker M. Pregnancy-related mortality in the United States, 1987–1990. Obstet Gynecol 1996;88: 161.

Bis KA, Waxman B. Rupture of the liver associated with pregnancy: a review of the literature and report of two cases. Obstet Gynecol Surv 1976;31:763–773.

Bletka M, Hlavaty V, Trnkova M, et al. Volume of whole blood and absolute amount of serum proteins in the early stage of late toxemia of pregnancy. Am J Obstet Gynecol 1970;106:10–13.

Bohman VR, Cotton DB. Supralethal magnesemia with patient survival. Obstet Gynecol 1990;76:984–985.

Borges LF, Gucer G. Effect of magnesium on epileptic foci. Epilepsia 1978;19:81–91.

Branch DW, Andres R, Digre KB, et al. The association of antiphospholipid antibodies with severe preeclampsia. Obstet Gynecol 1989;73:541–545.

Branch DW, Silver RM, Blackwell JL, et al. Outcome of treated pregnancies in women with antiphospholipid syndrome: an update of the Utah experience. Obstet Gynecol 1992;80:614–620.

Brown CEL, Cunningham FG, Pritchard JA. Convulsions in hypertensive proteinuric primiparas more than 24 hours after delivery: eclampsia or some other course. J Reprod Med 1987;32:449–503.

Browne JCM, Veall N. The maternal placental blood flow in normotensive and hypertensive women. J Obstet Gynaecol Br Emp 1953;60:141–147.

Bryant RD, Fleming JG. Veratrum viride in the treatment of eclampsia: II. JAMA 1940;115:1333–1339.

Burrows RF, Hunter DJS, Andrew M, Kelton JG. A prospective study investigating the mechanism of thrombocytopenia in preeclampsia. Obstet Gynecol 1987;70:334–338.

Chesley LC. Plasma and red cell volumes during pregnancy. Am J Obstet Gynecol 1972;112:440–450.

Chesley LC. A short history of eclampsia. Obstet Gynecol 1974;43: 599–602.

Chesley LC. Remote prognosis. In: Chesley LC, ed. Hypertensive Disorders in Pregnancy. New York: Appleton-Century-Crofts, 1978:421.

Chesley LC. Parenteral magnesium sulfate and the distribution, plasma levels, and excretion of magnesium. Am J Obstet Gynecol 1979;133:1–7.

Chesley LC. History and epidemiology of pre-eclampsia–eclampsia. Clin Obstet Gynecol 1984;27:801–820.

Chesley LC. Diagnosis of preeclampsia. Obstet Gynecol 1985;65: 423–425.

Chesley LC, Duffus GM. Preeclampsia, posture, and renal function. Obstet Gynecol 1971;38:1–5.

Chesley LC, Annitto JE, Cosgrove RA. The remote prognosis of eclamptic women. Am J Obstet Gynecol 1976;124:446–459.

Chien PF, Khan KS, Arnott N. Magnesium sulphate in the treatment of eclampsia and pre-eclampsia: an overview of the evidence from randomised trials. Br J Obstet Gynaecol 1996;103:1085–1091.

Clark SL, Cotton DB. Clinical indications for pulmonary artery catheterization in the patient with severe preeclampsia. Am J Obstet Gynecol 1988;158:453–458.

Clark SL, Horenstein JM, Phelan JP, et al. Experience with the pulmonary artery catheter in obstetrics and gynecology. Am J Obstet Gynecol 1985a;152:374–378.

Clark SL, Divon MY, Phelan JP. Preeclampsia/eclampsia: hemodynamic and neurologic correlations. Obstet Gynecol 1985b; 66:337–340.

Clark SL, Greenspoon JS, Aldahl D, Phelan JP. Severe preeclampsia with persistent oliguria: management of hemodynamic subsets. Am J Obstet Gynecol 1986a;154:490–494.

Clark SL, Phelan JP, Allen SH, Golde SH. Antepartum reversal of hematologic abnormalities with the HELLP syndrome. J Reprod Med 1986b;31:70–72.

Clark SL, Cotton DB, Lee W, et al. Central hemodynamic observations in normal third trimester pregnancy. Am J Obstet Gynecol 1989;161:1439–1442.

Coetzee EJ, Dommisse J, Anthony J. A randomised controlled trial of intravenous magnesium sulphate versus placebo in the management of women with severe pre-eclampsia. Br J Obstet Gynaecol 1998;105:300–303.

Coevoet B, Leuliet J, Comoy E, et al. Labetalol in the treatment of hypertension of pregnancy: clinical effects and interactions with plasma renin and dopamine betahydroxylase activities, and with plasma concentrations of catecholamine. Kidney Int 1980;17: 701.

Conde-Agudelo A, Belizan JM, Lede R, Bergel EF. What does an elevated mean arterial pressure in the second half of pregnancy predict – gestational hypertension or preeclampsia? Am J Obstet Gynecol 1993;169:509–514.

Conde-Agudelo A, Lede R, Belizan J. Evaluation of methods used in the prediction of hypertensive disorders of pregnancy. Obstet Gynecol Surv 1994;49:210–222.

Connell H, Dalgleish JG, Downing JW. General anaesthesia in mothers with severe preeclampsia/eclampsia. Br J Anaesth 1987;59: 1375–1380.

Cotton DB, Benedetti TJ. Use of the Swan–Ganz catheter in obstetrics and gynecology. Obstet Gynecol 1980;56:641–645.

Cotton DB, Gonik B, Spillman T, Dorman KF. Intrapartum to postpartum changes in colloid osmotic pressure. Am J Obstet Gynecol 1984a;149:174–177.

Cotton DB, Gonik B, Dorman KR. Cardiovascular alterations in severe pregnancy-induced hypertension: acute effects of intravenous magnesium sulfate. Am J Obstet Gynecol 1984b;148:162–165.

Cotton DB, Gonik B, Dorman K, Harrist R. Cardiovascular alterations in severe pregnancy-induced hypertension: relationship of central venous pressure to pulmonary capillary wedge pressure. Am J Obstet Gynecol 1985;151:762–764.

Cotton DB, Longmire S, Jones MM, et al. Cardiovascular alterations in severe pregnancy-induced hypertension: effects of intravenous nitroglycerin coupled with blood volume expansion. Am J Obstet Gynecol 1986a;154:1053–1059.

Cotton DB, Jones MM, Longmire S, et al. Role of intravenous nitroglycerin in the treatment of severe pregnancy-induced hypertension complicated by pulmonary edema. Am J Obstet Gynecol 1986b;154:91–93.

Cotton DB, Lee W, Huhta JC, Dorman KF. Hemodynamic profile of severe pregnancy-induced hypertension. Am J Obstet Gynecol 1988;158:523–529.

Cunningham FG, Gant NF. Management of eclampsia. Semin Perinatol 1994;18:103–113.

Cunningham FG, Pritchard JA. Hematologic considerations of pregnancy-induced hypertension. Semin Perinatol 1978;2:29–38.

Cunningham FG, Lowe T, Guss S, Mason R. Erythrocyte morphology in women with severe preeclampsia and eclampsia. Preliminary observations with scanning electron microscopy. Am J Obstet Gynecol 1985;153:358–363.

Cunningham FG, Fernandez CO, Hernandez C. Blindness associated with preeclampsia and eclampsia. Am J Obstet Gynecol 1995; 172:1291–1298.

Dadek C, Kefalides A, Sinzinger H, Weber G. Reduced umbilical artery prostacyclin formation in complicated pregnancies. Am J Obstet Gynecol 1982;144:792–795.

Dieckmann WJ, Michel HL. Vascular–renal effects of posterior pituitary extracts in pregnant women. Am J Obstet Gynecol 1937; 33:131–137.

Dildy GA. Antenatal surveillance in preeclampsia and chronic hypertension. In: Belfort MA, Thornton S, Saade GR, eds. Hypertension in Pregnancy. New York: Marcel Dekker, 2003.

Dildy GA, Cotton DB. Hemodynamic changes in pregnancy and pregnancy complicated by hypertension. Acute Care 1988–89;14–15: 26–46.

Dildy GA, Cotton DB. Management of severe preeclampsia and eclampsia. Crit Care Clin 1991;7:829–850.

Dixon HG, Brown JCM, Davey DA. Choriodecidual and myometrial blood flow. Lancet 1963;ii:369–373.

Donaldson JO. The case against magnesium sulfate for eclamptic convulsions. Int J Obstet Anesth 1992;1:159–166.

Dorsett L. The intramuscular injection of magnesium sulphate for the control of convulsions in eclampsia. Am J Obstet Gynecol 1926; 11:227–231.

Douglas KA, Redman CWG. Eclampsia in the United Kingdom. Br Med J 1994;309:1395–1399.

Downing I, Shepherd GI, Lewis PJ. Kinetics of prostacyclin synthetase in umbilical artery microsomes from normal and preeclamptic pregnancies. Br J Clin Pharmacol 1982;13:195–198.

Duley L, Gulmezoglu AM. Magnesium sulfate compared with lytic cocktail for women with eclampsia (Cochrane Review). In: The Cochrane Library. Oxford: Update Software, 2002, Issue 2.

Duley L, Henderson-Smart D. Magnesium sulphate versus diazepam for eclampsia (Cochrane Review). In: The Cochrane Library. Oxford: Update Software, 2002a, Issue 2.

Duley L, Henderson-Smart D. Magnesium sulphate versus phenytoin for eclampsia (Cochrane Review). In: The Cochrane Library. Oxford: Update Software, 2002b, Issue 2.

Duley L, Johanson R. Magnesium sulphate for pre-eclampsia and eclampsia: the evidence so far. Br J Obstet Gynaecol 1994;101:565–567.

Duley L, Gulmezoglu AM, Henderson-Smart DJ. Anticonvulsants for women with pre-eclampsia (Cochrane Review). In: The Cochrane Library. Oxford: Update Software, 2002, Issue 2.

Dunn R, Lee W, Cotton DB. Evaluation by computerized axial tomography of eclamptic women with seizures refractory to magnesium sulfate therapy. Am J Obstet Gynecol 1986;155:267–268.

Easterling TR, Benedetti TJ. Preeclampsia: a hyperdynamic disease model. Am J Obstet Gynecol 1989;160:1447–1453.

Eastman NJ, Steptoe PP. The management of pre-eclampsia. Can Med Assoc J 1945;52:562–568.

Eclampsia Trial Collaborative Group. Which anticonvulsant for women with eclampsia? Evidence from the Collaborative Eclampsia Trial. Lancet 1995;345:1455–1463.

Entman SS, Kambam JR, Bradley CA, Cousar JB. Increased levels of carboxyhemoglobin and serum iron as an indicator of increased red cell turnover in preeclampsia. Am J Obstet Gynecol 1987;156: 1169–1173.

Eskenazi B, Fenster L, Sidney S, Elkin EP. Fetal growth retardation in infants of multiparous and nulliparous women with preeclampsia. Am J Obstet Gynecol 1993;169:1112–1118.

Fein A, Grossman RF, Jones JG, et al. The value of edema fluid protein measurement in patients with pulmonary edema. Am J Med 1979;67:32–38.

Feliciano DV, Mattox KL, Jordan GL, et al. Management of 1,000 consecutive cases of hepatic trauma (1979–1984). Ann Surg 1986; 204:438–445.

Fenakel K, Fenakel G, Appleman ZVI, et al. Nifedipine in the treatment of severe preeclampsia. Obstet Gynecol 1991;77:331–336.

Ferris TF, Weir EK. Effect of captopril on uterine blood flow and prostaglandin E synthesis in the pregnant rabbit. J Clin Invest 1983;71:809–815.

Fisher KA, Luger A, Spargo BH, Lindheimer MD. Hypertension in pregnancy: Clinical–pathological correlations and remote prognosis. Medicine 1981;60:267–276.

Friedman SA. Preeclampsia: a review of the role of prostaglandins. Obstet Gynecol 1988;71:122–137.

Friedman SA, de Groot CJM, Taylor RN, et al. Plasma cellular fibronectin as a measure of endothelial involvement in preeclampsia and intrauterine growth retardation. Am J Obstet Gynecol 1994; 170;838–841.

Gallery EDM, Hunyor SN, Gyory AZ. Plasma volume contraction: a significant factor in both pregnancy-associated hypertension (preeclampsia) and chronic hypertension in pregnancy. Q J Med 1979;48:593–602.

Gallery ED, Ross M, Gyory AZ. Urinary red blood cell and cast excretion in normal and hypertensive human pregnancy. Am J Obstet Gynecol 1993;168:67–70.

Gant NF, Daley GL, Chand S, et al. A study of angiotensin II pressor response throughout primigravid pregnancy. J Clin Invest 1973;52: 2682–2689.

Gardner WJ, Storer J. The use of the G suit in control of intra-abdominal bleeding. Surg Gynecol Obstet 1966;123:792–798.

Gibson B, Hunter D, Neame PB, Kelton JG. Thrombocytopenia in preeclampsia and eclampsia. Semin Thromb Hemost 1982;8: 234–247.

Gilbert WM, Towner DR, Field NT, Anthony J. The safety and utility of pulmonary artery catheterization in severe preeclampsia and eclampsia. Am J Obstet Gynecol 2000;182:1397–1403.

Gonik B, Cotton DB. Peripartum colloid osmotic pressure changes: influence of intravenous hydration. Am J Obstet Gynecol 1984; 150:90–100.

Goodlin RC. Severe preeclampsia: another great imitator. Am J Obstet Gynecol 1976;125:747–753.

Goodlin RC. Preeclampsia as the great imposter. Am J Obstet Gynecol 1991;164:1577–1581.

Goodlin RC, Mostello D. Maternal hyponatremia and the syndrome of hemolysis, elevated liver enzymes, and low platelet count. Am J Obstet Gynecol 1987;156:910–911.

Goodlin RC, Anderson JC, Hodgson PE. Conservative treatment of liver hematoma in the postpartum period. A report of two cases. J Reprod Med 1985;30:368–370.

Govan ADT. The pathogenesis of eclamptic lesions. Pathol Microbiol (Basel) 1961;24:561–575.

Graham C, Goldstein A. Epidural analgesia and cardiac output in severe preeclamptics. Anaesthesia 1980;35:709–712.

Greenstein D, Henderson JM, Boyer TD. Liver hemorrhage: recurrent episodes during pregnancy complicated by preeclampsia. Gastroenterology 1994;106:1668–1671.

Grimes DA. The morbidity and mortality of pregnancy: still risky business. Am J Obstet Gynecol 1994;170:1489–1494.

Groenendijk R, Trimbos JBMJ, Wallenburg HCS. Hemodynamic measurements in preeclampsia: preliminary observations. Am J Obstet Gynecol 1984;150:232–236.

Grunfeld JP, Pertuiset N. Acute renal failure in pregnancy. Am J Kidney Dis 1987;9:359–362.

Gutsche B. The experts opine: is epidural block for labor and delivery and for cesarean section a safe form of analgesia in severe preeclampsia or eclampsia? Surv Anesth 1986;30:304–311.

Hallak M. Effect of parenteral magnesium sulfate administration on excitatory amino acid receptors in the rat brain. Magnes Res 1998;11:117–131.

Hallak M, Berman RF, Irtenkauf SM, Janusz CA, Cotton DB. Magnesium sulfate treatment decreases *N*-methyl-D-aspartate receptor binding in the rat brain: an autoradiographic study. J Soc Gynecol Invest 1994;1:25–30.

Hankins GDV, Wendell GD, Cunningham FG, Leveno KJ. Longitudinal evaluation of hemodynamic changes in eclampsia. Am J Obstet Gynecol 1984;150:506–512.

Hanssens M, Keirse MJ, Vankelecom F, Van Assche FA. Fetal and neonatal effects of treatment with angiotensin-converting enzyme inhibitors in pregnancy. Obstet Gynecol 1991;78:128–135.

Harbert GM, Claiborne HA, McGaughey HS, et al. Convulsive toxemia. Am J Obstet Gynecol 1968;100:336–342.

Hays PM, Cruikshank DP, Dunn LJ. Plasma volume determination in normal and preeclamptic pregnancies. Am J Obstet Gynecol 1985;151:958–966.

Head BB, Owen J, Vincent RD Jr, Shih G, Chestnut DH, Hauth JC. A randomized trial of intrapartum analgesia in women with severe preeclampsia. Obstet Gynecol 2002;99:452–457.

Henderson DW, Vilos GA, Milne KJ, Nichol PM. The role of Swan–Ganz catheterization in severe pregnancy-induced hypertension. Am J Obstet Gynecol 1984;148:570–574.

Henny CP, Lim AE, Brummelkamp WH, et al. A review of the importance of acute multidisciplinary treatment following spontaneous rupture of the liver capsule during pregnancy. Surg Gynecol Obstet 1983;156:593–598.

Herbert WNP, Brenner WE. Improving survival with liver rupture complicating pregnancy. Am J Obstet Gynecol 1982;142:530–534.

Herling IM. Intravenous nitroglycerin: clinical pharmacology and therapeutic considerations. Am Heart J 1984;108:141–149.

Heyborne KD, Burke MS, Porreco RP. Prolongation of premature gestation in women with hemolysis, elevated liver enzymes and low platelets: a report of five cases. J Reprod Med 1990;35:53–57.

Hibbard LT. Maternal mortality due to acute toxemia. Obstet Gynecol 1973;42:263–270.

Hill JA, Devoe LD, Elgammal TA. Central hemodynamic findings associated with cortical blindness in severe preeclampsia. A case report. J Reprod Med 1985;30:435–438.

Hinchey J, Chaves C, Appignani B, et al. A reversible posterior leukoencephalopathy syndrome. N Engl J Med 1996;334:494–500.

Hodgkinson R, Husain FJ, Hayashi RH. Systemic and pulmonary blood pressure during cesarean section in parturients with gestational hypertension. Can Anaesth Soc J 1980;27:389–394.

Hogg B, Hauth JC, Caritis SN, et al. Safety of labor epidural anesthesia for women with severe hypertensive disease. National Institute of Child Health and Human Development Maternal–Fetal Medicine Units Network. Am J Obstet Gynecol 1999;181:1096–1101.

Hunter SK, Martin M, Benda JA, Zlatnik FJ. Liver transplant after massive spontaneous hepatic rupture in pregnancy complicated by preeclampsia. Obstet Gynecol 1995;85:819–822.

Hurault de Ligny B, Ryckelynck JP, Mintz P, et al. Captopril therapy in preeclampsia. Nephron 1987;46:329–330.

Hurd WW, Miodovnik M, Herzberg V, Lavin JP. Selective management of abruptio placentae: a prospective study. Obstet Gynecol 1983;61:467–473.

Hutt R, Ogunniyi SO, Sullivan MHF, Elder MG. Increased platelet volume and aggregation precede the onset of preeclampsia. Obstet Gynecol 1994;83:146–149.

Hutton JD, James DK, Stirrat GM, et al. Management of severe preeclampsia and eclampsia by UK consultants. Br J Obstet Gynaecol 1992;99:554–556.

Hypertensive disorders in pregnancy. In: Cunningham FG, Gant NF, Leveno KJ, Gilstrap LC, Hauth JC, Wenstrom KD, eds. Williams Obstetrics. New York: McGraw-Hill, 2001.

Jones MM, Longmire S, Cotton DB, et al. Influence of crystalloid versus colloid infusion on peripartum colloid osmotic pressure changes. Obstet Gynecol 1986;68:659–661.

Jouppila P, Jouppila R, Hollman A, Koivula A. Lumbar epidural analgesia to improve intervillous blood flow during labor in severe preeclampsia. Obstet Gynecol 1982;59:158–161.

Jouppila P, Kirkinen P, Koivula A, Ylikorkala O. Effects of dihydralazine infusion on the fetoplacental blood flow and maternal prostanoids. Obstet Gynecol 1985;65:115–118.

Joyce TH, Debnath KS, Baker EA. Preeclampsia: relationship of central venous pressure and epidural anesthesia. Anesthesiology 1979; 51:S297.

Kaunitz AM, Hughes JM, Grimes DA, et al. Causes of maternal mortality in the United States. Obstet Gynecol 1985;65:605–612.

Killam AP, Dillard SH, Patton RC, Pederson PR. Pregnancy-induced hypertension complicated by acute liver disease and disseminated intravascular coagulation. Am J Obstet Gynecol 1975;123:823–828.

Kinsella CB, Milner M, McCarthy N, Walshe J. Sixth nerve palsy: an unusual manifestation of preeclampsia. Obstet Gynecol 1994; 83:849–851.

Kirby JC, Jaindl JJ. Cerebral CT findings in toxemia of pregnancy. Radiology 1984;154:114.

Kirshon B, Cotton DB. Invasive hemodynamic monitoring in the obstetric patient. Clin Obstet Gynecol 1987;30:579–590.

Kirshon B, Lee W, Mauer MB, Cotton DB. Effects of low-dose dopamine therapy in the oliguric patient with preeclampsia. Am J Obstet Gynecol 1988a;159:604–607.

Kirshon B, Moise KJ Jr, Cotton DB, et al. Role of volume expansion in severe preeclampsia. Surg Gynecol Obstet 1988b;167:367–371.

Klechner HB, Giles HR, Corrigan JJ. The association of maternal and neonatal thrombocytopenia in high risk pregnancies. Am J Obstet Gynecol 1977;128:235–238.

Koch-Weser J. Hydralazine. N Engl J Med 1976;295;320–323.

Koontz WLL, Reid KH. Effect of parenteral magnesium sulfate on penicillin-induced seizure in foci in anesthetized cats. Am J Obstet Gynecol 1985;153:96–99.

Krane NK. Acute renal failure in pregnancy. Arch Intern Med 1988;148:2347–2357.

Kupferminc MJ, Peaceman AM, Wigton TR, et al. Tumor necrosis factor-α is elevated in plasma and amniotic fluid of patients with severe preeclampsia. Am J Obstet Gynecol 1994;170:1752–1759.

Kuzniar J, Skret A, Piela A, et al. Hemodynamic effects of intravenous hydralazine in pregnant women with severe hypertension. Obstet Gynecol 1985;66:453–458.

Lamming GD, Symonds EM. Use of labetalol and methyldopa in pregnancy-induced hypertension. Br J Clin Pharmacol 1979;8:217S–222S.

Lazard EM. An analysis of 575 cases of eclamptic and pre-eclamptic toxemias treated by intravenous injections of magnesium sulphate. Am J Obstet Gynecol 1933;26:647–656.

Leduc L, Lederer E, Lee W, Cotton DB. Urinary sediment changes in severe preeclampsia. Obstet Gynecol 1991;77:186–189.

Lee W, Gonik B, Cotton DB. Urinary diagnostic indices in preeclampsia-associated oligura: correlation with invasive hemodynamic monitoring. Am J Obstet Gynecol 1987;156:100–103.

Lees MM. Central circulatory response to normotensive and hypertensive pregnancy. Postgrad Med J 1979;55:311–314.

Lewis PJ, Shepherd GI, Ritter J. Prostacyclin and preeclampsia. Lancet 1981;i:559.

Liedholm H, Wahlin-Boll E, Hanson A, et al. Transplacental passage and breast milk concentrations of hydralazine. Eur J Clin Pharmacol 1982;21:417–419.

Lin CC, Lindheimer MD, River P, Moawad AH. Fetal outcome in hypertensive disorders of pregnancy. Am J Obstet Gynecol 1982; 142:255–260.

Lindheimer MD, Katz AI. Current concepts. Hypertension in pregnancy. N Engl J Med 1985;313:675–680.

Lopez-Llera M. Complicated eclampsia: fifteen years experience in a referral medical center. Am J Obstet Gynecol 1982;142:28–35.

Lubarsky SL, Barton JR, Friedman SA, et al. Late postpartum eclampsia revisited. Obstet Gynecol 1994;83:502–505.

Lubbe WF. Hypertension in pregnancy: whom and how to treat. Br J Clin Pharmacol 1987;24:15S–20S.

Lucas CE, Ledgerwood AM. Prospective evaluation of hemostatic techniques for liver injuries. J Trauma 1976;16:442.

Lucas MJ, DePalma RT, Peters MT, et al. A simplified phenytoin regimen for preeclampsia. Am J Perinatol 1994;11:153–156.

Lucas MJ, Leveno KJ, Cunningham FG. A comparison of magnesium sulfate with phenytoin for the prevention of eclampsia. N Engl J Med 1995;333:201–205.

Lund-Johansen P. The haemodynamic pattern in mild and borderline hypertension. Acta Med Scand 1983;Suppl 686:15.

Lund-Johnson P. Short- and long-term (six year) hemodynamic effects of labetalol in essential hypertension. Am J Med 1983;75: 24–31.

Lunell NO, Hjemdahl P, Fredholm BB, et al. Circulatory and metabolic effects of a combined α- and β-adrenoceptor blocker (labetalol) in hypertension of pregnancy. Br J Clin Pharmacol 1981;12:345–348.

Lunell NO, Nylung LE, Lewander R, Sabey B. Uteroplacental blood flow in preeclampsia: measurements with indium-113m and a computer-linked gamma camera. Clin Exp Hypertens 1982;B1:105–107.

Lunell NO, Lewander R, Mamoun I, et al. Utero-placental blood flow in pregnancy-induced hypertension. Scand J Clin Lab Invest 1984;Suppl 169:28–35.

Mabie WC, Gonzalez AR, Sibai BM, Amon E. A comparative trial of labetalol and hydralazine in the acute management of severe hypertension complicating pregnancy. Obstet Gynecol 1987;70:328–333.

Mabie WC, Ratts TE, Sibai BM. The central hemodynamics of severe preeclampsia. Am J Obstet Gynecol 1989;161:1443–1448.

MacKenna J, Dover NL, Brame RG. Preeclampsia associated with hemolysis, elevated liver enzymes, and low platelets: an obstetric emergency? Obstet Gynecol 1983;62:751–754.

Magpie Trial Collaboration Group. Do women with pre-eclampsia, and their babies, benefit from magnesium sulphate? The Magpie Trial: a randomised placebo-controlled trial. Lancet 2002;359: 1877–1890.

Majoko F, Mujaji C. Maternal outcome in eclampsia at Harare Maternity Hospital. Cent Afr J Med 2001;47:123–128.

Martin JN, Blake PG, Perry KG, et al. The natural history of HELLP syndrome: patterns of disease progression and regression. Am J Obstet Gynecol 1991;164:1500–1513.

Masse J, Forest JC, Moutquin JM, et al. A prospective study of several potential biologic markers for early prediction of the development of preeclampsia. Am J Obstet Gynecol 1993;169:501–508.

Massobrio M, Benedetto C, Bertini E, et al. Immune complexes in preeclampsia and normal pregnancy. Am J Obstet Gynecol 1985; 152:578–583.

Messer RH. Symposium on bleeding disorders in pregnancy: observations on bleeding in pregnancy. Am J Obstet Gynecol 1987; 156:1419–1420.

Meyer NL, Mercer BM, Friedman SA, Sibai BM. Urinary dipstick protein: a poor predictor of absent or severe proteinuria. Am J Obstet Gynecol 1994;170:137–141.

Michael CA. Use of labetalol in the treatment of severe hypertension during pregnancy. Br J Clin Pharmacol 1979;8:211S–215S.

Michael CA. The evaluation of labetalol in the treatment of hypertension complicating pregnancy. Br J Clin Pharmacol 1982;13: 127S–131S.

Mikhail MS, Anyaegbunam A, Garfinkel D, et al. Preeclampsia and antioxidant nutrients: decreased plasma levels of reduced ascorbic acid, α-tocopherol, and beta-carotene in women with preeclampsia. Am J Obstet Gynecol 1994;171:150–157.

Miller JD. The management of cerebral edema. Br J Hosp Med 1979;21:152–165.

Mitchell SE, Clark RA. Complications of central venous catheterization. Am J Roentgenol 1979;133:467–476.

Morgan MA, Silavin SL, Dormer KJ, et al. Effects of labetalol on uterine blood flow and cardiovascular hemodynamics in the hypertensive gravid baboon. Am J Obstet Gynecol 1993;168:1574–1579.

Morris RH, Vassalli P, Beller PK, McCluskey RT. Immunofluorescent studies of renal biopsies in the diagnosis of toxemia of pregnancy. Obstet Gynecol 1964;24:32–46.

Mroczek WJ, Lee WR, Davidov ME. Effect of magnesium sulfate on cardiovascular hemodynamics. Angiology 1977;28:720–724.

Naden RP, Redman CWG. Antihypertensive drugs in pregnancy. Clin Perinatol 1985;12:521–538.

National High Blood Pressure Education Program Working Group. Report on high blood pressure in pregnancy. Am J Obstet Gynecol 1990;163:1689–1712.

Neiger R, Contag SA, Coustan DR. The resolution of preeclampsia-related thrombocytopenia. Obstet Gynecol 1991;77:692–695.

Newsome LR, Bramwell RS, Curling PE. Severe preeclampsia: hemodynamic effects of lumbar epidural anesthesia. Anesth Analg 1986;65:31–36.

Oates JA, Wood AJJ. Converting-enzyme inhibitors in the treatment of hypertension. N Engl J Med 1988;319:1517–1525.

Odendaal HJ, Pattinson RC, Bam R, et al. Aggressive or expectant management for patients with severe preeclampsia between 28–34 weeks' gestation: a randomized controlled trial. Obstet Gynecol 1990;76:1070–1074.

Onwuhafua PI, Onwuhafua A, Adze J, Mairami Z. Eclampsia in Kaduna State of Nigeria—a proposal for a better outcome. Niger J Med 2001;10:81–84.

Oosterhof H, Voorhoeve PG, Aarnoudse JG. Enhancement of hepatic artery resistance to blood flow in preeclampsia in presence or absence of HELLP syndrome (hemolysis, elevated liver enzymes, and low platelets). Am J Obstet Gynecol 1994;171:526–530.

Pasch T, Schulz V, Hoppelshauser G. Nitroprusside-induced formation of cyanide and its detoxification with thiosulfate during deliberate hypotension. J Cardiovasc Pharmacol 1983;5:77–85.

Phelan JP, Yurth DA. Severe preeclampsia. I. Peripartum hemodynamic observations. Am J Obstet Gynecol 1982;144:17–22.

Pickles CJ, Symonds EM, Pipkin FB. The fetal outcome in a randomized double-blind controlled trial of labetalol versus placebo in pregnancy-induced hypertension. Br J Obstet Gynaecol 1989;96: 38–43.

Pritchard JA. The use of magnesium iron in the management of eclamptogenic toxemias. Surg Gynecol Obstet 1955;100:131–140.

Pritchard JA. The use of magnesium sulfate in preeclampsia–eclampsia. J Reprod Med 1979;23:107–114.

Pritchard JA, Pritchard SA. Standardized treatment of 154 consecutive cases of eclampsia. Am J Obstet Gynecol 1975;123:543–552.

Pritchard JA, Weisman R, Ratnoff OD, Vosburgh GJ. Intravascular hemolysis, thrombocytopenia, and other hematologic abnormalities associated with severe toxemia of pregnancy. N Engl J Med 1954;150:89–98.

Pritchard JA, Cunningham FG, Mason RA. Coagulation changes in preeclampsia: their frequency and pathogenesis. Am J Obstet Gynecol 1976;124:855–864.

Pritchard JA, Cunningham FG, Pritchard SA. The Parkland Memorial Hospital protocol for the treatment of eclampsia: evaluation of 245 cases. Am J Obstet Gynecol 1984;148:951–963.

Pritchard JA, MacDonald PC, Grant NF. In: Williams Obstetrics, 17th edn. Norwalk, CT: Appleton-Century-Crofts, 1985:525.

Pritchard JA, Cunningham FG, Pritchard SA, Mason RA. How often does maternal preeclampsia–eclampsia incite thrombocytopenia in the fetus? Obstet Gynecol 1987;69:292–295.

Pruett KM, Krishon B, Cotton DB, et al. The effects of magnesium sulfate therapy on Apgar scores. Am J Obstet Gynecol 1988;159: 1047–1048.

Rademaker L. Spontaneous rupture of liver complicating pregnancy. Ann Surg 1943;118:396–401.

Rafferty TD, Berkowitz RL. Hemodynamics in patients with severe toxemia during labor and delivery. Am J Obstet Gynecol 1980; 138:263–270.

Ramos-Santos E, Devoe LD, Wakefield ML, Sherline DM, Metheny WP. The effects of epidural anesthesia on the Doppler velocimetry of umbilical and uterine arteries in normal and hypertensive patients during active term labor. Obstet Gynecol 1991;77:20–26.

Reck T, Bussenius-Kammerer M, Ott R, Muller V, Beinder E, Hohenberger W. Surgical treatment of HELLP syndrome-associated liver rupture: an update. Eur J Obstet Gynecol Reprod Biol 2001;99:57–65.

Redman CWG. Immunologic factors in the pathogenesis of preeclampsia. Contrib Nephrol 1981;25:120.

Redman CWG, Beilin LJ, Bonner J. Renal function in preeclampsia. J Clin Pathol 1976;10:94–96.

Repke JT, Friedman SA, Kaplan PW. Prophylaxis of eclamptic seizures: current controversies. Clin Obstet Gynecol 1992;35:365–374.

Report of the National High Blood Pressure Education Program Working Group on High Blood Pressure in Pregnancy. Am J Obstet Gynecol 2000;183:S1–S22.

Rey E, LeLorier J, Burgess E, Lange IR, Leduc L. Report of the Canadian Hypertension Society Consensus Conference: 3. Pharmacologic treatment of hypertensive disorders in pregnancy. Can Med Assoc J 1997;157:1245–1254.

Riley AJ. Clinical pharmacology of labetalol in pregnancy. J Cardiovasc Pharmacol 1981;3:S53–S59.

Robillard P, Hulsey TC, Perianin J, et al. Association of pregnancy-induced hypertension with duration of sexual cohabitation before conception. Lancet 1994;344:973–975.

Rodgers GM, Taylor RN, Roberts JM. Preeclampsia is associated with a serum factor cytotoxic to human endothelial cells. Am J Obstet Gynecol 1988;159:908–914.

Romero R, Lockwood C, Oyarzun E, Hobbins JC. Toxemia: new concepts in an old disease. Semin Perinatol 1988a;12:302–323.

Romero R, Vizoso J, Emamian M, et al. Clinical significance of liver dysfunction in pregnancy-induced hypertension. Am J Perinatol 1988b;5:146–151.

Romero R, Mazor M, Lockwood CJ, et al. Clinical significance, prevalence, and natural history of thrombocytopenia in pregnancy-induced hypertension. Am J Perinatol 1989;6:32–38.

Rote NS, Caudle MR. Circulating immune complexes in pregnancy, preeclampsia, and auto-immune diseases: evaluation of Raji cell enzyme-linked immunosorbent assay and polyethylene glycol precipitation methods. Am J Obstet Gynecol 1983;147:267–273.

Rubin AA, Roth FE, Taylor RM, Rosenkilde H. Pharmacology of

diazoxide, an antihypertensive, non-diuretic benzothiadiazine. J Pharmacol Exp Ther 1962;136:344–352.

Saftlas AF, Olson DR, Franks AL, Atrash HK, Pokras R. Epidemiology of preeclampsia and eclampsia in the United States, 1979–1986. Am J Obstet Gynecol 1990;163:460–465.

Sakala EP, Moore WD. Successful term delivery after previous pregnancy with ruptured liver. Obstet Gynecol 1986;68:124–126.

Savelieva GM, Efimov VS, Grishin VL, et al. Blood coagulation changes in pregnant women at risk of developing preeclampsia. Int J Gynecol Obstet 1995;48:3–8.

Schubiger G, Flury G, Nussberger J. Enalapril for pregnancy-induced hypertension: acute renal failure in a neonate. Ann Intern Med 1988;108:215–216.

Schwartz ML, Brenner W. Severe preeclampsia with persistent postpartum hemolysis and thrombocytopenia treated by plasmapheresis. Obstet Gynecol 1985;65:53S–55S.

Seidman DS, Serr DM, Ben-Rafael Z. Renal and ocular manifestations of hypertensive disease of pregnancy. Obstet Gynecol Surv 1991;46:71–76.

Sheehan HL. Pathological lesions in the hypertensive toxemias of pregnancy. In: Hammond J, Browne FJ, Walstenholme GEW, eds. Toxemias of Pregnancy, Human and Veterinary. Philadelphia: Blakiston, 1950:16–22.

Sheehan HL. Renal morphology in preeclampsia. Kidney Int 1980;18:241–252.

Shelley WC, Gutsche BB. Magnesium and seizure control. Am J Obstet Gynecol 1980;136:146–147.

Shukla PK, Sharma D, Mandal RK. Serum lactate dehydrogenase in detecting liver damage associated with preeclampsia. Br J Obstet Gynaecol 1978;85:40–42.

Sibai BM. Pitfalls in diagnosis and management of preeclampsia. Am J Obstet Gynecol 1988;159:1–5.

Sibai BM. Eclampsia. VI. Maternal–perinatal outcome in 254 consecutive cases. Am J Obstet Gynecol 1990;163:1049–1054.

Sibai BM. Treatment of hypertension in pregnant women. N Engl J Med 1996;335:257.

Sibai BM, Ramadan MK. Acute renal failure in pregnancies complicated by hemolysis, elevated liver enzymes, and low platelets. Am J Obstet Gynecol 1993;168:1682–1690.

Sibai BM, Schneider JM, Morrison JC, et al. The late postpartum eclampsia controversy. Obstet Gynecol 1980;55:74–78.

Sibai BM, Spinnato JA, Watson DL, et al. Effect of magnesium sulfate on electroencephalographic findings in preeclampsia–eclampsia. Obstet Gynecol 1984a;64:261–266.

Sibai BM, Graham JM, McCubbin JH. A comparison of intravenous and intramuscular magnesium sulfate regimens in preeclampsia. Am J Obstet Gynecol 1984b;150:728–733.

Sibai BM, Saslimi M, Abdella TN, et al. Maternal and perinatal outcome of conservative management of severe preeclampsia in midtrimester. Am J Obstet Gynecol 1985a;152:32–37.

Sibai BM, Spinnato JA, Watson DL, et al. Eclampsia. IV. Neurological findings and future outcome. Am J Obstet Gynecol 1985b;152:184–192.

Sibai BM, El-Nazer A, Gonzalez-Ruiz A. Severe preeclampsia–eclampsia in young primigravid women: subsequent pregnancy outcome and remote prognosis. Am J Obstet Gynecol 1986a;155: 1011–1016.

Sibai BM, Taslimi MM, El-Nazer A, et al. Maternal–perinatal outcome associated with the syndrome of hemolysis, elevated liver enzymes, and low platelets in severe preeclampsia–eclampsia. Am J Obstet Gynecol 1986b;155:501–509.

Sibai BM, Abdella TN, Spinnato JA, et al. Eclampsia. V. The incidence of non-preventable eclampsia. Am J Obstet Gynecol 1986c;154; 561–566.

Sibai BM, Mabie BC, Harvey CJ, Gonzalez AR. Pulmonary edema in severe preeclampsia–eclampsia: analysis of thirty-seven consecutive cases. Am J Obstet Gynecol 1987;156:1174–1179.

Sibai BM, Mercer B, Sarinoglu C. Severe preeclampsia in the second trimester: recurrence risk and long-term prognosis. Am J Obstet Gynecol 1991;165:1408–1412.

Sibai BM, Sarinoglu C, Mercer BM. Pregnancy outcome after eclampsia and long term prognosis. Am J Obstet Gynecol 1992;166:1757.

Sibai BM, Ramadan MK, Usta I, et al. Maternal morbidity and mortality in 442 pregnancies with hemolysis, elevated liver enzymes, and low platelets (HELLP syndrome). Am J Obstet Gynecol 1993;169: 1000–1006.

Sibai BM, Mercer BM, Schiff E, Friedman SA. Aggressive versus expectant management of severe preeclampsia at 28 to 32 weeks' gestation: a randomized controlled trial. Am J Obstet Gynecol 1994;171:818–822.

Sibai BM, Ramadan MK, Chari RS, Friedman SA. Pregnancies complicated by HELLP syndrome (hemolysis, elevated liver enzymes, and low platelets): subsequent pregnancy outcome and long-term prognosis. Am J Obstet Gynecol 1995;172:125–129.

Smith LG, Moise KJ, Dildy GA, Carpenter RJ. Spontaneous rupture of liver during pregnancy: current therapy. Obstet Gynecol 1991;77:171–175.

Sorensen JD, Olsen SF, Pederson AK, et al. Effects of fish oil supplementation in the third trimester of pregnancy on prostacyclin and thromboxane production. Am J Obstet Gynecol 1993;168:915–922.

Spinnato JA, Sibai BM, Anderson GD. Fetal distress after hydralazine therapy for severe pregnancy-induced hypertension. South Med J 1986;79:559–562.

Stahnke E. Über das verhalten der blutplättchen bie eklampsie. Zentralbl Gynäk 1922;46:391.

Stone JL, Lockwood CJ, Berkowitz GS, et al. Risk factors for severe preeclampsia. Obstet Gynecol 1994;83:357–361.

Strauss RG, Keefer JR, Burke T, Civetta JM. Hemodynamic monitoring of cardiogenic pulmonary edema complicating toxemia of pregnancy. Obstet Gynecol 1980;55:170–174.

Sullivan CA, Magann EF, Perry KG, et al. The recurrence risk of the syndrome of hemolysis, elevated liver enzymes, and low platelets (HELLP) in subsequent gestations. Am J Obstet Gynecol 1994;171:940–943.

Swan HJC, Ganz W, Forrester JS, et al. Catheterization of the heart in man with the use of flow-directed balloon-tipped catheter. N Engl J Med 1970;283:447–451.

Thien T, Koene RAP, Schijf C, et al. Infusion of diazoxide in severe hypertension during pregnancy. Eur J Obstet Gynecol Reprod Biol 1980;10:367–374.

Thiagarajah S, Bourgeois FJ, Harbert GM, Caudle MR. Thrombocytopenia in preeclampsia: associated abnormalities and management principles. Am J Obstet Gynecol 1984;150:1–7.

Van Dam PA, Reiner M, Baekelandt M, et al. Disseminated intravascular coagulation and the syndrome of hemolysis, elevated liver enzymes, and low platelets in severe preeclampsia. Obstet Gynecol 1989;73:97–102.

Vardi J, Fields GA. Microangiopathic hemolytic anemia in severe preeclampsia. Am J Obstet Gynecol 1974;119:617–622.

Vermillion ST, Scardo JA, Newman RB, Chauhan SP. A randomized, double-blind trial of oral nifedipine and intravenous labetalol in hypertensive emergencies of pregnancy. Am J Obstet Gynecol 1999; 181:858–861.

Villar MA, Sibai BM. Clinical significance of elevated mean arterial blood pressure in second trimester and threshold increase in systolic or diastolic blood pressure during third trimester. Am J Obstet Gynecol 1989;160:419.

Waisman GD, Mayorga LM, Camera MI, et al. Magnesium plus nifedipine: potentiation of hypotensive effect in preeclampsia? Am J Obstet Gynecol 1988;159:308–309.

Ward K, Hata A, Jeunemaitre X, et al. A molecular variant of angiotensinogen associated with preeclampsia. Nature Genetics 1993;4:59–61.

Wasserstrum N, Cotton DB. Hemodynamic monitoring in severe pregnancy-induced hypertension. Clin Perinatol 1986;13:781–799.

Wasserstrum N, Kirshon B, Willis RS, et al. Quantitive hemodynamic effects of acute volume expansion in severe preeclampsia. Obstet Gynecol 1989;73:546–550.

Weenink GH, Treffers PE, Vijn P, Smorenberg-Schoorl ME, Ten Cate JW. Antithrombin III levels in preeclampsia correlate with maternal and fetal morbidity. Am J Obstet Gynecol 1984;148:1092–1097.

Weil MN, Henning RJ, Puri VK. Colloid osmotic pressure: clinical significance: Crit Care Med 1979;7:113–116.

Weiner CP, Kwaan HC, Xu C, et al. Antithrombin III activity in women with hypertension during pregnancies. Obstet Gynecol 1985; 65:301–306.

Weinstein L. Syndrome of hemolysis, elevated liver enzymes, and low platelet count: a severe consequence of hypertension in pregnancy. Am J Obstet Gynecol 1982;142:159–167.

Weinstein L. Preeclampsia/eclampsia with hemolysis, elevated liver enzymes, and thrombocytopenia. Obstet Gynecol 1985;66:657–660.

Weiss MH. Cerebral edema. Acute Care 1985;11:187–204.

Whalley PJ, Everett RB, Gant NF, et al. Pressor responsiveness to angiotensin II in hospitalized primigravid women with pregnancy-induced hypertension. Am J Obstet Gynecol 1983;145:481–483.

Wheeler TC, Graves CR, Troiano NH, Reed GW. Base deficit and oxygen transport in severe preeclampsia. Obstet Gynecol 1996;87: 375–379.

Worley RJ. Pathophysiology of pregnancy-induced hypertension. Clin Obstet Gynecol 1984;27:821–823.

Young BK, Weinstein HM. Effects of magnesium sulfate on toxemic patients in labor. Obstet Gynecol 1977;49:681–685.

Zimmerman JL. Hypertensive crisis: emergencies and urgencies. In: Ayers SM, ed. Textbook of Critical Care. Philadelphia: WB Saunders, 1995.

Zuspan FP. Treatment of severe preeclampsia and eclampsia. Clin Obstet Gynecol 1966;9:945–972.

Zuspan FP. Problems encountered in the treatment of pregnancy-induced hypertension. Am J Obstet Gynecol 1978;131:591–597.

34 Anaphylactoid syndrome of pregnancy (amniotic fluid embolism)

Gary A. Dildy III
Steven L. Clark

Amniotic fluid embolism (AFE) is an uncommon obstetric disorder with a mortality of 60–70% and is a leading cause of maternal mortality in western industrialized countries (Morgan, 1979; Kaunitz et al., 1985; Grimes, 1994; Hogberg et al., 1994; Clark et al., 1995). It is classically characterized by hypoxia, hypotension or hemodynamic collapse, and coagulopathy. Despite numerous attempts to develop an animal model, AFE remains incompletely understood. Nevertheless, during the past decade, there have been several significant advances in our understanding of this enigmatic condition. A recent population-based study of over one million deliveries in California during 1994–95 reported a 1 in 20,000 incidence (Gilbert & Danielsen, 1999).

Historic considerations

The earliest written description of AFE is attributed to Meyer in 1926. The condition was not widely recognized, however, until the report of Steiner and Luschbaugh in 1941. These investigators described autopsy findings in eight pregnant women with sudden shock and pulmonary edema during labor. In all cases, squamous cells or mucin, presumably of fetal origin, were found in the pulmonary vasculature. In a follow-up report in 1969 by Liban and Raz, cellular debris was also observed in the kidneys, liver, spleen, pancreas, and brain of several such patients. Squamous cells also were identified in uterine veins of several control patients in this series, a finding confirmed in a report of Thompson and Budd (1963) in a patient without AFE. It should be noted, however, that in the initial description of Steiner and Luschbaugh (1941), seven of the eight patients carried clinical diagnoses other than AFE (including sepsis and unrecognized uterine rupture) and were not materially different from the diagnoses of their control patients without these specific histologic findings. Only one of the eight patients in the classic AFE group died of "obstetric shock" without an additional clinical diagnosis. Thus, the relevance of this original report to patients presently dying of AFE after the exclusion of other diagnoses is questionable.

Since the initial descriptions of AFE, more than 300 case reports have appeared in the literature. Although most cases were reported during labor, sudden death in pregnancy has been attributed to AFE under many widely varying circumstances, including cases of first- and second-trimester abortion (Resnik et al., 1976; Guidotti et al., 1981; Cromley et al., 1983; Meier & Bowes, 1983). In 1948, Eastman, in an editorial review, stated, "Let us be careful not to make [the diagnosis of AFE] a waste basket for cases of unexplained death in labor." Fortunately, increased understanding of the syndrome of AFE makes such errors less likely today.

Experimental models

The first animal model of AFE was that of Steiner and Luschbaugh (1941), who showed that rabbits and dogs could be killed by the intravenous injection of heterologous amniotic fluid and meconium. Several subsequent reports of AFE in experimental animals have yielded conflicting results (Table 34.1) (Steiner & Luschbaugh, 1941; Cron et al., 1952; Schneider, 1955; Jaques et al., 1960; Halmagyi et al., 1962; Attwood & Downing, 1965; Reis et al., 1965; Stolte et al., 1967; MacMillan, 1968; Dutta et al., 1970; Adamsons et al., 1971; Kitzmiller & Lucas, 1972; Reeves et al., 1974; Spence & Mason, 1974; Azegami & Mori, 1986; Richards et al., 1988; Hankins et al., 1993; Petroianu et al., 1999). In most series, experimental injection of amniotic fluid had adverse effects, ranging from transient alterations in systemic and pulmonary artery pressures in dogs, sheep, cats, and calves to sudden death in rabbits. Only two of these studies, however, involved pregnant animals, and in most, heterologous amniotic fluid was used. In several studies, the effects of whole or meconium-enriched amniotic fluid were contrasted with those of filtered amniotic fluid. A pathologic response was obtained only in particulate-rich amniotic fluid in four such studies, whereas three reports demonstrated physiologic changes with filtered amniotic fluid as well. Data produced with the models involving particulate-enriched amniotic fluid may have little relevance to the human model, because the con-

Table 34.1 Animal models of amniotic fluid embolism

					Effects					
Reference	**Year**	**Animal**	**Anesthetized**	**Pregnant**	**Filtered AF**	**Whole AF**	**AF species**	**Hemodynamic changes**	**Coagulopathy**	**Autopsy**
Steiner & Luschbaugh	1941	Rabbit/ dog	No	No	No	Yes	Human	NE (death)	No	Debris in PA
Cron et al.	1952	Rabbit	No	No	NE	Yes	Human	NNE (death)	No	Debris in PA
Schneider	1953	Dog	No	No	NE	Yes	Human	NE (death)	5 of 8	Debris in PA
Jacques et al.	1960	Dog	Yes	No	NE	Yes	Human/ dog	Yes	Fibrinogen 12 of 13	Debris in PA
Halmagyi et al.	1962	Sheep	Yes	No	No	Yes	Human	Yes	No	NE
Attwood & Downing	1965	Dog	Yes	No	Yes	Yes	Human	Yes	4 of 12	NE
Stolte et al.	1967	Monkey	Yes	Yes	No	No	Human/ monkey	No	1 of 12	NE
Macmillan	1968	Rabbit	No	No	No	Yes	Human	NE (death)	2 of 12	Minimal debris, hemorrhage
Reis et al.	1969	Sheep	Yes	Yes	Yes	Yes	Sheep	Yes	No	Normal
Dutta et al.	1970	Rabbit	Yes	No	NE	Yes	Human	NE (death)	No	Minimal debris, massive infarction
Adamsons et al.	1971	Monkey	Yes	Yes	NE	No	Monkey	No	No	NE
Kitzmiller & Lucas	1972	Cat	Yes	No	No	Yes	Human	Yes	No	NE
Spence & Mason	1974	Rabbit	No	Yes	No	No	Rabbit	No	No	NE
Reeves et al.	1974	Calf	No	No	NE	Yes	Calf	Yes		
Azegami & Mori	1986	Rabbit	No	No	No	Yes	Human	NE (death)	No	Pulmonary edema, debris in PA
Richards et al.	1988	Rat*	Yes	No	Yes	NE	Human	Coronary flow		
Hankins et al.	1993	Goat	Yes	Yes	Yes	Yes	Goat	Yes	No	NE
Petroianu et al.	1999	Mini-pig	Yes	Yes	Yes	Yes	Mini-pig		Yes	Debris in PA

* Isolated heart preparation.

AF, amniotic fluid; BP, blood pressure; CO, cardiac output; CVP, central venous pressure; LAP, left atrial pressure; NE, not examined; P, pulse; PA, pulmonary artery; PAP, pulmonary artery pressure; PCWP, pulmonary capillary wedge pressure; PVR, pulmonary vascular resistance; RR, respiratory rate; SVR, systemic vascular resistance.

centration of particulate matter injected has been many times greater than that present in human amniotic fluid, even in the presence of meconium. In the four studies in which injections of amniotic fluid into the arterial and venous systems were compared, three showed toxic effected with both arterial and venous injection, implying a pathologic humoral substance or response. In studies in which autopsy was performed, pulmonary findings ranged from massive vascular plugging with fetal debris (after embolization with particulate-enriched amniotic fluid) to normal.

In contrast, the only two studies carried out in primates showed the intravenous injection of amniotic fluid to be entirely innocuous without effects on blood pressure, pulse, or respiratory rate (Stolte et al., 1967; Adamsons et al., 1971). In one study, the volume of amniotic fluid infused would, in the human, represent 80% of the total amniotic fluid volume. More recently, a carefully controlled study in the goat model using homologous amniotic fluid demonstrated hemodynamic and clinical findings similar to that seen in humans, including an initial transient rise in pulmonary and systemic vascular resistance and myocardial depression (Hankins et al., 1993). These findings were especially prominent when the injectate included meconium. Importantly, the initial phase of pulmonary hypertension in all animal models studied has been transient and in survivors has resolved within 30 minutes (Clark, 1990). Because most attempts at the development of an animal model of AFE have involved the injection of tissue from a foreign species, the resultant physiologic effects may have limited clinical relevance to the human condition and must be interpreted with caution.

Clinical presentation

Hemodynamic alterations

In humans, an initial transient phase of hemodynamic change involving both systemic and pulmonary vasospasm leads to a more often recognized secondary phase involving principally hypotension and depressed ventricular function (Clark et al., 1985, 1988, 1995; Girard et al., 1986).

Figure 34.1 demonstrates in a graphic manner the depression of left ventricular function seen in five patients monitored with pulmonary artery catheterization. The mechanism of left ventricular failure is uncertain. Work in the rat model by Richards et al. (1988) suggests the presence of possible coronary artery spasm and myocardial ischemia in animal AFE. On the other hand, the global hypoxia commonly seen in patients with AFE could account for left ventricular dysfunction. The in vitro observation of decreased myometrial contractility in the presence of amniotic fluid also suggests the possibility of a similar effect of amniotic fluid on myocardium (Courtney, 1970).

Pulmonary manifestations

Patients suffering AFE typically develop rapid and often profound hypoxia, which may result in permanent neurologic impairment in survivors of this condition. This hypoxia is likely due to a combination of initial pulmonary vasospasm and ventricular dysfunction. A recent case report of transesophageal echocardiography findings during the hyperacute stage of AFE revealed acute right ventricular failure and suprasystemic right-sided pressures (Shechtman et al., 1999). In both animal models and human experience, however, this initial hypoxia is often transient. Figure 34.2 details arterial blood gas findings in a group of patients with AFE for whom paired data are available. Initial profound shunting and rapid recovery are seen. In survivors, primary lung injury often leads to acute respiratory distress syndrome and secondary oxygenation defects.

Coagulopathy

Patients surviving the initial hemodynamic insult may succumb to a secondary coagulopathy (Clark et al., 1995; Porter et al., 1996). The exact incidence of the coagulopathy is unknown. Coagulopathy was an entry criterion for inclusion in the initial analysis of the National AFE Registry; however, several patients submitted to the registry who clearly had AFE did not have clinical evidence of coagulopathy (Clark et al., 1995). In a similar manner, a number of patients have been observed who developed an acute obstetric coagulopathy alone in the absence of placental abruption and suffered fatal exsanguination without any evidence of primary hemodynamic or pulmonary insult (Porter et al., 1996).

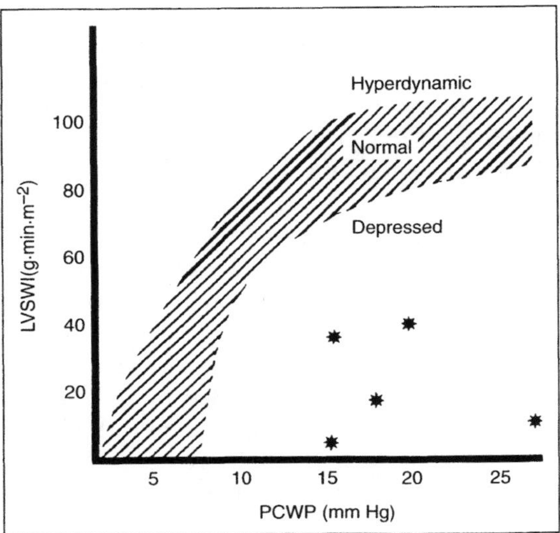

Fig. 34.1 Modified Starling curve, demonstrating depressed left ventricular function in five patients with amniotic fluid embolism. LVSWI, left ventricular stroke work index; PCWP, pulmonary capillary wedge pressure.

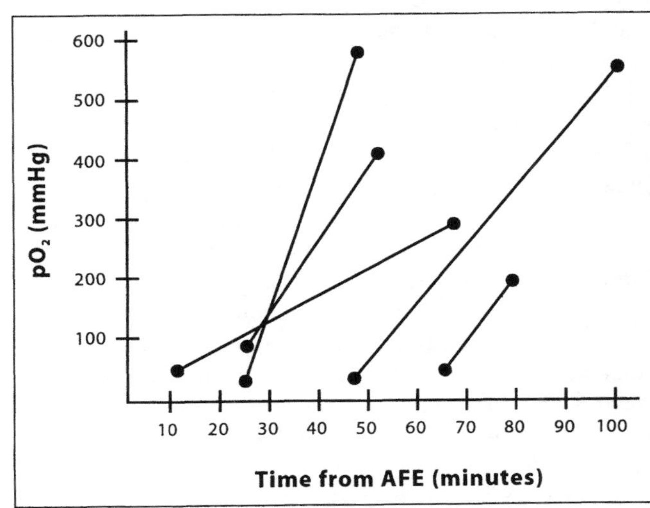

Fig. 34.2 Resolution of hypoxia after amniotic fluid embolism (AFE).

As with experimental investigations into hemodynamic alterations associated with AFE, investigations of this coagulopathy has yielded contradictory results. Amniotic fluid has been shown in vitro to shorten whole blood clotting time, to have a thromboplastin-like effect, to induce platelet aggregation and release of platelet factor III, and to activate the compliment cascade (Ratnoff & Vosbugh, 1952; Beller et al., 1963). In addition, Courtney and Allington (1972) showed that amniotic fluid contains a direct factor X-activating factor. Although confirming the factor X-activating properties of amniotic fluid, Phillips and Davison (1972) concluded that the amount of procoagulant in clear amniotic fluid is insufficient to cause significant intravascular coagulation, a finding disputed by the studies of Lockwood et al. (1991) and Philips and Davidson (1972).

In the experimental animal models discussed previously, coagulopathy has likewise been an inconsistent finding. Thus, the exact nature of the consumptive coagulopathy demonstrated in humans with AFE is yet to be satisfactorily explained. The powerful thromboplastin effects of trophoblast are well established. The coagulopathy associated with severe placental abruption and that seen with AFE are probably similar in origin and represent activation of the coagulation cascade following exposure of the maternal circulation to a variety of fetal antigens with varying thromboplastin-like effects (Clark et al., 1995).

Pathophysiology

In an analysis of the National AFE Registry, a marked similarity was noted between the clinical, hemodynamic, and hematologic manifestations of AFE and both septic and anaphylactic shock (Clark et al., 1995). Clearly, the clinical manifestations of this condition are not identical; fever is unique to septic shock, and cutaneous manifestations are more common in anaphylaxis. Nevertheless, the marked similarities of these conditions suggest similar pathophysiologic mechanisms.

Detailed discussions of the pathophysiologic features of septic shock and anaphylactic shock are presented elsewhere in this text. Both of these conditions involve the entrance of a foreign substance (bacterial endotoxin or specific antigens) into the circulation, which then results in the release of various primary and secondary endogenous mediators (Fig. 34.3). Similar pathophysiology has also been proposed in nonpregnant patients with pulmonary fat embolism. It is the release of these mediators that results in the principal physiologic derangements characterizing these syndromes. These abnormalities include profound myocardial depression and decreased cardiac output, described in both animals and humans; pulmonary hypertension, demonstrated in lower primate models of anaphylaxis; and disseminated intervascular coagulation, described in both human anaphylactic reactions and septic shock (Parker, 1980; Smith et al., 1980; Smedegard et al., 1981; Enjeti et al., 1983; Silverman et al., 1984; Kapin & Ferguson, 1985; Lee et al., 1988; Raper & Fisher, 1988; Wong et al., 1990; Parillo, 1993). Further, the temporal sequence of hemodynamic decompensation and recovery seen in experimental AFE is virtually identical to that described in canine anaphylaxis (Kapin & Ferguson, 1985). An anaphylactoid response is also well described in humans and involves the nonimmunologic release of similar mediators (Parker, 1980). It is also intriguing that, on admission to hospital, 41% of patients in the AFE registry gave a history of either drug allergy or atopy (Clark et al., 1995).

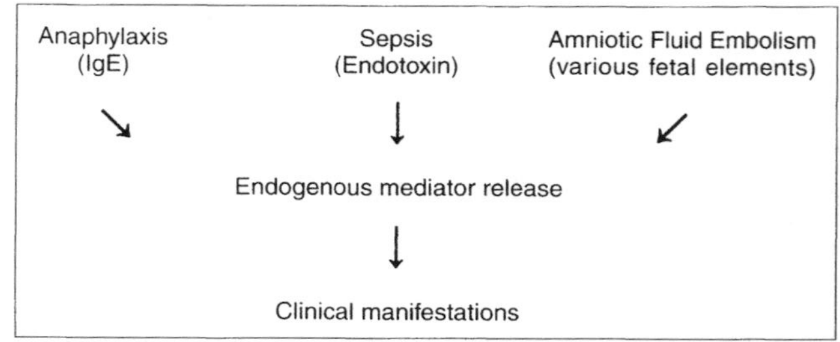

Fig. 34.3 Proposed pathophysiologic relation between AFE, septic shock, and anaphylactic shock. Each syndrome also may have specific direct physiologic effects. (Reproduced by permission from Clark SL, Hankins GVD, Dudley DA, et al. Amniotic fluid embolism: analysis of the national registry. Am J Obstet Gynecol 1995;172:1158–1169.)

The ability of arachidonic acid metabolites to cause the same physiologic and hemodynamic changes observed in human AFE has been noted (Clark, 1985). Further, in the rabbit model of AFE, pretreatment with an inhibitor of leukotriene synthesis has been shown to prevent death (Azegami & Mori, 1986). These experimental observations further support the clinical conclusions of the National AFE Registry analysis that this condition involves the anaphylactoid release of endogenous mediators, including arachidonic acid metabolites, which result in the devastating pathophysiologic sequence seen in clinical AFE (Clark et al., 1995).

Earlier anecdotal reports suggested a possible relationship between hypertonic uterine contractions or oxytocin use and AFE. Although disputed on statistical grounds by Morgan (1979), this misconception persisted in some writings until recently. The historic anecdotal association between hypertonic uterine contractions and the onset of symptoms in AFE was made clear by the analysis of the National Registry (Clark et al., 1995). These data demonstrated that the hypertonic contractions commonly seen in association with AFE appear to be a result of the release of catecholamines into the circulation as part of the initial human hemodynamic response to any massive physiologic insult. Under these circumstances, norepinephrine, in particular, acts as a potent uterotonic agent (Paul et al., 1978; Clark et al., 1995). Thus, while the association of hypertonic contractions and AFE appears to be valid, it is the physiologic response to AFE that cause the hypertonic uterine activity rather than the converse. Indeed, there is a complete cessation of uterine blood flow in the presence of even moderate uterine contractions; thus, a tetanic contraction is the least likely time during an entire labor process for any exchange between maternal and fetal compartments (Towell, 1976). Oxytocin is not used with increased frequency in patients suffering AFE compared with the general population, nor does oxytocin-induced hyperstimulation commonly precede this condition (Clark et al., 1995). Thus, several authorities, including the American College of Obstetricians and Gynecologists, have concluded that oxytocin use has no relationship to the occurrence of AFE (Morgan, 1979; ACOG, 1993; Clark et al., 1995).

The syndrome of AFE appears to be initiated after maternal intravascular exposure to various types of fetal tissue. Such exposure may occur during the course of normal labor and delivery; after potentially minor traumatic events, such as appropriate intrauterine pressure catheter placement; or during cesarean section. Because fetal-to-maternal tissue transfer is virtually universal during the labor and delivery process, actions by health-care providers, such as intrauterine manipulation or cesarean delivery, may affect the timing of the exposure; no evidence exists, however, to suggest that exposure itself can be avoided by altering clinical management. Simple exposure of the maternal circulatory system to even small amounts of amniotic fluid or other fetal tissue may, under the right circumstances, initiate the syndrome of AFE. This understanding explains the well-documented occurrence of fatal AFE during first-trimester pregnancy termination at a time when neither the volume of fluid nor positive intrauterine pressure could be contributing factors (Guidotti et al., 1981). Whereas much has been written about the importance to the fetus of an immunologic barrier between the mother and the antigenically different products of conception, little attention has been paid to the potential importance of this barrier to maternal well-being. The observations of the National Registry as well as cumulative data for the past several decades suggest that breaches of this barrier may, under certain circumstances and in susceptible maternal–fetal pairs, be of immense significance to the mother as well (Clarke et al., 1995).

Previous experimental evidence in animals and humans unequivocally demonstrates that the intravenous administration of even large amounts of amniotic fluid per se is innocuous (Sparr & Pritchard, 1958; Stolte et al., 1967; Adamsons et al., 1971). Further, the clinical findings described in the National Registry are not consistent with an embolic event as commonly understood (Table 34.2). Thus, the term "amniotic fluid embolism" itself appears to be a misnomer. In the National Registry analysis, the authors suggested, that the term "amniotic fluid embolism" be discarded and the syndrome of acute peripartum hypoxia, hemodynamic collapse, and coagulopathy should be designated in a more descriptive manner, as "anaphylactoid syndrome of pregnancy."

Table 34.2 Signs and symptoms noted in patients with amniotic fluid embolism

Sign or symptom	No. of patients (%)
Hypotension	43 (100)
Fetal distress*	30 (100)
Pulmonary edema or ARDS†	28 (93)
Cardiopulmonary arrest	40 (87)
Cyanosis	38 (83)
Coagulopathy‡	38 (83)
Dyspnea§	22 (49)
Seizure	22 (48)
Atony	11 (23)
Bronchospasm¶	7 (15)
Transient hypertension	5 (11)
Cough	3 (7)
Headache	3 (7)
Chest pain	1 (2)

* Includes all live fetuses in utero at time of event.
† Eighteen patients did not survive long enough for these diagnoses to be confirmed.
‡ Eight patients did not survive long enough for this diagnosis to be confirmed.
§ One patient was intubated at the time of the event and could not be assessed.
¶ Difficult ventilation was noted during cardiac arrest in six patients, and wheezes were auscultated in one patient.
(Reproduced by permission from Clark SL, Hankins GVD, Dudley DA. Amniotic fluid embolism: analysis of a national registry. Am J Obstet Gynecol 1995;172:1158–1169.)

Clinical presentation

Clinical signs and symptoms noted in patients with AFE are described in Table 34.2. In a typical case, a patient in labor, having just undergone cesarean delivery or immediately following vaginal delivery or pregnancy termination, suffers the acute onset of profound hypoxia and hypotension followed by cardiopulmonary arrest. The initial episode often is complicated by the development of a consumptive coagulopathy, which may lead to exsanguination, even if attempts to restore hemodynamic and respiratory function are successful. It must be emphasized, however, that in any individual patient any of the three principal phases (hypoxia, hypotension, or coagulopathy) may either dominate or be entirely absent (Clark et al., 1995; Porter et al., 1996; Gilbert & Danielsen, 1999). Clinical variations in this syndrome may be related to variations in either the nature of the antigenic exposure or maternal response.

Maternal outcome is dismal in patients with AFE syndrome. The overall maternal mortality rate appears to be 60–80% (Clark, 1990; Clark et al., 1995). Only 15% of patients, however, survive neurologically intact. In a number of cases, following successful hemodynamic resuscitation and reversal of disseminated intravascular coagulation, life-support systems were withdrawn because of brain death resulting from the initial profound hypoxia. In patients progressing to cardiac arrest, only 8% survive neurologically intact (Clark et al., 1995). In the National Registry data, no form of therapy appeared to be consistently associated with improved outcome. A recent large series of patients in whom the diagnosis of AFE was obtained from the discharge summary reported a 26% mortality rate. Notably, however, many patients in this series lacked one or more potentially lethal clinical manifestation of the disease classically considered mandatory for diagnosis, thus casting the diagnosis into doubt. However, if one assumes that the discharge diagnosis of these patients was accurate, these data suggest improved outcome for those women with milder forms of the disease (Gilbert & Danielsen, 1999).

Neonatal outcome is similarly poor. If the event occurs prior to delivery, the neonatal survival rate is approximately 80%; only half of these fetuses survive neurologically intact (Clark et al., 1995). Fetuses surviving to delivery generally demonstrate profound respiratory acidemia. Although at the present time no form of therapy appears to be associated with improved maternal outcome, there is a clear relationship between neonatal outcome and event-to-delivery interval in those women suffering cardiac arrest (Table 34.3) (Clark et al., 1995). Similar findings were reported by Katz et al. (1986) in patients suffering cardiac arrest in a number of different clinical situations.

Diagnosis

In the past, histologic confirmation of the clinical syndrome of AFE was often sought by the detection of cellular debris of presumed fetal origin either in the distal port of a pulmonary artery catheter or at autopsy (Clark, 1990). Several studies conducted during the past decade, however, suggest that such findings are commonly encountered, even in normal pregnant women (Fig. 34.4) (Plauche, 1983; Covone et al., 1984; Clark et al., 1986; Lee et al., 1986). In the analysis of the National AFE Registry, fetal elements were found in roughly 50% of cases in which pulmonary artery catheter aspirate was analyzed and in roughly 75% of patients who went to autopsy (Clark et al., 1995). The frequency with which such findings are encountered varies with the number of histologic sections obtained. In addition, multiple special stains often are required to document such debris (Clark, 1990). Thus, the diagnosis of AFE remains a clinical one; histologic findings are neither sensitive nor specific. It is interesting to note that similar conclusions have been drawn regarding the diagnostic significance of histologic findings in patients with pulmonary fat embolism (Gitin et al., 1993).

Table 34.3 Cardiac arrest-to-delivery interval and neonatal outcome

Interval (min)	Survival	Intact survival
5	3/3	2/3 (67%)
5–15	3/3	2/3 (67%)
16–25	2/5	2/5 (40%)
26–35	3/4	1/4 (25%)
36–54	0/1	0/1 (0%)

(Reproduced by permission from Clark SL, Hankins GVD, Dudley DA. Amniotic fluid embolism: analysis of the national registry. Am J Obstet Gynecol 1995;172:1158–1169.)

Treatment

For the mother, the end-result of therapy remains disappointing, with an overall mortality rate of 60–80%. In the National Registry, we noted no difference in survival among patients suffering initial cardiac arrest in small rural hospitals attended by family practitioners compared with those suffering identical clinical signs and symptoms in tertiary-level centers attended by board-certified anesthesiologists, cardiologists, and maternal–fetal medicine specialists. Nevertheless, several generalizations can be drawn.

1 The initial treatment for AFE is supportive. Cardiopulmonary resuscitation is performed if the patient is suffering from a lethal dysrhythmia. Oxygen should be provided at high concentrations.

2 In the patient who survives the initial cardiopulmonary insult, it should be remembered that left ventricular failure is

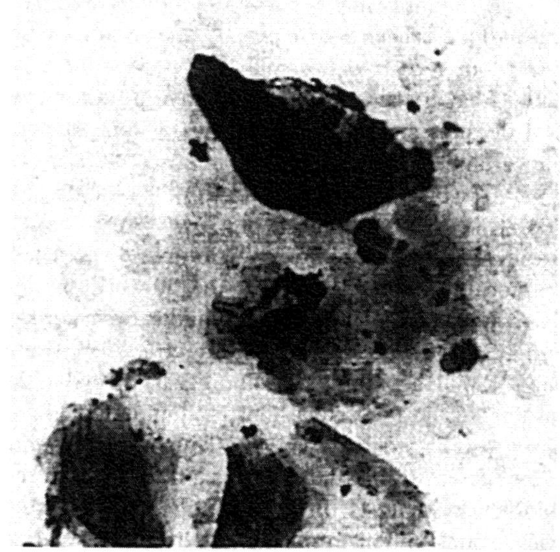

Fig. 34.4 Squamous cells recovered from the pulmonary arterial circulation of a pregnant patient with class IV rheumatic mitral stenosis (magnification, ×1,000).

commonly seen. Thus, volume expansion to optimize ventricular preload is performed, and if the patient remains significantly hypotensive, the addition of an inotropic agent such as dopamine seems most appropriate. In patients who remain unstable following the initial resuscitative efforts, pulmonary artery catheterization may be of benefit to guide hemodynamic manipulation.

3 Although no evidence exists to document the benefit of corticosteroids in patients with AFE, the similarities between AFE and anaphylaxis proposed in the National Registry suggest that the administration of high doses of corticosteroids could potentially be a consideration. In the absence of any data to suggest the benefit of this, however, steroid treatment is not mandated by standard of care; in fact since the original suggestion of corticosteroid therapy by the authors of the National Registry report, we have reviewed several cases where death resulted despite early high-dose steroid treatment.

4 In antepartum cases of AFE, careful attention must be paid to the fetal condition. In a mother who is hemodynamically unstable but has not yet undergone cardiorespiratory arrest, maternal considerations must be weighed carefully against those of the fetus. The decision to subject such an unstable mother to a major abdominal operation (cesarean section) is a difficult one, and each case must be individualized. However, it is axiomatic in these situations that where a choice must be made, maternal well-being must take precedence over that of the fetus.

5 In mothers who have progressed to frank cardiac arrest, the situation is different. Under these circumstances, maternal survival is extremely unlikely, regardless of the therapy rendered. In such women, it is highly unlikely that the imposition of cesarean section would significantly alter the maternal outcome. Even properly performed cardiopulmonary resuscitation (difficult at best in a pregnant woman) provides only a maximum of 30% of normal cardiac output. Under these circumstances, it is fair to assume that the proportion of blood shunted to the uterus and other splanchnic distributions approaches zero. Thus, the fetus will be, for practical purposes, anoxic at all times following maternal cardiac arrest, even during ideal performance of cardiopulmonary resuscitation. Because the interval from maternal arrest to delivery is directly correlated with newborn outcome, perimortum cesarean section should be initiated immediately on the diagnosis of maternal cardiac arrest in patients with AFE, assuming sufficient personnel are available to continue to provide care to the mother and deliver the baby (Katz et al., 1986; Clark et al., 1995). For the pregnant patient, the standard ABC of cardiopulmonary resuscitation should be modified to include a fourth category, D: delivery.

There are limited data on risk of recurrence in a subsequent pregnancy for women who experience AFE; at present, fewer than 10 cases are reported in the published literature (Clark, 1992; Stiller et al., 2000). New modalities for the treatment of AFE, such as extracorporeal membrane oxygenation with intra-aortic balloon counterpulsation (Hsieh et al., 2000) and continuous hemodiafiltration (Kaneko et al., 2001), have been reported in survivors but are thus far of limited cumulative experience or demonstrated benefit.

Despite many advances in the understanding of this condition, AFE or anaphylactoid syndrome of pregnancy remains enigmatic and in most cases is associated with dismal maternal and fetal outcomes, regardless of the quality of care rendered. Thus, AFE remains unpredictable, unpreventable, and, for the most part, untreatable. It is anticipated that new insight into the pathophysiology of AFE suggested by the US Registry data may allow future advances in the treatment of this condition. Recently, a new AFE Registry has been initiated in the United Kingdom, which should provide further understanding of this most feared obstetric complication (de Swiet, 2000; Tuffnell & Johnson, 2000).

References

ACOG. Prologue. Amniotic fluid embolism syndrome. In: Obstetrics, 3rd edn. Washington, DC: American College of Obstetricians and Gynecologists, 1993;94.

Adamsons K, Mueller-Heubach E, Myer RE. The innocuousness of amniotic fluid infusion in the pregnant rhesus monkey. Am J Obstet Gynecol 1971;109:977.

Attwood HD, Downing SE. Experimental amniotic fluid embolism. Surg Gynecol Obstet 1965;120:255.

Azegami M, Mori N. Amniotic fluid embolism and leukotrienes. Am J Obstet Gynecol 1986;155:1119.

Beller FK, Douglas GW, Debrovner CH, et al. The fibrinolytic system in amniotic fluid embolism. Am J Obstet Gynecol 1963;87:48.

Clark SL. Arachidonic acid metabolites and the pathophysiology of amniotic fluid embolism. Semin Reprod Endocrinol 1985;3:253.

Clark SL. New concepts of amniotic fluid embolism: a review. Obstet Gynecol Surv 1990;45:360.

Clark SL. Successful pregnancy outcomes after amniotic fluid embolism. Am J Obstet Gynecol 1992;167:511.

Clark SL, Montz FJ, Phelan JP. Hemodynamic alterations in amniotic fluid embolism: a reappraisal. Am J Obstet Gynecol 1985;151:617.

Clark SL, Pavlova Z, Horenstein J, et al. Squamous cells in the maternal pulmonary circulation. Am J Obstet Gynecol 1986;154:104.

Clark SL, Cotton DB, Gonik B, et al. Central hemodynamic alterations in amniotic fluid embolism. Am J Obstet Gynecol 1988;158:1124.

Clark SL, Hankins GDV, Dudley DA, et al. Amniotic fluid embolism: analysis of a national registry. Am J Obstet Gynecol 1995;172:1158.

Courtney LD. Coagulation failure in pregnancy. Br Med J 1970;1:691.

Courtney LD, Allington LM. Effect of amniotic fluid on blood coagulation. Br J Haematol 1972;113:911.

Covone AE, Johnson PM, Mutton D, et al. Trophoblast cells in peripheral blood from pregnant women. Lancet 1984;i:841.

Cromley MG, Taylor PJ, Cummings DC. Probable amniotic fluid embolism after first trimester pregnancy termination. J Reprod Med 1983;28:209.

Cron RS, Kilkenny GS, Wirthwein C, et al. Amniotic fluid embolism. Am J Obstet Gynecol 1952;64:1360.

De Swiet M. Maternal mortality: confidential enquiries into maternal deaths in the United Kingdom. Am J Obstet Gynecol 2000;182: 760.

Dutta D, Bhargava KC, Chakravarti RN, et al. Therapeutic studies in experimental amniotic fluid embolism in rabbits. Am J Obstet Gynecol 1970;106:1201.

Eastman NJ. Editorial comment. Obstet Gynecol Surv 1948;3:35.

Enjeti S, Bleecker ER, Smith PL, et al. Hemodynamic mechanisms in anaphylaxis. Circ Shock 1983;11:297.

Gilbert WM, Danielsen B. Amniotic fluid embolism: decreased mortality in a population-based study. Obstet Gynecol 1999;93:973.

Girard P, Mal H, Laine JR, et al. Left heart failure in amniotic fluid embolism. Anesthesiology 1986;64:262.

Gitin TA, Seidel T, Cera PJ, et al. Pulmonary microvascular fat: the significance? Crit Care Med 1993;21:664.

Grimes DA. The morbidity and mortality of pregnancy: still a risky business. Am J Obstet Gynecol 1994;170:1489.

Guidotti RJ, Grimes DA, Cates W. Fatal amniotic fluid embolism during legally induced abortion in the United States, 1972–1978. Am J Obstet Gynecol 1981;141:257.

Halmagyi DFJ, Starzecki B, Shearman RP. Experimental amniotic fluid embolism: mechanism and treatment. Am J Obstet Gynecol 1962;84:251.

Hankins GDV, Snyder RR, Clark SL, et al. Acute hemodynamic and respiratory effects of amniotic fluid embolism in the pregnant goat model. Am J Obstet Gynecol 1993;168:1113.

Hogberg U, Innala E, Sandstrom A. Maternal mortality in Sweden, 1980–1988. Obstet Gynecol 1994;84:240.

Hsieh YY, Chang CC, Li PC, Tsai HD, Tsai CH. Successful application of extracorporeal membrane oxygenation and intra-aortic balloon counterpulsation as lifesaving therapy for a patient with amniotic fluid embolism. Am J Obstet Gynecol 2000;183:496–497.

Jacques WE, Hampton JW, Bird RM, et al. Pulmonary hypertension and plasma thromboplastin antecedent deficiency in dogs. Arch Pathol 1960;69:248.

Kaneko Y, Ogihara T, Tajima H, Mochimaru F. Continuous hemodiafiltration for disseminated intravascular coagulation and shock due to amniotic fluid embolism: report of a dramatic response. Intern Med 2001;40:945–947.

Kapin MA, Ferguson JL. Hemodynamic and regional circulatory alterations in dog during anaphylactic challenge. Am J Physiol 1985;249:H430.

Katz VJ, Dotters DJ, Droegemueller W. Perimortem cesarean delivery. Obstet Gynecol 1986;68:571.

Kaunitz AM, Hughes JM, Grimes DA. Causes of maternal mortality in the United States. Obstet Gynecol 1985;65:605.

Kitzmiller JL, Lucas WE. Studies on a model of amniotic fluid embolism. Obstet Gynecol 1972;39:626.

Lee W, Ginsburg KA, Cotton DB, Kaufman RH. Squamous and trophoblastic cells in the maternal pulmonary circulation identified by invasive hemodynamic monitoring during the peripartum period. Am J Obstet Gynecol 1986;155:999.

Lee WP, Clark SL, Cotton DB, et al. Septic shock during pregnancy. Am J Obstet Gynecol 1988;159:410.

Liban E, Raz S. A clinicopathologic study of fourteen cases of amniotic fluid embolism. Am J Clin Pathol 1969;51:477.

Lockwood CJ, Bach R, Guha A, et al. Amniotic fluid contains tissue factor, a potent initiator of coagulation. Am J Obstet Gynecol 1991;165:1335.

MacMillan D. Experimental amniotic fluid embolism. J Obstet Gynaecol Br Comwlth 1968;75:8.

Meier PR, Bowes WA. Amniotic fluid embolus-like syndrome presenting in the second trimester of pregnancy. Obstet Gynecol 1983;61(Suppl):31.

Meyer JR. Embolia pulmonar amniocaseosa. Bras/Med 1926;2:301–303.

Morgan M. Amniotic fluid embolism. Anaesthesia 1979;34:29.

Parker CW. In: Clinical Immunology. Philadelphia: WB Saunders, 1980;1208.

Parrillo JE. Pathogenic mechanisms of septic shock. N Engl J Med 1993;328:1471.

Paul RH, Koh BS, Bernstein SG. Changes in fetal heart rate: uterine contraction patterns associated with eclampsia. Am J Obstet Gynecol 1978;130:165.

Petroianu GA, Altmannsberger SH, Maleck WH, et al. Meconium and amniotic fluid embolism: effects on coagulation in pregnant minipigs. Crit Care Med 1999;27:348.

Phillips LL, Davidson EC. Procoagulant properties of amniotic fluid. Am J Obstet Gynecol 1972;113:911.

Plauche WC. Amniotic fluid embolism. Am J Obstet Gynecol 1983;147:982.

Porter TF, Clark SL, Dildy GA, Hankins GDV. Isolated disseminated intravascular coagulation and amniotic fluid embolism. Society of Perinatal Obstetricians 16th Annual Meeting, Poster Presentation, Kona, Hawaii, January 1996.

Raper RF, Fisher MM. Profound reversible myocardial depression after anaphylaxis. Lancet 1988;i:386.

Ratnoff OD, Vosbugh GJ. Observations of the clotting defect in amniotic fluid embolism. N Engl J Med 1952;247:970.

Reeves JT, Daoud FS, Estridge M, et al. Pulmonary pressor effects of small amounts of bovine amniotic fluid. Respir Physiol 1974;20:231.

Reis RL, Pierce WS, Behrendt DM. Hemodynamic effects of amniotic fluid embolism. Surg Gynecol Obstet 1965;129:45.

Resnik R, Swartz WH, Plumer MH, Benirschke K, Stratthaus ME. Amniotic fluid embolism with survival. Obstet Gynecol 1976; 47:295–298.

Richards DS, Carter LS, Corke B, et al. The effect of human amniotic fluid on the isolated perfused rat heart. Am J Obstet Gynecol 1988;158:210.

Schneider CL. Coagulation defects in obstetric shock: meconium embolism and defibrination. Am J Obstet Gynecol 1955;69:748.

Shechtman M, Ziser A, Markovits R, Rozenberg B. Amniotic fluid embolism: early findings of transesophageal echocardiography. Anesth Analg 1999;89:1456.

Silverman HJ, Van Hook C, Haponik EF. Hemodynamic changes in human anaphylaxis. Am J Med 1984;77:341.

Smedegard G, Revenas B, Lundberg C, Arfors KE. Anaphylactic shock in monkeys passively sensitized with human reaginic serum. I. Hemodynamics and cardiac performances. Acta Physiol Scand 1981;111:239.

Smith PL, Kagey-Sobotka A, Bleecker ER, et al. Physiologic manifestations of human anaphylaxis. J Clin Invest 1980;66:1072.

Sparr RA, Pritchard JA. Studies to detect the escape of amniotic fluid into the maternal circulation during parturition. Surg Gynecol Obstet 1958;107:550.

Spence MR, Mason KG. Experimental amniotic fluid embolism in rabbits. Am J Obstet Gynecol 1974;119:1073.

Steiner PE, Luschbaugh CC. Maternal pulmonary embolism by amniotic fluid. JAMA 1941;117:1245.

Stiller RJ, Siddiqui D, Laifer SA, Tiakowski RL, Whetham JC. Successful pregnancy after suspected anaphylactoid syndrome of pregnancy (amniotic fluid embolus). A case report. J Reprod Med 2000;45:1007.

Stolte L, van Kessel H, Seelen J, et al. Failure to produce the syndrome of amniotic fluid embolism by infusion of amniotic fluid and meconium into monkeys. Am J Obstet Gynecol 1967;98:694.

Thomson WB, Budd JW. Erroneous diagnosis of amniotic fluid embolism. Am J Obstet Gynecol 1963;91:606.

Towell ME. Fetal acid–base physiology and intrauterine asphyxia. In: Goodwin JW, Godden JO, Chance GW, eds. Perinatal Medicine. Baltimore: Williams and Wilkins, 1976:200.

Tuffnell DJ, Johnson H. Amniotic fluid embolism: the UK register. Hosp Med 2000;61:532–534.

Wong S, Dykewicz MS, Patterson R. Idiopathic anaphylaxis: a clinical summary of 175 patients. Arch Intern Med 1990;150:1323.

35 Systemic lupus erythematosus and the antiphospholipid syndrome

T. Flint Porter
D. Ware Branch

Systemic lupus erythematosus (SLE) is a chronic inflammatory condition affecting virtually every organ system of the body. With an increased prevalence among women of reproductive age, it is the autoimmune disease most commonly encountered during pregnancy. The majority of women with stable uncomplicated SLE tolerate pregnancy well, with relatively few serious obstetric complications. However, women with uncontrolled disease and/or serious SLE-related comorbidities are at substantial risk for serious morbidity and even mortality, as well as several adverse obstetric outcomes. Antiphospholipid syndrome (APS) is another autoimmune disorder that may lead to serious maternal and perinatal morbidity. Though anticoagulation prophylaxis in pregnancy may reduce the risk of thromboembolism and fetal death, the incidence of preeclampsia, uteroplacental insufficiency, and preterm birth remain high.

Pregnancy appears to influence the expression SLE and APS and disease activity may be related to alterations in estrogen and progesterone levels (Doria et al., 2002). Occasionally, life-threatening catastrophic exacerbations may occur. Management of both SLE and APS during pregnancy requires vigilance for signs and symptoms of disease exacerbation, aggressive immunosuppressive treatment when needed, and careful assessment of fetal well-being. For these reasons, obstetricians should be familiar with SLE and APS, how they influence and are influenced by pregnancy, and what special medical risks may be in store for mother and the fetus.

Systemic lupus erythematosus in pregnancy

Epidemiology

The prevalence of SLE varies depending on the population under study but is generally 5–125 per 100,000 and affects women 5–10 times more often than men (Ruiz-Irastorza et al., 2001). While no specific gene mutation for SLE has been identified, 5–12% of affected individuals have another relative with SLE (Arnett et al., 1984; Lawrence et al., 1987) and 25–50% of affected monozygotic twins are concordant for the disease (Block et al., 1975; Deapen et al., 1986). Several alterations in the human leukocyte antigen (HLA) system have been linked to the development of SLE, including those involving HLA-B8, HLA-DR3, and HLA-DR2 (Howard et al., 1986; Welch et al., 1988; Hartung et al., 1989; Eroglu & Kohler, 2002). Homozygous carriers of inherited complement deficiency disorders also appear to be predisposed to SLE (Glass et al., 1976; Howard et al., 1986).

SLE exacerbation (flare) during pregnancy

There is considerable debate regarding the incidence and severity of SLE flare during pregnancy. All studies on the subject have been hampered by the fact that many of the signs and symptoms typically associated with SLE flare are often considered routine during pregnancy. Some investigators have reported higher rates of SLE flare in pregnant women compared to nonpregnant controls, even when disease is inactive at the time of conception (Petri et al., 1991; Wong et al., 1991; Ruiz-Irastorza et al., 1996; Petri, 1997; Johns et al., 1998; Kleinman et al., 1998). In contrast, Lockshin et al. (1984) reported SLE flare in fewer than 25% of untreated pregnant and nonpregnant women, all of whom had well-controlled SLE. Mintz et al. (1986) reported similar results in women who received prophylactic treatment with 10 mg of prednisone daily. Other trials have also reported no difference in the rate of SLE flare during pregnancy though SLE flare occurred at higher rates in both pregnant women (35–65%) and in nonpregnant controls (35–60%) (Urowitz et al., 1993; Derksen et al., 1994; Le Huong et al., 1997; Aggarwal et al., 1999; Georgiou et al., 2000). Importantly, in almost all studies of pregnant women with SLE, most flares have been mild to moderate in nature and easily treated with glucocorticoids (Lockshin et al., 1984; Mintz et al., 1986; Urowitz et al., 1993; Ruiz-Irastoraz et al., 1996; Huong et al., 1997; Aggarwal et al., 1999; Georgiou et al., 2000).

Women at greatest risk for SLE flare during pregnancy and obstetric complications are undoubtedly those with preexisting lupus nephritis (LN) (Johns et al., 1998). Approximately half of all SLE patients eventually develop LN as a result of immune complex deposition in the kidney, with subsequent complement activation and inflammatory tissue damage. Patients typically present with proteinuria, hematuria, aseptic pyuria, and urinary sediment. Renal biopsy is necessary to confirm the diagnosis and is important for determining the prognosis and providing appropriate treatment. Histologically, LN can be grouped into four basic histologic and clinical categories.

1 *Diffuse proliferative glomerulonephritis* is most common (40%) and most severe with a 10-year survival around 60%. Patients typically present with hypertension, moderate to heavy proteinuria and nephrotic syndrome, hematuria, pyuria, casts, hypocomplementemia, and circulating immune complexes.
2 *Focal proliferative glomerulonephritis* is usually associated with mild hypertension and proteinuria and serious renal insufficiency is uncommon.
3 *Membranous glomerulonephritis* typically presents with moderate to heavy proteinuria, but lacks the active urinary sediment and does not cause renal insufficiency.
4 *Mesangial nephritis* is the least severe lesion clinically and carries the best long-term prognosis.

Women with LN are at increased risk for maternal and fetal morbidity and mortality. Those with preexisting proteinuria are likely to have worsening proteinuria during gestation as physiologic changes in renal blood flow occur. Pregnancy may predispose to deterioration of renal function, especially for women with active nephritis and/or renal insufficiency (Hayslett & Lynn, 1980; Bobrie et al., 1987). However, based on the experience in the most recent, large series of women with LN during pregnancy, the course of renal disease in most pregnant women with mild LN may not be so serious (Devoe & Taylor, 1979; Hayslett & Lynn, 1980; Fine et al., 1981; Jungers et al., 1982; Imbasciati et al., 1984; Bobrie et al., 1987; Julkunen et al., 1993a; Huong et al., 2001). About one-third of women with LN experience flare during pregnancy, fewer than 25% have worsening renal function, and only 10% of have permanent deterioration. The incidence of maternal death attributed to renal failure during pregnancy is less than 2%.

Disease activity at the onset of pregnancy has been assessed in several studies and in all the rate of SLE flare is lower among women with SLE in remission prior to conception. Renal deterioration is also less severe in women with inactive LN in the 6 months prior to conception (Hayslett & Lynn, 1980; Bobrie et al., 1987; Johns et al., 1998; Georgiou et al., 2000). In two recent series, embryonic and fetal losses were less common in women with well-controlled disease at conception (Johns et al., 1998; Georgiou et al., 2000). In another report, women with planned pregnancies after disease remission appeared to have outcomes similar to those of the general population (Le Huong et al., 1997). Thus, it seems reasonable to recommend that SLE patients achieve remission before considering pregnancy.

Obstetric complications in women with SLE

Women with SLE are at risk for several obstetric complications including preeclampsia, uteroplacental insufficiency, preterm delivery, and pregnancy loss. The risk of these complications is magnified for women who also have secondary APS (Lockshin et al., 1987; Ramsey-Goldman et al., 1993). Between 20 and 30% of women with SLE have pregnancies complicated by preeclampsia (Hayslett & Lynn, 1980; Kleinman et al., 1998). Important predisposing factors appear to be secondary APS, underlying renal disease, chronic hypertension, and chronic steroid use (Hayslett & Lynn, 1980; Fine et al., 1981; Oviasu et al., 1991; Packham et al., 1992; Julkunen et al., 1993; Ramsey-Goldman et al., 1993; Kleinman et al., 1998). Uteroplacental insufficiency resulting in intrauterine growth restriction (IUGR) or small-for-gestational-age neonates has been reported in 12–40% of pregnancies complicated by SLE (Packham et al., 1992; Ruiz-Irastorza et al., 1996; Johns et al., 1998; Aggarwal et al., 1999; Yasmeen, 2001). The risk of uteroplacental insufficiency is highest for women with renal insufficiency and/or hypertension (Julkunen et al., 1993; Rahman et al., 1998). Most series have also reported that preterm birth is more common among women with SLE (Johns et al., 1998; Kleinman et al., 1998; Aggarwal et al., 1999; Yasmeen, 2001). In multiparous women, the rate is higher after the diagnosis of SLE is made (24% vs. 6%) (Petri, 1993). Much of the preterm birth occurring in pregnancies complicated by SLE can probably be attributed to iatrogenic delivery secondary to maternal or fetal complications. However, one group reported preterm rupture of membranes in 39% of pregnancies complicated by SLE.

Pregnancy loss is thought to be more prevalent among women with SLE, with rates ranging from 10 to 50% (Mintz et al., 1986; Wong et al., 1991; Le Thi Huong et al., 1994; Rahman et al., 1998). However, few studies have distinguished between first-trimester miscarriage and later fetal death. In one series, 20% of losses occurred during the second or third trimester. Disease activity increases the likelihood of pregnancy loss (Johns et al., 1998) with one study reporting live births in 64% of women with active disease within 6 months of conception, compared to 88% in women with quiescent disease (Hayslett & Lynn, 1980). Accordingly, pregnancy loss is more likely if SLE is diagnosed during the index pregnancy (Jungers et al., 1982; Imbasciati et al., 1984). Renal insufficiency is also important; one group reported fetal loss in 50% of pregnancies complicated by moderate to severe renal insufficiency as defined by serum creatinine >1.5 mg/dL (Hayslett & Lynn, 1980) and in 40% with preexisting proteinuria as defined by >300 mg/24 hours or a creatinine clearance <100 mL/min (Fine et al., 1981). Not surprisingly, the most important risk factor for pregnancy loss in women with SLE is coexisting APS. In one series of pregnant women with SLE, the presence of antiphospholipid antibodies had a positive predictive value for pregnancy loss of 50% (Englert et al., 1988). In another, positive predictive value increased to over 85% if women with SLE also had a fetal death in a prior pregnancy (Ramsey-Goldman et al., 1993).

Neonatal lupus erythematosus

Neonatal lupus erythematosus (NLE) is a rare condition of the fetus and neonate, occurring in 1 of 20,000 of all live births and in fewer than 5% of all women with SLE (Lockshin et al., 1988). Dermatologic NLE is most common and is described as erythematous, scaling annular or elliptical plaques occurring on the face or scalp, analogous to the subacute cutaneous lesions in adults. Lesions appear in the first weeks of life, probably induced by exposure of the skin to ultraviolet light, and may last for up to 6 months (Neiman et al., 2000). Hypopigmentation may persist for up to 2 years. A small percentage of affected infants will go on to have other autoimmune diseases later in life (Neiman et al., 2000). Hematologic NLE is rare and may be manifest as autoimmune hemolytic anemia, leukopenia, thrombocytopenia, and hepatosplenomegaly.

Cardiac NLE lesions include congenital complete heart block (CCHB) and the less frequently reported endocardial fibroelastosis. Endomyocardial fibrosis caused by NLE leads to interruption of the conduction system, especially in the area of the atrioventricular node. The diagnosis is typically made around 23 weeks of gestation (Buyon et al., 1998) when a fixed bradycardia, in the range of 60–80 bpm is detected during a routine prenatal visit. Fetal echocardiography reveals complete atrioventricular dissociation with a structurally normal heart. The prognosis varies, but in the most severe cases hydrops fetalis develops in utero. Because the endomyocardial damage is permanent, a pacemaker may be necessary for neonatal survival. In the largest series of 113 cases diagnosed before birth, 19% died, of which 73% died within 3 months of delivery (Buyon et al., 1998). In that same series, the 3-year survival was 79%. Cutaneous manifestations of NLE have also been reported in infants with CCHB (Neiman et al., 2000).

Not all women who give birth to babies with NLE have been previously diagnosed with an autoimmune disorder (Laurence et al., 2000; Neiman et al., 2000). However, in one study, seven of 13 previously asymptomatic mothers who delivered infants with dermatologic NLE were later diagnosed with one of several autoimmune disorders (Neiman et al., 2000). Surprisingly, asymptomatic women who deliver infants with CCHB are less likely to later develop an autoimmune disorder than those with dermatologic manifestations alone (Lawrence et al., 2000).

Fetal immunologic damage is probably caused by maternal autoantibodies that cross the placenta and bind to fetal tissue (Scott et al., 1983; Taylor et al., 1986; Lee et al., 1989; Buyon et al., 1993; McCauliffe, 1995). Anti-Ro/SSA antibodies are found in 75–95% mothers who deliver babies with NLE (Buyon et al., 1993, 1998; Lee et al., 1994). A smaller percentage has anti-La/SSB, and some have both (Lee et al., 1994). Dermatologic NLE has also been associated with anti-U1RNP without anti-Ro/SSA or anti-La/SSB (Provost et al., 1987; Lee et al., 1994). Of mothers with SLE who are serologically positive for anti-Ro/SSA antibodies, 15% will have infants affected with dermatologic SLE; the proportion who deliver infants with CCHB is much smaller. However, once a women with SLE and anti-Ro/SSA antibodies delivers one infant with CCHB, her risk for recurrence is at least twofold to threefold higher than other women with anti-SSA/Ro-SSB/La antibodies who have never had an affected child (Buyon et al., 1998).

There is no known in utero therapy which completely reverses fetal CCHB secondary to SLE. However, there is some evidence that treatment with glucocorticoids, plasmapheresis, intravenous immune globulin, or some combination thereof may slow the progression of prenatally diagnosed CCHB or at least prevent recurrence in a future pregnancy (Kaaja et al., 1991). In utero treatment with dexamethasone was felt to slow disease progression in one case report of hydrops secondary to CCHB (Carreira et al., 1993). In one retrospective study, maternally administered dexamethasone appeared to prevent progression from second-degree block to third-degree block (Saleeb et al., 1999). In a large series of 87 pregnancies at risk for NLE, mothers who received corticosteroids before 16 weeks of gestation were less likely to deliver infants with CCHB compared to mothers who received no therapy. However, there was no benefit to treatment when CCHB was diagnosed in utero. In utero treatment with digoxin is not beneficial for prenatally diagnosed CCHB (Eronen et al., 2001).

Diagnosis of SLE and detection of SLE exacerbation (flare)

Thorough and frequent clinical assessment remains essential for the timely and accurate detection of SLE flare. In pregnancy, detection is more difficult because many of the typical signs and symptoms associated with flare are considered normal. The most common presenting symptom in both flare and new-onset disease is extreme fatigue (Table 35.1). Fever, weight loss, myalgia, and arthralgia are also very common. In pregnancy, skin rashes are more frequent than musculoskeletal manifestations (Petri et al., 1996). Patients with LN exhibit worsening proteinuria along with pyuria, hematuria, and urinary casts. Not surprisingly, SLE flare in pregnant women with LN is easily confused with the development of preeclampsia–eclampsia syndromes.

Serologic evaluation of SLE disease activity may be beneficial in confirming flare in confusing cases. However, no study has found serial laboratory testing superior to thorough clinical assessment. Most specific are elevations in anti-double-stranded DNA (anti-dsDNA) titers, which precede lupus flare in more than 80% of patients (ter Borg et al., 1990; Bootsma et al., 1995). In pregnancy, elevated anti-dsDNA titers have also been shown to correlate with the need for preterm delivery (Tomer et al., 1996). In combination with anticardio-

Table 35.1 Approximate frequency of clinical symptoms in SLE

Symptoms	Patients (%)
Fatigue	80–100
Fever	80–100
Arthralgia, arthritis	95
Myalgia	70
Weight loss	>60
Skin	
Butterfly rash	50
Photosensitivity	60
Mucous membrane lesions	35
Renal involvement	50
Pulmonary	
Pleurisy	50
Effusion	25
Pneumonitis	5–10
Cardiac (pericarditis)	10–50
Lymphadenopathy	50
CNS	
Seizures	15–20
Psychosis	<25

Table 35.2 Suggested methods for tapering prednisone

1 Consolidate to a single morning dose of prednisone. Reduce the daily dose by 10% per week, as tolerated. When a dose of 20–30 mg/day is reached, reduce by 2.5-mg increments per week. If the patient remains asymptomatic at a dose of 15 mg/day, reduce the dose by 1-mg increments per week to a dose of 5–10 mg/day

2 Consolidate to a single morning dose of prednisone. Taper to 50–60 mg/day by reducing the dose 10% per week. Thereafter eliminate the alternate-day dose by tapering it 10% per week, as tolerated. Thereafter, taper the remaining every-other-day dose by 10% per week, as tolerated

lipin antibodies, elevated levels of anti-dsDNA are associated with an increased risk of fetal loss.

Serial evaluation of complement levels has also been suggested as method of predicting SLE flare during pregnancy. Devoe and Loy (1984) reported that SLE flare was signaled by a decline of C3 and C4 into the subnormal range and Buyon et al. (1986) reported that the physiologic rise in C3 and C4 levels normally seen during pregnancy did not occur in women with active disease. The same group reported that activation of the alternative complement pathway accompanies flare during pregnancy (Buyon et al., 1992) and that a combination of low C3, C4, or CH50 levels accompanied by an elevation in complement split products is useful in detecting flare during pregnancy (Buyon et al., 1992). The results of other studies of complement activation in pregnant women with SLE have been either inconsistent or not predictive of SLE flare (Adelsberg, 1983; Wong et al., 1991; Abramson & Buyon, 1992). Lockshin et al. (1986) reported normal concentrations of the C1s–C1 inhibitor complex in pregnant patients with hypocomplementemia, which suggests poor synthesis of complement components rather than excessive consumption.

Laboratory confirmation of SLE flare is probably most helpful in women with active LN in whom proteinuria, hypertension, and evidence of multiorgan dysfunction may easily be confused with preeclampsia. Both elevated anti-dsDNA titers and urinary sediment with cellular casts and hematuria weigh in favor of active LN. Preeclampsia is more likely in women with decreased levels of antithrombin III (Weiner & Brandt, 1982; Weiner et al., 1985). Complement concentrations are not helpful because activation may also occur in women with preeclampsia (Mellembakken et al., 2001). In the most severe and confusing cases, the diagnosis can be confirmed only with renal biopsy. However, in reality, concerns about maternal and fetal well-being often prompt delivery, rendering the distinction between SLE flare and preeclampsia clinically moot.

Medications used for SLE during pregnancy

Glucocorticoids

The group of drugs most commonly given to pregnant women with SLE is the glucocorticoid preparations, both as maintenance therapy and in "bursts" to treat suspected SLE flares. The doses used in pregnancy are the same as those used in nonpregnant patients (see Table 35.2). Pregnancy per se is not an indication to reduce the dose of glucocorticoids, though a carefully monitored reduction in dosage may be reasonable in appropriately selected women whose disease appears to be in remission. Some groups have recommended prophylactic glucocorticoid therapy during pregnancy (Mintz et al., 1986; Tincani et al., 1992; Le Huong et al., 1997) but no controlled studies have shown this practice to be prudent or necessary in women with inactive SLE. Moreover, good maternal and fetal outcomes are achieved without prophylactic treatment of women with stable disease (Derksen et al., 1994). In contrast, glucocorticoid treatment of women with active disease and/or elevated anti-dsDNA titers has been shown to result in fewer relapses and better pregnancy outcomes (Bootsma et al., 1995; Georgiou et al., 2000).

While glucocorticoids have a low potential for teratogenesis (Brooks & Needs, 1990), they are not without risk during pregnancy. Patients requiring chronic maintenance therapy are best treated with prednisolone or methylprednisolone because of their conversion to relatively inactive forms by the abundance of 11βol dehydrogenase found in the human placenta. Glucocorticoids with fluorine at the 9α position (dexamethasone, betamethasone) are considerably less well metabolized by the placenta and chronic use during pregnancy should be avoided. Both have been associated with untoward fetal effects (NIH statement). Maternal side effects of chronic glucocorticoid therapy are the same as in nonpregnant patients and include weight gain, striae, acne, hirsutism, immunosuppression, osteonecrosis, and gastrointestinal ulceration. During pregnancy, chronic glucocorticoid therapy has also been associated with an increased risk of preeclampsia (Lockshin et al., 1987; Laskin et al., 1997; Vaquero et al., 2001), uteroplacental insufficiency (Rayburn, 1998), and glucose intolerance (Laskin et al., 1997; Vaquero et al., 2001). Women chronically treated with glucocorticoids should be screened for gestational diabetes at 22–24, 28–30, and 32–34 weeks of gestation.

Antimalarials

An accumulating body of evidence suggests that antimalarial drugs, such as hydroxychloroquine, may be used safely for the treatment of SLE during pregnancy (Buchanan et al., 1996; Khamashta et al., 1996; Klinger et al., 2001; Motta et al., 2002). In the past, many patients and their physicians have discontinued antimalarials during pregnancy because of concerns about teratogenicity including ototoxicity (Hart & Naughton, 1964) and eye damage (Nylander, 1967). The latter was of particular concern because of the affinity of these drugs for melanin-containing tissues such as the eye. However, antimalarials have been used safely in women considered at risk for malaria for years without any reported adverse fetal effects. This experience has been confirmed in recent large series showing hydroxychloroquine to be safe during pregnancy (Buchanan et al., 1996; Khamashta et al., 1996; Klinger et al., 2001; Motta et al., 2002). Furthermore, antimalarials may be more beneficial than glucocorticoids for women who need maintenance therapy during pregnancy. In a recent randomized controlled trial, women who continued hydroxychloroquine during pregnancy experienced a significant reduction in SLE disease activity compared to women who changed to glucocorticoid therapy (Levy et al., 2001).

Cytotoxic agents

Cytotoxic agents, including azathioprine, methotrexate, and cyclophosphamide, are used to treat only the most severely affected patients with SLE. Limited data suggest that azathioprine, a derivative of 6-mercaptopurine, is not a teratogen in humans but has been associated with fetal growth impairment (Armenti et al., 1994, 1998) and impaired neonatal immunity (Cote et al., 1974). Women who require azathioprine to control SLE disease activity should not necessarily be discouraged from becoming pregnant, though the benefits of treatment should clearly outweigh the risks of medication. Cyclophosphamide is reportedly teratogenic in both animals (Ujhazy et al., 1993) and humans (Kirshon et al., 1998; Enns et al., 1999) and should be avoided during the first trimester. Thereafter, cyclophosphamide should be used only in unusual circumstances such as in women with severe, progressive, proliferative glomerulonephritis (Ruiz-Irastorza et al., 2001). Methotrexate is well known for killing chorionic villi and causing fetal death and its use should be scrupulously avoided.

Nonsteroidal anti-inflammatory drugs

The most common types of analgesics used in the treatment of SLE are nonsteroidal anti-inflammatory drugs (NSAIDs). Unfortunately, their use in pregnancy should be avoided after the first trimester because they readily cross the placenta and block prostaglandin synthesis in a wide variety of fetal tissues. Maternal ingestion of normal adult doses of aspirin in the week prior to delivery has been associated with intracranial hemorrhage in preterm neonates (Rumack et al., 1981; Stuart et al., 1982). Though short-term tocolytic therapy with indomethacin appears to be safe (Macones & Robinson, 1997; Vermillion & Newman, 1999), chronic use has been associated with a number of untoward fetal effects and, when used after 32 weeks, may result in constriction or closure of the fetal ductus arteriosus (Pryde et al., 2001). Long-term use of all NSAIDs has been associated with decreased fetal urinary output and oligohydramnios as well as neonatal renal insufficiency (Ostensen & Villiger, 2001). Given these risks, chronic use of adult dosages of aspirin and other NSAIDs should be avoided during pregnancy. Acetaminophen and narcotic-containing preparations are acceptable alternatives if analgesia is needed during pregnancy.

Other treatments

Several new treatment regimens, including cyclosporin, high-dose intravenous immune globulin (IVIG), mycophenolate mofetil, and thalidomide, have been studied in the treatment of nonpregnant patients with SLE (Ruiz-Irastorza et al., 2001). Only IVIG has been used during pregnancy without reports of adverse fetal effects. Obviously, thalidomide is strictly contraindicated during pregnancy because of its known potent teratogenicity. Complete immunoablative therapy followed by bone marrow stem cell transplantation has also been studied in patients with the most severe unresponsive SLE (Ruiz-Irastorza et al., 2001).

Treatment of SLE flare during pregnancy

Mild-to-moderate symptomatic exacerbations of SLE without CNS or renal involvement may be treated with initiation of glucocorticoids or an increase in the dose of glucocorticoids. Relatively small doses of prednisone (e.g. 15–30 mg/day) will result in improvement in most cases. For severe exacerbations without CNS or renal involvement, doses of 1.0–1.5 mg/kg/day of prednisone in divided doses should be used, and a good clinical response can be expected in 5–

10 days. Thereafter, glucocorticoids may be tapered by several different approaches (Table 35.2).

Severe exacerbations, expecially those involving the CNS or kidneys, are treated more aggressively. In recent years, intravenous pulse glucocorticoid therapy has become popular. The initial regimen involves a daily intravenous dose of methylprednisolone at 10–30 mg/kg (about 500–1,000 mg) for 3–6 days. Thereafter, the patients is treated with 1.0–1.5 mg/kg/day of prednisone in divided doses and rapidly tapered over the course of 1 month. One can expect that 75% of patients will respond favorably to this approach. This regimen may be repeated every 1–3 months in severe cases as an alternative to cytotoxic drugs.

In nonpregnant patients, both azathioprine and cyclophosphamide may be used in severe SLE exacerbations to control disease, reduce irreversible tissue damage, and reduce glucocorticoid doses (Sesso et al., 1994; Austin & Balow, 2000; Nossent & Koldingsnes, 2000). In particular, severe proliferative LN may be treated more effectively with cyclophosphamide, usually in combination with glucocorticoids (Austin & Balow, 2000). The drug may be given either orally or intravenously, but the most effective cyclophosphamide regimen is uncertain. Cyclophosphamide appears to be useful in the treatment of severe cerebral lupus as well. Azathioprine is perhaps less effective than cyclophosphamide, though it is also less toxic.

Plasmapheresis and IVIG have been used for treatment of severe cases of SLE flare unresponsive to standard treatments. Plasmapheresis should be considered in life-threatening disease that is unresponsive to other treatments. A cytotoxic agent should also be administered soon after plasmapheresis is initiated (days 5 through 10 of therapy) if the patients is no longer pregnant. IVIG has been used for "salvage" treatment of recalcitrant SLE flare with neuropsychiatric or renal involvement (Rauova et al., 2001).

Antiphospholipid syndrome in pregnancy

The diagnosis of APS is based on the presence of one or more characteristic thrombotic or obstetric features of the condition; laboratory testing for antiphospholipid antibodies (aPL) is ued to confirm or refute the diagnosis. The 1999 International Consensus Statement provides simplified criteria for the diagnosis of APS (Wilson et al., 1999). Patients with bona fide APS must manifest at least one of two clinical criteria (vascular thrombosis or pregnancy morbidity) and at least one of two laboratory criteria, namely positive lupus anticoagulant (LAC) or medium-to-high titers of β_2-glycoprotein I-dependent IgG or IgM isotype anticardiolipin (aCL) antibodies, confirmed on two separate occasions, at least 6 weeks apart. Thrombosis may be either arterial or venous and must be confirmed by an imaging or Doppler study or by histopathology. Pregnancy morbidity is divided into three categories: (i) otherwise unexplained fetal death (10 weeks' gestation); (ii) preterm birth (34 weeks' gestation) for severe preeclampsia or placental insufficiency; or (iii) otherwise unexplained recurrent preembryonic or embryonic pregnancy loss. Autoimmune thrombocytopenia and amaurosis fugax are often associated with APS but are not considered sufficient diagnostic criteria. APS may exist as an isolated immunologic derangement (primary APS) or in combination with other autoimmune diseases (secondary APS), most commonly SLE.

Pathogenesis of APS

The mechanism(s) by which aPL cause thrombosis most likely involves interference with normal hemostasis by interaction with phospholipids or phospholipid-binding protein components such as β_2-glycoprotein-GPI (which has anticoagulant properties), prostacyclin, prothrombin, protein C, annexin V, and tissue factor (Levine et al., 2002). Antiphospholipid antibodies also appear to activate endothelial cells, indicated by increased expression of adhesion molecules, secretion of cytokines, and production of arachidonic acid metabolites (Meroni et al., 2000). The findings that some aCL cross-react with oxidized low-density lipoprotein (Vaarala et al., 1993) and that human aCL bind to oxidized, but not reduced, cardiolipin (Hörkkö et al., 1996) imply that aPL may participate in oxidant-mediated injury of the vascular endothelium. However, aPL do bind perturbed cells, such as activated platelets (Shi et al., 1993) or apoptotic cells (Price et al., 1996), which typically lose normal membrane symmetry and express anionic phospholipids on their surface.

Whether aPL per se are the cause of adverse obstetric outcomes is also a matter of debate. Investigators working with murine models have found that passive transfer of aPL results in clinical manifestations of APS, including fetal loss and thrombocytopenia (Blank et al., 1991; Chamley et al., 1994). One group has used a murine pinch-induced venous thrombosis model to demonstrate that human polyclonal and murine monoclonal aPL are associated with larger and more persistent thrombi compared to mice treated with control antibodies. Recent work points to the complement system as having a major role in APS-related pregnancy loss, showing that C3 activation is required for fetal loss in a murine model (Holers et al., 2002). In humans, APS-related pregnancy complications are probably related to abnormal placental function. Some authorities have focused on abnormalities in the decidual spiral arteries as the immediate cause of fetal loss in APS pregnancies. Some investigators have found narrowing of the spiral arterioles, intimal thickening, acute atherosis, and fibrinoid necrosis (De Wolf et al., 1982; Erlendsson et al., 1993; Rand et al., 1997). In addition, placental histopathology demonstrates extensive necrosis, infarction, and thrombosis (De Wolf et al., 1982). These abnormalities might result from thrombosis during the development of normal materno-placental circulation via interference with trophoblastic annexin V (Rand et al.,

1997) or by impairing trophoblastic hormone production or invasion (di Somone et al., 2000).

Clinical features of APS during pregnancy

In the original description of APS, the sole obstetric criterion for diagnosis was fetal loss (>10 menstrual weeks of gestation) (Harris, 1987; Asherson et al., 1989). At least 40% of pregnancy losses reported by women with LAC or medium-to-high positive IgG aCL occur in the fetal period (Branch, 1987; Branch et al., 1992; Pattison et al., 1993; Oshiro et al., 1996). More recently, APS-related pregnancy loss has been extended to include women with early recurrent pregnancy loss (RPL), including those occurring in the preembryonic (<6 menstrual weeks of gestation) and embryonic (6–9 menstrual weeks of gestation) periods (Wilson et al., 1999). In serologic evaluation of women with RPL, 10–20% have detectable aPL (Clifford et al., 1994; Kutteh, 1996; Yetman & Kutteh, 1996; Branch et al., 1997; Rai et al., 1997; Pattison et al., 2000). Women with APS followed prospectively also have demonstrated high rates of premature delivery for gestational hypertension or preeclampsia and uteroplacental insufficiency as manifested by fetal growth restriction, oligohydramnios, and nonreassuring fetal surveillance (Branch et al., 1992; Lima et al., 1996; Huong et al., 2001). Obstetric complications other than pregnancy loss appear to persist in spite of treatment.

Fetal death and early RPL are seen by some as two points along the same continuum of APS-related pregnancy loss. However, women with APS identified because of a prior fetal death and/or thromboembolism seem to have more serious complications in subsequent pregnancies than those with early RPL (Branch, 1998). Recent prospective treatment trials of APS during pregnancy have been comprised mainly of women with early RPL and no other APS-related medical problems (Cowchock et al., 1992; Silver et al., 1993; Kutteh, 1996; Granger & Farquharson, 1997; Rai et al., 1997; Pattison et al., 2000). Accordingly, the rates of obstetric complications were relatively low with fetal death, preeclampsia, and preterm birth, occurring in 4.5% (0–15%), 10.5% (0–15%), and 10.5% (5–40%), respectively. Only 1 of 300 women suffered a thrombotic event and no neonatal deaths due to complications of prematurity were reported. Based on these data, it seems unlikely that early RPL, fetal death, and preterm birth resulting from severe preeclampsia or placental insufficiency are a result of the same pathophysiologic mechanism. Certainly, hypercoagulability causing defective uteroplacental circulation resulting in diminished intervillous blood flow might be responsible for later pregnancy complications. Women with early RPL probably represent a different patient population with pregnancy losses due to different mechanisms, perhaps relating to different aPL specificities or aPL operating on a fundamentally different pathophysiologic background.

Treatment of APS during pregnancy

The end-results of APS treatment during pregnancy should include (i) improvement in maternal and fetal–neonatal outcome by preventing pregnancy loss, preeclampsia, placental insufficiency, and preterm birth, and (ii) reduction or elimination of risk of thromboembolism. Early enthusiasm for treatment with glucocorticoids to reduce the risk of pregnancy loss waned after publication of a small randomized trial found maternally administered heparin to be as effective as prednisone (Cowchock et al., 1992). At present, maternally administered heparin is considered the treatment of choice, usually initiated in the early first trimester after ultrasonographic demonstration of a live embryo. In most case series and trials, daily low-dose aspirin is included in the treatment regimen (Cowchock et al., 1992; Silver et al., 1993; Kutteh, 1996; Granger & Farquharson, 1997; Rai et al., 1997; Pattison et al., 2000; Empson et al., 2002). In a recent meta-analysis of treatment trials (Empson et al., 2002), the live birth rate was improved by 54%.

The safe and effective dose of heparin for pregnant women with APS is debated but should probably depend on individual patient history. Women with APS and a history of thromboembolism should probably receive full anticoagulation with heparin during pregnancy because of their substantial risk of recurrent thromboembolism (Rosove & Brewer, 1992; Rivier et al., 1994; Khamashta et al., 1995). Most authorities recommend full, adjusted-dose anticoagulation (ACOG, 2000; Ginsberg et al., 2001). In contrast, women diagnosed with APS *without* a history of thromboembolic disease may have less risk of thromboembolism during pregnancy. Women with early RPL alone, without a history of thromboembolism, have been treated with both low-dose prophylaxis and adjusted-dose anticoagulation regimens (Empson et al., 2002). Live rates have exceeded 70% using either strategy (Cowchock et al., 1992; Kutteh, 1996). Women with a history of fetal death alone may be at higher risk for thromboembolism during pregnancy (Erkan et al., 2001) and should probably receive higher doses of heparin prophylaxis. It is our practice to treat such women with generous thromboprophylaxis (e.g. 15,000–20,000 units of standard heparin or 60 mg of enoxaparin in divided doses daily) (Branch et al., 1992; Cowchock et al., 1992; Welch, 1997).

Women with APS should be counseled about the potential risks of heparin therapy during pregnancy, including heparin-induced osteoporosis and heparin-induced thrombocytopenia (HIT). Osteoporosis resulting in fracture occurs in 1–2% of women treated during pregnancy (Dahlman, 1993). Women treated with heparin should be encouraged to take daily supplemental calcium and vitamin D (e.g. prenatal vitamins). It also seems prudent to encourage daily axial skeleton weight-bearing exercise (e.g. walking). Immune-mediated HIT is much less common but potentially more serious. Most cases have their onset 3–21 days after heparin initiation and are relatively mild in nature (Kelton, 2002). A more severe form of HIT paradoxically involves venous and arterial thromboses, resulting in limb ischemia, cerebrovascular accidents, and myocardial infarctions, as well as venous thromboses (Warkentin & Kelton, 2001). It may occur in up to 0.5% of patients treated with unfractionated sodium heparin (Kelton, 2002). Low-molecular-weight heparin is much less likely to be associated with HIT compared with unfractionated sodium heparin (Warkentin et al., 1995).

Other pregnancy complications associated with APS occur in spite of appropriate treatment (Branch et al., 1992; Backos et al., 1999). In a recent observational study of 107 pregnancies complicated by APS, preeclampsia occurred in 20%, preterm birth in 24%, and growth restriction in 15% of treated women (Backos et al., 1999).

Pregnancy losses continue to occur in 20–30% of cases even when heparin prophylaxis is given (Branch et al., 1992; Cowchock et al., 1992; Empson et al., 2002). Several alternative therapies have been tried in so-called refractory cases. Glucocorticoids, often in high doses, have sometimes been added to regimens of heparin and low-dose aspirin. While there are anecdotal reports of success, this practice has never been studied in appropriately designed trials and the combination of glucocorticoids and heparin may increase the risk of osteoporotic fracture. IVIG has also been used in pregnancies complicated by APS, especially in women with particularly poor past histories or recurrent pregnancy loss during heparin treatment (Wapner et al., 1989). However, a small, randomized, controlled, pilot study of IVIG treatment found no benefit to this expensive therapy compared to heparin and low-dose aspirin (Clark et al., 1999). Hydroxychloroquine has been shown to diminish the thrombogenic properties of aPL in a murine thrombosis model (Edwards et al., 1997). There are few case reports and no trials of APS patients being treated during pregnancy with hydroxychloroquine.

Healthy women with recurrent embryonic and preembryonic loss and low titers of aPL do not require treatment (Cowchock & Reece, 1997). The controlled trial of Pattison et al. (2000) included a majority of such women and found no difference in live birth rates using either low-dose aspirin or placebo.

Postpartum and catastrophic APS

Catastrophic APS is a rare but devastating syndrome characterized by multiple simultaneous vascular occlusions throughout the body, often resulting in death. The diagnosis should be suspected if at least three organ systems are affected and confirmed if there is histolopathologic evidence of acute thrombotic microangiopathy affecting small vessels. Renal involvement occurs in 78% of patients. Most have hypertension and 25% eventually require dialysis. Other common manifestations described by Asherson (1999) include adult respiratory distress syndrome (66%), cerebral microthrombi and microinfarctions (56%), myocardial microthrombi (50%), dermatologic abnormalities (50%), and disseminated intravascular coagulation (25%). Death from multiorgan failure occurs in 50% of patients (Asherson, 1999). The pathophysiology of catastrophic APS is poorly understood. However, the onset may be presaged by several factors including infection, surgical procedures, discontinuation of anticoagulant therapy, and use of drugs such as oral contraceptives (Asherson, 1999; Schaar et al., 1999; Camera et al., 2000).

Table 35.3 Proposed protocol for acute treatment of catastrophic APS

1 Intravenous heparin should be initiated and adjusted to achieve an activated partial thromboplastin time (aPTT) two to three times greater than the mean. Heparin levels may be necessary for women with the LAC because they demonstrate a prolonged aPTT without anticoagulation
2 Intravenous methylprednisolone should be initiated at a dosage of 10–30 mg/kg/day
3 Plasmapheresis should be initiated with the replacement of 40 mL of plasma per kilogram of body weight or up to 3 L per exchange. This should be repeated three times weekly for 2–6 weeks. The simultaneous administration of immunosuppressive agents may block potential rebound in production of autoantibodies

Early and aggressive treatment of catastrophic APS is necessary to avoid death. Patients should be transferred to an intensive care unit where supportive care can be provided. Hypertension should be aggressively treated with appropriate antihypertensive medication. While no treatment has been shown to be superior to another, a combination of anticoagulants (usually heparin) and steroids plus either plasmapheresis or IVIG has been successful in some patients (Asherson, 1999; Schaar et al., 1999) (Table 35.3). Streptokinase and urokinase have also been used to treat acute vascular thrombosis (Asherson, 1999). Women suspected of catastrophic APS during pregnancy should probably be delivered.

References

Abramson SB, Buyon JP. Activation of the complement pathway: comparison of normal pregnancy, preeclampsia, and systemic lupus erythematosus during pregnancy. Am J Reprod Immunol 1992;28:183–187.

ACOG. Thromboembolism in pregnancy. ACOG Practice Bulletin 19. Washington, DC: American College of Obstetricians and Gynecologists, 2000.

Adelsberg BR. The complement system in pregnancy. Am J Reprod Immunol 1983;4:38–44.

Aggarwal N, Sawhney H, Vasishta K, Chopra S, Bambery P. Pregnancy in patients with systemic lupus erythematosus. Aust N Z J Obstet Gynaecol 1999;39:28–30.

Armenti VT, Ahlswede KM, Ahlswede BA, et al. National transplantation pregnancy registry: outcomes of 154 pregnancies in cyclosporine-treated female kidney transplant recipients. Transplantation 1994;57:502–506.

Armenti VT, Moritz MJ, Davison JM. Drug safety issues in pregnancy following transplantation and immunosuppression: effects and outcomes. Drug Saf 1998;19:219–232.

Arnett FC, Reveille JD, Wilson RW, et al. Systemic lupus erythematosus: current state of the genetic hypothesis. Semin Arthritis Rheum 1984;14:24–35.

Asherson RA, Khamashta MA, Ordi-Ros J, et al. The "primary" antiphospholipid syndrome: major clinical and serological features. Medicine (Baltimore) 1989;68:366–374.

Austin HA, Balow JE. Treatment of lupus nephritis. Semin Nephrol 2000;20:265–276.

Backos M, Rai R, Baxter N, Chilcott IT, Cohen H, Regan L. Pregnancy complications in women with recurrent miscarriage associated with antiphospholipid antibodies treated with low dose aspirin and heparin. Br J Obstet Gynaecol 1999;106:102–107.

Blank M, Cohen J, Toder V, et al. Induction of anti-phospholipid syndrome in naive mice with mouse lupus monoclonal and human polyclonal anti-cardiolipin antibodies. Proc Natl Acad Sci USA 1991;88:3069–3073.

Block SR, Winfield JB, Lockshin MD, et al. Studies of twins with systemic lupus erythematosus. A review of the literature and presentation of 12 additional sets. Am J Med 1975;59:533–552.

Bobrie G, Liote F, Houillier P, Grunfeld JP, Jungers P. Pregnancy in lupus nephritis and related disorders. Am J Kidney Dis 1987;9:339–343.

Bootsma H, Spronk PE, Derksen R, et al. Prevention of relapses in systemic lupus erythematosus. Lancet 1995;345:1595–1599.

Branch DW. Immunologic disease and fetal death. Clin Obstet Gynecol 1987;30:295–311.

Branch DW. Antiphospholipid antibodies and reproductive outcome: the current state of affairs. J Reprod Immunol 1998;38:75–87.

Branch DW, Silver RM, Blackwell JL, et al. Outcome of treated pregnancies in women with antiphospholipid syndrome: an update of the Utah experience. Obstet Gynecol 1992;80:614–620.

Branch DW, Silver R, Pierangeli S, van Leeuwen I, Harris EN. Antiphospholipid antibodies other than lupus anticoagulant and anticardiolipin antibodies in women with recurrent pregnancy loss, fertile controls, and antiphospholipid syndrome. Obstet Gynecol 1997;89:549–555.

Brooks PM, Needs CJ. Antirheumatic drugs in pregnancy and lactation. Baillieres Clin Rheumatol 1990;4:157–171.

Buchanan NM, Toubi E, Khamashta MA, Lima F, Kerslake S, Hughes GR. Hydroxychloroquine and lupus pregnancy: review of a series of 36 cases. Ann Rheum Dis 1996;55:486–488.

Buyon JP, Cronstein BN, Morris M, Tanner M, Weissman G. Serum complement values (C3 and C4) to differentiate between systemic lupus activity and preeclampsia. Am J Med 1986;81:194–200.

Buyon JP, Hiebert R, Copel J, et al. Autoimmune-associated congenital heart block: demographics, mortality, morbidity and recurrence rates obtained from a national neonatal lupus registry. J Am Coll Cardiol 1998;31:1658–1666.

Buyon JP, Tamerius J, Ordorica S, Young B, Abramson SB. Activation of the alternative complement pathway accompanies disease flares in systemic lupus erythematosus during pregnancy. Arthritis Rheum 1992;35:55–61.

Buyon JP, Winchester RJ, Slade SG, et al. Identification of mothers at risk for congenital heart block and other neonatal lupus syndromes in their children: comparison of enzyme-linked immunosorbent asay and immunoblot for measurement of anti-SS-A/Ro and anti-SS-B/La antibodies. Arthritis Rheum 1993;36:1263–1273.

Camera A, Rocco S, De Lucia D, et al. Reversible adult respiratory distress in primary antiphospholipid syndrome. Haematologica 2000;85:208–210.

Carreira PE, Gutierrez-Larraya F, Gomez-Reino JJ. Successful intrauterine therapy with dexamethasone for fetal myocarditis and heart block in a woman with systemic lupus erythematosus. J Rheumatol 1993;20:1204–1207.

Chamley LW, Pattison NS, McKay EJ. The effect of human anticardiolipin antibodies on murine pregnancy. J Reprod Immunol 1994;27:123–134.

Clark AL, Branch DW, Silver RM, Harris EN, Pierangeli S, Spinnato JA. Pregnancy complicated by the antiphospholipid syndrome: outcomes with intravenous immunoglobulin therapy. Obstet Gynecol 1999;93:437–441.

Clifford K, Rai R, Watson H, Regan L. An informative protocol for the investigation of recurrent miscarriage: preliminary experience of 500 consecutive cases. Hum Reprod 1994;9:1328–1332.

Cote CJ, Meuwissen HJ, Pickering RJ. Effects on the neonate of prednisone and azathioprine administered to the mother during pregnancy. J Pediatr 1974;85:324–328.

Cowchock S, Reece EA. Do low-risk pregnant women with antiphospholipid antibodies need to be treated? Organizing Group of the Antiphospholipid Antibody Treatment Trial. Am J Obstet Gynecol 1997;176:1099–1100.

Cowchock FS, Reece EA, Balaban D, Branch DW, Plouffe L. Repeated fetal losses associated with antiphospholipid antibodies: a collaborative randomized trial comparing prednisone with low-dose heparin treatment. Am J Obstet Gynecol 1992;166:1318–1323.

Dahlman TC. Osteoporotic fractures and the recurrence of thromboembolism during pregnancy and the puerperium in 184 women undergoing thromboprophylaxis with heparin. Am J Obstet Gynecol 1993;168:1265–1270.

Deapen DM, Weinrib L, Langholz B, et al. A revised estimate of twin concordance in SLE: a survey of 138 pairs. Arthritis Rheum 1986;29(Suppl 4):S26.

Derksen RH, Bruinse HW, de Groot PG, Kater L. Pregnancy in systemic lupus erythematosus: a prospective study. Lupus 1994;3:149–155.

Devoe LD, Loy GL. Serum complement levels and perinatal outcome in pregnancies complicated by systemic lupus erythematosus. Obstet Gynecol 1984;63:796–800.

Devoe LD, Taylor RL. Systemic lupus erythematosus in pregnancy. Am J Obstet Gynecol 1979;135:473–479.

De Wolf F, Carreras LO, Moerman P, Vermylen J, Van Assche A, Renaer M. Decidual vasculopathy and extensive placental infarction in a patient with repeated thromboembolic accidents, recurrent fetal loss, and a lupus anticoagulant. Am J Obstet Gynecol 1982;142:829–834.

di Somone N, Meroni PL, del Papa N, et al. Antiphospholipid antibodies affect trophoblast gonadotropin secretion and invasiveness by binding directly and through adhered beta2-glycoprotein I. Arthritis Rheum 2000;43:140–150.

Doria A, Cutolo M, Ghirardello A, et al. Steroid hormones and disease activity during pregnancy in systemic lupus erythematosus. Arthritis Rheum 2002;47:202–209.

Edwards MH, Pierangeli S, Liu X, Barker JH, Anderson G, Harris EN. Hydroxychloroquine reverses thrombogenic properties of antiphospholipid antibodies in mice. Circulation 1997;96:4380–4384.

Empson M, Lassere M, Craig JC, Scott JR. Recurrent pregnancy loss with antiphospholipid antibody: a systematic review of therapeutic trials. Obstet Gynecol 2002;99:135–144.

Englert HJ, Derue GM, Loizou S, et al. Pregnancy and lupus: prognostic indicators and response to treatment. Q J Med 1988;66:125–136.

Enns GM, Roeder E, Chan RT, Ali-Khan Catts Z, Cox VA, Golabi M. Apparent cyclophosphamide (cytoxan) embryopathy: a distinct phenotype? Am J Med Genet 1999;86:237–241.

Erkan D, Merrill JT, Yazici Y, Sammaritano L, Buyon JP, Lockshin MD. High thrombosis rate after fetal loss in antiphospholipid syndrome: effective prophylaxis with aspirin. Arthritis Rheum 2001;44: 1466–1467.

Erlendsson K, Steinsson K, Johannsson JH, et al. Relation of antiphospholipid antibody and placental bed inflammatory vascular changes to the outcome of pregnancy in successive pregnancies of 2 women with systemic lupus erythematosus. J Rheumatol 1993;20:1779–1785.

Eroglu GE, Kohler PF. Familial systemic lupus erythematosus: the role of genetic and environmental factors. Ann Rheum Dis 2002;61: 29–31.

Eronen M, Heikkila P, Teramo K. Congenital complete heart block in the fetus: hemodynamic features, antenatal treatment, and outcome in six cases. Pediatr Cardiol 2001;22:385–392.

Fine LG, Barnett EV, Danovitch GM, et al. Systemic lupus erythematosus in pregnancy. Arch Intern Med 1981;94:667–677.

Georgiou PE, Politi EN, Katsimbri P, Sakka V, Drosos AA. Outcome of lupus pregnancy: a controlled study. Rheumatology (Oxford) 2000;39:1014–1019.

Ginsberg JS, Greer I, Hirsh J. Use of antithrombotic agents during pregnancy. Chest 2001;119(1 Suppl):122S–131S.

Glass D, Raum D, Gibson D, et al. Inherited deficiency of the second component of complement. Rheumatic disease associations. J Clin Invest 1976;58:853–861.

Granger KA, Farquharson RG. Obstetric outcome in antiphospholipid syndrome. Lupus 1997;6:509–513.

Harris EN. Syndrome of the black swan. Br J Rheumatol 1987;26: 324–326.

Hart C, Naughton RF. The ototoxicity of chloroquine phosphate. Arch Otolaryngol 1964;80:407.

Hartung K, Fontana A, Klar M, et al. Association of class I, II, and III MHC gene products with systemic lupus erythematosus. Results of a Central European multicenter study. Rheumatol Int 1989; 9:13–18.

Hayslett JP, Lynn RI. Effect of pregnancy in patients with lupus nephropathy. Kidney Int 1980;18:207–220.

Holers VM, Girardi G, Mo L, et al. Complement C3 activation is required for antiphospholipid antibody-induced fetal loss. J Exp Med 2002;195:211–220.

Hörkkö S, Miller E, Dudl E, et al. Antiphospholipid antibodies are directed against epitopes of oxidized phospholipids: recognition of cardiolipin by monoclonal antibodies to epitopes of oxidized low density lipoprotein. J Clin Invest 1996;98:815–825.

Howard PF, Hochberg MC, Bias WB, et al. Relationship between C4 null genes, HLA-D region antigens, and genetic susceptibility to SLE in Caucasian and black Americans. Am J Med 1986;81:187–193.

Huong DL, Wechsler B, Vauthier-Brouzes D, Beaufils H, Lefebvre G, Piette JC. Pregnancy in past or present lupus nephritis: a study of 32 pregnancies from a single centre. Ann Rheum Dis 2001;60:599–604.

Imbasciati E, Surian M, Bottino W, et al. Lupus nephropathy and pregnancy. Nephron 1984;36:46–51.

Johns KR, Morand EF, Littlejohn GO. Pregnancy outcome in systemic lupus erythematosus (SLE): a review of 54 cases. Aust N Z J Med 1998;28:18–22.

Julkunen H, Jouhikainen T, Kaaja R, et al. Fetal outcome in lupus pregnancy: a retrospective case-control study of 242 pregnancies in 112 patients. Lupus 1993a;2:125–131.

Julkunen H, Kaaja R, Palosuo T, et al. Pregnancy in lupus nephropathy. Acta Obstet Gynecol Scand 1993b;72:258–263.

Jungers P, Dougados M, Pelissier C, et al. Lupus nephropathy and pregnancy. Arch Intern Med 1982;142:771–776.

Kaaja R, Julkunen H, Ammala P, et al. Congenital heart block: successful prophylactic treatment with intravenous gamma globulin and corticosteroid therapy. Am J Obstet Gynecol 1991;165:1333–1334.

Kelton JG. Heparin-induced thrombocytopenia: an overview. Blood Rev 2002;16:77–80.

Khamashta MA, Cuadrado MJ, Mujic F, Taub NA, Hunt BJ, Hughes GR. The management of thrombosis in the antiphospholipid-antibody syndrome. N Engl J Med 1995;332:993–997.

Khamashta MA, Buchanan NM, Hughes GR. The use of hydroxychloroquine in lupus pregnancy: the British experience. Lupus 1996;5(Suppl 1):S65–S66.

Kirshon B, Wasserstrum N, Willis R, Herman GE, McCabe ER. Teratogenic effects of first-trimester cyclophosphamide therapy. Obstet Gynecol 1988;72:462–464.

Kleinman D, Katz VL, Kuller JA. Perinatal outcomes in women with systemic lupus erythematosus. J Perinatol 1998;18:178–182.

Klinger G, Morad Y, Westall CA, et al. Ocular toxicity and antenatal exposure to chloroquine or hydroxychloroquine for rheumatic diseases. Lancet 2001;358:813–814.

Kutteh WH. Antiphospholipid antibody-associated recurrent pregnancy loss: treatment with heparin and low-dose aspirin is superior to low-dose aspirin alone. Am J Obstet Gynecol 1996;174:1584–1589.

Laskin CA, Bombardier C, Hannah ME, et al. Prednisone and aspirin in women with autoantibodies and unexplained recurrent fetal loss. N Engl J Med 1997;337:148–153.

Lawrence JS, Martins CL, Drake G. A family survey of lupus erythematosus. I. Heritability. J Rheumatol 1987;14:913–921.

Lawrence S, Luy L, Laxer R, Krafchik B, Silverman E. The health of mothers of children with cutaneous neonatal lupus erythematosus differs from that of mothers of children with congenital heart block. Am J Med 2000;108:705–709.

Lee LA, Gaither KK, Coulter SN, et al. Pattern of cutaneous immunoglobulin G deposition in subacute cutaneous lupus erythematosus is reproduced by infusing purified anti-Ro (SSA) autoantibodies into human skin-grafted mice. J Clin Invest 1989;83:1556–1562.

Lee LA, Frank MB, McCubbin VR, Reichlin M. Autoantibodies of neonatal lupus erythematosus. J Invest Dermatol 1994;102:963–966.

Le Huong D, Wechsler B, Vauthier-Brouzes D, et al. Outcome of planned pregnancies in systemic lupus erythematosus: a prospective study on 62 pregnancies. Br J Rheumatol 1997;36:772–777.

Le Thi Huong D, Wechsler B, Piette JC, Bletry O, Godeau P. Pregnancy and its outcome in systemic lupus erythematosus. Q J Med 1994;87:721–729.

Levine J, Branch DW, Rauch J. The antiphospholipid syndrome. N Engl J Med 2002;346:752–763.

Levy RA, Vilela VS, Cataldo MJ, et al. Hydroxychloroquine (HCQ) in lupus pregnancy: double-blind and placebo-controlled study. Lupus 2001;10:401–404.

Lima F, Khamashta MA, Buchanan NM, Kerslake S, Hunt BJ, Hughes GR. A study of sixty pregnancies in patients with the antiphospholipid syndrome. Clin Exp Rheumatol 1996;14:131–136.

Lockshin MD, Reinitz E, Druzin ML, Murrman M, Estes D. Lupus pregnancy. Case-control prospective study demonstrating absence of lupus exacerbation during or after pregnancy. Am J Med 1984;77:893–898.

Lockshin MD, Qamar T, Redecha P, Harpel PC. Hypocomplementemia with low C1s–C1 inhibitor complex in systemic lupus erythematosus. Arthritis Rheum 1986;29:1467–1472.

Lockshin MD, Qamar T, Druzin ML. Hazards of lupus pregnancy. J Rheumatol 1987;14(Suppl 13):214–217.

Lockshin MD, Bonfa E, Elkon D, Druzin ML. Neonatal lupus risk to newborns of mothers with systemic lupus erythematosus. Arthritis Rheum 1988;31:697–701.

McCauliffe DP. Neonatal lupus erythematosus: a transplacentally acquired autoimmune disorder. Semin Dermatol 1995;14:47–53.

Macones GA, Robinson CA. Is there justification for using indomethacin in preterm labor? An analysis of neonatal risks and benefits. Am J Obstet Gynecol 1997;177:819–824.

Mellembakken JR, Hogasen K, Mollnes TE, Hack CE, Abyholm T, Videm V. Increased systemic activation of neutrophils but not complement in preeclampsia. Obstet Gynecol 2001;97:371–374.

Meroni PL, Raschi E, Camera M, et al. Endothelial activation by aPL: a potential pathogenetic mechanism for the clinical manifestations of the syndrome. J Autoimmun 2000;15:237–240.

Mintz R, Niz J, Gutierrez G, Garcia-Alonso A, Karchmer S. Prospective study of pregnancy in systemic lupus erythematosus: results of a multidisciplinary approach. J Rheumatol 1986;13:732–739.

Motta M, Tincani A, Faden D, Zinzini E, Chirico G. Antimalarial agents in pregnancy. Lancet 2002;359:524–525.

Neiman AR, Lee LA, Weston WL, Buyon JP. Cutaneous manifestations of neonatal lupus without heart block: characteristics of mothers and children enrolled in a national registry. J Pediatr 2000;137:674–680.

Nossent HC, Koldingsnes W. Long-term efficacy of azathioprine treatment for proliferative lupus nephritis. Rheumatology (Oxford) 2000;39:969–974.

Nylander U. Ocular damage in chloroquine therapy. Acta Ophthalmol (Copenh) 1967;45(Suppl 92):1–71.

Oshiro BT, Silver RM, Scott JR, et al. Antiphospholipid antibodies and fetal death. Obstet Gynecol 1996;87:489–493.

Ostensen M, Villiger PM. Nonsteroidal anti-inflammatory drugs in systemic lupus erythematosus. Lupus 2001;10:135–139.

Oviasu E, Hicks J, Cameron JS. The outcome of pregnancy in women with lupus nephritis. Lupus 1991;1:19–25.

Packham DK, Lam SS, Nichols K, et al. Lupus nephritis and pregnancy. Q J Med 1992;83:315–324.

Pattison NS, Chamley LW, McKay EJ, et al. Antiphospholipid antibodies in pregnancy: prevalence and clinical associations. Br J Obstet Gynaecol 1993;100:909–913.

Pattison NS, Chamley LW, Birdsall M, Zanderigo AM, Liddell HS, McDougall J. Does aspirin have a role in improving pregnancy outcome for women with the antiphospholipid syndrome? A randomized controlled trial. Am J Obstet Gynecol 2000; 183:1008–1012.

Petri M. Hopkins Lupus Pregnancy Center: 1987 to 1996. Rheum Dis Clin North Am 1997;23:1–13.

Petri M, Howard D, Repke J. Frequency of lupus flare in pregnancy. The Hopkins lupus pregnancy center experience. Arthritis Rheum 1991;34:1538–1545.

Price BE, Rauch J, Shia MA et al. Anti-phospholipid autoantibodies manner. J Immunol 1996;157:2201–2208.

Provost TT, Watson R, Ganmmon WR. Neonatal lupus syndrome associated with U_1RNP (nRNP) antibodies. N Engl J Med 1987; 316:1135–1138.

Pryde PG, Besinger RE, Gianopoulos JG, Mittendorf R. Adverse and beneficial effects of tocolytic therapy. Semin Perinatol 2001;25:316–340.

Rahman P, Gladman DD, Urowitz MB. Clinical predictors of fetal outcome in systemic lupus erythematosus. J Rheumatol 1998; 25:1526–1530.

Rai R, Cohen H, Dave M, Regan L. Randomised controlled trial of aspirin and aspirin plus heparin in pregnant women with recurrent miscarriage associated with phospholipid antibodies (or antiphospholipid antibodies). BMJ 1997;314:253–257.

Ramsey-Goldman R, Kutzer JE, Kuller LH, Guzick D, Carpenter AB, Medsger TA. Pregnancy outcome and anti-cardiolipin antibody in women with systemic lupus erythematosus. Am J Epidemiol 1993;138:1057–1069.

Rand JH, Wu X-X, Andree HAM, et al. Pregnancy loss in the antiphospholipid-antibody syndrome: a possible thrombogenic mechanism. N Engl J Med 1997;337:154–160. [Erratum, N Engl J Med 1997;337:1327.]

Rauova L, Lukac J, Levy Y, Rovensky J, Shoenfeld Y. High-dose intravenous immunoglobulins for lupus nephritis: a salvage immunomodulation. Lupus 2001;10:209–213.

Rayburn WF. Connective tissue disorders and pregnancy. Recommendations for prescribing. J Reprod Med 1998;43:341–349.

Rivier G, Herranz MT, Khamashta MA, Hughes GR. Thrombosis and antiphospholipid syndrome: a preliminary assessment of three antithrombotic treatments. Lupus 1994;3:85–90.

Rosove MH, Brewer PM. Antiphospholipid thrombosis: clinical course after the first thrombotic event in 70 patients. Ann Intern Med 1992;117:303–308.

Ruiz-Irastorza G, Lima F, Alves J, et al. Increased rate of lupus flare during pregnancy and the puerperium: a prospective study of 78 pregnancies. Br J Rheumatol 1996;35:133–138.

Ruiz-Irastorza G, Khamashta MA, Castellino G, Hughes GR. Systemic lupus erythematosus. Lancet 2001;357:1027–1032.

Rumack CM, Guggenheim MA, Rumack BH, et al. Neonatal intracranial haemorrhage and maternal use of aspirin. Obstet Gynecol 1981;58(Suppl 5):S52–56.

Saleeb S, Copel J, Friedman D, Buyon JP. Comparison of treatment with fluorinated glucocorticoids to the natural history of autoantibody-associated congenital heart block: retrospective review of the research registry for neonatal lupus. Arthritis Rheum 1999; 42:2335–2345.

Schaar CG, Ronday KH, Boets EP, van der Lubbe PA, Breedveld FC. Catastrophic manifestation of the antiphospholipid syndrome. J Rheumatol 1999;26:2261–2264.

Scott JS, Maddison PJ, Taylor MV, et al. Connective tissue disease, antibodies to ribonucleoprotein and congenital heart disease. N Engl J Med 1983;309:209–212

Sesso R, Monteiro M, Sato E, Kirsztajn G, Silva L, Ajzen H. A controlled trial of pulse cyclophosphamide versus pulse methylprednisolone in severe lupus nephritis. Lupus 1994;3:107–112.

Shi W, Chong BH, Chesterman CN. β2-Glycoprotein I is a requirement for anticardiolipin antibodies binding to activated platelets: differences with lupus anticoagulants. Blood 1993;81:1255–1262.

Silver RK, MacGregor SN, Sholl JS, Hobart JM, Neerhof MG, Ragin A. Comparative trial of prednisone plus aspirin versus aspirin alone in the treatment of anticardiolipin antibody-positive obstetric patients. Am J Obstet Gynecol 1993;169:1411–1417.

Stuart JJ, Gross SJ, Elrad H, et al. Effects of acetylsalicylic acid ingestion on maternal and neonatal hemostasis. N Engl J Med 1982;307:909–912.

Taylor PV, Scott JS, Gerlis LM, Path FRC, Esscher E, Scott O. Maternal antibodies against fetal cardiac antigens in congenital complete heart block. N Engl J Med 1986;315:667–672.

ter Borg EJ, Horst G, Hummel EJ, Limburg PC, Kallenberg CG. Measurement of increases in anti-double-stranded DNA antibody levels as a predictor of disease exacerbation in systemic lupus erythematosus. A long-term, prospective study. Arthritis Rheum 1990;33:634–643.

Tincani A, Faden D, Tarantini M, et al. Systemic lupus erythematosus and pregnancy: a prospective study. Clin Exp Rheumatol 1992; 10:439–446.

Tomer Y, Viegas, OAC, Swissa M, Koh SCL, Shoenfeld Y. Levels of lupus autoantibodies in pregnant SLE patients: correlations with disease activity and pregnancy outcome. Clin Exp Rheumatol 1996;14:275–280.

Ujhazy E, Balonova T, Durisova M, et al. Teratogenicity of cyclophosphamide in New Zealand white rabbits. Neoplasma 1993;40:45–49.

Urowitz MB, Gladman DD, Farewell VT, Stewart J, McDonald J. Lupus and pregnancy studies. Arthritis Rheum 1993;36:1392–1397.

Vaarala O, Alfthan G, Jauhiainen M, Leirisalo-Repo M, Aho K, Palosuo T. Crossreaction between antibodies to oxidised low-density lipoprotein and to cardiolipin in systemic lupus erythematosus. Lancet 1993;341:923–925.

Vaquero E, Lazzarin N, Valensise H, et al. Pregnancy outcome in recurrent spontaneous abortion associated with antiphospholipid antibodies: a comparative study of intravenous immunoglobulin versus prednisone plus low-dose aspirin. Am J Reprod Immunol 2001;45:174–179.

Vermillion ST, Newman RB. Recent indomethacin tocolysis is not associated with neonatal complications in preterm infants. Am J Obstet Gynecol 1999;181:1083–1086.

Wapner RJ, Cowchock FS, Shapiro SS. Successful treatment in two women with antiphospholipid antibodies and refractory pregnancy losses with intravenous immunoglobulin infusions. Am J Obstet Gynecol 1989;161:1271–1272.

Warkentin TE, Kelton JG. Delayed-onset heparin-induced thrombocytopenia and thrombosis. Ann Intern Med 2001;135:502–506.

Warkentin TE, Levine MN, Hirsh J, et al. Heparin-induced thrombocytopenia in patients treated with low-molecular-weight heparin or unfractionated heparin. N Engl J Med 1995;332:1330–1335.

Weiner CP, Brandt J. Plasma antithrombin III activity: an aid in the diagnosis of preeclampsia–eclampsia. Am J Obstet Gynecol 1982;142:275–281.

Welch TR, Beischel LS, Balakrishnan K, et al. Major histocompatibility complex extended haplotypes in systemic lupus erythematosus. Dis Markers 1988;6:247–255.

Wilson WA, Gharavi AE, Koike T, et al. International consensus statement on preliminary classification criteria for definite antiphospholipid syndrome: report of an international workshop. Arthritis Rheum 1999;42:1309–1311.

Wong KL, Chan FY, Lee CP. Outcome of pregnancy in patients with systemic lupus erythematosus. A prospective study. Arch Intern Med 1991;151:269–273.

Yetman DL, Kutteh WH. Antiphospholipid antibody panels and recurrent pregnancy loss: prevalence of anticardiolipin antibodies compared with other antiphospholipid antibodies. Fertil Steril 1996;66:540–546.

36 Trauma in pregnancy

James W. Van Hook
Alfredo F. Gei
Luis Diego Pacheco

Major trauma affects up to 8% of pregnant patients, with life-threatening maternal injuries complicating 3–4 per 1,000 deliveries (Lavery & Staten-McCormick, 1995). Trauma is the leading cause of nonobstetric maternal death in the United States (Varner, 1989; Moise & Belfort, 1997). The maternal death rate secondary to trauma is 1.9 per 1,000 live births (Sachs et al., 1987). Trauma caused by battering or abuse occurs in as many as 10% of pregnant women (Helton et al., 1987; Satin et al., 1991). Thus trauma is a very significant cause of both maternal and fetal morbidity and mortality. The appropriate multidisciplinary treatment of trauma during pregnancy is of great importance for any provider who cares for pregnant women. In this chapter, we will discuss trauma during pregnancy and underscore issues unique in the care of the pregnant trauma victim.

Maternal physiologic adaptations applicable to trauma during pregnancy

Normal maternal physiologic changes during pregnancy have a significant influence on the pathophysiologic responses the mother and her fetus manifest as a result of trauma. Furthermore, the physiologic changes of pregnancy may alter the clinician's ability to accurately diagnose trauma and may either favorably or adversely influence maternal outcome. The most important physiologic changes, as applicable to the pregnant trauma victim, are summarized in Table 36.1.

Cardiovascular alterations

Several maternal adaptations to pregnancy have the potential to affect trauma management. One of the most extensive and important physiologic adaptations to pregnancy that affects trauma care and pregnancy outcome is the associated increase in blood and plasma volume. Plasma volume increases by up to 50% during pregnancy. Increase in volume occurs toward the end of the first trimester with maximal expansion completed by 28–32 weeks of gestation (Scott, 1972; Whittaker et al., 1996). Red cell mass, also expanded during pregnancy, increases relatively less than plasma volume. The end result is a dilutional anemia of pregnancy with a small decrease in hematocrit (Pritchard, 1965; Whittaker et al., 1996). Consequently normal pregnancy imparts a natural buffer to the expected 500–1,000 mL blood loss of normal vaginal or cesarean delivery (Cunningham et al., 2001a). Additionally, during blood loss associated with trauma, the pregnant woman is apt to display relative physiologic stability until massive blood loss ensues (Kuhlmann & Cruikshank, 1994).

Table 36.2 categorizes hemorrhage according to the amount of blood loss and related manifestations (Ramenofsky et al. 1993). In pregnancy, due to the blood volume changes described above plus the fact that most pregnant patients are young and otherwise healthy, signs and symptoms of profound blood loss are usually attenuated and the diagnosis of ongoing blood loss may be missed or delayed until profound hemodynamic collapse occurs. Conversely, providers who do not normally care for pregnant women could be incorrectly misled by the normal dilutional anemia of pregnancy if they compare hematocrit values to normal nonpregnant values. Recognition of the volume changes evident during pregnancy must be considered during evaluation of the pregnant trauma patient.

In addition to the blood volume changes, blood pressure and cardiac output also change during normal pregnancy. Systolic and diastolic blood pressure decrease to nadir values by approximately 28 weeks of gestation (Wilson et al., 1980). Heart rate increases by approximately 15–20% over nonpregnancy levels. Cardiac output increases by 30–50% over control values by the late second trimester, secondary to increases in both heart rate and stroke volume (Clark et al., 1989). The etiology of the increase in cardiac output may be hormonal, volume related, or secondary to the functional 20–30% arteriovenous shunt produced by the low resistance placental circuit. Despite an increase in stroke volume, left ventricular filling pressures are not increased during pregnancy. Systemic vascular resistance decreases during gestation, with a partial return toward prepregnancy values by late pregnancy. An often unrecognized pregnancy-associated cardiovascular

Table 36.1 Maternal adaptation to pregnancy and relevance to trauma

Parameter	Change	Implications
Plasma volume	Increases by 45–50%	Relative maternal resistance to limited blood loss
Red cell mass	Increases by 30%	Dilutional anemia
Cardiac output	Increases by 30–50%	Relative maternal resistance to limited blood loss
Uteroplacental blood flow	20–30% shunt	Uterine injury may predispose to increased blood loss Increased uterine vascularity
Uterine size	Dramatic increase	Increased incidence of uterine injury with abdominal trauma Change in position of abdominal contents Supine hypotension
Minute ventilation	Increases by 25–30%	Diminished P_aco_2 Diminished buffering capacity
Functional residual volume	Decreased	Predisposition to atelectasis and hypoxemia
Gastric emptying	Delayed	Predisposition to aspiration

See text for sources of data.

Table 36.2 Categorization of acute hemorrhage

	Class 1	Class 2	Class 3	Class 4
Blood loss (% blood volume)	15%	15–30%	30–40%	>40%
Pulse rate	<100	>100	>120	>140
Pulse pressure	Normal	Decreased	Decreased	Decreased
Blood pressure	Normal or increased	Decreased	Decreased	Decreased

(From Ramenofsky, et al., eds. Advanced Trauma Life Support (R) for Doctors—1993 Instructor Manual. American College of Surgeons. Chicago: First Impressions, 1993.)

effect is the profound hypotension that can occur with supine positioning of the pregnant woman. Supine hypotension results from aortocaval compression by the enlarged gravid uterus and can have profound effects on both normal and hemodynamically-compromised patients (Lees et al., 1967). Avoidance of supine hypotension can often be accomplished by proper patient positioning (Vaizey et al., 1994), using a wedge placed under the right hip or by placing the operating room table on tilt.

Labor itself imposes additional cardiovascular demands on the pregnant patient. In healthy pregnant subjects, cardiac output increases by an additional 40% over basal third-trimester values. This increase is partially attenuated by pain relief and the provision of conduction anesthesia (Ueland & Hansen, 1969a,b). Immediately after delivery, cardiac output is often at its peak. Cardiac output and stroke volume may increase by nearly 60% and over 70%, respectively. Ventricular filling pressure and pulmonary artery pressure also increase immediately postpartum (Ueland & Metcalfe, 1975). Progressive diuresis and resolution of hormonal changes produce normalization of hemodynamic parameters by about 6 weeks postpartum (Chesley et al., 1959).

Pulmonary and respiratory changes

Several mechanical and metabolic changes in respiratory physiology occur during pregnancy. Minute ventilation increases by some 40%, predominantly secondary to an increase in tidal volume, but also with a much smaller increase in respiratory rate. As a consequence of increased minute volume, the arterial partial pressure of CO_2 (P_aco_2) diminishes to approximately 30 mmHg (Prowse & Gaensler, 1965; de Swiet, 1991). The resulting compensated respiratory alkalosis causes pH to trend to the alkalemic range of normal. Concomitantly, serum bicarbonate (HCO_3) decreases to 18–22 mEq/L and serum buffering capacity is thereby reduced (Hankins et al., 1995). Finally, it is important to remember that other derangements (e.g. hypoxia, sepsis, ketoacidosis, etc.) exert an additive effect on underlying blood gas changes of pregnancy. Hyperventilation from moderately high altitude has been shown to reduce P_aco_2 in the third-trimester gravida to values as low as 25–26 mmHg (Hankins et al., 1995; Hankins & Van Hook, 1999). Therefore any pathophysiologic acid–base derangement in pregnancy should be interpreted in light of the fact that a primary acid–base disturbance normally exists.

Functional residual volume (FRV) is decreased during pregnancy (Alaily & Carrol, 1978). Tidal breathing may be at or near critical closing volume, potentially predisposing the pregnant patient to hypoxemia, particularly in situations that normally reduce FRV anyway (e.g. supine positioning, intrinsic pulmonary disease, chest wall trauma) (Garrard et al., 1978; Van Hook, 1997). The diaphragm is elevated by about 4 cm during pregnancy, making injury during thoracostomy tube placement potentially more likely (Lavery & Staten-McCormick, 1995).

Gastrointestinal changes

The mechanical effect of the enlarged uterus as pregnancy progresses causes displacement of the small bowel into the upper abdomen (Kuhlmann & Cruikshank, 1994). As will be discussed in the section on abdominal trauma, the change in position of the abdominal viscera has impact on mechanisms, diagnosis, and treatment of abdominal trauma. Hormonal and metabolic factors both result in delayed gastric emptying and increased gastrointestinal transit time. Consequently, pulmonary aspiration of stomach contents is more likely during pregnancy (Mendelson, 1946; Davison et al., 1977).

Genitourinary changes

The progestational effect of smooth muscle relaxation, along with mechanical compression from the gravid uterus, cause dilation of the ureters and the renal pelvises. Consequently, radiographic imaging of the genitourinary system may show some degree of "physiologic" hydronephrosis (Lindheimer & Katz, 1970; Bellina et al., 1976; Kuhlmann & Cruickshank, 1994). Ureteropelvical dilation may also predispose the urinary collecting system to stasis. Bacteriuria and pyelonephritis are more common during pregnancy (Cunningham et al., 2001b). Creatinine clearance is increased in normal pregnancy. Simplistically, the increase in creatinine clearance is due to a cardiac output mediated increase in renal blood flow. Therefore, in pregnancy, a serum creatinine at the upper limit of what is considered normal when not pregnant may reflect diminished renal function (Lindheimer & Katz, 1970; Cunningham et al., 2001a). The urinary bladder is "abdominalized" after the first trimester of pregnancy, increasing the propensity for the female bladder to become injured during abdominal trauma.

Hematological changes

As discussed previously, normal pregnancy is associated with a relative dilutional anemia despite an increase in overall red cell mass. A mild leukocytosis is also noted during pregnancy (Taylor et al., 1981). Factors VII, VIII, IX, X, and fibrinogen are elevated during pregnancy. Factor IX, factor XIII, and platelet count are unchanged or minimally decreased during pregnancy (Burrows & Kelton, 1988; Cunningham et al., 2001a). Despite these somewhat conflicting changes, pregnancy is a hypercoagulable state. Consequently, pregnancy accentuates other predisposing factors leading to the development of deep venous thrombosis (Rutherford & Phelan, 1991; Witlin et al., 1999). Coagulation factor changes in pregnancy are summarized in Table 36.3.

Table 36.3 Hemostatic changes during pregnancy

Factor	Change	Normal in late pregnancy
Fibrinogen	50% increase	300–600 mg/dL
Factor II	Slight increase	Variable
Factor VII	Increased	Variable
Factor IX	Increased	Variable
Factor X	Increased	Variable
Factor IX	Minimal decrease	Variable
Factor XIII	Minimal decrease	Variable
Platelet count	Normal or slightly lower	Variable

See text for source of data.

Uterus

By 12 weeks of gestation, the uterus becomes an abdominal organ. Prior to 12 weeks' gestation, the small size and the pelvic location of the uterus make it resistant to injury (Crosby & Costiloe, 1971). Conversely, late in pregnancy, the abdominal location of the uterus predisposes it to injury from blunt or penetrating abdominal trauma (Kuhlmann & Cruickshank, 1994). Perhaps even more important is the dramatic increase in uteropelvic blood flow during pregnancy. By late pregnancy, a volume equivalent to the mother's entire circulating blood volume passes through the uterus at least every 10 minutes (Vaizey et al., 1994). The dramatic increase in uterine blood flow, coupled with the abdominalization of the dramatically larger gravid organ pose a synergistic propensity for hemorrhage in the face of uterine trauma (Esposito, 1994). Fortunately, uterine rupture is an infrequent complication of multiorgan trauma during pregnancy. Rupture of the uterus is found in less than 1% of pregnant trauma victims (Davison et al., 1977; Hankins et al., 1995). Uterine rupture is most usually associated with direct and substantial abdominal impact or other predisposing obstetric factors such as gestational age or previous uterine surgery (Williams et al., 1990). Fetal death usually occurs with uterine rupture. Maternal death from uterine rupture is reported to occur in 10% of cases with traumatic uterine rupture (Pearlman & Tintinalli, 1991). Often, however, death is from other severe injuries that tend to occur in patients with uterine rupture.

Management of trauma

The American College of Surgeons has long advocated a standardized approach to the management of trauma (Committee on Trauma, 1999). Resuscitation is based upon a systematic survey and intervention method. Some review of this philosophy as it relates to pregnant patients is justified. A modified basic algorithm for initial resuscitation of the pregnant trauma patient is provided in Fig. 36.1.

Primary survey

The primary survey encompasses the immediate evaluation of the pregnant or nonpregnant trauma patient. The initials "A-B-C-D-E" are used to describe the steps of the primary survey (Fig. 36.1) (Moore, 1990; Trunkey & Lewis, 1991; Ramenofsky et al., 1993; Vaizey et al., 1994; Lavery & Staten-McCormick, 1995). Little is different in performing the primary survey

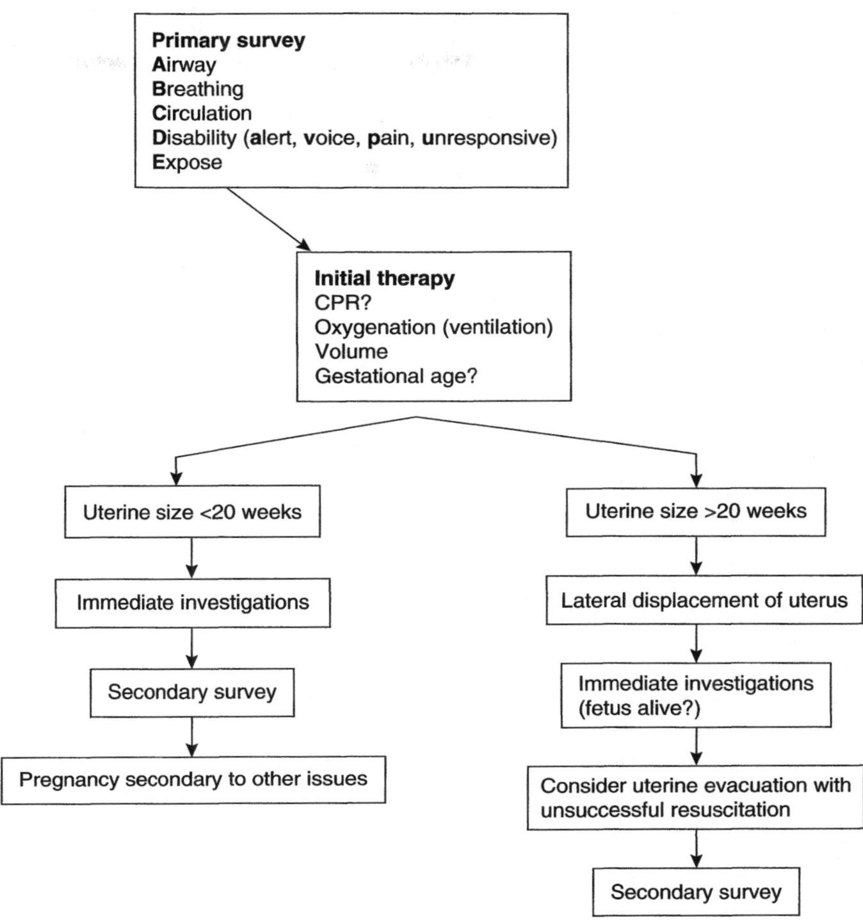

Fig. 36.1 Initial resuscitation of the pregnant trauma patient. CPR, cardiopulmonary resuscitation. (See text for sources of data.)

during pregnancy as compared to the nonpregnant individual. Foremost in the primary survey is stabilization of a proper airway ("A"). If an adequate functioning airway is not present, chin lift (with a stabilized neck and cervical spine) and oral or nasal airway insertion may be necessary. Early endotracheal intubation by qualified personnel must be performed if the just-described measures fail. Because of a potential for aspiration, intubation should be more aggressively pursued in the pregnant trauma victim than in her nonpregnant counterpart (Kuhlmann & Cruickshank, 1994). After airway stabilization, adequate respiration ("B") must be established. Supplemental oxygen is given as necessary and its adequacy assessed via pulse oximetry. Arterial blood gas determination, if obtained, must be interpreted in reference to what is normally found during pregnancy. A decreased serum bicarbonate level may be indicative of significant risk for fetal loss. One series reported that initial serum bicarbonate levels were significantly lower (16.4 ± 3.0 mEq/L versus 20.3 ± 2.2 mEq/L) in pregnant major trauma victims in which fetal loss was noted (Scorpio et al., 1992).

"C" refers to circulation. Pulse quality, blood pressure, and capillary refill are basic clinical determinants of the adequacy of perfusion. As mentioned earlier, clinical evaluation of maternal intravascular homeostasis is altered by the underlying physiologic changes of pregnancy. Also, fetal effects from maternal hypovolemia are not addressed by basic hemodynamic physical diagnosis (Greiss, 1966; Dilts et al., 1967; Hoff et al., 1991; Scorpio et al., 1992). In any case, because of the ongoing hemorrhage often present in any severely-injured trauma patient, immediate assessment and treatment of hypovolemia must be provided. In nearly all trauma cases, a large-bore (14 or 16 G) intravenous (IV) access should be established. It is our custom in the multiple trauma patients to insert large-bore IV in both an upper and lower extremity. Central venous access is not immediately indicated, provided adequate peripheral access can be established. An appropriately sized peripheral IV (14 or 16 G) will provide the ability to rapidly instill large amounts of volume. Hypotension in the trauma patient is assumed to be hypovolemia until proven otherwise. Because of the blood-volume changes described previously, it is not uncommon for pregnant patients to seemingly "tolerate" 1,500–2,000 mL of blood loss with only subtle hemodynamic changes (Lavery & Staten-McCormick, 1995). Splanchnic and uterine blood flow is none the less compromised (Greiss, 1966;

Dilts et al., 1967) and deterioration of the patient can develop rapidly with any further blood loss. *Initial* therapy for hypotension found during the primary survey is rapid infusion of up to 2,000 mL of crystalloid solution and preparation for blood transfusion as necessary. Cardiopulmonary resuscitation in the pregnant trauma victim, discussed in subsequent sections of this chapter, is begun if pulses are not palpated.

Up to this point in the primary survey, obstetric and nonobstetric management is very similar. However, at this stage of the resuscitation process, attention to great vessel compression by the gravid uterus must be addressed in pregnancies beyond 20 weeks' gestation. In multiple-trauma, because of potential vertebral injury, patients are generally placed on a rigid spinal "board" and usual methods for avoiding aortocaval compression (e.g. lateral roll, lateral tilt, etc.) are not possible. Manual lateral displacement of the uterus is therefore performed. Alternatively, if the gravid trauma patient is on a trauma backboard, the entire board can be tilted 15 degrees, providing stabilization of the vertebral column is maintained (Ramenofsky et al., 1993; Hankins et al., 1995).

The letter "D" in the sequence stands for "disability." With any trauma, early neurological evaluation is undertaken. A rapid assessment is by the "A-V-P-U" method (*A*lert; *V*oice; *P*ain; *U*nresponsive) (Ramenofsky et al., 1993). The Glasgow Coma Scale (GCS) can also be used (Table 36.4) (Teasdale & Jennett, 1974; Jennett et al., 1979). A GCS of 8 or less may be indicative of significant ongoing neurologic pathology (Baxt & Moody, 1987; Rutherford & Nelson, 1995). Use of the GCS allows general prognostication regarding the rate of craniotomy. In one nonobstetric study of level one trauma patients, subjects with a GCS of less than 8 had a 19% rate of craniotomy, those with GCS between 8 and 13 had a 9% rate of craniotomy, and victims who presented with a GCS of greater than 13 had a 3% need for craniotomy (Trunkey & Lewis, 1991; Winchell et al., 1995).

Table 36.4 Glascow Coma Scale

	Points
Eye-opening response (E-score)	
Spontaneous (already open and blinking)	4
Opens in response to speech	3
Opens in response to pain (not to face)	2
No response	1
Verbal response (V-score)	
Oriented and appropriate response	5
Confused response	4
Inappropriate wording	3
Incomprehensible words	2
No response	1
Motor response (M-score)	
Obeys command	6
Localizes pain	5
Withdraws to pain	4
Flexion response to pain	3
Extension response to pain	2
No response	1

Glasgow Coma Scale is the sum of scores in the three areas listed. A GCS score ≤8 is consistent with coma. Caregivers need to consider the intubated patient's inability to speak.
(From Teasdale G, Jennett B. Assessment of coma and impaired consciousness: a practical scale. Lancet 1974;1:81.)

Assessment of the patient with trauma in the fashion just described will immediately identify significant cardiovascular or central nervous system dysfunction. The next step in the evaluation is to expose ("E") the patient. "Expose" means completely undressing the patient and examining her from head to toe. The back is examined for entrance or exit wounds, the extremities are briefly palpated, and any obvious visible injuries are noted. At this stage, the pregnant patient must undergo some preliminary determination of gestational age, the presence or absence of labor, and attempted measurement of fetal heart rate. Because of both the potential for fetal viability and for the supine hypotension effects previously described, pregnancies greater than 20–24 weeks' gestation evoke different management concerns than do gestations at less than the midpoint of pregnancy. For the patient undergoing CPR, perimortem cesarean section may be necessary. However, it should be emphasized that *initial* management of the pregnant patient should be the same as in the nonpregnant individual. Maternal resuscitation *initially* takes precedence over fetal evaluation. Always remember that the leading cause of fetal mortality in trauma is maternal mortality and rapid recognition and resuscitation reduces maternal mortality.

Inflatable military antishock trousers ("MAST" trousers) have enjoyed some past popularity in the resuscitation or transport of the hypotensive trauma patient. MAST trousers are less frequently used in general adult trauma, with the device's most compelling indication being stabilization of the severely fractured pelvis. Conventional wisdom holds that if used in pregnancy, MAST trousers should only have the lower (leg) compartments inflated. The abdominal compartment should probably not be inflated in any patient with a potentially salvageable gestation as uteroplacental blood flow is not preserved (Pearlman et al., 1990a; Esposito, 1994). Other potential obstetric and gynecologic indications for MAST trousers include temporary stabilization of unremitting vaginal bleeding from uterine inversion, advanced reproductive tract malignancy, and recalcitrant uterine atony remote from a medical facility. Data supporting MAST application in such circumstances is anecdotal at best. Therefore, generally speaking, MAST trousers should not be used in the pregnant *trauma* patient except under special circumstances. In the prehospital management of nonpregnant trauma patients, the majority of major trauma centers have abandoned MAST application for hypotensive trauma patients (Neufield, 1993).

Investigations

At the conclusion of the primary survey, critical resuscitation is underway, major injuries are identified, and a general idea about the status of the pregnancy itself is known. At this juncture in management, diagnostic testing is ordered. *Immediate investigations* include necessary imaging studies, laboratory evaluation, and ancillary examination (Liberman et al., 2000). "Fingers and/or tubes" should be placed in every orifice. Particular attention should be paid to the maternal bladder. Catheterization is undertaken and if gross hematuria is noted, consideration of bladder, urethral, ureteral, renal, or uterine trauma is essential. Evaluation for ruptured amniotic membranes, cervical dilatation, vaginal bleeding, and fetal malpresentation is accomplished at this time. Cervical spine and other necessary radiographs are not contraindicated in the pregnant trauma patient. If otherwise indicated, pregnant trauma patients with multiple injuries should be considered candidates for chest and cervical vertebral radiographs. Other immediate investigations may include blood gas analysis, complete blood count, coagulation studies, serum electrolytes, and serum glucose determinations.

Measurement of fetomaternal hemorrhage (FMH) is indicated during the immediate investigation stage (Neufield, 1993). The Kleihauer-Betke acid elution stain (KB) can identify as little as 0.1 mL of fetal cells in the maternal circulation. The incidence of FMH is 4–5-fold higher in pregnant women who have experienced trauma than in uninjured controls. Therefore, 10–30% of pregnant trauma cases have some evidence of fetal–maternal admixture of blood (Goodwin & Breen, 1990; Pearlman et al., 1990b). The Rh-negative gravida who may be carrying an Rh-positive fetus requires Rh-immune globulin (RhIG). In order to calculate the appropriate dose of RhIG in the Rh-negative patient with evidence of FMH (Rose et al., 1985; Lavery & Staten-McCormick, 1995), the following formula may be useful to calculate the volume of fetal cells in maternal circulation:

(Number of fetal cells/number of adult cells) × Maternal red cell volume

One milliliter of RhIG (300 μg) is given for each 15 mL of fetal cells (30 mL of fetal whole blood) detected. The mean volume of FMH is usually less than 15 mL of blood and over 90% exhibit less than 30 mL of FMH. Therefore, in the majority of such patients, 300 μg of RhIG will suffice. Measurement of RhIG in the maternal circulation on the day following administration via indirect Coombs assay should be weakly positive, thereby reflecting some residual "unused" RhIG. If the follow-up indirect Coombs is negative, additional RhIG may be needed (Bowman, 1978, 1994; Bowman et al., 1978; Laml et al., 2001). Finally, even in the absence of detectable fetal cells in the Rh-negative and previously non-immunized trauma victim, administration of a 300 μg dose of RhIG should be considered anyway, given the significant risk of FMH in the presence of trauma coupled with the relatively small amount of fetal blood required to sensitize the Rh-negative mother (Hankins et al., 1995). FMH may also be a marker for occult or active placental abruption or uterine rupture, albeit less reliably than fetal heart rate monitoring or clinical signs (Goodwin & Breen, 1990; Pearlman et al., 1990b).

Secondary survey and treatment

At the conclusion of the primary survey, a second "top to bottom" physical assessment is made. This point in the resuscitation is ideal for a more extensive fetal evaluation. Earlier efforts were aimed at: (i) general evaluation of fetal age and presence of life; (ii) ascertainment of the appropriateness of perimortem cesarean during unsuccessful CPR; (iii) minimizing the effects of uterine compression on maternal resuscitation; and (iv) indirect fetal resuscitation through successful maternal hemodynamic resuscitation. During the secondary survey, however, specific fetal investigations are indicated. Identification of vaginal bleeding, ruptured amniotic membranes, preterm labor, placental abruption, direct uterine or fetal injury, and fetal distress are accomplished.

Fetal evaluation

Fetal injury or death from maternal trauma occurs by several mechanisms. Pearlman and colleagues (1990) noted a 41% fetal loss rate with life-threatening maternal injuries and a 1.6% fetal loss rate with nonlife-threatening maternal injuries. Generally fetal loss is correlated with the severity of maternal injury; but unfortunately, lethal fetal injury can readily occur in absence of significant maternal injury (Fries & Hankins, 1989).

Placental abruption complicates up to 5% of otherwise minor injuries and up to 50% of major injuries during pregnancy (Pearlman et al., 1990a; Neufield, 1993; Esposito, 1994; Vaizey et al., 1994; Hankins et al., 1995). Placental abruption is a frequent cause of fetal death from trauma. The relatively inelastic placenta is thought to shear secondary to deformation of the much more elastic myometrium. Another possible mechanism is that placental abruption from traumatic injury may be a manifestation of placental fracture or laceration —again from decelerative force and/or direct injury (Cunningham et al., 2001a). Uterine tenderness, uterine contractions, vaginal bleeding, and fetal heart rate abnormalities are clinical hallmarks of placental abruption. The association of contractions with placental abruption is a significant one. Williams et al. (1990) studied pregnant trauma patients with electronic fetal monitoring. Placental abruption did not occur in women who did not have uterine contractions, or who had contractions at a frequency of less than one every 10 minutes after 4 hours of fetal monitoring. In patients with more frequent contractions, nearly 20% had placental abruption. Other fetal heart rate abnormalities, such as bradycardia, late decelerations, and tachycardia, were also frequently seen in patients who had experienced abruption. Current evidence suggests that a period of continuous fetal monitoring is usually advisable in most cases of trauma during pregnancy of greater than 22–24 weeks' gestation. In those patients who are clinically unstable, prolonged monitoring is usually indicated (Williams et al., 1990; Hankins et al., 1995; ACOG, 1998). Finally, placental abruption may be associated with a consumptive coagulopathy and, if so, it will be additive to other trauma-associated coagulopathies (Pritchard & Brekken, 1967).

Confident recommendations regarding the duration of electronic fetal heart rate monitoring after maternal trauma are unclear. Delayed manifestation of catastrophic abruption has been reported over 48 hours after trauma (Higgins & Garite, 1987). Fortunately, the majority of catastrophic events occur much sooner. Patients with regular uterine contractions or fetal heart rate abnormalities should be monitored until resolution of such findings. In patients without uterine contractions, or fetal heart rate abnormalities, or other objective signs or symptoms of abruption, it is suggested that a period of 2–6 hours of monitoring will suffice (ACOG, 1998). Electronic fetal monitoring is probably the best tool for detection of abruption in the trauma patient of sufficient gestational age to warrant fetal monitoring. In one large series no abruption was identified unless uterine activity was noted within the first 4 hours of monitoring (Pearlman et al., 1990a). Ultrasonography is not a sensitive enough modality to diagnose many cases of placental abruption (Dahmus & Sibai, 1993; ACOG, 1998).

In the woman actively undergoing resuscitation, continuous electronic fetal monitoring of the potentially viable fetus is a useful indicator of fetal response to and adequacy of resuscitation. Fetal heart rate monitoring has been demonstrated to be an indicator of maternal hypovolemia (Katz et al., 1976). Given the relatively large uteroplacental perfusion requirements during pregnancy, coupled with poor placental autoregulation in the face of hypotension, the fetoplacental unit often may manifest pathophysiologic alterations in the absence of any obvious maternal manifestations of hypovolemia. The risk of fetal loss is directly related to the degree of maternal hemorrhagic shock (Scorpio et al., 1992). Hence, aggressive volume replacement and shock treatment, coupled with continuous electronic fetal monitoring, is indicated in the gravid trauma patient who is otherwise a candidate for fetal monitoring.

The fetal patient

Direct fetal injuries and fractures complicate less than 1% of blunt traumatic injury during pregnancy. Fetal injury is more common in late pregnancy in gravidas with appreciable injuries (Hartl & Ko, 1996; Evrard et al., 1998). The uterus of the early pregnant and nonpregnant patient is well-protected by the bony pelvis. Direct fetal injury from blunt abdominal trauma often involves the fetal skull and brain and is seen in the third trimester in patients with pelvic fractures (Esposito, 1994). This mechanism of injury may be due to the frequent occurrence of engagement of the fetal head within the confines of the bony pelvis late in pregnancy (Palmer & Sparrow, 1994). Decelerative injury to the unengaged fetal head may also occur (Weyerts et al., 1992).

Very few diagnostic or therapeutic interventions are *absolutely* contraindicated in the pregnant trauma victim with life-threatening injuries. While the effects of high doses of ionizing radiation on the fetus may be pronounced, the degree and amount of fetal exposure from routinely obtained conventional or computed tomography (CT) radiography is considerably less. While an absolute lower threshold of safe exposure to ionizing radiation is not known, animal and human data show little or no risk to the fetus from up to 0.1 Gy or more of ionizing radiation (Shepard, 1992; Briss et al., 1994). A single pelvic film delivers less than 0.01 Gy to the fetus. Although fetal exposure is higher with CT scans or pyelography, they should not be avoided if needed to evaluate and treat the mother (Esposito, 1994). Despite the requirement to use fluoroscopy in conjunction with the technique, angiography may also be relatively beneficial to the pregnant trauma patient because of its ability to assist hemostasis (Ben-Menachem et al., 1985). As a general guideline for the practitioner, the maximum recommended dose by the National Council on Radiation Protection During Pregnancy is 0.5 cGy. Exposure levels of less than 5–15 cGy appear to have a relatively low risk of teratogenicity (Bruddage, 2000).

Few medications produce harmful fetal effects, and most teratogens impact only early pregnancy. With the supposition that fetal survival and well-being is directly related to maternal survival and well-being, most medically necessary interventions applied to the pregnant trauma patient are indicated for both maternal and fetal well-being. As a general guide, we would recommend an assessment of the risk versus benefit of medical therapy, and would consult available sources on whatever medications are to be used. One such source is referenced for the reader (Briggs et al., 1998). Tetanus toxoid administration and tetanus immune globulin are not contraindicated in the gravid trauma patient. Administration should be identical to that of the nonpregnant trauma patient.

Most obstetricians are familiar with the benefits and limitations of ultrasound. As stated previously in this chapter, diagnostic ultrasound is not as sensitive as electronic fetal monitoring in the diagnosis of abruption (Fries & Hankins, 1989; Pearlman et al., 1990a; Dahmus & Sibai, 1993). Obstetric ultrasound is useful during the secondary evaluation of the pregnant trauma patient for measurement of fetal biometric indices, screening for direct trauma, and to aid in the biophysical assessment of the fetus. Abdominal ultrasound is very useful in the evaluation of trauma patients. Detection of free fluid or air is possible through the use of ultrasound (Bode et al., 1993). In nonpregnant trauma patients, abdominal ultrasonography demonstrates a sensitivity of 85–99% and a specificity from 97 to 100% for the diagnosis of hemoperitoneum (Healy et al., 1996; Hoyt et al., 2001). At least one recent study suggests that the sensitivity and specificity of abdominal ultrasound for the evaluation of trauma in pregnancy is similar to that in nonpregnant subjects (Goodwin et al., 2001).

Volume resuscitation in pregnancy

Volume replacement in pregnancy merits special consideration. By virtue of young age, and the volume changes inherent in normal pregnancy, the pregnant woman may not exhibit clinically significant symptomatology of blood loss until 1,500–2,000 mL are lost. Blood loss greater than 2,000 mL often produces rapid maternal deterioration. Because fetal status is a sensitive indicator of maternal hemodynamic homeostasis, fetal compromise may occur at maternal blood losses significantly less than 2,000 mL. Fetal heart rate changes may be an early indicator of maternal hypovolemia. Initial treatment of suspected hypovolemia should consist of rapid infusion of isotonic crystalloid solution (normal saline or lactated Ringer's solution). Blood products should be considered in trauma with ongoing hemorrhage greater than 1,000 mL (Esposito, 1994; Mighty, 1994). Type and Rh-specific blood should be available as soon as possible. Until blood is available, isotonic crystalloid solution is replaced at a rate of 3 mL for each milliliter of estimated blood loss. While whole blood may be preferable to packed red blood cells, it is generally not available. Component therapy should not be given empirically, except perhaps in the case of massive exsanguination. Initial resuscitation goals include restoration of maternal vital signs, normalization of fetal heart rate, and resumption of normal urine output. It should be re-emphasized that up to a 20% reduction in uteroplacental blood flow can occur without changes in maternal blood pressure. Maternal resuscitation should be taken in the context of fetal resuscitation during pregnancy (Boba et al., 1966; Jennett et al., 1979).

Perimortem cesarean delivery

Under normal circumstances, cesarean delivery in the trauma patient is reserved for the usual obstetric indications and is performed at gestational ages consistent with fetal viability. Unique clinical circumstances may alter these guidelines somewhat when perimortem cesarean delivery is considered during unsuccessful maternal CPR. Uterine evacuation may be indicated for either maternal or fetal reasons, or both. Due to the inefficiency of CPR in the provision of adequate cerebral and coronary blood flow, prolonged CPR in the nonpregnant individual is rarely successful. Because of aortocaval compression from the uterus after 20–24 weeks' gestation, the significant circulatory shunt produced by the uteroplacental circuit, and the force-vector-mediated degradation of chest compression effectiveness in the laterally-tilted pregnant patient, CPR is likely to be even less effective in the 20+ week pregnant patient (Kuhlmann & Cruikshank, 1994; Moise & Belfort, 1997). This supposition is supported by bupivicaine-induced arrest in animals with aortocaval compression (Kasten & Martin, 1986; Moise & Belfort, 1997). Therefore, during CPR of the 20+ week gravid female, uterine evacuation after 5–10 minutes of unsuccessful resuscitation may be therapeutic for the mother. In Katz's (1986) review of fetal outcome from perimortem cesarean, intact fetal survival was excellent if delivery was accomplished within 5 minutes of arrest. All surviving infants delivered within 5 minutes of maternal arrest were noted to be neurologically intact. Survival and intact survival rates diminished steadily as the interval from arrest or death to delivery increased. Therefore, when there is a living fetus at a potentially viable gestational age, perimortem cesarean delivery should be strongly considered after 4 minutes of unsuccessful CPR (Fig. 36.2). This strategy would potentially allow delivery to occur close to the 5 minute window of intact survival noted by Katz, affording perhaps the best overall balance of risk and benefit to the fetus and mother. Other investigators have made similar recommendations (Morris et al., 1996). Bedside laparotomy and delivery should always be considered during the CPR of any advanced-gestation-age trauma patient. Little equipment beyond gloves and a scalpel is needed. The hypotension from the arrest often results in minimal blood loss from the surgery. Perimortem cesarean delivery should not be delayed to take the patient to an operating room, although a qualified physician should perform the surgery.

Manifestations of trauma during pregnancy

Blunt abdominal trauma

Motor vehicle accidents account for a large portion of severe blunt obstetric trauma. Other causes of blunt abdominal trauma include accidental falls and intentional trauma (violence) (Goodwin & Breen, 1990; Pearlman et al., 1990a; Morris et al., 1996; ACOG, 1998). The fetus is more vulnerable to injury during the third trimester of pregnancy due to the thinning of the uterine wall and a reduction in the amniotic fluid volume (Rothenberger et al., 1978). Fetal head engagement into the maternal pelvis predisposes the fetus to head trauma associated with pelvic lesions (Kimball, 2001).

Motor vehicle accidents produce blunt abdominal trauma in addition to other forms of maternal injury. A recent large retrospective study revealed motor vehicle accidents to be the leading cause of fetal death related to maternal trauma (Weiss, 2001). In motor vehicle accidents, the most common cause of fetal death is maternal death (Crosby & Costiloe, 1971). Expulsion from the vehicle and the presence of coexisting head trauma portend poor maternal and fetal outcome. The value of automobile passenger restraint systems is evident from both fetal and maternal trauma data. Crosby and Costiloe (1971)

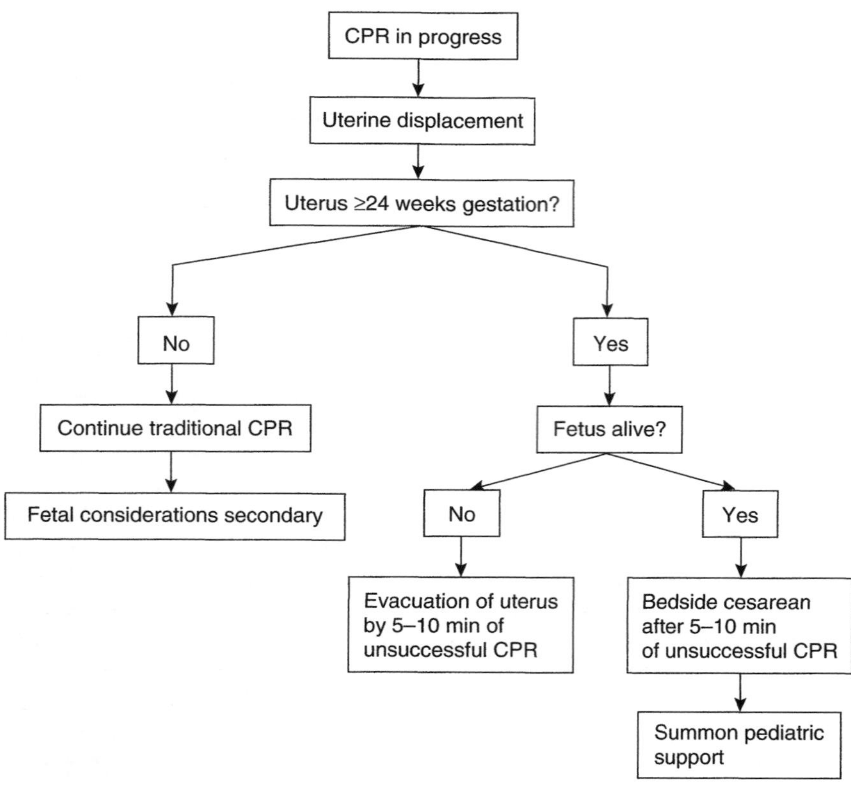

Fig. 36.2 Perimortem cesarean section. CPR, cardiopulmonary resuscitation. (Produced permission from Katz VL, Dotters DJ, Droegemueller W. Perimortem cesarean delivery. Obstet Gynecol 1986;68:571.)

noted a 33% mortality in unrestrained gravid automobile accident victims compared to a 5% mortality in those pregnant victims using two-point restraints (traditional lap belt). The fetal death rate was also lower in the restraint group. The three-point restraint system (lap and shoulder belt) limits "jack-knifing" of the gravid abdomen during sudden deceleration. In a more recent study of motor vehicle accident trauma during pregnancy in which a large majority of restrained victims were using three-point restraint belts, Pearlman and associates (2000) noted that the proper use of seat belts was the best predictor of maternal and fetal outcome in crashes controlled for severity of collision. The impact of air bags is expected to be positive on both maternal and fetal outcome, but thus far there are no data to address this. Overall, it is felt that the use of airbags, in conjunction with proper positioning of the mother, along with correctly placed and used three-point restraints affords the best protection to the pregnant mother and her unborn child. At present, the National Highway Traffic Safety Administration does not consider pregnancy as an indication for deactivation of airbags (NHTSA, 1997). The majority of fetal deaths occur in conjunction with relatively minor maternal injury, and most are due to placental abruption (Agran et al., 1987; Stafford et al., 1988; Lane, 1989; Pearlman, 1995; ACOG, 1998). In addition to abruption, fetal death is also often associated with fetal skull fracture and intracranial hemorrhage (Kimball, 2001). Lap belts should be positioned low across the bony pelvis instead of over the mid or upper uterine fundus. Incorrect placement of the lap belt over the uterine fundus results in an increase in direct force transmission to the uterus during decelerative trauma. The transmission of direct force may result in placental abruption (Bunai et al., 2000). Shoulder belts should be adjusted for comfort to lie across the gravid uterus and be located between the breasts (ACOG, 1998). Although fetal injury and death have been attributed to lap belts, restraint systems are still recommended and in most states are mandatory (Crosby & Costiloe, 1971; Griffiths et al., 1991; Pearce, 1992). Available data from crash test dummy simulations of restrained collision during pregnancy suggests that there does not appear to be extraordinary force transmission to the pregnant uterus when seat belts are properly placed (Pearlman & Viano, 1996).

Up to 40% of severe blunt abdominal trauma is associated with placental abruption but a 2.6% rate of abruption is seen with otherwise "minor" abdominal trauma (Agran et al., 1987; Fries & Hankins, 1989; Lane, 1989; Hankins et al., 1995). Preterm labor is seen *de novo* in approximately 1% of nonlife-threatening abdominal trauma, and is probably more frequent in severe abdominal trauma. As stated earlier in this chapter, contractions are frequently associated with the eventual manifestation of placental abruption. Most patients without clinical evidence of abruption eventually cease to contract (Pearlman, 1995). Severity and mechanism of injury may not directly correlate with the incidence or severity of fetomaternal hemorrhage. Relatively minor direct blunt abdominal trauma may cause placental abruption and/or fetomaternal hemorrhage.

Evaluation of the pregnant patient with blunt abdominal trauma generally is similar to evaluation in the nonpregnant patient, although the presence of the gravid uterus does alter the typical patterns of injury seen in blunt trauma. Bowel injury is less frequent in the pregnant blunt trauma patients when compared to their nonpregnant counterparts (Goodwin & Breen, 1990). Conversely, hepatic and splenic injury are more frequent during pregnancy. Up to 25% of severe blunt trauma patients suffer hemodynamically significant hepatic and/or splenic injuries (Kuhlmann & Cruikshank, 1994). Upper abdominal pain, referred shoulder pain, sudden onset of pain, and elevated transaminases are consistent with injuries to the liver or spleen. Abdominal ultrasound may be an important tool in the evaluation of the gravid patient with blunt abdominal trauma. Ultrasound is particularly useful in the identification of intraperitoneal fluid collections secondary to hemorrhage. The sensitivity and specificity of abdominal ultrasonography to detect intraperitoneal fluid associated with intra-abdominal lesions have been demonstrated to be similar to those seen in nonpregnant individuals. Patients with no intraperitoneal fluid visible by ultrasound are usually at low risk of having intra-abdominal lesions requiring immediate operative management. CT scanning may aid diagnosis in less obvious cases. Hemodynamically stable patients with ultrasound-identified abdominal fluid may have characterization of the fluid source and nature through use of CT scanning (Goodwin et al., 2001; Sirlin et al., 2001). Embolization or hepatic lobe resection, coupled with packing and local control may ameliorate hepatic hemorrhage. Splenectomy is generally the preferred treatment for splenic rupture. Other indications for exploratory laparotomy in the pregnant patient with blunt abdominal trauma include hemodynamic instability with suspected active bleeding, viscus perforation, infection, and fetal distress in the viable gestation. In less severe cases, diagnostic peritoneal lavage (DPL) is as useful in pregnancy as in nonpregnant abdominal trauma patients. During pregnancy, an open technique (analogous to open laparoscopy) in which the lavage catheter is placed in the abdomen to help the operator avoid the enlarged uterus is recommended. Guidelines for a positive DPL are included in Table 36.5. Fetal outcome is not adversely affected by the performance of a DPL during pregnancy.

An important caveat does exist in the evaluation of the pregnant patient with blunt abdominal trauma. Because of maternal volume changes and pregnancy-associated intra-abdominal anatomical alternations, many pregnant patients who ultimately require a laparotomy for intra-abdominal injuries present without significant abdominal signs or symptoms. In one series, 44% of those patients who eventually required laparotomy for intra-abdominal pathology were initially asymptomatic. If maternal hypotension (systolic blood pressure <90 mmHg) and tachycardia are present, they may represent late findings. Consequently, the risk of pregnancy loss is much higher in such cases (Baerga et al., 2000). Rib or pelvic fractures in the pregnant trauma patient should heighten one's suspicion for hepatic, splenic, genitourinary, uterine, or other abdominal injury (Davis et al., 1976; Lavery & Staten-McCormick, 1995). Uterine rupture may occur as a result of abdominal blunt trauma. Patients with other predispositions to uterine rupture (previous cesarean delivery) may be at increased risk. In patients without a surgically scarred uterus, uterine rupture often involves the posterior aspect of the uterus (Kimball, 2001).

Table 36.5 Diagnostic peritoneal lavage

	Positive	Equivocal	Negative
Aspirate			
Blood	>10 mL	>5 mL but <10 mL	<5 mL
Fluid	Enteric fluid	—	—
Lavage		No response	1
RBCs	>100,000/μL	>50,000/μL	>50,000/μL
WBCs	>500/μL	>200/μL but <500/μL	<200/μL
Amylase	>20 IU/L	—	—
Bile	Present	—	—

Open technique recommended during pregnancy. Ten milliliters per kilogram (approximately 1 L) of warmed Ringer's lactate or isotonic normal saline infused and allowed to return to IV base. "Negative" findings must be interpreted in clinical context.
(From McAnena OJ, Moore EE, Marx JA. Initial evaluation of the patient with blunt abdominal trauma. Surg Clin North Am 1990;70:495; and Esposito TJ, Gens DR, Smith CG, Scorpio R. Evaluation of blunt abdominal trauma occurring during pregnancy. J Trauma 1989;29:1628.)

Blunt abdominal trauma is one of the more common results of physical abuse during pregnancy. Between one in six and one in 10 pregnant women will experience physical or sexual abuse during pregnancy. In addition to blunt abdominal trauma, other injuries commonly occur on the face, neck, and proximal extremities. Providers must maintain an index of suspicion for physical or sexual abuse during pregnancy (Satin et al., 1991; Newberger et al., 1992; Parker et al., 1994).

Uterine rupture is a relatively infrequent complication of blunt traumatic injury during pregnancy. The incidence does tend to increase with advancing gestational age and the severity of direct traumatic abdominal force of injury. Most traumatic uterine rupture involves the uterine fundus. Other locations and degrees of uterine injury may be found. At least one case of complete transection of the gravid uterus has been reported as a result of blunt vehicular trauma combined with incorrect seat belt positioning (McCormick, 1968). Principles of management and repair of uterine rupture secondary to trauma are similar to those used in treatment of nontraumatic uterine rupture. Pelvic fractures as a result of blunt trauma during pregnancy may result in significant retroperitoneal bleeding. Regarding delivery route in a future pregnancy, the past presence of a pelvic fracture is not an absolute contraindication for vaginal delivery. Provided pelvic architecture is not substantially disrupted and the old fracture is not unstable, safe vaginal delivery is often possible (Fries & Hankins, 1989).

Penetrating abdominal trauma

The two most common types of penetrating abdominal injury are stab and gunshot wounds. As with blunt trauma, pregnancy often changes the usual manifestations of penetrating abdominal injury. The gravid uterus displaces lower abdominal organs cephalad. Therefore, after the first trimester, the gravid uterus is somewhat protective of other intra-abdominal organs. Accordingly, reported maternal mortality is lower from abdominal gunshot wounds than it is in nonpregnant adults (3.9% versus 12.5%). Fetal mortality (71%), however, is high (Sandy & Koerner, 1989). Reported data from abdominal stab wounds was similar in that fetal mortality was high (42%) and maternal mortality was not seen (Sakala & Kost, 1988). The reduced maternal mortality, yet high fetal loss, from penetrating abdominal injury are probably due to the gravid uterus shielding other abdominal contents from the force of the penetrating projectile when the impact of the shell or penetrating object is below the uterine fundus (Sakala & Kost, 1988; Sandy & Koerner, 1989; Esposito, 1994; Lavery & Staten-McCormick, 1995). Contrawise, upper abdominal penetrating injuries are more likely to produce small bowel injury in advanced gestation than would occur in nonpregnant patients.

Management of gunshot wounds to the pregnant abdomen includes general resuscitation measures outlined previously. Particular attention should be paid to the pathway of the projectile. Entry and exit wounds must both be identified. If the missile has not exited the abdomen, radiographic localization aids bullet location and injury prognostication. Gunshot projectiles that enter into the uterus often will remain in utero. Penetrating trauma occurring anteriorly and above the uterine fundus or from the maternal back carries a high risk of extrauterine visceral injuries. Patients in whom the missile entered anteriorly and below the uterine fundus often do not have maternal visceral involvement (Stone, 1999). Fetal death may be direct or indirect. Most authors recommend abdominal exploration for all extrauterine intra-abdominal gunshot wounds and most intrauterine wounds. Experience from the Middle East conflict and other reports suggests an individualized approach to intrauterine injuries (Del Rossi, 1990; Awwad et al., 1994; Kuhlmann & Cruikshank, 1994). Awwad and colleagues advocate conservative management in anterior abdominal entry wound which enter below the uterine fundus. Posterior abdominal wounds, upper abdominal wounds, fetal or maternal compromise, or uterine location of projectile in cases of gunshot wound are not, according to Awwad, optimal for expectant management. We generally advocate surgical exploration of the pregnant intra-abdominal gunshot wound patients (Grubb, 1992).

Abdominal stab wounds generally are less serious than gunshot wounds. Because of less likelihood for "collateral damage", many pregnant stab wound patients will not have abdominal organ damage that requires surgical repair. Because of the compartmentalization that occurs with advanced pregnancy, the mechanism of injury changes with abdominal stab wounds during pregnancy. Small bowel involvement is more frequent with upper abdominal stab wounds during pregnancy (Stone, 1999; Cunningham et al., 2001a). Also, the upper abdomen is the most frequent site of abdominal stab wounds during pregnancy, comprising some two out of three anterior abdominal penetrating wounds (Kuhlmann & Cruikshank, 1994). Because of the propensity for small intestinal injury and the potentially catastrophic effects of diaphragmatic involvement with up to a 66% mortality with thoracic herniation and strangulation of small intestine, most recommend exploration of upper abdominal stab wounds during pregnancy.

Lower abdominal stab wounds during pregnancy may involve the uterus, fetus, uteropelvic vessels, or urinary bladder. An individualized approach to management is suggested. DPL is useful to evaluate intra-abdominal bleeding (Esposito, 1994). Amniocentesis and ultrasound help in the evaluation of intrauterine bleeding (Esposito, 1994). Urinary bladder involvement may be determined by radiographic evaluation (Kuhlmann & Cruikshank, 1994). Actual abdominal cavity entry can be determined through direct exploration of the wound or the performance of a wound fistulogram (Cornell et al., 1976). While not all lower abdominal stab wounds need to be explored, a very high index of suspicion for the need to explore the abdomen should be maintained.

During exploratory laparotomy for penetrating abdominal trauma, the uterus must be carefully inspected for injury. If direct uterine perforation is noted in the presence of a living term fetus, abdominal delivery is probably warranted. Less extensive uterine or adnexal injury or the presence of intrauterine fetal death does not necessarily dictate evacuation of the uterus (Franger et al., 1989). Likewise, the uterus should not necessarily be emptied via cesarean section or hysterectomy during surgery for nonuterine injuries. In cases in which direct uterine injury is found and the fetus is alive, premature, but potentially viable, cesarean section may be obvious for fetal or maternal hemorrhage or intrauterine infection (Kuhlmann & Cruikshank, 1994; Lavery & Staten-McCormick, 1995; Edwards et al., 2001). These are incredibly difficult cases and will require an assessment of the risk : benefit ratio of expectant management versus delivery by cesarean section specific to the best estimate of gestational age, of fetal injury, and of both the maternal and fetal prognosis if left undelivered.

Other obstetric considerations for delivery also apply in that direct uterine injury to the active uterine segment probably necessitates eventual cesarean section as the preferred route of delivery. Injury to the lower uterine segment with delayed delivery probably needs to be approached on an individual case-by-case basis.

In cases of direct uterine injury, preterm labor may be treated with tocolytics, although betasympathomimetics and nonsteroidal anti-inflammatory agents generally should be avoided because of their effects upon maternal hemodynamics and platelet function, respectively (Hankins, 1991; Caritis et al., 1992). Magnesium sulfate is probably the drug of choice for treatment of preterm labor in the circumstance of maternal trauma. The usual precautions for administration of magnesium sulfate are to be considered with its use in trauma.

Victims of penetrating trauma should receive tetanus prophylaxis as needed. In the previously immunized patient with no booster within the last 5 years, 0.5 mL of tetanus toxoid is administered. If the patient has not been previously immunized, the toxoid is administered in conjunction with tetanus immunoglobulin at a dose of 500 U intramuscularly (Moise & Belfort, 1997).

Chest trauma

Thoracic trauma represents a particular challenge to the clinician caring for the pregnant trauma patient. There is a paucity of information regarding thoracic trauma (or its management) during pregnancy. In the United States, chest trauma accounts for one in four trauma deaths annually. Recognition and stabilization of chest trauma is vital, because less than 10% of blunt chest trauma and less than 30% of penetrating chest injuries require immediate thoracotomy (Ramenofsky et al., 1993; Hoyt et al., 2001). Most cases of thoracic trauma initially respond to nonsurgical stabilization. Effective stabilization ultimately results in improved operative outcome if surgery is required. A basic understanding of the types of chest trauma will help the obstetric member of the trauma team function more effectively in the overall resuscitation of the injured gravida.

Chest trauma can be classified functionally or mechanistically. Mechanistically, thoracic trauma is subdivided into blunt and penetrating injuries (much like abdominal trauma). More immediately important is the recognition of immediately life-threatening chest trauma, with differentiation of life-threatening trauma from potentially serious, but less immediately life-threatening subtypes of chest trauma. In this discussion we will generally divide chest trauma into immediately life-threatening and nonlife-threatening subtypes (Del Rossi, 1990; Ramenofsky et al., 1993).

The primary survey of a trauma patient will identify several types of life-threatening thoracic trauma. When identified, life-threatening injuries require expedient management. Fortunately, many immediately life-threatening injuries can be initially managed by oxygen administration, mechanical ventilation, needle pneumothoracocentesis, or tube thoracostomy (chest tube) placement. Life-threatening chest injuries include airway obstruction, open pneumothorax, massive hemothorax, tension pneumothorax, flail chest, cardiac tamponade, and trauma-mediated severe myocardial dysfunction (Table 36.6) (Ramenofsky et al., 1993).

Airway obstruction should be managed initially as described elsewhere in this text with CPR, and then systematically with early intubation or cricothyroidotomy, if required. Cervical spine protection by neck stabilization and jaw thrust is vital during intubation of any patient with an unevaluated cervical spine. In pregnancy, the additional increased risk of aspiration of gastric contents may necessitate the more aggressive use of endotracheal intubation or surgical airway control. The requirement for oxygenation and effective pulmonary gas exchange precedes all other aspects of resuscitation (Barone et al., 1986; Winchell et al., 1995).

Tension pneumothorax develops when a one-way flow of gas collects in the pleural space. Intrapleural pressure increases progressively with each inspiration. When intrapleural pressure increases to a level higher than great vessel pressures, hemodynamic instability results. The clinical diagnosis of tension pneumothorax is made by a combination of respiratory distress, hypotension, tachycardia, diminished or absent breath sounds, possible jugular venous distention, and tracheal deviation. The differential diagnosis of tension pneumothorax includes massive hemothorax (similar thoracic pathophysiology and treatment) and pericardial tamponade (much less common) (Wilson, 1995). Radiographic confirmation of a suspected tension pneumothorax is usually only useful for postmortem correlation (Weaver et al., 1986).

In addition to trauma, other causes of tension pneumothorax include central line placement, bullous emphysema, and mechanical ventilation. Regardless of its etiology, immediate recognition and treatment of a tension pneumothorax or massive hemothorax is vital. Needle thoracostomy, performed in the second intercostal space–mid-clavicular line, will convert a tension pneumothorax to a simple pneumothorax. Defini-

Table 36.6 Life-threatening chest injuries

Immediately life threatening	Initial treatment
Airway obstruction	Airway control
Open pneumothorax	Injury site control and thoracotomy tube
Tension pneumothorax	Needle thoracostomy
Flail chest	Supportive (± intubation)
Cardiac tamponade	Volume therapy and pericardiocentesis
Severe myocardiac damage	Inotropic support and treatment of dysrhythmias

Qualified consultants should be involved in the care of any chest trauma patient. These treatment recommendations are guidelines. Each case should be individualized.

(Reproduced by permission from American College of Surgeons' Committee on Trauma, from Ramenofsky, et al., eds. Advanced Trauma Life Support (R) for Doctors—1993 Instructor Manual. American College of Surgeons. Chicago: First Impressions, 1993.)

tive treatment is by insertion of a thoracostomy tube in the affected hemithorax. For this indication, a thoracostomy tube is usually placed in the fifth intercostal space (nipple level), anterior to the mid-axillary line (Feliciano, 1992). Additional care during pregnancy must be taken, because of the normally elevated diaphragm (Lavery & Staten-McCormick, 1995). Inadvertent abdominal insertion of a chest tube with the resultant diaphragmatic, hepatic, or splenic injury is potentially more likely during pregnancy. Particular attention to this potentially catastrophic complication must be heeded if additional thoracostomy tubes are placed in locations other than the anterior mid-axillary fifth intercostal space, and especially if such tubes are placed in lower intercostal spaces. To reduce the chance of abdominal placement, consideration should be taken to place the thoracostomy tube at least one interspace higher than usual.

Massive hemothorax is initially treated by thoracostomy tube placement as described. In order to facilitate drainage of thoracic blood, the chest tube should be directed inferiorly (after its insertion in the mid-axillary fifth intercostal space). Once again, care should be taken to avoid abdominal entry. A large chest tube (i.e. No. 38 French) is usually recommended. If the initial volume of blood drained from the tube is ≥1,500 mL, early thoracotomy is probably necessary. Continued loss of 300 mL or more per hour from the chest tube may also indicate the need of a thoracotomy. Other temporizing measures such as volume replacement, transfusion, and potential use of cell-saving autotransfusion should be initiated until the patient is evaluated by a qualified thoracic trauma surgeon (Mattox, 1989; Mansour et al., 1992; Wilson, 1995).

Open pneumothorax is often referred to as a "sucking chest wound." If the size of the opening to the hemothorax is near to or greater than the size of the tracheal diameter, physics dictates that air will preferentially enter the chest through the chest wall rather than through the trachea during inspiratory attempts. Consequently, to temporarily restore effective ventilation, a large occlusive dressing is placed upon the open injury. Ultimately, thoracostomy tube placement at a site distal to the thoracic entry would and surgical repair is required (Hoyt et al., 2001).

Cardiac tamponade has been mentioned previously in our discussion of tension pneumothorax. Tamponade usually occurs with penetrating injuries, and is less common than tension pneumothorax. Catastrophic hypotension and ultimately, pulseless electrical activity (electromechanical disassociation) result from cardiac tamponade. Because of noncompliance of the pericardial sac, a relatively small amount of rapidly collected blood will cause hemodynamic compromise. Diagnosis is possible in some cases by clinical features of Beck's triad (venous pressure elevation, decreased arterial pressure, and muffled heart tones), radiographic examination (enlarged cardiac silhouette), or echocardiography. Unfortunately, as with tension pneumothorax, time is often not available to definitively diagnose cardiac tamponade. Pericardiocentesis by a qualified operator is a lifesaving temporizing measure. Rapid volume infusion will also often temporarily alleviate the problem. As with thoracostomy tube placement, pericardiocentesis should be undertaken with recognition of the fact that the pregnant patient's diaphragm is normally elevated. Definitive treatment of pericardiocentesis is usually by the opening of the pericardium by a qualified thoracic trauma surgeon (Shoemaker et al., 1970; Shoemaker, 1975).

Flail chest is secondary to trauma-mediated separation of a part of the bony chest wall from the remaining thorax. Respiratory failure from pain-induced atelectasis and underlying pulmonary contusion is produced by flail chest (Reul et al., 1973). Paradoxical movement of part of the chest during respiration, direct physical examination of the chest, and radiographic evaluation lead to the diagnosis of this condition. Intubation and mechanical ventilation may be required in the flail chest patient with intractable hypoxemia or other injuries (Trinkle et al., 1975; Sankaran & Wilson, 1976).

Massive chest trauma can produce intrinsic myocardial damage. Myocardial contusion, myocardial ischemia from hypoperfusion, or underlying substance abuse all may cause or contribute to myocardial injury (Paone et al., 1993). Although usually diagnosed during the secondary survey, potentially lethal dysrhythmias can also be noted during the primary survey. These dysrhythmias may be produced by the initial injury or from reperfusion of injured myocardium. Standard treatment of such dysrhythmias it recommended to reduce the likelihood of malignant degeneration of the rhythm or cardiac arrest (Sankaran & Wilson, 1976; Frazee et al, 1986; Mattox et al., 1992).

The secondary survey may also uncover evolving life-threatening thoracic injuries, albeit *usually* the progression of such injuries is less fulminant than when they are diagnosed during the primary survey. Potentially lethal secondary survey injuries include pulmonary contusion, myocardial contusion, aortic disruption, esophageal disruption, tracheal or bronchial rupture, and traumatic diaphragmatic rupture (Ramenofsky et al., 1993).

Pulmonary contusion is a very frequent complication of blunt chest trauma (Hoyt et al., 2001). Progressive hypoxemia results from the secondary effects of the contusion. Typically, respiratory failure from pulmonary contusion progresses insidiously and is often not immediately present. A diffuse radiographic injury pattern is characteristic of pulmonary contusion. Careful clinical monitoring, frequent blood gas analysis, and a low threshold for intubation and mechanical ventilation in the patient with a severe pulmonary contusion help reduce mortality (Stellin, 1981; Ramenofsky et al., 1993).

Myocardial contusion may initiate malignant dysrhythmias as a delayed event. Ischemia, new onset bundle branch block, presence of ventricular or supraventricular dysrhythmias, and pure myocardial pump failure in the victim of severe thoracic trauma should heighten the suspicion for myocardial contusion (Mattox et al., 1992; Paone et al., 1993). Continuous ECG monitoring is suggested in any patient felt to be predisposed to the sequelae of myocardial contusion (Wilson, 1995). Prompt recognition and treatment may prevent hemodynamic deterioration. Diagnosis is by electrocardiogram or echocardiography.

The increased frequency of traumatic diaphragmatic rupture in association with upper abdominal injury during pregnancy needs to be considered in any pregnant chest or upper abdominal trauma patient (Ramenofsky et al., 1993).

Traumatic aortic rupture frequently occurs in conjunction with motor vehicle accidents or falls from great heights (Ramenofsky et al., 1993; Stone, 1999). Aortic rupture mechanistically occurs from the relative fixation of the aorta, thereby reducing its ability to move or flex with sudden deceleration. Tearing of one or more of the layers of the vessel is produced. Aortic rupture is often initially associated with only modest hypotension, especially with lesions near the ligamentum arteriosum. With aortic rupture, those patients with unconfined lesions or transection usually exsanguinate before or shortly after arrival to the hospital while patients with contained hematomas are more frequently alive at hospital presentation. Diagnosis of the contained aortic rupture may be difficult. Mediastinal widening, obliteration of the aortic knob, or first or second rib fractures suggest an increased probability of aortic rupture (Mattox, 1989). Ultrasound, magnetic resonance imaging, or CT may assist in the diagnosis of aortic rupture, but angiography is ultimately the diagnostic procedure for traumatic aortic rupture (Ramenofsky et al., 1993). Once again, any needed radiographic studies are not to be deferred in the severely-ill pregnant trauma patient.

Tracheobronchial tree injuries (TBI) may produce sudden airway obstruction. A high clinical index of suspicion, especially in cases of refractory pneumothorax, subcutaneous emphysema, or blast injuries is necessary for timely diagnosis. Operative intervention is frequently necessary in patients with TBI (Taskinen et al., 1989; Scorpio et al., 1992; Wilson, 1995).

Esophageal trauma is often an insidious feature of chest trauma. It is usually, but not always, associated with penetrating chest trauma. Esophageal rupture is suspected in any patient with severe epigastric injury, substernal trauma, pneumothorax without chest wall injury, and/or in patients with continued particulate material in their thoracostomy tube drainage. Esophagoscopy or contrast studies confirm the diagnosis. Death may result directly from hemorrhage or from unrelenting mediastinitis (Tilanus et al., 1991; Jones & Ginsberg, 1992).

While thoracic trauma should be evaluated by a thoracic specialist familiar with chest trauma management, an understanding of the ramifications of potentially lethal chest trauma often will allow the obstetrician to recognize and stabilize the chest trauma patient.

Head trauma

Approximately 50% of all trauma deaths are associated with head injury. Over 60% of motor vehicle associated trauma deaths occur as a result of head trauma (Scorpio et al., 1992). In a recent review of pregnant trauma deaths in Cook County (Illinois), approximately 10% of maternal trauma deaths were directly due to head injury (Fildes et al., 1992).

Several aspects of cranial and cerebral physiology and pathophysiology are very important in head trauma patients. The brain is one of the most carefully protected organs of the body; the calvarium and cerebrospinal fluid cushion the brain from minor trauma. However, in severe trauma, these two otherwise protective features may contribute to or precipitate brain injury. The brain, with limited metabolic reserve, has poor tolerance of diminished perfusion. Global cerebral oxygen consumption of at least 1.5 mL/100 g/min must be maintained to prevent injury. Oxygen delivery to the brain is determined by blood pressure, blood oxygen content, blood flow distribution, and relative perfusion pressure. Because the closed space of the calvarium is occupied by blood, cerebrospinal fluid, and brain volume, intracranial pressure is a function of all three components, referred to as the Monro-Kellie doctrine. Cerebral edema results in increased brain volume, thereby producing elevated intracranial pressure. Traumatic collections of blood in the cranial vault will similarly increase intracranial pressure. Often, both of these mechanisms are present in the head trauma patient (Hayek & Veremakis, 1991).

Cerebral autoregulation is normally maintained over a wide range of blood pressure. Extremes of blood pressure, such as hypotension found in the multiple trauma patient, tax the brain's ability to autoregulate. When coupled with cerebral edema and/or intracranial bleeding, hypotension further aggravates the inability of the brain to autoregulate. Furthermore, the injured brain may lose its ability to autoregulate, yet another mechanism for self-perpetuation of brain injury. Finally, because the cranium is a closed system, propagation of elevated extravascular cerebral pressure transmurally causes the driving pressure in the cerebral circulation to be significantly decreased. In that flow is directly determined by a change in pressure, diminished cerebral perfusion pressure (mean arterial blood pressure – intracranial pressure) causes decreased effective cerebral blood flow. Cerebral mass lesions will therefore diminish cerebral perfusion pressure in proportion to their size even in the face of normal blood pressure. It should thus be obvious that acute brain injury is often self-perpetuating and in evolution and is poorly tolerated by the fastidious neuronal cells. Cell death and permanent injury may result. The therapeutic goal of acute cerebral resuscitation is to limit cell death by regulated reperfusion to nonfunctioning, but still viable brain tissue (*ischemic penumbra*). The clinician's ability to accomplish this goal is often limited (Maset et al., 1987; Hayek & Veremakis, 1991; Robertson et al., 1992).

Another feature of brain injury is the concept of secondary, or reperfusion, injury. An initial insult produces the loss of autoregulation described above. Unfortunately, reperfusion of the injured area may occur in the presence of absent or diminished autoregulation. Injury is either mechanically (through edema) or metabolically (through inappropriate substrate production) produced through reperfusion (Bruce et al., 1973; Smith et al., 1990; Hayek & Veremakis, 1991).

In order to avoid or limit permanent cerebral injury, specific cerebral resuscitation must be carried out in the head trauma patient. The sooner resuscitation is begun, the greater the chance injured, but living, neuronal tissue will survive.

Penetrating head injuries produce injury by obvious mechanisms. With blunt head trauma, especially in deceleration events, movement of the brain occurs first in one direction with a secondary rebound movement in the opposite direction producing a *coup–countercoup* effect. Closed head injuries can occur without significant injury of the cutaneous tissues and calvarium through bruising or contusion of the brain at *coup* or *countercoup* sites. Intracerebral hemorrhage from traumatic brain injury often results from severe contusion. Subdural or epidural hematomas are produced by direct laceration or tearing of subdural or epidural vessels, respectively (Scorpio et al., 1992).

Initial management of suspected brain injury starts with the basic "ABCs" discussed previously. Profound hypotension, defined as systolic blood pressure less than 60 mmHg in non-pregnant individuals, may cause or contribute to altered consciousness. Correction of hypotension is important. While possible, hypotension as a result of the neurologic insult is uncommon. Until proven otherwise, hypotension in the presence of head injury is from other causes. Severe hypertension in the comatose trauma patient may be centrally mediated. This "Cushing Response" is also characterized by bradycardia and a diminished respiratory rate (Hayek & Veremakis, 1991). Altered levels of consciousness may also be produced by alcohol or drug ingestion. Toxicological assessment is recommended in most trauma patients with altered levels of consciousness. Conversely, an altered level of consciousness should never be totally attributed to alcohol or other drug ingestion alone unless completely proven otherwise. Finally, other medical conditions such as hypoglycemia may occasionally be seen coincidental with trauma.

A baseline and ongoing mental assessment is necessary as a frame of reference in all trauma patients (Scorpio et al., 1992). The "A-V-P-U" mini exam (Fig. 36.1) is a brief primary survey tool. In the secondary survey, more extensive evaluation, such as by the GCS is recommended (Table 36.4) (Teasdale & Jennett, 1974). A score of 8 or less is indicative of the diagnosis of coma and is classified as severe head injury (Baxt & Moody, 1987; Rutherford & Nelson, 1995). If the GCS is from 9 to 12, the injury is classified as moderate. GCS scores greater than 12 are classified as minor head injuries (Jordan, 1994). Once again, the GCS and other neurologic examinations need to be performed frequently so trends in neurologic response can be identified. A decrease in the GCS score of 2 or more points is indicative of deterioration (Scorpio et al., 1992; Kuhlmann & Cruikshank, 1994). Irrespective of the GCS score, unequal pupils, unequal motor findings, open head injury with leaking cerebrospinal fluid or exposed brain tissue, and/or the presence of a depressed skull fracture also indicate severe head injury. Finally, if headache severity dramatically increases, pupillary size increases unilaterally, or lateralizing weakness is noted to develop, particular concern is warranted.

Appropriate immediate investigations of the head trauma victim may include roentgenograms (X-ray), CT and neurologic or neurosurgical consultation. Sedation and/or paralysis is delayed until the consultant examines the patient, if possible. Generally, all patients with moderate or severe head injury should be radiographically evaluated for cervical spine fracture. Conversely, skull roentgenograms are often not helpful (Scorpio et al., 1992) as physical examination or CT imaging provides higher quality data. CT imaging is a vital tool in the evaluation of head injuries and except for women with minor injuries, all head-injured patients require CT imaging. Severe injury dictates imaging as soon as possible. However, it is important to adequately monitor the patient while she undergoes imaging. Once C-spine fractures are ruled out, the 20+ week gestation pregnant patient is placed in left lateral tilt during the scanning (Kuhlmann & Cruikshank, 1994). Head injuries can be simply classified into the categories of diffuse brain injury, focal brain injury, and skull fractures (Table 36.7) (Scorpio et al., 1992).

Diffuse brain injury can be classified as a concussion or diffuse axonal injury. Concussion is produced from widespread brief interruption of global brain function. Although confusion, headache, dizziness, etc., are often present in the recovering concussion victim, any persistent neurological abnormalities in the patient with a presumed concussion must be investigated for other etiologies. Many authors feel that the

Table 36.7 Classification of acute head trauma

- I Diffuse brain injury
  - A Concussion
  - B Diffuse axonal injury
- II Focal brain injury
  - A Contusion
  - B Hemorrhage/hematoma
    - 1 Parenchymal hemorrhage
    - 2 Meningeal hemorrhage/hematoma
      - a Acute epidural hemorrhage/hematoma
      - b Subarachnoid hemorrhage/hematoma
- III Skull fractures
  - A Simple fracture
  - B Basilar skull fracture
  - C Depressed skull fracture

patient with 5 minutes or more of lost consciousness should be observed in the hospital for at least 24 hours (Hoff et al., 1991; Jordan, 1994). Diffuse axonal injury (DAI), more commonly known as "closed head injury" is produced by widespread global brain injury or the cerebral edema resulting from diffuse brain injury (Adams et al., 1982). Prolonged coma is the hallmark of DAI. CT imaging will show cerebral edema without focal lesions. Nearly 50% of coma-producing brain injuries are caused by DAI. DAI is classified clinically into mild, moderate, and severe categories (Judy, 2001). Severe DAI carries a 50% mortality. Long-term supportive care and control of intracranial hypertension are the only treatment for the condition. Partial or complete recovery is possible, but permanent coma ("chronic vegetative state") is often an inexorable consequence of severe DAI (Hoff et al., 1991).

Focal brain injuries are those in which damage occurs in a relatively local area. Types of focal brain injury include contusions, hemorrhages, and hematomas. Because focal injuries may produce a mass effect and damage underlying normal brain tissue, rapid diagnosis and treatment of focal brain injuries may improve outcome and recovery.

Contusions are usually caused by deceleration *coup–countercoup* trauma as previously described. Although contusions can occur anywhere, they are most commonly found in the tips of the frontal and temporal lobes. In addition to producing deficits from focal injury, delayed bleeding and edema can produce injury from mass effects (Kuhlmann & Cruikshank, 1994). Prolonged observation is recommended. If neurologic deterioration is detected and is thought to be from a mass effect, surgery may be indicated.

Hemorrhages and hematomas can be functionally classified into those occurring in the meningeal or parenchymal regions of the brain. Parenchymal hemorrhage includes intracerebral hematomas, impalement injuries and missile (bullet) wounds. Meningeal hemorrhage is further classified as acute epidural hemorrhage, acute subdural hematoma, or subarachnoid hemorrhage.

Acute epidural hemorrhage (AEH) usually occurs from tears in the middle meningeal artery. Although found in 1% or less of coma-producing acute brain injuries, AEH can be rapidly progressive and fatal. Figure 36.3 describes the usual sequence of events associated with AEH. It is important to note that the patient with AEH may display an intervening period of lucidity prior to a rapid deterioration from massive rebleeding of the lesion (Adams et al., 1982). If surgically treated early, the prognosis is good (91% survival) (Scorpio et al., 1992). If not evacuated until hemiparesis and pupil fixation, the prognosis is poor. AEH is, in effect, "the vasa previa" of acute brain injury. Rapid recognition and treatment yields markedly improved results.

Subarachnoid hemorrhage (SAH) produces bleeding in the subarachnoid space. Meningeal irritation occurs with the resulting symptoms of headache and/or photophobia. Because the subarachnoid space is much larger than the epidural space, bleeding does not usually rapidly progress to death. Although bloody spinal fluid is a hallmark of SAH, CT scanning has basically replaced lumbar puncture in the diagnosis of SAH. Evacuation is rarely required; treatment is supportive. Meningeal irritation can produce unwanted cerebral artery vasospasm. Treatment of cerebral artery vasospasm involves volume loading and control of hypertension with calcium-channel blocker therapy (nimodipine). Refractory treatment of vasospasm has been advocated by the use of angiographically instilled papaverine or direct balloon angioplasty (American Nimodipine Study Group, 1992; Judy, 2001).

Acute subdural hematoma (SDH) is one of the more common causes of serious brain hemorrhage and commonly occurs from rupture of bridging veins between the cerebral cortex and dura. Direct laceration of the brain or cortical arteries also can produce SDH (Gennarelli & Thibault, 1982). The clinical presentation of SDH often depends upon the rapidity of expansion of the hematoma. Rapidly expanding hematomas carry a poorer prognosis than do stable, chronic SDHs. Early evacuation of rapidly growing SDHs may favorably impact the 60% mortality that SDH carries (Scorpio et al., 1992). Others advocate early (within 4 hours of injury) evacuation of subdural hematomas greater than 1 cm in diameter that are associated with shift of midline brain structures. Patients with subdural hematomas of less than 5 mm with only mild or absent neurologic symptoms may be candidates for expectant management.

Intracerebral hematomas can develop anywhere in the brain. Symptoms and outcome depend upon the size and location. Intraventricular and intracerebellar hemorrhages portend poor outcome. With impalement injuries the missile or projectile should be left in place until neurosurgical evaluation is obtained. Bullet wounds should be mapped as to entrance and potential exit. Skull films may help the localization process of any remaining missile fragments. Non-penetrating bullet wounds may result in significant blunt trauma (Bullock & Teasdale, 1990).

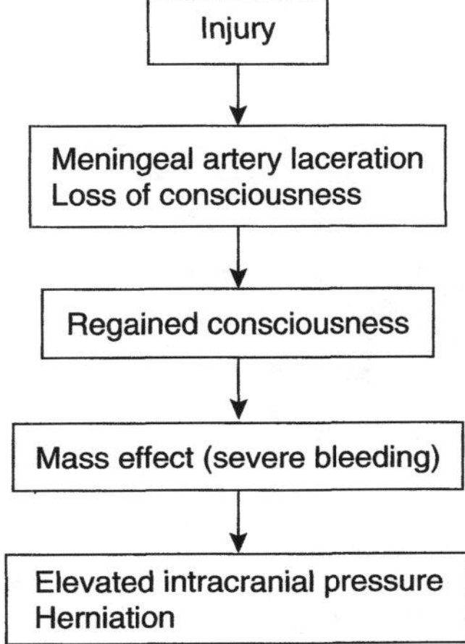

Fig. 36.3 Sequence of events associated with acute epidural hemorrhage.

Skull fractures are relatively common and may or may not be associated with severe brain injury. Because skull fractures may be an indicator that significant energy dispersal occurred on the cranial vault, most patients with seemingly uncomplicated skull fractures should still be observed in the hospital with serial neurosurgical evaluations.

Different types of skull fractures deserve specific considerations. Linear nondepressed skull fractures that traverse suture lines or vascular arterial grooves may be associated with epidural hemorrhage. Depressed skull fractures may require operative elevation of the bony fragment. Open skull fractures nearly always require early operative intervention. Basilar skull fractures may not immediately be apparent. Anterior basilar skull fractures may predispose to inadvertent placement of a nasogastric tube into the intracranial space (Scorpio et al., 1992).

Skull fractures are evaluated initially with cranial CT and physical exam. Skull X-rays may subsequently be useful. Attempt at precise delineation of skull fractures should not delay recognition and treatment of other head injuries.

Mainstays in the treatment of head trauma include maintenance of brain perfusion, reduction of cerebral edema, elimination or reduction of hemorrhage, and prevention of infection. Patients with evolving symptomatology or unremitting coma need to be evaluated immediately for potential neurosurgical intervention. Maintenance of normal arterial blood pressure will aid the often impaired cerebral autoregulation seen with head trauma. Normalization of blood glucose will help supply cerebral metabolic needs. Hyperglycemia is to be avoided, as it is as undesirable as hypoglycemia (Bullock & Ward, 1995).

Figure 36.4 outlines a general schemata for severe head injury triage and features of high-, moderate-, and low-risk lesions. It should be noted that a lateralizing defect and GCS ≤ 8 requires immediate evaluation for surgical treatment. Intracranial pressure (ICP) monitoring has been long advocated as a measure to improve outcome in traumatic brain injury. Controversies regarding indications and effectiveness of ICP monitoring are evident. Current consensus recommendations propose ICP monitoring be used in comatose patients with GCS scores of ≤8 after resuscitation who also demonstrate pathologic CT radiographic abnormalities. In those patients with a GCS of ≤8 without CT abnormalities, ICP monitoring is indicated if two or more of the following are present: age >40 years, unilateral or bilateral posturing, and systolic blood pressure less than 90 mmHg at any time since injury (Muizelaar et al., 1983; Brain Trauma Foundation, 2000b). Abnormal ICP is medically treated with controlled hyperventilation, mannitol administration, barbiturate coma, loop diuretics, volume restriction, and head up positioning (Scorpio et al., 1992; Bullock & Ward, 1995; Brain Trauma Foundation, 2000a). When ICP monitoring is employed,

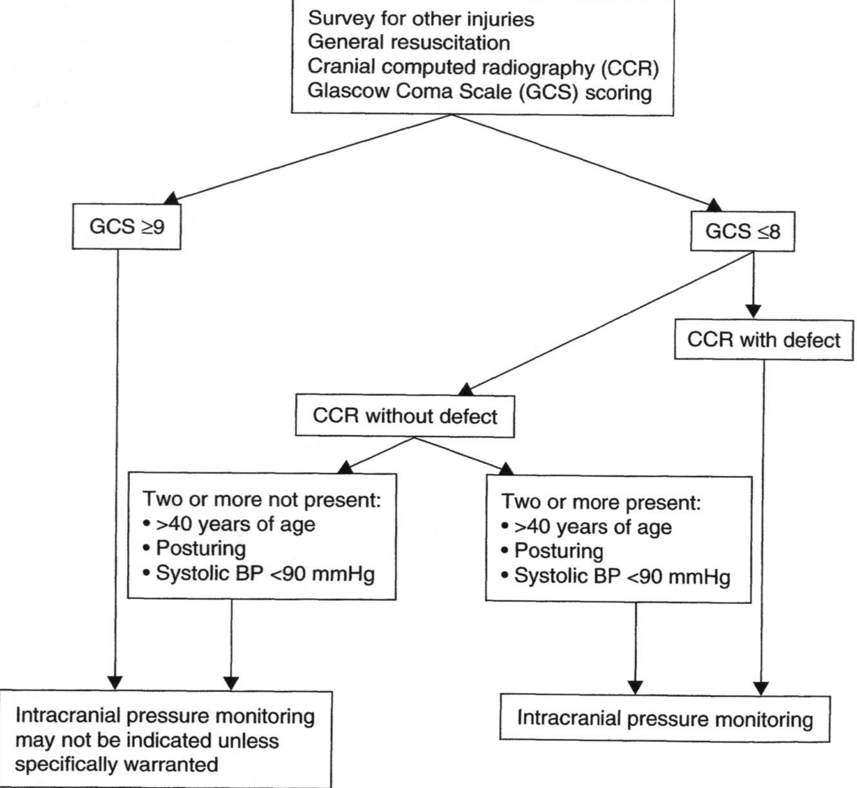

Fig. 36.4 Initial evaluation of the comatose trauma patient. Neurosurgical consultation is liberally indicated during the evaluation of the comatose trauma patient. A lateralizing defect with GCS ≤8 may necessitate expedited surgical exploration (sources as referenced in text).

measurements above 20–25 mmHg generally necessitate treatment strategies to lower ICP (Gennarelli & Thibault, 1982; Durbin, 2001).

Hyperventilation works to transiently decrease ICP by reducing cerebral blood flow. If used, hyperventilation should be undertaken to a $P_{a}CO_2$ endpoint of 26–28 mmHg (Enevoldsen & Jensen, 1978), although the appropriate level for pregnancy is not established. Hyperventilation is *not* effective in "prophylaxis" against elevated ICP (Muizelaar et al., 1991). If hyperventilation is abruptly discontinued, ICP may rise rapidly. Current data refutes the long-held clinical practice of using aggressive hyperventilation for the treatment or prevention of intracranial hypertension. In nonpregnant patients, sustained hyperventilation is associated with worse outcome which is probably mediated through reduction in cerebral blood flow in normal brain parenchyma surrounding damaged neural tissue. Hyperventilation is no longer recommended; the modality should be avoided, if possible, within the first 24 hours following acute brain injury. If used at all, the technique is reserved for temporary treatment of severe intractable intracranial hypertension (Brain Trauma Foundation, 2000b). The effects of normal pregnancy (compensated respiratory alkalosis) on CO_2-mediated regulation of cerebral blood flow are not known.

Mannitol functions as a hyperosmotic diuretic. Doses of 0.5–1.0 g/kg body weight are typically used as primary treatment of intracranial hypertension (Muizelaar et al., 1983). Frequent monitoring of serum osmolality is needed and mannitol should be withheld if osmolality is greater than 315–320 mosmol/L. Treatment may be directed at maintaining ICP at less than 20–25 mmHg. Alternatively, cerebral perfusion pressure (CPP = mean arterial pressure – ICP) directed treatment may be instituted using mannitol and peripheral vasoconstrictors to increase mean peripheral arterial pressure. At present, there is no standard recommendation for CPP nor is there a recommendation as to the most effective way for achieving a particular CPP treatment endpoint (Durbin, 2001). Mannitol can theoretically affect uteroplacental perfusion and/or fetal volume homeostasis. However, given the grave circumstances for which mannitol is used in severe head trauma, the benefits of its administration far outweigh these risks (Kuhlmann & Cruikshank, 1994). Diuresis with furosemide or other loop diuretics may also be used. Overhydration, especially with hypotonic solutions, should be avoided. Head-up positioning at 20° may marginally reduce hydrostatic pressure (Bullock & Ward, 1995).

Barbiturate coma has been utilized as a treatment of refractory intracranial hypertension. The technique probably works by reducing cerebral oxygen consumption (Bullock & Ward, 1995; Brain Trauma Foundation, 2000c; Durbin, 2001). Corticosteroids are not indicated for therapy of cerebral edema from trauma (Dearden et al., 1986; Rutherford & Nelson, 1995). Other less successful treatments of refractory intracranial hypertension include hypothermia, decompressive craniotomy, hypertonic saline, and a variety of investigational neuroprotective agents. Research is ongoing in this area of neurotrauma.

The best route of delivery in the patient with acute brain injury is controversial. The only large series of data germane to the delivery of the pregnant head trauma patient without surgical correction of a specific bleeding site involves uncorrected ruptured cerebral aneurysms (Hunt et al., 1974). The investigation of 142 cases of *nontraumatic* subarachnoid hemorrhage led to the conclusion that vaginal delivery was not contraindicated. Importantly, stable *nontraumatic* cerebral injuries may behave quite differently from cases in which acute brain injury occurs (Hunt et al., 1974). We generally favor ICP monitoring for the at-risk head trauma patient undergoing labor and vaginal or cesarean delivery. We also liberally use cesarean section in such patients with team management by obstetricians, neurosurgeons, and obstetric anesthesiologists.

Rapid diagnosis, early neurosurgical intervention, and meticulous attention to support measures offer the best hope for a good outcome in patients with severe brain injuries. Co-management with consultants, appropriate and timely use of cranial CT, and serial neurologic examination may reduce mortality and morbidity in brain trauma. Improvement in maternal outcome offers the best hope for improved fetal outcome.

Conclusion

Trauma during pregnancy poses a special and immediate challenge to the obstetrician and to the emergency room provider. Generally speaking, most diagnostic and therapeutic modalities relating to trauma care should not be avoided or modified during pregnancy. Co-management, with input from obstetric and nonobstetric services, functions to insure appropriate care of the pregnant trauma patient and her fetus.

References

Adams J, Graham D, Murray L, et al. Diffuse axonal injury due to nonmissile head injury in humans: An analysis of 45 cases. Ann Neurol 1982;12:557–563.

Agran PF, Dunkle DE, Winn DG, Kent D. Fetal death in motor vehicle accidents. Ann Emerg Med 1987;16:1355–1358.

Alaily AB, Carrol KB. Pulmonary ventilation in pregnancy. Br J Obstet Gynaecol 1978;85:518–524.

American College of Obstetricians and Gynecologists. Obstetric aspects of trauma management. Technical Bulletin Number 251;1998.

American Nimodipine Study Group. Clinical trial of nimodipine in acute ischemic stroke. Stroke 1992;23:3–8.

Astarita DC, Feldman B. Seat belt placement resulting in uterine rupture. J Trauma 1997;42:738–740.

Awwad JT, Azar GB, Seoud MA, Mroueh AM, Karam KS. High-velocity penetrating wounds of the gravid uterus: Review of 16 years of civil war. Obstet Gynecol 1994;83:259–264.

Baerga VY, Zietlow S, Scott P, Bannom M, Harsem W, Illstrup D. Trauma in Pregnancy. Mayo Clinic Proc 2000;75(12):1243–1248.

Barone JE, Pizzi WS, Nealon TF Jr, et al. Indications for intubation in blunt chest trauma. J Trauma 1986;26:334–338.

Baxt WG, Moody P. The differential survival of trauma patients. J Trauma 1987;27:602–606.

Bellina JH, Dougherty CM, Mickal A. Pyeloureteral dilatation and pregnancy. Am J Obstet Gynecol 1976;108:356–363.

Ben-Menachem Y, Handel SF, Ray RD, et al. Embolization procedures in trauma, a matter of urgency. Semin Intervent Radiol 1985;2:107.

Boba A, Linkie DM, Plotz EJ. Effects of vasopressor administration and fluid replacement on fetal bradycardia and hypoxia induced by maternal hemorrhage. Obstet Gynecol 1966;27:408–413.

Bode PJ, Niezen RA, van Vost AB, et al. Abdominal ultrasound as a reliable indicator for conclusive laparotomy in blunt abdominal trauma. J Trauma 1993;34:27–31.

Bowman JM. Management of Rh-isoimmunization. Obstet Gynecol 1978;52:1–16.

Bowman JM. Hemolytic disease (erythroblastosis fetalis). In: Creasy RK, Resnik R, eds. Maternal Fetal Medicine—Principles and Practice, 3rd edn. Philadelphia: WB Saunders, 1994:711–743.

Bowman JM, Chown B, Lewis M, et al. Rh-isoimmunization during pregnancy: Antenatal prophylaxis. Can Med Assoc J 1978; 118:623–627.

Brain Trauma Foundation. The American Association of Neurological Surgeons. The joint section on neurotrauma and critical care. Intracranial pressure treatment threshold. J Neurotrauma 2000a;17: 493–495.

Brain Trauma Foundation. The American Association of Neurological Surgeons. The joint section on neurotrauma and critical care. Hyperventilation. J Neurotrauma 2000b;17:513–520.

Brain Trauma Foundation. The American Association of Neurological Surgeons. The joint section on neurotrauma and critical care. Critical pathway for the treatment of established intracranial hypertension. J Neurotrauma 2000c;17:537–538.

Briggs GG, Freeman RK, Yaffe SJ. Drugs In Pregnancy and Lactation, 5th edn. Philadelphia: Lippincott Williams & Wilkins, 1998.

Briss GG, Freeman RK, Jaffe SJ. A Reference Guide to Fetal and Neonatal Risk—Drugs in Pregnancy and Lactation, 4th edn. Baltimore: Williams and Wilkins, 1994.

Bruce DA, Langfitt TW, Miller JD, et al. Regional cererbral blood flow, intracranial pressure, and brain metabolism in comatose patients. J Neurosurg 1973;38:131–144.

Bruddage SI, Davies JK, Jurkovich GJ. Trauma to the pregnant patient. In: Grenvik A, Ayers SM, Holbrook PR, Shoemaker WC, eds. Critical Care, 4th edn. Philadelphia: WB Saunders, 2000:383–391.

Bullock R, Teasdale GM. Surgical management of traumatic intracranial hematomas. In: Breakman R, ed. Handbook of Clinical Neurology—Head Injury. Amsterdam: Elsevier, 1990:259–297.

Bullock R, Ward JD. Management of head trauma. In: Ayres SM, Granuik A, Holbrook PR, Shoemaker WC, eds. Textbook of Critical Care. Philadelphia: WB Saunders, 1995:1449–1457.

Bunai Y, Nagai A, Nakamura I, Ohya I. Fetal death from abruptio placentae associated with incorrect use of a seatbelt. Am J Forensic Med Pathol 2000;21(3):207–209.

Burrows RF, Kelton JG. Incidentally detached thrombocytopenia in healthy mothers and their infants. N Engl J Med 1988;319:142–145.

Caritis SN, Kuller JA, Watt-Morse ML. Pharmacologic options for treating preterm lator. In: Rayburn WF, Zuspan FP, eds. Drug Therapy in Obstetrics and Gynecology, 3rd edn. St Louis: Mosby Year Book, 1992:74–89.

Chesley LC, Valenti C, Uichano L. Alterations in body fluid compartments and exchangeable sodium in early puerperium. Am J Obstet Gynecol 1959;77:1054.

Clark SL, Cotton DB, Lee W, et al. Central hemodynamic assessment of normal term pregnancy. Am J Obstet Gynecol 1989;161:1439.

Committee on Trauma: Resources for optimal care of the injured patient. Chicago, American College of Surgeons, 1999.

Cornell WP, Ebert PA, Zuidema GD. X-ray diagnosis of penetrating wounds of the abdomen. J Surg Res 1976;5:142.

Crosby WM, Costiloe JP. Safety of lap belt restraints for pregnant victims of automobile collisions. N Engl J Med 1971;284:632–636.

Cunningham FG, Gant N, Leveno KJ, Gilstrap LC, Hauth JC, Wenstrom KD. Maternal adaptations to pregnancy. In: Williams Obstetrics, 21st edn. Norwalk, CT: Appleton and Lange, 2001a:167–200.

Cunningham FG, Gant N, Leveno KJ, Gilstrap LC, Hauth JC, Wenstrom KD. Renal and urinary tract disorders. In: Williams Obstetrics, 21st edn. Norwalk, CT: Appleton and Lange, 2001b:1251–1272.

Dahmus MA, Sibai BM. Blunt abdominal trauma: Are there predictive factors for abruptio placentae or maternal-fetal distress? Am J Obstet Gynecol 1993;169:1054–1059.

Davis JJ, Cohn I, Nance FC. Diagnosis and management of blunt abdominal trauma. Ann Surg 1976;183:672–678.

Davison JS, Davison MC, Hay DM. Gastric emptying time in late pregnancy and labor. J Obstet Gynaecol Br Commonw 1977;77:37–41.

Dearden NM, Gibson JS, McDowell DG, et al. Effect of high dose dexamethasone on outcome from severe head injury. J Neurosurg 1986;64:81–88.

Del Rossi AJ (ed.). Blunt thoracic trauma. Trauma Quarterly 1990;6(3):1.

Dilts PV, Brinkman CR 3rd, Kirschbaum TH, et al. Uterine and systemic hemodynamic interrelationships and their response to hypoxia. Am J Obstet Gynecol 1967;103:138–157.

Durbin, CG. Management of traumatic brain injury: Have we learned what works. Critical Care Alert 2001;9(6):63–68.

Edwards R, Bennet B, Ripley D, et al. Surgery in the pregnant patient. Curr Probl Surg 2001;38(4):274–281.

Enevoldsen EM, Jensen FT. Autoregulation and CO_2 responses of cerebral blood flow in patients with acute severe head injury. J Neurosurg 1978;48:689–703.

Esposito TJ. Trauma during pregnancy. Emerg Med Clin North Am 1994;12:167–199.

Evrard JR, Sturner WQ, Murray EJ. Fetal skull fracture from an automobile accident. Am J Forensic Med Pathol 1998;10:232–234.

Feliciano DV. Tube thoracostomy. In: Benumof JL, ed. Clinical Procedures in Anesthesia and Intensive Care. Philadelphia: JB Lippincott, 1992:305–314.

Fildes J, Reed L, Jones N, Martin M, Barrett J. Trauma: The leading cause of maternal death. J Trauma 1992;32:643–645.

Franger AL, Buchsbaum HJ, Peaceman AM. Abdominal gunshot wounds in pregnancy. Am J Obstet Gynecol 1989;160:1124–1128.

Frazee RC, Mucha P, Farnell MB, et al. Objective evidence of blunt cardiac trauma. J Trauma 1986;26:510–520.

Fries MH, Hankins GDV. Motor vehicle accident associated with minimal maternal trauma, but subsequent fetal demise. Ann Emerg Med 1989;18:301–304.

Garrard BS, Littler WA, Redman CWG. Closing volume during pregnancy. Thorax 1978;33:488–492.

Gennarelli TA, Thibault LE. Biomechanics of acute subdural hematoma. J Trauma 1982;22:680–686.

Goodwin H, Holmes JF, Wisner DH. Abdominal ultrasound examination in pregnant blunt trauma patients. J Trauma 2001;50:689–693.

Goodwin TM, Breen MT. Pregnancy outcome and fetomaternal hemorrhage after noncatastrophic trauma. Am J Obstet Gynecol 1990;162:665–671.

Greiss F. Uterine vascular response to hemorrhage during pregnancy. With observations on therapy. Obstet Gynecol 1966;27:549–554.

Griffiths M, Hillman G, Usherwood M. Seat belt injury in pregnancy resulting in fetal death. A need for education? Case reports. Br J Obstet Gynaecol 1991;98:320–321.

Grubb DK. Non-surgical management of penetrating uterine trauma in pregnancy—a case report. Am J Obstet Gynecol 1992;166:583–584.

Hankins GD. Complications of beta-sympathomimetic tocolytic agents. In: Clark SL, Cotton DB, Hankins GD, Phelan JP, eds. Critical Care Obstetrics, 2nd edn. Boston: Blackwell Scientific, 1991: 223–250.

Hankins GD, Van Hook JW. Maternal oxygen transport variables during the third trimester of normal pregnancy. Am J Obstet Gynecol 1999;180:406–409.

Hankins GD, Barth WH, Satin AJ. Critical care medicine and the obstetric patient. In: Ayres SM, Grenuik A, Holbrook PR, Shoemaker WC, eds. Textbook of Critical Care, 3rd edn. Philadelphia: WB Saunders, 1995:50–64.

Hartl R, Ko K. In utero skull fracture: case report. J Trauma 1996;41:549–552.

Hayek DA, Veremakis C. Intracranial pathophysiology of brain injury. Probl Crit Care 1991;5:135.

Healy MA, Simons RK, Winchell RJ, et al. A prosepective evaluation of abdominal ultrasound in blunt trauma: Is it useful? J Trauma 1996;40:875–883.

Helton AS, McFarlane J, Anderson ET. Battered and pregnant: A prevalence study. Am J Public Health 1987;77:1337–1339.

Higgins SD, Garite TJ. Late abruptio placentae in trauma patients: Implications for monitoring. Obstet Gynecol 1987;63(Suppl 3): S10–13.

Hoff WS, D'Amelio LF, Tinkhoff GH, et al. Maternal predictors of fetal demise during pregnancy. Surg Gynecol Obstet 1991;172:175–180.

Hoyt DB, Coimbra R, Winchell RJ. Management of acute trauma. In: Townsend CM, Beauchamp RD, Evers BM, Mattox KL, eds. Sabiston Textbook of Surgery, 16th edn. Philadelphia: WB Saunders, 2001:311–344.

Hunt HB, Schifrin BS, Suzuki K. Ruptured berry aneurysms and pregnancy. Obstet Gynecol 1974;43:827–837.

Jennett B, Teasdale G, Braakman R, et al. Prognosis of patients with severe head injury. Neurosurgery 1979;4:283–289.

Jones WG, Ginsberg RJ. Esophageal perforation: A continuing challenge. Ann Thorac Surg 1992;53:534–543.

Jordan BD. Maternal head trauma during pregnancy. In: Devinsky O, Feldman E, Hainlinc B, eds. Neurologic Complications of Pregnancy. New York: Raven Press, 1994:131–138.

Judy KD. Craniotomy. In: Lanken PN, Hanson CW, Manaker S, eds. The Intensive Care Unit Manual. Philadelphia: WB Saunders, 2001:979–986.

Kasten GW, Martin ST. Resuscitation from bupivicaine-induced cardiovascular toxicity during partial inferior vena cava occlusion. Anesth Analg 1986;65:341–344.

Katz JD, Hook R, Baragh PG. Fetal heart rate monitoring in pregnant patients undergoing surgery. Am J Obstet Gynecol 1976;125:267–269.

Kimball IM. Maternal fetal trauma. Semin Pediatr Surg 2001;10(1): 32–34.

Kuhlmann RS, Cruikshank DP. Maternal trauma during pregnancy. Clin Obstet Gynecol 1994;37:274–293.

Laml T, Egermann R, Lapin A, Zekert M, Wagenbichler P. Feto-maternal hemorrhage after a car accident: a case report. Acta Obstet Gynecol Scand 2001;80:480–481.

Lane PL. Traumatic fetal deaths. J Emerg Med 1989;7:433–435.

Lavery JP, Staten-McCormick M. Management of moderate to severe trauma in pregnancy. Obstet Gynecol Clin North Am 1995;22:69–90.

Lees M, Scott D, Carr MG, et al. The circulatory effects of recumbent postural changes in late pregnancy. Clin Sci 1967;32:453–465.

Liberman M, Mulder D, Sampalis J. Advanced or basic life support for trauma: Meta-analysis and critical review of the literature. J Trauma 2000;49:584–589.

Lindheimer M, Katz H. Current concepts. The kidney in pregnancy. N Engl J Med 1970;283:1095–1097.

McCormick RD. Seat belt injury: case of complete transection of pregnant uterus. J Am Osteopathic Assoc 1968;67:1139–1141.

Mansour MA, Moore EE, Moore FA, et al. Exingent post-injury thoracotomy. Analysis of blunt versus penetrating trauma. Surg Gynecol Obstet 1992;175:97–101.

Maset AL, Marmarou A, Ward JD, et al. Pressure-volume index in head injury. J Neurosurg 1987;67:832–840.

Mattox KL. Approaches to trauma involving the major vessels of the thorax. Surg Clin North Am 1989;69:77.

Mattox KL, Flint LM, Carrico CJ, et al. Blunt cardiac injury (formerly termed "myocardiac contusion") (Editorial). J Trauma 1992;33: 649–650.

Mendelson CL. The aspiration of stomach contents into the lungs during obstetric anesthesia. Am J Obstet Gynecol 1946;52:191.

Mighty H. Trauma in pregnancy. Crit Care Clin 1994;10:623–624.

Moise KJ, Belfort MA. Damage control for the obstetric patient. Surg Clin North Am 1997;77:835–852.

Moore EE (ed.). Early Care of the Injured Patient, 4th edn. Philadelphia: BC Decker, 1990.

Morris JA, Rosenbower TJ, Jurkovich GJ, et al. Infant survival after cesarean section for trauma. Ann Surg 1996;223:481–488.

Muizelaar JP, Wei EP, Kontos HA, et al. Mannitol causes compensatory cerebral vasoconstriction and vasodilation in response to blood viscosity changes. J Neurosurg 1983;59:822–828.

Muizelaar JP, Marmarou A, Ward JD, et al. Adverse effects of prolonged hyperventilation in patients with severe head injury: A randomized clinical trial. J Neurosurg 1991;75:731–739.

Neufield JDG. Trauma in pregnancy, what if . . . ? Emerg Med Clin North Am 1993;11:207.

Newberger EH, Barkan SE, Lieberman ES, et al. Abuse of pregnant women and adverse birth outcomes. Current knowledge and implications for practice. JAMA 1992;267:2370–2372.

NHTSA. National Conference on Medical Indications for Air Bag Disconnection. George Washington University Medical Center.

Final Report. 1997. [NHTSA (National Highway Traffic Safety Administration) web site]. Available at: *http://www.nhtsa.gov/airbags/air%20bag%20conference%20final%20report.doc.* Accessed September 12, 2001.

Palmer JD, Sparrow OC. Extradural hematoma following intrauterine trauma. Injury 1994;25:671–673.

Paone RF, Peacock JB, Smith DL. Diagnosis of myocardiac contusion. South Med J 1993;86:867–870.

Parker B, McFarlane J, Soeken K. Abuse during pregnancy: Effects on maternal complications and birth weight in adult and teenage women. Obstet Gynecol 1994;84:323–328.

Pearce M. Seat belts in pregnancy. BMJ 1992;304:586–587.

Pearlman MD. Trauma. In: Hankins GDV, Clark SL, Cunningham FG, Gilstrap LC, eds. Operative Obstetrics. Norwalk, CT: Appleton & Lange, 1995:651–666.

Pearlman MD, Tintinalli JE. Evaluation and treatment of the gravida and fetus following trauma during pregnancy. Obstet Gynecol Clin North Am 1991;18:371–381.

Pearlman MD, Viano D. Automobile crash simulation with first pregnant crash test dummy. Am J Obstet Gynecol 1996;175:977–981.

Pearlman MD, Tintinalli JE, Lorenz RP. A prospective controlled study of outcome after trauma during pregnancy. Am J Obstet Gynecol 1990a;162:1502–1507.

Pearlman MD, Tintinalli JE, Lorenz RP. Blunt trauma during pregnancy. N Engl J Med 1990b;323:1609–1613.

Pearlman MD, Klinich KD, Schneider LW, et al. A comprehensive program to improve safety for pregnant women and fetuses in motor vehicle crashes: a preliminary report. Am J Obstet Gynecol 2000;182:1554–1564.

Pritchard JA. Changes in blood volume during pregnancy and delivery. Anesthesiology 1965;26:393.

Pritchard JA, Brekken AL. Clinical and laboratory studies on severe abruptio placentae. Am J Obstet Gynecol 1967;97:681–700.

Prowse CM, Gaensler EA. Respiratory and acid base changes during pregnancy. Anesthesiology 1965;26:381.

Ramenofsky ML, Alexander RH, Ali J, et al, (eds.). Advanced Trauma Life Support (R) for Doctors—1993 Instructor Manual. American College of Surgeons. Chicago: First Impressions, 1993.

Reul G, Mattox K, Beall A, et al. Recent advances in the operative management of massive chest trauma. Ann Thorac Surg 1973;16: 52–66.

Robertson CS, Contant CF, Gokaslan ZL, et al. Cerebral blood flow, arteriovenous oxygen difference and outcome in head injured patients. J Neurol Neurosurg Psychiatry 1992;55:594–603.

Rose PG, Strohm PL, Zuspan FP. Fetomaternal hemorrhage following trauma. Am J Obstet Gynecol 1985;153:844–847.

Rothenberger D, Quattlebaum FW, Perry JF Jr, et al. Blunt maternal trauma: A review of 103 cases. J Trauma 1978;18:173–179.

Rutherford EJ, Nelson LD. Initial assessment of the multiple trauma patient. In: Ayres SM, Grenvitz A, Holbrook PR, Shoemaker WC, eds. Textbook of Critical Care, 3rd edn. Philadelphia: WB Saunders, 1995:1382–1389.

Rutherford SE, Phelan JP. Deep venous thrombosis and pulmonary embolus. In: Clark SL, Cotton DG, Hantins EDV, Phelan JP, eds. Critical Care Obstetrics, 2nd ed. Boston: Blackwell Scientific, 1991: 150–179.

Sachs BP, Brown DAT, Driscoll SG, et al. Maternal mortality Massachusetts: Trends and prevention. N Engl J Med 1987;316: 667–672.

Sakala EP, Kost DD. Management of stab wounds to the pregnant uterus. A case report and review of the literature. Obstet Gynecol Surv 1988;43:319–324.

Sandy EA, Koerner M. Self-inflicted gunshot wound to the pregnant abdomen: Report of a case and review of the literature. Am J Perinatol 1989;6:30–31.

Sankaran S, Wilson RF. Factors affecting prognosis in patients with flail chest. J Thorac Cardiovasc Surg 1976;60:402–410.

Satin A, Hemsell DL, Stone IC, et al. Sexual assault in pregnancy. Obstet Gynecol 1991;77:710–714.

Scorpio RJ, Esposito TJ, Smith LG, Gens DR. Blunt trauma during pregnancy: Factors affecting fetal outcome. J Trauma 1992;32: 213–216.

Scott DE. Anemia during pregnancy. Obstet Gynecol Annu 1972;1: 219–244.

Shepard TH. Catalog of Teratogenic Agents, 7th edn. Baltimore: Johns Hopkins, 1992.

Shoemaker WC. Algorithm for early recognition and management of cardiac tamponade. Crit Care Med 1975;3:59–63.

Shoemaker WC, Carey JS, Yao ST, et al. Hemodynamic alterations in acute cardiac tamponade after penetrating injuries of the heart. Surgery 1970;67:754–764.

Sirlin C, Casola G, Brown M, et al. US of blunt abdominal trauma: importance of free pelvic fluid in women of reproductive age. Radiology 2001;219:229–235.

Smith DS, Levy W, Maris M, et al. Reperfusion hyperoxia in brain after circulatory arrest in humans. Anesthesiology 1990;73:12–19.

Stafford PA, Biddinger PW, Zumwalt RE. Lethal intrauterine fetal trauma. Am J Obstet Gynecol 1988;159:485–489.

Stellin G. Survival in trauma victims with pulmonary contusion. Am Surg 1981;57:780–784.

Stone IK. Trauma in the obstetric patient. Obstet Gynecol Clin North Am 1999;26:459–467.

de Swiet M. The respiratory system. In: Hytten F, Chamberlain G, eds. Clinical Physiology in Obstetrics, 2nd edn. London: Blackwell Scientific, 1991:83–100.

Taskinen SO, Salo JA, Halttunen PEA, et al. Tracheobronchial rupture due to blunt chest trauma: A follow-up study. Ann Thorac Surg 1989;48:846–849.

Taylor DJ, Phillips P, Lind T. Puerperal hematological indices. Br J Obstet Gynaecol 1981;88:601–606.

Teasdale G, Jennett B. Assessment of coma and impaired consciousness: A practical scale. Lancet 1974;2:81–84.

Tilanus HW, Bossuyt P, Schattenkeck ME, et al. Treatment of oesophageal perforation: A multivariate analysis. Br J Surg 1991;78:582–585.

Trinkle JK, Richardson JD, Franz JL, et al. Management of flail chest without mechanical ventilation. Ann Thorac Surg 1975;19: 355–363.

Trunkey DD, Lewis FR Jr (ed.). Current Therapy of Trauma, 3rd edn. Philadelphia: BC Decker, 1991.

Ueland K, Hansen JM. Maternal cardiovascular dynamics, II. Posture and uterine contractions. Am J Obstet Gynecol 1969a; 103:1–7.

Ueland K, Hansen JM. Maternal cardiovascular dynamics, III. Labor and delivery under local and caudal anesthesia. Am J Obstet Gynecol 1969b;103:8–18.

Ueland K, Metcalfe J. Circulatory changes in pregnancy. Clin Obstet Gynecol 1975;18:41–50.

Van Hook JW. Acute Respiratory Distress Syndrome in Pregnancy. Sem Perinatol 1997;21:4:320–327.

Vaizey CJ, Jacobson MJ, Cross FW. Trauma in pregnancy. Br J Surg 1994;81:1406–1415.

Varner MW. Maternal mortality in Iowa from 1952 to 1986. Surg Obstet Gynecol 1989;168:555–562.

Weaver WD, Cobb LA, Hallstrom AP, et al. Factors influencing survival after out of hospital cardiac arrest. J Am Coll Cardiol 1986;7:752–757.

Weiss HB, Songer TJ, Fabio A. Fetal deaths related to maternal injury. JAMA 2001;286:1863–1868.

Weyerts LK, Jones MC, James HE. Paraplegia and congenital fractures as a consequence of intrauterine trauma. Am J Med Genet 1992;43:751–752.

Whittaker PG, MacPhail S, Lind T. Serial hematologic changes and pregnancy outcome. Obstet Gynecol 1996;88:33–39.

Williams JK, McClain L, Rosemursy AS, Colorado NM. Evaluation of blunt abdominal trauma in the third trimester of pregnancy: Obstet Gynecol 1990;75:33–37.

Wilson M, Morganti AA, Zervoudakis I, et al. Blood pressure, the renin-aldosterone system, and sex steroids throughout normal pregnancy. Am J Med 1980;68:97–104.

Wilson RF. Thoracic injuries. In: Ayres SM, Grenvik A, Holbrook PR, Shoemaker WC, eds. Textbook of Critical Care. Philadelphia: WB Saunders, 1995:1429–1438.

Winchell RJ, Hoyt DB, Simons RK. Use of computed tomography of the head in the hypotensive blunt-trauma patient. Ann Emerg Med 1995;25:737–742.

Witlin AG, Mattar FM, Saade GR, Van Hook JW, Sibai BM. Presentation of venous thromboembolism during pregnancy. Am J Obstet Gynecol 1999;181:1181–1121.

37 Thermal and electrical injury

Cornelia R. Graves

Most burns are caused by exposure to a thermal, chemical, or electrical source. Recent studies have estimated that approximately 7% of women of reproductive age are seen for treatment of major burns. Maternal and perinatal morbidity and mortality increase as the total body surface area burned increases (Caine & Lefcourt, 1993; Akhtar et al., 1994) (Fig. 37.1). In the nonpregnant population, recent advances in treatment have reduced mortality rates and improved the quality of life in burn survivors. This has been translated into improved survival for both mother and fetus. Due to the complicated clinical nature of the process, a multidisciplinary approach is required to achieve the best results.

Classification

Burns are classified by degree based on the depth of the burn into the skin and also by the amount of surface area involved. Partial-thickness injury includes first- and second-degree burns; third-degree burns are full-thickness.

First-degree or superficial burns involve the epidermis only. The skin is erythematous and painful to touch. The best example of this type of burn is a sunburn. These types of burns require topical treatment only.

Second-degree burns involve death and destruction of portions of the epidermis and part of the corium or dermis. A superficial burn is typically characterized by fluid-filled blisters. A deep partial-thickness burn may form eschar. On initial evaluation, it may be difficult to assess the depth of the injury. These burns are painful, but enough viable tissue is left for healing to take place without grafting.

Third-degree or full-thickness burns involve the dermis and the corium (dermis) and extend into the fat layer or further. The skin has a thick layer of eschar and may or may not be painful depending on the amount of damage done to the surrounding nerves (Caine & Lefcourt, 1993).

In addition to the thickness of the burn, the part of the body burned, concurrent injuries, and past medical history may also affect outcome.

Estimation of total body surface area (TBSA) involved in a burn may be determined in two way: "the rule of nines" or the Lund–Browder chart. The rule of nines divides the body into sections that allows for quick estimation of the burn area and is especially useful in emergency situations (Table 37.1). The Lund–Browder chart also divides the body into sections but is more accurate as it takes into account changes in body surface area related to patient age. In both methods only second- and third-degree burns are estimated. A chart specific to pregnancy has not been developed (Demling, 1991).

Minor burns involve less than 10% of TBSA, are no more than partial thickness in depth, and are otherwise uncomplicated. Burns are considered major if the patient has a history of chronic illness, if the burn involves the face, hands, or perineum, if there is concurrent injury, or if the burn is caused by electrical injury (Polko & McMahon, 1999). Critical burns encompass greater than 40% of TBSA and are associated with major morbidity and mortality. Severe burns involve 20–39% of TBSA; moderate burns involve 10–19% of TBSA (Reiss, 1994).

Thermal burns

Thermal injuries during pregnancy usually occur at home and are most often caused by flame burns or hot scalding liquids. This type of burn commonly involves smoke inhalation injury. The burn only involves the area of the body that was in direct contact with the cause of the injury. Thermal burns are classified based on the degree of injury as described above (Gang et al., 1992; Caine & Lefcourt, 1993).

Chemical burns

The amount of injury to the skin from a chemical burn is dependent on several factors: (i) the concentration of the chemical; (ii) the length of exposure to the chemical; (iii) the amount of chemical involved; (iv) the type of chemical; and (v) the effect of the chemical on the skin or exposed area. Unlike thermal burns, the degree of injury is directly related to the length of

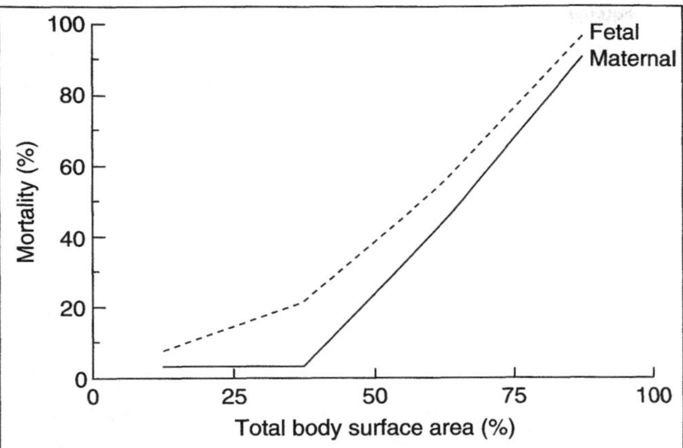

Fig. 37.1 Maternal and perinatal morbidity and mortality increase as the total body surface area burned increases. (From Polko LE, McMahon MJ. Burns in pregnancy. Obstet Gynecol Surv 1999;54:131.)

Table 37.1 Small burns are classified as less than 20% of TBSA

Anatomic area	Percent of body surface area
Head	9
Upper extremities	9 (each)
Lower extremities	9 (each)
Anterior trunk	18
Posterior trunk	18
Neck	1

exposure. Flushing of the skin or exposed area should be accomplished as soon as possible after exposure. While water is usually the flushing medium of choice, a careful history should be taken as water may actually potentiate the injury when used with certain chemicals such as phosphorus.

Electrical burns

The passage of high-voltage electrical energy through tissues results in thermal injury (Holliman et al., 1982) and a burn that not only involves the skin and subcutaneous tissues but also all other tissue in the path of the current. The amount of damage to the tissues depends on the characteristics of the electrical current.

The burn area usually involves an entry and an exit site. The amount of underlying tissue, muscle, and nerve damage can be extremely difficult to assess. Electrical current may be delivered as a wave or alternating pattern called alternating current (AC) or as direct current (DC). Current is created when the flow of electricity, measured by voltage, meets resistance. When this flow encounters resistance it generates current, measured by amperage. The higher the current, the more severe the injury.

Alternating current is more dangerous than direct current as it can cause tonic muscle contractions and the victim may be unable to release the source of electrical energy. Since different parts of the body provide varying degrees of resistance, the damage caused by electricity can vary. As the same current can generate varying amounts of heat, damage is based on the resistance it encounters (Caine & Lefcourt, 1993).

Electrical injury can occur through four mechanisms. Direct contact with the electrical source results in injury to the skin in contact with the source and the surrounding subcutaneous tissues. Arcing of electricity usually occurs across joint areas as electrical charge is transferred. This results in cutaneous burns in areas not involved with entry or the exit site. Conduction burns occur when the current is conducted through another medium such as water to another body area. Secondary ignition burns occur when the electrical source ignites a flammable material.

The most common causes of electrical burns include occupational hazards, household appliances, and lightning.

There is scarce information regarding fetal outcome after accidental electric shock in pregnancy. A prospective cohort study noted that in most cases accidental electric shock occurring during day-to-day life during pregnancy does not pose a major fetal risk (Einarson et al., 1997).

Maternal concerns

There are a number of physiologic changes that occur during pregnancy. These changes can make the management of the burn patient especially challenging. This section will address these changes and their relationship to maternal complications.

Cardiovascular system

During pregnancy, cardiac output and plasma volume are increased. Systemic vascular resistance is decreased to compensate for the increased circulatory volume. Colloid osmotic pressure is decreased in the vascular spaces. This high-flow, low-resistance state is essential for maintaining perfusion to the uterus and for increasing oxygen delivery to the fetus. A loss of integrity of the skin results in a loss of body water. This loss is more exaggerated in pregnancy due to the decreased colloid osmotic pressure. Therefore, the pregnant burn patient is at increased risk of losing cardiac output and circulatory volume, which are essential for maintaining a stable hemodynamic profile.

Pulmonary system

Increased oxygen delivery and consumption are the hallmark changes in the pulmonary system during pregnancy. Respiratory rate, tidal volume, and minute volume are increased. These changes lead to a state of relative hyperventilation. Arterial blood gases reflect higher resting oxygen tension and resting carbon dioxide tension (<30 mmHg) than that seen in the nonpregnant state.

Oxygen delivery is facilitated by the increased cardiac output and circulating red cell volume. Oxygen needs of the placenta and fetus increase oxygen consumption, making the patient susceptible to hypoxemia if oxygen delivery decrease.

As many thermal and chemical inhalation injuries involve the pulmonary system, early evaluation is warranted. Burns involving the face, neck, or chest may also involve damage to the respiratory passages, leading to compromise of the airway. As the trachea tends to be more edematous, especially during the third trimester of pregnancy, consideration should be given to early intubation in any case where there is potential damage to the airway.

Integumentary system

The skin is the organ system most often involved in burns. The skin serves as a barrier to infection and a regulator of fluid, electrolyte, and thermal balance. During pregnancy, the skin is also expected to adapt to changes in body habitus. Severe burns involving the trunk of the patient before or during early pregnancy may lead to problems with skin expansion, especially during the second and third trimester when the abdomen must expand to accommodate the growing fetus (Widgerow et al., 1991). A longitudinal study of seven patients with circumferential truncal burns sustained during childhood reveal one case of scar tissue breakdown in the third trimester. Burn treatment of all seven patients included excision and split-thickness skin grafts (McCauley et al., 1991). Cultured epidermal autograft has also been used successfully in pregnancy in the case of severe burns over a large surface area when the patient has a shortage of skin suitable for grafting (Barillo et al., 1992). A recent case report described using the naturally expanded skin of pregnancy to reconstruct the abdominal wall to allow for future pregnancies to proceed without discomfort (Webb et al., 1995).

Management strategies

Management of burns in the nonpregnant patient can be divided into four periods: the resuscitation period (0–36 hours post injury), the postresuscitation period (2–5 days post injury), the inflammation–infection period (from 6 days to post wound closure), and rehabilitation (Demling, 1995).

Resuscitation period

The primary treatment goal of the patient suffering a large burn is the avoidance of complications related to fluid and electrolyte deficits in the period immediately after the burn. Cardiovascular and pulmonary support is crucial.

Estimation of TBSA and the severity of the burns are the first steps toward management. While there are many formulas for calculating fluid replacement based on TBSA, the modified Brooke formula and the Parkland formula are two of the most frequently used. Initial management includes placement of a Foley catheter to monitor renal perfusion. In patients with a history of cardiac or pulmonary disease, those with combined cutaneous and pulmonary injury, or in patients unresponsive to initial resuscitative efforts, a pulmonary artery catheter should be considered to help with management of fluid balance.

Early intubation is recommended in those patients with suspected inhalation injury as inflammation and development of tissue edema in the airway may make intubation difficult. Chemical damage of the respiratory passages may require intubation to provide the adequate pulmonary toilet necessary for healing. Pulmonary injury in a pregnant woman adds to the complexity of managing a burn patient since hypoxia may lead to uterine contractions and fetal compromise and these concerns must be anticipated (Pimental, 1991).

Serial chemical and electrolyte studies should be performed. Care should be taken to monitor glucose carefully since hypoglycemia can occur as the patient tries to regulate her body temperature. Arterial blood gases should be obtained immediately, as should a complete blood cell count, blood cultures when indicated, and a coagulation panel. When X-ray examinations are indicated abdominal shielding should be used when possible. Tetanus toxoid is not contraindicated in pregnancy and should be given if indicated.

Crystalloid is given in the form of lactated Ringers at a rate of 4 mL/kg per percent of body burn during the first 24 hours. For example, in a 65-kg patient with TBSA burn of 50%, 13,000 mL of fluid would be required. Half of this volume should be given over the first 8 hours, the remaining half over the next 16 hours in divided increments (Georgiade & Pederson, 1987). Red cell replacement may be required and can be used for volume expansion as well as for increasing oxygen-carrying capacity. The hematocrit may be falsely elevated in the face of volume depletion and is not a reliable indicator of volume status. The use of more sophisticated methods of fluid volume monitoring is usually indicated. Urinary output should be maintained at approximately 100 mL/hr by judicious volume expansion. Hypoproteinemia secondary to losses from the burn area and the decreased colloid osmotic pressure of pregnancy may be associated with massive tissue edema during the resuscitation period.

The wound should be treated daily with debridement, cleansing, and topical antibacterial creams. External fetal monitoring should be instituted at a viable gestational age, usually around 24–26 weeks (Kuhlmann & Cruikshank, 1994). This may be difficult in cases where the abdomen is burned.

Postresuscitation period

This period typically begins 2–5 days after the injury has taken place. If the patient is hemodynamically stable and oxygen delivery is adequate, operative management of the wound can begin. It is important to accomplish excision of the burned tissue and closure of the skin at this time before inflammation and infection occur. This usually takes the form of a series of short surgical procedures since hypothermia is always a concern. To combat infection, topical antibiotic administration and frequent wound cultures (to determine specific bacterial colonization) are carried out. Intravenous antibiotics are specifically targeted to those organisms identified in culture. A consumptive coagulopathy may occur during this period requiring blood component therapy replacement. When interpreting the coagulation profile during pregnancy, it should be remembered that fibrinogen levels are increased and that fibrinogen in the normal range may be a sign of an early coagulopathy.

Inflammation–infection period

The hypermetabolic response to injury begins at about 4–5 days after injury and peaks at about 7–10 days (Alexander, 1987). Cardiac output is often more than doubled in order to keep pace with the necessary increase in oxygen demand. Carbon dioxide production is also increased, and this can lead to rapid deterioration in respiratory status as the injured lung may be unable to exchange gases satisfactorily. The difficulty in differentiating a hypermetabolic state from sepsis or pregnancy-related processes can make diagnosis during this period extremely difficult. The injured lung is also at increased risk for pneumonia secondary to hypoxia, atelectasis, mucous plugging, and increased tissue edema. In addition to all of the pathologic processes, the decreased colloid osmotic pressure of pregnancy further contributes to the development of acute respiratory distress syndrome (ARDS).

Adequate nutritional support is crucial during this period. Supplementation via the gastrointestinal route is optimal. Parenteral nutrition may also be needed to meet caloric demands. When calculating nutritional needs it is important to remember that the metabolic demands of pregnancy are increased and early nutritional assessment is recommended. A true measurement of caloric needs can be obtained from indirect calorimetry and this technique may be required to adequately address the nutritional situation.

The burn wound is best managed by the use of topical antibiotics. Silver sulfadiazine is most commonly used and is not contraindicated in pregnancy. *Staphylococcus aureus* is the most common bacterium responsible for wound infection; however, Gram-negative organisms, especially *Pseudomonas aeruginosa*, may also be cultured (Boss et al., 1985). Once infection has been ruled out or treated, skin grafting can take place if needed. This is usually accomplished 2–3 weeks after the injury.

Rehabilitation

Active range of motion exercises in the burn patient should be instituted as soon as possible to prevent loss of muscle and loss of joint function. In the parturient, movement of the lower extremities and early ambulation is important for another reason as well, since it can prevent the formation of deep venous thrombosis. Some authors recommend the use of mini-dose heparin for the prevention of thromboembolism (Mabrouk & EL-Feky, 1997). Left lateral recumbent positioning helps to increase blood flow to the fetus and avoid maternal hypotension The route of delivery should be based on obstetric considerations. Some authors advocate proceeding with urgent delivery at term in those patients who have critical burns (Ullmann et al., 1997; Guo et al., 2001).

Maternal complications

Acute renal failure

Acute renal failure presenting as oliguria or anuria is not uncommon in the burn patient. Prerenal azotemia occurs frequently because underestimation of the extent of the injury may lead to an underestimation of volume status. In the pregnant patient, assessment of vital signs alone may be insufficient as the increased maternal cardiac output and increased volume status associated with pregnancy may mask signs of hemodynamic compromise. Treatment should be aimed at maintaining adequate intravascular volume. In the patient who is unresponsive to reasonable fluid replacement, hemodynamic monitoring should be instituted to assist in aggressive fluid replacement. Low-dose dopamine is not contraindicated in pregnancy.

In the electrical burn patient, deep tissue injury may not be readily apparent. Massive muscle injury, common in the electrical burn patient, may lead to the production of myoglobin. Myoglobin, a breakdown product of necrotic muscle, is directly toxic to the renal tubule. Hypovolemia may assist in potentiating renal injury in patients with myoglobinuria. Hyperkalemia can accompany myoglobinuria and may be life-threatening. The diagnosis of myoglobinuria can be easily performed at the bedside. The presence of reddish-brown urine and a negative urine dipstick for hemoglobin confirms the presence of myoglobin. Treatment should be undertaken to maintain urine output through volume replacement. Mannitol may also be used to aid in increasing urinary output. This is one condition in which the use of bicarbonate should be considered in all intravenous fluids in order to alkalize the urine and assist in the excretion of myoglobin.

Sepsis/ARDS

Sepsis is major cause of death in burn patients. It has been estimated that approximately half of all deaths from burns are due to complications from infection and pneumonia. The most common causes of infection include *S. aureus*, *Enterococcus*, *Candida albicans*, and *Pseudomonas* species. The regular use of wound biopsies as well as tissue and blood cultures has allowed for the more specific and controlled use of systemic antimicrobial and antifungal agents. Aggressive efforts are needed to prevent sepsis since this may lead to multisystem end-organ failure.

Multisystem end-organ failure in the burn patient has a mortality rate of nearly 100%. The immunosuppressive effects of pregnancy, as well as host compromise secondary to injury, may make the parturient especially susceptible to the development of septic complications. Recognition of appropriate treatment is crucial. In interpreting pulmonary artery catheter values, the hyperdynamic state of pregnancy must be considered and taken into account, and this is certainly an area where obstetricians can assist their critical care colleagues.

During pregnancy, the development of sepsis frequently leads to the development of ARDS. As mentioned above, changes in the respiratory system during pregnancy may make the lung susceptible to injury. Smoke inhalation injury associated with massive fluid shifts during the postresuscitation period may predispose the patient to bacterial colonization and the development of pneumonia. As respiratory failure is the leading cause of death in the burn patient, early recognition of respiratory distress is imperative. Early intubation and the use of positive end-expiratory pressure may prevent further injury. While parameters have not been established for pregnancy, it is my opinion that intubation be strongly considered in patients with a respiratory rate of greater than 40/minute, a P_ao_2 of less than 80 mmHg, or a P_aco_2 of greater than 40 mmHg. Given the physiologic changes of pregnancy, P_ao_2 and P_aco_2 levels that would be otherwise tolerated in a nonpregnant individual are unacceptable in pregnancy. A sustained P_ao_2 of less than 60 mmHg will lead to fetal distress, and a sustained P_aco_2 of greater than 40 mmHg will affect placental gas exchange and lead to fetal acidosis. The frequently employed strategies of permissive hypoventilation and hypoxia/hypercapnia may not be possible in a pregnant woman if there is concern about fetal health. Obviously the maternal condition takes precedence and fetal outcome may in some cases be disregarded, especially in nonviable fetuses. In other cases, however, early delivery may be required in order to allow institution of permissive ventilation strategies for the mother. This is another area where the obstetrician is often of great value to the critical care team.

Fractures

Evaluation for skeletal trauma should occur early in the assessment in patients experiencing electrical injury. Increased tetany of the muscles during electrocution may result in long bone fractures as well as fractures of the vertebral column. Appropriate radiologic investigation should not be delayed or avoided because of the pregnant state.

Mortality

Maternal mortality following burn injury is related to the severity of the injury and the potential for complications. Maternal mortality is lower than 5% when less than 50% of TBSA is involved, and greater than 100% when more than 80% of TBSA is involved.

Fetal complications

Preterm labor

Preterm labor and delivery usually ensue within the first few days after significant thermal injury. Prostaglandin levels are uniformly increased in the burn patient. Inadequate volume resuscitation may also lead to a decrease in uteroplacental perfusion and tissue hypoxia. These factors combine to increase the incidence of preterm labor and delivery. As burn patients are at great risk for complications from tocolytic therapy, care should be taken to individualize care for each patient. Because β-mimetics are associated with increased capillary permeability and electrolyte imbalances, it has been suggested that the safest tocolytic agent in these patients may be parenteral magnesium sulfate (Unsur et al., 1996). Corticosteroids should be administered to those patients between 24 and 34 weeks if appropriate and infection is not a major concern. In a retrospective review, 100% of patients with critical burns delivered their fetus within the first 7 days after their injury (Rayburn et al., 1984).

Pregnancy loss

Several authors have noted an increase in the spontaneous abortion rate in patients who experience burns during the first trimester. In one study, four of six patients who were injured during this period miscarried (Jain & Garg, 1993). Some authors have advocated therapeutic terminations in patients with severe burns in the first trimester; however, there are no data to associate this with improved maternal outcome (Lippin et al., 1993).

Fetal distress and stillbirths

Fetal distress secondary to hypoxia and uteroplacental insufficiency may necessitate the need for emergent delivery. For this reason, all parturients with a viable fetus should have fetal monitoring instituted if at all possible. Perinatal morbidity is directly related to the severity of the burn. When less than 40% of TBSA is involved, the perinatal mortality rate is approximately 25%; when 50% of TBSA is involved, the perinatal mortality rate increases to 50%; and when greater than 80% of TBSA is involved, 100% of fetuses are usually lost (Fig. 37.1).

Conclusions

While massive burn injury is relatively uncommon during pregnancy, it is associated with significant maternal and neonatal morbidity and mortality. Aggressive resuscitation and therapeutic measures aimed at stabilizing the mother and the fetus as well as collaborative care between the surgical and obstetric team are necessary to optimize outcome.

References

Akhtar MA, Mulawkar PM, Kulkarni HR. Burns in pregnancy: effect on maternal and fetal outcomes. Burns 1994;20:351–355.

Alexander J. The role of infection in the burn patient. In: Boswick J, ed. The Art and Science of Burn Care. Rockville, MD: Aspen Publishers, 1987;103.

Barillo DJ, Nangle NE, Farrell K. Preliminary experience with cultured epidermal autograft in a community hospital burn unit. J Burn Care Rehabil 1992;13:158–165.

Boss WK, Brand DA, Acampora D, et al. Effectiveness of prophylactic antibiotics in the outpatient treatment of burns. J Trauma 1985;25:244–247.

Caine R, Lefcourt N. Patients with burns. In: Clochesy J, Breu C, Cardin S, et al., eds. Critical Care Nursing. Philadelphia: WB Saunders, 1993:183.

Demling RH. Burn management. In: Wilmore D, ed. Pre- and Postoperative Care. New York: Scientific American, 1991.

Demling RH. Management of the burn patient. In: Grenvik A, Holbrook PR, Shoemaker WC, eds. Textbook of Critical Care, 3rd edn. Philadelphia: WB Saunders, 1995:1499.

Einarson, A, Bailey B, Inocencion G, et al. Accidental electric shock in pregnancy: a prospective cohort study. Am J Obstet Gynecol 1997;176:678–681.

Gang RK, Bajec J, Tahboub M. Management of thermal injury in pregnancy: an analysis of 16 patients. Burns 1992;18:317–320.

Georgiade G, Pederson C. Burns. In: Sabiston DC, ed. Essentials of Surgery. Philadelphia: WB Saunders, 1987:122.

Guo S, Greenspoon JS, Kahn AM. Management of burn injuries during pregnancy. Burns 2001;27:394–397.

Holliman CJ, Saffle JR, Kravitz M, et al. Early surgical decompression in the management of electrical injuries. Am J Surg 1982;144:733–739.

Jain ML, Garg AK. Burns with pregnancy: a review of 25 cases. Burns 1993;19:166–167.

Kuhlmann RS, Cruikshank DP. Maternal trauma during pregnancy. Clin Obstet Gynecol 1994;37:274–293.

Lippin Y, Shvoron A, Tsur H. Therapeutic abortion in a severely burned woman. J Burn Care Rehabil 1993;14:398.

Mabrouk AR, El-Feky AE. Burns during pregnancy: a gloomy outcome. Burns 1997;23:596–600.

McCauley RL, Stenberg BA, Phillips LG, et al. Long-term assessment of the effects of circumferential truncal burns in pediatric patients on subsequent pregnancies. J Burn Care Rehabil 1991;12:51–53.

Pimental L. Mother and child trauma in pregnancy. Emerg Med Clin North Am 1991;9:549.

Polko LE, McMahon MJ. Burns in pregnancy. Obstet Gynecol Surv 1999;54:131.

Rayburn W, Smith B, Feller I, Varner, M, Cruikshank D. Major burns during pregnancy: effects on fetal well-being. Obstet Gynecol 1984;63:392–395.

Reiss G. Thermal injuries. In: Lopez-Veigo MA, ed. The Parkland Trauma Handbook. St Louis: Mosby, 1994;389.

Ullmann Y, Blumenfield Z, Hakim M, et al. Urgent delivery, the treatment of choice in term pregnant women with extended burn injury. Burns 1997;23:157–159.

Unsur V, Oztopcu C, Atalay C, et al. A retrospective study of 11 pregnant women with thermal injuries. Eur J Obstet Gynecol Reprod Biol 1996;64:55–58.

Webb JC, Baack BR, Osler TM, et al. A pregnancy complicated by mature abdominal burns scarring and its surgical solution: a case report. J Burn Care Rehabil 1995;16:276–279.

Widgerow AD, Ford TD, Botha M. Burn contracture preventing uterine expansion. Ann Plast Surg 1991;27:269–271.

38 Overdose, poisoning, and envenomation

Alfredo F. Gei
Victor R. Suárez

All substances are poisons.

Paracelsus (1493–1541)

Definitions

Although the terms of poisoning and overdose are frequently used interchangeably, poisoning denotes the morbid state produced by the exposure of a toxic agent (poison), that because of its chemical action, causes a functional disturbance (e.g. renal failure or hepatitis) and/or structural damage (e.g. chemical burn) (Clark et al., 1992). The terms overdose or overdosage refer to a state produced by the excess or abuse of a drug or substance (Clark et al., 1992). Consequently overdoses can be considered as a particular type of poisoning. Whereas the former suggests an intentional exposure, and the second connotes unintentional or unknown toxic exposure, in the following text we will use the terms poisoning or overdose relative to the ingestion of chemical agents or drugs and medications, respectively. Envenomations are a particular type of toxic exposure resulting from the human contact with biologic substances (venoms or toxins) produced in specialized glands or tissues from animals, usually by cutaneous or transdermal (parenteral) injection (bee and scorpion stings, snake bites, etc.). This definition is in contrast to poisoning or intoxication, which refer to the oral ingestion of toxins produced or accumulated in nonspecialized glands or tissues.

Scope of the problem

Toxic exposures

It is estimated that every year 4.6 million poisonings occur in the United States, at a rate of approximately 9 exposures per 1,000 population (Litovitz et al., 2000). A little over 50% of those toxic exposures occur in women, and more than 300,000 of the poisonings take place in women of reproductive age. Additionally, although toxic exposures are overall more frequent in children, the age distribution of the fatal exposures peaks in the late reproductive years (Litovitz et al., 2000). In addition, studies performed in emergency departments have shown that up to 6.3% of female patients may have an unrecognized pregnancy, even when the patient's history is not suggestive of such (Stengel et al., 1994). For this reason, it has been recommended that a pregnancy test should be part of the evaluation of any woman of child-bearing age presenting with an overdose or poisoning (Jones et al., 1997).

Pregnancy and medications

Independently of comorbid conditions, pregnancy increases the average intake of medications among women (UNICEF, 1992). This period in a woman's life should therefore be considered a predisposing condition for adverse effects of medications, including overdose. As shown in Table 38.1, the incidence of poisoning during pregnancy is fortunately low, likely due to an increased awareness of potentially adverse side effects of medications upon the fetus and to a quoted healthier emotional state of bringing a new life to the world (Greenblatt, 1997; Gei & Saade, 2001).

Toxic exposures during pregnancy

Despite being only a fraction of the national exposures in 2000, 8,438 cases of toxic exposures during pregnancy were reported to the 65 Poison Control Centers in this country. The temporal distribution during pregnancy is approximately equal along the different trimesters, with a slight predominance of the second trimester (Table 38.1) (Litovitz et al., 2000). Since 1993, the number of toxic exposures accounted for by pregnant patients has increased in a parallel manner to the total number of exposures reported (Table 38.1) (Litovitz et al., 2000; Gei & Saade, 2001). The majority of the toxic exposures occurring during pregnancy are acute (87% for 1999) and to a single substance (91%). The most frequent route of exposure is oral (50%), followed by inhalation (30%) and dermal (10%). Although the

Table 38.1 Toxic exposures during pregnancy reported to the Poison Control Centers in the United States: 1993–2000. Between 1993 and 2001, the number of toxic exposures during pregnancy represent only a fraction of the exposures reported nationwide (0.3–0.4%). Overall, during this time period, both the total number of exposures and the ones reported by pregnant women have increased steadily by a factor of 1.6–10% per year. The distribution of toxic exposures per trimester of pregnancy has been stable over the past 9 years, with a slightly higher predominance of the second over the other two trimesters

			Trimester*		
Year	Total	Pregnant *N* (%)	First (%)	Second (%)	Third (%)
1993	1,751,476	6,443 (0.36)	32	38	30
1994	1,926,438	6,147 (0.32)	31	38	31
1995	2,023,089	6,484 (0.32)	30	39	31
1996	2,155,952	7,103 (0.33)	30	39	31
1997	2,192,088	7,250 (0.33)	31	38	31
1998	2,241,082	8,120 (0.36)	32	38	30
1999	2,201,156	8,980 (0.40)	32	38	30
2000	2,168,248	8,438 (0.38)	32	38	31
2001	2,267,979	7,588 (0.33)	32	38	30

* Of those with known gestational age.
(Source: 1993, 1994, 1995, 1996, 1997, 1998, 1999, 2000 and 2001 (in press) Annual Reports of the American Association of Poison Control Centers Toxic Exposure Surveillance System.)

majority of patients were treated on site, 5% of the exposures resulted in moderate to major effects and 3% required admission to a critical care facility. No deaths were reported in this series (Gei et al., 2001a).

During pregnancy, drug overdose frequently is part of a suicide gesture (Rogers & Lee, 1988; Gilstrap & Little 1992; Broughan & Soloway, 2000). Less frequently, it is the result of an attempt to induce an abortion. Even though most of the exposures during pregnancy are accidental (78% for 1999), almost one-fifth (18%) are intentional, either related to a suicide attempt (or gesture) or as the result of drug abuse or misuse (Gei et al., 2001a; Litovitz et al., 2001). More than 95% of suicide gestures involve ingestion of a combination of drugs. In a series of more than 1,000 pregnant women where the exposure reported occurred with more than one substance, the risk of a suicide attempt (as the mechanism for the exposure) was three times higher than when the exposure was to a single substance (odds ratio (OR): 3.1; 95% CI: 2.75–3.49) (Gei et al., 2001b). The risk for suicidal exposure was also three times higher for pregnant teenagers than for other age groups (OR: 3.1%; 95% CI: 2.79–3.49) (Gei et al., 2001b). Approximately 1% of suicide gestures in a gravid woman will result in a maternal death (Bayer, 1983). The consideration of a suicide attempt as the mechanism of the poisoning or overdose is extremely important when evaluating and treating these patients.

Toxicologic considerations in pregnancy

The poisoned pregnant woman poses particular challenges to the obstetrician as well as to the emergency department physicians and toxicology experts. Most of these challenges are the result of the variable effects with which the physiologic changes of pregnancy may influence the absorption, distribution and metabolic disposition of different potentially toxic agents (see Table 38.2) (Gei & Saade, 2001).

It is fair to say that overall, there is little information on the appropriate treatment of poisoning in pregnancy, and the use of antidotes raises ethical and medicolegal questions (McElhatton, 1997). Several instances have been reported where treatment has been withheld to women because of the gravid condition, with catastrophic results for both mother and fetus (Richards & Brooks, 1966; Strom et al., 1976; Olenmark et al., 1987).

A developing fetus brings forth the considerations and concerns for latent and delayed effects, including teratogenesis and developmental issues on the conceptus. Up to a certain extent, although the pregnant patient goes through an episode of overdose or poisoning during pregnancy, the fetus would continue to be exposed to the toxic agent and environment sometimes for several weeks. Once the acute compromise of the pregnant patient resolves, a specific discussion on those regards is in many cases warranted and proper follow-up needs to be considered (Gei & Saade, 2001).

Evaluation of the poisoned pregnant patient

Although both the poisoning and the pregnancy can be concealed or unknown at the time of patient presentation or initial consult, the most common scenario is that of a pregnant woman in her second trimester with a history of an acute exposure to a known toxic agent. The ideal setting for the evaluation of these patients is the emergency department, as the situation can range from a very straightforward one of no consequence to a complex life-threatening one, requiring a multidisciplinary team and elaborate forms of treatment. The algorithms presented in Figs 38.1 and 38.2 summarize guidelines of evaluation and management of pregnant patients with a known or suspected toxic exposure, regardless of the agent(s) in question. Specific comments are made on the most relevant aspects (Gei & Saade, 2001).

Initial evaluation (Figs 38.1, 38.2)

The initial assessment should determine in a matter of seconds if the patient is conscious or unconscious and if so, if she is in cardiac or respiratory arrest (Fig. 38.1). The management of the latter conditions in pregnancy differs very little from the ones on nonpregnant patients with the exception of two additional considerations.

Table 38.2 Physiological changes of pregnancy and their toxicological impact

System/gestational change	Toxicological implication
Digestive Pica Decreased intra-esophageal pressure Delayed gastric emptying Delayed transit time Hepatic flow unchanged Reduced hepatic enzymatic activity	*Pros:* • Window of opportunity for gastric lavage potentially longer *Cons:* • Increased risk of exposure • Increased gastric absorption • Increased risk of aspiration • Increased enteral absorption • Increased risk of hepatotoxicity
Respiratory Hyperemia of upper respiratory tract Increased minute ventilation Decreased residual lung volume Increased diffusing capacity	*Pros:* • Higher sensitivity to hypoxemia and hypercarbia (protective against respiratory depression) *Cons:* • Increased absorption of inhaled agents
Circulatory 30–50% increase in cardiac output 50% increase in plasma volume 25% decrease in serum albumin Increased oxygen consumption	*Pros:* • Dilutional effect *Cons:* • Higher concentrations in organs with rich perfusion (uterus, placental bed, kidneys, skin) • Higher free fraction of toxins and higher placental passage
Renal Increase in glomerular filtration rate Increased tubular reabsorption	*Pros:* • Increased renal clearance of protein bound and unbound substances *Cons:* • Increased nephrotoxicity potential
Skin Increased surface Increased blood flow	*Cons:* • Increased absorption of contact agents
Uterus/placenta Volume increased by 2,000% at term Increased blood perfusion Pronounced liposolubility	*Pros:* • Maternal protection for certain exposures *Cons:* • Fetal exposure to toxic agents
Others Body mass: • Increased by 25% at term Oxygen consumption: • Increased by 20% Fat: • Increased storage • Third-trimester mobilization	*Pros:* • Larger distribution volumes *Cons:* • Potential for re-exposure during third trimester

(Reproduced by permission from Gei AF, Saade GR. Poisoning during pregnancy and lactation. In: Yankowitz J, Niebyl J., eds. Drug Therapy in Pregnancy, 3rd edn. Philadelphia: Lippincott, Williams and Wilkins, 2001.)

1 Special positioning with a pelvic tilt or wedge to the left and/or the manual displacement of the uterus off the midline to the left is recommended, to relieve the aortocaval compression by the gravid uterus and improve venous blood return.
2 If evaluated by emergency department physicians, a prompt consult to the obstetric service is recommended, as these patients require expert assessment of the gestational age and eventually the capability to proceed with a bedside cesarean section if the resuscitative efforts are not successful (see Fig. 38.2, unconscious algorithm) (Kloeck et al., 1997).

The rapid removal of all clothes (including footwear) is critical. The personnel involved in the patient care should handle the clothes with gloves and set them aside in a labeled

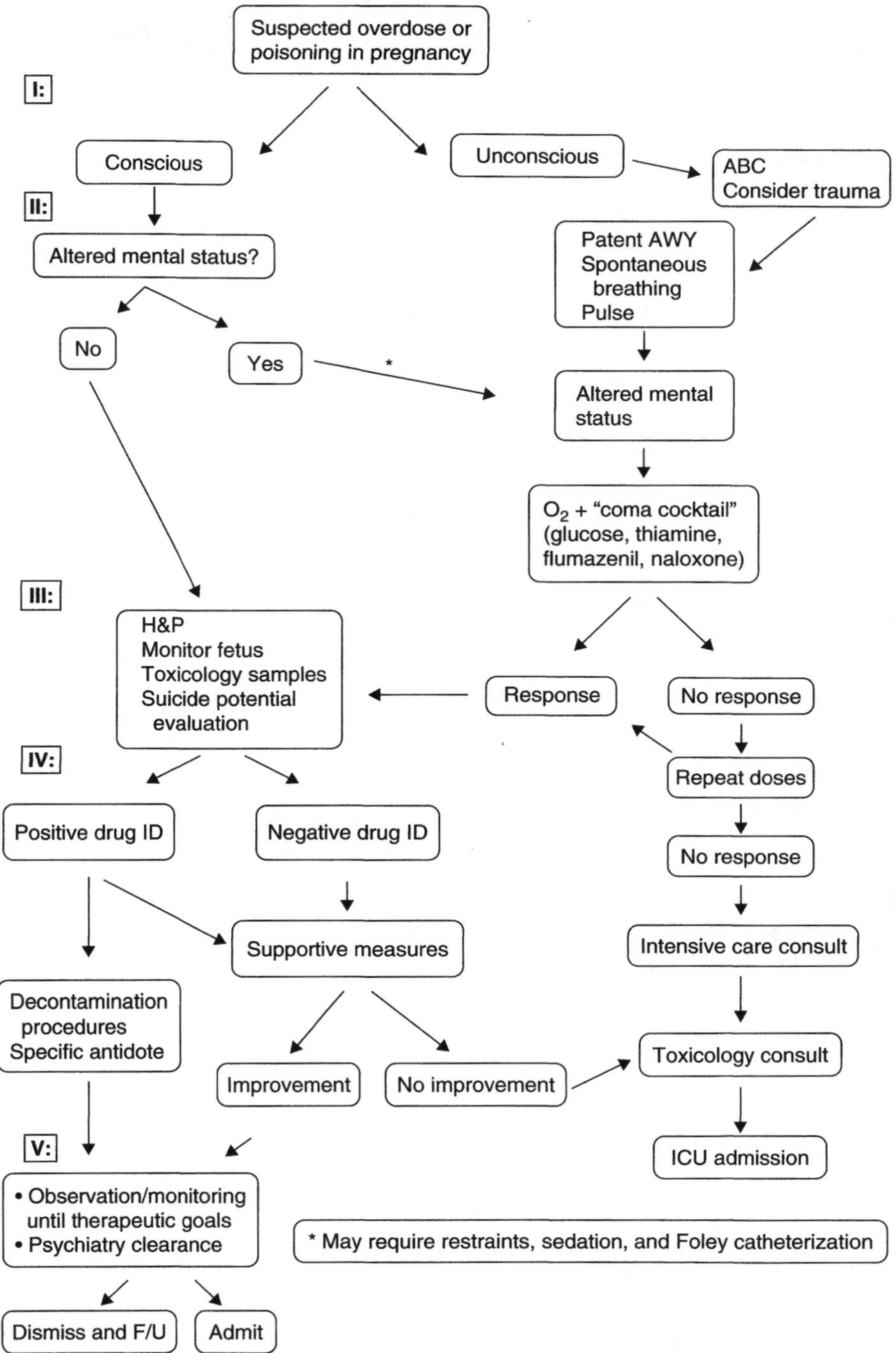

Fig. 38.1 Guidelines for evaluation and management of pregnant patients with a known or suspected toxic exposure. ABC, airway/breathing/circulation; AWY, airway; F/U, follow-up; H&P, history and physical; ICU, intensive care unit.

plastic bag. Absorption through the skin of toxins, organic chemicals, and industrial compounds is generally the rule rather than the exception. Garments can potentially be used for sampling later and should not be disposed of.

In the unconscious patient with suspected toxic exposure, trauma should be strongly considered and cervical spine injury should be stabilized until it can be evaluated and cleared by the trauma physicians.

Altered mental status

If the patient is unconscious but hemodynamically stable, or conscious but disoriented, the diagnosis of "altered mental status" is made.

Hypoxemia and hypoglycemia should immediately be considered as possible etiologies; supplemental oxygen and parenteral glucose infusion (50 g of 50% glucose) are started

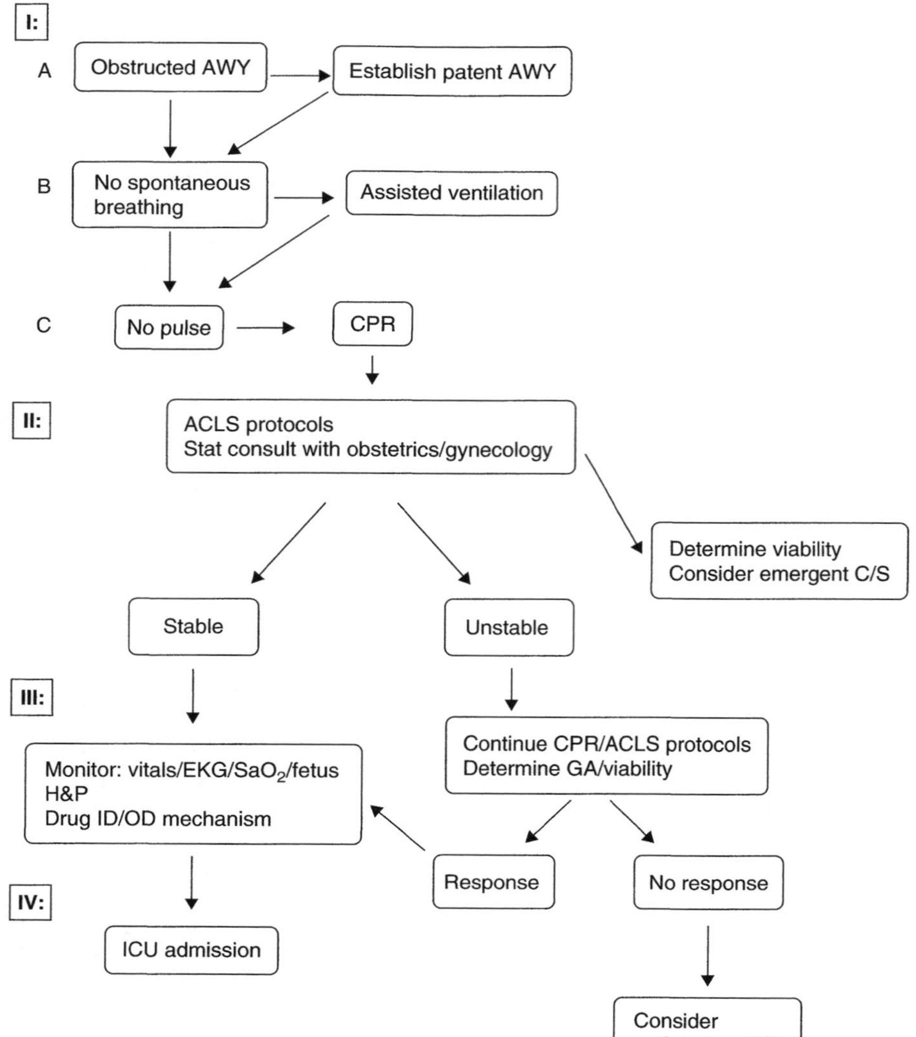

Fig. 38.2 Guidelines for the evaluation of the unconscious pregnant patient with a known or suspected toxic exposure. ACLS, advanced cardiac life support; AWY, airway; CPR, cardiopulmonary resuscitation; C/S, cesarean section; EKG, electrocardiogram; GA, gestational age; H&P, history and physical; OD, overdose.

without delay, even before the diagnosis is confirmed, through an arterial blood gas and a glucose determination. Forcing oral intake in a patient with altered mental status is discouraged.

The use of padded restraints, the insertion of an indwelling bladder catheter and intravenous sedation may be required for the management of uncooperative and belligerent patients. The use of sedatives should ideally be delayed until the toxic agent(s) of exposure is identified to avoid unforeseeable interactions and possibly further CNS depression. Most institutions have special policies regarding the documentation of indications, the extent and the duration for physical restraints.

Other components of the so-called coma-cocktail (thiamine, naloxone, and flumazenil) should not be given routinely but selectively and as considered appropriate by the treating physicians. Specific recommendations for the use of these medications can be seen in Table 38.3.

Secondary evaluation

History taking is of fundamental importance and every effort should be made to obtain as much information from as many sources as possible (patient, her relatives or friends, and the paramedic personnel if she was brought to the emergency department). Besides the obstetric and general history, specific questions that need to be asked regarding the toxic exposure are: the time of exposure, substances exposed to, the amount of exposure (including strength of prescription, if pills or medications), route of exposure, treatment prior to arrival (including emetics, dilutants, and adsorbants), vomit (number and content) or diarrhea (number and content), and symptoms.

A high degree of caution needs to be exercised with the interpretation of the histories, as the information obtained can be contradictory, and in the case of suicide attempts/gestures,

Table 38.3 Altered mental status: indications for antidote treatment in pregnancy

Medication	Indication	Dose/route/interval/cautions
Naloxone (Narcan)	Altered mental status (AMS) associated with: • miosis • respiratory rate less than 12 or • circumstantial evidence of opioid use/abuse	2 mg (IV, IM, ET, IL); onset of action: 1–3 min. May repeat if no response is noted after 3–5 min (maximal effect is observed within 5–10 min) • An IV drip or repeated doses are given as needed • Higher doses may be necessary to reverse methadone, diphenoxylate, propoxyphene, butorphanol, pentazocine, nalbuphine, designer drugs, or veterinary tranquilizers • Caution in cardiovascular disease; may precipitate withdrawal symptoms in patients with opiate addiction
Thiamine (vitamin B_1, thiamilate)	AMS in patient with risk factors for B_1 deficiency: • ethanol abuse • malnutrition • hyperemesis gravidarum • eating disorder • total parenteral nutrition • AIDS • cancer • dialysis requirement	100 mg daily IV/IM for up to 2 weeks • Administer before or with dextrose-containing fluids (100 mg/L of fluid)
Flumazenil (Romazicon)	AMS with: • suspected or known benzodiazepine exposure and no contraindication for antidote use (hypersensitivity, use of benzodiazepine for control of life-threatening condition, intracranial pressure or seizure disorder), coexposure to tricyclic antidepressant or chronic benzodiazepine use • check EKG to rule out conduction disturbances, which would suggest the presence of tricyclics	0.2 mg (2 mL) given IV over 30 sec; a second dose of 0.3 mg (3 mL) can be given over another 30 sec • Further doses of 0.5 mg (5 mL) can be given over 30 sec at 1-min intervals up to a total dose of 3 mg (although some patients may require up to 5 mg) • If the patient has not responded 5 min after receiving a cumulative dose of 5 mg, the major cause of sedation is probably not due to benzodiazepines and additional doses of flumazenil are likely to have no effect • For resedation, repeated doses may be given at 20-min intervals; no more than 1 mg (given as 0.5 mg/min) at any one time and no more than 3 mg in any 1 hr should be administered

deceitful. As a rule of thumb, the most severe history of exposure obtained should be used as a clinical parameter to guide the initial treatment (Gei et al., 1997).

Some groups of agents produce a complex of signs and symptoms that can be recognized as a typical syndrome (toxidrome) (see Table 38.4) (Noji & Kelen, 1989; Briggs & Freeman, 1994; Doyon & Roberts, 1994). Knowledge of such toxidromes is particularly useful when information about the substance is not available. Other physical findings that are useful in the recognition of a toxic exposure are outlined in Table 38.5.

Pregnant victims have particular issues to be considered in the interpretation and treatment of overdose and poisoning (see Table 38.6).

Toxic identification

The collection of samples for toxicology is of paramount importance in the identification of the toxic agent(s), to predict the severity and to implement and monitor specific treatment/antidotes. As a general rule, at least one sample of all biologic fluids obtained should be held for toxicology analysis. Depending on the clinical circumstances, these will include blood, urine, saliva, vomit, gastric lavage fluid, feces, CSF, amniotic fluid if collected, and even meconium if the patient delivers soon after admission. Ideally, specimens sent to the laboratory should include 10–15 mL of serum (whole blood for certain toxic substances), 50–100 mL of urine, and 100 mL of initial gastric aspirate or emesis (Shannon et al., 1995) (see Tables 38.7 and 38.8).

The main treatments for all poisonings are supportive measures. For some toxic agents, three additional strategies can be implemented to: (i) decrease the exposure (decontamination procedures); (ii) enhance elimination (diuresis, hemofiltration, hemoperfusion, hemodialysis, plasmapheresis); or (iii) counteract the toxicity of the agent (antidotes or immunotherapy) (Pond, 1990). Measures to enhance elimination and the use of antidotes is specific for every toxic substance and will be discussed later as appropriate (see Tables 38.9, 38.10, 38.11).

Table 38.4 The most common toxic syndromes

Class of drug	Common signs	Common causes
Anticholinergics	Dementia with mumbling speech Tachycardia Dry flushed skin Dilated pupils (mydriasis) Myoclonus Temperature slightly elevated Urinary retention Decreased bowel sounds Seizures/dysrhythmias (severe cases)	Antihistamines Antiparkinsonian medications Atropine Scopolamine Amantadine Antipsychotics Antidepressants Antispasmodics Mydriatics Skeletal muscle relaxants Some plants (i.e. jimson weed)
Sympathomimetics	Delusions Paranoia Tachycardia Hypertension Hyperpyrexia Diaphoresis Piloerection Mydriasis Hyperreflexia Seizures/dysrhythmias (severe cases)	Cocaine Amphetamines Methamphetamines and derivatives Over-the-counter decongestants (phenylpropanolamine, ephedrine, pseudoephedrine) NB: Caffeine and theophylline overdoses have similar findings, except for organic psychiatric signs
Opiate/sedatives	Coma Respiratory depression Constricted pupils (miosis) Hypotension Bradycardia Hypothermia Pulmonary edema Decreased bowel sounds Hyporeflexia Needle marks	Narcotics Barbiturates Benzodiazepines Ethchlorvynol Glutethimide Methyprylon Methaqualone Meprobamate
Cholinergics	Confusion/CNS depression Weakness Salivation Lacrimation Urinary and fecal incontinence Gastrointestinal cramping Emesis Diarrhea Diaphoresis Muscle fasciculations Bronchospasm	Organophosphate and carbamate insecticides Physostigmine Edrophonium Some mushrooms (*Amanita muscaria*; *Amanita pantherina*, *Inocybe* spp., *Clitocybe* spp.)

(From Briggs GG, Freeman RK, eds. Drugs in pregnancy and lactation, 4th edn. Baltimore: Williams and Wilkins, 1994; and Doyon S, Roberts JR. Reappraisal of the "coma cocktail". Dextrose, flumazenil, naloxone and thiamine. *Emerg Clin of North Am*, 1994;12:301–316.)

Decontamination procedures

Skin

Substances that can cause significant systemic toxicity through transdermal absorption include: organophosphate insecticides, organochlorines, nitrates, and industrial aromatic hydrocarbons. Organophosphates in particular can pass through intact skin at a remarkable speed, without causing any specific skin sensation of burning or itching. In theory, pregnancy, as shown earlier in Table 38.2 predisposes to such toxicity, given the physiologic increase in skin perfusion throughout gestation.

The skin should be flushed thoroughly with warm soapy water. It may be worthwhile to use an industrial shower (as is used for corrosive exposure) as higher flow and volumes are desirable to thoroughly rinse the entire body.

A rare exception to immediate skin decontamination would be exposure to agents that react violently with water (e.g. the chemical may ignite, explode, or produce toxic fumes with water). Examples include chlorosulfonic acid, titanium tetrachloride, and calcium oxide.

Gastrointestinal

Several strategies can be useful (Smilkstein, 1998).

Dilution

Lacking alternatives (see below), 200–300 mL of milk may be given orally (not through gastric tubes) for caustic ingestions (acids or alkalis).

Table 38.5 Physical findings in poisoning

Pupils		
Dilation		
Alkaloids	Ergot	Phenytoin
Aminophylline	Ethanol	Quinine
Anticholinergics	Ethylene glycol	Reserpine
Antihistaminics	Glutethimide	Sympathomimetics
Barbiturates	LSD	Toluene
Carbon monoxide	Methaqualone	Tricyclics
Cocaine	Mushrooms	Withdrawal states
Cyanide	Phenothiazines	
Constriction		
Acetone	Cholinesterase inhibitors	Organophosphates
Barbiturates	Clonidine	Phencyclidine
Benzodiazepines	Codeine	Phenothiazines
Caffeine	Ethanol	Propoxyphene
Chloral hydrate	Meprobamate	Sympatholytics
Cholinergics	Opiates (except meperidine)	
Breath odor		
Acetone:	Acetone, chloroform, ethanol, isopropyl alcohol, salicylates	
Acrid or pear-like:	Chloral hydrate, paraldehyde	
Bitter almonds:	Cyanide	
Carrots:	Cicutoxin (water hemlock)	
Garlic:	Arsenic, organophosphates, phosphorus, selenium, thallium	
Mothballs:	Camphor, naphthalene, paradichlorobenzene	
Pungent aromatic:	Ethchlorvynol (Placidyl)	
Violets:	Turpentine	
Wintergreen:	Methyl salicylate	
Reflexes		
Depressed		
Antidepressants	Ethanol	Narcotics
Barbiturates	Ethchlorvynol	Phenothiazines
Benzodiazepines	Glutethimide	Tricyclic antidepressants
Chloral hydrate	Meprobamate	Valproic acid
Clonidine		
Hyperreflexia		
Amphetamines	Haloperidol	Propoxyphene
Carbamazepine	Methaqualone	Propranolol
Carbon monoxide	Phencyclidine	Strychnine
Cocaine	Phenothiazines	Tricyclic antidepressants
Cyanide	Phenytoin	

(Data for "Breath odor" from Olson K. Poisoning and drug overdose, 2nd edn. Norwalk, CT: Appleton and Lange, 1994.)

Induction of emesis

This is considered the second choice after lavage as the preferred method for gastric emptying. The dose in adults is 30 mL of ipecac with water and repeated in 15–30 minutes if vomiting is not induced. Indicated in ingestions of drugs that can form gastric concretions: salicylates, meprobamate, barbiturates, glutethimide or drugs that can delay the gastric emptying: tricyclics, narcotics, salicylates or conditions producing adynamic ileus (Table 38.12).

Its use is controversial for the following reasons:

1 Not immediately effective.
2 The effect may persist for 2 hours, delaying the administration of adsorbants.
3 Unlikely to be effective within several hours after the ingestion (more than 1–2 hours with exceptions).
4 Not proven to be better than lavage.
5 Has several contraindications: caustic ingestion; altered mental status; inability to protect airway; seizures or seizure potential; hemorrhagic diathesis; hematemesis; ingestion of drugs that can lead to rapid change in the patient's condition (tricyclics, β-blockers, phencyclidine (PCP), isoniazid).
6 Has no value in ethanol intoxication and certain hydrocarbon ingestions.
7 In case of failure to induce emesis (about 5% of cases), the stomach should be evacuated by other means, since ipecac can be cardiotoxic (theoretical risk).

Table 38.6 Factors to consider in the clinical management of the pregnant poison patient

Supine hypotensive syndrome
Lower potential to resist acidosis in pregnancy
Need for preservation of a maternal P_aO_2 of at least 60–70 mmHg for fetal oxygenation
Increased maternal cardiac output and oxygen consumption
Increased renal clearance of antidotes and therapeutic drugs
Different "normal" values of blood tests such as BUN and creatinine
Effects of various resuscitative drugs on the uteroplacental circulation and myometrium
Increased potential for gastric aspiration in pregnant women and heightened need for airway protection

Table 38.7 Quantitative toxicology testing

Test	Time to sample postingestion	Repeat sample	Implication positive test
Acetaminophen	4 hr	None	Blood level Nomogram and N-acetylcysteine
Carbamazepine	2–4 hr	2–4 hr	Repetitive doses of activated charcoal/hemoperfusion
Carboxyhemoglobin	Immediate	2–4 hr	100% oxygen
Cholinesterase blood RBC	Immediate	12–24 hr	Confirm exposure to insecticide
Digoxin	2–4 hr	2–4 hr	Digoxin antibody fragments (Fab)
Ethanol	0.5–1 hr	Not necessary	If negative, not ethanol intoxication; if positive, inconclusive (tolerance)
Ethylene glycol	0.5–1 hr	2 hr	Ethanol therapy, hemodialysis, sodium bicarbonate
Heavy metals	First 24 hr	2–4 hr	Chelation therapy, dialysis
Iron	2–4 hr (chewable/liquid preparation absorbed faster)	2–4 hr	Serum iron 350 μg use deferoxamine
Isopropanol	0.5–1 hr	2 hr	Supportive-care hemodialysis
Lithium	2–4 hr	4 hr	Hemodialysis
Methanol	0.5–1 hr	2 hr	Ethanol therapy folinic acid, $NaHCO_3$, hemodialysis
Methemoglobin	Immediate	1–2 hr	Methylene blue
Phenobarbital	1–2 hr	4–6 hr	Alkaline diuresis Repeated activated charcoal; hemoperfusion
Phenytoin	1–2 hr	4–6 hr	Supportive care Repeated activated charcoal
Salicylates	2–4 hr	2–4 hr	Serum and urine alkalinization Repeated activated charcoal, hemodialysis
Theophylline	1-hr peak at 12–36 hr	1–2 hr	Repeat activated charcoal, hemoperfusion

2-PAM, pralidoxime; ABGs, arterial blood gases; Fab, fragment antigen-binding; PT, prothrombin time; PTT, partial thromboplastin time.
(Reproduced by permission from Mowry JB, Furbee RB, Chyka PA. Poisoning. In: Chernow B, Borater DC, Holaday JW, et al., eds. The Pharmacological Approach to the Critically Ill Patient, 3rd edn. Baltimore: Williams and Wilkins, 1995.)

Table 38.8 Time intervals for detecting drugs in urine after use

Drug	Detectable after use
Alcohol	24 hr
Amphetamines	48 hr
Barbiturates	
Short-acting	48 hr
Long-acting	7 days
Benzodiazepines	72 hr
Cocaine	72 hr
Marijuana	
Single use	72 hr
Chronic use	30 days

(Reproduced by permission from Thorp J. Management of drug dependency, overdose, and withdrawal in the obstetric patient. Obstet Gynecol Clin North Am 1995;22).

Gastric lavage

Gastric lavage is indicated when emesis is inappropriate or contraindicated, the patient is comatose or mentally altered, the substance ingested has the potential for seizures or when the substance ingested is lethal and/or rapidly absorbed (i.e. delay for emesis can result in death). This measure is contraindicated in ingestion of caustics and in hemorrhagic diathesis. It has the advantages that it can be performed immediately on arrival, takes only 15–20 minutes to complete, and facilitates the administration of charcoal.

A large gastric tube (Ewald, Lavaculator, and others), size 36–40 French, should be passed orally with lubricant. Consideration for intubation needs to be made in patients with depressed mental status, altered gag reflex, and seizures or seizure potential. The patient needs to be placed in Trendelenburg position or sitting position and aspiration prior to lavage

Table 38.9 Compounds for which hemoperfusion is appropriate

Acetaminophen	Chloroquine	Heptabarbital	Procainamide
Amanita toxins	Creatinine	Meprobamate	Quinalbital
Ammonia	Cyclobarbital	Methaqualone	Quinidine
Amobarbital	Demeton	Methotrexate	Salicylates
Barbital	Digoxin	Methyprylon	Secobarbital
Bromide	Dimethoate	Nitrostigmine	Theophylline
Butabarbital	Diquat	Paraquat	Thyroxine
Camphor	Diisopyramide	Parathion	Tricyclic antidepressant
Carbon tetrachloride	Ethanol	Pentobarbital	Triiodothyronine
Carbamazepine	Ethchlorvynol	Phenobarbital	Uric acid
Chloral hydrate	Glutethimide	Phenytoin	

Table 38.10 Compounds for which dialysis is an appropriate consideration

Acetaminophen	Chloride	Gallamine	Nitrofurantoin
Aluminum	Chromate	Gentamicin	Ouabain
Amanita toxin	Cimetidine	Glutethimide	Paraquat
Amikacin	Cisplatin	Hydrogen ions	Penicillin
Ammonia	Citrate	Iodide	Phenobarbital
Amobarbital	Colistin	Iron desferrioxamine	Phosphate
Amoxicillin	Creatinine	Isoniazid	Potassium
Amphetamines	Cyclobarbital	Isopropyl alcohol	Primidone
Ampicillin	Cyclophosphamide	Kanamycin	Procainamide
Aniline	Cycloserine	Lactate	Quinidine
Arsenic	Demeton	Lead edetate	Quinine
Azathioprine	Diazoxide	Lithium	Salicylates
Barbital	Dimethoate	Magnesium	Sodium
Borate	Diquat	Mannitol	Streptomycin
Bromide	Diisopyramide	Meprobamate	Strontium
Butabarbital	Ethambutol	Methanol	Sulfonamides
Calcium	Ethanol	Methaqualone	Theophylline
Camphor	Ethchlorvynol	Methotrexate	Thiocyanate
Carbenicillin	Ethionamide	Methyldopa	Ticarcillin
Carbon tetrachloride	Ethylene glycol	Methylprednisolone	Tobramycin
Cephalosporins	Flucytosine	Methyprylon	Trichloroethylene
Chloral hydrate	Fluoride	Metronidazole	Urea
Chloramphenicol	5-Fluorouracil	MAO inhibitors	Uric acid
Chlorate	Fosfomycin	Neomycin	Water

Table 38.11 Antidotes

Poison	Antidote	Dosage
Acetaminophen	N-Acetylcysteine	140 mg/kg PO, followed by 70 mg/kg/4 hr × 17 doses
Anticholinergics (atropine)	Physostigmine salicylate	0.5–2.0 mg IV (IM) over 2 min every 30–60 min prn
Anticholinesterases (organophosphates)	Atropine sulfate	1–5 mg IV (IM, SQ) every 15 min prn
	Pralidoxime (2-PAM) chloride	1 g IV (PO) over 15–30 min every 8–12 hr × 3 doses prn
Benzodiazepines	Flumazenil (British data)	1–2 mg IV (for respiratory arrest)
Carbon monoxide	Oxygen	100%, hyperbaric
Cyanide	Amyl nitrite	Inhalation pearls for 15–30 sec every minute
	Sodium nitrite	300 mg (10 mL of 3% solution) IV over 3 min, repeated in half dosage in 2 hr if persistent toxicity
	Sodium thiosulfate	12.5 g (50 mL of 25% solution) IV over 10 min, repeated in half dosage in 2 hr if persistent toxicity
Digoxin	Antidigoxin Fab fragments	—
Ethylene glycol	Ethanol	0.6 g/kg ethanol in D5W IV (PO) over 30–45 min, followed initially by 110 mg/kg/hr to maintain blood level of 100–150 mg/dL
Extrapyramidal signs	Diphenhydramine HCl	25–50 mg IV (IM, PO) prn
	Benztropine mesylate	1–2 mg IV (IM,PO) prn
Heavy metals (arsenic, copper, gold, lead, mercury)	Chelator	
	Calcium disodium edetate (EDTA)	1 g IV (IM) over 1 hr every 12 hr
	Dimercaprol (BAL)	2.5–5.0 mg/kg IM every 4–6 hr
	Penicillamine	250–500 mg PO every 6 hr
Heparin	Protamine	1 mg/100 units heparin and for every 60 min after heparin, halved dose
Iron	Desferrioxamine mesylate	1 g IM (IV at a rate of ≤15 mg/kg/hr if hypotension) every 8 hr prn (maximum 80 mg/kg in 24 hr)
Isoniazid	Pyridoxine	Gram per gram ingested; 5 g, if INH dose unknown
Magnesium sulfate	Calcium glutamate	2–3 g IV over 5 min (in 30-mL D10)
Methanol	Ethanol	See ethylene glycol
Methemoglobinemia (nitrites)	Methylene blue	1–2 mg/kg (0.1–0.2 mL/kg 1% solution) IV over 5 min, repeated in 1 hr prn
Opiates/narcotics	Naloxone HCl	0.4–2.0 mg IV (IM, SQ, ET) prn
Warfarin	Phytonadione/vitamin K	0.5 mg/min IV (in NS or D5W)

2-PAM, pralidoxime; ET, endotracheal; IM, intramuscularly; INH, isoniazid; NS, normal saline; PO, by mouth; prn, as circumstances may require; SQ, subcutaneously.
(From Thorp J. Management of drug dependency, overdose, and withdrawal in the obstetric patient. Obstet Gynecol Clin North Am 1995;22:222–228; and Roberts JM. Pregnancy related hypertension. In: Creasy RK, Resnick R, eds. Maternal-fetal Medicine: Principles and Practice, 3rd edn. Philadelphia: WB Saunders, 1994:804–843.)

Table 38.12 Indications for ipecac syrup

Gastric concretion formation
Salicylates
Meprobamate
Barbiturates
Glutethimide
Gastric emptying delay (pregnancy)
Tricyclics
Narcotics
Salicylates
Conditions producing adynamic ileus

needs to be made to confirm placement of the tube (collect sample for analysis). Lavage is made with normal saline or water in runs of 1.5 mL/kg (up to 200 mL) until clear and then with at least one more liter. Some recommend slight movement changes of the patient or position changes to dislodge potential residues of medications or nondissolved pills.

Adsorption (activated charcoal)
Activated charcoal is a finely divided powder made by pyrolysis of carbonaceous material. It consists of small particles with an internal network of pores that adsorb substances. It is indicated after gastric emptying procedures (successful or not) and in repeated doses (2–4 hours) for drugs with enterohepatic circulation (theophylline, digoxin, nortryptiline and

amitryptiline, salicylates, benzodiazepines, phenytoin and phenobarbital, for example). This effect has been called gastrointestinal dialysis. Activated charcoal may be used immediately after ipecac (does nor interfere with its action; some authors actually think it is the best way to administer) and N-acetylcysteine. It is contraindicated in caustic ingestions and ineffective in ingestion of elemental metals (e.g. iron), some pesticides (malathion; DDT), cyanide, ethanol, and methanol.

The typical dose is 30–100 g in adults (or 1 g/kg) and is usually given with a cathartic (50 mL of 70% sorbitol or 30 g of magnesium sulfate) in order to accelerate the transit time of the complex toxin–charcoal. A superactivated charcoal formulation, capable of adsorbing 2–3 times the conventional capacity of the charcoal is available.

Neutralizing agents

In some poisonings a neutralizing agent instead of charcoal is preferable for instillation (see Table 38.13).

Table 38.13 Poisoning in which a specific neutralizing agent is preferable to activated charcoal

Mercury	Sodium formaldehyde (20 g) converts HgCl to less soluble metallic mercury
Iron	Iodium bicarbonate (200–300 mL) converts ferrous iron to ferrous carbonate
iodine	Starch solution (75 g of starch in 1 L of water; continue until aspirate is no longer blue)
Strychnine, nicotine, quinine, physostigmine	Pótassium permanganate (1 : 10,000)

Cathartics

Cathartics are used as adjunctive treatment with charcoal. These agents should be used only when needed. They are contraindicated in diarrhea, dehydration, electrolyte imbalances, abdominal trauma, intestinal obstruction, and ileus. The agent most frequently used in poisoning treatment is sorbitol because of the onset of action (less than an hour), duration of effect (8–12 hours), and no interaction with charcoal. Oil cathartics are contraindicated because they can be aspirated and can increase the absorption of hydrocarbons. Complications can result from over-aggressive use (fluid and electrolyte imbalances).

Whole bowel irrigation

This consists of the administration of polyethylene-glycol at a rate of 500–2,000 mL/hr orally or through a nasogastric tube with the purpose of cleaning the bowel of whole or undissolved pills. It may be helpful in clearing the GI tract of iron, delayed-release formulations not adsorbed by charcoal, or very delayed onset of treatment. The procedure takes 3–5 hours and may be complicated by bowel perforation or obstruction, ileus, or gastrointestinal hemorrhage.

Specific agents

More than 250,000 drugs and commercial products are available for ingestion (Weisman et al., 1990; Olson, 1994). Table 38.14 lists the most frequent causes of morbidity and mortality from poisoning in the United States (Litovitz et al., 2000). Figure 38.3 details the classes of drugs most frequently used in suicide attempts among 1,085 pregnant women in 1999. The general characteristics and management of selected toxic exposures during pregnancy is discussed in further detail in their alphabetical order for ease of access. Since

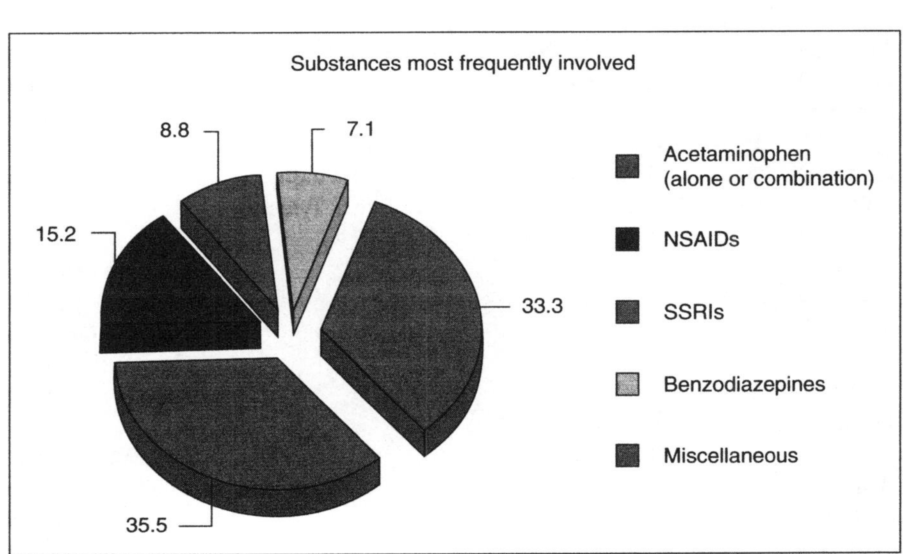

Fig. 38.3 Suicide attempts during pregnancy by poisoning or overdose. During 1999 1,085 suicidal toxic exposures were reported to American Poison Control Centers among pregnant women. This represents 12% of the toxic exposures reported during pregnancy for that year and less than 1% of the suicide attempts by poisoning reported to the AAPCC. The substances most frequently involved were: acetaminophen (alone or in combination with decongestants and antihistamines) (35.5%), NSAIDs (15.2%), SSRIs (8.8%), and benzodiazepines (7.1%). (From American Association of Poison Control Centers (AAPCC). Toxic Exposure Surveillance System (TESS) exposures in pregnant women 1999 special report. Washington DC.)

Table 38.14 Substances most frequently involved in adult exposures (>19 years)

Substance	No.	% of all adult exposures	As cause of mortality
Analgesics	92,245	13.3	1
Sedatives / hypnotics / antipsychotics	67,946	9.8	3
Cleaning substances	66,384	9.5	12
Antidepressants	55,429	8.0	2
Bites/envenomations	55,145	7.9	19
Alcohols	37,451	5.4	6
Food products, food poisoning	35,860	5.2	20
Cosmetics and personal care products	33,511	4.8	18
Chemicals	31,738	4.6	10
Pesticides	31,285	4.5	15
Cardiovascular drugs	28,941	4.2	5
Fumes / gases / vapors	27,486	3.9	9
Hydrocarbons	27,419	3.9	16
Antihistamines	19,570	2.8	11
Anticonvulsants	17,851	2.6	7
Antimicrobials	17,683	2.5	14
Stimulants and street drugs	17,423	2.5	4
Plants	17,261	2.5	17
Cough and cold preparations	16,866	2.4	18

(From Litovitz TL, Klein-Schwartz W, White S, et al. 2000. Annual report of the American Association of Poison Control Centers Toxic Exposure Surveillance System. Am J Emerg Med 2001;19(5):337–95.)

the publication of the previous edition, the different regional Poison Control Centers in the United States have adopted a universal phone number for reports and consults: 1-800-222-1222.

Acetaminophen (Horowitz et al., 1997; Jones & Prescott, 1997; McElhatton et al., 1997; Wang et al., 1997; Erickson & Neylan, 1998; Goldfrank et al., 1998; Rutherfoord-Rose, 1998)

Toxicology

Common proprietary names
Alka-Seltzer (some presentations), Anacin, Benadryl (some presentations), Comtrex, Contac, Coricidin, Darvocet, Dimetapp, Drixoral, Esgic, Excedrin (aspirin-free), Fioricet, Goody's Body Pain Relief, Lortab, Midol, Midrin, Nyquil, Pamprin, Panadol, Parafon R, Percocet, Phenaphen, Robitussin, Sudafed, Tavist, Thera-Flu, Triaminic, Tylenol, Tempra, Unisom, Vicodin, Wygesic.

FDA classification
B.

As a cause of morbidity
1 (other analgesics included) (Litovitz et al., 1999).

As a cause of mortality
1 (other analgesics included) (Litovitz et al., 1999).

Most frequent route of exposure
Ingestion.

Most frequent reason for exposure
Unintentional overdose.

Metabolism
Acetaminophen is metabolized in the liver to nontoxic sulfate (52%) and glucuronide (42%) forms and then excreted by the kidneys. Approximately 4% is metabolized by the hepatic cytochrome oxidase P-450 system, resulting in a toxic reactive intermediate. This toxic metabolite is conjugated with glutathione and excreted in the urine as nontoxic mercaptourate. Two percent of acetaminophen is excreted unchanged. In an overdose, the hepatic glutathione stores are depleted and the toxic intermediates become covalently bound to hepatic cellular proteins, resulting in hepatocellular necrosis (Peterson, 1978).

Serum half-life
In pregnancy the serum half-life is 3.7 hours, and the pharmacokinetics (absorption, metabolism, and renal clearance) are similar in the pregnant and nonpregnant states (Rayburn et al., 1986; Reynolds et al., 1990).

Lethal dosage
The lethal dosage is in excess of 140 mg/kg and primarily involves hepatotoxicity (Peterson, 1978). The lethality of acetaminophen is not related directly to the dose, and other factors

such as age, nutritional status, and other compounds ingested may affect the amount of cytochrome P-450 present and, thus, its toxicity. Renal failure, myocardial depression, and pancreatitis also have been observed in acute overdoses.

Maternal considerations

In general, the primary short-term problem of acetaminophen overdose is hepatocellular necrosis, which peaks at 72–96 hours. Cardiac, renal, and pancreatic complications rarely occur, but appropriate monitoring should be instituted. Perhaps the most serious long-term consequence is residual liver damage.

Symptoms
Nausea; vomiting; anorexia; right upper quadrant pain. The symptoms of acetaminophen toxicity have been divided into four stages (Table 38.15).

Signs
Icterus; right upper abdominal tenderness; lethargy; evidence of bleeding.

Diagnostic tests
Blood: acetaminophen level (at 4 or more hours of ingestion). A level drawn less than 4 hours after ingestion may reflect a partially absorbed and falsely low level; transaminases (elevated); lactic dehydrogenase (LDH) (elevated); prothrombin time (PT) (prolonged); amylase (elevated); lipase (elevated); creatinine (elevated); urinalysis. Plot acetaminophen values in the Rumack–Matthew nomogram (Fig. 38.4) to assess risk of hepatotoxicity. EKG: Nonspecific ST/T changes.

Short-term problems
Oliguria; pancreatitis; hypotension; myocardial ischemia and necrosis. Premature contractions; potential for premature delivery.

Long-term problems
Diffuse hepatic necrosis (potential for 1–2% late mortality).

Table 38.15 Stages of acetaminophen toxicity

Phase	Time	Symptoms
I	0–24 hr	Gastrointestinal symptoms (anorexia, nausea, vomiting), malaise, diaphoresis
II	24–48 hr	Clinical improvement, but abnormal liver function tests
III	72–96 hr	Peak hepatotoxicity with encephalopathy, coagulopathy, and hypoglycemia
IV	7–8 days	Death, or recovery from hepatic failure (begins within 5 days and usually progresses to complete resolution within 3 months)

Fetal and neonatal considerations

General
Crosses the placenta; fetus at risk of poisoning, particularly late in pregnancy. Unless severe maternal toxicity develops, acetaminophen overdose does not appear to increase the risk for adverse pregnancy outcome (Kozer & Koren, 2001). Placental transfer of therapeutic levels of N-acetylcysteine in humans has been documented and provides evidence of a direct antidotal effect of N-acetylcysteine in the fetus (Horowitz et al., 1997).

Signs
Decreased fetal movements; decreased beat to beat variability; absence of fetal heart rate accelerations; falling baseline heart rate.

Teratogenic potential
No support for association; potential for fetal liver damage (hepatocellular necrosis); increased risks of spontaneous abortion and stillbirth. None of the reported studies has shown an increase in fetal anomalies after an overdose (Rumack & Matthew, 1975; McElhatton et al., 1997).

Fetal distress potential
Yes; reported. There is a relationship between pregnancy outcome and the interval between drug exposure and administra-

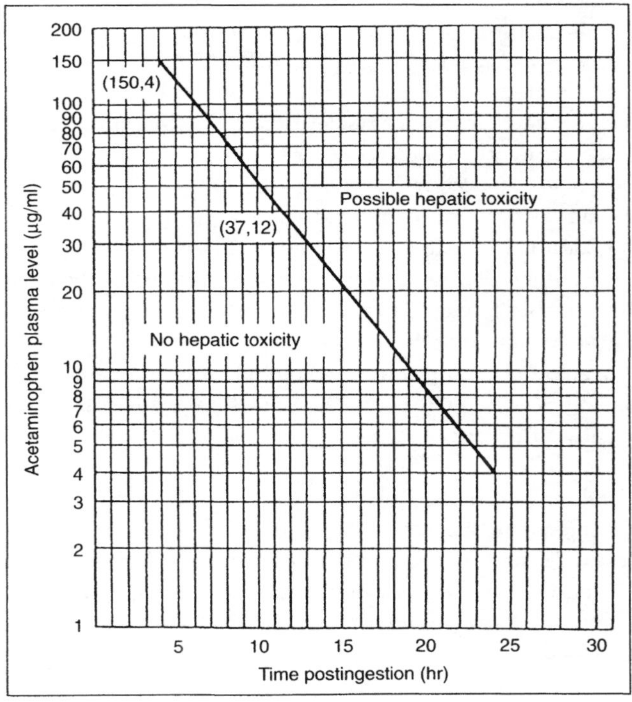

Fig. 38.4 Nomogram for acetaminophen toxicity. (Reproduced by permission of Pediatrics from Rumack RH, Matthew H. Acetaminophen poisoning and toxicity. Pediatrics 1975;55:871.)

tion of N-acetylcysteine, with an increase in the incidence of spontaneous abortion and stillbirth as the interval increases (Ludmir et al., 1986; Riggs et al., 1989).

Indications for delivery
Nonreassuring fetal condition.

Neonatal period
Hyperbilirubinemia.

Management guidelines

In regards to acetaminophen poisoning, pregnant patients should be managed no differently from nonpregnant patients.

Supportive measures
Induced emesis may be indicated for home treatment of a large dose (>100 mg/kg or ~6 g). Gastric lavage + activated charcoal (1 g/kg in water or sorbitol).

Specific measures / antidotes
Available. Indications for antidotal use are:
1 Ingestion greater than 6 g (or 100 mg/kg).
2 Acetaminophen levels (at 4 or more hours after exposure) of 150 μg/mL or greater (993 μmol/L),
3 History of exposure to other hepatotoxics or history of liver disease associated with the acetaminophen exposure (including ethanol, carbamazepine, and isoniazide).
4 If the results of the acetaminophen levels will not be available by 7–8 hours after the exposure.

Oral: methionine (2.5 g every 4 hours × 4 doses) or N-acetylcysteine (category B) (140 mg/kg loading followed by 70 mg/kg every 4 hours for 17 doses).
Parenteral (preferred in pregnancy): N-acetylcysteine: 150 mg/kg in 200 mL of 5% dextrose over 15 min or 100 mg/kg in 1,000 mL 5% dextrose over 16 hours. The best results are obtained when therapy is started within 16 hours of the overdose, but N-acetylcysteine is still indicated up to 24 hours after ingestion of the overdose (Rumack et al., 1981).

In selected circumstances, hemoperfusion and hemodialysis have been found to be effective, but these techniques are not usually indicated.

Monitoring
Vital signs/mental status/intake and output. *Blood:* transaminases, PT, and acetaminophen level every 4 hours (first 24 hours), then daily or as indicated. Other tests if originally abnormal or drawn less than 4 hours since exposure. *EFM:* indicated.

Therapeutic goals
Asymptomatic patient; normal liver function tests (transaminases and PT).

Disposition considerations
ICU admission if hepatic failure or encephalopathy (see Table 38.16). Consider psychiatric evaluation for all exposures. Contemplate induction of labor in third-trimester exposures in severe exposures. May discharge after 72–96 hours from exposure if therapeutic goals met.

Follow-up
Caution the patient about possibility of spontaneous abortion, premature delivery, and risk of stillbirth. Counsel against the use potential hepatotoxics. Consider serial biophysical profiles in viable pregnancies and severe exposure (value not established). Clinical follow-up may include a social worker, obstetrician, hepatologist, and psychiatrist.

Amphetamines

Toxicology

Amphetamines are a group of sympathomimetic drugs used to stimulate the CNS via norepinephrine- and dopamine-mediated pathways. Although the precise mechanism of action is unknown, proposed mechanisms have included presynaptic release of catecholamines, direct postsynaptic stimulation, and inhibition of monoamine oxidase. These drugs are used frequently for appetite suppression, to treat narcolepsy, or for illicit recreational reasons.

Examples/other names
Amphetamine sulfate (Benzedrine) (Briggs & Freeman, 1994), dextroamphetamine (Dexedrine), methamphetamine (Methedrine); "ecstasy," "X," "E," "XTC," "Adam;" "hug;" "beans;" "love drug."

FDA classification
C(M).

As a cause of morbidity
17 (Litovitz et al., 2000).

Table 38.16 Criteria for consideration of admission to the intensive care unit

Mechanical ventilation required
Vasopressor support necessary
Arrhythmia management or need for hemodialysis
Signs of severe poisoning
Worsening signs of toxicity
Predisposing underlying medical conditions
Potential for prolonged absorption of toxin
Potential for delayed onset of toxicity
Invasive procedures or monitoring needed
Antidotes with potential for serious side effects
Suicidal patients requiring observation

As a cause of mortality
4 (Litovitz et al., 2000).

Most frequent route of exposure
Oral; occasionally mucous membranes (snorting and suppositories); rarely injected.

Most frequent reason for exposure
Unintentional overdose.

Metabolism
Amphetamines are weak bases with a p*K*a of 9.9 and are metabolized in the liver. Both active metabolites and free amphetamines are excreted in the urine. Chronic abusers develop tolerance to amphetamines and may ingest lethal doses without effect. Thus, most cases of fatal intoxication seen are of people who are not chronic abusers.

Lethal dosage
The lethal dose in adults is 20–25 mg/kg. Smaller doses, however, have been known to be fatal (Haddad & Winchester, 1990).

Maternal considerations

Pregnant women who use "ecstasy" (3,4-methylenedioxy-methamphetamine, MDMA) tend to be young, single, and report psychological morbidity, and have a clustering of risk factors that may compromise the pregnancy and fetus. Smoking, heavy alcohol intake, and polydrug use, combined with a higher than expected rate of unplanned pregnancies, increases the risk of fetal exposure to potentially harmful substances (Ho et al., 2001).

Symptoms (See Table 38.17)

Signs
Tachycardia; hypertension; muscle tension; involuntary teeth clenching.

Diagnostic tests
Blood levels correlate partly with both clinical status and mortality risk, secondary to the development of tolerance.

Short-term problems
Short-term problems are manifested by cardiovascular changes such as severe hypertension, tachyarrhythmias, and cardiovascular collapse. Strokes have been reported.

Long-term problems
The potential long-term consequence of chronic abuse is psychosis and Parkinsonism.

Table 38.17 Signs and symptoms of amphetamine overdose

Mild toxicity
Respiratory (tachypnea)
Cardiovascular (tachycardia, mild hypertension, chest pain, palpitations)
Gastrointestinal (abdominal cramping, nausea, vomiting, diarrhea)
Sympathetic stimulation (mild hyperpyrexia, dry mouth, mydriasis, diaphoresis, hyperreflexia)
Central nervous system symptoms (dizziness, hyperactivity, irritability, confusion, and panic)
Severe toxicity
Cardiovascular (severe hypertension with intracranial hemorrhage, tachyarrhythmias, ventricular tachycardia or fibrillation, hypotension, and cardiovascular collapse)
Severe hyperthermia (associated with coagulopathies, rhabdomyolysis, and renal failure)
Metabolic (systemic acidosis)
Central nervous system (convulsions, delirium, psychosis, usually in chronic abusers with paranoia, delusions, and hallucinations, coma)

Fetal and neonatal considerations

Signs
Intrauterine growth restriction. Neonatal amphetamine and methamphetamine withdrawal syndromes have been described (Sussman, 1965; Neuberg, 1970; Oro & Dixon, 1987).

Teratogenic potential
The teratogenic potential of amphetamines depends on the type and teratogenic category (Briggs & Freeman, 1994). Presently, there is no evidence that amphetamines are associated with an increase in the frequency of major and/or minor congenital malformations (Biggs et al., 1975; Little et al., 1989). Correcting for confounding factors (tobacco, alcohol), however, babies of amphetamine abusers have significantly decreased birth weight, length, and head circumference (Little et al., 1989). Nevertheless, a prospective follow-up of 136 babies exposed to ecstasy in utero indicated that the drug may be associated with a significantly increased risk of congenital defects (15.4% [95% CI 8.2–25.4]). Cardiovascular anomalies (26 per 1,000 liver births [3.0–90.0]) and musculoskeletal anomalies (38 per 1,000 [8.0–109.0]) were predominant. Data suggest that exposure to MDMA in utero during the maturation phase does not produce damage to 5-HT nerve terminals in the fetal rat brain, in contrast to the damage seen in the brains of the mothers. This may be due to MDMA being metabolized to free-radical producing entities in the adult brain but not in the immature brain or, alternatively, to more effective or more active free-radical scavenging mechanisms being present in the immature brain (Colado et al., 1997).

Fetal distress potential
Controversial. Some found that infants exposed to methamphetamine and/or cocaine have significantly greater fre-

quency of prematurity, intrauterine growth retardation, placental hemorrhage, and anemia (Rayburn et al., 1984; Oro & Dixon, 1987). To others, the incidence of fetal distress, preterm labor, and premature rupture of membrane is reduced in these women (Matera et al., 1990; Gillogley et al., 1990).

Indications for delivery
Obstetric indications.

Management consideration

Supportive
With amphetamine overdose, the therapeutic goal is to provide primarily supportive care until the patient is stabilized. Then, the patient should be placed in a cool, quiet environment to diminish external stimulation.

Specific measures/antidotes
The first step is gastric emptying, followed by charcoal instillation and cathartic administration for oral overdoses. Forced acid diuresis is indicated in severe toxicity to enhance renal excretion. In addition, symptomatic therapy for psychosis and agitation can best be treated with haloperidol (chlorpromazine may increase the half-life of amphetamines and cause greater respiratory depression) or diazepam. Along with these complications, seizures may be terminated with diazepam, and recurrent seizures may be treated with phenytoin. Cardiovascular complications such as arrhythmias and hypertension can be managed with propranolol and haloperidol or chlorpromazine, respectively.

Severe or refractory hypertension may require phentolamine or nitroprusside. Hypotension may be treated initially with IV fluids. Refractory hypotension may be due to catecholamine depletion and may require a direct-acting agent such as norepinephrine.

Hyperthermia is an ominous sign. Haloperidol or chlorpromazine and active cooling should be used to manage temperatures in excess of 102° F.

Hemodialysis may be useful for life-threatening cases that are unresponsive to supportive care or in patients with renal compromise.

Monitoring
As part of patient management, appropriate patient monitoring is essential. This includes EKG, BP, respiratory rate and blood gases, electrolytes, temperature, urine myoglobin levels, and fetal heart rate and uterine activity, when applicable.

Therapeutic goals
Asymptomatic patient.

Discharge considerations
When the patient is considered ready for discharge, she should be considered for drug rehabilitation.

Follow-up
Clinical follow-up may include a social worker, obstetrician, and psychiatrist. Subsequently, she should be monitored for evidence of preterm labor, placental hemorrhage, and intrauterine growth restriction.

Antidepressants (Martin et al., 1974; Vree & Zwart, 1985; Levine et al., 1991; Gossel, 1994; Gimovsky, 1995; Perrone & Hoffman, 1997, 1998; Erickson & Neylan, 1998; PDR Electronic Library, 1999)

Toxicology

The safety profile of SSRIs in overdose is very favorable. SSRIs' efficacy for both mood and anxiety disorders, relatively weak effect on the cytochrome P-450 system, ad tolerability profile and safety in overdose are factors that contribute to make it a first-line agent during pregnancy (Mourilhe & Stokes, 1998; MacQueen et al., 2001).

Bupropion hydrochloride is a new antidepressant that differs clinically and pharmacologically from the tricyclic antidepressants and the monoamine oxidase inhibitors. Bupropion is devoid of cardiovascular effects (e.g. impaired intracardiac conduction, reduced myocardial contractility, decreased peripheral resistance, orthostatic hypotension) in both human and animal studies. The drug is nonsedating and antagonizes the effects of commonly used sedatives, such as alcohol and diazepam. Given this profile, bupropion should be less toxic than conventional antidepressants when taken in overdoses; however, overdose experience with the drug is limited (Preskorn & Othmer, 1984).

Examples/other names
Imipramine, amitriptyline, doxepin, trimipramine, trazadone, fluoxetine, Anafranil, Asendin, Celexa, Desyrel, Effexor, Elavil, Etafron, Limbitrol, Luvox, Nardil, Norpramin, Parnate, Pamelor, Paxil, Prozac, Remeron, Serzone, Sinequan, Surmontil, Tofranil, Triavil, Vivactil, Wellbutrin, Zoloft.

FDA classification
D.

As a cause of morbidity
4 (Litovitz et al., 2000).

As a cause of mortality
2 (Litovitz et al., 2000).

Most frequent route of exposure
Ingestion.

Most frequent reason for exposure
Unintentional overdose.

Maternal considerations

Antidepressant drugs (imipramine, amitriptyline, Doxepin, trimipramine, trazadone, fluoxetine) may produce three major toxidromes: anticholinergic crisis, cardiovascular failure, or seizure activity. A patient may experience one or all three of these toxic effects, depending on the dose and the drug taken.

Symptoms
Dry mouth; urinary retention; delirium (Table 38.18).

Signs
No evident toxicity; agitation; mydriasis; hyperthermia; tachycardia; dry axilla; myoclonus; rapid loss of consciousness; seizures; cardiac dysrrhythmias (Table 38.18).

Diagnostic tests
In patients with an overdose, an EKG is the most helpful diagnostic test. Here, the clinician is looking for a sinus tachycardia with prolonged PR, QRS, and QT intervals. Prolongation of the QRS segment greater than 0.12 is a reliable indicator of serious cardiovascular and neurologic toxicity (with the exception of amoxapine). In addition, bradyarrhythmias carry a bad prognosis. Additional ECG changes include atrioventricular block and ventricular tachycardia. Although drug levels can be obtained, these are not generally useful in the acute management of an overdose. Arterial blood gases, electrolytes, glucose, and complete blood count also are helpful laboratory tests.

Short-term problems
Short-term problems include cardiac dysrhythmias, seizures, urinary retention, gastrointestinal hypomotility, aspiration pneumonitis, and acute respiratory distress syndrome (ARDS).

Table 38.18 Signs and symptoms of antidepressant overdose

Signs	Symptoms
Tachycardia	Blurred vision
Dry skin and mucous membranes	Dysarthria
Blisters	Visual hallucinations
Mydriasis	Sedation
Divergent strabismus	Delirium
Decreased bowel sounds	Sedation
Urinary retention	Coma
Increased muscular tone	
Hyperreflexia	
Myoclonic activity	
Rapid loss of consciousness	
Seizures	
Cardiac dysrhythmias	
Hypotension	
Pulmonary edema	

Long-term problems
Long-term problems include rhabdomyolysis, brain damage, and multisystem failure.

Fetal and neonatal considerations

The effects of antidepressants on the fetus are variable.

Teratogenic potential
The teratogenic potential appears to involve an increased risk of cardiovascular defects in exposed fetuses

Fetal distress potential
Yes due to maternal seizures, hypotension, or dysrhythmias.

Indications for delivery
Usual obstetric indications.

Postnatal
Postnatally, the neonate may be predisposed to tachypnea, cyanosis, irritability, urinary retention, and paralytic ileus.

Management considerations

Supportive
With antidepressant overdose, the therapeutic goal is to prevent complications in the first 24 hours after a significant ingestion. During therapy, 12 hours of maternal and fetal cardiac monitoring is recommended in asymptomatic pregnant patients. If there are signs of significant maternal toxicity, 24 hours in an intensive care setting appears warranted. Because painful interventions and patient movement can precipitate seizures, such stimuli should be avoided. Agitation, seizures, hyperthermia, hypotension, and arrhythmias should be treated.

Specific measures / antidotes
The first step is decontamination with activated charcoal and a cathartic. Induced emesis is contraindicated because of the risk of sudden onset of seizures. A gastric lavage also should be performed, after which the orogastric or nasogastric tube is connected to continuous suctions).

Forced diuresis, dialysis, and hemoperfusion are generally ineffective.

If the patient manifests coma, seizures, QRS greater than 0.1 second, ventricular arrhythmias, or hypotension, alkalinization therapy with IV sodium bicarbonate is indicated. To alkalinize the patient, one ampule (44–50 mEq) of sodium bicarbonate should be given IV slowly over 1–5 minutes. This is followed by an infusion at 0.5 mEq/kg/hr to maintain an arterial pH of 7.45–7.55. If perfusion is compromised or there is hypotension despite bicarbonate therapy, phenytoin 100 mg over 3 minutes should be considered. Antiarrhythmics are used to control dysrhythmias.

Controversy exists regarding the use of physostigmine salicylate (usually given as a 2 mg bolus over 2 min) because it may precipitate convulsions or ventricular tachycardia. In situations in which there is doubt as to the cause of the coma, or in patients with altered mental status and serious respiratory compromise, physostigmine may be considered.

If seizures are not immediately controlled with anticonvulsants, muscle relaxation with a nondepolarizing long-acting agent (pancuronium, norcuronium) should be instituted to avoid hyperthermia and lactic acidosis. An EEG may be required to evaluated the effectiveness of the anticonvulsant therapy.

Monitoring
At least 6 hours of cardiac monitoring is recommended. Patients who initially are awake may abruptly lose consciousness and/or develop seizures without warning. Once decontamination has been initiated, supportive therapy is warranted to maintain the airway, and, if necessary, mechanical ventilation should be instituted.

Therapeutic goals
Asymptomatic patient. Normal EKG. Observe (or make arrangements for outpatient monitoring) for 72 hours, because deaths from the original overdose have been reported up to 3 days after ingestion.

Discharge considerations
Prior to the discharge of the patient, a final dose of charcoal should be considered. In addition, the patients will need to be evaluated for suicide potential.

Follow-up
Clinical follow-up may include a social worker, obstetrician, and a psychiatrist.

Aspirin (Rejent & Baik, 1985; Balaskas, 1992; Chan 1996; Erickson & Neylan, 1998; Goldfrank et al., 1998; Kerns, 1998; Palatrick & Tenenbein, 1998; White & Wong, 1998; PDR Electronic Library, 1999)

Common proprietary names
Alka-Seltzer, Ascriptin, BC Powder, Bufferin, Darvon, Ecotrin, Excedrin, Fiorinal, Goody's Body Pain Relief, Norgesic, Pepto-Bismol, Percodan, Soma, Talwin.

FDA classification
C (D if full dose used in third trimester).

As a cause of morbidity
1 (other analgesics included) (Litovitz et al., 1999).

As a cause of mortality
1 (other analgesics included) (Litovitz et al., 1999).

Main route of exposure
Oral.

Main mechanism of exposure
Intentional.

Maternal considerations

Symptoms
None; nausea, vomiting; abdominal pain; tinnitus; decreased audition; dyspnea.

Signs
Hyperventilation; altered mental status; flushing; diaphoresis; hyperpirexia; gastrointestinal bleeding; petechiae; bruising; hypovolemia; pulmonary edema; seizures; ARDS; coma.

Diagnostic tests
Blood: *arterial blood gases*: respiratory alkalosis; compensated metabolic acidosis or metabolic acidosis; increased anion gap (greater than 14 mEq/L; see Table 38.19); salicylate levels; creatinine; blood urea nitrogen; electrolytes, glucose; complete blood count; prothrombin and partial thromboplastin times; *urinalysis*: specific gravity, volume and ferric chloride test (beside colorimetric test: add 10% ferric chloride ($FeCl_3$) in equal amounts to a 1 mL of urine at least 2 hours after ingestion: purple to purple brown indicates salicylate presence). *Chest X ray*: edema.

Short-term problems
Volume depletion; shock; hemorrhage; seizures.

Long-term problems
Prolonged pregnancy; prolonged labor; higher risk of peripartum hemorrhage.

Fetal considerations

Salicylates cross the placenta freely and concentrate within the fetus, particularly in the CNS.

Signs
Constriction of ductus arteriosus; growth restriction.

Teratogenic potential
No.

Table 38.19 Causes for an increased or decreased anion gap

Increased anion gap
Lactic acidosis:
Beta-adrenergic drugs
Caffeine
Carbon monoxide
Cyanide
Hydrogen sulfide
Ibuprofen
Iron
Isoniazid
Phenformin
Salicylates
Seizures
Theophylline
Other:
Benzyl alcohol
Ethanol (ketoacidosis)
Ethylene glycol
Exogenous organic and mineral acids
Formaldehyde
Methaldehyde
Methanol
Toluene
Decreased anion gap
Bromates
Lithium
Nitrites

Fetal distress potential
Yes.

Indications for delivery
Nonreassuring fetal condition. Avoidance of instrumental delivery is recommended (risk for cephalohematomata and intracranial bleeding).

Neonatal period
Hyperbilirrubinemia; clinical evidence of thrombocytopenia.

Management considerations

Supportive
Generous IV fluid (glucose containing solutions) replacement; if hypotension is refractory, may use plasma or blood. May need central hemodynamic monitoring to manage fluid administration. If assisted ventilation required, hyperventilation (16–20/min) as needed to keep Pco_2 around 35 mmHg. Keep glycemia above 90 mg/dL.

Specific measures/antidotes
Induced emesis not recommended.

Gastric lavage is recommended (even if more than 4 hours have elapsed since ingestion).

Forced alkaline diuresis (0.45% saline solution + 5% glucose + 44 mEq of bicarbonate and 20 mEq of KCl added per liter); goal: 5–10 mL/min of urine with pH of 7.5.

Administer *vitamin K* 10 mg IV or IM (aspirin inhibits vitamin K).

Hemodyalisis may be indicated (severe CNS symptoms; pulmonary edema; renal failure; salicylate level greater than 90 mg/dL (6.6 mmol/L); inability to alkalinize urine and/or no improvement with decontamination and urine alkalinization).

Monitoring
Vital signs/mental status/intake and output/EKG/oxymetry. *Blood*: arterial blood gases and potassium every 2–4 hours (monitor alkalinization). Serial determination of salicylate levels (every 2 hours) until declining trend noted and levels fall below 30 mg/dL (2.2 mmol/L). Serial blood glucose. Urine: pH every hour. If fetus is viable consider informing the neonatology or pediatrics service of the potential delivery of a salicylate-exposed infant.

Therapeutic goals
Asymptomatic patient; level under 30 mg/dL (2.2 mmol/L) more than 2 hours after exposure.

Disposition considerations
Contemplate induction of labor in third trimester exposures in severe exposures. May discharge if asymptomatic, appropriate treatment administered, decreasing serum levels and absence of electrolyte or acid–base imbalance.

Follow-up
Establish. Consider evaluation of fetal growth. Consider psychiatric evaluation of all ingestions.

Barbiturates (Martin et al., 1974; Mazurek & Mazurek, 1975; Nicholson, 1983; Coupey, 1997; Erickson & Neylan, 1998; McFarland, 1998; PDR Electronic Library, 1999)

Toxicology

Barbiturates (Table 38.20) (Winchester et al., 1977) are weak acids with pKa values ranging between 7.2 and 8.0. The more lipid-soluble drugs have a faster onset but shorter duration of action (see Table 38.20). Barbiturates cause CNS depression and in toxic doses depress other excitable tissues (skeletal, cardiac, and smooth muscle) (Stine & Marcus, 1983). The short-acting agents cause more potent CNS depression, are more toxic, and are more commonly abused.

Common names and examples
Amobarbital, barbital, butabarbital, pentobarbital, phenobarbital, secobarbital, thiamylal, thiopental, Amytal, Arco-Lase,

Table 38.20 Barbiturates commonly associated with overdose*

Type	Duration of action	Drug
Ultra-short-acting (methohexital)	20 min	Thiopental, thiamylal
Short-acting	3 hr	Pentobarbital, secobarbital, hexobarbital
Intermediate-acting	3–6 hr	Amobarbital, butabarbital, aprobarbital,
Long-acting	6–12 hr	Barbital, phenobarbital, mephobarbital Primidone

* Lethal dosage: short-acting, ingestion of 3 g (lethal level, 3.5 mg/dL); long-acting, ingestion of 5 g (lethal level, 8 mg/dL) (Winchester et al., 1977).

Butisol, Donnatal, Esgic, Fioricet, Fiorinal, Luminal, Membaral, Nembutal, Phrenilin, Sedapap, Tuinal, Veronal.

FDA classification
D (most of them).

As a cause of morbidity
2 (sedatives, hypnotics and antipsychotics) (Litovitz et al., 2000).

As a cause of mortality
3 (sedatives, hypnotics and antipsychotics) (Litovitz et al., 2000).

Most frequent route of exposure
Ingestion.

Most frequent reason for exposure
Unintentional overdose; acute or chronic.

Maternal considerations

Barbiturate use by adolescents has increased gradually in the past several years, often used to treat unpleasant effects of illicit stimulants, to reduce anxiety, and to get "high."

Symptoms
Weakness; fatigue; sleepiness.

Signs
Sedation; altered mental status; miosis; bradypnea; respiratory depression; ataxia; nystagmus; extraocular muscle palsies; dysarthria; hyporeflexia; decreased bowel sounds; hypothermia; hypotension; cardiovascular collapse (see Table 38.21).

Table 38.21 Signs and symptoms of barbiturate overdose

Central nervous system
Mild intoxication: drowsiness
Moderate intoxication: CNS depression, slurred speech, ataxia, nystagmus, and miosis
Severe intoxication: extraocular motor palsies, absent corneal reflexes, sluggish pupillary reaction, mydriasis, absent deep tendon reflexes, absent Babinski sign, and coma. A flatline EEG has been reported
Respiratory system
Respiratory depression (typically three times the hypnotic dose) (Stine, 1983; Roberts, 1994)
Aspiration pneumonia, atelectasis, pulmonary edema, and bronchopneumonia also have been reported
Cardiovascular system
Hypotension, low cardiac output, and direct myocardial depression (Stine & Marcus, 1983; Roberts, 1994)
Other
Hypothermia due to depressed thermal regulation in the brainstem
Cutaneous bullae (barb-burns) over pressure points (Roberts, 1994)
Decreased GI motility
Renal failure due to cardiovascular shock or rhabdomyolysis

Diagnostic tests
Blood: complete blood cell count; electrolytes; glucose; creatinine and blood urea nitrogen; PT and PTT; phenobarbital level (levels may not correlate with symptoms). *Urinalysis*: drug screen; pH.

Short-term problems
Respiratory failure; coma; anoxic encephalopathy (interpretation of EEGs is unreliable with abnormal levels of barbiturates).

Long-term problems
Withdrawal syndrome is chronic user/abuser (insomnia; excitement; delirium; psychosis; seizures; hypotension).

Fetal considerations

Signs
Potential for decreased beat to beat variability; bradycardia; abnormal biophysical profile in severe maternal poisoning.

Teratogenic potential
Controversial. Because barbiturates cross the placenta, the teratogenic potential depends on the agent and the category (B/C/D/Y) (Briggs & Freeman, 1994). Epileptic pregnant women taking phenobarbital in combination with other anticonvulsants have a two-to-threefold greater risk of minor congenital defects in the fetus (Briggs & Freeman, 1994). A recent large cohort study found a significant increase of major malformations, microcephaly, growth retardation, midface hypoplasia and hypoplasia of the fingers among infants born to mothers receiving phenobarbital as antiepileptic (Holmes, 2001).

Fetal distress potential
The potential for fetal distress depends on maternal clinical status. In severe intoxication, cardiopulmonary depression (respiratory depression, hypoxemia, or cardiovascular collapse) may lead to fetal compromise.

Indications for delivery
Obstetric indications. Caution is suggested when interpreting fetal assessment techniques (electronic fetal monitoring and biophysical profile).

Postnatal
Fetal and neonatal addiction have been reported (Shubert & Savage, 1994). Neonatal withdrawal complications may occur 3–14 days after delivery and may require treatment (Desmond et al., 1972). Phenobarbital and other anticonvulsant agents also have been associated with early hemorrhagic disease of the newborn (Bleyer & Skinner, 1982). May cause neonatal sedation of some breastfed infants (caution patients about it).

Management considerations

With barbiturate overdose, the initial therapeutic goal is stabilization of maternal cardiopulmonary status. Gradual detoxification is then instituted to prevent abrupt withdrawal complications.

Supportive
Respiratory support is the priority; measures needed may range from supplemental oxygen to endotracheal intubation and mechanical ventilation. Maintaining an adequate volume expansion and diuresis is critical. Forced alkaline diuresis recommended for symptomatic patients (add potassium to the bicarbonate infusion).

Specific measures/antidotes
Induced emesis may be indicated if no significant depression; gastric lavage (even after 8 hours after the exposure) followed by activated charcoal and catharsis is recommended. Multiple doses of activated charcoal (every 4 hours) are recommended. Alkaline diuresis through the combination of sodium bicarbonate, intravenous fluids, and diuretics enhances elimination (goal: 5–10 mL/min of urine with a pH ~8.0) and may be indicated in stage III or IV coma induced by long-acting barbiturates (Stine & Marcus, 1983).

Because phenobarbital may form gastric concretions, endoscopic removal (Shannon et al., 1995) may be surgically necessary.

Hypotension may be supported by oxygen and IV fluids. With severe hypotension, dopamine or norepinephrine may be required.

In chronic overdose, a decremental dosage regimen, beginning with 200 mg of phenobarbital every 6 hours should be used to prevent withdrawal complications in both mother and fetus (Shubert & Savage, 1994; Shannon et al., 1995). Hemoperfusion (resin over charcoal) or hemodialysis may be indicated in cases of toxic/lethal exposures (phenobarbital level of 100 μg/mL or 430 μmol/L), if uremia develops or when the exposure is to long-acting barbiturates.

No specific antidote is available.

Monitoring
Vital signs/mental status/airway/blood pressure/EKG/oxygen saturation; electrolytes and serum calcium levels need to be followed. Severe toxicity requires management in an ICU (Stine & Marcus, 1983). In cases of suspected barbiturate overdose, blood levels may be useful for confirming the identity of the drug, although the quantitative level may not reflect the clinical status of the patient. The patient's clinical condition is the best predictor of morbidity and mortality in cases of barbiturate toxicity. Death occurs from cardiopulmonary depression and is seen only in deeply comatose patients. The quantity of drug ingested and the blood level may not correlate with the clinical status, because chronic abusers develop tolerance (Stine & Marcus, 1983).

Therapeutic goals
Asymptomatic patient; no need for supplemental oxygen or volume expansion; therapeutic or subtherapeutic level.

Discharge considerations
Dose adjustment if patient is epileptic. Psychiatry consult recommended if mechanism of exposure is deemed intentional. Barbiturate withdrawal is characterized by insomnia, excitement, delirium, hallucinations, toxic psychosis, tremors, nausea and vomiting, orthostatic hypotension, and seizures. This condition may not present until 48–72 hours after the last dose but must be considered whenever managing a chronic abuser, because deaths have been reported with severe withdrawal reactions (see Table 38.22) (Victor & Adams, 1980).

Follow-up
Follow phenobarbital levels. Notify primary physician (obstetrician and neurologist) before discharge. Consider folate supplementation in chronic users. Clinical follow-up with a social worker, obstetrician, and psychiatrist is warranted. As part of the patient's ongoing care, drug rehabilitation should be considered.

Benzodiazepines (Cerqueira et al., 1988; Gaudreault et al., 1991; Stahl et al., 1993; Doyon & Roberts, 1994; Hoffman & Goldfrank, 1995; Sakai et al., 1996; Gei et al., 1997; Weinbrown et al., 1997; Dixon et al., 1998; Erickson & Neylan, 1998; Goldfrank et al., 1998; Schauben, 1998; PDR Electronic Library, 1999)

Toxicology

Benzodiazepines are CNS depressants and are widely pre-

Table 38.22 Therapy for maternal drug withdrawal

Drugs	Therapy
Alcohol	Barbiturates Pentobarbital sodium (short-acting) followed by phenobarbital (longer-acting) Benzodiazepines (cleared slowly by fetus)
Amphetamines	Tricyclic antidepressants (severe depression)
Barbiturates	Barbiturates: 200 mg pentobarbital sodium IV or by mouth to test for physical dependence (short-acting), followed by phenobarbital (withdrawal equivalent, 30 mg phenobarbital/100 mg of short-acting). Estimated dose of phenobarbital is administered by mouth every 8 hr (maximum daily dose, 500 mg; if toxicity, daily dose is halved; if withdrawal symptoms, 200 mg phenobarbital intramuscularly). Once stable, decrease daily dose by 30 mg
Benzodiazepine	Benzodiazepine: slow tapering over a 1–2-week period Barbiturates (see Barbiturates in text) Withdrawal equivalents: 30 mg phenobarbital/100 mg chlordiazepoxide or 50 mg diazepam
Opiates	Librium 10–25 mg by mouth every 8 hr ± compazine, as warranted, for nausea/vomiting Methadone 10–20 mg intramuscularly Refractory withdrawal may require short-acting narcotics (morphine, meperidine, hydromorphine)

(From Stine RJ, Marcus RH. Toxicologic emergencies. In: Haddad LM, Winchester JF, eds. Clinical management of poisoning and drug overdose. Philadelphia: WB Saunders, 1983:297–342; and Thorp J. Management of drug dependency, overdose, and withdrawal in the obstetric patient. Obstet Gynecol Clin North Am 1995;22:131.)

scribed for their anxiolytic, muscle relaxant, anticonvulsant, and hypnotic effects. These drugs have a wide therapeutic index therefore a low lethal potential if the exposure is isolated. Suspect coingestion (particularly with alcohol and tricyclics).

Common names and examples
Lorazepam, oxazepam, clonazepam, diazepam, temazepam, chlordiazepoxide, Ativan, Centrax, Dalmane, Diastat, Halcion, Klonopin, Librium, Limbitrol, ProSom, Restoril, Serax, Tranxene, Valium, Versed, Xanax.

FDA classification
C, D, Y (depending of the drug).

As a cause of morbidity
2 (sedatives, hypnotics and antipsychotics) (Litovitz et al., 2000).

As a cause of mortality
3 (sedatives, hypnotics and antipsychotics) (Litovitz et al., 2000).

Most frequent route of exposure
Ingestion.

Most frequent reason for exposure
Unintentional overdose.

Metabolism
Benzodiazepines are metabolized in the liver by desmethylation (active metabolites) and/or conjugation (inactive metabolites) and are excreted in the urine (predominantly) and in the bile (Hardman & Limbird, 1996). Gastrointestinal absorption is rapid and complete, while intramuscular absorption is erratic (Shannon et al., 1995). Benzodiazepines have a wide therapeutic index (Shannon et al., 1995) and are relatively safe when taken orally and as a single agent (Stine & Marcus, 1983). Intravenous administration, however, has been associated with a 2% mortality from respiratory or cardiac arrest (Shannon et al., 1995).

Maternal considerations

Symptoms
Mild overdose is manifested by drowsiness, nystagmus, dysarthria, ataxia, dizziness, weakness, and confusion. Occasionally, paradoxical irritability, excitation, or delirium may occur (MacGregor & Keith, 1992). Coma is the manifestation of severe overdose. Uncommonly, respiratory and/or circulatory depression may be present.

Signs
Lethargy, altered mental status; slurred speech; ataxia; brady- or tachycardia; decreased bowel sounds; respiratory depression; hypotension; dyskinesia; acute dystonic reactions; coma (rare in the absence of co-ingestants).

Diagnostic tests
Blood: complete blood count; electrolytes and glucose; toxicology screen (detects most of them except clonazepam). Of note, drug levels do not correlate with clinical status. Calculation of osmolal and anion gaps recommended if suspicion of coingestants and severe clinical manifestations (see Tables 38.19 or 38.23). *Urinalysis*: drug screen; specific gravity.

Short-term problems
Respiratory depression; hypotension; anoxic encephalopathy (interpretation of EEG is unreliable with abnormal levels of benzodiazepines).

Long-term problems
Withdrawal syndrome (anxiety; insomnia; dysphoria; nausea; palpitations; fatigue; confusion; delirium; muscle twitching; seizures; psychosis) may appear after 1–7 days after abrupt cessation of benzodiazepines.

Fetal and neonatal considerations

Signs
Potential for decreased beat-to-beat variability; bradycardia; abnormal biophysical profile in severe maternal poisoning.

Teratogenic potential
There is some evidence that a cause-and-effect relationship exists between benzodiazepines and congenital fetal anomalies. In one study, chlordiazepoxide (category D) was associated with a fourfold increase in congenital anomalies (mental deficiency, diplegia and deafness, duodenal atresia, and Meckel's diverticulum) (Milkovich & van den Berg, 1974). However, there was no such association noted in the Collaborative Perinatal Project with first-trimester exposure (Hartz et al., 1975). Diazepam (category D) has been reported to be associated with oral clefts (Safra & Oakley, 1975; Saxen & Saxen, 1975). This association, however, has not been confirmed (Rosenberg et al., 1983; Shiono & Mills, 1984). Laegreid et al. (1987) reported on seven children who were prenatally exposed to benzodiazepines and developed minor anomalies, growth deficiency, and CNS abnormalities, including mental retardation.

Table 38.23 Causes of increased osmolal gap

Methanol (mol. wt = 32)
Ethanol (mol. wt = 46)
Acetone (mol. wt = 58)
Isopropyl alcohol (mol. wt = 60)
Ethylene glycol (mol. wt = 62)
Propylene glycol (mol. wt = 76)
Mannitol (mol. wt = 182)
Ethyl ether
Magnesium
Renal failure without dialysis
Severe alcoholic or lactic ketoacidosis

Fetal distress potential
Only in the presence of severe maternal toxicity and secondary to maternal hypovolemia or hypoxemia.

Indications for delivery
Obstetric indications. Caution is suggested when interpreting fetal assessment techniques (electronic fetal monitoring and biophysical profile).

Postdelivery
High-dose or recent use prior to delivery has been associated with birth depression and withdrawal stigmata in neonates, needing resuscitation measures; risk of neonatal withdrawal may produce seizures 2–6 days after delivery (Athinarayanan et al., 1976). Inform pediatrician of perinatal exposure. Use in lactating women is in general not recommended.

Management considerations

Supportive
If severe toxicity is present, respiratory and cardiovascular support may be required; crystalloid infusion to maintain adequate volume; dopamine and norepinephrine infusions may be required in refractory hypotension.

Specific measures/antidotes
Induced emesis not recommended; gastric lavage recommended in pregnancy followed by activated charcoal (50–60) in sorbitol (1 g/kg) and repeated (25–30 g) every 4 hours (the sorbitol added only every 12 hours)

Flumazenil (Romazicon; category C); give if vital signs are not stable, tricyclic coingestion excluded and if no history of chronic use or abuse on benzodiazepines (possibility of inducing seizures). If the patient develops seizures, IV injection of benzodiazepine may be required to terminate withdrawal seizures, followed by a gradual withdrawal of the agent (MacGregor & Keith, 1992). An alternative treatment is phenobarbital for seizure control.

Monitoring
Vital signs/mental status/oximetry/intermittent fetal heart rate monitoring. Repeat drug levels not indicated.

Therapeutic goals
Asymptomatic patient; normal mental status without benzodiazepine antagonism (at least more than 4 hours since last dose of flumazenil); normal bowel sounds; completed decontamination procedures; no evidence of coingestion; reassuring fetal condition; consults completed.

Discharge considerations
Investigate chronic use/abuse of benzodiazepines. Consider drug counselor, psychiatry and social worker evaluations. Seizures have been reported up to 12 days after withdrawal in chronic users (MacGregor & Keith, 1992).

Follow-up
Notify primary care physician (obstetrician, psychiatry). Clinical follow-up with a social worker, obstetrician, and psychiatrist is warranted. As part of the patient's ongoing care, drug rehabilitation should be considered.

Carbon monoxide (Longo, 1977; Silvers & Hampson, 1995; Koren, 1996; Abramovich et al., 1997; Rubio & García, 1997; Silverman & Montano, 1997; Erickson & Neylan, 1998; Goldfrank et al., 1998; Kopelman & Plaut, 1998; Tomaszewski, 1999)

Toxicology

Carbon monoxide is a colorless, odorless gas. It is a by-product of cigarette smoking (the most common source of carbon monoxide exposure), automobile exhaust, faulty heating systems, and fire (Balaskas, 1992). It is absorbed rapidly through the respiratory tract. Hemoglobin's affinity for carbon monoxide is 250–300 times greater than for oxygen.

Examples
Fires, motor vehicle fumes, heat stoves.

As a cause of morbidity
11th (Litovitz et al., 1999).

As a cause of mortality
8th (Litovitz et al., 1999).

Main route of exposure
Inhalation.

Reasons for exposure
Unintentional; intentional (suicide attempt).

Maternal considerations

Symptoms
Depends on concentration (% COHb): headache; shortness of breath; nausea; dizziness; dim vision; weakness (see Table 38.24).

Signs
Vasodilation; disturbed judgement; collapse; coma; convulsions; Cheyne–Stokes respirations (see Table 38.24).

Table 38.24 Signs and symptoms of carbon monoxide overdose*

Signs	Symptoms
Vasodilation	Headache
Disturbed judgment	Shortness of breath
Collapse	Nausea
Coma	Dizziness
Convulsions	Visual disturbances
Cheyne–Stokes respiration	Weakness

* Signs and symptoms will vary depending on the concentration of carboxyhemoglobin.

Diagnostic tests
EKG: sinus tachycardia, ST depression, atrial fibrillation, prolonged PR and QT intervals; AV or bundle branch block; *Arterial blood gas:* % COHb (correlating with symptoms and signs). *Others:* complete blood count, transaminases, electrolytes, creatinine and urinalysis. If patient rescued from a fire, consider a cyanide level.

Short-term problems
Myocardial ischemia/infarction; rhabdomyolysis; renal failure; pulmonary edema; blindness; hearing loss.

Long-term problems
Delayed CNS toxicity (perivascular infarction; demyelinition of basal ganglia) on comatose of acidotic patients on arrival.

Fetal and neonatal considerations

CO crosses the placenta; higher affinity for fetal than adult hemoglobin results in 10–15% higher levels than maternal levels and higher risk of mortality for fetus (Athinarayanan et al., 1976).

Teratogenic potential
Potential for fetal brain damage; subsequent development delays.

Fetal distress potential
Yes; high.

Indications for delivery
Obstetric indications; fetal distress.

Management considerations

Short-term concerns with carbon monoxide poisoning include myocardial ischemia or infarction, rhabdomyolysis, renal failure, pulmonary edema, blindness, and hearing loss. Delayed problems include CNS toxicity due to perivascular infarction and demyelination of basal ganglia. This is usually seen in patients who are comatose or acidotic on arrival to the hospital.

Supportive
Remove the patient from contaminated environment; absolute rest to decrease oxygen consumption.

Specific measures/antidotes
Oxygen at 100% via tight-fitted non-rebreather mask; some authorities recommend the administration of oxygen for five times as long as it is expected for the maternal levels to normalize (Longo, 1977). Hyperbaric oxygen is recommended if COHb is greater than 20 (versus greater than 40 in the nonpregnant state), signs of nonreassuring fetal condition and any unfavorable neurologic signs in the mother (Haddad & Winchester, 1990).

Monitoring
Additionally, the patient's mental state and acid–base status should be monitored. Diagnostic tests focus on oxygen-sensitive structures such as the heart, lungs, kidneys, and brain. Cardiac evaluation will include an EKG; sinus tachycardia, ST depression, atrial fibrillation, and prolonged PR and QT intervals, and atrioventricular or bundle branch block can be seen. Additionally, arterial blood gases and a COHb level are helpful. The latter correlates with the patient's signs and symptoms. Finally, a complete blood count, transaminases, electrolytes and creatinine, and urinalysis are recommended. If cardiovascular complications are present, the patient should be admitted to be ICU. Such complications are expected in nonpregnant patients with a COHb greater than 15%. This level is lower in pregnant women (COHb 10%).

Admit if impaired mentation or metabolic acidosis are present on arrival.

Therapeutic goals
COHb < 5% and no symptoms. During therapy, any pregnant woman who is exposed to carbon monoxide and has a potentially viable fetus should be monitored for a minimum of 12 hours.

Discharge considerations
Prior to discharge, the identification and avoidance of the source of exposure should be done (social works consult may be helpful). Suicidal potential evaluation (psychiatry consult) if circumstances suggest such possibility. Counsel on discussion of long-term effects on fetus.

Follow-up
Establish. Consider follow-up of intrauterine growth. Clinical follow-up should include ultrasound assessment for possible intrauterine growth evaluation.

Cocaine (Greenland, 1989; Cohen et al., 1991; Lovejoy et al., 1992; Nair et al., 1994; Emery et al., 1995; Miller et al., 1995; Wehbeh et al., 1995; Martinez et al., 1996; Gei et al., 1997; Jackson, 1997; Delaney et al., 1997; Erickson & Neylan, 1998; Goldfrank et al., 1998; PDR Electronic Library, 1999)

Toxicology

Cocaine is naturally occurring agent that is legally available for use as a topical anesthetic. It is more commonly used illegally as a CNS stimulant with a street-sample purity 15–60% (Gay, 1982). It is principally used in one of two forms: either as the hydrochloride salt ("snorted" intranasally or IV) or as an alkaloid ("crack," "free base"). Illegally produced cocaine is frequently adulterated with foreign substances such as lactose, mannitol, lidocaine, and/or procaine (Gay, 1982). It is a sympathomimetic with direct cardiovascular stimulant activity that causes hypertension and vasoconstriction. Cocaine has both direct and indirect cardiotoxic effects (sensitizing the myocardium to epinephrine and norepinephrine) (Zuckerman et al., 1989).

Prevalence rates as high as 10–18% have been reported in indigent pregnant women seen in an inner-city hospital population. The cocaine abuse rate among fee-for-service patients is reported to be 1.4% (Riggs et al., 1989; Zuckerman et al., 1989).

Examples / other names
"Crack," "rock," "blow," "snow," "liquid lady": alcohol + cocaine, "speedball": heroine + cocaine.

FDA classification
X (C if used as a local anesthetic).

As a cause of morbidity
N/A.

As a cause of mortality
4 (street drugs and other stimulants) (Litovitz et al., 2000).

Most frequent route of exposure
Inhalation. Absorbed through mucous membranes; can be inhaled; smoked; swallowed; injected IV, intramuscularly, or subcutaneously; or placed in the vagina or rectum (Grinspoon & Bakalar, 1981).

Most frequent reason for exposure
Unintentional overdose.

Metabolism
It is detoxified by liver and plasma cholinesterase. The fetus and pregnant woman experience slower metabolism and elimination (Bingol et al., 1987; Moore et al., 1989). The peak effects of cocaine in nonpregnant women occur within 3–5 minutes IV or at 60–90 minutes orally. The plasma half-life is 1 hour.

Lethal dose

The lethal dosage of cocaine is approximately 1,400 mg taken orally or 750 mg taken parenterally or inhaled (Gay, 1982). Lethal overdoses can be taken via any route but are more likely with parenteral use of "freebasing" (smoking purified cocaine).

Maternal considerations

Symptoms and signs are secondary to adrenergic stimulation and depend on the severity of the toxicity.

Symptoms

Anxiety; chest pain; respiratory difficulty; palpitations; dizziness; headache; nausea.

Signs

Agitation; altered mental status (up to frank psychosis); tachycardia; hypertension; hyperthermia; mydriasis; tachypnea; diaphoresis; hyperactive bowel sounds; pulmonary edema; uterine contractions (up to tetany); vaginal bleeding. Rectal and vaginal exams indicated to rule out occult drug packing.

Diagnostic tests

Blood: complete blood count; electrolytes and glucose; creatinine and blood urea nitrogen; creatine phosphokinase (CPK) and isofractions; myoglobin; troponine I; amylase; lipase. Urine: microhematuria; myoglobinuria. *EKG*: tachycardia; ischemia; ST elevation; acute myocardial infarction. *Chest X-ray*: pulmonary edema, pulmonary infarction. Consider other X-rays surveys if history of recent travel (possibility of body packing). *Computed tomography* and *lumbar puncture* if seizures.

Short-term problems

Arrhythmias; myocardial infarction; seizures; pulmonary infarction; intracranial hemorrhage or infarcts; visceral infarcts; preterm delivery; abruptio placentae. Cerebral infarction is more common among alkaloidal cocaine users, and hemorrhagic stroke is seen more frequently in IV cocaine hydrochloride use. Cerebral catastrophes can occur within minutes of the use of cocaine (Levine et al., 1991). Death may occur rapidly from respiratory depression and/or circulatory collapse (Balaskas, 1992). In pregnancy, there is a significant increase in the incidence of preterm labor (25–30% vs 12–17%) (Gillogley et al., 1990; Matera et al., 1990).

Long-term problems

Malnutrition; sexually transmitted diseases; preeclampsia; others include the aftermath of intracranial hemorrhage or infarction and rhabdomyolysis.

Fetal and neonatal considerations

Cocaine has high water and lipid solubility, a low molecular weight, and a low degree of ionization, all of which facilitate its passage across the placenta and into the fetus (Bingol et al., 1987). Cocaine infusion is associated with a decrease in uterine blood flow, leading to fetal hypoxic damage in the short term and to intrauterine growth retardation over time (Neerhof et al., 1989; Zucherman et al., 1989).

Signs

Fetal tachycardia; decreased beat to beat variability; bradycardia; late decelerations.

Teratogenic potential

Controversial data; no strong evidence to support it. Urinary tract malformations (hydronephrosis, hypospadias, prune-belly syndrome), congenital heart defects (transposition of the great vessels, hypoplastic right heart, ventricular septal defect, patent ductus arteriosus), and skull defects (exencephaly, encephalocele) (Briggs & Freeman, 1994) are associated with cocaine use in pregnancy.

Fetal distress potential

Yes secondary to uterine hyperstimulation, uterine vasoconstriction, placental abruption (×10 risk; Bingol et al., 1987) and maternal seizures. Up to 13% of women who used cocaine during pregnancy develop an abruption, which may be sudden, unpredictable, and catastrophic (Chasnoff et al., 1987, 1989).

Indications for delivery

Nonreassuring fetal condition; acute abruptio placentae and severe growth restriction.

Postnatal

Meconium aspiration, premature rupture of membranes, and fetal distress are all increased (Gillogley et al., 1990; Matera et al., 1990); neonatal hypotonia and significantly lower 5-minute Apgar scores (Chasnoff & MacGregor, 1987). There is risk of withdrawal syndrome (seizures; cardiovascular collapse); antenatal notification of the Neonatology Service recommended. Postnatally, perinatal or newborn cerebrovascular accidents may be found in neonates with a positive cocaine screening test (Chasnoff et al., 1987; Chasnoff & MacGregor, 1987). The pathology of such cocaine-induced injury may include, in addition to hypoxic ischemic encephalopathy, hemorrhagic infarction, cystic lesions, posterior fossa hemorrhage, absent septum pellucidum, atrophy, and brain edema (Dixon & Bejar, 1988). Necrotizing enterocolitis also has been described in neonates exposed to cocaine (Telsey et al., 1988).

Management considerations

With cocaine overdose, the initial therapeutic goal is to stabilize and support the patient for 24 hours.

Supportive
Hydration (forced alkaline diuresis if myoglobinuria detected or if creatinine elevated on arrival).

Specific measures / antidotes
Activated charcoal and whole bowel irrigation may decrease absorption if history of ingestion ("stuffing").

Benzodiazepines (diazepam 5–10 mg IV or lorazepam 2–4 mg IV) are the first line of treatment for supraventricular arrhythmias, hypertension, ischemic chest pain, anxiety, and seizures.

Lidocaine (1.5 mg/kg IV bolus followed by infusion of 2 mg/min) and alkalinization are the treatments of choice for ventricular arrhythmias. Use β-blockers with caution (may worsen coronary vasoconstriction and induce seizures); occasionally propranolol or esmolol may be used to block adrenergic stimulation in cases of arrhythmias associated with hypertension. In severe cases of hypertension, nitroprusside or phentolamine may be needed for control. In cases of hypotension, treatment with IV fluids should be initiated. For refractory hypotension, dopamine or norepinephrine may be required.

When seizures occur, diazepam can be used. Phenobarbital is the second choice for seizures. If the patient has recurrent seizures, phenobarbital or phenytoin are indicated. Status epilepticus may require neuromuscular blockade and ventilation.

In ischemic chest pain, may also use nitroglycerine (0.4 mg SL every 5 min and IV continuous drip thereafter) and in refractory cases phentolamine 1 mg IV (repeat in 5 min).

Heparinize if ischemic chest pain (5,000 IU IV bolus + 1,000 IU/h infusion).

Rhabdomyolysis is treated with maintenance and alkalinization of urine with IV fluids and sodium bicarbonate infusion.

Hyperthermia is managed with external cooling. This is especially important in pregnancy to protect the fetus (neuromuscular blockade may be needed in severe cases).

Hemodialysis may be indicated for renal failure secondary to myoglobinuria.

No specific antidote available.

Monitoring
Vitals/mental status/oximetry/cardiac for at least 24 hours after the exposure. Consider repeat EKG and cardiac enzymes every 6 hours if significant exposure, risk factors for coronary artery disease or chest pain on arrival. Cocaine is detectable in blood within 24 hours of ingestion and in urine for several days. In addition to a drug screen, evaluation may include blood gases, chest X-ray, complete blood count, renal and liver function tests, prothrombin and partial thromboplastin times, and urinalysis for myoglobin.

Therapeutic goals
Asymptomatic patient; normal laboratory values; no contractions or bleeding; reassuring fetal condition; more than 24 hours of observation. Consults obtained (see below).

Disposition considerations
Admit to an ICU if seizures, ventricular arrhythmias or hyperthermia. Drug counselor, psychiatry, and social worker consults recommended. Evaluate for sexually transmitted diseases.

Follow-up
Establish since most of these patients do not have prenatal care. Consider follow-up of fetal growth. On discharge, the patient will need clinical follow-up with a social worker, obstetrician, or psychiatric service. Fetal follow-up will require ultrasound evaluations to monitor fetal growth and anatomy. Once the fetus is potentially viable, assessment of fetal wellbeing is warranted. In addition, evaluation of the newborn for cerebral, urologic, and gastrointestinal sequelae is indicated.

Ethanol (Streissguth et al., 1989; Brien & Smith, 1991; Gossel & Bricker, 1994; Koren, 1994; Stewart & Streiner, 1994; Barinov et al., 1997; Goldfrank et al., 1998; Morgan & Ford, 1998; Levine, 1999)

According to the National Natality Survey, 39% of women admitted to alcohol use during their pregnancies. The prevalence of heavy or problem drinkers has been estimated to be 6–11% (Andres & Jones, 1994). Clinical presentation may vary with acute and/or chronic ethanol abuse or withdrawal. Only acute overdosage is considered here.

Toxicology

Examples/other names
Alcohol; ethilic alcohol; booze.

FDA classification
D (X if used in large amounts or for prolonged periods).

As a cause of morbidity
6th (Litovitz et al., 2000).

As a cause of mortality
6th (Litovitz et al., 2000).

Most frequent route of exposure
Ingestion.

Most frequent reason for exposure
Unintentional overdose.

Maternal considerations

Clinical presentation may vary with acute and/or chronic ethanol abuse or withdrawal.

We will consider here the acute overdose.

Symptoms
Euphoria, incoordination, impaired judgment, and reflexes. Social inhibitions are loosened. Aggressive or boisterous behavior is common. Hypoglycemia may occur.

Signs
As above plus ataxia, nystagmus, altered mental status, small pupils, characteristic breath smell. In severe overdoses: decreased temperature, pulse, blood pressure, respiratory depression, respiratory distress, and coma. Aggressive or boisterous behavior is commonly seen.

Diagnostic tests
Glucose, electrolytes, BUN, creatinine, transaminases, PT, magnesium, arterial blood gases or pulse oxymetry, chest X-ray if aspiration is suspected.

Short-term problems
Respiratory depression, pulmonary aspiration, hypoglycemia, coma. Less frequently gastrointestinal bleeding or rhabdomyolisis.

Long-term problems
Long-term problems are both organic and social. Organic problems include pancreatitis, hepatitis, cirrhosis, hepatic encephalopathy, portal hypertension, gastrointestinal bleeding, anemia, thiamine deficiency, alcoholic ketoacidosis, decreased resistance to infection, hypomagnesemia, hypokalemia, and hypophosphatemia. Social problems are manifested by malnutrition, isolation, depression, or suicide attempts.

Fetal and neonatal considerations

Signs
The fetal signs of acute maternal alcohol ingestion are a decrease in fetal heart rate accelerations and variability, suppression of fetal breathing movements, and lower fetal weight. In the neonate, suppression of neonatal electrocorticographic activity and electrooculographic activity (Brien & Smith, 1991) is seen.

Teratogenic potential
The major teratogenic potential of alcohol involves fetal alcohol syndrome (FAS), characterized by craniofacial dysmorphology (short palpebral fissures, ptosis, strabismus, epicanthal folds, myopia, microphthalmia, hypoplastic philtrum and maxilla, short upturned nose, posterior rotation of ears, poorly formed concha), prenatal growth deficiencies (body length more than weight), and CNS dysfunction (mild-to-moderate retardation, hypotonia, poor coordination, microcephaly). Other abnormalities, mainly cardiac, renogenital, and hemangiomas, are seen in at least 30–40% of exposed infants. Of note, the neonatal diagnosis of FAS may be delayed until 9–12 months of age.

Fetal distress potential
Not likely unless the acute intoxication is complicated by trauma. Transient no reactivity to fetal movements or to external stimuli has been described in acute intoxications.

Indications for delivery
Obstetric indications. Allow metabolism of alcoholic load before acting upon nonreassuring tracings of electric fetal monitoring.

Postnatally
Potential for withdrawal syndrome in neonates. Ethanol passes freely into breast milk; potential for sedation and dose-related psychomotor development delay in breastfed infants. Postnatally, the potential for withdrawal syndrome in neonates should be considered and the infant carefully monitored. In infants with FAS, the literature suggests an increased risk for the development of acute nonlymphocytic leukemia (Van Duijn et al., 1994) and possibly other neoplasias. For ethanol, which cannot be measured in hair or meconium, accumulation of its fatty acid ethyl esters in meconium is emerging as a promising test for heavy maternal drinking in the second part of pregnancy (Koren et al., 2002).

Management considerations

With ethanol overdose, the therapeutic goal is to prevent acute complications in the first 6–8 hours following admission. Elimination occurs at a fixed rate.

Decontamination
Emesis is not indicated unless a substantial ingestion has occurred within minutes of presentation or other drug ingestion is suspected. Gastric lavage indicated if intake of large amounts within 30–45 minutes of presentation. Charcoal does not efficiently adsorb ethanol; useful if other drugs were (or suspected to be) ingested.

Supportive
The airway should be protected because of the possibility of gastric aspiration. Treatment of coma and seizures if they occur.

Specific measures/antidotes
No specific antidote; flumazenil and naloxone may alleviate respiratory depression (anecdotal arousal after use of naloxone). Give glucose and thiamine.

Monitoring
To assess the patient with an acute ethanol overdose, blood glucose, electrolytes, BUN, creatinine, transaminases, PT, magnesium, arterial blood gases, or noninvasive oximetry are obtained. If aspiration is suspected, a chest X-ray should be obtained. During therapy, continuous pulse oximetry should be used if the patient is asleep or if the initial reading is abnormal.

Therapeutic goals
Sobriety; no acute complications in 6–8 hours of observation.

Discharge considerations
Ponder admission for social reasons. Social worker, drug counseling, and psychiatry evaluations may be helpful. Consider folate supplementation.

Follow-up
Establish. Upon discharge, clinical follow-up may involve a social worker, drug counselor, or obstetrician, and/or psychiatrist. Fetal follow-up will require ultrasound evaluations to monitor fetal growth.

Iron (Balaskas, 1992; Lacoste et al., 1992; Erickson & Neylan, 1998; Goldfrank et al., 1998; PDR Electronic Library, 1999; Rayburn et al., 1984; Tran et al., 2000)

Toxicology

Examples/common names
Ferrous gluconate, ferrous fumarate, ferrous sulfate/Chromagen, Feosol, Fergon, Ferro-Folic, Ferro-Grad, Ferlecit, Iberet, Irospan, Megadose, Nephrofer, Nephrovite, Prenate, Slow Fe, Trinsicon.

FDA classification
A.

As a cause of morbidity
2 (Rayburn).

As a cause of mortality
Rare.

Most frequent route of exposure
Ingestion.

Most frequent reason for exposure
Intentional overdose; suicidal gesture.

Maternal considerations

Symptoms
Abdominal pain; indigestion; nausea; vomiting; hematemesis; diarrhea.

Signs
As above + bloody stools; fever; shock and acidosis in severe cases.

Diagnostic tests
Complete blood count: leukocytosis; *serum iron levels:* (<18 μmol/L = nontoxic; 18–59 μmol/L = minimal toxicity; 60–89 μmol/L = moderate toxicity; >90 μmol/L = severe toxicity). *Other tests:* glucose: mild hyperglycemia; liver function tests; arterial blood gases if in shock or patient's mental status is altered.

Short-term problems
Shock; hemorrhage; hepatic failure; pulmonary edema/hemorrhage; disseminated intravascular coagulation. In a metanalysis of 61 cases of obstetric iron overdose it was found that the peak iron level ⩾400 μg/dL was not associated with increased risk of spontaneous abortion, preterm delivery, congenital anomalies, or maternal death.

Long-term problems
Gastrointestinal scarring; small intestine infarction; hepatic necrosis; achlorhydria. Patients with evidence of organ failure due to iron toxicity were more likely to spontaneously abort, deliver preterm, or experience maternal death (Tran et al., 2000).

Fetal and neonatal considerations

Signs
Uterine contractions.

Teratogenic potential
None specific.

Fetal distress potential
None unless associated maternal acidosis or bleeding.

Indications for delivery
Obsteric indications.

Management considerations

Pregnancy should not alter therapy for acute iron overdose. Deferoxamine administered in the third trimester is not associated with perinatal complications and is potentially lifesaving (McElhatton et al., 1991; Tran et al., 1998).

Supportive
Vigorous IV hydration and gastric lavage. Ipecac emesis recommended within the first hour in the conscious patient if lavage and bicarbonate not available.

Specific measures/antidotes
1% Sodium bicarbonate (200–300 mL) after lavage or induced emesis: converts the ferrous ion to ferrous carbonate which is less soluble. Deferoxamine (category C medication) at a dose of 1 g IM followed by 500 mg IM every 4 hours for 2 doses is recommended for patients with serum iron levels of 300 µg/dL or greater or a calculated ingestion of 30 mg/kg of elemental iron. Intravenous infusion at the same doses is preferred in patients in shock (infusion no greater than 15 mg/kg/hr).

Monitoring
Serum iron levels every 4–6 hours until within normal range.

Therapeutic goals
Normal serum iron levels.

Discharge considerations
Evaluate suicidal potential (psychiatry consult).

Follow-up
Establish. Upon discharge, clinical follow-up may involve a social worker, obstetrician, and/or psychiatrist.

Organophosphates*

(Dmochowska-Mroczek et al., 1972; Saadeh et al., 1996; Bailey, 1997; Gei et al., 1997; Okumura, 1997; Sancewicz et al., 1997; Erickson & Neylan, 1998; PDR Electronic Library, 1999)

Examples/other names
Dichlorvos, Diazinon, Dimethoate, Malathion, Parathion, Quinalphos, Sarin (nerve gas).

As a cause of morbidity
10 (Litovitz et al., 2000).

As a cause of mortality
15 (Litovitz et al., 2000).

Most frequent route of exposure
Ingestion.

Most frequent reason for exposure
Intentional overdose.

*The insecticides belonging to the family of the *carbamates* (e.g. Carboryl and Bendiocarb) have the same mechanisms of poisoning, clinical manifestations and therapy.

Maternal consideration

Symptoms
Nausea; vomiting; blurred vision; headache; dizziness; respiratory difficulty; abdominal pain (cramping usually); diarrhea; urinary incontinence; coma.

Signs
Agitation; altered mental status; fever; miosis; fasciculations or tremors; sialorrhea; bronchorrhea; bronchospasm; pulmonary edema; tachy- or bradycardia; hypo- or hypertension; respiratory arrest.

Diagnostic tests
Blood: decrease of 80–90% of erythrocyte cholinesterase (serum pseudocholinesterase is less specific). *Urine:* drug screen (intentional use can coexist with cocaine).

Short-term problems
Respiratory failure; aspiration pneumonia; ventricular arrhythmias; ARDS.

Long-term problems
Hepatic failure; relapse after apparent recovery is a well-described phenomenon in organophosphate poisoning: the "intermediate syndrome" has been described 24–96 hours after exposure and manifesting as muscular paralysis developing after recovery from the cholinergic phase. Another form of delayed toxicity is explained by the hepatic metabolism to more toxic compounds within 72 hours of the exposure.

Fetal considerations

Crosses the placenta.

Teratogenic potential
Not enough evidence (one case reported of multiple anomalies after exposure to oxydemeton-methyl at 4 weeks).

Fetal distress potential
Yes; from maternal hypoxia.

Indications for delivery
Obstetric indications. Fetal distress.

Management considerations

Supportive
Respiratory support.

Specific measures/antidotes
Pralidoxime chloride (2-PAM chloride) (category C) 1 g IV over several minutes is effective in reversing the action on cholinesterases if given within 24-hour of the exposure; it can

be repeated twice in 24-hour period if needed. Atropine (category C) 2 mg IV in repeated doses controls muscarinic effects. Diazepam IV can be used for seizures.

Monitoring
Pulse oximetry; respiratory frequency.

Therapeutic goals
Asymptomatic patient with normal levels of erythrocyte cholinesterase.

Discharge considerations
More than 72 hours after significant exposure; easy accessibility to hospital.

Follow-up
Establish. Upon discharge, clinical follow-up may involve a social worker, obstetrician, and/or psychiatrist.

Envenomations during pregnancy

During 1999, 524 cases of bites or stings during pregnancy were reported to the American Poison Control Centers. This represents 6% of all the toxic exposures occurring during pregnancy reported nationally in 1999. Moderate effects (more pronounced or prolonged than minor effects, usually requiring some form of treatment) were seen in only 5%; however, the rate increased to 13% when the envenomation was by a spider bite. No major effects (life-threatening or resulting in residual disability or disfigurement) were reported in this series (Gei et al., 2001c).

Snakebites

Snakebites during pregnancy are fortunately an uncommon event. In 1998, ophidic accidents represented 3.5% of all the stings and bites reported to American Poison Control Centers (Litovitz et al., 1999). The majority of snakebites during pregnancy cases arise from envenomation by snakes in the Crotalidae family (pit viper) (see Table 38.25). Common pit vipers in the United States include the rattle snakes (*Sistrusus* and *Crotalus* spp.) and the moccasins snakes: cotton-mouths (*Agkistrodon piscivorus*) and copperheads (*Agkistrodon contortrix*). Overall, rattlesnakes cause two-thirds of all bites by identified venomous snakes in the United States.

Venom usually is injected into subcutaneous tissue via fangs; occasionally, intramuscular or intravenous injection can occur. Dry bites (no envenomation) occur in as many as 50% of strikes. Venom generally is composed of several digestive enzymes and spreading factors, which result in local and systemic injury. In general, viper venom is mainly cytotoxic, whereas elapid venom is mainly neurotoxic, colubrid venom predominantly hemotoxic, and sea snake venom chiefly myotoxic (Pantanowitz & Guidozzi, 1996). Clinically, local effects most commonly predominate, progressing from pain and edema to ecchymosis and bullae. Hematologic abnormalities, including benign defibrination with or without thrombocytopenia, may result, but severe generalized bleeding is uncommon. Local or diffuse myotoxicity may result in complications such as compartment syndrome or rhabdomyolysis. Other rare general effects include cardiotoxicity, fasciculations, and shock.

Local measures include positive identification of the type of snake (venomous snakes generally have a triangle-shaped head) and rapid transport to definitive medical care. Because venom may be transported, a loose constriction bandage may be used to delay spread of the venom. If care is available within 60 minutes, wound incision and suctioning is not recommended. Unfortunately negative pressure venom extraction devices have shown no benefit (Bush et al., 2000). Tourniquets are not recommended. Local and supportive measures for poisonous snakebite include careful cleaning of the wound, maintaining the extremity in neutral position, supportive care, potential use of antibiotics, and tetanus prophylaxis (Pennell et al., 1987). Tetanus prophylaxis is not contraindicated in any pregnant snakebite or trauma victim who otherwise would be a candidate for the toxoid booster or antiglobulin.

Table 38.25 Snake envenomation during pregnancy by type of snake and maternal effects, US: 1999

Type of snake	No.	Minor effect	Moderate effects	Major effects	No. follow-up
Copperhead	2	2 (100%)	0	0	0
Rattlesnake	3	2 (67%)	0	1(33%)	0
Nonpoisonous	8	3 (37%)	0	0	5 (63%)
Unknown snake	5	3 (60%)	1 (20%)	0	1 (20%)
Total	18	10 (56%)	1 (5%)	1 (5%)	6 (34%)

Minor effects are signs or symptoms developing from the exposure but minimally bothersome and generally resolving without residual disability. A *moderate effect* is one that is more pronounced or prolonged than minor effects, usually requiring some form of treatment. *Major effects* are life-threatening signs or symptoms of the exposure that result in significant disability or disfigurement.
(Reproduced by permission from Toxic Exposure Surveillance System (TESS). Exposures in Pregnant Women, 1999. AAPCC 2000.)

Equine-derived antivenom is considered the standard of care; however, a promising new treatment is sheep-derived antigen binding fragment ovine (CroFab), which is much less allergenic. Although there is no universal grading system for snakebites, a I–IV grading scale is clinically useful as a guide to antivenom administration (Table 38.26) (Wood et al., 1955; Dunnihoo et al., 1992). When considering the use of antivenom, the risk of adverse reaction to antivenom must be weighed against the benefits of reducing venom toxicity. Antivenom should not be given in the field because of the risk of severe allergic complications.

With pit viper poisoning, antivenom is usually recommended for grade III or IV bites. Because copperheads carry a lesser potent venom, their bites usually do not require antivenom. Hypersensitivity reactions are common with antivenom use. Skin testing and careful monitoring must be available and used when antivenom is given.

In their review of snakebites during pregnancy, Dunnihoo et al. (1992) reported an overall fetal wastage of 43% and a maternal mortality of 10%. Bleeding diathesis results from pit viper envenomation. Fetal and placental effects from the anticoagulation are postulated to produce the fetal wastage. Although the specific effects of venom on the human fetus are unknown, there is evidence that snake venom may cross the placenta affecting the fetus even without evidence of envenomation in the mother (James, 1985). Snake venom has uterotonic properties (Osman & Gumaa, 1974) and fetal wastage during early gestation may be due to intrauterine bleeding, hypoxia and pyrexia (Parrish & Kahn, 1996).

We were unable to find any English-language reports of Elapidae (e.g. coral snake) envenomation during pregnancy. Snakes of the Elapidae family are much less efficient in injecting venom into their prey; thus, their poor efficiency at envenomation, coupled with their relatively small size and shy nature, may play a role in the paucity of information concerning coral snake bites during pregnancy. Coral snake bites often show little local reaction. Systemic effects may be delayed for several hours. Because of the neurotoxicity of coral snake venom, coral snake antivenom is usually recommended for victims of Elapidae bites.

Occasionally, a patient will present with the bite of a rare, exotic snake. Most zoos or poison control centers have specific information on unusual breeds of snakes. Timely consultation is highly recommended.

Spider bites

In the United States, spider bites during pregnancy are reported twice as frequently as snake bites (see Table 38.27). In the US only two types of poisonous spider bites are of concern,

Table 38.26 Grading of snakebite poisoning

Grade	Envenomation	Skin effects	Symptoms	Lab abnormalities
I	None	1 inch of edema or erythema, puncture wounds	None	None
II	Minimal	1–5 inch of edema or erythema within first 12 hr	None	None
III	Moderate	6–12 inch of edema or erythema within first 12 hr	Minimal (nausea, vomiting, paresthesias, metallic taste, and fasciculations)	Platelets < 90,000/μL Fibrinogen < 100 mg/dL) PT > 14 sec CK > 500–1,000 U/L
IV	Severe	Rapidly involves the entire part; potential compartment syndrome	Systemic effects may include shock, diffuse or life-threatening bleeding, renal failure, respiratory difficulty, and altered mental status	Platelets < 20,000/μL Any abnormal coagulation parameter associated with potentially life-threatening bleeding Rhabdomyolysis Myoglobinuric renal failure

PT, prothrombin time; CK, creatine kinase.

(From Wood JT, Moback WW, Green TW. Poisonous snakebites resulting in lack of venom poisoning. Va Med Monthly 1955;82:130; and Dunnihoo DR, Rush BM, Wise RB, Brooks GG, Otterson WN. Snake bite poisoning in pregnancy: a review of the literature. J Reprod Med 1992;37:653–658.)

Table 38.27 Insect and arthropod envenomation by category of exposure and maternal effects, US: 1999

Category of exposure	Total	No effect	Minor effects	Moderate effects	No follow-up
Ants/fire ants	14	1 (7.1%)	3 (21.4%)	3 (21.4%)	7 (50%)
Bee/wasp/hornet	66	1 (1.5%)	23 (34.8%)	1 (1.5%)	41 (62.1%)
Miscellaneous insects	97	6 (6.1%)	31 (31.9%)	3 (3.1%)	56 (57.7%)
Caterpillar/centipede	9	1 (11.1%)	4 (44.4%)	0	4 (44.4%)
Scorpion	165	1 (0.6%)	67 (40.6%)	3 (1.8%)	94 (56.9%)
Ticks	11	0	5 (45.4%)	0	6 (54.5%)
Black widow spider	22	2 (9.1%)	11 (50%)	5 (22.7%)	4 (18.1%)
Brown recluse spider	23	0	7 (30.4%)	3 (13.0%)	13 (56.5%)
Other spiders	77	0	20 (25.9%)	8 (10.3%)	49 (63.6%)
Miscellaneous arthropods	41	0	13 (31.7%)	1 (2.4%)	27 (65.8%)
Total:	524	12 (2.3%)	184 (35.1%)	27 (5.1%)	301 (57.4%)

Minor effects are signs or symptoms developing from the exposure but minimally bothersome and generally resolving without residual disability. A *moderate effect* is one that is more pronounced or prolonged than minor effects, usually requiring some form of treatment. *Major effects* (exposure resulting in life-threatening signs or symptoms or results in significant disability or disfigurement) were not reported in this series.
(From Gei AF, Van Hook JW, Olson GL, Saade GR, Hankins GDV. Arthropod envenomations during pregnancy. Report from a national database—1999. (Abstract no. 0662). Annual Meeting of the Society for Maternal–Fetal Medicine, Reno, Nevada, 2001.)

the black widow and the brown recluse. These spiders bite only when trapped or crushed against the skin (Wilson & King, 1990).

The adult female black widow spider (*Latrodectus mactans*) has a highly neurotoxic venom (alpha-latrotoxin), which destabilizes the cell membranes and degranulates the nerve terminals resulting in massive noradrenaline (norepinephrine) and acetylcholine release into synapses causing excessive stimulation and fatigue of the motor end plate and muscle.

Recently, alpha-latrotoxin-binding membrane receptors have been identified: neurexin and latrophilin/CIRL (calcium-independent receptor for alpha-latrotoxin). Although the nervous system is the primary target of low doses of alpha-latrotoxin, cells of other tissues (placenta, kidney, spleen, ovary, heart, and lung) are also susceptible to the toxic effects of alpha-latrotoxin because of the presence of CIRL-2, a low affinity receptor of the toxin (Ichtchenko et al., 1999). Although it is known that this venom does not affect the central nervous system due to its inability to cross the blood–brain barrier, it is not known whether it crosses the placenta or has direct fetal effects.

The diagnosis of a black widow spider bite is mainly clinical. Within about 1 hour of the incident, patients develop an autonomic and neuromuscular syndrome characterized by hypertension, tachycardia and diaphoresis, abdominal pain and tenderness, and back, chest, or lower extremity pain (painful muscle spasms and cramping), and weakness within minutes to hours of envenomation (Rauber, 1983; Pennell et al., 1987; Binder, 1989; Wilson & King, 1990). These neuromuscular symptoms progress over several hours and then subside over 2–3 days (Binder, 1989). Severe *Latrodectus* envenomation is characterized by: generalized muscular pain in the back, abdomen, and chest refractory to analgesics, diaphoresis remote from envenomation site, abnormal vital signs (BP >140/90 mmHg, pulse >100), nausea, vomiting, and headache (Bush & Gerardo, 2002). Unlike the dermonecrotic effects of the *Loxosceles* bite, the site lesion secondary to *Latrodectus* is unremarkable (similar to coral snake's bite). The evaluation of these patients may include a complete blood count, abdominal ultrasound or CT, EKG and creatine phosphokinase to evaluate acute abdominal and chest pain syndromes.

General supportive management (airway protection, breathing, and circulation per ACLS protocols) must be instituted promptly. Most widow spider envenomations may be managed with opioid analgesics and sedative-hypnotics. A specific antivenom for black widow bites is available. Although it results in resolution of most symptoms 30 min after administration and has been shown to decrease the need for hospitalization significantly, it should be cautiously restricted for severe envenomations, due to hypersensitivity, anaphylaxis, and serum sickness reactions (Binder, 1989; Heard et al., 1999). Antivenom should be considered when envenomation seriously threatens pregnancy or precipitates potentially limb- or life-threatening effects such as severe hypertension or unstable angina (Bush, 2002). As is the case with snake antivenoms, it should be given only in the hospital setting. The antivenom must be diluted and administered slowly (200 mL over an hour) after skin testing and antihistamine (Benadryl) administration, to reduce acute adverse reactions to the antivenom. Symptoms have been shown to improve within 1 hour of antivenom administration and for as long as 48 hours after envenomation (Bush, 2002).

Analgesics (morphine) and benzodiazepines (midazolam) are effective adjuvant treatment for the neuromuscular symptoms (Rauber, 1983). Calcium gluconate is no longer recommended for widow spider envenomation (Clark et al., 1992). Studies suggest benzodiazepines are more efficacious than muscle relaxants for treatment of widow spider envenomation. Antibiotics are not indicated. Tetanus immunization should be instituted following a black widow spider bite.

In the particular case of pregnancy, black widow envenomations can mimic acute intra-abdominal processes (Torregiani & La Cavera, 1990; Scalzone & Wells, 1994) and preeclampsia (abdominal pain, headache, hypertension, and proteinuria) (Sherman et al., 2000). Hospitalization and treatment with specific antivenom is recommended given that maternal mortality has been postulated to be as high as 5% (Scalzone & Wells, 1994). In 1999, 22 bites by black widow spiders were reported to Poison Control Centers in the US (Table 38.27). Half of the women reported only minor effects and another five women (19%) reported effects requiring some form of treatment. The outcome was not known in four cases (Gei et al., 2001c).

Loxosceles reclusa, also known as the brown recluse spider, enjoys a nationwide distribution in the US. Characteristic violin-shaped markings on their backs have led brown recluses to also be known as fiddleback spiders. In South America, the more potent venom of the species *Loxosceles laeta* is responsible for several deaths each year. The venom of these spiders contains at least eight enzymes, consisting of various lysins (facilitating venom spread) and sphingomyelinase D, which causes cell membrane injury and lysis, thrombosis, local ischemia, and chemotaxis.

The usual habitat of the brown recluse is in dark closet corners and the sides of cardboard boxes. Although not aggressive, the spider will bite when trapped.

Although most bites are asymptomatic, envenomation can begin with pain and itching that progresses to vesiculation (single clear or hemorrhagic vesicle) with violaceous necrosis and surrounding erythema, and ultimately ulcer formation and necrosis (dermonecrotic arachnidism) (see Fig. 38.5). Differential diagnosis includes herpes simplex, Stevens–Johnson syndrome, and toxic epidermal necrolysis. Treatment of local envenomations is conservative (local wound care, cryotherapy, elevation, tetanus prophylaxis, and close follow-up). Severe brown recluse spider bites produce dermonecrosis within 72–96 hours, which should be treated with rest, ice compresses, antibiotics, dapsone, and surgery delayed for several weeks. Skin grafting may be necessary after 4–6 weeks of standard therapy or until the lesion borders are well defined. Although large areas of necrosis require debridement and skin grafing, most cases of arachnidism cause self-limited wounds that require only local care (Fig. 38.5) (Pennell et al., 1987; Wright et al., 1997). Loxoscelism is the term used to describe the systemic clinical syndrome caused by envenomation from the brown spiders. Systemic involvement, although uncommon, occurs more frequently in children than in adults. These systemic envenomations may be life-threatening, and present with fever, constitutional symptoms, petechial eruptions, thrombocytopenia, and hemolysis with hemoglobinuric renal failure, seizures, or coma, usually associated with minimal skin changes (Forks, 2000). Systemic envenomation requires supportive care and treatment of arising complications, corticosteroids to stabilize red blood cell membranes, and support of renal function.

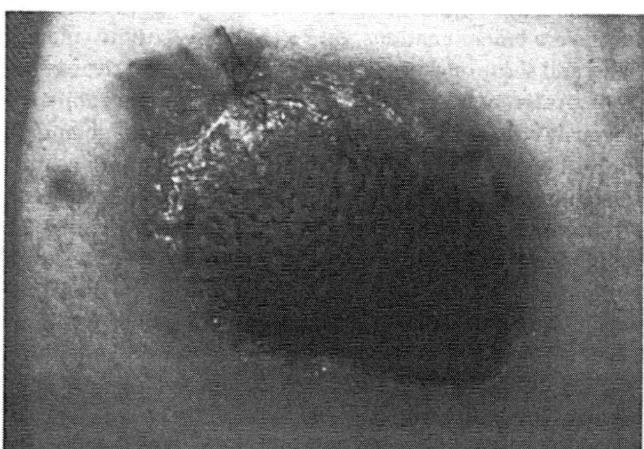

Fig. 38.5 Effects of *Loxosceles reclusa* bite. (Photograph courtesy of Dr Ramon L. Sanchez Galveston, Texas.)

Given its leukocyte-inhibiting properties, dapsone has frequently been recommended by authorities for the treatment of local lesions. However, because of the potential for adverse effects associated with dapsone use, especially in the setting of G-6-PD deficiency, hypersensitivity, and methemoglobinemia, appropriate caution should be exercised if using this medication. To date, no well-controlled studies have shown dapsone to affect clinical outcome in human brown recluse envenomations; therefore, it is not routinely recommended (Arnold, 2002).

Other treatments, such as colchicine, steroids, antivenom, nitroglycerin patches, and surgical excision, have been reported but insufficient data exist to support their clinical use today (Arnold, 2002). Intradermal anti-loxosceles Fab fragments have been shown to attenuate dermonecrotic arachnidism in a rabbit model when given up to 4 hours after venom inoculation (Gomez et al., 1999). Antivenom is not commercially available for *Loxosceles reclusa*. The only commercially available antivenom is for *Loxosceles laeta* in South America.

Anderson (1991) reported five cases of envenomation by *Loxosceles reclusa* in pregnant patients. He concluded that no special risks or complications resulted from being bitten by the brown recluse during pregnancy when managed conservatively only with low-dose prednisone. No episodes of hemolysis, disorders of coagulation, or renal damage were reported in this case series. In 1999, 23 bites by brown recluse spiders were reported to Poison Control Centers nationwide. Of those bites, the outcome is unknown in the majority (13) and moderate effects (more pronounced or prolonged than minimal; usually requiring some form of treatment) were reported in three cases (Gei et al., 2001c).

Scorpions

Over 650 species of scorpions are known to cause envenomation. They are endemic mostly in arid and tropical areas. Venoms and clinical presentations vary across the different species. The most important clinical effects of envenomations are neuromuscular, neuroautonomic, or local tissue effects (Bush & Gerardo, 2002). Grade I is limited to local reactions. Grade II is characterized by remote pain and/or paresthesias at the site of sting (envenomation). Grade III is characterized by either cranial/autonomic or somatic skeletal neuromuscular dysfunction, including blurred vision, roving eye movements, hypersalivation, tongue fasciculations, dysphagia, dysphonia, and problems with upper airway; restlessness and severe involuntary shaking or jerking of extremities that may be mistaken for a seizure. Grade IV combines cranial/autonomic and somatic nerve dysfunction (Bush & Gerardo, 2002).

Most commonly, an inflammatory local reaction occurs with envenomation, which is treated with wound debridement and cleaning, tetanus prophylaxis, and antihistamines (Binder, 1989). Antivenom is recommended for grade III and IV envenomations. In 1999, 165 pregnant women reported scorpion envenomations. In those patients with known outcome, minor symptoms were predominant. No life-threatening symptoms or signs were reported (Gei et al., 2001c).

Summary

- Poisoning during pregnancy represents a third of a percent of all toxic exposures reported in the United States.
- The number of reported toxic exposures has increased by about 25% over the past 6 years both in the pregnant and nonpregnant population.
- Although slightly more frequent during the second trimester, toxic exposures during pregnancy are reported with similar frequency in all trimesters.
- The emergency treatment and stabilization of the mother should take priority over the monitoring and treatment of the fetus.
- A prompt consultation with the obstetric service is recommended in the emergent management of the compromised poisoned pregnant patient. The goals of this consult are : (i) the assessment of fetal viability; and (ii) the decision/skill to proceed with an emergent or perimortem cesarean section if the patient's condition worsens or the resuscitative efforts are not successful.
- The mechanism of exposure needs to be sought and established, since intentional toxic exposure usually indicates severe social, emotional, and/or psychiatric pathology. When identified, the need for additional and aggressive intervention (hospital admission, social and psychiatry consults, etc.) may prevent a potentially fatal recurrence.
- Insect and arthropod exposures are not uncommon during pregnancy. The majority of these envenomations resulted in minor or no effects. Moderate effects are more likely when the cause of the exposure is a spider bite than with other arthropod exposures, including scorpion and bee stings.
- Regardless of their severity, all toxic exposures need to be reported to the respective Poison Control Center (Tel. 1-800-222-1222).

References

Abramovich A, Shupak A, Ramon Y, et al. Hyperbaric oxygen for carbon monoxide poisoning. Harefuah 1997;132:21–24.

Anderson PC. Loxoscelism threatening pregnancy: five cases. Am J Obstet Gynecol 1991;165:1454–1456.

Andres RL, Jones KL. Social and elicit drug use in pregnancy. In: Creasy RK, Resnik R, eds. Maternal-fetal medicine: principles and practice, 3rd edn. Philadelphia: WB Saunders, 1994:182.

Arnold T. Spider Envenomations, Brown Recluse. http://www.emedicine.com/emerg/topic547.htm (accessed 6/7/02).

Athinarayanan P, Pieroy SH, Nigan SK, Glass L. Chlordiazepoxide withdrawal in the neonate. Am J Obstet Gynecol 1976;124:212–213.

Bailey B. Organophosphate poisoning in pregnancy. (Letter) Ann Emerg Med 1997;29:299.

Balaskas TN. Common poisons. In: Gleicher N, Elkayam U, Galgraith RM, et al., eds. Principles and practice of medical therapy in pregnancy, 2nd edn. Norwalk, CT: Appleton and Lange, 1992.

Barinov EK, Burago II, Bulanakova AB. The death of a newborn infant from ethanol poisoning. Sud Med Ekspert, 1997;40:45.

Bayer MJ, Rumack BH. Poisoning and overdose. Rockville, MD. Aspen Systems, 1983.

Berg MJ, Berlinger WG, Goldberg MJ, et al. Acceleration of the body clearance of phenobarbital by oral activated charcoal. N Engl J Med 1982;507:642–644.

Biggs GG, Samaon JH, Crawford DJ. Lack of abnormalities in a newborn exposed to amphetamine during gestation. Am J Dis Child 1975;129:249–250.

Binder LS. Acute arthropod envenomation. Incidence, clinical features and management. Med Toxicol 1989;4:163–173.

Bingol N, Fuchs M, Diaz V. Teratogenicity of cocaine in humans. J Pediatr 1987;110:93–96.

Bleyer WA, Skinner AL. Fatal neonatal hemorrhage after maternal anticonvulsant therapy. JAMA 1976;235:826–827.

Bolgiano EB, Barish RA. Use of new and established antidotes. Emerg Med Clin North Am 1994;12:22–27.

Brien JF, Smith GN. Effects of alcohol (ethanol) on the fetus. J Dev Physiol 1991;15:21.

Briggs GG, Freeman RK, eds. Drugs in pregnancy and lactation, 4th edn. Baltimore: Williams and Wilkins, 1994.

Broughan TA, Soloway RD. Acetaminophen hepatoxicity. Dig Dis Sci 2000;45:1553–1558.

Bunikowski R, Grimmer I, Heiser A, Metze B, Schafer A, Obladen M.

Neurodevelopmental outcome after prenatal exposure to opiates. Eur J Pediatr 1998;157(9):724–730.

Bush SP. Spider envenomations: Widow. http://www.emedicine.com/emerg/topic546.htm (accessed 6/5/02).

Bush SP, Gerardo C. Scorpion envenomations. http://www.emedicine.com/emerg/topic524.htm (accessed 6/5/02).

Bush SP, Hegewald KG, Green SM, Cardwell MD, Hayes WK. Effects of a negative pressure venom extraction device (Extractor) on local tissue injury after artificial rattlesnake envenomation in a porcine model. Wilderness Environ Med 2000;11:180–188.

Byer AJ, Taylor TR, Semmer JR. Acetaminophen overdose in the third trimester of pregnancy. JAMA 1982;247:3114–3115.

Cerqueira MJ, Olle C, Bellart J, et al. Intoxication by benzodiazepines during pregnancy. Lancet 1988;1(8598):1341.

Chan TYK. Potential dangers from topical preparations containing methyl salicylate. Hum Exp Toxicol 1996;15:747–750.

Chasnoff IJ, MacGregor S. Maternal cocaine use and neonatal morbidity. Pediatr Res 1987;21:356.

Chasnoff IJ, Burns KA, Burns WJ. Cocaine use in pregnancy: perinatal morbidity and mortality. Neurotoxicol Teratol 1987;9:291–293.

Chasnoff IJ, Griffith DR, MacGregor S, et al. Temporal patterns of cocaine use in pregnancy: perinatal outcome. JAMA 1989;261: 1741–1744.

Clark RF, Wethern-Kestner S, Vance MV, Gerkin R. Clinical presentation and treatment of black widow spider envenomation: a review of 163 cases. Ann Emerg Med 1992;21:782-787.

Cohen HR, Green JR, Crombleholme WR. Peripartum cocaine use: estimating risk of adverse pregnancy outcome. Int J Gynecol Obstet 1991;35:51–54.

Colado MI, O'Shea E, Granados R, Misra A, Murray TK, Green AR. A study of the neurotoxic effect of MDMA ('ecstasy') on 5-HT neurones in the brains of mothers and neonates following administration of the drug during pregnancy. Br J Pharmacol 1997;121:827–833.

Coupey SM. Barbiturates. Pediatr Rev 1997;18:260–264.

Delaney DB, Larrabee KD, Monga M. Preterm premature rupture of the membranes associated with recent cocaine use. Am J Perinatol 1997;14:285–288.

Desmond MM, Schwanecke PP, Wilson GS, et al. Maternal barbiturate utilization and neonatal withdrawal symptomatology. J Pediatr 1972;80:190–197.

Dickson PH, Lind A, Studts P, et al. The routine analysis of breast milk for drugs of abuse in a clinical toxicology laboratory. J Forensic Sci 1994;39:207–214.

Dixon JC, Speidel BD, Dixon JJ. Neonatal flumazenil therapy reverses maternal diazepam. Acta Paediatr 1998;87:225–226.

Dixon SD, Bejar R. Brain lesions in cocaine and methamphetamine exposed neonates. Pediatr Res 1988;23:405.

Dmochowska-Mroczek H, Lebensztejn W, Tolwinski K. Severe intoxication with Dipterex in a pregnant woman. Polski Tygodnik Lekarski 1972;27:1406–1407.

Doyon S, Roberts JR. Reappraisal of the "coma cocktail". Dextrose, flumazenil, naloxone and thiamine. Emerg Clin North Am 1994;12:301–316.

Dunnihoo DR, Rush BM, Wise RB, Brooks GG, Otterson WN. Snake bite poisoning in pregnancy: a review of the literature. J Reprod Med 1992;37:653–658.

Elliott JP, O'Keeffe DF, Schon DA, Cheron LB. Dialysis in pregnancy: a critical review. Obstet Gynecol Survey 1991;46:319–324.

Emery CL, Morway LF, Chung-Park M, et al. The Kleihauer-Betke test. Clinical utility, indication, and correlation in patients with placental abruption and cocaine use. Arch Path Lab Med 1995;119:1032-1037.

Erickson TB, Neylan VD. Management principles of overdose in pregnancy. In: Haddad LM, Shannon MW, Winchester JF, eds. Clinical Management of Poisoning and Drug Overdose, 3rd edn. Philadelphia: WB Saunders, 1998.

Forks TP. Brown recluse spider bites. J Am Board Family Pract 2000;13:415–423.

Gaudreault P, Guay J, Thivierge RL, et al. Benzodiazepine poisoning. Clinical and pharmacological considerations and treatment. Drug Safety 1991;6:247–265.

Gay GR. Clinical management of acute and chronic cocaine poisoning. Ann Emerg Med 1982;11:562–572.

Gei AF, Saade GR. Poisoning during pregnancy and lactation. In: Yankowitz J, Niebyl J, eds. Drug Therapy in Pregnancy, 3rd edn. Philadelphia: Lippincott, Williams and Wilkins, 2001.

Gei AF, Wen T, Belfort MA. Overdose and poisoning. In: Clark SL, Cotton DB, Hankins GDV, Phelan JP, eds. Critical Care Obstetrics, 3rd edn. Malden: Blackwell Science, 1997:636–669.

Gei AF, Locksmith GJ, Saade GR, Hankins GD. Toxic exposures during pregnancy: Report from a national database—1999. (Abstract # 0146). Annual Meeting of the Society for Maternal-Fetal Medicine, Reno, Nevada, 2001a.

Gei AF, Suarez VR, Goodrum L, Saade GR, Hankins GD. Suicide attempts during pregnancy by poisoning or overdose. Report from a national database—1999. (Abstract # 0623). Annual Meeting of the Society for Maternal-Fetal Medicine, Reno, Nevada, 2001b.

Gei AF, Van Hook JW, Olson GL, Saade GR, Hankins GD. Arthropod envenomations during pregnancy. Report from a national database—1999. (Abstract # 0662). Annual Meeting of the Society for Maternal-Fetal Medicine, Reno, Nevada, 2001c.

Gillogley KM, Evans AT, Hansen RL, et al. The perinatal impact of cocaine, amphetamine and opiate use detected by universal intrapartum screening. Am J Obstet Gynecol 1990;163:1535–1542.

Gilstrap L III, Little BB. Drugs and Pregnancy. New York: Elsevier, 1992.

Gimovsky ML. Fetal heart rate monitoring casebook. J Perinatol 1995;15:246–249.

Goldfrank LR, Flomenbaum NE, Lewin NA, et al., eds. Goldfrank's Toxicologic Emergencies, 6th edn. Stamford: Appleton & Lange, 1998.

Gomez HF, Miller MJ, Trachy JW, Marks RM, Warren JS. Intradermal anti-Loxosceles Fab fragments attenuate dermonecrotic arachnidism. Acad Emerg Med 1999;6:1195–1202.

Gossel TA, Bricker JD, eds. Principles of Clinical Toxicology, 3rd edn. New York: Raven Press, 1994.

Greenblatt JF, Dannenberg AL, Johnson CJ. Incidence of hospitalized injuries among pregnant women in Maryland, 1979–1990. Am J Prevent Med 1997;13:374–379.

Greenland VC, Delke I, Minkoff HL. Vaginally administered cocaine overdose in a pregnant woman. Obstet Gynecol 1989;740(3 Pt 2):476–477.

Grinspoon L, Bakalar JB. Adverse effects of cocaine: selected issues. Ann NY Acad Sci 1981;326:125–131.

Haddad LM, Winchester JF, eds. Clinical Management of Poisoning and Drug Overdose, 2nd edn. Philadelphia: WB Saunders, 1990.

Haibach H, Akhter JE, Muscato MS. Acetaminophen overdose with fetal demise. Am J Clin Pathol 1984;82:240–242.

Hardman JG, Limbird LE, eds. Goodman & Gilman's the Pharmacological Basis of Therapeutics, 9th edn. New York: McGraw-Hill, 1996.

Hartz SC, Heinonen OP, Shapiro S, et al. Antenatal exposure to meprobamate and chlordiazepoxide in relation to malformations, mental development and childhood mortality. N Engl J Med 1975;292:726–728.

Heard K, O'Malley GF, Dart RC. Antivenom therapy in the Americas. Drugs 1999;58:5–15.

Ho E, Karimi-Tabesh L, Koren G. Characteristics of pregnant women who use ecstasy (3,4-methylenedioxymethamphetamine). Neurotoxicol Teratol 2001;23(6):561–567.

Hoffman RS, Goldfrank LR. The poisoned patient with altered consciousness. Controversies in the use of a "coma cocktail". JAMA 1995;274:562–569.

Horowitz RS, Dart RC, Jarvie DR, et al. Placental transfer of N-Acetylcysteine following human maternal acetaminophen toxicity. Clin Toxicol 1997;35:447–451.

Houston H, Jacobson L. Overdose and termination of pregnancy: an important association? Br J Gen Practice 1996;46:737–738.

Ichtchenko K, Bittner MA, Krasnoperov V, Little AR, Chepurny O, Holz RW, Petrenko AG. A novel ubiquitously expressed alpha-latrotoxin receptor is a member of the CIRL family of G-protein-coupled receptors. J Biol Chem 1999;274:5491–5498.

Jackson LD. Different presentations of cocaine intoxication: four cases studies. J Emerg Nursing 1997;23:232–234.

Jackson T, Lorenz R, Menor KMJ, et al. Successful outcome of pregnancy requiring dialysis: effects on serum progesterone and estrogen. J Reprod Med 1979;22:217.

James RF. Snake bites in pregnancy. Lancet 1985;2(8457):731.

Jones AL, Prescott LF. Unusual complications of paracetamol poisoning. Q J Med, 1997;90:161–168.

Jones KL. Effects of therapeutic, diagnostic and environmental agents. In: Creasy RK, Resnik R, eds. Maternal-fetal Medicine: Principles and Practice, 3rd edn. Philadelphia: WB Saunders, 1994:171–181.

Jones JS, Dickson K, Carlson S. Unrecognized pregnancy in the overdosed or poisoned patient. Am J Emerg Med 1997;15:538–541.

Kerns II W. Salicylate and nosteroidal anti-inflammatory drug poisoning. In: Howell JM, Altieri M, Jagoda AS, et al., eds. Emergency Medicine. Philadelphia: Saunders, 1998.

Kim E, Brion LP, Meenan G, et al. Perinatal toxicology screening: comparison of carious maternal and neonatal samples. J Perinatol 1998;18:116–121.

Kloeck A, Cummins RO, Chamberlain D, et al. Special Resuscitation Situations. An Advisory Statement from the International Liaison Committee on Resuscitation. Circulation 1997;95:2196–2210.

Kopelman AE, Plaut TA. Fetal compromise caused by maternal carbon monoxide poisoning. J Perinatol 1998;18:74–77.

Koren G, ed. *Maternal-Fetal Toxicology*, 2nd edn. New York: Marcel Dekker Inc., 1994.

Koren G. Carbon monoxide poisoning in pregnancy. Can Fam Phys 1996;42:854–855.

Koren G, Chan D, Klein J, Karaskov T. Estimation of fetal exposure to drugs of abuse, environmental tobacco smoke, and ethanol. Ther Drug Monitor 2002;24(1):23–25 Feb.

Kozer E, Koren G. Management of paracetamol overdose: current controversies. Drug Safety 2001;24:503–512.

Kurtz GG, Michael OF, Morosi HJ, et al. Hemodialysis during pregnancy: report of a case of glutethamide poisoning complicated by acute renal failure. Arch Intern Med 1996;118:30.

Lacoste H, Goyert GL, Goldman LS, et al. Acute iron intoxication in pregnancy: Case report and review of the literature. Obstet Gynecol 1992;80:500–501.

Laegreid L, Olegard R, Wahlstrom J, et al. Abnormalities in children exposed to benzodiazepines in utero. Lancet 1987;1:108–109.

Levine B, ed. Principles of Forensic Toxicology. Washington DC: American Association of Clinical Chemistry, 1999.

Levine SR, Brust JC, Futrell N, et al. A comparative study of the cerebrovascular complications of cocaine: alkaloid versus hydrochloride—a review. Neurology 1991;41:1173–1177.

Levy G, Garretson LK, Socha DM. Evidence of placental transfer of acetaminophen. Pediatrics 1975;55:895.

Litovitz TL, Felberg L, Soloway RA, et al. 1994 Annual report of the American Association of Poison Control Centers Toxic Exposure Surveillance System. Am J Emerg Med 1995;13:551–597.

Litovitz TL, Klein-Schwartz W, Martin E, et al. 1998 American Annual Report of the American Association of Poison Control Centers Toxic Exposure Surveillance System. Am J Emerg Med 1999;17:435–487.

Litovitz TL, Klein-Schwartz W, White S, et al. 2000 Annual report of the American Association of Poison Control Centers Toxic Exposure Surveillance System. Am J Emerg Med 2001 Sep;19(5):337–395.

Little BB, Snell LM, Klein VR, Gilstrap LC. Cocaine abuse during pregnancy: maternal and fetal implication. Obstet Gynecol 1989;72:157–160.

Longo LD. The biological effects of carbon monoxide on the pregnant woman, fetus, and newborn infant. Am J Obstet Gynecol 1977;129:69–103.

Lovejoy FH, Shannon M, Woolf AD. Recent advances in clinical toxicology. Curr Prob Pediatr 1992;March:119–128.

Ludmir J, Main DM, Landon MB, Gabbe SG. Maternal acetaminophen overdose at 15 weeks of gestation. Obstet Gynecol 1986;67:750–751.

McElhatton PR, Roberts JC, Sullivan FM. The consequences of iron overdose and its treatment with desferrioxamine in pregnancy. Hum Exp Toxicol 1991;10:251–259.

McElhatton PR, Sullivan FM, Volans GN. Paracetamol overdose in pregnancy analysis of the outcomes of 300 cases referred to the Teratology Information Service. Reprod Toxicol 1997;11:85–94.

McElhatton PR, Bateman DN, Evans C, Pughe KR, Thomas SH. Congenital anomalies after prenatal ecstasy exposure. Lancet 1999;23:354(9188):1441–1442.

McFarland III AK. Anticonvulsants. In: Howell JM, Altieri M, Jagoda AS, et al, eds. *Emergency Medicine*. Philadelphia: WB Saunders, 1998.

MacGregor SN, Keith LG. Drug abuse during pregnancy. In: Rayburn RF, Zuspan FP, eds. Drug therapy in obstetrics and gynecology. 3rd ed. St. Louis: Mosby Year Book, 1992:164–189.

MacQueen G, Born L, Steiner M. The selective serotonin reuptake inhibitor sertraline: its profile and use in psychiatric disorders. CNS Drug Rev 2001;7:1–24.

Marchand LL. Trends in birth defects for a Hawaiian population exposed to heptachlor and for the United States. Arch Environ Health 1986;41:145.

Martin Cl, Babib JL, Demarquez B, et al. Intoxication Néo-natale par certaines thérapeutiques psychotropes maternelles. Aspects cliniques et physiopathologiques. Pédiatrie 1974;29:147–157.

Martinez A, Larrabee K, Monga M. Cocaine is associated with intrauterine fetal death in women with suspected preterm labor. Am J Perinatol 1996;13:163–166.

Matera C, Warren WB, Moomjy M, et al. Prevalence of use of cocaine and other substances in an obstetric population. Am J Obstet Gynecol 1990;163:797–801.

Mazurek A, Mazurek J. Acute barbiturate poisoning in the 39th week of pregnancy. Case report. Anaesth Resusc Intensive Ther 1975;3:193–196.

Milkovich L, van den Berg BJ. Effects of prenatal meprobamate and chlordiazepoxide, hydrochloride in human embryonic and fetal development. N Engl J Med 1974;291:1268–1271.

Miller JM, Boudreaux MC, Regan FA. A case-control study of cocaine use in pregnancy. Am J Obstet Gynecol 1995;172:180–185.

Moore TR, Sorg J, Miller L. Hemodynamic effects of intravenous cocaine on the pregnant ewe and fetus. Am J Obstet Gynecol 1989;155:883–888.

Morgan BW, Ford MD. Ethanol. In: Howell JM, Altieri M, Jagoda AS, et al., eds. Emergency Medicine. Philadelphia: WB Saunders, 1998.

Mourilhe P, Stokes PE. Risks and benefits of selective serotonin reuptake inhibitors in the treatment of depression. Drug Safety 1998; 18:57–82.

Mowry JB, Furbee RB, Chyka PA. Poisoning. In: Chernow B, Borater DC, Holaday JW, et al., eds. The Pharmacological Approach to the Critically Ill Patient, 3rd edn. Baltimore: Williams and Wilkins, 1995.

Nair P, Rothblim S, Hebel R. Neonatal outcome in infants with evidence of fetal exposure to opiates, cocaine, and canabinoids. Clin Pediatr 1994;May:280–285.

Neerhof MG, MacGregor SN, Retzky SS, Sullivan JP. Cocaine abuse during pregnancy: peripartum prevalence and perinatal outcome. Am J Obstet Gynecol 1989;161:633–638.

Neuberg R. Drug dependence and pregnancy: a review of the problems and their management. J Obstet Gynaecol Br Cmwlth 1970;66:1117–1122.

Nicholson DP. The immediate management of overdose. Med Clin North Am 1983;67:1279–1293.

Noji E, Kelen G. Manual of Toxicologic Emergencies. St. Louis: Year Book Medical, 1989.

Okumura T. Organophosphate poisoning in pregnancy. (Reply) Ann Emerg Med 1997;29:299.

Olenmark M, Biber B, Dottori O, et al. Fatal iron intoxication in late pregnancy. Clin Toxicol 1987;25:347–359.

Olson K. Poisoning and Drug Overdose, 2nd edn. Norwalk, CT: Appleton and Lange, 1994.

Oro AS, Dixon SD. Perinatal cocaine and methamphetamine exposure: maternal and neonatal correlates. J Pediatr 1987;111:571–578.

Osman OH, Gomaa KA. Pharmacological studies of snake (bitis arietans) Venom. Toxicon 1974;12:569–75.

Palanick W, Tenenbein M. Aspirin poisoning during pregnancy: increased fetal sensitivity. Am J Perinatol 1998;15:39–41.

Pantanowitz L, Guidozzi F. Management of snake and spider bite in pregnancy. Obstet Gynecol Surv 1996;51:615–20.

Parrish HM. Khan MS. Snakebite during pregnancy. Report of 4 cases. Obstet Gynecol 1996;27:468–471.

PDR[R] Electronic Library. Version 5.1.0a. Montvale: Medical Economics Company, Inc., 1999.

Pennell TC, Babu SS, Meredith JW. The management of snake and spider bites in the southeastern United States. Am Surg 1987;53:198–204.

Perrone J, Hoffman RS. Toxic ingestions in pregnancy: abortifacient use in a case series of pregnant overdose patients. Acad Emerg Med 1997;4:206–209.

Perrone JM, Hoffman RS. Antidepressants. In: Howell JM, Altieri M, Jagoda AS, et al., eds. Emergency Medicine. Philadelphia: WB Saunders, 1998.

Peterson RG, Rumack BH. Toxicity of acetaminophen overdose. JACEP 1978;7:202–205.

Pond SM. Principles of techniques used to enhance elimination of toxic compounds. In: Goldfrank LR, Flomenbaum NE, Lewin NA, et al., eds. Goldfrank's Toxicologic Emergencies, 4th edn. Norwalk, CT: Appleton and Lange, 1990:21–28.

Preskorn SH, Othmer SC. Evaluation of bupropion hydrochloride: the first of a new class of atypical antidepressants. Pharmacotherapy, 1984;4:20–34.

Rauber A. Black widow spider bites. J Toxicol Clin Toxicol 1983–84;21: 473–485.

Rayburn W, Anonow R, Delay B, Hogan MJ. Drug overdose during pregnancy: an overview from a metropolitan poison control center. Obstet Gynecol 1984;64:611.

Rayburn W, Shukla U, Stetson P, et al. Acetaminophen pharmacokinetics: comparison between pregnant and nonpregnant women. Am J Obstet Gynecol 1986;155:1353–1356.

Rejent TA, Baik S. Fatal in utero salicylism. J Forensic Sci 1985; 30:942–944.

Reynolds JR, Howland MA, Weisman RS. Pharmacokinetic and toxicokinetic principles. In: Goldfrank LR, Flomenbaum NE, Lewin NA, et al., eds. Goldfrank's Toxicologic Emergencies, 4th edn. Norwalk, CT: Appleton and Lange, 1990:29–38.

Richards S, Brooks SHE. Ferrous sulphate poisoning in pregnancy (with apofibrinogenaemia as a complication). West Indian Med J 1966;15:134–140.

Riggs BS, Bronstein AC, Kuling K, et al. Acute acetaminophen overdose during pregnancy. Obstet Gynecol 1989;74:247–253.

Roberts JM. Pregnancy related hypertension. In: Creasy RK, Resnik R, eds. Maternal-fetal Medicine: Principles and Practice, 3rd edn. Philadelphia: WB Saunders, 1994:804–843.

Rogers BD, Lee RV. Drugs abuse. In: Burrow GN, Ferris TF, eds. Medical Complications During Pregnancy, 3rd edn. Philadelphia: WB Saunders, 1988:570–581.

Rosenberg L, Mitchell AA, Parsells JL, et al. Lack of relation of oral clefts to diazepam use during pregnancy. N Engl J Med 1983; 309:1282–1285.

Rubio S, García ML. Intoxicación por monóxido de carbono. Medicina Clínica 1997;108:776–778.

Rumack BH, Matthew H. Acetaminophen poisoning and toxicity. Pediatrics 1975;55:871–876.

Rumack BH, Peterson RC, Koch GG, Amara IA. Acetaminophen overdose: 662 cases with evaluation of oral acetylcysteine treatment. Arch Intern Med 1981;141:380–385.

Russell FE, Marcus P, Streng JA. Black widow spider envenomation during pregnancy. Report of a case. Toxicon 1979;17:188–189.

Rutherfoord-Rose S. Acetaminophen. In: Howell JM, Altieri M, Jagoda AS, et al., eds. Emergency Medicine. Philadelphia: WB Saunders, 1998.

Saadeh AM, Al-Ali MK, Farsakh NA, et al. Clinical and sociodemographic features of acute carbamate and organophosphate poisoning: a study of 70 adult patients in North Jordan. Clin Toxicol 1996;34:45–51.

Safra MJ, Oakley JP. Association between cleft lip with and without cleft palate and prenatal exposure to diazepam. Lancet 1975;2:478–480.

Sakai T, Matsuda H, Watanabe N. Triazolam (Halcion) intoxication in a neonate—a first report. Eur J Pediatr 1996;155:1065–1068.

Sancewicz K, Groszek B, Pach D, et al. Acute pesticides poisonings in pregnant women. Przeglad Lekarski 1997;54:741–744.

Sancewicz-Pach K, Chmiest W, Lichota E. Suicidal paracetamol poisoning of a pregnant woman just before a delivery. Przeglad Lekarski 1999;56(6):459–462.

Sánchez-Casajus, Ramos I, Sánchez M. Hemodiálisis durante el embarazo. Rev Clin Esp 1978;149:187–188.

Saxen I, Saxen L. Letter: association between maternal intake of diazepam and oral clefts. Lancet 1975;2:498.

Scalzone JM, Wells SL. Latrodectus mactans (black widow spider) envenomation: an unusual cause for abdominal pain in pregnancy. Obstet Gynecol 1994;83:830–831.

Schauben JL. Benzodiazepines. In: Howell JM, Altieri M, Jagoda AS, et al., eds. Emergency Medicine. Philadelphia: WB Saunders, 1998.

Shannon BE, Jenkins JL, Loscalzo J. Poisoning and ingestion. In: Jenkins JL, Loscalzo J, eds. Manual of Emergency Medicine—Diagnosis and Treatment, 2nd edn. Boston: Little, Brown, 1995:417–469.

Shannon MW, Haddad LM. The emergency management of poisoning. In: Haddad LM, Shannon MW, Winchester JF, eds. Clinical Management of Poisoning and Drug Overdose, 3rd edn. Philadelphia: WB Saunders, 1998.

Sherman RP, Groll JM, Gonzalez DI, Aerts MA. Black widow spider (Latrodectus mactans) envenomation in a term pregnancy. Curr Surg 2000;57:346–348.

Shiono PH, Mills JL. Oral clefts and diazepam use during pregnancy. N Engl J Med 1984;311:919–920.

Shubert PJ, Savage B, Smoking, alcohol and drug abuse. In: James DK, Stein RJ, Weiner CP, Gonik B, eds. High risk pregnancy management options. Philadelphia: WB Saunders, 1994:51–66.

Silversman RK, Montano J. Hyperbaric oxygen treatment during pregnancy in acute carbon monoxide poisoning. A case report. J Reprod Med 1997;42:309–311.

Silvers SM, Hampson NB. Carbon monoxide poisoning among recreational boaters. JAMA 1995;274:1614–1616.

Sim MR, McNeil JJ. Monitoring chemical exposure using breast milk: a methodological review. Am J Epidemiol 1992;136:1–11.

Smilkstein MJ. Techniques used to prevent gastrointestinal absorption of toxic compounds. In: Goldfrank LR, Flomenbaum NE, Lewin NA, et al., eds. *Goldfrank's Toxicologic Emergencies*, 6th edn. Stamford: Appleton & Lange, 1998.

Stahl MM, Saldeen P, Vinge E. Reversal of fetal benzodiazepine intoxication using flumazenil. Br J Obstet Gynaecol 1993;100:185–188.

Stengel CL, Seaburg DC, MacLeod BA. Pregnancy in the emergency department: Risk factors and prevalence among all women. Ann Emerg Med 1994;24:697–700.

Stewart DE, Streiner D. Alcohol drinking in pregnancy. Gen Hosp Psychiat 1994;16:406–412.

Stine RJ, Marcus RH. Toxicologic emergencies. In: Haddad LM, Winchester JF, eds. Clinical Management of Poisoning and Drug Overdose. Philadelphia: WB Saunders, 1983:297–342.

Stokes IM. Paracetamol overdose in the second trimester of pregnancy—case report. Br J Obstet Gynaecol 1984;91:286–288.

Streissguth AP, Sampson PD, Barr HM. Neurobehavioral dose-response effects of prenatal alcohol exposure in humans from infancy to adulthood. Ann N Y Acad Sci 1989;562:145–158.

Storm RL, Schiller P, Seeds AE, et al. Fatal iron poisoning in a pregnant female: case report. Minnesota Med 1976;59:483–489.

Sussman S. Narcotic and methamphetamine use during pregnancy: effect on newborn and infants. Am J Dis Child 1965;106:325–330.

Telsey AM, Merrit TA, Dixon SD. Cocaine exposure in a term neonate: necrotizing enterocolitis as a complication. Clin Pediatr 1988;27: 547–550.

Tenenbein M. Methanol poisoning during pregnancy-prediction of risk and suggestions for management. Clin Toxicol 1997;35:193–194.

Thorp J. Management of drug dependency, overdose, and withdrawal in the obstetric patient. Obstet Gynecol Clin North Am 1995:22.

Tímár L, Czeizel AE. Birth weight and congenital anomalies following poisonous mushroom intoxication during pregnancy. Reprod Toxicol 1997;11:861–866.

Tomaszewski C. Carbon monoxide poisoning. Early awareness and intervention can save lives. Postgrad Med 1999;105:39–50.

Torregiani F, La Cavera C. Differential diagnosis of acute abdomen and latrodectism. Minerva Chirurgica 1990;45:303–305.

Tran T, Wax JR, Steinfeld JD, Ingardia CJ. Acute intentional iron overdose in pregnancy. Obstet Gynecol 1998;92:678–680.

Tran T, Wax JR, Philput C, Steinfeld JD, Ingardia CJ. Intentional iron overdose in pregnancy—management and outcome. J Emerg Med 2000;18:225–228.

UNICEF. Drug Use in Pregnancy. The Prescriber, 1992.

Unzelman RF, Alderfer GR, Chojnacki RE. Pregnancy and chronic hemodialysis. Trans Am Soc Artif Intern Organs 1973;19:144–149.

Van Duijn CM, vanSteensel-Moll HA, Coebergh JW, et al. Risk factors for childhood acute non-lymphocytic leukemia association with maternal alcohol consumption during pregnancy. Cancer Epidemiol Biomarkers Prev 1994;3:457–460.

Victor M, Adams RD. Barbiturates. In: Isselbacher KS, Adams RD, Braunswald E, et al., eds. Principles of Internal Medicine, 9th edn. New York: McGraw-Hill, 1980:982–985.

Vree PH, Zwart P. A newborn infant with amitriptyline poisoning. Nederlands Tijdschrift voor Geneeskunde 1985;129:910–912.

Wang PH, Yang MJ, Lee WL, et al. Acetaminophen poisoning in late pregnancy. A case report. J Reprod Med 1997;42:367–371.

Wehbeh H, Matthews RP, McCalla S, et al. The effect of recent cocaine use on the progress of labor. Am J Obstet Gynecol 1995;172: 1014–1018.

Weinbroum AA, Flaishon R, Sorkine P, et al. A risk-benefit assessment of flumazenil in the management of benzodiazepine overdose. Drug Safety 1997;17:181–196.

Weisman RS, Howland MA, Flomenbaum NE. The toxicology laboratory. In: Goldfrank LR, Flomenbaum NE, Lewin NA, et al. Goldfrank's Toxicologic Emergencies, 4th edn. Norwalk, CT: Appleton and Lange, 1990:45–46.

White S, Wong SHY. Standards of laboratory practice: analgesic drug monitoring. Clin Chem 1998;44:1110–1123.

Wilson DC, King LE Jr. Spiders and spider bites. Dermatol Clin 1990;8:277–286.

Winchester JF, Gelfand MC, Knepshield JH, Schreiner GE. Dialysis and hemoperfusion of poisons and drugs update. Trans Am Soc Artif Intern Organs 1977;23:762–842.

Wood JT, Hoback WW, Green TW. Poisonous snakebites resulting in lack of venom poisoning. Va Med Monthly 1955;82:130.

Wright SW, Wrenn KD, Murray L, Seger D. Clinical presentation and outcome of brown recluse spider bite. Ann Emerg Med 1997;30: 28–32.

Yasin SY, BeyDoun SW. Hemodialysis in pregnancy. Obstet Gynecol Survey 1988;43:655–668.

Zed PJ, Krenzelok EP. Treatment of acetaminophen overdose. Am J Health-System Pharm 1999;56:1081–1091.

Zuckerman B, Frank DA, Hingson R, et al. Effects of maternal marijuana and cocaine use on fetal growth. N Engl J Med 1989;320: 762–768.

39 Hypovolemic and cardiac shock

Scott Roberts

Hemorrhage is the leading cause of pregnancy-related mortality in the United States (Table 39.1) and abruptio placentae is the overall leading cause of pregnancy-related death due to hemorrhage (Chichakli et al., 1999). The specific causes of pregnancy-related deaths due to hemorrhage differ by pregnancy outcome. For women who die after live births, the leading cause is uterine atony and postpartum bleeding. For those whose pregnancies end in stillbirth, the leading cause of maternal death is abruptio placentae. Genital tract laceration and uterine rupture are the leading causes of death among women whose pregnancies end in abortion, as well as in women who are undelivered at the time of death (Chichakli et al., 1999).

Of the approximately 500,000 pregnancy-related deaths that occur each year worldwide, postpartum hemorrhage remains a significant problem, contributing to 30% of these deaths in the developing world (AbouZahr & Royston, 1991). Hemorrhage resulting from rupture of the ectopic site accounts for almost 95% of deaths associated with ectopic pregnancies (Koonin et al., 1997).

These deaths are mediated through hypovolemic shock which is also responsible for a number of other serious nonfatal complications, including acute renal failure, acute respiratory distress syndrome (ARDS), and, more rarely, postpartum pituitary necrosis. The parturient undergoes several important physiologic adaptations during pregnancy to protect herself from the bleeding expected at the time of delivery. Peripartum complications can occur quickly and since the uterus receives a blood flow of 450–650 mL/min (Edman et al., 1981), quick, definitive, and coordinated action on the part of the practitioner and supporting staff can be life saving. Shock is perhaps best defined as reduced tissue oxygenation resulting from poor perfusion (Shoemaker, 2000). Low flow or unevenly distributed flow from hypovolemia and disproportionate vasoconstriction are major causes of inadequate tissue perfusion in the acutely ill patient with circulatory dysfunction or shock. In hemorrhagic shock, the disparity is a result of blood loss that leads to both compensatory neurohormonal activation as well as the release of various endogenous mediators, which may aggravate the primary physiologic effects of hypovolemia (Pullicino et al., 1990; Abraham, 1991; Hoch et al., 1993). Because the purpose of the circulation is to provide oxygen and oxidative substrates for metabolic requirements, insufficient tissue perfusion and oxygenation to support body metabolism is the common circulatory problem of acute critical illness. This inadequate perfusion leads to local tissue hypoxia, organ dysfunction, multiple organ failure, and death.

Blood flow to the capillary beds of various organs is controlled by arterioles, which are resistance vessels that in turn are controlled by the CNS. On the other hand, 70% of the total blood volume is contained in venules, capacitance vessels controlled by humoral factors. Hypovolemic shock evolves through several pathophysiologic stages as body mechanisms combat acute blood volume loss (Table 39.2). The diagnosis of shock is most often made by the presence of hypotension, oliguria, acidosis, and collapse in the late stage, when therapy is frequently ineffective. Early in the course of massive hemorrhage, there are decreases in mean arterial pressure (MAP), cardiac output (CO), central venous pressure (CVP) and pulmonary capillary wedge pressure (PCWP), stroke volume and work, mixed venous oxygen saturation, and oxygen consumption. Increases are seen in systemic vascular resistance (SVR) and arteriovenous oxygen content differences. These latter changes serve to improve tissue oxygenation when blood flow is reduced (Bassin et al., 1971). Catecholamine release also causes a generalized increase in venular tone, resulting in an autotransfusion effect from the capacitance reservoir. These changes are accompanied by compensatory increases in heart rate, SVR and pulmonary vascular resistance, and myocardial contractility.

Nonsurvivors tend to have greater initial reduction in MAP, CO, oxygen delivery (Do_2), and oxygen consumption (Vo_2) with the initial hemorrhage, and less complete return of these factors to normal within the first 24 hours after resuscitation (Bishop et al., 1991, 1993). In addition, redistribution of CO and blood volume occurs via selective arteriolar constriction mediated by the CNS. This results in diminished perfusion to the kidneys, gut, skin, and uterus, with relative maintenance of blood flow to the heart, brain, and adrenal glands. In the

Table 39.1 Pregnancy-related mortality (deaths per 100,000 live births) in the United States, 1987–1990

	Outcome of pregnancy (% distribution)						All outcomes		
Cause of death	**Live birth**	**Stillbirth**	**Ectopic**	**Abortion**	**Molar**	**Undelivered**	**Unknown**	**%**	**PRMR**
Hemorrhage	21.1	27.2	94.9	18.5	16.7	15.7	20.1	28.8	2.6
Embolism	23.4	10.7	1.3	11.1	0	35.2	21.1	19.9	1.8
Pregnancy-induced hypertension	23.8	26.2	0	1.2	0	4.6	16.3	17.6	1.6
Infection	12.1	19.4	1.3	49.4	0	13	9	13.1	1.2
Cardiomyopathy	6.1	2.9	0	0	0	2.8	13.9	5.7	0.5
Anesthesia complication	2.7	0	1.9	8.6	0	1.8	1	2.5	0.2
Other/unknown	11.1	13.6	0.6	11.1	83.3	27.5	19.3	12.8	1.2
Total	100	100	100	100	100	100	100	100	9.2

(From Koonin LM, et al. Pregnancy-related mortality surveillance—United States, 1987–1990. MMWR 1997;46:17.)

Table 39.2 Clinical classification of maternal hemorrhage

Class	Blood loss (mL)	Volume deficit (%)	Signs and symptoms
I	≤1,000	15	Orthostatic tachycardia (↑ 20 bpm)
II	1,001–1,500	15–25	↑ HR 100–120 bpm Orthostatic changes (↓ 15 mmHg) Cap refill > 2 sec Mental changes
III	1,501–2,500	25–40	↑ HR (120–160 bpm) Supine ↓ BP ↑ RR (30–50 rpm) Oliguria
IV	>2,500	>40	Obtundation Oliguria-anuria CV collapse

BP, blood pressure; bpm, beats per minute; CV, cardiovascular; rpm, respiration per minute; RR, respiratory.
(From Eisenberg M, Copass MK, eds. Emergency Medical Therapy. Philadelphia PA: WB Saunders, 1982:40.)

pregnant patient, such redistribution may result in fetal hypoxia and distress, even before the mother becomes overtly hypotensive. In such situations, the uterus is, from a teleologic viewpoint, relatively less important than the essential lifesaving organ systems. Regardless of the absolute maternal BP, significant maternal shock is highly unlikely in the absence of fetal distress (Clark, 1990).

Peripheral vasoconstriction caused by the adrenomedullary stress response is an initial reaction to blood loss that maintains pressure in the presence of decreasing flow. This vasoconstriction, however, is disparate and leads to unevenly distributed microcirculatory flow. In nonsurvivors, these early changes precede the development of organ failure. In the presence of continued hypovolemia, the stress response may result in poor tissue perfusion, tissue hypoxia, covert clinical shock, organ dysfunction, ARDS, and other organ failure (Shoemaker et al., 1992, 1993). As the blood volume deficit approaches 25%, such compensatory mechanisms become inadequate to maintain CO and arterial pressure. At this point, small additional losses of blood result in rapid clinical deterioration, producing a vicious cycle of cellular death and vasoconstriction, organ ischemia, loss of capillary membrane integrity, and additional loss of intravascular fluid volume into the extravascular space (Shoemaker, 1973; Slater et al., 1973).

Increased platelet aggregation is also found in hypovolemic shock. Aggregated platelets release vasoactive substances, which cause small vessel occlusion and impaired microcirculatory perfusion. These platelet aggregates can embolize to the lungs and be a factor contributing to respiratory failure, which is often seen following prolonged shock.

Physiologic changes in preparation for pregnancy blood loss

The pregnant woman undergoes profound physiologic changes to prepare for the blood loss that will occur at the time of parturition. By the end of the second trimester of pregnancy, the maternal blood volume has increased by 1,000–2,000 mL (Pritchard, 1965). The maternal CO increases by 40–45% while total peripheral resistance decreases (Clark et al., 1989). This decreased peripheral resistance results from hormonal factors (progesterone, prostaglandin metabolites such as prostacyclin) that reduce overall vasomotor tone and from the development of a low-resistance arteriovenous shunt through the placenta. The decreased peripheral resistance is maximal in the second trimester. About 20–25% of the maternal CO goes to the placental shunt to yield a blood flow of approximately

500 mL/min. Placental blood flow is directly proportional to the uterine perfusion pressure, which in turn is proportional to systemic BP. Any decrease in maternal CO results in a proportionate decrease in placental perfusion. The uterine arterioles are very sensitive to exogenous vasopressor substances (Greiss, 1965), but, because of an incompletely understood pregnancy-related stimulus of the renin–angiotensin system, the vasopressor effect of angiotensin appears to be blunted during pregnancy.

Thus, during her pregnancy, the mother has been prepared for a blood volume loss of up to 1,000 mL. Following a normal spontaneous vaginal delivery, a first-day postpartum hematocrit usually is not altered significantly from the admission hematocrit. In practice, blood loss at delivery is often underestimated. Actual measurements show that the average blood loss after normal spontaneous vaginal delivery is over 600 mL. With a postpartum blood loss of less than 1,000 mL, the parturient's vital signs may not reflect acute blood loss (i.e. hypotension and tachycardia).

During the antepartum period, the obstetrician must be concerned with both of the patients. Fetal oxygenation decreases in proportion to the decrease in maternal CO. The catecholamine output from the mother's adrenal medulla may preferentially increase arteriolar resistance of the spiral arterioles in the placental bed, thus further decreasing oxygenation. Under such circumstances, the fetus may be in jeopardy, even though compensatory mechanisms maintain stable maternal vital signs. Thus, even in the absence of overt hypotension, for the well-being of the fetus, the health-care team must act quickly to expand the intravascular volume of an antepartum patient who has lost a significant amount of blood.

Although all vital organs receive increased blood flow during pregnancy, three (other than the placenta) are particularly susceptible to damage when perfusion pressure decreases as a result of hemorrhagic shock. These organs are the anterior pituitary gland, the kidneys, and the lungs. During pregnancy, the anterior pituitary enlarges and receives increased blood flow. Under the condition of shock, blood flow is shunted away from the anterior pituitary gland, which may undergo ischemic necrosis. Sheehan and Murdoch first described the syndrome of hypopituitarism secondary to postpartum hypotension as result of hemorrhage (Sheehan & Murdoch, 1938). This condition is now a rare complication in modern obstetrics. The clinical presentation can vary, but secondary amenorrhea resulting from loss of pituitary gonadotrophs is usually present. In severe cases, thyrotropic and adrenotropic pituitary hormones also may be deficient. Atypical or partial deficiency syndromes of both anterior and posterior pituitary hormones have been reported. Hypovolemia from any cause leads to reduced renal perfusion, which can result in acute tubular necrosis. In one series, hemorrhage and hypovolemia were precipitating factors in 75% of obstetric patients with acute renal failure (Smith et al., 1968). Prompt blood and fluid replacement is essential in order to avoid such sequelae. Lung injury resulting from hypovolemic shock is discussed in Chapter 23. In the nonpregnant state, a critical cardiac output exists below which oxygen extraction becomes impaired, and this critical oxygen delivery has been implicated in the pathogenesis of ARDS in humans. The question of a critical oxygen delivery point in human pregnancy is unclear although it has been suggested as a component of the pathology of severe preeclampsia (Belfort et al., 1993). Evans and colleagues (1996) presented evidence that in the pregnant sheep model, such a critical cardiac output does not exist.

Causes of obstetric hemorrhage

Any disruption in the integrity of the maternal vascular system during pregnancy has the potential for devastating blood loss. As an overview, ectopic pregnancy is the leading cause of life-threatening obstetric hemorrhage in the first half of gestation (Koonin et al., 1991). Beyond the first trimester, antepartum obstetric hemorrhage usually results from a disruption of the placental attachment site (involving either a normally implanted placenta or placenta previa) or uterine rupture (spontaneous or trauma related). During the intrapartum period, the likelihood of clinical shock is enhanced in patients with preeclampsia. Because of the intravascular volume depletion associated with this condition, even the usual blood loss associated with delivery may result in clinical instability. Another pathophysiologic change often associated with preeclampsia is thrombocytopenia, which when severe, may contribute to postpartum blood loss (see Chapter 33).

Most serious obstetric hemorrhage occurs in the postpartum period. The most common cause is uterine atony following placental separation. Under normal conditions, shortening myometrial fibers act as physiologic ligatures around the arterioles of the placental bed. Thus, uterine atony with failure of myometrial contraction results in arterial hemorrhage. Factors that predispose a patient to uterine atony include either precipitous or prolonged labor, oxytocin augmentation, magnesium sulfate infusion, chorioamnionitis, enlarged uterus resulting from increased intrauterine contents, and operative deliveries (Clark, 1990; Naef et al., 1994). Obstetric trauma is another common cause of postpartum hemorrhage. Cervical and vaginal lacerations are more common with midpelvic operative deliveries, and as a consequence of an extension of a uterine incision for cesarean birth. Other causes of postpartum hemorrhage (Table 39.3) include uterine inversion, morbidly adherent placenta (accreta/percreta), amniotic fluid embolism, retroperitoneal bleeding from either birth trauma or episiotomy, and coagulopathies of various causes (Clark, 1990; Zelop et al., 1993; Naef et al., 1994).

Table 39.3 Common causes of obstetric hemorrhage

Antepartum and intrapartum
Placental abruption
Uterine rupture
Placenta previa
Postpartum
Retained placenta
Uterine atony
Uterine rupture
Genital tract trauma
Coagulopathy

Management of hypovolemic shock in pregnancy

Perhaps the most important aspect of treating shock of any etiology is to recognize that physiologic manifestations such as hypotension and oliguria are secondary problems; frequently they are approached by the administration of vasopressors or diuretics respectively, which, while effecting a temporary improvement in vital signs and urine output, may actually aggravate the underlying physiologic derangements and hasten the development of secondary organ damage and death. It also must be emphasized that in the initial resuscitation of the patient in hypovolemic shock, time is of the essence in restoring hemodynamic and oxygenation parameters to normal if survival is to be optimized (Bishop, 1991, 1993; Shoemaker, 1995). When invasive monitoring is started near the time of the acute precipitating event in hypovolemic shock, it is found that survivors started with low flow but promptly developed compensatory hyperdynamic states, whereas nonsurvivors continued to have normal or low flow, tissue hypoxia, organ failure, capillary leak, and finally death.

Oxygenation

The most frequent cause of death of a patient in shock is inadequate respiratory exchange leading to multiple organ failure (Shoemaker et al., 1992). The duration of relative tissue hypoxia is important in the accumulation of byproducts of anaerobic metabolism. Thus, increasing the partial pressure of oxygen across the pulmonary capillary membrane by giving 8–10 L of oxygen per minute by tight-fitting mask may forestall the onset of tissue hypoxia and is a logical first priority. Also, in a pregnant patient, increasing the partial pressure of oxygen in maternal blood will increase the amount of oxygen carried to fetal tissue (Dildy et al., 1994). If the airway is not patent, or the tidal volume is inadequate, the clinician should not hesitate to perform endotracheal intubation and institute positive-pressure ventilation to achieve adequate oxygenation. In patients who do not respond promptly to simple resuscitative measures, assessment of Do_2 and Vo_2 and aggressive efforts to restore these values to normal or supranormal are essential. A therapeutic goal of achieving Do_2 greater than 800 mL/m^2 and Vo_2 greater than 180 mL/m^2 has been suggested in the non-pregnant patient (Shoemaker et al., 1988). Studies in adult critical care indicate that tissue oxygen debt resulting from reduced tissue perfusion is the primary underlying physiologic mechanism that subsequently leads to organ failure and death (Thangathurai et al., 1996; Taylor, 1997). Two prospective, randomized trials, however, found no benefit to normalization of SVo_2, or to supraphysiologic goals of hemodynamic manipulation (Hayes et al., 1994; Gattinoni et al., 1995). However, significant outcome improvement was noted in seven other randomized studies when such aggressive therapy was given early or prophylactically (Boyd & Bennett, 1996).

It seems that early identification and treatment of hypovolemic shock and its inciting cause is imperative to improving outcome. One approach commonly used to assist the clinician is to classify the degree of hemorrhage from I to IV based on the patient's signs and symptoms (Table 39.2). One recent randomized clinical trial in patients with sepsis and septic shock demonstrated reduced mortality when an early definitive resuscitation strategy involved goal-oriented manipulation of cardiac preload, afterload, and contractility to achieve a balance between systemic oxygen delivery and oxygen demand (Rivers et al., 2001).

Volume replacement

Protracted shock appears to cause secondary changes in the microcirculation; and these changes affect circulating blood volume. In early shock, there is a tendency to draw fluid from the interstitial space into the capillary bed. As the shock state progresses, however, damage to the capillary endothelium occurs and is manifested by an increase in capillary permeability, which further accentuates the loss of intravascular volume. This deficit is reflected clinically by the disproportionately large volume of fluid necessary to resuscitate patients in severe shock. Sometimes, the amount of fluid required for resuscitation is twice the amount indicated by calculation of blood loss volume. Prolonged hemorrhagic shock also alters active transport of ions at the cellular level, and intracellular water decreases. Thus, replacement of intracellular fluid with crystalloid or colloid solutions may be considered the primary therapeutic goal.

The two most common crystalloid fluids used for resuscitation are 0.9% sodium chloride and lactated Ringer's solution. Both have equal plasma volume-expanding effects. As illustrated in Fig. 39.1, the large volumes of required crystalloids can markedly diminish the colloid osmotic pressure (COP). Because albumin is integral to the maintenance of plasma COP, a 5% or 25% albumin solution has been suggested as being useful to resuscitate patients with acute hypovolemia.

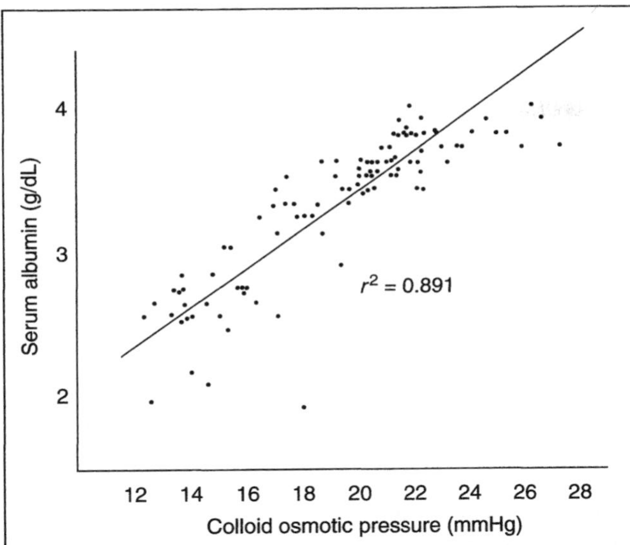

Fig. 39.1 Relationship between serum albumin and colloid oncotic pressure. The regression equation is calculated as follows: colloid oncotic pressure (mmHg) = 8.1 (serum albumin [g/dL]) − 8.2. (Reprinted with permission from the American College of Obstetricians and Gynecologists. Obstetrica and Gynecology, 1986;68:807.)

The intravascular effect of infused albumin lasts approximately 24 hours, much longer than that of infused crystalloids (Hauser et al., 1980). For a given infusion volume, colloids expand the plasma to a greater extent than do crystalloids. A randomized prospective clinical trial comparing 5% albumin, 5% hetastarch, and 0.9% saline for resuscitation of patients in hypovolemic or septic shock found that 2–4 times the volume of saline, compared with that of the albumin or hetastarch, was required to reach the same hemodynamic endpoint and that saline decreased the COP by 34% (Rackow et al., 1983). Albumin and hetastarch significantly increased the COP compared with baseline throughout the study period. In one report, only 20% of crystalloids remain in the intravascular space after 1 hour, and by 2 hours, virtually all of the infused fluid becomes interstitial (Shoemaker & Kram, 1991). In studies including critically ill patients, 500 mL of 5% albumin persisted in the intravascular space for approximately 4 hours, compared with 5–6 hours for a similar volume of hetastarch and 40 minutes for crystalloid (Hauser et al., 1980; Appel & Shoemaker, 1981). Fluid resuscitation in young, previously healthy patients can be accomplished safely with modest volumes of either colloid or crystalloid fluid and with little risk of pulmonary edema. The enormous volumes of crystalloids necessary to adequately resuscitate profound hypovolemic shock, however, will reduce the gradient between the COP and the PCWP and may contribute to the pathogenesis of pulmonary edema (Harms et al., 1981). This concept, however, remains unproven in actual clinical practice, and there continues to be a split of opinion on the use of crystalloid versus colloid solutions for initial resuscitation of patients in hypovolemic shock. The results of several randomized controlled trials, analyzed in a meta-analysis, do not support the conclusion that colloids achieve superior outcome, including survival, as a resuscitation fluid (Velanovich, 1989). The clinician must understand the effects and potential risk of such fluid therapy and must choose either or both for rapid repletion of intravascular volume and restoration of hemodynamic stability (Carey et al., 1970). Currently, the use of albumin and hetastarch in pregnant hypovolemic women is not regarded as first-line therapy and the initial fluid resuscitation carried out in most units is via crytalloid solutions.

Modern blood transfusion practice emphasizes the use of cell components or component hemotherapy rather than whole blood. Red blood cells are administered to improve oxygen delivery in patients with decreased red cell mass resulting from hemorrhage. A National Institutes of Health (NIH) consensus conference concluded that transfusion of fresh frozen plasma (FFP) was inappropriate for volume replacement or as a nutritional supplement (Consensus Conference, 1985). In the past, up to 90% of FFP use was for volume replacement. The other 10% was for the following conditions approved by the NIH consensus conference: replacement of isolated coagulation factor deficiencies, reversal of coumarin effect, antithrombin III deficiency, immunodeficiency syndromes, and treatment of thrombotic thrombocytopenic purpura. The current concern for excessive use of FFP is at least threefold. Firstly, the high profile of cost containment has caused blood banks to reevaluate use of blood products and the time involved in their preparation. Second, the routine use of FFP compromises the availability of raw material for preparation of factor VIII concentrates for hemophiliacs. Third, with regard to recipient safety, the risk of FFP includes disease transmission, anaphylactoid reactions, alloimmunization, and excessive intravascular volume (Oberman, 1985).

Massive blood replacement is defined as transfusion of at least one total blood volume within 24 hours. The NIH consensus conference report noted that pathologic hemorrhage in the patient receiving a massive transfusion is caused more frequently by thrombocytopenia than by depletion of coagulation factors. This finding was demonstrated in a prospective study of 27 massively transfused patients in whom levels of factors V, VII, and IX and fibrinogen could not be correlated with the number of units of whole blood transfused (Counts et al., 1979). A study of combat casualties suggested the thrombocytopenia was more important than depletion of coagulation factors as a cause of bleeding in massively transfused patients (Miller, 1971). In this report, restoration of the prothrombin times (PT) and partial thromboplastin times (PTT) to normal with FFP had little effect on abnormal bleeding; however, platelet transfusions were effective. There is no evidence that routine administration of FFP per a given number of units of RBCs decreases transfusion requirements in patients who are receiving multiple transfusion and who do not have documented coagulation defects (Mannucci, 1982). Thus, during massive blood replacement, correction of specific coagulation defects (fibrinogen levels < 100 mg/dL) and thrombocytopenia (platelet count < 30,000/mL) will minimize further transfusion requirements. In acute hemorrhagic shock, CVP or PCWP reflect intravascular volume status and may be useful in guiding fluid therapy. In the critically ill patient, however, CVP may be a less reliable indicator of volume status due to compliance changes in the vein walls (Shippy et al., 1984). Fortunately, in obstetrics, rapid recovery is the rule following prompt and adequate resuscitative measures, and such considerations are of less practical importance.

Pharmacologic agents

During the antepartum and intrapartum periods, only correction of maternal hypovolemia will maintain placental perfusion and prevent fetal compromise. Although vasopressors may temporarily correct hypotension, they do so at the expense of uteroplacental perfusion. Thus, vasopressors are not used in the treatment of obstetric hemorrhagic shock except as a last resort, because the uterine spiral arterioles are especially sensitive to these agents. In situations of acute circulatory failure, inotropic drugs such as dopamine may have a beneficial effect on hemodynamic function. Dopamine, however, has been demonstrated to decrease uterine blood flow (Fig. 39.2) in healthy and hypotensive pregnant sheep (Callender et al., 1978; Rolbin et al., 1979). In hypovolemic shock, vasopressors or inotropic agents are rarely indicated and should never be given until intravascular preload (PCWP) has been optimized. When given in equivalent doses to patients in shock, the vasopressor dopamine results in greater increases in MAP and PCWP than dobutamine. However, cardiac index, Vo_2, and Do_2 are improved to a much greater extent with dobutamine (Fig. 39.3). For this reason, the latter agent is preferred by some critical care specialists (Shoemaker et al., 1989).

Further evaluation

After the patient's oxygenation and expansion of intravascular volume have been accomplished and her condition is beginning to stabilize, it is essential for the health-care team to evaluate the patient's response to therapy, to diagnose the basic condition that resulted in circulatory shock, and to consider the fetal condition. Serial evaluation of vital signs, urine output, acid–base status, blood chemistry, and coagulation status aid in this assessment. In select cases, placement of a pulmonary artery catheter should be considered to assist in the assessment of cardiac function and oxygen transport variables. In general, however, central hemodynamic monitoring is not necessary in simple hypovolemic shock.

Evaluation of the fetal cardiotocograph may indicate fetal distress during the acute maternal episode. In general, however, only after the maternal condition is stabilized and there are persistent signs of fetal distress should the clinician

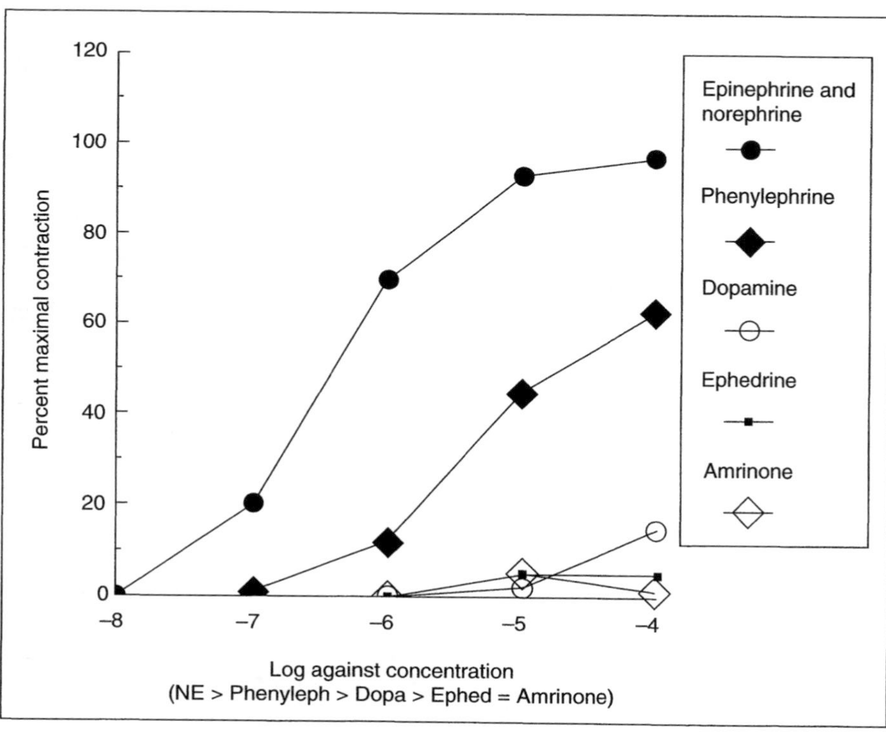

Fig. 39.2 Uterine artery response to vasopressors. (Courtesy of Dr Renee Bobrowski.)

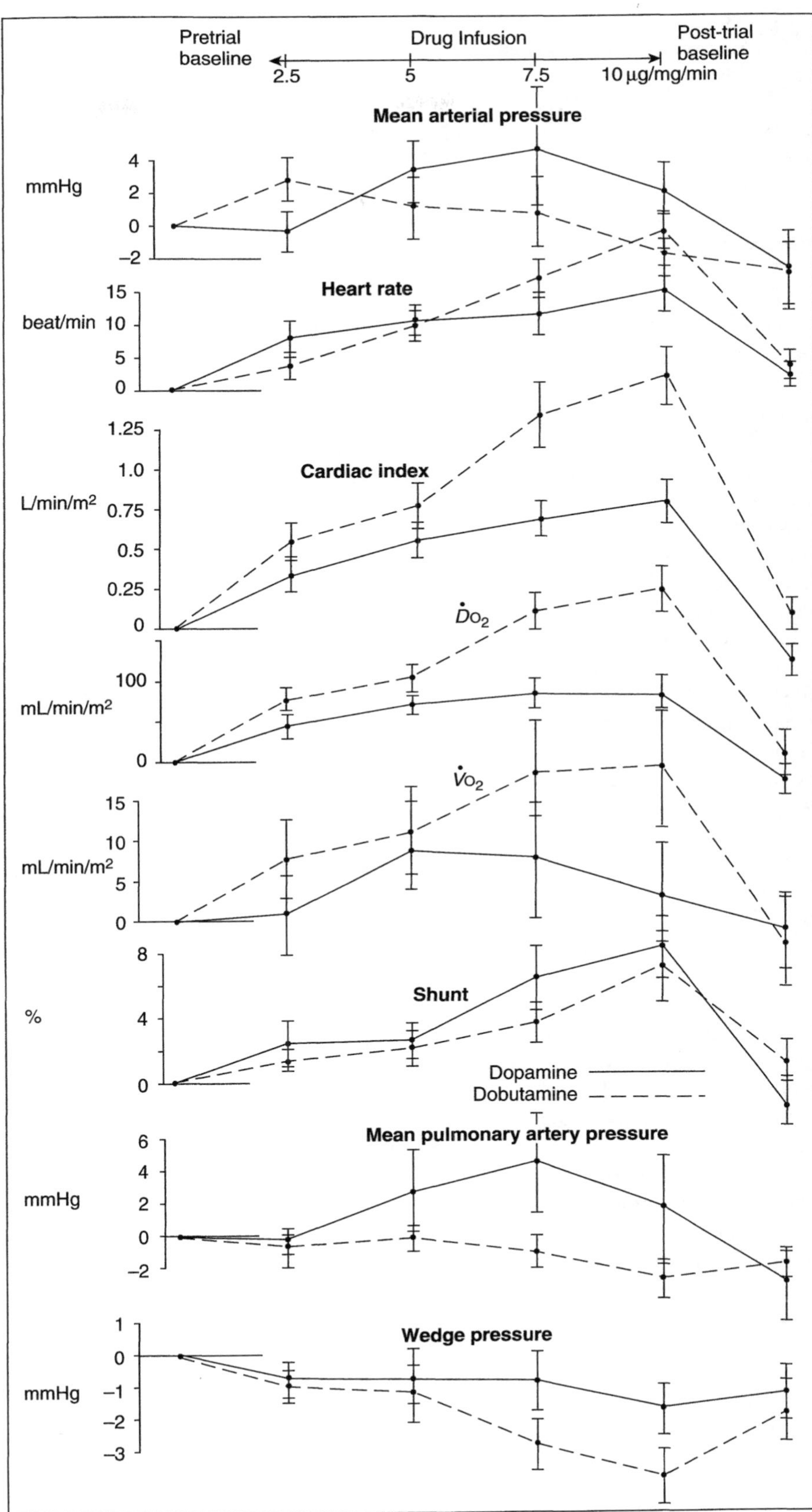

Fig. 39.3 Hemodynamic and oxygen transport effects of dobutamine (dashed line) and dopamine (solid line) in high-risk postoperative patients. (Reproduced by permission from Shoemaker WC. Diagnosis and treatment of the shock syndrome. In: Ayers SM, Grenvik A, Holbrook PR, Shoemaker WC, eds. Textbook of critical care. Philadelphia: WB Saunders, 1995.)

consider delivery. It is important to realize that as the maternal hypoxia, acidosis, and underperfusion of the uteroplacental unit are being corrected, the fetus may recover. Serial evaluation of the fetal status and in utero resuscitation are preferable to emergency delivery of a depressed infant from a hemodynamically unstable mother.

Hemostasis

In certain situation, such as uterine rupture with intraperitoneal bleeding, definitive surgical therapy may need to be instituted before stabilization can be achieved. With postpartum hemorrhage resulting from uterine atony that has not responded to the conventional methods of uterine compression and dilute intravenous oxytocin, the physician should consider intramuscular methergine or 15 methyl prostaglandin $F_{2\alpha}$. The latter is administered as a 250 μg dose, which may be repeated as necessary for up to five doses. In a small series of patients, rectal administration of misoprostol, a PGE_1 analogue, has been found effective in the treatment of uterine atony as well (O'Brien et al., 1998).

In cases of persistent vaginal bleeding, careful exploration of the vagina, cervix, and uterus is performed. The clinician looks for retained products of conception or lacerations. For hemorrhage resulting from uterine atony that has failed to respond to the previously described conservative measures, as well as in cases of extensive placenta accreta or uterine rupture not amenable to simple closure, laparotomy and hysterectomy may be indicated. If the patient does desire future fertility and is clinically stable, uterine artery ligation or stepwise uterine devascularization have been favorably described (AbdRabbo, 1994; O'Leary, 1995). The fundus compression suture as decribed by B-Lynch has also been reported to abate uterine hemorrhage in many cases (B-Lynch et al., 1997). Rarely, hypogastric artery ligation is surgically necessary.

Balloon occlusion and embolization of the internal iliac arteries have also been described in cases of placenta percreta (Dubois et al., 1997). A good discussion of many of these techniques, as well as a more comprehensive discussion of techniques for achieving medical and surgical hemostasis in patients with postpartum bleeding have been described elsewhere (Dildy, 2002; Gilstrap et al., 2002).

It should be emphasized that preventable surgical death in obstetrics may, on occasion, represent an error in judgment and a reluctance to proceed with laparotomy or hysterectomy, rather than deficiencies in knowledge or surgical technique. Proper management of serious hemorrhage requires crisp medical and surgical decision making as well as meticulous attention to the aforementioned principles of blood and volume replacement.

References

AbdRabbo SA. Stepwise uterine devascularization: a novel technique for management of uncontrolled postpartum hemorrhage with preservation of the uterus. Am J Obstet Gynecol 1994;171(3):694–700.

AbouZahr C, Royston E, eds. The global picture: the causes of maternal death. In: Maternal mortality: a global factbook. Geneva: World Health Organization, 1991:7.

Abraham E. Physiologic stress and cellular ischemia: relationship to immunosuppression and susceptibility to sepsis. Crit Care Med 1991;19:613–618.

Appel PL, Shoemaker WC. Fluid therapy in adult respiratory failure. Crit Care Med 1981;9:862.

B-Lynch C, Coker A, Lawal AH, Abu J, Cowen MJ. The B-Lynch surgical technique for the control of massive postpartum hemorrhage: an alternative to hysterectomy? Br J Obstet Gynecol 1997;104:372–375.

Bassin R, Vladeck B, Kim SI, et al. Comparison of hemodynamic responses of two experimental shock models with clinical hemorrhage. Surgery 1971;69:722–729.

Belfort MA, Anthony J, Saade GR, et al. The oxygen consumption: oxygen delivery curve in severe preeclampsia: evidence for a fixed oxygen extraction state. Am J Obstet Gynecol 1993;169:1448–1455.

Bishop MH, Jorgens J, Shoemaker WC, et al. Relationship between ARDS, hemodynamics, fluid balance and pulmonary infiltration in critically ill surgical patients. Am J Surg 1991;57:785–792.

Bishop MH, Shoemaker WC, Appel PL, et al. Influence of time optimal circulatory resuscitation in high-risk trauma. Crit Care Med 1993;221:56.

Boyd O, Bennett D. Enhancement of perioperative tissue perfusion as a therapeutic strategy for major surgery. New Horiz 1996;4:453–465.

Callender K, Levinson G, Shnider SM, et al. Dopamine administration in the normotensive pregnant ewe. Obstet Gynecol 1978;51:586–589.

Carey JS, Scharschmidt BF, Culliford AF, et al. Hemodynamic effectiveness of colloid and electrolyte solutions for replacement of simulated operative blood loss. Surg Gynecol Obstet 1970;131:679–686.

Chichakli LO, Atrash HK, Mackay AP, et al. Pregnancy-related mortality in the United States due to hemorrhage: 1979–1992. Obstet Gynecol 1999;94:721–725.

Clark SL. Shock in the pregnant patient. Semin Perinatol 1990;14:52–58.

Clark SL, Cotton DB, Lee W, et al. Central hemodynamic assessment of normal term pregnancy. Am J Obstet Gynecol 1989;161:1439–1442.

Consensus Conference. Fresh frozen plasma. Indications and risks. JAMA 1985;253:551–553.

Counts RB, Haisch C, Simon TL, et al. Hemostasis in massively transfused trauma patients. Ann Surg 1979;190:91–99.

Dildy GA. Postpartum hemorrhage: new management options. Clin Obstet Gynecol 2002;45(2):330–344.

Dildy GA, Clark SL, Loucks CA. Intrapartum fetal pulse oximetry: the effects of maternal hyperoxia on fetal arterial oxygen saturation. Am J Obstet Gynecol 1994;171:1120–1124.

Dubois J, Burel L, Brignon A, et al. Placenta percreta: Balloon occlusion and embolization of the internal iliac arteries to reduce intraoperative blood loss. Am J Obstet Gynecol 1997;176:723–726.

Edman CD, Toofanian A, MacDonald PC, Gant NF. Placental clearance rate of maternal plasma androstenedione through placental estradiol formation: An indirect method of assessing uteroplacental blood flow. Am J Obstet Gynecol 1981;141:1029–1037.

Evans W, Capelle SC, Edelstone DI. Lack of a critical cardiac output and critical systemic oxygen delivery during low cardiac output in the third trimester in the pregnant sheep. Am J Obstet Gynecol 1996;175:222–228.

Gattinoni L, Brazzi L, Pelosi P, et al. A trial of goal-oriented hemodynamic therapy in critically ill patients. N Engl J Med 1995;333:1025–1032.

Gilstrap LC, Cunningham FG, Vandorsten JP, eds. Operative obstetrics, 2nd edn. New York: McGraw-Hill, 2002.

Greiss FC. Uterine vascular response to hemorrhage during pregnancy and delivery. Anesthesiology 1965;26:393.

Harms BA, Kramer GC, Bodai BI, et al. The effect of hypoproteinemia and pulmonary and soft tissue edema formation. Crit Care Med 1981;9:503.

Hauser CJ, Shoemaker WC, Turpin I, et al. Hemodynamic and oxygen transport responses to body water shifts produced by colloids and crystalloids in critically ill patients. Surg Gynecol Obstet 1980;150:811.

Hayes MA, Timmins AC, Yau EHS, et al. Elevation of systemic oxygen delivery in the treatment of critically ill patients. N Engl J Med 1994;330:1717–1722.

Hoch RC, Rodriguez R, Manning T, et al. Effects of accidental trauma on cytokine and endotoxin production. Crit Care Med 1993;21:839–845.

Koonin LM, Atrash HK, Lawson HW, et al. Maternal mortality surveillance, United States 1979–1986. MMWR 1991;40:1–13.

Koonin LM, MacKay AP, Berg CJ, et al. Pregnancy-related mortality surveillance—United States, 1987–1990. MMWR 1997;46:17–36.

Mannucci PM, Federici AB, Sirchia G. Hemostasis testing during massive blood replacement: a study of 172 cases. Vox Sang 1982;42:113–123.

Miller RD, Robbins TO, Tong MJ, et al. Coagulation defects associated with massive blood transfusions. Ann Surg 1971;174:794–801.

Naef RW, Chauhan SP, Chevalier SP, et al. Prediction of hemorrhage at cesarean delivery. Obstet Gynecol 1994;83:923–926.

O'Brien P, El-Refaey H, Gordon A, et al. Rectally administered misoprostol for the treatment of postpartum hemorrhage unresponsive to oxytocin and ergotomine: a descriptive study. Obstet Gynecol 1998;92:212–214.

O'Leary JA. Uterine artery ligation in the control of postcesarean hemorrhage. J Reprod Med 1995;40:189–193.

Oberman HA. Uses and abuses of fresh frozen plasma. In: Garrity A, ed. Current concepts in transfusion therapy. Arlington, VA: American Association of Blood Banks, 1985.

Pritchard JA. Changes in the blood volume during pregnancy and delivery. Anesthesiology 1965;26:393.

Pullicino EA, Carli F, Poole S, et al. The relationship between cir ulating concentrations of interleukin-6, tumor necrosis factor, and the acute phase response to elective surgery and accidental injury. Lymphokine Res 1990;9:231–238.

Rackow EC, Falk JL, Fein IA. Fluid resuscitation in circulatory shock: a comparison of the cardiorespiratory effects of albumin, hetastarch and saline solutions in patients with hypovolemic and septic shock. Crit Care Med 1983;11:839–850.

Rivers E, Nguyen B, Havstad S, et al. Early goal-directed therapy in the treatment of severe sepsis and septic shock. N Engl J Med 2001; 345:1368–1377.

Rolbin SH, Levinson G, Shnider SM, et al. Dopamine treatment of spinal hypotension decreases uterine blood flow in the pregnant ewe. Anesthesiology 1979;51:37–40.

Sheehan HL, Murdoch R. Postpartum necrosis of the anterior pituitary: pathologic and clinical aspects. Br J Obstet Gynaecol 1938; 45:456.

Shippy CR, Appel PL, Shoemaker WC. Reliability of clinical monitoring to assess blood volume in critically ill patients. Crit Care Med 1984;12:107–112.

Shoemaker WC. Pathophysiologic basis for therapy for shock and trauma syndromes: use of sequential cardiorespiratory measurements to describe natural histories and evaluate possible mechanisms. Semin Drug Treat 1973;3:211–229.

Shoemaker WC. Diagnosis and treatment of the shock syndromes. In: Ayers SM, Grenvik A, Holbrook PR, Shoemaker WC, eds. Textbook of critical care, 3rd edn. Philadelphia: WB Saunders, 1995.

Shoemaker WC. Diagnosis and treatment of shock and circulatory dysfunction. In: Grenvik A, Ayers SM, Holbrook PR, Shoemaker WC, eds. Textbook of critical care, 4th edn. Philadelphia: WB Saunders, 2000.

Shoemaker WC, Kram HB. Comparison of the effects of crystalloids and colloids on homodynamic oxygen transport, mortality and morbidity. In: Simmon RS, Udeko AJ, eds. Debates in general surgery. Chicago: Year Book Medical, 1991.

Shoemaker WC, Appel PL, Kram HB, et al. Prospective trial of supranormal values of survivors as therapeutic goals in high risk surgical patients. Chest 1988;94:1176–1186.

Shoemaker WC, Appel PL, Kram HB, et al. Comparison of hemodynamic and oxygen transport effects of dopamine and dobutamine in critically ill surgical patients. Chest 1989;96:120–126.

Shoemaker WC, Appel PL, Kram HB. Role of oxygen debt in the development of organ failure, sepsis, and death in high risk surgical patients. Chest 1992;102:208–215.

Shoemaker WE, Appel PL, Kram HB. Hemodynamic and oxygen transport responses in survivors and nonsurvivors of high risk surgery. Crit Care Med 1993;21:977–990.

Slater G, Vladeck BA, Bassin R, et al. Sequential changes in the distribution of cardiac output in various stages of experimental hemorrhagic shock, Surgery 1973;73:714–722.

Smith K, Browne JCM, Shackman R, et al. Renal failure of obstetric origin. Br Med Bull 1968;24:49.

Taylor RW. Pulmonary Artery Catheter Consensus Conference Participants: Pulmonary Artery Catheter Consensus Conference Consensus Statement. Crit Care Med 1997;25:910.

Thangathurai D, Charbonnet C, Wo CCJ, Shoemaker WC, et al. Intraoperative maintenance of tissue perfusion prevents ARDS. New Horiz 1996;4:466–474.

Velanovich V. Crystalloid versus colloid fluid resuscitation: a meta-analysis of mortality. Surgery 1989;105(1):65–71.

Zelop CM, Harlow BL, Frigoletto FD, et al. Emergency peripartum hysterectomy. Am J Obstet Gynecol 1993;168:1443–1448.

40 Septic shock

Michael R. Leonardi
Bernard Gonik

Sepsis is a clinical syndrome that encompasses a variety of host responses to systemic infection. *Shock* is a morbid condition in which the patient's vascular bed is inadequately filled by the functional intravascular volume, resulting in hypotension and inadequate tissue perfusion. If the course of this pathologic process is left unaltered, cellular hypoxia, organ dysfunction, and death ensue (Bone et al., 1992a). *Septic shock* describes the constellation of clinical findings which result from the systemic inflammatory response to an infectious insult and are marked by alteration of the ability of the host to maintain vascular integrity and homeostasis, resulting in inadequate tissue oxygenation and circulatory failure. The spectrum of host response ranges from simple sepsis to septic shock with multiple-organ system dysfunction and death.

Septic shock accounts for approximately 10% of admissions to noncoronary intensive care units (ICUs) and is the thirteenth leading cause of death in the United States. Its incidence appears to be increasing (CDCP, 1993). After correcting for the increased age of the population, the rate of septic shock reported by the Centers for Disease Control (CDC) between 1979 and 1987 more than doubled. This increased rate of septic shock was observed regardless of age group or geographic area (Progress in Chronic Disease Progression, 1990). Despite optimal ICU care, the mortality rate from septic shock remains 40–50% in most series (Brun-Buisson et al., 1995). Although septic shock remains an uncommon event in the obstetric population, factors that contribute to the increased rate of sepsis in the general population are also more common in women of reproductive age. Additionally, because maternal mortality is so uncommon, sepsis will remain an important overall cause of maternal mortality (Gibbs & Locke, 1976).

Systemic inflammatory response syndrome

The systemic inflammatory response syndrome (SIRS) describes the general inflammatory response to a variety of insults. Its etiology is not limited to infection, since burns, trauma, and pancreatitis can elicit a similar clinical picture. It is characterized by two or more of the following: (i) body temperature less than 36°C or more than 38°C; (ii) pulse greater than 90 beats per minute (bpm); (iii) tachypnea manifested as respiratory rate exceeding 20 per minute or $Paco_2$ less than 32 mmHg; or (iv) leukocyte count less than 4,000/μL, greater than 12,000/μL, or more than 10% immature forms in the differential count. When SIRS is the result of documented infection, it is termed *sepsis*.

Severe sepsis is diagnosed when SIRS is associated with organ dysfunction, hypoperfusion, or hypotension. Useful indicators of hypoperfusion include lactic acidosis, oliguria, or acute alterations in mental status. If abnormalities of BP and perfusion persist despite adequate fluid resuscitation, *septic shock* is present. Hypotension is not necessary for the diagnosis if the patient requires vasopressor support. Multiple-organ system dysfunction syndrome (MODS) is the terminal phase of this spectrum, represented by the progressive physiologic deterioration of interdependent organ systems such that homeostasis cannot be maintained without active intervention. Commonly affected organ systems include the pulmonary and renal with acute respiratory distress syndrome (ARDS) and acute renal failure, respectively (Bone et al., 1992a).

Clincial presentation

The observed clinical spectrum of sepsis represents increasing severity of the host response to infection rather than increasing severity of infection (Bone, 1991). Because experimentally infused endogenous inflammatory mediators such as interleukins 1 and 2 (IL-1, IL-2) and tumor necrosis factor-alpha (TNF-α) reproduce this syndrome, an exaggerated host inflammatory response is felt to be central to its pathophysiology (Tracey et al., 1987; Okusawa et al., 1988; Sculier et al., 1988). Although various risk factors have been identified and scoring systems developed, no effective method to predict which patients will progress from bacteremia to septic shock and MODS has been identified (Bone, 1992b). The classification scheme has proven useful, however, in prognosticating the prevalence of infection as well as the risk of mortality. More severe inflammatory responses are accompanied by progressively greater mortality rates (Rangel-Frausto et al., 1995).

The clinical manifestations of septic shock fall into three broad categories, which correlate with progressive physiologic derangement. *Early (warm) shock* is characterized by a hyperdynamic circulation and decreased systemic vascular resistance (SVR). The hallmark of *late (cold) shock* is abnormal perfusion and oxygenation secondary to regional (peripheral) vasoconstriction and myocardial dysfunction. *Secondary (irreversible) shock* is frequently a terminal condition associated with multiple-organ system dysfunction (Table 40.1). Each phase represents a continued downward progression in the course of this disease process.

In the early phase of septic shock, bacteremia is heralded typically by shaking chills, sudden rise in temperature, tachycardia, and warm extremities. Although the patient may appear ill, the diagnosis of septic shock may be elusive until hypotension is documented. In addition, patients may present initially with nonspecific complaints such as malaise, nausea, vomiting, and at times, profuse diarrhea. Abrupt alterations in mental status also may herald the onset of septic shock; these behavior alterations have been attributed to the reductions in cerebral blood flow. Tachypnea or dyspnea may be present with minimal findings on physical examination. These findings may represent the endotoxin's direct effect on the respiratory center and may immediately precede the clinical development of ARDS.

Table 40.1 Presenting features of septic shock

Early (warm) shock
Altered mental status
Peripheral vasodilation (warm skin, flushing)
Tachypnea or shortness of breath
Tachycardia
Temperature instability
Hypotension
Increased cardiac output and decreased peripheral resistance
Late (cold) shock
Peripheral vasoconstriction (cool, clammy skin)
Oliguria
Cyanosis
ARDS
Decreased cardiac output and decreased peripheral resistance
Secondary (irreversible) shock
Obtundation
Anuria
Hypoglycemia
Disseminated intravascular coagulation
Decreased cardiac output and decreased peripheral resistance
Myocardial failure

Laboratory findings are quite variable during the early stages of septic shock. The WBC count may be depressed at first; soon afterward, a marked leukocytosis is usually evident. Although there is a transient increase in blood glucose level secondary to catecholamine release and tissue underutilization, hypoglycemia may prevail later when a reduction in gluconeogenesis occurs secondary to hepatic dysfunction. Early evidence of disseminated intravascular coagulation (DIC) may be represented by a decreased platelet count, decreased fibrinogen, elevated fibrin split products, and elevated thrombin time. Initial arterial blood gases may show a transient respiratory alkalosis secondary to tachypnea. These parameters later reflect an increasing metabolic acidosis, because tissue hypoxia and lactic acid levels increase.

Later clinical manifestations of untreated shock include cold extremities, oliguria, and peripheral cyanosis. As suggested previously, myocardial depression becomes a prominent feature of severe septic shock, with marked reductions in cardiac output and SVR (Parker & Parillo, 1983). Overt evidence of prolonged cellular hypoxia and dysfunction include profound metabolic acidosis, electrolyte imbalances, and DIC. If these symptoms are left untreated, rapid progression to irreversible shock is the rule.

Progressive cardiac dysfunction features prominently in the clinical presentation of septic shock. Cardiac output and cardiac index (CI) are initially increased due to increased heart rate and the profound decreases in SVR. The increased cardiac output, however, is inadequate to meet the patient's metabolic needs. Both the left and right ventricles dilate, and the ejection fractions decrease (Porembka, 1993). The limitation in cardiac performance and ejection fraction is greater than that seen in equally ill nonseptic patients (Parker et al., 1984). Ventricular compliance is also affected, as evidenced by a decrease in the ability to increase contractility in response to increase in preload (Ognibene et al., 1988).

Parker and Parillo (1983) studied 20 patients in septic shock. By conventional criteria, 95% of the patients would have been classified as hyperdynamic, but 10 of the 20 had abnormally depressed ejection fractions. These alterations in ejection fraction were not accounted for by differences in preload, afterload, or positive end-expiratory pressure (PEEP). In the acute phase of septic shock, the ability to dilate the left ventricle in order to maintain cardiac output in the face of declining ejection fraction appears to represent an adaptive response that confers a survival advantage (Parker et al., 1984). Two subsets of patients have been identified based on response to volume loading: those who respond with ventricular dilation and those who respond with increased pulmonary capillary wedge pressure (PCWP) rather than an increased cardiac output (Parrillo, 1985). Cardiac depression of similar magnitude and frequency has been reported in obstetric patients with septic shock managed with pulmonary artery (PA) catheters (Lee et al., 1988).

Extensive studies in humans and animal models points to a

circulating myocardial depressant factor rather than alterations in coronary flow or myocardial oxygenation as the etiology for myocardial dysfunction (Marksad et al., 1979). Alterations in ejection fraction observed with structural heart disease, in postinfarction patients, or in critically ill nonseptic patients are not associated with a similar circulating factor (Parrillo et al., 1985). Endotoxin infusion in humans produces comparable left ventricular dilation and decreases in performance (Porembka, 1993), suggesting that endotoxin plays some role in stimulating the production of this myocardial depressant factor.

Predisposing factors in obstetrics

Pregnancy is often considered an immunocompromised state, although little objective evidence exists comparing the ability of pregnant and nonpregnant individuals to process bacterial antigens and elicit an appropriate immune response. Pregnant women remain at risk for common medical and surgical illnesses such as pneumonia and appendicitis, as well as conditions unique to pregnancy, all of which may result in sepsis (Table 40.2). Although genital tract infections are common on an obstetric service (Gibbs et al., 1978; Duff, 1986; Balk & Bone, 1989), septic shock in this same population tends to be an uncommon event. When an obstetric patient has clinical evidence of local infection, the incidence of bacteremia is approximately 8–10% (Ledger et al., 1975; Monif & Baer, 1976; Blanco et al., 1981; Bryan et al., 1984; Reimer & Reller, 1984). Overall, rates of bacteremia of 7.5 per 1,000 admissions to the obstetrics and gynecology services at two large teaching hospitals have been reported (Ledger et al., 1975; Blanco et al., 1981). More striking is that patients with bacteremia rarely progress to develop more significant complications, such as septic shock. Ledger and colleagues (1975) identified only a 4% rate of shock in pregnant patients with bacteremia. This value agrees with that of other investigators, who have reported a 0–12% incidence of septic shock in bacteremic obstetric and gynecologic patients (Chow & Guze, 1974; Ledger et al., 1975; Monif & Baer, 1976; Blanco et al., 1981; Bryan et al., 1984; Reimer & Reller, 1984). Obstetric conditions that have been identified as predisposing to the development of septic shock are listed in Table 40.2 (Lowthian & Gillard, 1980; Mariona & Ismail, 1980; Blanco et al., 1981; Cavanagh et al., 1982; Lloyd et al., 1983; Chow et al., 1984; Duff, 1984).

Table 40.2 Bacterial infections associated with septic shock and found in the obstetric patient

	Incidence (%)
Chorioamnionitis	0.5–1.0
Postpartum endometritis	
Cesarean section	0.5–85.0
Vaginal delivery	<10
Urinary tract infections	1–4
Pyelonephritis	1–4
Septic abortion	1–2
Necrotizing fasciitis (postoperative)	<1
Toxic shock syndrome	<1

The physiologic changes that accompany pregnancy may place the gravida at greater risk for morbidity than her nonpregnant counterpart. Elevation of the diaphragm by the gravid uterus, delayed gastric emptying, and the emergent nature of many intubations in obstetrics dramatically increase the risk of aspiration pneumonitis. Although the pregnant patient has been previously identified as being at increased risk of pulmonary sequelae from systemic infection such as pyelonephritis, the pathophysiologic mechanisms have been known only for the past decade (Cunningham et al., 1987). Hemodynamic investigation in normal women using flow-directed PA catheters has quantified the physiologic alterations that place the patient at increased risk for pulmonary injury. Pregnancy decreases the gradient between colloid oncotic pressure and PCWP (Clark et al., 1989). This increases the propensity for pulmonary edema if pulmonary capillary permeability changes or the PCWP increases. In the critically ill, nonpregnant patient, decreases in the COP–PCWP gradient predict an increased propensity for pulmonary edema (Rackow et al., 1977, 1982; Weil et al., 1978a), and that gradient is already decreased by normal pregnancy. The intrapulmonary shunt fraction (Q_s/Q_T) is also increased (Hankins et al., 1996), which may increase the risk of pulmonary morbidity.

Fortunately, mortality from septic shock, which is extremely high in the face of bacteremia in other medical and surgical specialties, tends to be an infrequent event in obstetrics and gynecology. The incidence of death from sepsis is estimated at 0–3% in obstetric patients, as compared with 10–81% in nonobstetric patients (Ledger et al., 1975; Blanco et al., 1981; Cavanagh et al., 1982; Weinstein et al., 1983). Suggested reasons for these more favorable outcomes in the gravid woman include: (i) younger age group; (ii) transient nature of the bacteremia; (iii) type of organisms involved; (iv) primary site of infection (pelvis) more amenable to both surgical and medical intervention; and (v) lack of associated medical diseases that could adversely impact the prognosis for recovery. This fifth factor is echoed by Freid and Vosti (1968), who reported increased mortality in patients with underlying disease in addition to sepsis.

Pathophysiology of septic shock

The clinical manifestations of septic shock can be categorized as either systemic responses, including tachycardia, tachypnea, and hypotension, or end-organ dysfunction, such as ARDS and acute renal failure (Parrillo, 1993). The severity of the clinical presentation is felt to be determined by the vigor of the host inflammatory response rather than the virulence of the inciting infection (Lynn & Cohen, 1995). Once septic shock is established, the physiologic derangements induced by systemic activation of inflammatory mediators are more important than the microbial milieu in prognosticating outcome. In those patients who succumb, death is predominantly a function of the host response to the initiating insult (Brun-Buisson et al., 1995).

For the most part, Gram-negative sepsis has been the model used to study this phenomenon in experimental animals. Endotoxin, a complex lipopolysaccharide present in the cell wall of aerobic Gram-negative bacteria, appears to be the critical factor in producing the pathophysiologic derangements associated with septic shock (Gibbs & Locke, 1976). Endotoxin is released from the bacterium at the time of the organism's death. In patients with Gram-positive sepsis, shock can also develop and appears to be closely related to the release of an exotoxin (Kwaan & Weil, 1969). Cleary et al. (1992) demonstrated the production of exotoxin A by isolates of *Streptococcus pyogenes* associated with septic shock, whereas isolates from patients not in septic shock were unable to produce the exotoxin. From a clinical perspective, the overt physiologic alterations induced by either lipopolysaccharide endotoxins or exotoxins are the same.

Some investigators have suggested that differences may exist at the cellular level with regard to various Gram-positive bacterial toxins (Kwaan & Weil, 1969). Superantigenic toxins elaborated by some *Staphylococcus* and *Streptococcus* species, for example, can directly activate large numbers of T-lymphocytes without the need for intermediate antigen processing cells such as macrophages (Webb & Gascoigne, 1994). This abbreviated mechanism of lymphocyte activation may explain the rapidly progressive and particularly fulminant clinical course observed with some Gram-positive bacterial infections.

The ability of both Gram-positive and Gram-negative organisms to systematically activate the inflammatory cascade has particular relevance in the obstetric patient, in whom mixed polymicrobial infections are commonly identified (Monif & Baer, 1976). Although Gram-negative coliforms make up a significant portion of the organisms recovered in bacteremic obstetric patients, other organisms, including aerobic and anaerobic streptococci, *Bacteroides fragilis*, and *Gardnerella vaginalis*, are found frequently. Septic shock in pregnancy associated with legionella pneumonia has also been described (Tewari et al., 1997). As in other areas of medicine, the number of cases of obstetric sepsis associated with group A streptococcus appears to be increasing (Holm, 1996).

The series of events initiated by endotoxin is presented schematically in Fig. 40.1. Local activation of the immune system and its effector cells is important at the site of infection. The inflammatory process is normally tightly regulated and functions to locally confine the spread of infection. If the ability to regulate this response is lost, systemic activation of effector cells results in the elaboration of proinflammatory cytokines with widespread systemic effects (Pinsky & Matuschak, 1989). The syndrome of septic shock represents the culmination of overzealous activation of normal body defense mechanisms in an attempt to eradicate the invading pathogen (Sugerman et al., 1981).

Preliminary evidence suggests that an initial insult may cause simultaneous subclinical injury to multiple organ system. It is theorized that this initial insult primes the immune system for a disproportionate response to any subsequent insult (Van Bebber et al., 1989; Daryani et al., 1990; Moore et al., 1992; Poggetti et al., 1992). The immune system, as one of the affected organ systems, responds to a second insult with an outpouring of inflammatory mediators (Demling et al., 1994). Activation of the complement cascade also plays a central role in activation of the immune system (Fearon et al., 1975) and can produce the hemodynamic changes characteristic of sepsis in animal models (Schirmer et al., 1988).

Various proinflammatory mediators have been implicated in the pathogenesis of septic shock. Several lines of experimental evidence in both humans and animal models support the central role of lipopolysaccharide-induced secretion of the cytokine TNF-α in the pathophysiology of the sepsis syndrome (Tracey et al., 1988). Large amounts of TNF-α are produced in response to endotoxin administration in healthy human subjects (Hesse et al., 1988; Michie et al., 1988), and the administration of either endotoxin or TNF-α provokes similar physiologic derangements (Michie et al., 1988). Elevated levels of TNF-α in animals are associated with shock and lethality (Tracey, 1987a; Mayoral et al., 1990). The infusion of TNF-α into experimental animals produces the pulmonary, renal, and gastrointestinal (GI) histopathology observed at autopsy in septic patients (Tracey et al., 1986; Remick et al., 1987). In similar models, antibodies directed against TNF-α provide protection and decrease mortality if given early enough to provide adequate tissue levels (Beutler et al., 1985; Tracey, 1987b). At the cellular level, lipopolysaccharide bound to a carrier protein interacts with the CD14 receptor on cells of the monocyte line. The resulting monocyte activation leads to production of TNF-α and IL-1, either simultaneously or in parallel. Lipopolysaccharide also binds to soluble CD14 to facilitate interaction with tissues lacking the CD14 receptor, such as vascular endothelium (Lynn & Golenbock, 1992). The production of TNF-α stimulates the secretion of interleukins, prostaglandins, leukotrienes, and other inflammatory mediators. These inflammatory products cause the clinical symptoms associated with sepsis as well as capillary leak, hypotension, and activation of the coagulation system (Hageman & Caplan, 1995).

Vascular endothelium is a metabolically active tissue that exerts a pivotal role in the regulation of underlying vascular smooth muscle and maintenance of vessel integrity and the fluidity of blood, and in the regulation of leukocyte adhesion.

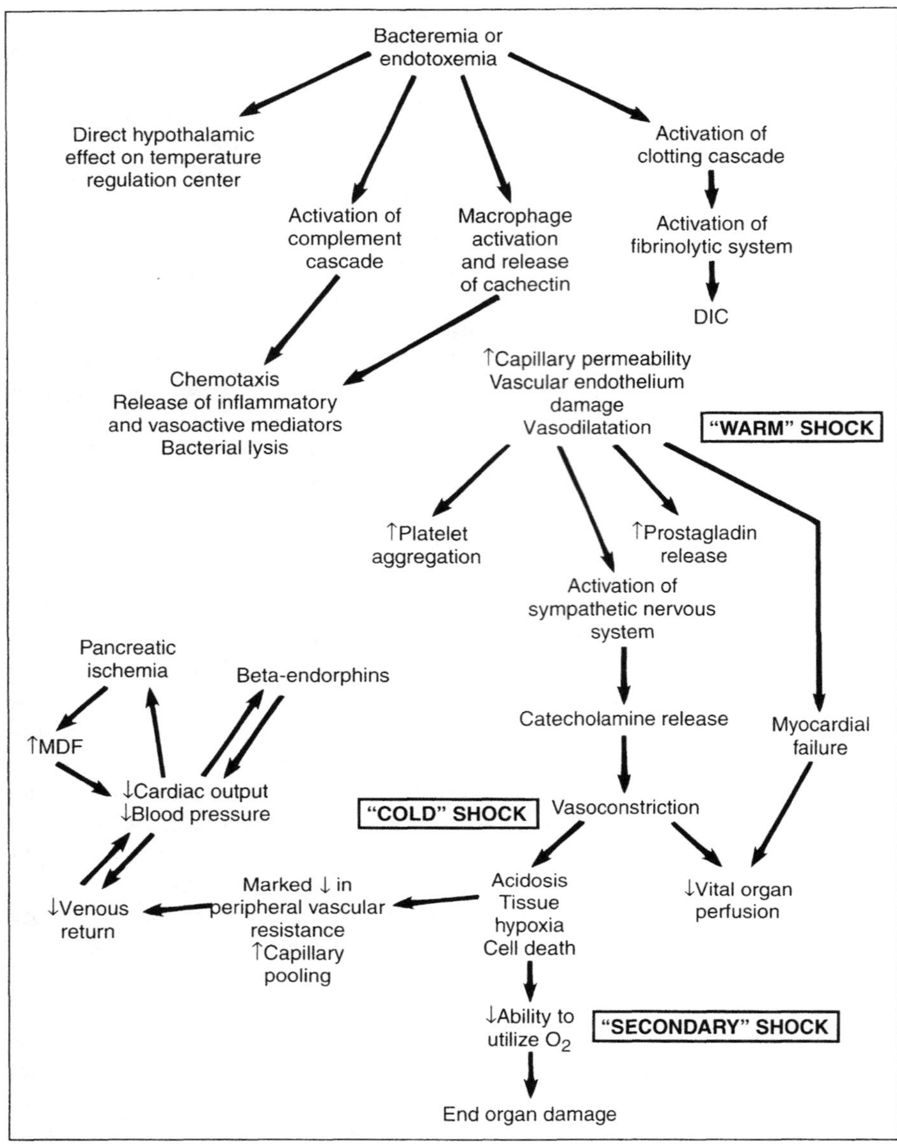

Fig. 40.1 Pathophysiology of septic shock. DIC, disseminated intravascular coagulation.

Maintenance of vascular homeostasis is regulated in large part by production of nitric oxide (endothelium-derived relaxing factor) (Hollenberg & Cunnion, 1994). TNF-α stimulation of macrophages causes a sustained increase in nitric oxide production, resulting in profound effects on vascular tone and permeability. Cyclo-oxygenase is also activated, and the elaboration of prostaglandins contributes to the misdistribution of blood flow (Dinerman et al., 1993).

Stimulation of endothelial cells by several cytokines including IL-1α, IL-1β, and TNF-α results in endothelial activation, and alters the structural and metabolic functions of the endothelium. Rather than its usual anticoagulant properties, the endothelial lining of blood vessels becomes a procoagulant surface, adhesion molecule production is upregulated, and production of chemoattractant and vasoactive substances increases. Endothelial expression of anticoagulants such as thrombomodulin and heparan sulfate is lost. Tissue factor is synthesized. Protein C is no longer activated by the endothelium, and the extrinsic pathway is activated. Phospholipid microparticles, which are normally buried within the cell membrane, are formed in the endothelium providing an anchoring substrate for vitamin K dependent coagulation factors.

In the normal state, few adhesion molecules are expressed on vascular endothelium. After activation, P-selectin, E-selectin, intercellular adhesion molecule-1, and other adhesions are produced. Leukocytes adhere and transmigrate into the surrounding tissues. When confined to the local area, this process promotes localization of infection. At some point, activation may progress to endothelial dysfunction with capillary leak. Systemic endothelial activation, with its associated outpouring of inflammatory mediators and cytokines, facilitates the inflammatory cascade and the clinical syndrome. As our understanding of this process grows, opportunities will be identified for targeted intervention to abort systemic inflammatory activation and progressive dysfunction (Hack & Zeerleder, 2001).

Clinically, disruption of the endothelium and vascular smooth muscle is a well-recognized component of septic shock, as is the blunting of response to vasoactive drugs. Because these effects are blocked in experimental models by treatment with inhibitors of nitric oxide synthesis, alterations in nitric oxide metabolism are felt to play a role in the development of refractoriness to endogenous catecholamines and exogenous vasopressors (Siegel et al., 1967). The elaboration of inflammatory mediators may also affect sympathetic vasomotor tone, resulting in impaired vasoconstriction to sympathetic stimulation. The combination of a leaky vasculature and loss of smooth muscle tone results in refractory hypotension (Siegel, 1967; Sibbald et al., 1991).

Tumor necrosis factor-alpha and activated complement fragments attract neutrophils whose products exacerbate endothelial injury (Sriskandan & Cohen, 1995). This results in altered ability of the host to maintain tissue perfusion through regulation of BP, cardiac output, and SVR (Parrillo, 1993). The production of IL-1β by macrophages has the added effect of producing procoagulant activity, which results in fibrin deposition in the microvasculature, leading to further perturbations of organ perfusion (Bonney & Humes, 1984; Goetzl et al., 1984; Jacobs & Tabor, 1989). Activation of the microvasculature endothelium by TNF-α and IL-1β produces capillary leak and increased leukocyte receptor expression.

Leukocyte migration and activation result in release of vasoactive substances such as histamine, serotonin, and bradykinin. These substances, in turn, increase capillary permeability, induce endothelial damage, and promote vasodilation (Sugerman et al., 1981). Neutrophil activation stimulates a respiratory burst with increased production and release of lysosomal enzymes and toxic oxygen species such as superoxide, hydroxyl, and peroxide radicals. This can have deleterious effects on the vasculature as well as other organs and is especially detrimental in the lung, where it is felt to play a key role in the pathogenesis of ARDS (Hollenberg & Cunnion, 1994). Stimulation of neutrophils by activated complement fragments also leads to leukotriene secretion, further affecting capillary permeability and blood flow distribution (Jacobs & Tabor, 1989). At the same time, the damage to the vascular endothelium stimulates platelet aggregation. Complement activation ensues, with microthrombus formation and fibrin deposition leading to further derangements of perfusion (Lee et al., 1989).

Intact reflex responses, via sympathetic activation, to what are initially local events may produce profound vasoconstriction in some organ systems; this vasoconstriction results in reduction in tissue perfusion (Sugerman et al., 1981). The local loss of control of vascular tone can also result in failure of arterioles and meta-arterioles to dilate in response to physiologic vasodilating substances such as histamine and bradykinin (Altura et al., 1985). Further capillary leak continues and leads to increased intravascular fluid loss. In addition, cellular hypoxia and acidosis disrupt the ability of individual cells to utilize available oxygen (Duff et al., 1969). Marked reduction in peripheral vascular resistance now appears, with extensive capillary pooling of blood.

In a rabbit model of IL-1β-induced hypotension, the lung was the primary organ injured. Although TNF-α produced more injury than IL-1β, pulmonary injury was massive when sublethal doses of both TNF-α and IL-1β were administered. The investigators concluded that TNF-α and IL-1 may act synergistically to disrupt vascular endothelium (Okusawa et al., 1988). Additional evidence for the role of cytokines in mediating lung injury in ARDS includes the increased production of IL-1 and TNF-α by lung macrophages in response to endotoxin administration (Tabor et al., 1988), and the in vivo observation that alveolar macrophages from ARDS patients produce increased amounts of IL-1 (Jacobs et al., 1988). Direct effects of bacterial immunologic complexes are also thought to play an important role in tissue injury (Knuppel et al., 1984). Immune complex precipitants have been identified within the lung vasculature, and they are thought to contribute to the development of ARDS. Likewise, focal areas of acute tubular necrosis seen in the kidney have been associated with the deposition of inflammatory infiltrates.

Disseminated intravascular coagulation frequently complicates septic shock. DIC involves activation of the coagulation cascade as well as fibrinolysis, with depletion of circulating coagulation factors. Tissue factor is released by TNF-α stimulation of monocytes and by exposure of subendothelially located tissue factor following injury to the vascular endothelium with activation of the extrinsic pathway. Microvasculature fibrin deposition compromises end-organ perfusion. At the same time, TNF-α also inhibits the production and action of regulatory proteins such as protein C, thereby amplifying the procoagulant state. Although its role in DIC is not significant, activation of the intrinsic pathway provides a powerful stimulus to the production of kinins, such as bradykinin, thus contributing to hypotension and disruption of vascular homeostasis. Derangements in the coagulation system are magnified by endotoxin's rapid activation and then suppression of fibrinolysis, which again appears to be mediated by TNF-α (Levi et al., 1993).

Pregnancy and septic shock

The peripartum host may be different from the traditional septic shock host in ways other than the difference in microbiologic pathogens involved. Physiologic adaptations to pregnancy designed to promote favorable maternal and fetal outcome occur in almost every organ system (Table 40.3)

(Clark et al., 1989; Hankins et al., 1996; Metcalfe & Ueland, 1974; Fletcher et al., 1979; Pritchard, 1997). Some of these changes, such as a dramatic increase in pelvic vascularity, promote maternal survival after infection. They also can influence the presentation and course of septic shock in the gravida, although such potential differences have received little attention in the literature. On the other hand, other physiologic adaptations to pregnancy (e.g. ureteral dilatation) may predispose the gravid female to more significant infectious morbidity than her nonpregnant counterpart.

In an animal model of endotoxin-induced septic shock, Beller and co-workers (1985) compared pregnant and nonpregnant responses to fixed doses of lipopolysaccharide. The pregnant animals had a much more pronounced respiratory and metabolic acidosis than did the controls, and they died secondary to cardiovascular collapse substantially faster than did nonpregnant controls. Although the increased susceptibility to endotoxin observed in pregnant animals is consistent (Bech-Jansen et al., 1972; Morishima et al., 1978; Beller et al., 1985), different animal species appear to succumb to different physiologic aberrations; thus, caution is warranted in applying the results of animal studies to critically ill pregnant women.

It is interesting to note that in the experimental model, the fetus and neonate are much more resistant to the direct deleterious effects of endotoxin than is the mother. Bech-Jansen et al. (1972) demonstrated that although blood flow to the uterus declined out of proportion to maternal hypotension, the fetus and the neonate were capable of tolerating endotoxin doses 10 times those proven to be lethal to the adult pregnant sheep. The fetal circulation was not affected until the adult's condition was terminal. The investigators hypothesize that these altered effects are related to the immature status of the fetal and neonatal vascular responsiveness. Morishima et al. (1978) administered endotoxin to pregnant baboons, and observed profound asphyxia and severe maternal and fetal acidemia with rapid deterioration in the fetus, evidenced by late decelerations and fetal death in utero during maternal circulatory collapse. These effects were thought to result primarily from maternal factors such as hypotension and increased myometrial activity, both of which contribute to a reduction in placental perfusion. Although the pathophysiologic basis for the increased susceptibility during gestation to endotoxin remains speculative, the results suggest that the gravida should be considered a compromised host. The response of the gravid female to infectious stimuli probably represents the combined effects of alterations in her physiology as well as enhanced responsiveness to the effects of endotoxin.

As would be expected in an uncommon condition, the available human data regarding septic shock in human pregnancy are limited. The data describing contemporary ICU management monitoring in the septic obstetric patient, including invasive hemodynamic monitoring, are even more scarce. The patient populations studied tend to be small and heterogenous and suffer from a variety of preexisting medical conditions, as well as some degree of ascertainment bias. The hemodynamic alterations seen in this patient population were described in a multi-institution review of women with sepsis in pregnancy whose management was guided by a PA catheter (Lee et al., 1988). In this series, maternal morbidity was 20%. Similar to the nonpregnant patient, septic shock in the pregnant women was accompanied by an overall decrease in peripheral SVR. The range of values for this hemodynamic variable was quite wide and was dependent on the stage of shock at which the PA catheter was initially inserted. At presentation, normal to increased cardiac output and decreased SVR were observed. Those patients who ultimately survived had an increase in their mean arterial pressure (MAP), SVR, and left ventricular stroke work index (LVSWI) in response to therapy. LVSWI appeared to be the best measure of cardiac function and predictor of outcome (Fig. 40.2). Longitudinal measurements of SVR also proved to be useful in monitoring the progress of therapy. Response to intervention was reflected in normalization of the SVR to intermediate values

Table 40.3 Hemodynamic and ventilatory parameters in pregnancy

	Nonpregnant	Pregnant	Relative change (%)
Cardiac output (L/min)	4.3	6.2	43
Heart rate (bpm)	71	83	17
Systemic vascular resistance (dyne/sec/cm^5)	1,530	1,210	21
Pulmonary vascular resistance (dyne/sec/cm^5)	119	78	34
COP (mmHg)	20.8	18.0	14
COP–PCWP gradient (mmHg)	14.5	10.5	18
Mean arterial pressure (mmHg)	86.4	90.3	No change
Central venous pressure (mmHg)	3.7	3.6	No change
PCWP (mmHg)	6.3	7.5	No change
Left ventricular stroke work index (g/m/m^2)	41	48	No change

(From Clark SL, Cotton DB, Lee W, et al. Central hemodynamic assessment of normal term pregnancy. Am J Obstet Gynecol 1989;161:1439–1442.)

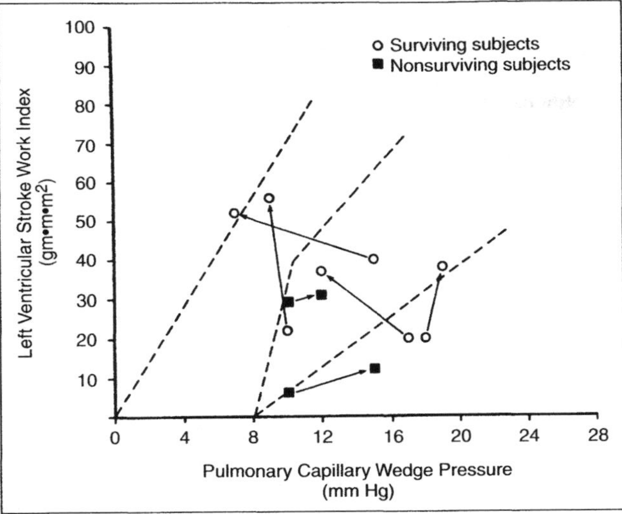

Fig. 40.2 Systemic vascular resistance index values measured serially in gravidas with septic shock.

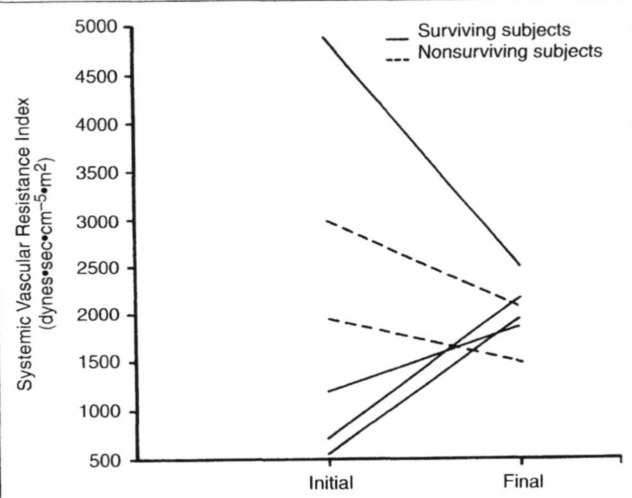

Fig. 40.3 Serial ventricular function determinations in gravidas with septic shock.

(Fig. 40.3) (Lee et al., 1988). These findings are consistent with physiologic patterns observed in nonpregnant septic shock patients (Shoemaker et al., 1973).

Treatment of septic shock

The resuscitation goals for the patient in septic shock have been directed toward the aggressive use of volume replacement and inotropes to treat hypotension. Contemporary management has modified these therapeutic goals and emphasizes oxygen delivery and organ perfusion as endpoints for hemodynamic intervention including normalization of mixed venous oxygenation, arterial lactate, and acid–base status. Future management algorithms will probably include recommendations for management of the effects of inflammatory mediators (Lindeborg & Pearl, 1993).

Initial intervention should be directed at the following general goals: (i) improvement in functional circulating intravascular volume; (ii) establishment and maintenance of an adequate airway to facilitate management of respiratory failure; (iii) assurance of adequate tissue perfusion and oxygenation; (iv) initiation of diagnostic evaluations to determine the septic focus; and (v) institution of empiric antimicrobial therapy to eradicate the most likely pathogens.

If the patient is pregnant, priorities should be directed toward maternal well-being first, even in the face of the potential deleterious effects of septic shock on the fetus. Because fetal compromise results primarily from maternal cardiovascular decompensation, improvements in the maternal status should have positive effects on the fetal condition. Furthermore, attempts at delivery of the fetus in a hemodynamically compromised mother may lead to increased risks of fetal distress and the need for more aggressive obstetric intervention. In a mother who is not adequately resuscitated or is unstable, further decreases in intravascular volume associated with blood loss at abdominal delivery may result in irrecoverable decompensation in maternal hemodynamic status. Maternal interests should take precedence, especially early in the course of resuscitation. This, of course, presumes that the fetal compartment is not the source of sepsis. Under such circumstances, therapy includes initiating delivery while stabilizing the mother.

Volume expansion

The mainstay of the acute management of septic shock involves volume expansion and correction of absolute or relative hypovolemia (Roberts & Laros, 1971; Hawkins, 1980; Packman & Rackow, 1983; Rackow et al., 1983; Kaufman et al., 1984; Knuppel et al., 1984). Such therapy is always needed and correlates closely with improvement in cardiac output, oxygen delivery, and survival (Weil & Nishijima, 1978). At times, considerable quantities of fluid are needed because of profound vasodilation, increased capillary permeability, and extravasation of fluid into the extravascular space. Blood pressure, heart rate, urine output, and hematocrit are conventionally used to assess the adequacy of intravascular volume. While these criteria are adequate for the initiation of volume resuscitation, they are unreliable in guiding optimal fluid and inotrope management in the patient with septic shock or multiple-organ system dysfunction (Shippy et al., 1984). The best means of monitoring this critical therapy is with the use of a flow-directed PA catheter (Swan et al., 1970; Shoemaker et al., 1990). Although central venous pressure (CVP) monitoring has been suggested as an alternative, available evidence suggesting erroneous information obtained with CVP monitoring supports the use of a flow-directed PA catheter (Cotton, 1985). In addition, PA catheterization allows determination of cardiac output and the calculation of variables related to oxygen delivery and utilization. These determinants cannot be made with standard CVP systems. Use of a PA catheter to optimize oxygen delivery and allow earlier intervention in the event of decompensation has been shown to decrease morbidity and mortality in high-risk surgical ICU patients (Shoemaker et al., 1990; Lindeborg & Pearl, 1993).

A common endpoint for volume replacement is a PCWP of 14–16 mmHg, a point at which, according to Starling's law, ventricular performance is optimal. Starling forces and ventricular performance are altered by sepsis, however, and a specific numerical value should not be chosen as an endpoint. Titration of therapy to optimize cardiopulmonary performance is preferable (Packman & Rackow, 1983; Rackow et al., 1987; Porembka, 1993). PCWP is used as an indicator of left ventricular end-diastolic pressure (LVEDP). Left ventricular end-diastolic volume (LVEDV) and circulating intravascular volume are inferred from the PCWP. For a given volume, LVEDP will vary with left ventricular compliance, which is influenced by a multitude of factors in the septic patient (Lewis & Gotsman, 1980; Packman & Rackow, 1983). Fluid resuscitation is a dynamic process, not an endpoint, and the value for PCWP that optimizes preload varies by patient. Therapy is optimized for the individual patient by sequentially expanding intravascular volume until a plateau is reached where further volume challenge produces no incremental increase in cardiac output (Porembka, 1993). An elevated PCWP may reflect an overexpanded intravascular space, a reduced left ventricular function, or both. The LVSWI can be used to differentiate between these two possibilities and select appropriate intervention. Information obtained from the PA catheter should be interpreted based on norms established for pregnancy rather than those derived from a nonpregnant population.

Controversy surrounds the debate about the optimal type of fluid to be used for volume expansion. Although isotonic crystalloid solutions such as normal saline are advocated most often, some investigators have recommended the use of colloid solutions (e.g. 5% normal human albumin) to maintain a normal COP–PCWP gradient (Haupt & Rackow, 1982). Rackow et al. (1983) have suggested that maintenance of the balance between COP and PCWP reduces the risk of pulmonary edema. Various colloid and crystalloid solutions have been studied. In one series, both were able to restore cardiac function and hemodynamic stability, but the use of crystalloid required 2–4 times as much volume to achieve the same hemodynamic endpoint. Crystalloids significantly decrease the COP and the COP–PCWP gradient, with a commensurate increase in the potential for pulmonary edema (Rackow et al., 1983). These findings are supported by the results of others who, in addition, found that the risk of pulmonary edema was lower in younger patients (Rackow et al., 1977; Weil et al., 1978). These authors concluded that younger, healthier patients are more able to tolerate crystalloid resuscitation. Colloids also have been shown to increase oxygen delivery and extraction (Shoemaker et al., 1991). Coupled with the decrease in COP and increased risk of pulmonary edema with massive infusion of crystalloids, further study in a homogenous group of patients is warranted. In clinical trials comparing crystalloid and colloid resuscitation, different endpoints and methodologies have been used, and the study groups were heterogenous, making comparisons between studies difficult (Wagner & D'Amelio, 1993). With appropriate caution, the use of either crystalloid or colloid solutions for volume resuscitation in septic shock is appropriate.

Vasoactive drug therapy

At times, fluid resuscitation proves inadequate in restoring optimal cardiovascular performance. After restoration of adequate intravascular volume guided by a PA catheter, the use of vasoactive agents is indicated. The most commonly used agent in this regard is dopamine hydrochloride. Dopamine is a drug with dose-dependent effects on dopaminergic, alpha-, and beta-adrenergic receptors (Rao & Cavanagh, 1982). In very low doses (5 μg/kg/min), a selective dopaminergic increase in mesenteric and renal blow flow occurs. As the dosage is increased, the predominant effect is to increase myocardial contractility and cardiac output. With doses exceeding 20 μg/kg/min, alpha effects predominate, with marked vasoconstriction and a further reduction in tissue perfusion. Dopamine is administered as a continuous infusion, starting at 2–5 μg/kg/min and titrated according to clinical and hemodynamic responses (Goldberg, 1974).

Dobutamine is an inotropic agent with fewer chronotropic effects than dopamine. It increases CI and oxygen delivery and decreases SVR, thereby improving perfusion (Bollaert et al., 1990). It is commonly combined with low-dose dopamine to improve myocardial performance and maintain renal perfusion in the ICU setting. Other vasoconstrictive drugs, including both norepinephrine (Desjars et al., 1987; Meadows et al., 1988) and epinephrine (Bollaert et al., 1990; MacKenzie et al., 1991; Lindeborg & Pearl, 1993; Moran et al., 1993), have been suggested as alternatives in dopamine-resistant shock. Epinephrine increases CI, oxygen delivery, BP, and contractility. Oxygen debt is increased, possibly reflecting decreased tissue oxygenation, but hypotension is reversed by a balanced effect on both SVR and cardiac output (Bollaert et al., 1990). These hemodynamic improvements come at the expense of increased myocardial work and oxygen requirement (Lindeborg & Pearl, 1993), which has limited the use of epinephrine. Significant vasoconstriction and end-organ hypoperfusion are also of concern.

Early experience using norepinephrine as a primary agent for inotropic support in septic shock was disappointing. Fears of excessive vasoconstriction and reversal of hypotension at the expense of organ perfusion limited its use. As newer catecholamines, such as dopamine, became available with more "favorable" side-effect profiles, they were used as first-line agents (Martin et al., 1993). Some now argue that norepinephrine's poor initial response related to inadequate monitoring and suboptimal volume replacement. This led to the subsequent need for excessively large vasopressor doses and development of hypoperfusion (Lucas, 1994). As a second-line drug reserved for cases of dopamine-resistant or refractory shock, additional adverse outcomes were reported (Desjars et al., 1987; Meadows et al., 1988).

Until recently, little attempt was made to compare the effects of dopamine and norepinephrine on hemodynamic parameters and oxygen delivery in septic shock in a randomized, controlled fashion. In one such study, Martin et al. (1993) demonstrated that norepinephrine more reliably reversed hypotension and oliguria than did dopamine. Likewise, oxygen delivery and consumption were more favorably improved with norepinephrine. Additionally, norepinephrine effectively reversed shock in those patients who failed dopamine therapy. Dopamine has also been demonstrated to adversely affect the balance between splanchnic oxygen delivery and utilization when compared with norepinephrine. Both agents comparably increased MAP, but dopamine decreased gastric intramucosal pH (pHi), suggesting detrimental effects on splanchnic perfusion (Marik & Mohedin, 1994).

Unfortunately, microvascular shunting and hypoperfusion associated with any vasoactive agent are at times difficult to recognize and only become apparent with deterioration of the patient's overall condition or with increased serum lactic acid concentrations (Porembka, 1993). Despite well-described limitations to this biochemical test, following lactic acid levels serially may be useful as an indicator of end-organ perfusion. Changes in calculated oxygen delivery and extraction are also helpful in assessing adequacy of tissue perfusion and response to therapy. Of note is the demonstration by Rolbin et al. (1979) that dopamine decreased uterine blood flow in hypotensive pregnant sheep. Therefore, dopamine (and the other vasoactive agents) may compromise fetal status while improving the maternal condition. This latter example suggests the need for continuous heart rate monitoring as a "marker" for end-organ perfusion in the gestationally viable fetus during resuscitation attempts with vasopressor therapy.

The ability to spontaneously generate a hyperdynamic state in response to sepsis is associated with lower mortality (Shoemaker et al., 1973; Parker & Parillo, 1983; Shippy et al., 1984; Moore et al., 1992). It is unclear whether the beneficial effect on mortality reflects the impact of therapeutic intervention or better underlying cardiovascular function in a host who is more responsive to intervention. Survivors are clearly more responsive to inotropic therapy (Shoemaker et al., 1991), but this may simply reflect underlying hemodynamic differences in survivors versus nonsurvivors.

The observation that better cardiovascular performance was associated with survival has prompted many intensivists to conclude that titration of inotropic support to supranormal values should improve outcome (Shoemaker et al., 1988, 1992; Tuchschmidt et al., 1992; Boyd et al., 1993; Yu et al., 1993; Bishop et al., 1995). The desired hemodynamic profile usually includes a CI greater than $4.5\,L/min/m^2$ and a Do_2 greater than $600\,mL/min/m^2$. These values are not prospectively derived; rather, they represent median values for survivors. This approach to management is controversial and has been questioned by two large prospective series. The controversy surrounding endpoints for inotropic support is, in part, attributable to differences in the populations studied and indication for ICU admission. This approach was initially evaluated as prophylaxis in high-risk surgical patients. In the more recent work, which questions this management scheme, patients were randomized after shock and organ failure were established. These prospective, randomized series found no benefits to normalization of SVo_2 or supraphysiologic goals for hemodynamic manipulation. Hayes et al. (1994) were unable to demonstrate a decrease in mortality as long as volume replacement was adequate and perfusion pressure was maintained. A large multicenter European trial also found that the targeted parameters were difficult to achieve, and the propensity to achieve them was a function of the patient's age. No decrease in mortality was found in patients who achieved supraphysiologic levels of cardiovascular performance regardless of group or reason for ICU admission (Gattinoni et al., 1995).

These series should not be interpreted as advocating a conservative approach to hemodynamic therapy in septic shock. The apparently contradictory findings may be viewed as complementary. In susceptible patients, oxygen delivery, intravascular volume, and perfusion should be optimized to prevent progression to organ failure. In patients who develop shock, inotropic therapy should be directed toward maintenance of adequate cardiac output and BP with inotropes to maintain perfusion and oxygenation (Hinds & Watson, 1995). Responsiveness to inotropic support and the ability to spontaneously generate a hyperdynamic state may allow some prognostication regarding outcome early in the clinical course.

Early, aggressive intervention is supported by the positive results of the most recent study of goal-directed therapy in the treatment of sepsis and septic shock. In fact, the in-hospital mortality was reduced from 46.5 to 35.5%. In contrast to earlier studies, aggressive resuscitation was begun as early as possible in the clinical course and while the patient was still in the emergency room. A specific management algorithm was used to direct therapy with specific clinical endpoints for gauging therapeutic response, and the interval between initial evaluation and initiation of therapy was extremely short (Rivers et al., 2001). This publication does not contradict earlier randomized studies where no benefit to supraphysiologic hemodynamic endpoints was demonstrable. Rather, it emphasizes the importance of intervening at the earliest possible time prior to systemic decompensation and cardiovascular collapse. The study of Rivers et al. (2001) also demonstrates the importance of continuous availability of on-site intensivists if the outcome of critically ill patients is to be optimized.

Oxygenation

Although oxygenation at the pulmonary level can be assessed easily by arterial blood gas determinations, oxygen consumption or utilization is a more difficult parameter to evaluate. The use of a PA catheter allows direct measurement and calculation of parameters relevant to oxygen delivery and consumption. Early in the course of shock, blood pressure may actually be normal due to peripheral vasoconstriction, because perfusion is disproportionately diverted from the renal and splanchnic circulations to maintain central BP. Impairment of splanchnic perfusion permits translocation of bacteria and toxins across the GI mucosa, thus worsening septic shock (Fiddian-Green et al., 1993; Demling et al., 1994). Oxygen delivery and tissue extraction are decreased in all forms of shock. Untreated, anaerobic metabolism and progressive oxygen debt develop and result in lactic acidemia, organ dysfunction, and death (Shoemaker et al., 1992).

Septic patients have increased metabolic needs for oxygen and, at the same time, a decreased ability to extract the oxygen that is delivered (Tuchschmidt et al., 1991). Peripheral tissue utilization of oxygen is frequently reduced, resulting in tissue hypoxia (Duff et al., 1969). Two possible mechanisms play a pivotal role in this phenomenon. First, there is evidence to suggest that cellular dysfunction during later stages of septic shock can lead to underextraction of delivered oxygen. Mitochondrial and cellular dysfunction decrease the ability to utilize oxygen (Rackow et al., 1988; Dantzker, 1989; Gutierrez et al., 1989). Second, microvascular shunting and loss of autoregulation of blood flow may decrease local availability of oxygen (Siegel et al., 1967; Duff et al., 1969). Additionally, hypophosphatemia, alkalosis, and multiple blood transfusions all shift the oxyhemoglobin dissociation curve to the left, resulting in a decrease in peripheral availability of oxygen.

Tissue oxygen extraction can be assessed indirectly. Elevation in mixed-venous oxygen saturation ($S\bar{V}O_2$) or reduced arteriovenous oxygen content difference reflect decreased tissue oxygen extraction (Tuchschmidt et al., 1991). Actual peripheral oxygen consumption can be calculated by using the Fick equation; the normal indexed nonpregnant range is 120–140 mL $O_2/min/m^2$ (Shoemaker et al., 1983). Oxygen consumption is normally independent of oxygen delivery, because delivery far exceeds consumption. In the septic patient, oxygen delivery should be increased until lactic acid concentrations return to normal (Shoemaker et al., 1991; Lindeborg & Pearl, 1993). Even in the absence of lactic acidosis, it is prudent to maintain excess oxygen delivery to avoid local reduction in tissue perfusion and subsequent organ dysfunction (Demling et al., 1994). In an animal model of sepsis, anaerobic metabolism (implying inadequate perfusion) was demonstrated in the gut despite supranormal cardiac output and oxygen delivery that was adequate for the rest of the body (Pinsky & Matuschak, 1989).

Acute respiratory distress syndrome

The diagnosis of ARDS is made on the basis of progressive hypoxemia, with a normal PCWP, diffuse infiltrates on chest X-ray, and/or decreased pulmonary compliance (Sugerman et al., 1981). These findings are consistent with a pathophysiological state in which increased capillary permeability leads to extravasation of fluid into interstitial spaces, with the development of progressive oxygen debt that contributes to multiple-organ system dysfunction and death.

The development of pulmonary hypertension increases the rate at which extravascular interstitial fluid collects and contributes to the progressive hypoxemia observed clinically. Pulmonary hypertension develops initially in response to neurohormonal mechanisms. Later, structural changes develop in the pulmonary microvasculature and parenchyma, probably in response to inflammatory byproducts in the lung parenchyma (Bersten & Sibbald, 1989). During this later inflammatory fibrotic phase, ARDS is commonly associated with fever, leukocytosis, and decreased SVR, making it exceedingly difficult to distinguish from pneumonia and worsening sepsis (Ashbaugh & Maier, 1985; Meduri et al., 1991).

The cornerstone of the treatment of ARDS involves intubation and ventilatory support to maintain adequate gas exchange at nontoxic levels of inspired oxygen. PEEP is often necessary to accomplish this goal, and serial monitoring of arterial blood gases is essential. The clinician must remember than even in the face of overt pulmonary capillary leakage, intravenous hydration should be continued and adequate intravascular volume maintained to promote systemic perfusion. Positive end-expiratory pressure generates increased intrathoracic pressure and may decrease venous return and consequently cardiac output, depending on volume status and amount of PEEP. When interpreting hemodynamic readings and assessing intravascular volume status, the clinician must keep in mind that PEEP can artificially increase PCWP measurements.

Recent advances in ventilator management and understanding of the role that overventilation plays in pulmonary injury and inflammation have improved outcome. Traditionally, supraphysiologic tidal volumes of 10–15 mL/kg of body weight were used to ventilate ICU patients. In patients with ARDS, this led to a high rate of stretch-induced lung injury, high airway pressures, and barotrauma. A recent randomized, multicenter trial demonstrated a 22% reduction in mortality with lower tidal volumes (6 mL/kg body weight). Higher levels of PEEP and F_iO_2 were required. Interestingly, the decrease in mortality was observed without any decrease in barotrauma. The lower tidal volume group demonstrated less lung inflammation. As our understanding of the pathophysiology of sepsis and ARDS evolves, incorporating into clinical practice measures to avoid iatrogenic lung injury and inflammation, such as limiting stretch-induced injury, will serve to improve patient outcome (Acute Respiratory Distress Syndrome Network, 2000).

Antimicrobial therapy

In concert with attempts at restoring normal cardiovascular function and tissue oxygenation, an aggressive investigation into the underlying etiology of sepsis should be initiated. Because the course of septic shock can be short and fulminant, such a work-up must be carried out without delay, and empiric antimicrobial therapy should be started. At times, the cause of sepsis in the parturient is obvious (e.g. chorioamnionitis or pyelonephritis). At other times, the etiology can be elusive (e.g. postpartum toxic shock syndrome, necrotizing fasciitis, septic pelvic thrombophlebitis). The diagnostic work-up may include the microbiologic evaluation of specimens from blood, urine, sputum, and wound. Because mixed flora are usually identified in transvaginal cultures, a careful sampling of the endometrial cavity is seldom clinically useful (Duff et al., 1983). In patients thought to have chorioamnionitis, transabdominal amniocentesis or cultures taken from a free-flowing internal pressure transducer catheter have been described, but are also of limited clinical utility (Gibbs et al., 1982).

Empiric therapy in the obstetric patient should include coverage for a wide variety of both aerobic and anaerobic Gram-negative and Gram-positive bacteria. Institution-specific sensitivities of common nosocomial pathogens and specific patient factors should be considered in the choice of empiric therapy until culture results are available. Parenteral therapy that includes a combination of ampicillin (2 g/6 hr), an aminoglycoside appropriately dosed for patient weight and renal function, and clindamycin phosphate (900 mg/8 hr) is generally recommended. Other treatment regimens are acceptable, and each clinician must be familiar with the administration and potential toxic effects of these drugs.

In patients who previously received cephalosporin therapy, additional coverage specifically directed against enterococci may be warranted. In addition, if *Staphylococcus aureus* is a suspected pathogen, a semisynthetic penicillin may be substituted for ampicillin. Because nephrotoxicity is a well-established complication of aminoglycoside usage and septic patients may already have or are prone for renal compromise, monitoring of peak and trough aminoglycoside levels is imperative. When available, culture results and organism sensitivities should be used to more selectively guide subsequent antimicrobial therapy.

The critically ill patient is at high risk for developing sources of infection not commonly encountered by obstetricians, and careful physical examination as well as selected imaging studies are important in excluding uncommon sources. Sinusitis may develop secondary to prolonged intubation or nasogastric suction, for example. Nosocomial pneumonia commonly develops in patients admitted to the ICU, and is independently associated with increased risk of mortality (Fagon et al., 1996). When broad-spectrum antibiotics are utilized, careful surveillance for resistant organisms and fungal infection is imperative.

Surgical therapy

Surgical extirpation of infected tissues (if possible) is important to ensure survival. In patients with suspected septic abortion, evacuation of the uterus should begin promptly after initiating antibiotics and stabilizing the patient. Septic shock in association with chorioamnionitis in a viable fetus is treated by delivery; this can be accomplished vaginally if maternal hemodynamic parameters are stable and delivery is imminent. Under certain circumstances, and after initial maternal resuscitation, cesarean section may be appropriate. This decision should be based on the chance of survival of the fetus and the risks to the mother if the nidus for infection is not removed rapidly. In the postpartum patient, hysterectomy may be indicated if microabscess formation is identified within myometrial tissues or if there is clinical evidence of deterioration in the patient's condition despite appropriate antibiotic therapy. When the diagnosis of septic pelvic thrombophlebitis is entertained, treatment with heparin in combination with broad-spectrum antibiotics is appropriate. If this proves unsuccessful, surgical evaluation may be necessary (Collins, 1970).

Coagulation system

Disseminated intravascular coagulation frequently complicates septic shock. Severe bleeding may result from the depletion of coagulation factors after activation of the coagulation system. Unless the patient has clinical evidence of bleeding, or surgical or invasive procedures are anticipated, aggressive attempt at correcting these laboratory defects is not usually recommended. The optimal management of DIC is treatment of the underlying condition, and spontaneous improvement will occur when the overall clinical picture improves. An exception to this approach is when the platelet count falls below 5,000–10,000/mL; platelet transfusion to prevent spontaneous hemorrhage may be indicated at this point.

Whenever thrombocytopenia occurs in the septic patient, the effect of heparin must be considered in the differential diagnosis. The use of heparin in the ICU is common, and it can cause thrombocytopenia via two mechanisms. The first, generally seen within 2–5 days after initiation of therapy, is usually mild and of little clinical significance. The second, immune-mediated heparin-induced thrombocytopenia, is less common but of considerably more importance and may cause profound thrombocytopenia. This phenomena occurs 7–15 days after initiation of therapy and is independent of dose or route of administration of heparin (Mei & Feeley, 1993). Rather than transfusing platelets, all sources of heparin must be eliminated, including subcutaneous injections for deep venous thrombosis prophylaxis, flushing solutions of indwelling lines, and total parenteral nutrition (TPN) solutions.

Since the last edition of this text, significant progress has been made in our understanding of the interaction between the coagulation system, circulating mediators of inflammation, and the clinical presentation of the systemic inflammatory response syndrome. Tissue hypoxia secondary to hypoperfusion mediated by the inflammatory response and plugging of the microvasculature by cellular and fibrinous debris causes further cellular injury and release of endogenous mediators of inflammation and chemokines. Concentrations of platelets, antithrombin III, protein C antigen and inhibitor, protein S, factors VII and XII are all decreased. Fibrinogen, thrombin-antithrombin, D-dimers, thrombomodulin, tPA activity and antigen, and others are increased. Together, the result is multiple perturbations in the coagulation and complement systems and further systemic activation of the inflammatory response (Marshall, 2001). Activation of the extrinsic pathway increases the coagulability of blood. Anticoagulation mediators are involved in the inflammatory process, and their depletion is frequently observed in patients with sepsis and ARDS. It is theorized that the lack of endogenous anticoagulants facilitates the production of microthrombi in the vasculature promoting hypoperfusion and tissue hypoxia. Experimental studies provide the rational for clinical trials of mediator replacement. Early studies have been promising. Large-scale, randomized trials are underway, but the results have been disappointing (Vincent, 2000). Unfortunately, our growing understanding of the inflammatory process and its systemic activation have not translated into an ability to manipulate or modulate it clinically.

Renal function

Renal function is best monitored with an indwelling catheter, and serial creatinine and BUN determinations. Although acute tubular necrosis most often presents with oliguria, it may present occasionally as a high-output state. Regardless, tests of tubular function will demonstrate increased fractional excretion of sodium and impaired concentrating ability, evidenced by a urinary sodium greater than 40 mEq/L and urine osmolality less than 400 mosmol/kg H_2O, respectively. Serum creatinine concentrations also rise at a rate of 0.5–1.5 mg/dL/day (Miller et al., 1978). Provided irreversible acute tubular necrosis has not occurred, correction of the hemodynamic and perfusion deficits should result in restoration of renal function. Table 40.4 lists various prognostic indicators of poor outcome in addition to renal parameters in patients with septic shock (Shoemaker et al., 1973, 1983; Weil & Nishijima, 1978; Hardaway, 1981; Sugerman et al., 1981; Kaufman et al., 1984).

Table 40.4 Prognostic indicators of poor outcome in septic shock

Delay in initial diagnosis
Underlying debilitation disease process
Poor response to intravenous fluid resuscitation
Depressed cardiac output
Reduced oxygen extraction
Presence of ARDS or renal failure
High serum lactate (<4 mmol/L)
Reduced COP (<15 mmHg)

Gastrointestinal tract and nutrition

Although often overlooked, the GI tract can be a reservoir of infection and a source of considerable morbidity to the ICU patient. Three interrelated areas requiring attention include provision for adequate nutrition, prevention or minimization of the effect of translocation of bacteria from the gut to the systemic circulation, and stress ulcer prophylaxis. All three relate directly to efforts aimed at maintaining adequate splanchnic circulation and the integrity of the GI mucosa.

Sepsis provokes a catabolic state, the effects of which are especially pronounced in skeletal muscle, loose connective tissue, and intestinal viscera (Pinsky & Matuschak, 1989). Metabolic alterations provoked by sepsis differ from starvation in that the compensatory mechanisms to preserve lean body mass in starvation are absent in sepsis (Wojnar et al., 1995). Provision for adequate nutrition early in the patient's ICU course is vital. In addition to providing adequate calories, carbohydrates, lipids, protein, vitamins, and trace elements to prevent catabolism, restoration of adequate nutritional support has other beneficial effects. Inadequate nutrition is associated with significant immune impairment, with suppression of both cellular and humoral immunity. The potential for alterations in immune function emphasizes the importance of providing adequate nutrition early in the course of sepsis. There are good animal evidence and preliminary human data to suggest that specific nutrients such as glutamine, arginine, and omega-3 fatty acids may have significant immunomodulatory functions (Mainous & Deitch 1994).

Malnutrition has additional deleterious effects. It alters gut mucosal integrity and promotes increases in endogenous gut flora. By itself, malnutrition does not promote translocation of bacteria and bacterial toxins into the circulation (Deitch et al., 1987). Sepsis increases the permeability of GI mucosa, and permeability increases with increasing severity of infection, an effect probably mediated by endotoxin (Deitch et al., 1987; Ziegler et al., 1988). When endotoxin is administered in the face of starvation or malnutrition, an increase in translocation of bacteria across the mucosa is observed, and this increase correlates with the duration of malnutrition (Deitch et al., 1987).

The mucosa is highly susceptible to injury from hypotension and reperfusion because of its high metabolic rate. It is affected early when perfusion is redirected away from the gut to maintain CNS and cardiac perfusion. Ischemia interferes with mucosal function to prevent bacterial translocation into the systemic circulation (Pinsky & Matuschak, 1989; Riddington et al., 1996). Several investigators have suggested that gastric tonometry be used to follow intramucosal pH as an indicator of GI and splanchnic perfusion. Mucosal pH has been correlated with perfusion, the propensity for mucosal injury, transmural migration of gut flora, and clinical outcome (Gys et al., 1988; Doglio et al., 1991; Fiddian-Green et al., 1993; Sauve & Cook, 1993). Clinical improvement in the patient's condition should be reflected in normalization of mucosal pH and no further increases in oxygen consumption with increased delivery.

When selecting the route to provide nutritional supplementation, the adage, "If the gut works, use it," should be borne in mind. Even in the face of nutritionally adequate replenishment, TPN is associated with impairment of host defenses and intrinsic gut immunity. Infectious complications are increased with TPN even when complications associated with central access and line sepsis are excluded (Mainous & Deitch, 1994). The enteral route slows atrophy and maintains integrity of the mucosal barrier, especially if glutamine is provided. If adequate caloric replacement cannot be provided enterally, even small-volume feeding with the remaining nutrition provided by TPN is better than TPN alone in promoting mucosal integrity and preventing atrophy (Wojnar et al., 1995). Enteral nutrition can be provided to the intubated patient either through a needle catheter jejunostomy or through a small nasogastric tube advanced well into the duodenum.

Alterations in splanchnic perfusion, the patient response to stress, and drugs administered to ICU patients can all promote ulceration and upper GI bleeding. Prophylaxis is commonly provided in the form of either regular administration of antacids, H_2-receptor antagonists, or cytoprotective agents such as sucralfate. More than 50 trials have been performed with various endpoints and have found a comparable protective effect regardless of which type of prophylaxis is used. A relative disadvantage of antacids and H_2-receptor antagonists is that they increase gastric pH, promoting overgrowth of the normally sterile stomach with Gram-negative enteric pathogens. The risk of aspiration and nosocomial pneumonia is increased significantly by their use and has led some to recommend sucralfate over antacids or H_2 blockers (Craven et al., 1986; Bresalier et al., 1987; Cannon et al., 1987; Driks et al., 1987; Tryba, 1987; Sauve & Cook 1993; Cook et al., 1996). Although sucralfate is associated with reductions in nosocomial pneumonias in intubated patients, adequate trials have not been conducted to demonstrate conclusively a reduction in mortality with sucralfate. Potential advantages of sucralfate in the gravid patient include poor GI absorption and lack of the potential systemic effects associated with H_2 blockers. It has no effect on fertility, does not cross the placenta, and is not teratogenic (Briggs, 1995). It should be considered a viable alternative for prophylaxis in the pregnant ICU patient who can tolerate nasogastric medications.

Additional measures that require the meticulous attention of the clinician include management of electrolyte imbalances, correction of metabolic acidosis, stabilization of coagulation defects, prophylaxis for deep venous thrombosis (with subcutaneous heparin, low molecular weight heparin, or pneumatic compression boots), and monitoring of renal function. Patients in septic shock may have either hypokalemia secondary to losses from the alimentary tract or hyperkalemia resulting from either acute cation shifts in the face of acidosis or from renal failure. Lactic acidosis from anaerobic metabolism should be monitored serially and treated aggressively by increasing oxygen delivery and perfusion to peripheral tissues. Half-normal saline infusions with one to two ampules of sodium bicarbonate can be administered periodically to help correct severe acidosis. Serum glucose levels may be elevated, normal, or depressed. If the serum glucose levels are depressed, some clinicians advocate the administration of glucose in combination with insulin to improve tissue uptake of the substrate.

Controversial treatment modalities

Historically, the most controversial modality in the treatment of septic shock was the use of high-dose steroids. Their use is theoretically appealing, with potential benefits that include stabilization of lysosomal membranes, inhibition of complement-induced inflammatory changes, and attenuation of the effects of cytokines and other inflammatory mediators. In an early trial, Sprung and co-workers (1984) reported reversal of shock when steroids were given early in the course of sepsis. Although there was some short-term improvement, ultimate in-hospital mortality was not changed and reversal of shock was not observed. Significantly, more than 25% of patients treated with steroids developed superinfections. Two large randomized, placebo-controlled, prospective studies subsequently demonstrated no benefit in the early administration of corticosteroids for either the treatment of severe sepsis and septic shock or for preventing progression to septic shock (Bone et al., 1987; Veterans Administration Systemic Sepsis Cooperative Study Group, 1987). Currently, there is no compelling reason to use corticosteroids in the therapy of septic shock; their use should be reserved for those patients with documented adrenal insufficiency.

Other potential roles for steroids in the management of the septic gravida may include their use in the late fibroproliferative phase of ARDS to prevent lung injury from evolving into fibrosis. Several small series have suggested that although progression from lung injury to ARDS is not prevented, steroids may be of some benefit in preventing pulmonary fibrosis and may accelerate recovery in patients with ARDS (Ashbaugh & Maier, 1985; Weigelt et al., 1985; Hooper & Kearl, 1990; Meduri et al., 1991). Transient suppression of maternal immune function has been described following betamethasone therapy for fetal pulmonary maturation (Cunningham & Evan, 1991). This effect is inconsequential and probably poses no maternal risk (Crowley, 1995).

Prostaglandins have long been thought to play a central role in septic shock, particularly in controlling regional blood flow distribution. Oettinger and colleagues (1983) demonstrated increased production and decreased degradation of prostaglandin F_2 in severe sepsis. Other researchers have suggested that these alterations are associated with known endotoxin-induced pulmonary vascular changes (Vada, 1984). Cefalo et al. (1980) used prostaglandin synthetase inhibitors to blunt these pathophysiologic responses in sheep. These same beneficial effects could be observed in other organ systems when experimental animals were pretreated with prostaglandin synthetase inhibitors prior to exposure to endotoxin (O'Brien et al., 1981; Rao et al., 1981; Makabali et al., 1983). Further clinical trials supporting the use of adjunctive antiprostaglandin therapy have not been forthcoming and their routine use cannot be recommended at this time.

Lachman et al. (1984) administered antilipopolysaccharide immunoglobulin to obstetric and gynecologic patients in septic shock. In treated patients, a reduction in both morbidity and mortality was observed. Despite this initial enthusiasm, antiendotoxin and anticytokine therapies are of questionable benefit in the therapy of septic shock. Preliminary studies showed that antibodies specifically directed against endotoxin or inflammatory mediators such as TNF-α reduced mortality in animal models and human septic shock patients (Beutler et al., 1985). Clinical trials have, unfortunately, produced inconsistent results. Although initially promising, the clinical experience has not been as good as expected (Greenman et al., 1991; Wenzel, 1991; Ziegler et al., 1991; Warren et al., 1992; Natanson et al., 1994). Circulating natural inhibitors of proinflammatory cytokines have been described. In animal models, these circulating inhibitors decrease mortality in endotoxic shock. The interactions between these circulating antagonists and the proinflammatory cytokines on the molecular level and their impact on the clinical course of sepsis are only beginning to be investigated. Their presence may explain the inconsistent results observed in clinical trials of exogenously administered inflammatory mediators (Goldie et al., 1995).

The results of a double-blind, placebo-controlled, multicenter phase 3 trial of antithrombin III replacement were recently published. Not only was no survival benefit demonstrated, there was a significant increase in the risk for hemorrhagic complications in patients receiving the study drug along with heparin (Warren et al., 2001). Recombinant activated protein C has also been studied. A significant reduction in mortality at the cost of an increased risk for bleeding, including two fatal intracranial hemorrhages, was reported. The authors calculated a rate of one serious bleeding event for every 66 patients treated in contrast to a calculated 28-day survival benefit for one patient out of every 16 treated (Bernard et al., 2001).

As these examples illustrate, manipulation of the coagulation, and inflammatory systems is not without risk. The patient groups studied are heterogenous, and we are as yet unable to optimally individualize therapy. Currently, standard therapy is reactive rather than proactive. Early intervention has obvious advantages, but attempts to manipulate or modulate the inflammatory cascade or abort systemic activation of the inflammatory response are in their infancy. The search for a magic bullet with which to treat sepsis and septic shock likely is overly simplistic. As the intricacies of the inflammatory cascade, its activation, the multiple feedback loops involved in its control, and the mechanisms resulting in loss of the ability to localize inflammation are elucidated, it becomes obvious that no single intervention or replacement of an individual coagulation factor can be expected to make dramatic differences in mortality.

References

Acute Respiratory Distress Syndrome Network. Ventilation with lower tidal volumes as compared with traditional tidal volumes for acute lung injury and the acute respiratory distress syndrome. N Engl J Med 2000;342:1301–1308.

Altura BM, Gebrewold A, Burton RW. Failure of microscopic metaarterioles to elicit vasodilator responses to acetylcholine, bradykinin, histamine and substance P after ischemic shock, endothelial cells. Microcirc Endothelium Lymphatics 1985;2:121–127.

Ashbaugh DG, Maier RV. Idiopathic pulmonary fibrosis in adult respiratory distress syndrome: diagnosis and treatment. Arch Surg 1985;120:530–535.

Balk RA, Bone RC. The septic syndrome: definition and clinical implications. Crit Care Clin 1989;5:1–8.

Bech-Jansen P, Brinkman CR 3rd, Johnson GH, et al. Circulatory shock in pregnant sheep. II: Effects of endotoxin on fetal and neonatal circulation. Am J Obstet Gynecol 1972;113:37–43.

Beller JF, Schmidt EH, Holzgreve W, et al. Septicemia during pregnancy: a study in different species of experimental animals. Am J Obstet Gynecol 1985;151:967–975.

Bernard GR, Vincent JL, Laterre PF, et al. Efficacy and safety of recombinant human activated protein C for severe sepsis. N Engl J Med 2001;344:699–709.

Bersten A, Sibbald WJ. Acute lung injury in septic shock. Crit Care Clin 1989;5:49–79.

Beutler B, Milsark IW, Cerami AC. Passive immunization against cachectin/tumor necrosis factor protects mice from lethal effect of endotoxin. Science 1985;229:869–871.

Bishop MH, Shoemaker WC, Appel PL, et al. Prospective, randomized trial of survivor values of cardiac index, oxygen delivery, and oxygen consumption as resuscitation endpoints in severe trauma. J Trauma 1995;38:780–787.

Blanco JD, Gibbs RS, Castaneda YS. Bacteremia in obstetrics: clinic course. Obstet Gynecol 1981;58:621–625.

Bollaert PE, Bauer P, Audibert G, et al. Effects of epinephrine on hemodynamics and oxygen metabolism in dopamine-resistant septic shock. Chest 1990;98:949–953.

Bone RC. Sepsis syndrome: new insights into its pathogenesis and treatment. Infect Dis Clin North Am 1991;5:793–805.

Bone RC, Fisher CJ Jr, Clemmer TP, et al. A controlled clinical trial of high-dose methylprednisolone in the treatment of severe sepsis and septic shock. N Engl J Med 1987;317:653–658.

Bone RC, Balk RA, Cerra FB, et al. Definitions for sepsis and organ failure and guidelines for the use of innovative therapies in sepsis. Chest 1992a;101:1644–1655.

Bone RC, Sibbald WJ, Sprung CL. The ACCP-SCCM consensus conference on sepsis and organ failure. Chest 1992b;101:1481–1483.

Bonney RJ, Humes JL. Physiological and pharmacological regulation of prostaglandin and leukotriene production by macrophages. J Leukoc Biol 1984;35:1–10.

Boyd O, Grounds RM, Bennett ED. A randomized clinical trial of the effect of deliberate perioperative increase of oxygen delivery on mortality in high-risk surgical patients. JAMA 1993;270:2699–2707.

Bresalier RS, Grendell JH, Cello JP, et al. Sucralfate suspension versus titrated antacid for the prevention of acute stress-related gastrointestinal hemorrhage in critically ill patients. Am J Med 1987;83:110.

Briggs GG, Freeman RK, Yaffe SJ, eds. Sucralfate: gastrointestinal agent. In: A reference guide to fetal and neonatal risk: drugs in pregnancy and lactation, 4th edn. Baltimore: Williams and Wilkins, 1995;792.

Brun-Buisson C, Doyon F, Carlet J, et al. Incidence, risk factors, and outcome of severe sepsis and septic shock in adults. A multicenter prospective study in intensive care units. JAMA 1995;274:968–974.

Bryan CS, Reynolds KL, Moore EE. Bacteremia in obstetrics and gynecology. Obstet Gynecol 1984;64:155–158.

Cannon LA, Heiselman D, Gardner W, et al. Prophylaxis of upper gastrointestinal tract bleeding in mechanically ventilated patients. A randomized study comparing the efficacy of sucralfate, cimetidine, and antacids. Arch Intern Med 1987;147:2101–2106.

Cavanagh D, Knuppel RA, Shepherd JH, et al. Septic shock and the obstetrician/gynecologist. South Med J 1982;75:809–813.

Cefalo RC, Lewis PE, O'Brien WF, et al. The role of prostaglandins in endotoxemia: comparisons in response in the nonpregnant, maternal, and fetal model. Am J Obstet Gynecol 1980;137:53–57.

Centers for Disease Control and Prevention. National Center for Health Statistics Mortality Patterns—United States, 1990. Monthly Vital Stat Rep 1993;41:5.

Chow AW, Guze LB. Bacteroidaceae bacteremia: clinical experience with 112 patients. Medicine 1974;53:93–126.

Clark SL, Cotton DB, Lee W, et al. Central hemodynamic assessment of normal term pregnancy. Am J Obstet Gynecol 1989;161:1439–1442.

Cleary PP, Kaplan EL, Handley JP, et al. Clonal basis for resurgence of serious Streptococcus pyogenes disease in the 1980s. Lancet 1992;339:518–521.

Collins CG. Suppurative pelvic thrombophlebitis. A study of 202 cases in which the disease was treated by ligation of the vena cava and ovarian vein. Am J Obstet Gynecol 1970;108:681–687.

Cook DJ, Reeve BK, Guyatt GH, et al. Stress ulcer prophylaxis in critically ill patients: resolving discordant meta-analyses. JAMA 1996;275:308–314.

Cotton DB, Gonik B, Dorman K, et al. Cardiovascular alterations in severe pregnancy-induced hypertension: relationship of central venous pressure to pulmonary capillary wedge pressure. Am J Obstet Gynecol 1985;151:762–764.

Craven DE, Kunches LM, Kilinshy V, et al. Risk factors for pneumonia and fatality in patients receiving continuous mechanical ventilation. Am Rev Respir Dis 1986;133:792–796.

Crowley PA. Antenatal corticosteroid therapy: a meta-analysis of the randomized trials, 1972 to 1994. Am J Obstet Gynecol 1995;173:322.

Cunningham DS, Evan EE. The effects of betamethasone on maternal cellular resistance to infection. Am J Obstet Gynecol 1991;165:610.

Cunningham FG, Lucas MJ, Hankins GD. Pulmonary injury complicating antepartum pyelonephritis. Am J Obstet Gynecol 1987; 156:797–807.

Dantzker D. Oxygen delivery and utlization in sepsis. Crit Care Clin 1989;5:81–98.

Daryani R, Lalonde C, Zhu D, et al. Effect of endotoxin and a burn injury on lung and liver lipid peroxidation and catalase activity. J Trauma 1990;30:1330–1334.

Deitch EA, Winterton J, Li M, et al. The gut as a portal of entry for bacteremia: role of protein malnutrition. Ann Surg 1987;195:681–692.

Demling RH, Lalonde C, Ikegami K. Physiologic support of the septic patient. Surg Clin North Am 1994;74:637–658.

Desjars P, Pinaud M, Poptel G, et al. A reappraisal of norepinephrine therapy in human septic shock. Crit Care Med 1987;15:134–137.

Dinerman JL, Lowenstein CJ, Snyder SH. Molecular mechanisms of nitric oxide regulation: potential relevance to cardiovascular disease. Circ Res 1993;73:217–222.

Doglio GR, Pusajo JF, Egurrola MA, et al. Gastric mucosal pH as a prognostic index of mortality in critically ill patients. Crit Care Med 1991;19:1037–1040.

Driks MR, Craven DE, Celli BR, et al. Nosocomial pneumonia in intubated patients given sucralfate as compared with antacids or histamine type 2 blockers. N Engl J Med 1987;317:1376–1382.

Duff JH, Groves AC, McLean AP, et al. Defective oxygen consumption in septic shock. Surg Gynecol Obstet 1969;128:1051–1060.

Duff P. Pyelonephritis in pregnancy. Clin Obstet Gynecol 1984;27: 17–31.

Duff P. Pathophysiology and management of postcesarean endomyometritis. Obstet Gynecol 1986;67:269–276.

Duff P, Gibbs RS, Blanco JD, et al. Endometrial culture techniques in puerperal patients. Obstet Gynecol 1983;61:217–222.

Fagon JY, Chastre J, Vuagnat A, et al. Nosocomial pneumonia and mortality among patients in intensive care units. JAMA 1996;275:866–869.

Fearon DT, Ruddy S, Schur PH, et al. Activation of the properdin pathway of complement in patients with gram-negative bacteremia. N Engl J Med 1975;292:937–940.

Fiddian-Green RG, Haglund U, Gutierrez G, et al. Goals for the resuscitation of shock. Crit Care Med 1993;21:S25–31.

Fletcher AP, Alkjaersig NK, Burstein R. The influence of pregnancy upon blood coagulation and plasma fibrinolytic enzyme function. Am J Obstet Gynecol 1979;134:743–751.

Freid MA, Vosti KL. The importance of underlying disease in patients with gram-negative bacteremia. Arch Intern Med 1968;121:418–423.

Gattinoni L, Brazzi L, Pelosi P, et al. A trial of goal-oriented hemodynamic therapy in critically ill patients. N Engl J Med 1995;333:1025–1032.

Gibbs CE, Locke WE. Maternal deaths in Texas, 1969 to 1973. A report of 501 consecutive maternal deaths from the Texas Medical Association's Committee on Maternal Health. Am J Obstet Gynecol 1976;126:687–692.

Gibbs RS, Jones PM, Wilder CJ. Antibiotic therapy of endometritis following cesarean section: treatment successes and failures. Obstet Gynecol 1978;52:31–37.

Gibbs RS, Blanco JD, Hrilica VS. Quantitative bacteriology of amniotic fluid from women with clinical intraamniotic infection at term. J Infect Dis 1982;145:1–8.

Goetzl EJ, Payan DG, Goldman DW. Immunopathogenic roles of leukotrienes in human diseases. J Clin Immunol 1984;4:79–84.

Goldberg LI. Dopamine: clinical uses of an endogenous catecholamine. N Engl J Med 1974;291:707–710.

Goldie AS, Fearon KCH, Ross JA, et al. Natural cytokine antagonists and endogenous antiendotoxin core antibodies in sepsis syndrome. JAMA 1995;274:172–177.

Greenman RL, Schein RMH, Martin MA, et al. A controlled clinical trial of E5 murine monoclonal IgM antibody to endotoxin in the treatment of gram-negative sepsis. JAMA 1991;266:1097–1102.

Gutierrez G, Lund N, Bryan-Brown CW. Cellular oxygen utilization during multiple organ failure. Crit Care Clin 1989;5:271–287.

Gys T, Hubens A, Neels H, et al. Prognostic value of gastric intramural pH in surgical intensive care patients. Crit Care Med 1988;16:1222–1224.

Hack CE, Zeerleder S. The endothelium in sepsis: Source of and a target for inflammation. Crit Care Med 2001;29:S21–27.

Hageman JR, Caplan MS. An introduction to the structure and function of inflammatory mediators for clinicians. Clin Perinatol 1995;22:251–261.

Hankins G, Clark S, Uckan E. Intrapulmonary shunt (QS/QT) and position in healthy third-trimester pregnancy. Am J Obstet Gynecol 1996;174:322A.

Hardaway RM. Prediction of survival or death of patients in a state of severe shock. Surg Gynecol Obstet 1981;152:200–206.

Haupt MT, Rackow EC. Colloid osmotic pressure and fluid resuscitation with hetastarch, albumin, and saline solutions. Crit Care Med 1982;10:159–162.

Hawkins DF. Management and treatment of obstetric bacteremia shcok. J Clin Pathol 1980;33:895–896.

Hayes MA, Timmins AC, Yau EH, et al. Elevation of systemic oxygen delivery in the treatment of critically ill patients. N Engl J Med 1994;330:1717–1722.

Hesse DG, Tracey KJ, Fong Y, et al. Cytokine appearance in human endotoxemia and primate bacteremia. Surg Gynecol Obstet 1988;166:147–153.

Hinds C, Watson D. Manipulating hemodynamic and oyxgen transport in critically ill patients. N Engl J Med 1995;333:1074–1075.

Hollenberg SM, Cunnion RE. Endothelial and vascular smooth muscle function in sepsis. J Crit Care 1994;9:262–280.

Holm SE. Invasive group A streptococcal infections. N Engl J Med 1996;335:590–591.

Hooper RG, Kearl RA. Established ARDS treated with a sustained course of adrenocortical steroids. Chest 1990;97:138–143.

Jacobs RF, Tabor DR. Immune cellular interactions during sepsis and septic injury. Crit Care Clin 1989;5:9.

Jacobs RF, Tabor DR, Lary CH, et al. Interleukin-1 production by alveolar macrophages and monocytes from ARDS and pneumonia patients compared to controls. Am Rev Respir Dis 1988;137: 228.

Kaufman BS, Rackow EC, Falk JL. The relationship between oxygen delivery and consumption during fluid resuscitation of hypovolemic and septic shock. Chest 1984;85:336–340.

Knuppel RA, Rao PS, Cavanagh D. Septic shock in obstetrics. Clin Obstet Gynecol 1984;27:3–10.

Kwaan HM. Weil MH. Differences in the mechanism of shock caused by infections. Surg Gynecol Obstet 1969;128:37–45.

Lachman E, Pitsoe SB, Gaffin SL. Antilipopolysaccharide immunotherapy in management of septic shock of obstetric and gynaecologic origin. Lancet 1984;1:981–983.

Ledger WJ, Norman M, Gee C, et al. Bacteremia on an obstetric-gynecologic service. Am J Obstet Gynecol 1975;121:205–212.

Lee W, Clark SL, Cotton DB, et al. Septic shock during pregnancy. Am J Obstet Gynecol 1988;159:410–416.

Lee W, Cotton DB, Hankins GDV, et al. Management of septic shock complicating pregnancy. Obstet Gynecol Surv 1989;16:431.

Levi M, ten Cate H, van der Poll T, et al. Pathogenesis of disseminated intravascular coagulation in sepsis. JAMA 1993;270:975–979.

Lewis BS, Gotsman MS. Current concepts of left ventricular relaxation and compliance. Am Heart J 1980;99:101–112.

Lindeborg DM, Pearl RG. Recent advances in critical care medicine: inotropic therapy in the critically ill patient. Int Anesthesiol Clin 1993;31:49–71.

Lloyd T, Dougherty J, Karlen J. Infected intrauterine pregnancy presenting as septic shock. Ann Emerg Med 1983;12:704–707.

Lowthian JT, Gillard LJ. Postpartum necrotizing faciitis. Obstet Gynecol 1980;56:661–663.

Lucas CE. A new look at dopamine and norepinephrine for hyperdynamic septic shock. Chest 1994;105:7–8.

Lynn WA, Cohen J. Science and clinical practice: management of septic shock. J Infect 1995;30:207–212.

Lynn WA, Golenbock DT. Lipopolysaccharide antagonists. Immunol Today 1992;13:271–276.

MacKenzie SJ, Kapadia F, Nimmo GR, et al. Adrenaline in treatment of septic shock: effects on hemodynamics and oxygen transport. Intensive Care Med 1991;17:36–39.

Mainous MR, Deitch EA. Nutrition and infection. Surg Clin North Am 1994;74:659–676.

Makabali GL, Mandal AK, Morris JA. An assessment of the participatory role of prostaglandins and serotonin in the pathophysiology of endotoxic shock. Am J Obstet Gynecol 1983;145:439–445.

Marik PE, Mohedin M. The contrasting effects of dopamine and norepinephrine on systemic and splanchnic oxygen utilization in hyperdynamic sepsis. JAMA 1994;272:1354–1357.

Mariona FG, Ismail MA. Clostridium perfringens septicemia following cesarean section. Obstet Gynecol 1980;56:518–521.

Marksad AK, Ona CJ, Stuart RC, et al. Myocardial depression in septic shock: physiologic and metabolic effect of a plasma factor on an isolated heart. Circ Shock 1979;1(Suppl):35.

Marshall JC. Inflammation, coagulopathy, and the pathogenesis of multiple organ dysfunction syndrome. Crit Care Med 2001; 29(Suppl):S99–S106.

Martin C, Papazian L, Perrin G, et al. Norepinephrine or dopamine for the treatment of hyperdynamic septic shock? Chest 1993;103: 1826–1831.

Mayoral JL, Schweich CJ, Dunn DL. Decreased tumor necrosis factor production during the initial stages of infection correlates with survival during murine gram-negative sepsis. Arch Surg 1990;125:24–27.

Meadows D, Edwards JD, Wilkins RG, et al. Reversal of intractable septic shock with norepinephrine therapy. Crit Care Med 1988;16:663–666.

Meduri GU, Belenchia JM, Estes RJ, et al. Fibroproliferative phase of ARDS: clinical findings and effects of corticosteroids. Chest 1991;100:943–952.

Mei CT, Feeley TW. Coagulopathies and the intensive care setting. Int Anesthesiol Clin 1993;31:97–117.

Metcalfe J, Ueland K. Maternal cardiovascular adjustments to pregnancy. Prog Cardiovasc Dis 1974;16:363–374.

Michie HR, Manogue KR, Spriggs DR, et al. Detection of circulating tumor necrosis factor after endotoxin administrations. N Engl J Med 1988a;318:1481–1486.

Michie HR, Spriggs DR, Manogue KB, et al. Tumor necrosis factor and endotoxin induce similar metabolic responses in human beings. Surgery 1988b;104:280–286.

Miller TR, Anderson RJ, Linas SL, et al. Urinary diagnostic indices in acute renal failure. Ann Intern Med 1978;89:47–50.

Monif GRG, Baer H. Polymicrobial bacteremia in obstetric patients. Obstet Gynecol 1976;48:167–169.

Moore FA, Haenel JB, Moore EE, et al. Incommensurate oxygen consumption in response to maximal oxygen availability predicts postinjury multiple organ failure. J Trauma 1992;33:58–65.

Moran JL, O'Fathartaigh MS, Peisach AR, et al. Epinephrine as an inotropic agent in septic shock: a dose-profile analysis. Crit Care Med 1993;21:70.

Morishima HO, Niemann WH, James LS. Effects of endotoxin on the pregnant baboon and fetus. Am J Obstet Gynecol 1978;131:899–902.

Natanson C, Hoffman WD, Suffredini AF, et al. Selected treatment strategies for shock based on proposed mechanisms of pathogenesis. Ann Intern Med 1994;120:771–783.

O'Brien WF, Cefalo RC, Lewis PE, et al. The role of prostaglandins in endotoxemia and comparisons in response in the nonpregnant, maternal, and fetal models. II. Alterations in prostaglandin physiology in the nonpregnant, pregnant, and fetal experimental animal. Am J Obstet Gynecol 1981;139:535–539.

Oettinger WK, Walter GO, Jensen UM, et al. Endogenous prostaglandin F2 alpha in the hyperdynamic state of severe sepsis in man. Br J Surg 1983;70:237–239.

Ognibene FP, Parker MM, Natanson C, et al. Depressed left ventricular performance: response to volume infusion in patients with sepsis and septic shock. Chest 1988;93:903–910.

Okusawa S, Gelfand JA, Ikejima T, et al. Interleukin 1 induces a shock-like state in rabbits: synergism with tumor necrosis factor and the effect of cyclooxygenase inhibition. J Clin Invest 1988;81:1162–1172.

Packman MI, Rackow EC. Optimum left heart filling pressure during fluid resuscitation of patients with hypovolemic and septic shock. Crit Care Med 1983;11:165–169.

Parker MM, Parillo JE. Septic shock: hemodynamics and pathogenesis. JAMA 1983;250:3324–3327.

Parker MM, Shelhamer JH, Bacharach SL, et al. Profound but reversible myocardial depression in patients with septic shock. Ann Intern Med 1984;100:483–490.

Parrillo JE. Cardiovascular dysfunction in septic shock: new insights into a deadly disease. Int J Cardiol 1985;7:314.

Parrillo JE. Pathogenetic mechanisms of septic shock. N Engl J Med 1993;328:1471–1477.

Parrillo JE, Burch C, Shelhamer JH, et al. A circulating myocardial depressant substance in humans with septic shock: septic shock patients with a reduced ejection fraction have a circulating factor that depresses in vitro myocardial cell performance. J Clin Invest 1985;76:1539.

Pinsky MR, Matuschak GM. Multiple systems organ failure: failure of host defense homeostasis. Crit Care Clin 1989;5:199–220.

Poggetti RS, Moore FA, Moore EE, et al. Liver injury is a reversible neutrophil-mediated event following gut ischemia. Arch Surg 1992;127:175–179.

Porembka DT. Cardiovascular abnormalities in sepsis. New Horiz 1993;2:324–341.

Pritchard JA, MacDonald PC, Gant NF, eds. Maternal adaption to pregnancy. In: Williams obstetrics, 20th edn. Norwalk, CT: Appleton-Century-Crofts, 1997.

Progress in Chronic Disease Prevention. Chronic disease reports: deaths from nine types of chronic disease—United States, 1986. MMWR 1990;39:30.

Rackow EC, Weil MK. Recent trends in diagnosis and management of septic shock. Curr Surg 1983;40:181–185.

Rackow EC, Fein IA, Leppo J. Colloid osmotic pressure as a prognostic indicator of pulmonary edema and mortality in the critically ill. Chest 1977;72:709–713.

Rackow EC, Fein IA, Siegel J. The relationship of the colloid osmotic-pulmonary artery wedge pressure gradient to pulmonary edema and mortality in critically ill patients. Chest 1982;82:433–437.

Rackow EC, Falk JL, Fein IA, et al. Fluid resuscitation in circulatory shock: a comparison of the cardiorespiratory effects of albumin, hetastarch, and saline solutions in patients with hypovolemic and septic shock. Crit Care Med 1983;11:839–850.

Rackow EC, Kaufman BS, Falk JL, et al. Hemodynamic response to fluid repletion in patients with septic shock: evidence for early depression of cardiac performance. Circ Shock 1987;22:11–22.

Rackow EC, Astiz ME, Weil MH. Cellular oxygen metabolism during sepsis and shock: the relationship of oxygen consumption to oxygen delivery. JAMA 1988;259:1989–1993.

Rangel-Frausto MS, Pittet D, Costigan M, et al. The natural history of the systemic inflammatory response syndrome (SIRS). JAMA 1995;273:117–123.

Rao PS, Cavanagh D. Endotoxic shock in the premate: some effects of dopamine administration. Am J Obstet Gynecol 1982;144:61–66.

Rao PS, Cavanagh D, Gaston LW. Endotoxic shock in the primate: effects of aspirin and dipyridamole administration. Am J Obstet Gynecol 1981;140:914–922.

Reimer LG, Reller LB. Gardnerella vaginalis bacteremia: a review of thirty cases. Obstet Gynecol 1984;64:170–172.

Remick DG, Kunkel RG, Larrick JW, et al. Acute in vivo effects of human recombinant tumor necrosis factor. Lab Invest 1987;56: 583–590.

Riddington DW, Venkatesh B, Boivin CM, et al. Intestinal permeability, gastric intramucosal pH, and systemic endotoxemia in patients undergoing cardiopulmonary bypass. JAMA 1996;275:1007–1012.

Rivers E, Nguyen B, Havstad S, Ressler J, Muzzin A, Knoblich B, et al. Early goal-directed therapy in the treatment of severe sepsis and septic shock. N Engl J Med 2001;345:1368–1377.

Roberts JM, Laros RK. Hemorrhagic and endotoxic shock: a pathophysiologic approach to diagnosis and management. Am J Obstet Gynecol 1971;110:1041–1049.

Rolbin SH, Levinson G, Shnider DM, et al. Dopamine treatment of spinal hypotension decreases uterine blood flow in the pregnant ewe. Anesthesiology 1979;51:37–40.

Sauve JS, Cook DJ. Gastrointestinal hemorrhage and ischemia: prevention and treatment. Int Anesthesiol Clin 1993;31:169–183.

Schirmer WJ, Schirmer JM, Naff GB, et al. Systemic complement activation produces hemodynamic changes characteristic of sepsis. Arch Surg 1988;123:316–321.

Sculier JP, Bron D, Verboven N, et al. Multiple organ failure during interleukin-2 and LAK cell infusion. Intensive Care Med 1988;14: 666–667.

Shippy CR, Appel PL, Shoemaker WC. Reliability of clinical monitoring to assess blood volume in critically ill patients. Crit Care Med 1984;12:107–112.

Shoemaker WC, Montgomery ES, Kaplan E, et al. Physiologic patterns in surviving and nonsurviving shock patients. Use of sequential cardiorespiratory variables in defining criteria for therapeutic goals and early warning of death. Arch Surg 1973;106:630–636.

Shoemaker WC, Appel PL, Bland R, et al. Clinical trial of an algorithm for outcome prediction in acute circulatory failure. Crit Care Med 1983;11:165.

Shoemaker WC, Appel PL, Kram HB, et al. Prospective trial of supranormal values of survivors as therapeutic goals in high-risk surgical patients. Chest 1988;94:1176–1186.

Shoemaker WC, Kram HB, Appel PL, et al. The efficacy of central venous and pulmonary artery catheters and therapy based upon them in reducing mortality and morbidity. Arch Surg 1990;125:1332–1337.

Shoemaker WC, Appel PL, Kram HB. Oxygen transport measurements to evaluate tissue perfusion and titrate therapy: dobutamine and dopamine effects. Crit Care Med 1991;19:672–688.

Shoemaker WC, Appel PL, Kram HB. Role of oxygen debt in the development of organ failure sepsis, and death in high-risk surgical patients. Chest 1992;102:208–215.

Sibbald WJ, Fox G, Martin C. Abnormalities of vascular reactivity in the sepsis syndrome. Chest 1991;100:S155–159.

Siegel JH, Greenspan M, Del Guercio LRM. Abnormal vascular tone, defective oxygen transport and myocardial failure in human septic shock. Ann Surg 1967;165:504–517.

Sprung CL, Caralis PV, Marcial EH, et al. The effects of high-dose corticosteroids in patients with septic shock. N Engl J Med 1984;311:1137–1143.

Sriskandan S, Cohen J. Science and clinical practice: the pathogenesis of septic shock. J Infect 1995;30:201–206.

Sugerman HJ, Peyton JWR, Greenfield LJ. Gram-negative sepsis. Curr Probl Surg 1981;18:405–475.

Swan HJ, Ganz W, Forrester J, et al. Catheterization of the heart in man with use of a flow-directed balloon-tipped catheter. N Engl J Med 1970;283:447–451.

Tabor DR, Burchett SK, Jacobs RF. Enhanced production of monokines by canine alveolar macrophages in response to endotoxin-induced shock (42681). Proc Soc Exp Biol Med 1988;187:408–415.

Tewari K, Wold SM, Asrat T. Septic shock in pregnancy associated with legionella pneumonia: Case report. Am J Obstet Gynecol 1997; 176:706–707.

Tracey KJ, Beutler B, Lowry SF, et al. Shock and tissue injury induced by recombinant human cachectin. Science 1986;234:470–474.

Tracey KJ, Lowry SF, Fahey TJ III, et al. Cachectin/tumor necrosis factor induces lethal shock and stress hormone responses in the dog. Surg Gynecol Obstet 1987a;164:415–422.

Tracey KJ, Fong Y, Hesse DG, et al. Anti-cachectin/TNF monoclonal antibodies prevent septic shock during lethal bacteriaemia. Nature 1987b;330:662–664.

Tracey KJ, Lowry SF, Cerami A. The pathophysiologic role of cachectin/TNF in septic shock and cachexia. Ann Institut Pasteur Immunol 1988;139:311–317.

Tryba M. Risk of acute stress bleeding and nosocomial pneumonia in ventilated intensive care unit patients: sucralfate versus antacids. Am J Med 1987;83:117–124.

Tuchschmidt J, Oblitas D, Fried JC. Oxygen consumption in sepsis and septic shock. Crit Care Med 1991;19:664–671.

Tuchschmidt J, Fried J, Astiz M, et al. Elevation of cardiac output and oxygen delivery improves outcome in septic shock. Chest 1992;102:216–220.

Vada P. Elevated plasma phospholipase A_2 levels: correlation with the hemodynamic and pulmonary changes in gram-negative septic shock. J Lab Clin Med 1984;104:873.

Van Bebber PT, Boekholz WKF, Goris RJ, et al. Neutrophil function and lipid peroxidation in a rat model of multiple organ failure. J Surg Res 1989;47:471–475.

Veterans Administration Systemic Sepsis Cooperative Study Group. Effect of high-dose glucocorticoid therapy on mortality in patients with clinical signs of systemic sepsis. N Engl J Med 1987;317:659.

Vincent JL. New therapeutic implications of anticoagulation mediatore replacement in sepsis and acute respiratory distress syndrome. Crit Care Med 2000;28:S83–85.

Wagner BKJ, D'Amelio LF. Pharmacologic and clinical considerations in selecting crystalloid, colloidal, and oxygen-carrying resuscitation fluids, part 2. Clin Pharm 1993;12:415–428.

Warren BL, Eid A, Singer P, et al. KyberSept Trial Study Group. Caring for the critically ill patients. High-dose antithrombin III in severe sepsis: a randomized controlled trial. JAMA 2001;286:1869–1878.

Warren HS, Danner RL, Munford RS. Anti-endotoxin monoclonal antibodies. N Engl J Med 1992;326:1153.

Webb SR, Gascoigne NRJ. T-cell activation by superantigens. Curr Opin Immunol 1994;6:467–475.

Weil MH, Henning RJ, Morissette M, et al. Relationship between colloid osmotic pressure and pulmonary artery wedge pressure in patients with acute cardiorespiratory failure. Am J Med 1978;64: 643–650.

Weil MN, Nishijima H. Cardiac output in bacterial shock. Am J Med 1978;64:920–922.

Wenzel RP. Monoclonal antibodies and the treatment of gram-negative bacteremia and shock. N Engl J Med 1991;324:486.

Weinstein MP, Murphy JR, Reller LB, et al. The clinical significance of positive blood cultures: a comparative analysis of 500 episodes of bacteremia and fungemia in adults. II. Clinical observations, with special reference to factors influencing prognosis. Rev Infect Dis 1983;5:54–70.

Wojnar MM, Hawkins WG, Lang CH. Nutritional support of the septic patient. Crit Care Clin 1995;11:717–733.

Yu M, Levy MM, Smith P, et al. Effect of maximizing oxygen delivery on morbidity and mortality rates in critically ill patients: a prospective, randomized, controlled study. Crit Care Med 1993;21: 830–838.

Ziegler EJ, Fisher CJ Jr, Sprung CL, et al. Treatment of gram-negative bacteremia and septic shock with HA-1A human monoclonal antibody against endotoxin. N Engl J Med 1991;324:429–436.

Ziegler TR, Smith RJ, O'Dwyer ST, et al. Increased intestinal permeability associated with infection in burn patients. Arch Surg 1988;123:1313–1319.

41 Anaphylactic shock

Donna Dizon-Townson

Historically, the first description of anaphylaxis may have been recorded in hieroglyphics circa 2640 BC in a depiction of a wasp sting leading to the sudden death of an Egyptian pharaoh (Fig. 41.1). The term anaphylaxis was first introduced in 1902 (Portier & Richet, 1902) and was used initially to denote a paradoxical effect that occurred with a particular experimental protocol. Attempting to induce improved tolerance or resistance to a toxin derived from the sea anemone, they repeatedly injected large but sublethal doses into dogs. After several weeks had passed, they observed unexpectedly that when reinjected with much smaller doses of the toxin, some dogs died within minutes. This dramatic and unexpected fatal response was the opposite (*ana* from Greek, meaning "back, backwards") of protection (*phylax* from Greek, meaning guard). Later, Richet was awarded the Nobel prize in medicine and physiology for his innovating work in this area.

Although anaphylaxis is a rare event, this dramatic syndrome may occur during a number of common obstetric procedures and treatments. Furthermore, with increased utilization of antibiotics for conditions such as group B *Streptococcus* colonization and preterm rupture of membranes, an increase in the incidence of anaphylactic reactions may be observed. Therefore, the obstetrician should be well versed in the diagnosis and management of this unexpected life-threatening condition.

Classification

Hypersensitivity is the term applied when an adaptive immune response occurs in an exaggerated or inappropriate form, causing cellular destruction and tissue damage. Four types of hypersensitivity reactions have been described (Roitt et al., 1985). Because these reactions are normal immune responses occurring in an exaggerated form, each type does not necessarily occur at the exclusion of another. Type I, or immediate hypersensitivity, occurs when antigen binds and cross-links immunoglobulin E (IgE)-sensitized mast cells and basophils, resulting in release of pharmacological mediators such as histamine, serine proteases, and cytokines. Types II, or antibody-dependent cytotoxic hypersensitivity, develops when antibody binds to antigen on cells, leading to phagocytosis, killer-cell activity, or complement-mediated lysis. Type III, or immune complex-mediated hypersensitivity, occurs when immune complexes are deposited in tissues, promoting complement activation and resulting in tissue damage. Finally, type IV, or delayed hypersensitivity, is produced when antigen-sensitized T-cells release lymphokines following a secondary contact with the same antigen, producing an exaggerated immune response.

Anaphylaxis is the cascade of events that occurs in a sensitized individual on subsequent exposure to the specific sensitized antigen. The spectrum of events ranges from a localized response to a catastrophic and life-threatening systemic reaction consisting of hypotension, tachycardia, and multisystem organ failure. Anaphylaxis most commonly refers to IgE-medicated, type I hypersensitivity response, produced by antigen-stimulated mast-cell mediator release. A clinically indistinguishable syndrome, anaphylactoid reaction, may occur, involving similar mediators but not requiring IgE antibody or previous exposure to the inciting substance. Anaphylaxis and anaphylactoid reactions have been classified further based on etiology. These classifications include IgE-mediated reactions, complement-mediated reaction, nonimmunologic mast-cell activation, exposure to modulators of arachidonic metabolism or sulfating agents, exercise-induced anaphylaxis, catamenial anaphylaxis, and idiopathic recurrent anaphylaxis (Atkinson & Kaliner, 1992).

IgE-mediated anaphylaxis

Common sources of antigens triggering IgE-mediated anaphylaxis include antibiotics, insulin, *Hymenoptera* venom, foods, seminal plasma, and latex proteins. IgE-mediated anaphylaxis represents the classic type I hypersensitivity reaction. Necessary components of this reaction include a sensitizing antigen; an IgE-class antibody reaction, resulting in the systemic sensitization of mast cells and basophils; reintroduction

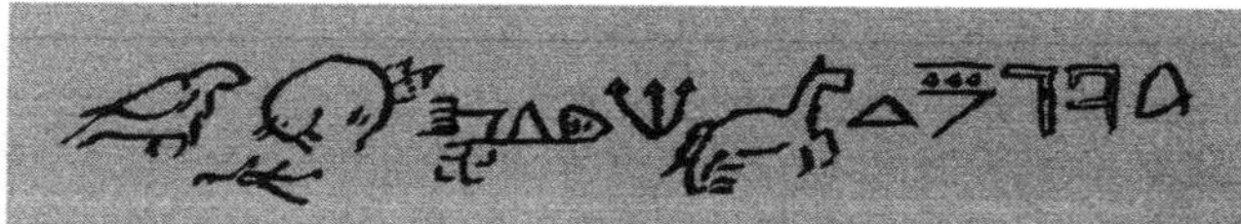

Fig. 41.1 Egyptian hieroglyphic describing the death of a pharaoh following a reaction to the sting of a wasp.

of the sensitizing antigen; and mediator release from mast cells and basophils (Atkinson & Kaliner, 1992). Either antigens or haptens may elicit IgE antibody production. Haptens are molecules too small to initiate an immune response independently. However, they may bind to other endogenous proteins and become antigenic. Penicillin and related antibiotics are probably the most important of all haptens. Typically, penicillin is metabolized to a major determinant, benzylpenicilloyl, and an additional series of minor determinants, including penicilloate, penilloate, penicilloyl-amine, and penicillin itself. These haptens elicit penicillin-specific IgE antibodies and may be found in 4–10% of persons who have received penicillin therapy. This common reaction is underscored due to increasing utilization of both penicillin and ampicillin for neonatal prophylaxis against maternal group B *Streptococcus* colonization.

Complement-mediated reactions

Various frequently administered blood products, including whole blood, serum, plasma, fractionated serum products, and immunoglobulins, are the inciting agents of other anaphylactic responses. A type III hypersensitive reaction with complement-mediated cellular destruction is one of the mechanisms causing these reactions. Complement activation with the generation of the anaphylatoxins, C3a, C4a, and C5a cause mast-cell degranulation, mediator generation and release, and the subsequent systemic reactions, including an increased vascular permeability and smooth muscle contraction. A cytotoxic antibody-mediated reaction, or type II hypersensitivity, with subsequent complement activation can also cause anaphylaxis in this setting. Mismatched blood transfusion may promote lysis of RBCs and mast-cell degranulation and result in a life-threatening reaction.

Nonimmunologic mast-cell activators (anaphylactoid reactions)

A myriad of agents, including radiocontrast media, narcotics, depolarizing agents, and dextrans, may directly cause mast-cell mediator release and anaphylactoid reactions. Radiocontrast media has long been recognized as a cause of anaphylactoid reaction (Lieberman et al., 1986, 1991a,b; Bush, 1990; Bush & Swanson, 1991; Weese et al., 1993; Keizur & Das, 1994). Mild reactions occur in approximately 5% of individuals receiving radiocontrast dyes; fatal reactions are less common (Grammar & Patterson, 1986; Lieberman et al., 1986). Two types of reactions to radiographic contrast have been described, including a dose-independent, unpredictable anaphylactoid reaction and a dose-dependent, predicable physicochemical reaction (Wittbrodt & Spinler 1994). The use of a lower-osmolar contrast media is associated with a lower incidence of reactions. Wittbrodt and Spinler recommend a lower osmolar contrast, pretreatment with a corticosteroid and an H_1-antagonist, and preparation for an anaphylactoid response in high-risk patients requiring a procedure with radiocontrast media. A high-risk patient was defined as one having a history of previous anaphylactoid reaction to radiographic contrast, asthma, and reaction to skin allergens or penicillin. More recently, Clark et al. (1995) documented the clinically anaphylactoid nature of amniotic fluid embolism.

Both immune- and nonimmune-mediated anaphylaxis involves the release of primary and secondary mediators. Those derived from mast cells and basophils are termed *primary mediators* and include histamine, prostaglandins (D_2, E_2, and F_2 alpha), leukotrienes (C_4, D_4, and E_4), and platelet-activating factor. Effects of these primary mediators include altered vascular tone, increased vascular permeability, bronchial smooth-muscle contraction, increased heart rate and contractility, and platelet aggregation. The effects of PGD_2 on vascular tone may be especially pronounced (Austen, 1994). These primary mediators also set into effect the cascading release of secondary mediators of anaphylaxis, which include components of the complement system, leading to further membrane injury, increased vascular permeability, and smooth-muscle contraction, as well as activation of the kinin system and intrinsic clotting cascade, the latter leading to disseminated intravascular coagulation. Myocardial depression is also seen in association with such mediator release; the marked coronary artery constriction seen with experimental administration of the cysteinyl leukotrienes may be involved in this process (Raper & Fisher, 1988; Austen, 1994).

Hemodynamic changes

Because the onset of anaphylactic shock has been observed in the setting of intense medical supervision, the hemodynamic evolution of this syndrome has been well delineated (Moss et al., 1981; Nicolas et al., 1984). Two phases have been observed: a hyperkinetic phase followed by a hypokinetic phase. The hyperkinetic phase lasts 2–3 minutes and involves a fall in systemic vascular resistance and hypotension. However, the combination of tachycardia and an increase in the systolic ejection volume results in a rapid rise in cardiac output. Central venous pressure and pulmonary capillary pressure initially remain stable. This is followed by a hypokinetic phase characterized by continued histamine-mediated vasodilation, hypotension, and tachycardia. The central venous pressure and pulmonary capillary wedge pressure decline.

Due to capillary stasis resulting from vasodilation, cardiac output eventually falls. These hemodynamic changes may be complicated further by the development of myocardial depression and disseminated intravascular coagulation (Silverman et al., 1984; Kapin & Ferguson, 1985; Wong et al., 1990; Austen, 1994).

Obstetric antecedents to anaphylaxis

More than 50 case reports describing the occurrence of anaphylaxis in association with common obstetric procedures and therapeutic regimens have been described. Anaphylaxis may occur at any time during gestation. Intravenous (IV) antibiotics, oxytocin, anesthetic agents, blood products, and latex exposure are some of the more common causes of anaphylaxis in pregnancy. Two case reports of anaphylaxis to laminaria used for a therapeutic abortion exist (Nguyen & Hoffman, 1995; Cole & Bruck, 2000). A rare, but potentially devastating allergy to seminal plasma may occur. Successful pregnancy in a woman with this type of allergy has been described (Iwahashi et al., 1999). The allergy was confirmed via a positive reaction to skin-prick test with whole semen. Pregnancy was achieved with artificial insemination following sperm washing three times using a continuous-step density gradient centrifugation method.

Antibiotics

Due to the rapid increase and diversification of antibiotic agents, there has been a concordant increase in the commendations for the usage of antibiotics for both prophylaxis and treatment of obstetric infections. Penicillin and its derivatives are the most common causes of drug reactions. From 0.6% to 10.0% of patients exhibit some form of hypersensitivity to penicillin. Fortunately, most reactions are mild; the incidence of anaphylaxis is reported as only 0.04–0.2% of patients receiving these drugs (Mandell & Sande, 1990). Approximately 0.001% of patients so treated die of anaphylaxis. Of those who experience fatal reactions, 15% have a history of other types of allergy. Seventy percent of patients with fatal reactions have received penicillin previously—two-thirds of these without a reaction. Disturbingly, one-third of patients succumbing to penicillin anaphylaxis have a history of prior reaction to these agents (Idsoe et al., 1968). Anaphylaxis may be seen following IV, oral, or subcutaneous administration of penicillin.

Up to 20% of patients with known penicillin allergy show immunologic cross-reactivity to cephalosporins (Levine, 1973), but only about 1% show actual clinical reaction to this class of drugs (Saxon et al., 1987). Such clinical cross-reactivity cannot be predicted on the basis of skin tests (Mandell & Sande, 1990). As a general rule, patients with a history of minor reactions to penicillin may be given cephalosporins when clinically indicated. In patients with a history of anaphylaxis, however, cephalosporin administration should be withheld unless no acceptable alternative antibiotic is available (Anderson, 1986; Konno & Nagase, 1995).

The incidence of penicillin-induced anaphylaxis has been reported to be 10–50 per 100,000 injections (Idsoe et al., 1968; Rudolph & Price, 1973). Fatal cases of penicillin-induced anaphylaxis have been estimated at 100–500 annually in the United States (Parker, 1963). There is no convincing evidence of risk factors such as age, sex, race, occupation, or geographic location for identifying individuals who are at increased risk. Most studies conclude that atopy does not predispose individuals to anaphylaxis from penicillin therapy or venom of a stinging insect (Austen, 1994).

Penicillin remains the treatment of choice for syphilis during pregnancy. If skin testing confirms the risk of IgE-mediated allergic reaction to penicillin, then penicillin desensitization is recommended and is followed by benzathine penicillin G treatment (Wendel et al., 1985). Selective prophylactic antibiotic usage for the prevention of neonatal group B streptococcal sepsis (ACOG, 1996) and for the prevention of endomyometritis after cesarean section (DePalma et al., 1982) are not uncommon. Dunn and colleagues (1999) reported a case of a serious anaphylactic reaction to penicillin in labor used for prophylaxis against group B *Streptococcus*. An emergency cesarean section resulted. Although the patient and infant were eventually discharged, the patient developed disseminated intravascular coagulation and suffered acute tubular necrosis that required dialysis. Gallagher (1988) reported a case of anaphylaxis in response to IV ampicillin for treatment of chorioamnionitis. Anaphylaxis secondary to IV cefotetan administered as surgical prophylaxis for cesarean section and transabdominal hysterectomy has been described (Bloomberg, 1998). As the use of antibiotics for an increasing number of obstetric indications becomes standard, the frequency of antibiotic-induced anaphylaxis may be encountered more commonly, thus emphisizing the importance of early recognition of symptomatology with subsequent aggressive fluid resuscitation and therapy.

Oxytocic agents

Syntocinon contains the active ingredient oxytocin and the inactive ingredients sodium acetate, chlorobutanol, ethanol, and acetic acid. Chlorobutanol is widely used for its bacteriostatic properties as a preservative for injectables such as oxytocin. Cases of anaphylactic shock from chlorobutanol-preserved oxytocin have been described (Slater et al., 1985; Hofmann et al., 1986; Maycock & Russell, 1993; Morriss et al., 1994). Hoffman et al. reported a case of anaphylactic shock that occurred after injection of oxytocin-containing chlorobutanol during an elective termination of pregnancy. Subsequent scratch testing on the forearm with both oxytocin and chlorobutanol yielded a positive reaction to chlorobutanol and no reaction to oxytocin. Maycock and Russell (1993) described a gravida who required an emergency cesarean section for fetal distress. Immediately after delivery of the infant, 5 units of syntocinon were given. This was followed by profound hypotension and laryngeal edema. Subsequent skin testing revealed chlorobutanol to be responsible for the reaction. A third case, reported by Morriss et al. (1994), detailed the occurrence of anaphylaxis during an elective cesarean for breech presentation. Anaphylactoid reaction due solely to oxytocin during cesarean was described by Kawarbayashi et al. (1988). In this case, an elective cesarean section under epidural anesthesia with mepivacaine was performed. Following delivery of the baby, 5 units of oxytocin were injected directly into the myometrium and another 5 units were added to the infusion bottle. Within minutes, the patient developed numbness, perioral and periorbital erythema, and edema. Severe and prolonged hypotension that failed to respond to 500 mg of hydrocortisone and 20 mg of ephedrine, but finally improved with 0.05 mg of epinephrine, was observed. Later, intradermal testing with 0.02 mL of oxytocin (5 units/mL) showed a markedly positive reaction at 15 and 30 minutes. Although reactions to syntocinon and oxytocin are rare, this possibility should be kept in mind by the practicing obstetrician.

Methotrexate

Methotrexate is sometimes used for the treatment of ectopic pregnancies in women who want to preserve fertility. In addition, methotrexate is the first line of therapy for persistent gestation trophoblastic disease. Systemic anaphylaxis from low-dose methotrexate has been reported (Cohn et al., 1993). These authors describe the acute onset of symptoms consisting of burning in the mouth followed by diffuse cutaneous erythema, dyspnea, cyanosis, hypotension, and respiratory arrest following the IV infusion of methotrexate as adjuvant chemotherapy for breast cancer. The patient required endotracheal intubation during the acute episode and subsequently recovered. Intradermal injection testing with methotrexate was done, which supported methotrexate as the offending agent. With this in mind, it seems of paramount importance to be familiar with the diagnosis and management of anaphylaxis when using this chemotherapeutic agent.

Latex

The combination of latex allergy and overt anaphylaxis is being reported with increasing frequency (ACAAI, 1995). Both delayed (type IV) hypersensitivity and immediate (type I) hypersensitivity reactions have been attributed to latex exposure (Tomazic et al., 1992). Nutter initially described latex-induced allergic reactions in 1979. Since that time, more severe reactions to latex gloves, Foley catheters, and endotracheal tubes have been reported (Zenarola, 1989; Gerber, 1990; Moneret-Vautrin et al., 1990; Swartz et al., 1990). Several case reports exist of anaphylaxis after latex contact during vaginal or cesarean delivery (Turjanmaa et al., 1988; Fisher, 1992; Diaz et al., 1996; Deusch et al., 1996; Porter et al., 1998; Ayeko & Smith, 1999; Eckhout & Ayad, 2001). Laurent and colleagues (1992) detailed a patient who developed an anaphylactic reaction following manual extraction of a placenta. This patient underwent a number of tests, including skin prick tests, intradermal tests, and IgE levels, which all confirmed latex contact as the triggering event. Infants with spina bifida are at increased risk for severe, systemic reactions to latex, and should be delivered and handled by medical personnel wearing and using nonlatex gloves and supplies (Ledger & Meripole, 1992; Kelly et al., 1994; Lu et al., 1995; Nieto et al., 1996).

Colloid solutions

The most commonly used colloid solutions, including human serum albumin, dextran, gelatin, and hydroxyethyl starch may evoke anaphylactic reactions (Blanloeil et al., 1982; Stafford et al., 1988; Guharoy & Barajas, 1991; Ring, 1991). In addition, dextran solutions are known for their antithrombotic effect. A number of case reports emphasize fetal morbidity due to anaphylactoid reactions associated with dextran (Ring & Messmer, 1977; Berg et al., 1991; Barbier et al., 1992). Barbier and colleagues describe a mother who fainted, developed urticaria, and had mild respiratory distress following dextran infusion. Hypotension was not observed. The infusion was stopped, and a dead neonate was delivered. Berg et al. (1991) described three severe cases of dextran-induced anaphylactoid reactions despite immunoprophylaxis with dextran-I hapten. In one of the cases, a patient was given dextran-70 prior to cesarean section and had a mild reaction, but, unfortunately, she gave birth to a child with serious brain damage. In both of these cases, it was observed that, despite apparently mild maternal reactions without hypotension, the fetuses were affected severely. Such observations are seen commonly in maternal shock of any etiology and reflect preferential maternal shunting of blood away from the splanchnic bed (including uterus) to maintain central pressure in shock states. Paull (1987) performed a prospective study of dextran-induced anaphylactoid reactions in 5,745 gynecologic and obstetric patients who received IV dextran-70 solution. In this study an incidence of 1 : 383 reactions per patient treated was observed; they concluded that the risks of dextran-70 treatment exceeded the risks of thromboembolism in this patient population.

Anesthetic agents

A number of anesthetic agents have been reported to cause anaphylaxis (Seigne, 1997). Often the obstetric patient will have received a number of potential anaphylactic agents intrapartum. It is important to review all anesthetic agents received, since this will have important implications for counseling regarding recurrence risks. Skin testing for the specific agent should not be overlooked. A case report of a pregnant woman with previous anaphylactic reaction to local anesthetics was reported (Browne & Birnbach, 2001). Skin testing confirming lidocaine allergy assisted in subsequent labor analgesia and obstetric management at term. Maternal anaphylactic reaction has been reported to occur due to general anesthesia during emergency cesarean section for fetal bradycardia (Stannard & Bellis, 2001).

Modulators of arachidonic acid metabolism

The "aspirin triad" includes chronic sinusitis, nasal polyposis, and asthma. Approximately 5–10% of patients with this condition will develop a reaction, which may include vasomotor collapse in response to nonsteroidal anti-inflammatory drugs. This appears to be a non-IgE-mediated anaphylactoid reaction similar to that seen with contrast medium.

Sulfiting agents and food allergy

Sulfiting agents are used commonly as preservatives to prevent food discoloration. These preservatives are added to leafy green salads, fruits, wine, beer, dehydrated soups, and fish. Intake of these agents may cause asthma and anaphylaxis in susceptible persons (Nicklas, 1989). Similar reactions may occur in susceptible women following ingestion of peanuts or shellfish (Fig. 41.2).

Exercise-induced anaphylaxis

Exercise-induced anaphylaxis is a well-recognized syndrome (Sheffer et al., 1983, 1985; Songsiridej & Busse, 1983; Sheffer & Austen, 1984; Kobayashi & Mellion, 1991; Briner & Sheffer, 1992; Nichols, 1992; Hough & Dec, 1994; Shadick et al., 1999) and has been diagnosed with increasing frequency during the past 20 years. The pathophysiology is somewhat controversial, but the most likely explanation is a combination of heat and water loss leading to endogenous mediator release. Smith (1985) described an interesting case of delivery as a cause of exercise-induced anaphylactoid reaction. This patient was a previously healthy 29-year-old woman whose medical history was significant for a severe anaphylactoid reaction following an intramuscular (IM) injection of ergometrine during her first delivery. During her second delivery, it was emphasized that "no drugs whatsoever more given." A few minutes after delivery of the placenta, the patient developed symptoms similar to her first episode of anaphylaxis. An extensive work-up, including testing for immune complexes, IgE levels, serum complement studies, and an estimation of C1 esterase inhibitor, failed to unmask the etiology. From a more in-depth history, it was revealed that as a teenager she had puffy eyes and urticaria most often associated with exercise. Of note, these episodes were not cyclical with menses, and it was concluded that the exertion of labor triggered the sequence of events.

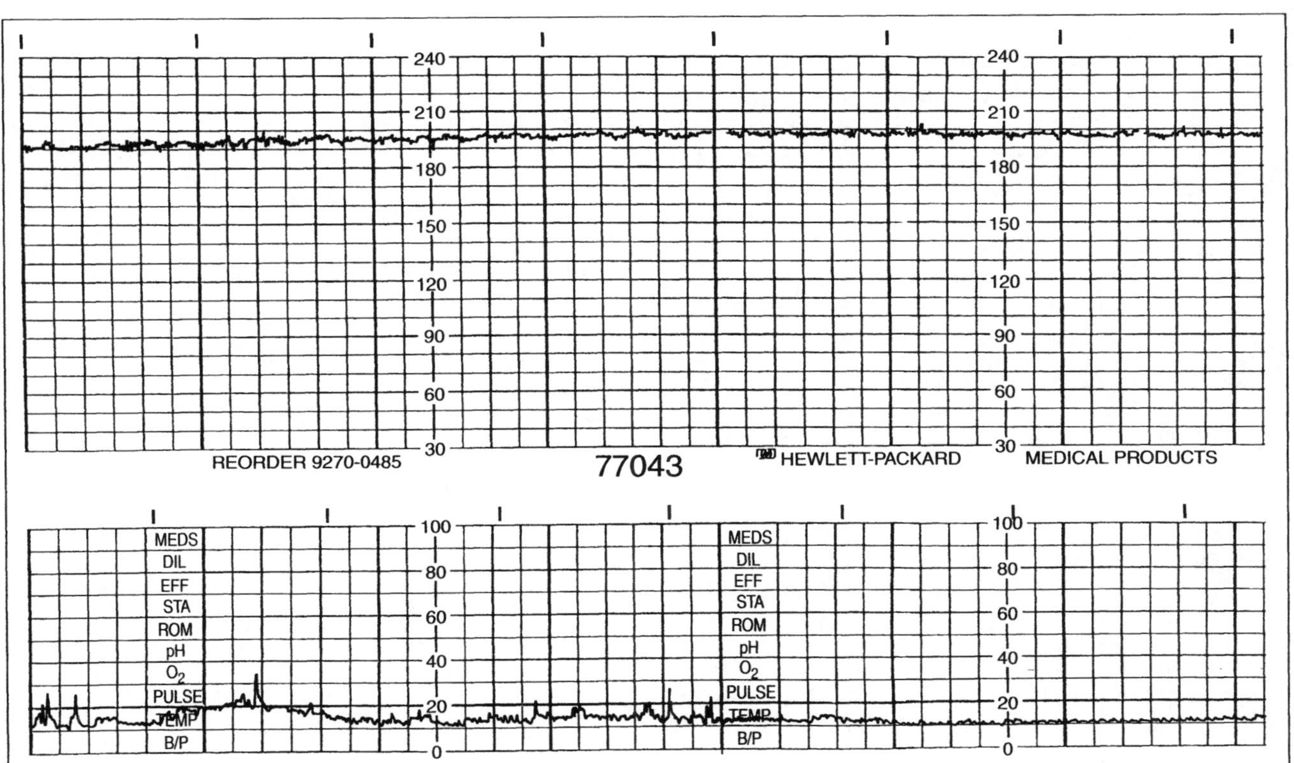

Fig. 41.2 Fetal heart rate tracing just prior to intrauterine death in a mother suffering an anaphylactic reaction to a peanut.

Clinical presentation

Early recognition of symptoms and prompt treatment of an anaphylactic reaction are the cornerstone for proper management. There are risk factors in addition to a previous history of anaphylaxis that can assist in early identification of individuals who may manifest the clinical spectrum of anaphylaxis. Organs primarily involved in humans include those of the cutaneous, gastrointestinal, respiratory, and cardiovascular systems (Table 41.1). Anaphylactic reactions have been classified according to severity of symptoms (Table 41.2). The hallmark of the anaphylactic reaction is the onset of some manifestation within seconds to minutes after introduction (either injection or ingestion) of the antigen substance. The patient may report a sense of impending doom that is coincident with flushing, tachycardia, and often pruritus. These symptoms may progress to signs that include urticaria, angioedema, rhinorrhea, bronchorrhea, nasal congestion, asthma, laryngeal edema, abdominal bloating, nausea, vomiting, cramps, arrhythmias, faintness, syncope, cardiovascular collapse, and ultimately death.

The clinical presentation of anaphylactic and anaphylactoid reactions has been reviewed (Moneret-Vautrin & Laxenaire, 1991). Mucocutaneous signs are often the first warning. Pruritus, burning, tingling, and numbness are commonly sensed by the patient. A maculopapular erythematous rash on the face and upper trunk may progress rapidly to generalized urticaria. Periorbital and perioral edema may accompany the rash. Associated symptoms include runny eyes, rhinorrhea, and conjunctival hyperemia.

Gastrointestinal disturbances consist of nausea, vomiting, diarrhea, and abdominal pains. A tendency for hypothermia is seen and rarely, hyperpyrexia may be manifest. Respiratory signs often present in the form of a dry cough, tachypnea, and wheezing secondary to bronchospasm. Laryngeal edema may make intubation difficult. Diffuse pulmonary edema causing severe respiratory distress hampers effective mechanical ventilation. Despite aggressive treatment, cardiovascular collapse is common. Hypotension and tachycardia are the rule. Rhythm and conduction disturbances are frequent and occur early. Cardiac arrest is most often of anoxic origin from irreversible bronchospasm and prolonged shock.

Table 41.1 Signs and symptoms produced by anaphylactic/anaphylactoid reactions

Organ system involved	Symptoms produced	Signs elicited
Cutaneous	Itching, burning tingling, numbness, flushing	Rash, swelling, hives
Cardiovascular	Faintness, malaise, weakness, palpitations, chest discomfort, collapse	Tachycardia, hypotension, arrhythmia, cardiac arrest
Respiratory	Congestion, dyspnea, choking, gasping, cough, hoarseness, lump in throat, difficulty swallowing or talking	Tachypnea, rhonchi, laryngeal swelling, pulmonary edema, respiratory arrest
Gastrointestinal	Abdominal bloating, cramps, nausea, vomiting, diarrhea, incontinence	Abdominal pain, metallic taste in mouth
Fetal	Decreased fetal movement	Late decelerations, tachycardia, diminished variability, bradycardia

Management

In addition to anaphylactic shock, the differential diagnosis includes amniotic fluid embolism, myocardial infarction, congestive heart failure, and pulmonary embolism. Initially, the source of the offending antigen should be removed. When possible, apply a tourniquet to obstruct the venous blood return from the source of the antigen or inciting medication. Release the tourniquet approximately every 15 minutes. Provide oxygen, place the patient in the recumbent position, and keep the patient warm. Aqueous epinephrine (0.3–0.5 mL of a 1:1,000 solution injected subcutaneously) is a mainstay of therapy. H_1 antihistamines (diphenhydramine 25–50 mg IM or IV) and H_2 antihistamines (cimetidine 300 mg or ranitidine 50 mg given slow IV over 3–5 minutes) should be given. Establish and maintain the airway. Aggressive use of IV fluids for maintaining blood pressure is recommended. A pressor agent such as dopamine hydrochloride (2–10 μg/kg/min) may be neces-

Table 41.2 Severity scale of anaphylactic reaction

Grade	Symptom
I	Skin symptoms and/or mild fever reaction
II	Measurable but not life-threatening cardiovascular reaction (tachycardia, hypotension) Gastrointestinal disturbance Respiratory disturbance
III	Shock, life-threatening spasm of smooth muscle, such as bronchi or uterus
IV	Cardiac or respiratory arrest

(From Ring J, Messmer K. Incidence and severity of anaphylactoid reactions to colloid volume substitutes. Lancet 1997;i:466.)

sary after intravascular preload has been optimized. If wheezing is present and is unresponsive to epinephrine, aminophylline (5–6 mg/kg) may be given over 20 minutes, followed by maintenance dose of 0.9 mg/kg/hr. Hydrocortisone (100 mg) or its equivalent should be administered every 6 hours. Epinephrine may be repeated every 20 minutes.

While treating the pregnant woman with anaphylaxis, fetal well-being also must be considered. For reasons outlined previously, fetal hypoxia, manifested by an abnormal fetal heart rate pattern, will virtually always accompany maternal shock or hypoxia of any etiology. Further, maternal blood pressure may be maintained at the expense of uterine (as well as other splanchnic) blood flow (Clark, 1990). Thus, the fetal heart rate should be monitored carefully in patients in anaphylactic shock. Heart rate abnormalities are often a sign of insufficient maternal oxygenation or relative hypovolemia and may be valuable clues to the underlying maternal condition (see Fig. 41.2). Cesarean section is rarely, if ever, indicated in such cases, and in fact may be detrimental to an unstable mother. Rather, abnormal fetal heart rate patterns can generally be alleviated by maternal positioning, maternal volume expansion, and increasing levels of oxygen administration in the borderline or frankly hypoxic mother. Unfortunately, fetal central nervous system damage may occur despite adequate therapy. Luciano and colleagues (Luciano et al., 1997) reported a case of fetal encephalopathy diagnosed via cerebral ultrasound and confirmed by magnetic resonance imaging at time of birth. The neonate suffered multicystic encephalomalacia and corpus callosum atrophy attributed to an episode of maternal anaphylactic shock which occurred at 27 weeks' gestation following an intravenous iron injection.

Concern has been raised regarding the use of epinephrine in pregnancy. During embryogenesis, epinephrine exposure was associated with an increased risk of umbilical hernia in the Collaborative Perinatal Project; however, it is difficult to distinguish potential drug effects from those of the condition for which epinephrine was administered (Briggs et al., 1994). Later in pregnancy, epinephrine may potentially decrease uterine blood flow. Terbutaline sulfate (0.25 mg subcutaneously), an agent devoid of such effects, has been advanced as an alternate agent in patients with asthma or anaphylaxis. In mild cases of anaphylaxis or asthma, a trial of terbutaline may be acceptable. In cases of life-threatening reactions or when terbutaline is not readily available, however, these theoretical disadvantages of epinephrine are far outweighed by its longstanding documented efficacy in combating maternal hemodynamic instability and respiratory compromise.

A variety of serum specimens may be obtained to further investigate the clinical presentation of anaphylaxis and search for a definite cause. An excellent review of markers and mechanisms of anaphylaxis was presented by Watkins (1992). In the past, several samples taken over a 20-minute period after the onset of the reaction and subsequent measurement of histamine levels were recommended. Histamine, however, has an extremely short half-life (2 min), and such an approach seems impractical. In contrast, the analysis of the histamine metabolite, methylhistamine, is of value, particularly when measured in the urine (Watkins & Wild, 1990). Another simpler analytical technique is to measure plasma tryptase release in serum or plasma samples taken sequentially during the immediate 24-hour period following the reaction (Watkins, 1989; Matsson et al., 1991). This serine protease is long-lived (approximately 2 hr) and is released exclusively from the mast cell in parallel with histamine. A radioimmunoassay based on the ELISA procedures is available. The knowledge of these markers may help confirm an anaphylactic reaction and assist future counseling.

References

American College of Allergy, Asthmas and Immunology. Position statement: latex allergy—an emerging healthcare problem. Ann Allergy Asthma Immunol 1995;75:2.

American College of Obstetricians and Gynecologists. Prevention of Early-Onset of Group B Streptococcal Disease in Newborns. ACOG Committee Opinion Number 173, June 1996.

Anderson JA. Cross-sensitivity to cephalosporins in patients allergic to penicillin. Pediatr Infect Dis 1986;5:557–561.

Atkinson TP, Kaliner MA. Anaphylaxis. Med Clin North Am 1992;76: 841–855.

Austen KF. Diseases of immediate hypersensitivity. In: Petersdorf RG, Adams RD, Braunwald E, et al., eds. Harrison's Principles of Internal Medicine, 13th edn. New York: McGraw-Hill, 1994.

Ayeko MO, Smith NJ. Coexisting allergies to latex and to muscle relaxants in a primigravida. Hosp Med 1999;60:311.

Barbier P, Jonville AP, Autret E. Fetal risks with dextrans during delivery. Drug Saf 1992;7:71–73.

Berg EM, Fasting S, Sellevold OFM. Serious complications with dextran-70 despite hapten prophylaxis. Is it best avoided prior to delivery? Anesthesia 1991;46:1033–1035.

Blanloeil Y, Pinaud M, Villers D, Nicolas F. Anaphylactic shock after infusion of a modified gelatin solution. Hemodynamic study (letter). Nouv Presse Med 1982;11:2847–2848.

Bloomberg RJ. Cefotetan-induced anaphylaxis. Am J Obstet Gynecol 1998;159:125–126.

Briggs GE, Freeman RK, Yaffe SJ. Drugs in pregnancy and lactation, 4th edn. Baltimore: Williams and Wilkins, 1994.

Briner WW, Sheffer AL. Exercise-induced anaphylaxis. Med Sci Sports Exerc 1992;92:849–850.

Browne IM, Birnbach DJ. A pregnant woman with previous anaphylactic reaction to local anesthetics: a case report. Am J Obstet Gynecol 2001;185:1253–1254.

Bush WH. Treatment of systemic reactions to contrast media. Urology 1990;35:145–150.

Bush WH, Swanson DP. Acute reactions to intravascular contrast media: types, risk factors, recognition, and specific treatment. AJR 1991;157:1153–1163.

Clark SL. Shock in the pregnant patient. Semin Perinatol 1990;14:52–58.

Clark SL, Hankins GD, Dudley DA, et al. Amniotic fluid embolism:

analysis of a national registry. Am J Obstet Gynecol 1995;172(4 Part 1):1158–1167.

Cohn JR, Cohn JB, Fellin R, Cantor R. Systemic anaphylaxis from low dose methotrexate. Ann Allergy 1993;70:384–385.

Cole DS, Bruck LR. Anaphylaxis after laminaria insertion. Obstet Gynecol 2000;95:1025.

DePalma RT, Cunningham FG, Leveno KJ, Roark ML. Continuing investigation of women at high risk for infection following cesarean delivery: the three-dose perioperative antimicrobial therapy. Obstet Gynecol 1982;60:53–59.

Deusch E, Reider N, Marth C. Anaphylactic reaction to latex during cesarean delivery. Obstet Gynecol 1996;88:727.

Diaz T, Martinez T, Antepara I, et al. Latex allergy as a risk during delivery. Br J Obstet Gynaecol 1996;103:173–175.

Dunn AB, Blomquist J, Khouzami V. Anaphylaxis in labor secondary to prophylaxis against group B Streptococcus. A case report. J Reprod Med 1999;44:381–384.

Eckhout GV Jr, Ayad S. Anaphylaxis due to airborne exposure to latex in a primigravida. Anesthesiology 2001;95:1034–1035.

Fisher A. Iatrogenic (intraoperative) rubber glove allergy and anaphylaxis. Cutis 1992;49:17–18.

Gallagher JS. Anaphylaxis in pregnancy. Obstet Gynecol 1988;71:491–493.

Gerber AC, Jorg W, Zbinden S, et al. Severe intraoperative anaphylaxis to surgical gloves: latex allergy, and unfamiliar condition. Anesthesiology 1990;73:556.

Grammar LC, Patterson R. Adverse reactions to radiographic contrast material. Clin Dermatol 1986;4:149.

Guharoy SR, Barajas M. Probable anaphylactic reaction to corn-derived dextrose solution. Vet Hum Toxicol 1991;33:609–610.

Hofmann H, Goerz G, Plewig G. Anaphylactic shock from chlorobutanol-preserved oxytocin. Contact Dermatitis 1986;15:241.

Hough DO, Dec KL. Exercise-induced asthma and anaphylaxis. Sports Med 1994;18:162–172.

Idsoe O, Guthe T, Wilcox RR, eds. Nature and extent of penicillin reactions with particular reference to fatalities from anaphylactic shock. Bull WHO 1968;38:159–188.

Iwahashi K, Miyazaki T, Kuji N, Yoshimura Y. Successful pregnancy in a woman with a human seminal plasma allergy. A case report. J Reprod Med 1999;44:391–393.

Kapin MA, Ferguson JL. Hemodynamic and regional circulatory alterations in dog during anaphylactic challenge. Am J Physiol 1985;249:H430–437.

Kawarabayashi T, Narisawa Y, Nakamura K, et al. Anaphylactoid reaction to oxytocin durin cesarean section. Gynecol Obstet Invest 1988;25:277–279.

Keizur JJ, Das S. Current perspectives on intravascular contrast agents for radiological imaging. J Urol 1994;151:1470–1478.

Kelly KJ, Pearson ML, Kurup VP, et al. A cluster of anaphylactic reactions in children with spina bifida during general anesthesia. Epidemiologic features, risk factors and latex hypersensitivity. J Allergy Clin Immunol 1994;94:53–61.

Kobayashi RH, Mellion MB. Exercise-induced asthma, anaphylaxis, and urticaria. Prim Care 1991;18:809–831.

Konno R, Nagase S. Anaphylactic reaction to cefazolin in pregnancy. J Obstet Gynaecol 1995;21:577–579.

Laurent J, Malet R, Smiejan JM, et al. Latex hypersensitivity after natural delivery. J Allergy Clin Immunol 1992;89:779–780.

Ledger R, Meripole A. Children at risk: latex allergies and spina bifida. J Pediatr Nurs 1992;7:371.

Levine BB. Antigenicity and cross reactivity of penicillins and cephalosportins. J Infect Dis 1973;128(Suppl):S364–366.

Lieberman P. Anaphylactoid reactions to radiocontrast. Ann Allergy 1991a;67:91.

Lieberman P. Anaphylactoid reactions to radiocontrast material. Clin Rev Allergy 1991b;9:319–338.

Lieberman P, Siegle RL, Treadwell G. Radiocontrast reactions. Clin Rev Allergy 1986;4:229–245.

Lu LJ, Kurup VP, Hoffman DR, et al. Characterization of a major latex allergen associated with hypersensitivity in spina bifida patients. J Immunol 1995;155:2721–2728.

Luciano R, Zuppa AA, Maragliano G, Gallini F, Tortorolo G. Fetal encephalopathy after maternal analphylaxis. Case Report. Biol Neonate 1997;71:190–193.

Mandell GL, Sande MA. Antimicrobial agents penicillins, cephalosporins and other beta lactam antibiotics. In: Gilman AG, Rall TW, Nies AS, Taylor P, eds. Goodman, the Pharmacologic Basis of Therapeutics. New York: Pergamon Press, 1990.

Matsson P, Enander I, Andersson AS, et al. Evaluation of mast cell activation (tryptase) in two patients suffering drug induced hypotensoid reactions. Agents Actions 1991;33:218–220.

Maycock EJ, Russell WC. Anaphylactoid reaction to syntocinon. Anaesth Intensive Care 1993;21:211–212.

Moneret-Vautrin DA, Laxenaire MC. Anaphylactic and anaphylactoid reactions. Clinical presentation. Clin Rev Allergy 1991;91:249–258.

Moneret-Vautrin DA, Laxenaire MC, Bavoux F. Allergic shock to latex and ethylene oxide during surgery from spina bifida. Anesthesiology 1990;73:556–558.

Morriss WW, Lavies NG, Anderson SK, Southgate HJ. Acute respiratory distress during cesarean section under spinal anaesthesia. A probable case of anaphylactoid reaction to syntocinon. Anaesthesia 1994;49:41–43.

Moss J, Fahmy NR, Sunder N, Beaven MA. Hormonal and hemodynamic profile of an anaphylactic reaction in man. Circulation 1981;63:210–213.

Nguyen MT, Hoffman DR. Anaphylaxis to laminaria. J Allergy Clin Immunol 1995;95:138–139.

Nichols AW. Exercise-induced anaphylaxis and urticaria. Clin Sports Med 1992;11:303.

Nicklas RA. Sulfites: a review with emphasis on biochemistry and clinical application. Allergy Proc 1989;10:349–356.

Nicolas R, Villers D, Blanloeil Y. Hemodynamic pattern in anaphylactic shock with cardiac arrest. Crit Care Med 1984;12:144–145.

Nieto A, Estornell F, Mazoon A, et al. Allergy to latex in spina bifida: a multivariate study of associated factors. J Allergy Clin Immunol 1996;98:501–507.

Nutter AF. Contact urticaria to rubber. Br J Dermatol 1979;101:597–598.

Parker CW. Penicillin allergy. Ann Intern Med 1963;34:747.

Paull J. A prospective study of dextran-induced anaphylactoid reactions in 5745 patients. Anaesth Intensive Care 1987;15:163–167.

Porter BJ, Acharya U, Ormerod AD, Herriot R. Latex/chlorhexidine-induced anaphylaxis in pregnancy. Allergy 1998;53:455–457.

Portier P, Richet C. Del'l'action anaphylactique de certians venins. Crit Rev Soc Biol 1902;6:170.

Raper RF, Fisher MM. Profound reversible myocardial depression after anaphylaxis. Lancet 1988;i:386–388.

Ring J. Anaphylactoid reactions to intravenous solutions used for volume substitution. Clin Rev Allergy 1991;9:397–414.

Ring J, Messmer K. Incidence and severity of anaphylactoid reactions to colloid volume substitutes. Lancet 1977;1:466–469.

Roitt IM, Brostoff J, Male DK, eds. Immunology. St. Louis: Mosby: 1985.

Rudolph AH, Price EV. Penicillin reactions among patients in venereal disease clinics: a national survey. JAMA 1973;223:499–501.

Saxon A, Beall GN, Rohr AS, et al. Immediate hypersensitivity reaction to beta lactam antibiotics. Ann Intern Med 1987;107:204–215.

Shadick NA, Liang MH, Partridge AJ, et al. The natural history of exercise-induced anaphylaxis: survey results from a 10-year follow-up study. J Allergy Clin Immunol 1999;104:123–127.

Sheffer AL, Soter NA, McFadden ER. Exercise induced anaphylaxis: a distinct form of physical allergy. JAMA 1983;250:2049.

Sheffer AL, Austen KF. Exercise-induced anaphylaxis. J Allergy Clin Immunol 1984;73:699–703.

Sheffer AL, Tong AKF, Murphy GF, et al. Exercise-induced anaphylaxis: a serious form of physical allergy associated with mast cell degranulation. J Allergy Clin Immunol 1985;75:479–484.

Seigne R. Allergies and anaesthesia. Br J Anaesth 1997;78:778.

Silverman HJ, Van Hook C, Haponik EF. Hemodynamic changes in human anaphylaxis. Am J Med 1984;77:341–344.

Slater RM, Bowles BJM, Pumphrey RSH. Anaphylactoid reaction to oxytocin in pregnancy. Anaesthesia 1985;40:655–656.

Smith HS. Delivery as a cause of exercise-induced anaphylactoid reaction: case report. Br J Obstet Gynaecol 1985;92:1196–1198.

Songsiridej V, Busse WW. Exercise-induced anaphylaxis. Clin Allergy 1983;13:317–321.

Stafford CT, Lobel SA, Fruge BC, et al. Anaphylaxis to human serum albumin. Ann Allergy 1988;61:85–88.

Stannard L, Bellis A. Maternal anaphylactic reaction to a general anaesthetic at emergency caesarean section for fetal bradycardia. Br J Obstet Gynaecol 2001;108:539–540.

Swartz JS, Gold M, Braude BM, et al. Intraoperative anaphylaxis to latex: an identifiable population at risk. Can J Anaesth 1990;37:S131.

Tomazic VJ, Withrow TJ, Fisher BR, Dillard SF. Latex associated allergies and anaphylactic reactions. Clin Immunol Immunopathol 1992;64:89–97.

Turjanmaa K, Reunala T, Tuimala R, Karkkainen T. Allergy to latex gloves: unusual complication during delivery. Br Med J 1988;297: 1029.

Watkins J. Heuristic decision-making in diagnosis and management of adverse drug reactions in anaesthesia and surgery: the case of muscle relaxants. Theor Surg 1989;4:212.

Watkins J. Markers and mechanisms of anaphylactoid reactions. Clin Basic Aspects Monogr Allergy 1992;30:108.

Watkins J, Wild G. Problems of mediator measurement for a national advisory service to UK anesthetists. Agents Actions 1990;30:247–249.

Weese DL, Greenberg HM, Zimmern PE. Contrast media reactions during voiding cystourethrography or retrograde pyelography. Urology 1993;41:81–84.

Wendel GD, Stark RJ, Jamison RR, et al. Penicillin allergy and desensitization in serious infections during pregnancy. N Engl J Med 1985;312:1229–1232.

Wittbrodt ET, Spinler SA. Prevention of anaphylactoid reactions in high-risk patients receiving radiographic contrast media. Ann Pharmacother 1994;28:236–241.

Wong S, Dykewicz MS, Patterson R. Idiopathic anaphylaxis—a clinical summary of 175 patients. Arch Intern Med 1990;150:1323–1328.

Zenarola P. Rubber latex allergy: unusual complications during surgery. Contact Dermatitis 1989;21:197–198.

V Special considerations

42 Fetal considerations in the critically ill gravida

Jeffrey P. Phelan
Cortney Kirkendall
Shailen S. Shah

Unlike any other medical or surgical specialty, obstetrics deals with the simultaneous management of two—and sometimes more—individuals. Under all circumstances, the obstetrician must delicately balance the impact of each treatment decision on the pregnant woman and her fetus, seeking, when possible, to minimize the risks of harm to each. Throughout this text, the primary focus has been on the critically ill obstetric patient and, secondarily, her fetus. Although the fetal effects of those illnesses were reviewed in part, the goal of this chapter is to highlight, especially for the nonobstetric clinician, the important clinical fetal considerations encountered when caring for these complicated pregnancies. To achieve that objective, this chapter reviews: (i) current techniques for assessing fetal well-being; (ii) fetal considerations in several maternal medical and surgical conditions; and (iii) the role of perimortem cesarean delivery in modern obstetrics.

Detection of fetal distress in the critically ill obstetric patient

More than three decades ago, Hon and Quilligan (1968) demonstrated the relationship between certain fetal heart rate (FHR) patterns and fetal condition by using continuous electronic FHR monitoring. Since then, continuous electronic FHR monitoring has become a universally accepted method of assessing fetal well-being (Paul et al., 1980; Shenker et al., 1980), with the goal of permitting the clinician to promptly identify fetuses at a greater likelihood of fetal death and to intervene when certain FHR abnormalities are present.

Although the presence of a reassuring FHR tracing is virtually always associated with a well-perfused and oxygenated fetus (Phelan, 1994; Skupski et al., 2002), an "abnormal tracing" is not necessarily predictive of an adverse fetal outcome. While it was anticipated that the detection of abnormal FHR patterns during labor and expeditious delivery of such fetuses would impact the subsequent development of cerebral palsy, this expectation has not been realized. However, with the ubiquitous use of electronic FHR monitoring during labor and a rise in the cesarean delivery rate for the past two decades from 5% to over 25%, a decline in the rate of asphyxial induced cerebral palsy among singleton term infants has been observed (Rosen & Dickinson, 1992; Smith et al., 2000). The latter report (Smith et al., 2000) documented a 56% decline over two decades in the incidence of hypoxic ischemic encephalopathy (HIE) among singleton term infants from 1 per 8,000 to 1 per 12,5000 births.

While the specific entity of cerebral palsy is, in many cases, related to prenatal developmental events, infection, or complications of prematurity, the basic physiologic observations relating to specific FHR patterns remain, for the most part, valid. The critically ill mother will shunt blood from the splanchnic bed (including the uterus) in response to shock. Because of this and the fact that the fetus operates on the steep portion of the oxyhemoglobin dissociation curve, any degree of maternal hypoxia or hypoperfusion may first be manifested as an abnormality of the FHR. In this sense, the late second- and third-trimester fetus serves as a physiologic oximeter and cardiac output computer. Observation of FHR changes, thus, may assist or alert the clinician to subtle degrees of physiologic instability, which would be unimportant in a nonpregnant adult but may have potentially detrimental effects to the fetus (Clark, 1990).

The next few pages present an overview of FHR patterns pertinent to the critically ill gravida. Interpretation of FHR patterns, like all diagnostic tests, depend on the index population, and consequently, certain of these observations may not generally apply to the laboring but otherwise well mother. For a more detailed description of antepartum and intrapartum FHR tracings associated with fetal brain injury the reader is referred to the classic descriptions by Phelan and Ahn (1994, 1998) and Phelan and Kim (2000).

Baseline fetal heart rate

The baseline FHR is the intrinsic heart rate of the fetus. A normal baseline FHR is between 110 beats per minute (bpm) and

160 bpm. A baseline FHR less than 110 bpm is termed a bradycardia, and 160 bpm or higher is considered a tachycardia.

Bradycardia

Bradycardia is defined as the intrinsic heart rate of the fetus of less than 110 bpm, as opposed to a prolonged FHR deceleration which is a drop in the rate to 60 bpm, for example, from a previously normal or tachycardic rate. As such, a FHR bradycardia can be associated with an underlying congenital fetal abnormality, such as a structural defect of the fetal heart. In addition, congenital bradyarrhythmias may involve fetal heart block secondary to a prior maternal infection, a structural defect of the fetal heart, or systemic lupus erythematosus with anti-Ro/SS-A antibodies (Lockshin et al., 1988). In these circumstances, the FHR bradycardia is not usually a threat to the fetus. But, alternative methods of fetal assessment, such as the fetal biophysical profile (FBP) (Manning et al., 1980), are necessary in this select group of patients to assure fetal well-being prior to and during labor.

Prolonged fetal heart rate deceleration

Prolonged FHR deceleration is distinctly different from a bradycardia. In the former, the fetal monitor strip is typically reactive with a normal or tachycardic baseline rate; but, due to a sentinel event, such as those depicted in Table 42.1, the FHR suddenly drops and remains at a lower level unresponsive to remedial measures and terbutaline therapy. In the critically ill obstetric patient with underlying hypertension, a prolonged FHR deceleration may arise from a partial or complete abruption or an aggressive lowering of maternal BP with antihypertensive agents (Rigg & McDonough, 1981). Additionally, an acute, prolonged FHR deceleration may herald sudden maternal hypoxia in conditions such as amniotic fluid embolus syndrome (Clark et al., 1995), acute respiratory insufficiency, or an eclamptic seizure (Paul et al., 1978). These decelerations have also been described during operative procedures such as cardiopulmonary bypass with inadequate maternal flow rates (Koh et al., 1975; Korsten et al., 1989), and brain surgery during hypothermia (Strange & Malldin, 1983).

In a patient with a prior normal baseline FHR, the abrupt occurrence and persistence of a fetal heart rate of less than 110 bpm for an extended period of time unresponsive to remedial measures and terbutaline therapy constitutes an obstetric emergency. Under these circumstances, and assuming the pregnant woman is hemodynamically stable and the fetus is potentially viable, these patients should be managed as if the fetus has had a cardiac arrest and be delivered as rapidly as it is technically feasible for the level of the institution.

Table 42.1 Sentinel events associated with a reactive fetal admission test and a subsequent prolonged FHR deceleration 60 bpm unresponsive to remedial measures, terbutaline therapy and lasting until delivery

Umbilical cord prolapse
Uterine rupture
Placental abruption
Maternal arrest, e.g. AFE syndrome
Fetal exsanguination

Tachycardia

Fetal tachycardia is defined as a baseline FHR of 160 bpm or greater. Most commonly, this type of baseline FHR abnormality is associated with prematurity, maternal pyrexia, or chorioamnionitis. In addition, betamimetic administration, hyperthyroidism, or fetal cardiac arrhythmias may also be responsible. The clinical observation of a FHR tachycardia, in and of itself, is probably not an ominous finding but probably reflects a normal physiologic adjustment to an underlying maternal or fetal condition. Although operative intervention is rarely required, a search for the underlying basis for the tachycardia and a review of the admission FHR pattern may be helpful.

For example, the patient with a previously reactive FHR pattern with a normal baseline rate (Fig. 42.1) who develops a substantial rise in the baseline rate often to a level of tachycardia (Figs 42.2, 42.3) in association with a loss of accelerations or nonreactivity, repetitive FHR decelerations, with or without a loss FHR variability is at risk for hypoxic ischemic brain injury (Phelan & Ahn, 1994, 1998; Phelan et al., 2001). As before, assessment of the usual causes of FHR tachycardia should be undertaken. If the mother does not have a fever to account for the change in fetal status, assessment of fetal acid–base status with scalp or acoustic stimulation (Phelan & Kim, 2000; Skupski et al., 2002) or delivery as soon as it is practical, in keeping with capability of the hospital, should be considered. If the gravida has a fever, she should be cultured, and treated with antibiotics and antipyretics. If the FHR pattern does not return to normal, i.e. normal baseline FHR and reactive, within approximately an hour of the initiation of medical therapy and regardless of whether the FHRV is average (Phelan & Ahn, 1998; Kim et al., 2000), the patient should be delivered as expeditiously as possible.

Fetal heart rate variability

Fetal heart rate variability (FHRV) is defined as the beat-to-beat variation in the FHR resulting from the continuous interaction of the parasympathetic and sympathetic nervous systems on the fetal heart. For clinical purposes, normal FHRV may be viewed as a beat-to-beat variation of the FHR of 6 bpm or more above and below the baseline FHR.

Decreased FHRV, in and of itself, is not an ominous observation. In most cases, the diminished FHRV represents normal

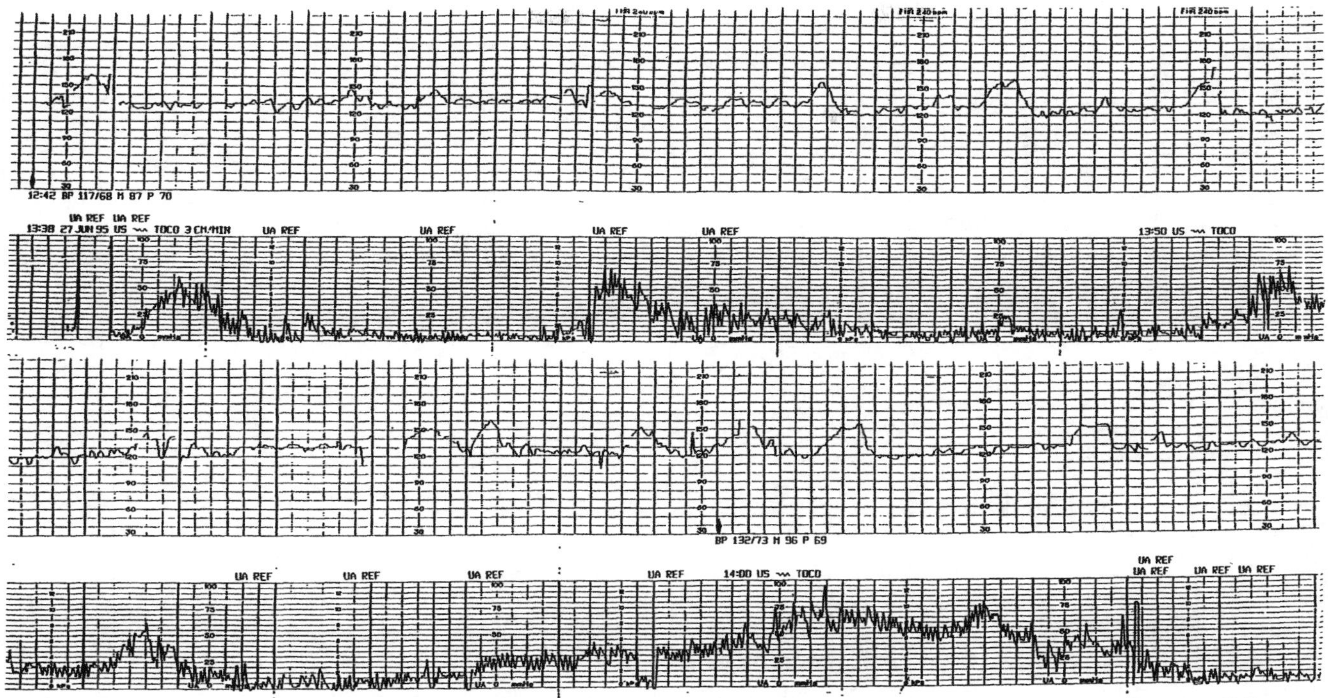

Fig. 42.1 Admission FHR of this term pregnancy with spontaneously ruptured membranes exhibits a baseline rate around 120 bpm and numerous FHR accelerations or a reactive FHR pattern.

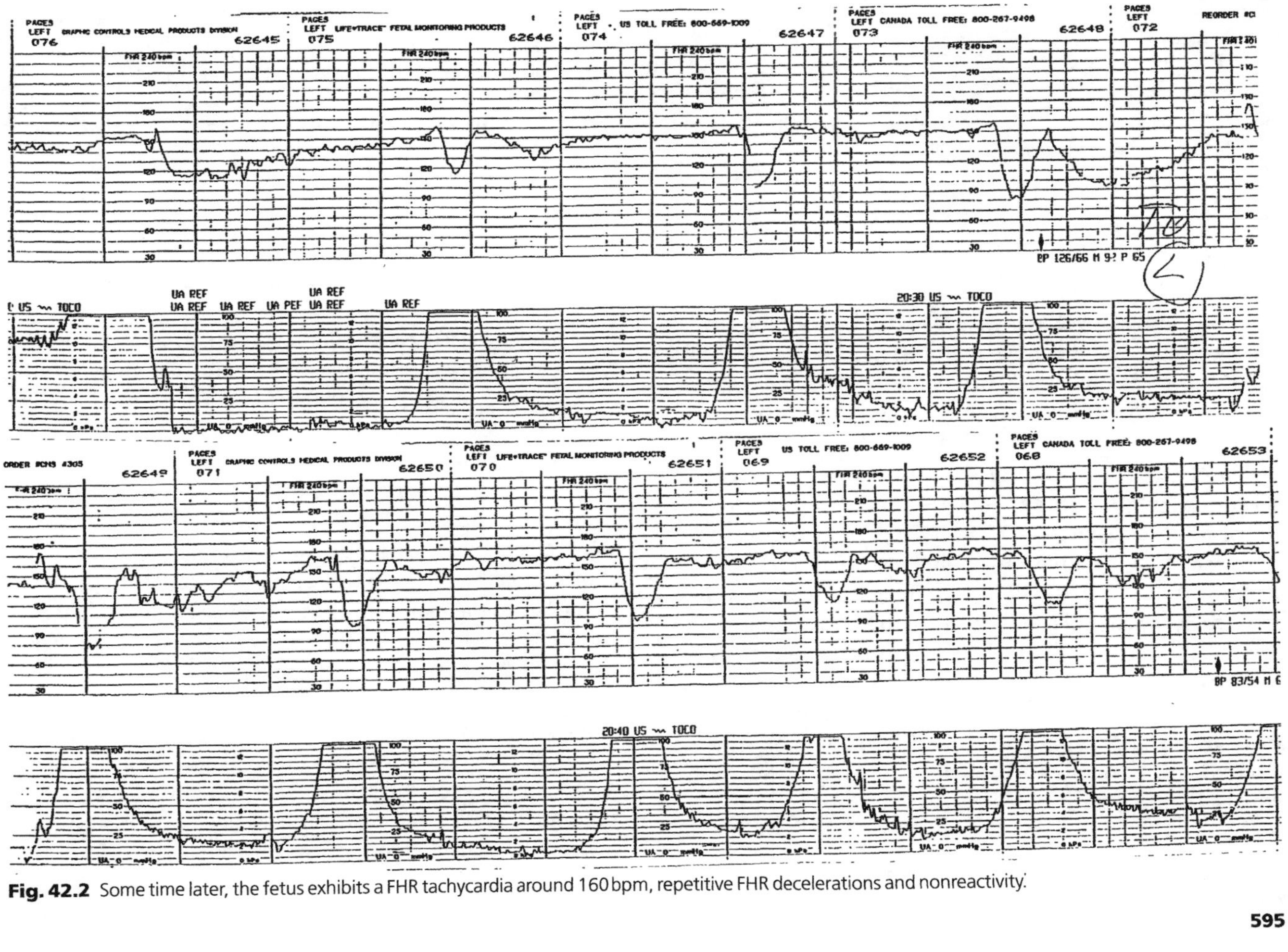

Fig. 42.2 Some time later, the fetus exhibits a FHR tachycardia around 160 bpm, repetitive FHR decelerations and nonreactivity.

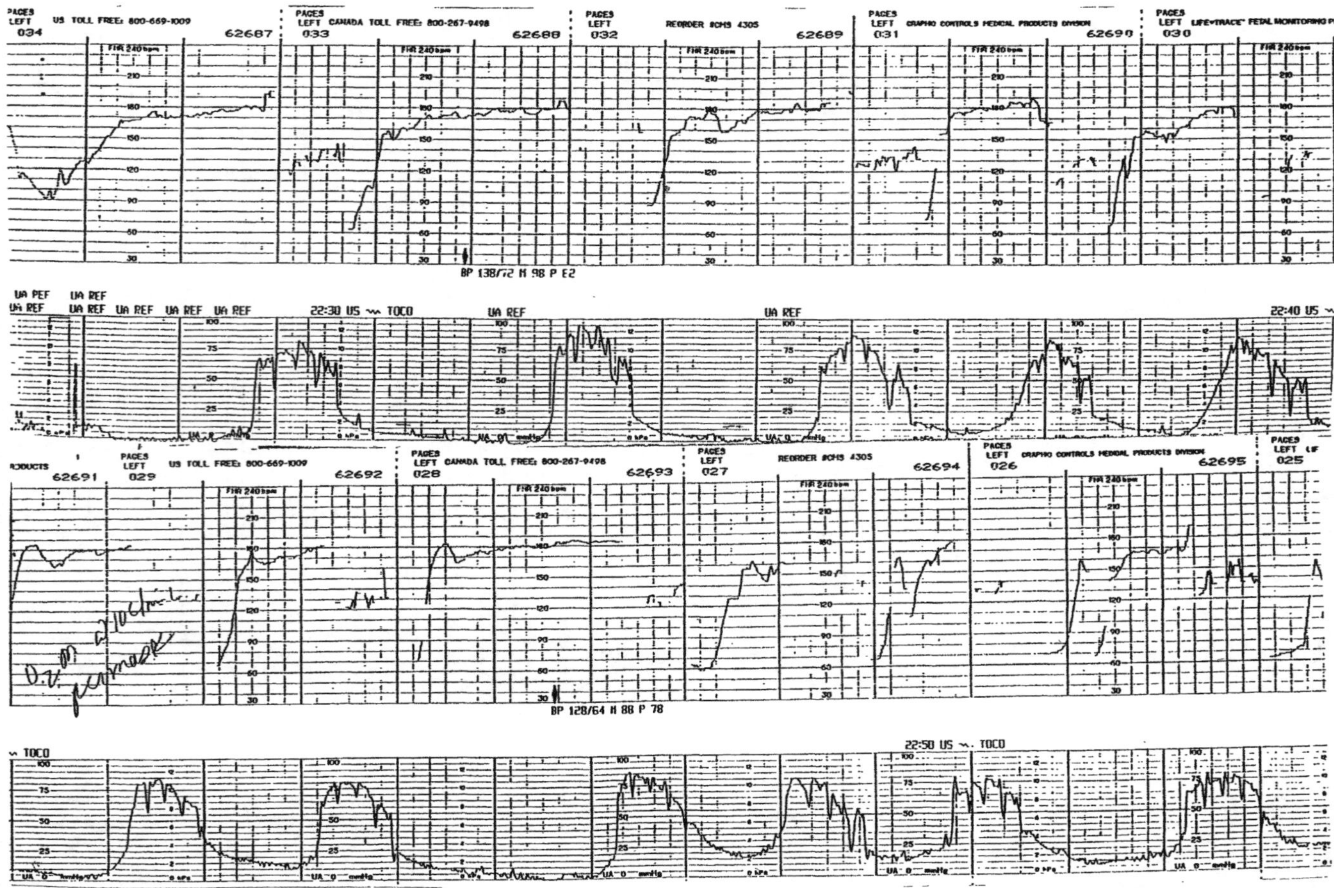

Fig. 42.3 Later in the labor, the baseline FHR reaches 180 bpm and continues to exhibit repetitive FHR decelerations, nonreactivity, and diminished variability. The fetus was born with hypoxic ischemic encephalopathy.

fetal physiologic adjustments to a number of medications, illicit substances or simply behavioral state changes such as 1F to 4F (Smith, 1994). For example, narcotic administration (Petrie et al., 1978) or magnesium sulfate infusion (Babakania & Niebyl, 1978) can alter FHRV by inducing a change in the behavioral state of the fetus to one of a sleep state or behavioral state 1F. Clinically, diminished FHRV appears to have meaning solely in the Hon pattern of intrapartum asphyxia (Phelan & Ahn, 1994, 1998; Phelan & Kim, 2000; Phelan et al., 2001). As observed herein (Figs 42.1, 42.2, 42.3), the FHR pattern was first reactive and exhibited a normal baseline rate. Subsequently, the FHR pattern changed. Then, the diminished FHRV was associated with a loss of FHR reactivity, a substantial rise in the baseline FHR, a FHR tachycardia, and repetitive FHR decelerations. Under these circumstances, the potential for fetal asphyxia is increased. Additionally, HIE, in this circumstance of diminished FHRV (Kim et al., 2000), is associated with significantly higher rates of neonatal cerebral edema.

Sinusoidal fetal heart rate pattern

A sinusoidal FHR pattern is defined as a persistent regular sine wave variation of the baseline FHR that has a frequency of 3–6 cycles per minute (Clark & Miller, 1984). The degree of oscillation correlates with fetal outcome (Katz et al., 1984). For instance, infants with oscillations of 25 bpm or more have a significantly greater perinatal mortality rate than do infants whose oscillations are less than 25 bpm (67% vs 1%). A favorable fetal outcome also is associated with the presence of FHR accelerations and/or nonpersistent sinusoidal FHR pattern.

The key to the management of a persistent sinusoidal FHR pattern is recognition. Once this FHR pattern is identified, a search for the underlying cause should be undertaken. Nonpersistent or an intermittent sinusoidal FHR pattern is commonly related to maternal narcotic administration (Epstein et al., 1982; Modanlou & Freeman, 1982). In the absence of maternal narcotic administration, the presence of a persistent sinusoidal FHR pattern and a lack of FHR accelerations suggests the potential for fetal anemia.

Fetal anemia may be associated with a number of obstetric conditions such as placental abruption or previa, fetomaternal hemorrhage, vasa previa, Rh sensitization, and nonimmune hydrops (Modanlou & Freeman, 1982). If, for example, a persistent sinusoidal FHR pattern is observed in a patient who recently has been involved in a motor vehicle accident, placental abruption is one consideration. Evidence of an abruption or other forms of fetal hemorrhage may also be suggested by a positive Kleihauer-Betke test for fetal RBCs in the maternal circulation. Finally, as suggested by Katz and associates (1984), a persistent sinusoidal FHR pattern in the absence of accelerations is a sign of potential fetal compromise. In this latter circumstance, a Kleihauer-Betke test with either delivery or some form of fetal acid–base assessment with scalp or acoustic stimulation should be considered (Theard et al., 1984; Kirhendall et al., 2001). Often, patients with a persistent sinusoidal FHR pattern will have a history of reduced fetal activity and, occasionally, an abnormal Kleihauer-Betke test (Kosasa et al., 1993; Kirkendall et al., 2001).

Periodic changes

The focus of this section is on periodic changes such as FHR accelerations and variable and late decelerations. FHR decelerations, in and of themselves, are not associated with an increased risk of perinatal morbidity and mortality (Phelan & Ahn, 1994, 1998; Phelan et al., 2001).

Accelerations

A FHR acceleration is defined as an abrupt increase in the FHR above baseline, spontaneously or in relation to uterine activity, fetal body movement, or fetal breathing. Criteria for FHR accelerations (i.e. a "reactive" tracing) include a rise in the FHR of at least 15 bpm from baseline, lasting at least 15 seconds from the time it leaves baseline until it returns (Phelan, 1994). Since the acceleration does not need to remain at 15 bpm or higher for 15 seconds, accelerations are in the form of a triangle rather than a rectangle. Whenever spontaneous or induced FHR accelerations are present, a healthy and nonacidotic fetus is present. This is true, regardless of whether otherwise "worrisome" features of the FHR tracing are present (Shaw & Clark, 1988; Phelan, 1994; Skupski et al., 2002). The presence of FHR accelerations is the basis to assess fetal well-being both antepartum and during labor (Phelan, 1994; Skupski et al., 2002).

The presence of FHR accelerations is a sign of fetal well-being with a low probability of fetal compromise (Phelan, 1994), brain damage (Ahn et al., 1998b), or death within several days to a week of fetal surveillance testing (Phelan, 1994). This observation persists irrespective of whether the acceleration is spontaneous or induced (Phelan, 1994). In contrast, the findings of a persistent nonreactive FHR pattern lasting longer than 120 minutes from admission to the hospital or the physician's office is a sign of preexisting compromise due to a preadmission to the hospital or pre-NST fetal brain injury (Phelan & Ahn, 1994, 1998; Phelan et al., 2001), structural (Garite et al., 1979) or chromosomal abnormality (Slomka & Phelan, 1981), fetal infection due to cytomegalovirus or toxoplasmosis (Phelan & Smith, 1989), or maternal substance abuse.

Briefly, the clinical approach to assessing fetal health begins with monitoring the baseline FHR for a reasonable period to determine the presence of FHR accelerations or reactivity. If the NST is considered nonreactive after a 40-minute monitoring period, several options are available to the clinician. These include, but are not limited to the following: to continue fetal monitoring, a contraction stress test, fetal biophysical profile, or some form of fetal stimulation. If, after acoustic stimulation, the fetus has a persistent nonreactive pattern, a contraction stress test (Phelan & Smith, 1989) or the FBP (Manning et al., 1980, 1990; Phelan, 1988) can be used to evaluate fetal status.

In the critical care setting, the FBP (Table 42.2) is the easiest approach to use after fetal monitoring. Since the introduction of the FBP, this technique has been modified to include the amniotic fluid index to estimate the amniotic fluid volume (Phelan et al., 1987a, b; Rutherford, 1987). Based on the work of Phelan and associates (1987a, b, 1994), an amniotic fluid index (AFI) of ≤5.0 cm is considered oligohydramnios. Consequently, if a patient has an AFI ≤5.0 cm, her FBP score for that component will be 0. Additional components of the FBP include fetal breathing movements, fetal limb movements, fetal tone, and reactivity on an NST. Based on the presence or absence of each component, the patient receives 0 or 2 points.

An FBP score of 8 or 10 is considered normal. In patients whose score is 6, the test is considered equivocal or suspicious. In such patients, a repeat FBP is recommended in 12–24 hours. If the patient is considered to be term, she should be evaluated for delivery (Phelan, 1988). The patient with a biophysical pro-

Table 42.2 Fetal biophysical profile (FBP) components required over a 30-minute period*

Components	Normal result	Score
Nonstress test	Reactive	2
Fetal breathing movements	Duration ≥1 min	2
Fetal movement	≥3 movements	2
Fetal tone	Flexion and extension of limb	2
Amniotic fluid volume	Amniotic fluid index >5.0 cm	2
Maximum score		10

Components of the FBP (Phelan & Lewis, 1981), which includes the modification for determining the amniotic fluid volume using the amniotic fluid index (Phelan, 1987a,b 1988).

* This represents one approach to the FBP.

file score of 0, 2, or 4 is considered for delivery; but this FBP score does not mandate a cesarean. A trial of labor is reasonable whenever the cervix is favorable for induction, the amniotic fluid volume is normal (AFI > 5.0 cm) and the fetus is not growth impaired.

Variable decelerations

Variable FHR decelerations have a variable or non-uniform shape and bear no consistent relationship to a uterine contraction. In general, the decline in rate is rapid and is followed by a quick recovery. Umbilical cord compression leading to an increased fetal BP and baroreceptor response is felt to be the most likely etiology. Umbilical cord compression is more likely to occur in circumstances of nuchal cords, knots, cord prolapse (Phelan & Lewis, 1981), or a diminished amniotic fluid volume (Gabbe et al., 1976; Phelan, 1989).

To simplify intrapartum management, investigators such as Kubli et al. (1969) and Krebs et al. (1983) have attempted to classify variable decelerations. For example, Kubli and associates have correlated fetal outcome with mild, moderate, or severe variable decelerations. Kubli's criteria, however, are cumbersome and do not lend themselves to easy clinical use. In contrast, Krebs et al. (1983) criteria rely on the visual characteristics of the variable decelerations rather than on the degree or amplitude of the FHR deceleration. Krebs has shown that when repetitive, atypical variable decelerations (Fig. 42.4) are present over a prolonged period in a patient with a previously normal FHR tracing, the risk of low Apgars is increased. Atypical variables, in and of themselves, are clinically insignificant.

However, these atypical features in the circumstance of a Hon pattern of intrapartum asphyxia (Phelan & Ahn, 1994a, 1998a; Phelan et al., 2001; Greenberg et al., 2001) can be associated with fetal brain injury. When persistent, atypical variable FHR decelerations arise in association with a substantial rise in the baseline FHR to a level of tachycardia, an absence of FHR accelerations or nonreactivity and with or without a loss of FHRV, expeditious delivery should be considered.

Late decelerations

Late decelerations are a uniform deceleration pattern with onset at the peak of the uterine contraction, the nadir in heart rate at the offset of the uterine contraction, and a delayed return to baseline. To be clinically significant, late decelerations must be repetitive (i.e. occur with each contraction of similar

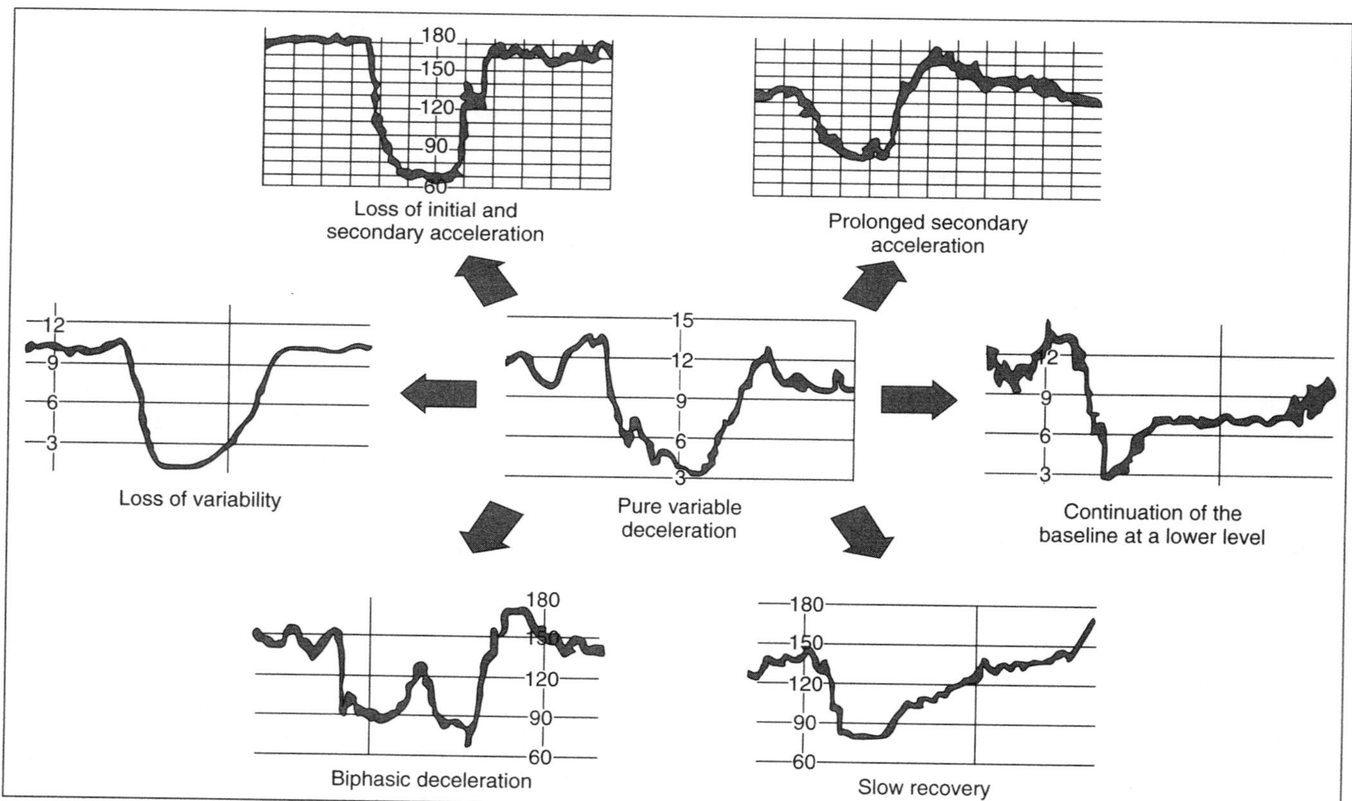

Fig. 42.4 Atypical variable FHR decelerations. (From Krebs HB, Peters RE, Dunn LH. Intrapartum fetal heart rate monitoring. VII. Atypical variable decelerations. Am J Obstet Gynecol 1983;145:305–310. Reproduced with permission from CV Mosby Co, St. Louis, MO.)

magnitude, and be associated with a substantial rise in baseline FHR, a loss of reactivity, with or without a loss of FHRV (Phelan & Ahn, 1994a, 1998b; Phelan et al., 2001). Nonpersistent or intermittent late decelerations are probably variables, and consequently, appear to have no bearing on fetal outcome (Nelson, 1996). In fact, Nelson and associates (1996) found that 99.7% of late decelerations observed on a fetal monitor strip were associated with favorable fetal outcome.

Whenever a patient with a reactive admission FHR pattern develops repetitive late decelerations in association with a fetal tachycardia and a loss of reactivity, traditional maneuvers of intrauterine resuscitation such as maternal repositioning, oxygen administration, and increased intravenous fluids are warranted. If this pattern persists, assessment of the fetal ability to accelerate its heart rate (Phelan, 1994; Skupski et al., 2002) or delivery should be considered.

In the critical care setting reversible, late decelerations can be seen in a number of settings such as diabetic ketoacidosis (LoBue & Goodlin, 1978; Rhodes & Ogburn, 1984), sickle cell crisis (Cruz et al., 1979), or anaphylaxis (Witter & Niebyl, 1983; Klein et al., 1984; Dunn et al., 1999; Stannard & Bellis, 2001). With correction of the underlying maternal metabolic abnormality, the FHR abnormality usually will resolve, and operative intervention is often unnecessary. Persistence of the FHR pattern after maternal metabolic recovery, however, may suggest an underlying fetal diabetic cardiomyopathy (Sheehan et al., 1986) or preexisting fetal compromise (Phelan & Ahn, 1994, 1998; Greenberg et al., 2001; Phelan et al., 2001) and should, when accompanied by the aformentioned additional signs of fetal compromise, lead to assessment for fetal reactivity or delivery.

Fetal acid–base assessment

Fetal acid–base assessment has no role in the contemporary practice of obstetrics. In the past, fetal acid–base status was thought to be an important part of labor management. This practice stemmed from the work of Saling (1964). In that work, Saling found that infants with a pH less than 7.2 were more likely to be delivered physiologically depressed. Conversely, a normal fetal outcome was more likely to be associated with a nonacidotic fetus (pH ≥ 7.20) (Saling & Schneider, 1967). Even at the peak of its popularity, fetal scalp blood sampling was used in a limited number of pregnancies (~3%) (Clark & Paul, 1985). Notwithstanding, Goodwin and associates (1994) recently concluded that fetal scalp blood sampling "... has been virtually eliminated without an increase in the cesarean rate for fetal distress or an increase in indicators of perinatal asphyxia. [Its continued role] in clinical practice is questioned."

If the clinical circumstances suggest the need for fetal acid–base assessment and the clinician is concerned about fetal status, the clinician should look alternatively for the presence of FHR accelerations. In key studies, Phelan (1994) and Skupski and colleagues (2002) have demonstrated with labor stimulation tests such as scalp or acoustic stimulation, that FHR accelerations were associated with a significantly greater likelihood of normal fetal acid–base status and a favorable fetal outcome. If the fetus fails to respond to the sound or scalp stimulation, delivery should be considered.

As with fetal scalp blood sampling, umbilical cord blood gas data do not appear to be useful in predicting long-term neurologic impairment. It is interesting to note that of 314 infants with severe umbilical artery acidosis identified in the world literature, 27 (8.6%) children were subsequently found to be brain damaged (Kirkendall & Phelan, 2001). In the Fee study (1990), for example, minor developmental delays or mild tone abnormalities were noted at the time of hospital discharge in 9 of 110 (8%) singleton term infants. When 108 of these infants were seen on long-term follow-up, all were considered neurologically normal, and none of these infants, which included a neonate with an umbilical artery pH of 6.57 at birth, demonstrated major motor or cognitive abnormality. In contrast, the neonatal outcomes for 113 infants in the Goodwin study (1992) were known. Of these, 98 (87%) had normal outcomes. In the remaining 15 infants with known outcomes, five neonates died and 10 infants were brain damaged. Of interest, Dennis and colleagues (1989) commented in their series of patients that "the very acidotic children did not perform worse than [the nonacidotic children]. Thus, the finding of severe fetal acidosis on an umbilical artery cord gas does not appear to be linked to subsequent neurologic deficits."

In contrast, the absence of severe acidosis does not ensure a favorable neurologic outcome. For example, Korst and associates (1997, 1999b) had previously shown that neonates with sufficient intrapartum asphyxia to produce persistent brain injury did not have to sustain severe acidosis (umbilical arterial pH ≤ 7.00). When her two studies are combined, 42 (60%) fetuses did not have severe acidosis, and all were neurologically impaired. Of 94 infants with reported permanent brain damage, Dennis and associates (1989) also noted that children without acidosis appeared to fare worse than acidotic children. Thus, it appears that factors other than the presence of severe acidosis are probably responsible for fetal brain injury.

It is interesting to note that severe acidosis may not be a proper endpoint to study intrapartum asphyxia (Garite et al., 2000) nor to define whether a fetus has sustained intrapartum brain damage (ACOG, 1992; MacLennan, 1999). These findings suggest that the pathophysiologic mechanisms responsible for fetal brain damage appear to operate independently of fetal acid/base status and to be more likely related to the adequacy of cerebral perfusion (Phelan & Kim, 2000). Thus, umbilical cord blood gases as with fetal scalp blood sampling to define brain damage or the quality of care may not have a role in the contemporary practice of obstetrics.

FHR patterns in the brain damaged infant

Term infants found to be brain damaged do not manifest a uniform FHR pattern (Phelan & Ahn, 1994, 1998; Phelan & Kim, 2000; Greenberg et al., 2001; Phelan et al., 2001). However, these fetuses do manifest distinct FHR patterns intrapartum that can be easily categorized and identified based on the admission FHR pattern and subsequent changes in the baseline rate.

Reactive admission test and subsequent fetal brain damage

When a pregnant woman is admitted to hospital, the overwhelming number of obstetric patients will have a reactive FHR pattern. Of these, more than 98% will go through labor uneventfully and most will deliver vaginally. In the few patients (typically 1–2%) that develop intrapartum "fetal distress" (Krebs et al., 1982; Ingemarsson et al., 1986), the characteristic "fetal distress" is usually, but not always, acute and manifested by a sudden prolonged FHR deceleration that is unresponsive to remedial measures and terbutaline therapy and lasts until delivery. Of these, an even smaller number of fetuses will ultimately experience a CNS injury. So, while unusual, fetal brain injury in the fetus with a reactive fetal admission test may arise, in the absence of trauma, as a result of a sudden prolonged FHR deceleration or a Hon pattern of intrapartum asphyxia.

Acute fetal brain injury

In this group (Table 42.1) the FHR pattern is reactive on admission, and, as a result of a sudden catastrophic event, a sudden prolonged FHR deceleration to approximately 60 bpm occurs and lasts until the time of delivery. This FHR deceleration is unresponsive to remedial measures and subcutaneous or intravenous terbutaline. The CNS injury in this group is primarily located in the basal ganglia and thalami (Myers, 1972; Roland et al., 1998; Phelan et al., 2001) and is due to sudden and prolonged reductions in fetal cardiac output (Myers, 1972; Roland et al., 1998; Phelan et al., 2001). The prolonged FHR decelerations is associated with a wide array of patient groups (Table 42.1) such as uterine rupture, placental abruption, and cord prolapse. Given the acute nature of this FHR pattern, limited time is available to preserve normal CNS function.

Time as it relates to fetal neurologic injury in this group is a function of multiple factors (Table 42.3). Each variable plays a role in determining the length of time required to sustain fetal brain damage. For example, the admission FHR pattern provides an indicator of fetal status prior to the catastrophic event. If, for example, the FHR pattern is reactive with a normal baseline rate and a sudden prolonged FHR deceleration occurs, the window to fetal brain injury will be longer than in the patient with a tachycardic baseline (Leung et al., 1993). As with the baseline rate, the other variables also play a role. But, it is not within the scope of this chapter to detail this information. The reader is referred to the work of Phelan and Kim (2000). Regardless, our experience (Phelan & Ahn, 1994, 1998; Phelan et al., 2001) would suggest an even shorter time to neurologic injury of 16 minutes or less whenever the placenta has completely separated. If the placenta remains intact, a longer period of time appears to be available before the onset of CNS injury. Thus, the intactness of the placenta plays a pivotal role in determining fetal outcome.

Hon pattern of asphyxia

The Hon pattern of intrapartum asphyxia (Figs 42.1, 42.2, 42.3) is uniquely different and evolves over a period of time (Phelan & Ahn, 1994, 1998; Phelan & Kim, 2000; Greenberg et al., 2001; Phelan et al., 2001). This FHR pattern begins with a reactive fetal admission test. Subsequently during labor, the fetus develops a nonreactive FHR pattern or loses its ability to accelerate its heart rate (Phelan & Ahn, 1994, 1998; Phelan et al., 2001). As the labor continues, a substantial rise in baseline heart rate from admission (135 ± 10 bpm) to a mean maximum (186 ± 15 bpm) baseline heart rate is seen (Phelan & Ahn, 1998). The maximum FHR ranged from 155 bpm to 220 bpm. This constituted a 39 ± 13% mean percent rise in baseline heart rate from admission and ranged from 17% to 82% (Phelan & Ahn, 1998). This rise in baseline FHR is usually not accompanied by maternal pyrexia. When a substantial rise in baseline FHR is encountered, the FHR pattern is also associated with repetitive FHR decelerations but not necessarily late decelerations and ultimately a loss of FHR variability (Phelan & Ahn, 1994, 1998; Greenberg et al., 2001; Phelan et al., 2001). "As labor progresses and the fetus nears death, the slopes become progressively less steep until the FHR does not return to its baseline rate and ultimately terminates in a profound bradycardia" (Hon & Lee, 1963) or a stairsteps-to-death pattern (Phelan & Ahn, 1994, 1998; Golditch et al., 1998; Phelan et al.,

Table 42.3 Five factors useful in determining the timing of fetal brain injury in the situation of a reactive admission test followed by a catastrophic event resulting in a sudden prolonged FHR deceleration to 60 bpm and lasting until delivery

Prior FHR pattern
Fetal growth pattern
Degree of fetal vasoconstriction
Duration of the FHR deceleration
Intactness of the placenta

FHR, fetal heart rate.
(Reproduced by permission from Phelan, JP, Kim, JO. Fetal heart rate observations in the brain-damaged infant. Semin Perinatal 2000;24:221–229.)

2001). Once a FHR tachycardia begins, the subsequent FHR pattern (Phelan & Ahn, 1998) does one of the following: (i) the FHR pattern remains tachycardic and/or continues to rise until delivery; (ii) a prolonged FHR deceleration that lasts until delivery occurs; or (iii) a stairsteps-to-death pattern or a progressive bradycardia are seen. Of particular clinical relevance is that all patients manifested a substantial rise in their baseline heart rates, lost their ability to generate FHR accelerations, became nonreactive and exhibited repetitive FHR decelerations. Of note, the repetitive FHR decelerations were not necessarily late decelerations and were frequently variable decelerations (Phelan & Ahn, 1994, 1998; Phelan et al., 2001).

In this group, FHR variability does not appear to be a reliable indicator of fetal status (Phelan & Ahn, 1998). For example, many brain damaged fetuses, upwards of 30%, exhibited average FHR variability at the time of their deliveries (Phelan & Ahn, 1998). In the neonatal period, brain damaged fetuses who had the Hon pattern of intrapartum asphyxia with average FHR variability had significantly less cerebral edema (Kim et al., 2000). Kim's cerebral edema (Kim et al., 2000) findings suggest that the use of diminished FHR variability as an endpoint for the Hon pattern of intrapartum asphyxia to decide the timing of operative intervention is probably not reasonable. This means that prior to a loss of FHR variability, the fetal brain has already been injured but is unlikely to develop cerebral edema.

The primary pathophysiologic mechanism responsible for the Hon and the persistent nonreactive patterns appears to be progressive fetal vasoconstriction (Fig. 42.5) and ultimately ischemia (Phelan & Kim, 2000). As stated previously the triggering mechanism may be meconium (Altschuler & Hyde, 1989; Altschuler et al., 1992) or infection (Yoon et al., 1995; Perlman et al., 1996) but is not uterine contractions (Phelan & Ahn, 1994). The resultant vasoconstriction or intrafetal shunting probably results in impaired renal perfusion and oligohydramnios. This is probably one explanation why amniotic fluid volume assessment in combination with a NST (Phelan, 1988, 1994) or biophysical profile (Manning et al., 1990) accounts for the reported reduction in cerebral palsy (Manning et al., 1998). Nevertheless, once the fetus develops ischemia or is unable to perfuse its brain cells, cellular hypoxia or injury occurs. Thus, the hypoxia encountered in the fetus is cellular rather than systemic. By the time fetal systemic hypoxia develops, the fetus, in our opinion, has already been brain injured and is probably near death (Phelan & Kim, 2000). Thus, cerebral perfusion deficits due to intrafetal and intracerebral shunting rather than fetal systemic hypoxia are most likely responsible for fetal brain injury (Visser et al., 2001).

This means, for example, that a fetus who develops the Hon pattern of intrapartum asphyxia would appear to move to ischemia or from point C to point D (Fig. 42.5). During this transition, a progressive and substantial rise in FHR is observed in an effort to preserve cerebral perfusion and cellular oxygenation. At the same time, fetal systemic oxygenation and oxygen saturation is maintained. In our opinion (Phelan & Kim, 2000), only after progressive and prolonged ischemia and brain injury do central fetal oxygen saturations begin to fall.

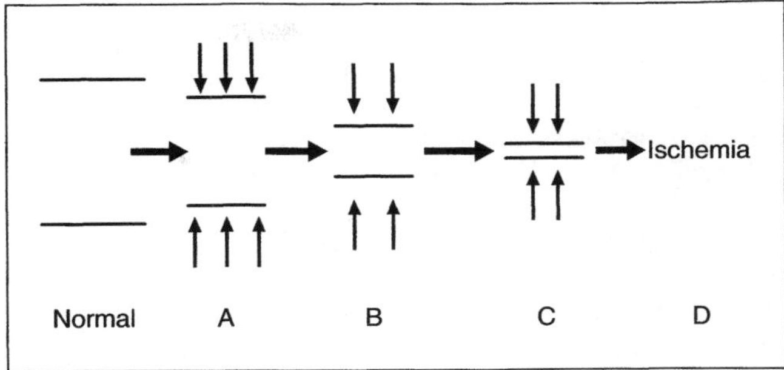

Fig. 42.5 Persistent fetal vasonconstriction over time or intrafetal shunting leads to progressive narrowing of the fetal vascular tree leading ultimately to ischemia.

The persistent nonreactive FHR pattern

The persistent nonreactive FHR pattern from admission to the hospital or a nonstress test accounts for 45% of the FHR patterns observed in a population of 300 brain damaged babies (Phelan & Ahn, 1998) and 33% of an updated population of 423 singleton term brain damaged children (Phelan et al., 2001). This population is typically, but not always characterized by the presence of reduced fetal activity prior to admission to the hospital, male fetuses, old meconium, meconium sequelae such as meconium aspiration syndrome and persistent pulmonary hypertension, and oligohydramnios (Phelan & Ahn, 1994). Along with these observations, these fetuses usually but not always have elevated nucleated red blood cell counts (Phelan et al., 1995; Korst et al., 1996; Phelan et al., 1998a; Blackwell et al., 2000), prolonged NRBC clearance times (Phelan et al., 1995; Korst et al., 1996; Phelan et al., 1998a), low initial platelet counts (Korst et al., 1999a), multiorgan system dysfunction (Korst et al., 1997, 1999b; Phelan, 1998b), delayed onset of seizures from birth (Ahn, 1998a; Kirkendall et al., 2000), and cortical or hemispheric brain injuries (Phelan et al., 2001). The typical FHR pattern is nonreactive with a fixed baseline rate that normally does not change from admission until delivery (Phelan & Ahn, 1994, 1998; Phelan & Kim, 2000; Phelan et al., 2001) in association with diminished or average variability.

When looking at the admission FHR pattern, the persistent nonreactive FHR pattern group can be divided into three phases (Table 42.4). These three phases, in our opinion, represent a post-CNS insult compensatory response in the fetus. Moreover, this FHR pattern, in our opinion, does not represent ongoing asphyxia or worsening of the CNS injury (Phelan & Ahn, 1994, 1998; Phelan et al., 2001). For a fetus to have ongoing fetal asphyxia, a FHR pattern similar to the Hon pattern of intrapartum asphyxia would have to be seen. There (Figs 42.1,

Table 42.4 Fetuses with preadmission central nervous system injury exhibit a persistent nonreactive FHR pattern intrapartum and can be divided into three phases based on the baseline FHR and the FHR variability

Phase	Baseline rate (bpm)	Variability	Incidence (%)
I	>160	Diminished	19
II	110–160	Diminished	39
III	110–160	Average	43

(Reproduced by permission from Phelan, JP, Ahn, MO. Fetal heart rate observations in 300 term brain damaged infants. J Mat Fetal Invest 1998;8:1–5.)

42.2, 42.3), a progressive and substantial rise in baseline heart rate in association with repetitive FHR decelerations is observed in response to ongoing fetal asphyxia. In contrast, the FHR baseline in the nonreactive group usually but not always remains fixed. Infrequently, a FHR tachycardia is seen; however, the rise in baseline rate is usually insubstantial. Thus, the phase of recovery appears to equate with the length of time from the fetal CNS insult. Thus, phase I would appear to be closer to the time of the insult, and phase III would appear to be more distant in time from the injury-producing event (Phelan & Kim, 2000).

The persistent nonreactive FHR pattern is not, in our opinion, a sign of ongoing fetal asphyxia but rather represents a static encephalopathy (Phelan & Ahn, 1994, 1998; Phelan et al., 2001). This means that earlier intervention in the form of a cesarean on admission to the hospital would not, in our opinion, substantially alter fetal outcome.

Fetal monitoring made simple

In light of the lessons learned from the children damaged in utero prior to and during labor, current fetal monitoring interpretation will need to change to reflect and include the significance of the initial fetal monitoring period. When a patient presents to labor and delivery, the initial fetal assessment should include an initial fetal monitoring period to assess reactivity (the presence of FHR accelerations) and to ascertain from the patient the quality and quantity of fetal movement. In the patient with a reactive FHR pattern and normal fetal movement, the key to clinical management prior to and during labor is to follow the baseline rate.

This means that the physician and nurse will need to watch for persistent elevations or falls of the baseline rate. To assist with the identification of the Hon pattern, medical and nursing personnel should try to compare the current tracing with the one obtained on admission. If the characteristics of the Hon pattern of intrapartum asphyxia develops, subsequent clinical management will depend on whether the gravida is febrile and as previously outlined in this chapter. In the nonreactive group, clinical management is directed towards keeping the fetus on the EFM until fetal status is clarified with prolonged fetal monitoring, fetal stimulation tests, a contraction stress test, or a biophysical profile. Once fetal status is clarified in the nonreactive group, the subsequent management with respect to the route of delivery will depend on the discussion with the family and the clinical findings.

Maternal and surgical conditions

Anaphylaxis

Anaphylaxis is an acute allergic reaction to food ingestion or drugs. It is generally associated with rapid onset of pruritus and urticaria and may result in respiratory distress, edema, vascular collapse, and shock. Medicines, primarily penicillins (Gallagher, 1998; Dunn et al., 1999), food substances, such as shellfish, exercise, contrast dyes, laminaria (Cole & Bruck, 2000), and latex (Deusch et al., 1996) are common causes of anaphylaxis (Van Arsdel, 1981; Reisman, 1989).

When an anaphylactic reaction occurs during pregnancy, the accompanying maternal physiologic changes may result in fetal distress. In a case described by Klein and associates (1984), a woman at 29 weeks' gestation presented with an acute allergic reaction after eating shellfish. On admission, she had evidence of regular uterine contractions and repetitive, severe late decelerations. The fetal distress was believed to be the result of maternal hypotension and relative hypovolemia, which accompanied the allergic reaction. Prompt treatment of the patient with intravenous fluids and ephedrine corrected the fetal distress. Subsequently, the patient delivered a healthy male infant at term with normal Apgar scores.

As suggested by these investigators and by Witter and Niebyl (1983), while acute maternal allergic reactions do pose a threat to the fetus, treatment directed at the underlying cause often remedies the accompanying fetal distress. To afford the fetus a wider margin of safety, efforts should be directed at maintaining maternal systolic BP above 90 mmHg. In addition, oxygen should be administered to correct maternal hypoxia; in the absence of maternal hypovolemia, a maternal P_aO_2 in excess of 60–70 mmHg will assure adequate fetal oxygenation (Klein et al., 1984; Witter & Niebyl, 1983). A persistent fetal tachycardia, bradycardia (Dunn et al., 1999), or other abnormal FHR patterns suggest the need for additional maternal hemodynamic support or oxygenation, even in the nominally "stable" mother.

Eclampsia

Maternal seizures are a well-known but infrequent sequel of preeclampsia. Although the maternal hemodynamic findings in patients with eclampsia are similar to those with severe preeclampsia (Clark et al., 1985), maternal convulsions require prompt attention to prevent harm to both mother and fetus (Lucas et al., 1995; Naidu et al., 1996). During a seizure, the fetal response usually is manifested as an abrupt, prolonged FHR deceleration (Boehm & Growdon, 1974; Paul et al., 1978). During the seizure, which generally lasts less than 1–2 minutes (Paul et al., 1978), transient maternal hypoxia and uterine artery vasospasm occur and combine to produce a decline in uterine blood flow. In addition, uterine activity increases secondary to the release of norepinephrine, resulting in additional reduction in uteroplacental perfusion. Ultimately, the reduction of uteroplacental perfusion causes the FHR deceleration. Such a deceleration may last up to 9 minutes (Paul et al., 1978). Following the seizure and recovery from the FHR deceleration, a loss of FHRV and a compensatory rise in baseline FHR are characteristically seen. Transient late decelerations are not uncommon but resolve once maternal metabolic recovery is complete.

The cornerstone of patient management during an eclamptic seizure is to maintain adequate maternal oxygenation and to administer appropriate anticonvulsants. After a convulsion occurs, an adequate airway should be maintained and oxygen administered. To optimize uteroplacental perfusion, the mother is repositioned onto her side. Anticonvulsant therapy with intravenous magnesium sulfate (Pritchard et al., 1984; Lucas et al., 1995; Naidu et al., 1996) to prevent seizure recurrence is recommended. In spite of adequate magnesium sulfate therapy, adjunctive anticonvulsant therapy occasionally may be necessary (Paul et al., 1978; Pritchard et al., 1984). In the event of persistent FHR decelerations, intrauterine resuscitation with a betamimetic (Barrett, 1984) or additional magnesium sulfate (Reece et al., 1984) may be helpful in relieving eclampsia-induced uterine hypertonus. Continuous electronic fetal monitoring should be used to follow the fetal condition. After the mother has been stabilized, and if the fetus continues to show signs of distress after a reasonable recovery period, assessment of fetal acid–base status (Phelan, 1994; Skupski et al., 2002) and/or delivery would be indicated.

Disseminated intravascular coagulopathy

Disseminated intravascular coagulopathy (DIC) occurs in a variety of obstetric conditions, such as abruptio placenta, amniotic fluid embolus syndrome, and the dead fetus syndrome. The pathophysiology of this condition is discussed in greater detail in Chapter 30.

Infrequently, DIC may be advanced to a point of overt bleeding (Porter et al., 1996). Under these circumstances, laboratory abnormalities accompany the clinical evidence of consumptive coagulopathy. In the rare circumstance of overt fetal distress and a clinically apparent maternal coagulopathy, obstetric management requires prompt replacement of deficient coagulation components before attempting to deliver the distressed fetus. This frequently requires balancing the interests of the pregnant woman with those of her unborn child.

For example, a 34-year-old woman presented to the hospital at 33 weeks's gestation with the FHR tracing illustrated in Fig. 42.6. Real-time sonography demonstrated asymmetric intrauterine growth retardation. Oxygen was administered, and the patient was repositioned on her left side. Appropriate laboratory studies were drawn, and informed consent for a cesarean was obtained. When a Foley catheter was inserted, grossly bloody urine was observed. The previously drawn blood did not clot, and she was observed to be bleeding from the site of her intravenous line. The abnormal FHR pattern persisted.

In this circumstance, the interests of the mother and fetus are at odds with one another, and a difficult clinical decision must now be made. Whose interest does the obstetrician protect in this instance? Immediate surgical intervention without blood products would lessen the mother's chances of survival. If the clinician waits for fresh frozen plasma and platelets infusion before undertaking surgery, the fetus will be at significant risk of death or permanent neurologic impairment. Ideally, the mother and/or her family should participate in such decisions. In reality, because of the unpredictable nature of these dilemmas and the need for rapid decision making, family involvement often is not always possible. Under such circumstances, it is axiomatic that maternal interests take precedence over those of the fetus.

Because blood products were not readily available, the decision was made to stabilize the mother and to move the patient to the operating room. Once she was in the operating room, the clinical management would include, but is not limited to, the following: to continue to oxygenate the mother; to maintain her in the left lateral recumbent position; to have an anesthesiologist, operating room personnel, and surgeons present; and to be prepared to operate. As soon as the blood products are available, and the fetus is alive, transfuse with fresh frozen plasma, platelets, and packed cells. Then, the clinician should begin the cesarean under general anesthesia. In this case, maternal and fetal outcomes were ultimately favorable.

In summary, the cornerstone of management of the patient with full-blown DIC and clinically apparent fetal distress is to stabilize the mother by correcting the maternal clotting abnormality before initiating surgery. While waiting for the blood products to be infused, the patient should be prepared and ready for immediate cesarean delivery. If the fetus dies in the interim, the cesarean should not be performed; and, the patient should be afforded the opportunity to deliver vaginally, to reduce maternal hemorrhagic risks.

The burn victim

Although burn victims are uncommonly encountered in high-risk obstetric units, the pregnant burn patient is sufficiently complex to require a team approach to enhance maternal and perinatal survival (Polko & McMahon, 1998; Guo et al., 2001). In most cases, this will require maternal–fetal transfer to a facility skilled to handle burn patients. Transfer will depend

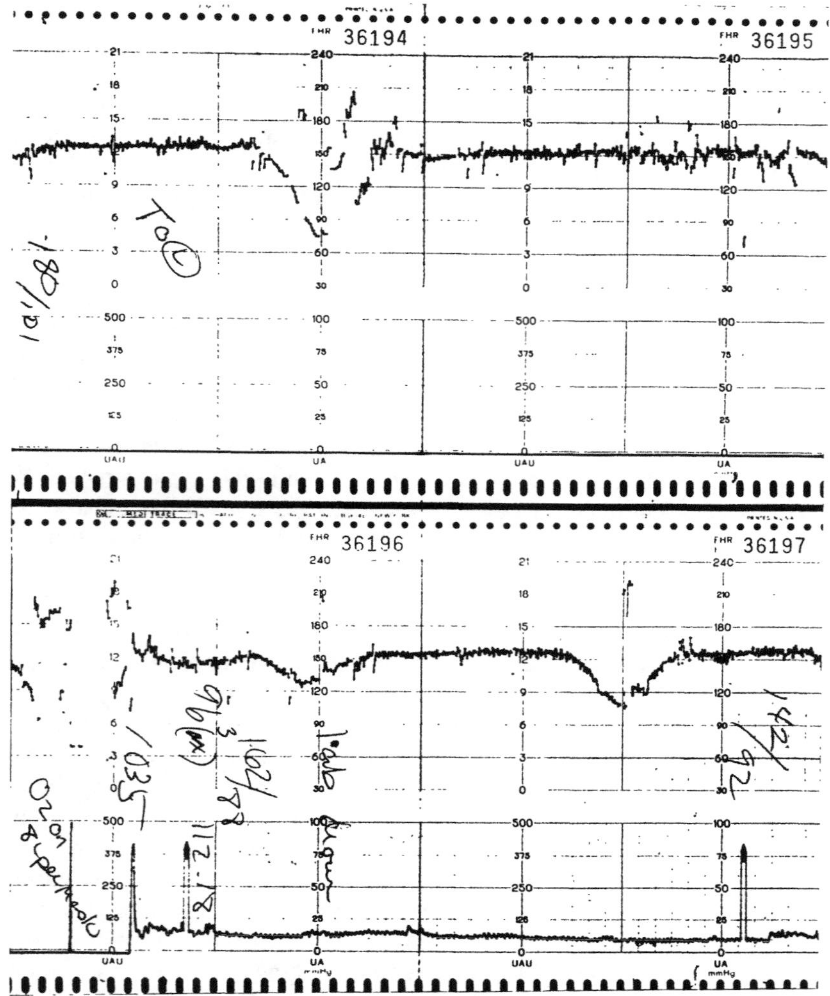

Fig. 42.6 The FHR pattern from a 33-week fetus with asymmetric intrauterine growth impairment whose mother presented with clinical DIC.

primarily on the severity of the burn and the stability of the pregnant woman and her fetus.

The first step in the management of the pregnant burn patient is to determine the depth and size of the burn. The depth of a burn may be partial or full thickness. A full-thickness burn, formerly called a third-degree burn, is the most severe and involves total destruction of the skin. As a result, regeneration of the epithelial surface is not possible.

The second element of burn management is to determine the percent of body surface area involved (Table 42.5). The percentage of maternal total body surface area covered by the burn is linked to maternal and perinatal outcome. The more severe the maternal burn, the higher is the maternal and perinatal mortality (Polko & McMahon, 1998; Guo et al., 2001). The risk of mortality becomes significant whenever 60% or more of the maternal total body surface area is burned (Polko & McMahon, 1998).

The subsequent clinical management of the pregnant burn patient will depend on the patient's burn phase (e.g. acute, convalescent, or remote). Each phase has unique problems. For example, the acute phase is characterized by premature labor, electrolyte and fluid disturbances, maternal cardiopulmonary instability, and the potential for fetal compromise. In contrast, the convalescent and remote periods are unique for their problems of sepsis and abdominal scarring, respectively. Because the potential for fetal compromise is greatest during

Table 42.5 Classification of burn patients based on the percent of body surface area involved

Classification	Body surface area (%)
Minor	<10
Major	
Moderate	10–19
Severe	20–39
Critical	≥40

the window of time immediately following the burn, the focus in this chapter is on acute-phase burn patients.

In the acute phase of a severe burn, the primary maternal focus centers on stabilization (Guo et al., 2001). Here, electrolyte disturbances due to transudation of fluid and altered renal function mandate close attention to the maternal intravascular volume and prompt and aggressive fluid resuscitation. At the same time, these patients are also potentially compromised from airway injury and/or smoke inhalation, and ventilator support may be necessary to maintain cardiopulmonary stability. Additionally, a high index of suspicion for venous thrombosis and sepsis with early and aggressive treatment should be considered. Given the complexities of these patients, invasive hemodynamic monitoring may be necessary. Because most of these patients will be in an intensive care unit (ICU), appropriate medical consultation and intensive nursing care for the mother and fetus are essential.

Assessing fetal well-being in the burn patient may be difficult. The ability to determine fetal status with ultrasound or fetal monitoring will depend on the size and location of the burn. If, for example, the burn involves the maternal abdominal wall, alternative methods of fetal assessment, such as fetal kick counts (alone or in response to acoustic stimulation) (Smith, 1994) or a modified FBP (Manning et al., 1980, 1990; Phelan, 1988) using vaginal ultrasound, may be necessary. In the absence of a maternal abdominal burn, continuous electronic fetal monitoring can generally be used. Because of such monitoring difficulties and the direct relationship between the size of the maternal burn and perinatal outcome (see Fig. 42.7), Matthews (1982) and Polko and McMahon (1998) have recommended immediate cesarean delivery (assuming maternal stability) in any pregnant burn patient with a potentially viable fetus and a burn that involves 50% or more of the maternal body surface area. In contrast, Guo (2001) recommends early delivery if the pregnancy is in the third trimester. As a reminder, burn patients with electrolyte disturbances may exhibit alterations in fetal status similar to those of a patient in sickle cell crisis (Cruz et al., 1979) or diabetic ketoacidosis (LoBue & Goodlin, 1978; Rhodes & Ogburn, 1984). Once the maternal electrolyte disturbance is corrected, fetal status may return to normal and intervention often can be avoided.

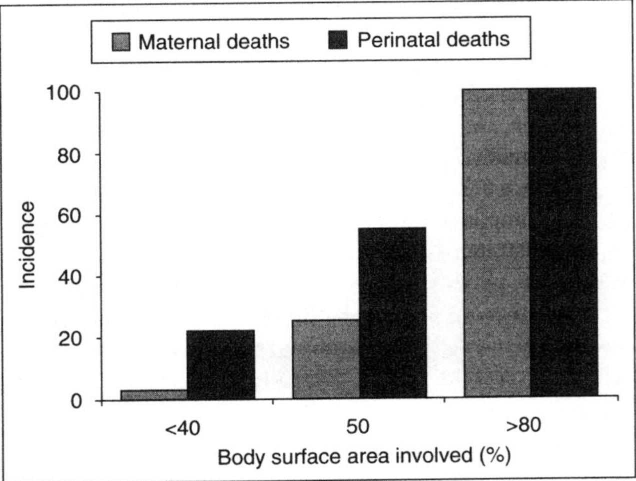

Fig. 42.7 Estimated maternal and perinatal mortality rates following maternal burn injuries according to the amount of body surface area involved.

Fetal considerations specific to cardiac bypass procedures and electrical shock are discussed in Chapters 13 and 37.

Maternal brain death or persistent vegetative state

With the advent of artificial life-support systems, prolonged viability of the brain-dead pregnant woman or one in a persistent vegetative state (PVS) is now a reality (Dillon et al., 1982; Gdansky & Schenker, 1998). As a consequence, an increasing number of obstetric patients on artificial life support will be encountered in the medical community. Maternal brain death poses an array of medical, legal, and ethical dilemmas for the obstetric health-care provider (Black, 1978; Bernat et al., 1981; Field et al., 1988; Gdansky & Schenker, 1998; Feldman et al., 2000). Should extraordinary care for the brain-dead mother be initiated to preserve the life of her unborn child, and if so, at what gestational age? If artificial life support is elected, how should the pregnancy be managed? When should the fetus be delivered? When should maternal life support be terminated? Is consent required to maintain the pregnancy? If so, from whom should it be obtained? Such questions illustrate the complexities of these cases.

It is not within the scope of this chapter to deal with the ethical, moral, and legal issues related to the obstetric care of the brain-dead gravida or the gravida with PVS. Rather, the emphasis is on the clinical management of these patients when a decision has been made to maintain artificial life support for the benefit of her unborn child. The key distinction between brain death and PVS is that in PVS, the brain stem may or may not be functioning normally. In the initial phases, it is arguably difficult to separate the two entities. With time, the distinction becomes clearer. Thus, clinical management is similar initially.

To date, 12 cases of maternal brain death during pregnancy have been reported (Table 42.6). In one, life support was terminated after a discussion between the patient's physician and family at 19 weeks' gestation. In the other cases, the pregnancies were maintained from 2 days (Iriye et al., 1995) to 27 weeks (Sampson & Peterson, 1979). Infants were delivered by classical cesarean and ultimately had favorable outcomes. For optimal care of such patients and fetuses, a cooperative effort among various health-care providers is essential. The goal is to maintain maternal somatic survival until the fetus is viable and reasonably mature. To achieve this goal, a number of ma-

Table 42.6 Perinatal outcome in eight reported cases of maternal brain death during pregnancy

Reference	Gestation age (weeks)		Indication for delivery	Mode of delivery	Apgar score at 5 min	Weight (g)
	Brain death	Delivery				
Sampson & Peterson (1979)	6	33	—	Forceps	—	1,640
Dillon et al. (1982)						
Case I	25	26	Fetal distress	Cesarean	8	390
Case II	18	Life support terminated 19 weeks				
BenAderet & Cohen (1984)	17	35	—	Cesarean	—	2,450
Heikkinen et al. (1985)	21	31	Maternal hypotension	Cesarean	7	1,600
Field et al. (1988)	22	31	Growth impaired Sepsis	Cesarean	8	1,440
Bernstein et al. (1989)	15	32	Fetal distress	Cesarean	9	1,555
Iriye et al. (1995)	30	30	Maternal hypotension FHR decelerations	Cesarean	8	1,610
Vives et al. (1996)	27	27	Fetal distress	Cesarean	10	1,150
Catanzarite et al. (1997)	25	29	Amnionitis	Cesarean	7	1,315
Lewis & Vidovich (1997)	25	31	—	Cesarean	—	—
Feldman et al. (2000)	15	31	Seizures Hypertension	Cesarean	9	1,506

Table 42.7 Medical and obstetric considerations in providing artificial life support to the brain-dead gravida

Maternal considerations	Fetal considerations
Mechanical ventilation	Fetal surveillance
Cardiovascular support	Ultrasonography
Temperature lability	Steroids
Hyperalimentation	Timing of delivery
Panhypopituitarism	
Infection surveillance	
Prophylactic anticoagulation	

ternal and fetal considerations must be addressed (Field et al., 1988) (Table 42.7).

As pointed out by Field and associates (1988), maternal medical considerations involve the regulation of most, if not all, maternal bodily functions. For example, the loss of the pneumotaxic center in the pons, which is responsible for cyclic respirations, and the medullary center, which is responsible for spontaneous respirations, make mechanical ventilation mandatory. Ventilation, under these circumstances, is similar to that for the nonpregnant patient. In contrast to the nonpregnant patient, the desirable gas concentrations are stricter due to the presence of the fetus. As such, the maternal P_aCO_2 should be kept between 28 mmHg and 32 mmHg and the maternal P_aO_2 greater than 60–70 mmHg, to avoid deleterious effects on uteroplacental perfusion.

Maternal hypotension occurs frequently in these patients and may be due to a combination of factors, including hypothermia, hypoxia, and panhypopituitarism. Maintenance of maternal BP can often be achieved with the infusion of low-dose dopamine, which elevates BP without affecting renal or splanchnic blood flow.

With maternal brain death, the thermoregulatory center located in the ventromedian nucleus of the hypothalamus does not function, and maternal body temperature cannot be maintained normally. As a result, maternal hypothermia is the rule. Maintenance of maternal euthermia is important and usually can be accomplished through the use of warming blankets and the administration of warm, inspired, humidified air.

Maternal pyrexia suggests an infectious process and the need for a thorough septic work-up. If the maternal temperature remains elevated for a protracted period, cooling blankets may be necessary to avoid potentially deleterious effects on the fetus (Edwards & Wanner, 1977).

Nutritional support, usually in the form of enteral or parenteral hyperalimentation, is required for maternal maintenance and fetal growth and development (see Chapter 11). Because of poor maternal gastric motility, parenteral rather than enteral hyperalimentation is often preferred (Field et al.,

1988). The use of hyperalimentation during pregnancy does not appear to have deleterious effects on the fetus (Smith et al., 1981). As a rule, the amount of hyperalimentation should be in keeping with the caloric requirements of pregnancy.

In such patients, panhypopituitarism frequently occurs. As a result, a variety of hypoendocrinopathies, such as diabetes insipidus, secondary adrenal insufficiency, and hypothyroidism, may develop, each mandating therapy to maintain the pregnancy. Treatment of these conditions requires the use of vasopressin, corticosteroids, and thyroid replacement, respectively.

Because of the hypercoagulable state of pregnancy and the immobility of the brain-dead gravida, these patients also are at an increased risk for thromboembolism. Therefore, to minimize the potential for deep venous thrombosis or pulmonary embolus, heparin prophylaxis (5,000–7,500 units twice or three times a day) and/or intermittent pneumatic calf compression are recommended (Clark-Pearson et al., 1993).

By artificially supporting the maternal physiologic system, the intrauterine environment can be theoretically maintained to allow for adequate fetal growth and development (Table 42.7). Obstetric management should focus on monitoring fetal growth with frequent ultrasound evaluations, antepartum FHR assessment, and the administration of corticosteroids between 24 and 34 weeks' gestation to enhance fetal lung maturation (Field et al., 1988; NIH, 1995). For stimulation of fetal lung maturity, the National Institutes of Health (1995) recommends betamethasone, 12 mg, initially and then a second dose 24 hours later. A weekly injection of betamethasone, 12 mg, is not currently recommended due to the concern over the effect of repeated steroid injections on fetal brain growth, and the absence of proven additive benefit.

The timing of delivery is based on the deterioration of maternal or fetal status or the presence of fetal lung maturity. Classical cesarean is the procedure of choice (Field et al., 1988) and is the least traumatic procedure for the fetus. To assure immediate cesarean capability, a cesarean pack and neonatal resuscitation equipment should be immediately available in the intensive care unit.

Perimortem cesarean delivery

For centuries, postmortem cesarean delivery has been described as an attempt to preserve the life of the unborn child (Weber, 1971). In 237 AD, Pliny the Elder described the first successful postmortem cesarean delivery, that of Scipio Africanus. Subsequently, in 1280, the Catholic Church at the Council of Cologne decreed that postmortem cesarean delivery must be performed to permit the unborn child to be baptized and to undergo a proper burial. Failure to perform the delivery was considered a punishable offense. This law mandated postmortem cesarean delivery only in women whose pregnancies were advanced beyond 6 months. To date, there have been 269 cases of postmortem cesarean delivery reported in the English literature, with 188 (70%) surviving infants (Katz & Dotters, 1986).

Since Weber's monumental review of the subject in 1971, the causes of maternal death leading to a postmortem cesarean delivery have not changed substantially (Katz & Dotters, 1986). These include hypertension, hemorrhage, and sepsis. With unanticipated or sudden death, such as amniotic fluid embolus syndrome, pulmonary embolus, or acute respiratory failure, the timing of cesarean delivery becomes an especially critical issue.

If a pregnant woman does sustain a cardiopulmonary arrest, cardiopulmonary resuscitation (CPR) should be initiated immediately (see Chapter 6). Optimal performance of CPR results in a cardiac output of 30–40% of normal in the nonpregnant patient. For best efficiency, the patient should be placed in the supine position. In this position, however, dextrorotation of the uterus may impede venous return and may further compromise this effort. Lateral uterine displacement may help to remedy this problem; but CPR in this position is extremely awkward. Ultimately, a cesarean may be necessary to alleviate this impedance to CPR.

If maternal and fetal outcomes are to be optimized, the timing of the cesarean delivery is critical. Katz and associates (1986) have suggested that "cesarean delivery should be begun within 4 minutes, and the baby delivered within 5 minutes of maternal cardiac arrest." Care must be taken to continue maternal CPR, not only until the birth of fetus, but also after the delivery. Similar results were presented in a series of patients undergoing cardiac arrest in association with amniotic fluid embolism; if delivery occurred within 15 minutes, most fetuses survived and were neurologically intact. However, poor neonatal outcome was seen occasionally, even with delivery within 5 minutes of maternal cardiac arrest (Clark et al., 1995).

As demonstrated in Table 42.8, fetal survival is linked closely to the interval between maternal arrest and delivery. Although the probability of a surviving, normal infant dimin-

Table 42.8 Perimortem cesarean delivery with the outcome of surviving infants from the time of maternal death until delivery

Time interval (min)	Surviving infants (no.)	Intact neurologic status of survivors (%)
0–5	45	98
6–15	18	83
16–25	9	33
26–35	4	25
36+	1	0

(From Katz VL, Dotters DJ, Droegemueller W. Perimortem cesarean delivery. Obstet Gynecol 1986;68:571–576; and Clark SL, Hankins GD, Dudley DA, et al. Amniotic fluid embolism: analysis of the National Registry. Am J Obstet Gynecol 1995;172:1158.)

ishes the longer the time interval from maternal death, the potential exists for a favorable fetal outcome even beyond 20 minutes of maternal cardiac arrest (Katz et al., 1986). Although delivery within 5 minutes of maternal cardiac arrest is ideal, in reality this rarely can be accomplished in a clinical setting, even with optimal care. Perhaps, the most realistic guideline would be to perform a cesarean as soon as possible following maternal cardiac arrest. In late second- or third-trimester pregnant patients, the standard ABCs of cardiopulmonary resuscitation (airway, breathing, circulation) should be expanded to include D (delivery).

While the timing of cesarean delivery is a major determinant of subsequent fetal outcome, the gestational age of the fetus also is an important consideration. The probability of survival is related directly to the neonatal birth weight and gestational age (Ferrara et al., 1989, 1994; Robertson et al., 1992; Copper et al., 1993). At what gestational age should a postmortem cesarean delivery be considered? Is there a lower limit? It becomes obvious immediately that there are no clear answers to these questions. As a general rule, intervention appears prudent whenever the fetus is potentially viable or is "capable of a meaningful existence outside the mother's womb" (Roe vs Wade, 1973). According to Gdansky and Schenker (1998), the gray zone rests between 23 and 26 weeks' gestation. But, this threshold is continually pushed to earlier gestational ages in keeping with the advances in neonatal care. Ideally, criteria for intervention in such circumstances should be formulated with the aid of an institution's current neonatal survival statistics and guidance from its bioethics committee. In light of the continual technologic advances in neonatology, care must be taken to periodically review these criteria because the gestational age and weight criteria may be lowered in the future (Roe vs Wade, 1973; Ferrara et al., 1989, 1994; Robertson et al., 1992; Copper et al., 1993).

When maternal death is an anticipated event, is informed consent necessary? For instance, patients hospitalized with terminal cancer, class IV cardiac disease, pulmonary hypertension, or previous myocardial infarction are at an increased risk of death during pregnancy. Although these cases are infrequent, it seems reasonable to prepare for such an eventuality. Decisions regarding intervention should be made in advance with the patient and family. When intervention has been agreed to, one consideration is to have a cesarean delivery pack and neonatal resuscitation equipment immediately available in the ICU.

In the unforeseeable, sudden, unexpected maternal death, consent to deliver the potentially viable fetus does not appear to be required (Katz et al., 1986). When maternal death is foreseeable, however, maternal consent for cesarean delivery in the event of death is desirable.

References

Ahn MO, Korst LM, Phelan JP, Martin GI. Does the onset of neonatal seizures correlate with the timing of fetal neurologic injury. Clin Pediatr 1998a;37:673–676.

Ahn MO, Korst LM, Phelan JP. Normal fetal heart rate patterns in the brain-damaged infant: A failure of intrapartum fetal monitoring? J Matern Fetal Invest 1998b;8:58–60.

Altschuler G, Hyde S. Meconium induced vasoconstriction: A potential cause of cerebral and other fetal hypoperfusion and of poor pregnancy outcome. J Child Neurol 1989;4:1337–1342.

Altschuler G, Arizawa M, Molnar-Nadasy G. Meconium-induced umbilical cord vascular necrosis and ulceration: A potential link between the placenta and poor pregnancy outcome. Obstet Gynecol 1992;79:760–766.

American College of Obstetricians and Gynecologists. Fetal and Neonatal Injury. Technical Bulletin No. 163. Washington, DC: American College of Obstetricians and Gynecologists, 1992.

Babakania A, Niebyl R. The effect of magnesium sulfate on fetal heart rate variability. Obstet Gynecol 1978;51(Suppl):2S–4S.

Barrett JM. Fetal resuscitation with terbutaline during eclampsia-induced uterine hypertonus. Am J Obstet Gynecol 1984;150:895.

BenAderet N, Cohen I, Abramowicz JS. Traumatic coma during pregnancy with persistent vegetative state. Case report. Br J Obstet Gynecol 1984;91:939–941.

Bernat JL, Culver CM, Gert B. On the definition and criterion of death. Ann Intern Med 1981;94:389–394.

Bernstein IM, Watson M, Simmons GM, Catalano PM, Davis G, Collings R. Maternal brain death and prolonged fetal survival. Obstet Gynecol 1989;74:434–437.

Black PM. Brain death. N Engl J Med 1978;229:338–344, 393–401.

Blackwell SC, Refuerzo JS, Wolfe HM, et al. The relationship between nucleated red blood cell counts and early-onset neonatal seizures. Am J Obstet Gynecol 2000;182:1452–1457.

Boehm FH, Growdon JH. The effect of eclamptic convulsions of the fetal heart rate. Am J Obstet Gynecol 1974;120:851–853.

Catanzarite VA, Willms DC, Holdy KE, et al. Brain death during pregnancy: tocolytic therapy and aggressive maternal support on behalf of the fetus. Am J Perinatol 1997;14:431–434.

Clark SL. Shock in the pregnant patient. Semin Perinatol 1990; 14:52–58.

Clark SL, Miller FC. Sinusoidal fetal heart rate pattern associated with massive fetomaternal transfusion. Am J Obstet Gynecol 1984; 149:97–99.

Clark SL, Paul RH. Intrapartum fetal surveillance: The role of fetal scalp sampling. Am J Obstet Gynecol 1985;153:717–720.

Clark SL, Divon M, Phelan JP. Preeclampsia/eclampsia: hemodynamic and neurologic correlations. Obstet Gynecol 1985;66:337–340.

Clark SL, Hawkins GD, Dudley DA, et al. Amniotic fluid embolism: analysis of the National Registry. Am J Obstet Gynecol 1995; 172:1158–1167.

Clark-Pearson DL, Synan IS, Dodge R, et al. A randomized trial of low-dose heparin and intermittent pneumatic calf compression for the prevention of deep venous thrombosis after gynecologic oncology surgery. Am J Obstet Gynecol 1993;168:1146–1154.

Cole DS, Bruck LR. Anaphylaxis after laminaria insertion. Obstet Gynecol 2000;95:1025.

Copper RL, Goldenberg RL, Creasy RK, et al. A multicenter study of preterm birth weight and gestational age specific neonatal mortality. Am J Obstet Gynecol 1993;168:78–84.

Cruz AC, Spellacy WN, Jarrell M. Fetal heart rate tracing during sickle cell crisis: a cause for transient late decelerations. Obstet Gynecol 1979;54:647–649.

Dennis J, Johnson A, Mutch L, et al. Acid-base study birth and neurodevelopmental outcome at four and one-half years. Am J Obstet Gynecol 1989;161:213–220.

Deusch E, Reider N, Marth C. Anaphylactic reaction to latex during cesarean delivery. Obstet Gynecol 1996;88:727.

Dillon WP, Lee RV, Tronolone MJ, et al. Life support and maternal brain death during pregnancy. JAMA 1982;248:1089–1091.

Dunn AB, Blomquist J, Khouzami V. Anaphylaxis in labor secondary to prophylaxis against group B Streptococcus: A case report. J Reprod Med 1999;44:381–384.

Edwards MJ, Wanner RA. Extremes of temperature. In: Wilson JG, Graser FC, eds. Handbook of teratology, vol. 1. New York: Plenum, 1977:421.

Epstein H, Waxman A, Fleicher N, et al. Meperidine-induced sinusoidal fetal heart rate pattern and its reversal with naloxone. Obstet Gynecol 1982;59(Suppl):22–25.

Fee SC, Malee K, Deddish R, et al. Severe acidosis and subsequent neurologic status. Am J Obstet Gynecol 1990;162:802–806.

Feldman DM, Borgida AF, Rodis JF, Campbell WA. Irreversible maternal brain injury during pregnancy: A case report and review of the literature. Obstet & Gynecologic Surv 2000;55:708–714.

Ferrara TB, Hoekstra RE, Gaziano E, et al. Changing outcome of extremely premature infants (26 weeks gestation and 750 gm): survival and follow-up at a tertiary center. Am J Obstet Gynecol 1989;161:1114–1118.

Ferrara TB, Hoekstra RE, Couser RJ, et al. Survival and follow-up of infants born at 23–26 weeks of gestational age: effects of surfactant therapy. J Pediatr 1994;124:119–124.

Field DR, Gates EA, Creasy RK, et al. Maternal brain death during pregnancy: medical and ethical issues. JAMA 1988;260:816–822.

Gabbe SG, Ettinger RB, Freeman RK, et al. Umbilical cord compression with amniotomy: laboratory observations. Am J Obstet Gynecol 1976;126:353–355.

Gallagher JS. Anaphylaxis in pregnancy. Obstet Gynecol 1988;71: 491–493.

Garite TJ, Linzey EM, Freeman RK, et al. Fetal heart rate patterns and fetal distress in fetuses with congenital anomalies. Obstet Gynecol 1979;53:716–720.

Garite TJ, Dildy GA, McNamara H, et al. A multicenter controlled trial of fetal pulse oximetry in the intrapartum management of nonreassuring fetal heart rate patterns. Am J Obstet Gynecol 2000;183: 1049–1058.

Gdanski E, Schenker G. Management of pregnancy in women with circulatory and brain death. Prenat Neonat Med 1998;3:327–333.

Golditch BD, Ahn MO, Phelan JP. The fetal admission test and intrapartum fetal death. Am J Perinatol 1998;15:273–276.

Goodwin TM, Belai I, Hernandez P, et al. Asphyxial complications in the term newborn from umbilical acidemia. Am J Obstet Gynecol 1992;162:1506–1512.

Goodwin TM, Milner-Masterson L, Paul RH. Elimination of fetal scalp blood sampling on a large clinical service. Obstet Gynecol 1994;83: 971–974.

Greenberg J, Economy K, Mark A, et al. In search of "True" birth asphyxia: Labor characteristics associated with the asphyxiated term infant. Am J Obstet Gynecol 2001;185:S94.

Guo SS, Greenspoon JS, Kahn AM. Management of burn injuries during pregnancy. Burns 2001;27:394–397.

Heikkinen JE, Rinne RI, Alahuhta SM, et al. Life support of 10 weeks with successful fetal outcome after fatal maternal brain damage. Br Med J Clin Res Ed 1985;290:1237–1238.

Hon EH, Lee ST. Electronic evaluation of the fetal heart rate: VIII. Patterns preceding fetal death, further observations. Am J Obstet Gynecol 1963;87:814–826.

Hon EH, Quilligan EJ. Electronic evaluation of the fetal heart rate. Clin Obstet Gynecol 1968;11:145–155.

Ingemarsson I, Arulkumaran S, Paul RH, et al. Admission test: A screening test for fetal distress in labor. Obstet Gynecol 1986;68: 800–806.

Iriye BK, Asrat T, Adashek JA, Carr MH. Intraventricular hemorrhage and maternal brain death associated with antepartum cocaine abuse. Br J Obstet Gynaecol 1995;102:68–69.

Katz M, Meizner I, Shani N, et al. Clinical significance of sinusoidal fetal heart rate pattern. Br J Obstet Gynaecol 1984;149:97–100.

Katz VL, Dotters DJ, Droegemueller W. Perimortem cesarean delivery. Obstet Gynecol 1986;68:571–576.

Kim JO, Martin G, Kirkendall C, Phelan JP. Intrapartum fetal heart rate variability and subsequent neonatal cerebral edema. Obstet Gynecol 2000;95:75S.

Klein VR, Harris AP, Abraham RA, Niebyl JR. Fetal distress during a maternal systemic allergic reaction. Obstet Gynecol 1984;64(Suppl): 15S–17S.

Kirkendall C, Phelan JP. Severe acidosis at birth and normal neurological outcome. Prenat Neonat Med 2001;6:267–270.

Kirkendall C, Ahn MO, Martin G, Korst L, Phelan JP. The brain injured baby, neonatal seizures, and the intrapartum fetal heart rate pattern: Is there a relationship? Am J Obstet Gynecol 2000;182: S184.

Kirkendall C, Romo M, Phelan JP. Fetomaternal hemorrhage in fetal brain injury. Am J Obstet Gynecol 2001;185(6):S153.

Koh KD, Friesen RM, Livingstone RA, et al. Fetal monitoring during maternal cardiac surgery with cardiopulmonary bypass. Can Med Assoc J 1975;112:1102–1106.

Kosasa TS, Ebesugawa I, Nakayama RT, Hale R. Massive fetomaternal hemorrhage preceded by decrease fetal movement and a nonreactive feta heart rate pattern. Obstet Gynecol 1993;82:711–714.

Korst LM, Phelan JP, Ahn MO, Martin GI. Nucleated red blood cells: An update on the marker for fetal asphyxia? Am J Obstet Gynecol 1996;175:843–846.

Korst LM, Phelan JP, Ahn MO, Martin GI. Can persistent brain injury resulting from intrapartum asphyxia be predicted by current criteria? Prenat Neonat Med 1997;2:286–293.

Korst LM, Phelan JP, Wang YM, Ahn MO. Neonatal platelet counts in fetal brain injury. Am J Perinatol 1999a;16:79–83.

Korst L, Phelan JP, Wang YM, Martin GI, Ahn MO. Acute fetal asphyxia and permanent brain injury: A retrospective analysis of current indicators. J Maternal-Fetal Med 1999b;8:101–106.

Korsten HHM, Van Zundert AAJ, Moou PNM, et al. Emergency aortic valve replacement in the 24th week of pregnancy. Acta Anaestesiol Belg 1989;40:201–205.

Krebs HB, Petres RE, Dunn LH, et al. Intrapartum fetal heart rate monitoring: VI. Prognostic significance of accelerations. Am J Obstet Gynecol 1982;142:297–305.

Krebs HB, Petres RE, Dunn LH, et al. Intrapartum fetal heart rate monitoring: VII. Atypical variable decelerations. Am J Obstet Gynecol 1983;145:297–305.

Kubli FW, Hon EH, Hhazin AF, et al. Observations in heart rate and pH in the human fetus during labor. Am J Obstet Gynecol 1969;104:1190–1206.

Leung A, Leung EK, Paul RH. Uterine rupture after previous cesarean delivery: Maternal and feta consequences. Am J Obstet Gynecol 1993;169:945–950.

Lewis DD, Vidovich RR. Organ recovery following childbirth in a brain-dead mother: A case report. J Transpl Coord 1997;7:103–105.

LoBue C, Goodlin RC. Treatment of fetal distress during diabetic ketoacidosis. J Reprod Med 1978;20:101–104.

Lockshin MD, Bonfa E, Elkon D, Druzin ML. Neonatal lupus risk to newborns of mother with systemic lupus erythematosus. Arthritis Rheum 1988;31:697–701.

Lucas MJ, Leveno KJ, Cunningham FG. A comparison of magnesium sulfate with phenytoin for the prevention of eclampsia. N Engl J Med 1995;333:201–205.

MacLennan A. A template for defining a causal relation between acute intrapartum events and cerebral palsy: International consensus statement. Br Med J 1999;319:1054–1059.

Manning FA, Platt LD, Sipos L. Antepartum fetal evaluation: development of a fetal biophysical profile. Am J Obstet Gynecol 1980;136:787–795.

Manning FA, Morrison I, Harman CR, Menticoglou SM. The abnormal fetal biophysical profile score V: predictive accuracy according to score composition. Am J Obstet Gynecol 1990;162:918–927.

Manning FA, Bondaji N, Harman CR, et al. Fetal assessment based on fetal biophysical profile scoring VIII. The incidence of cerebral palsy in tested and untested perinates. Am J Obstet Gynecol 1998;178: 696–706.

Matthews RN. Obstetric implications of burns in pregnancy. Br J Obstet Gynaecol 1982;89:603–609.

Modanlou HD, Freeman RK. Sinusoidal fetal heart rate pattern: its definition and clinical significance. Am J Obstet Gynecol 1982;142: 1033–1038.

Myers RE. Two patterns of perinatal brain damage and their conditions of occurrence. Am J Obstet Gynecol 1972;112:246–277.

Naidu S, Payne AJ, Moodley J, et al. Randomised study assessing the effect of phenytoin and magnesium sulfate on maternal cerebral circulation in eclampsia using transcranial doppler ultrasound. Br J Obstet Gynaecol 1996;103:111–116.

Nelson KB, Dambrosia JM, Ting TY, Grether JK. Uncertain value of electronic fetal monitoring in predicting cerebral palsy. N Engl J Med 1996;334:613–618.

NIH Consensus Conference on Effect of Corticosteroids for Fetal Maturation on Perinatal Outcomes. JAMA 1995;273:413–418.

Paul RH, Koh KS, Bernstein SG. Change in fetal heart rate: uterine contraction patterns associated with eclampsia. Am J Obstet Gynecol 1978;130:165–169.

Paul RH, Gauthier RJ, Quilligan EJ. Clinical fetal monitoring: the usage and relationship to trends in cesarean delivery and perinatal mortality. Acta Obstet Gynecol Scand 1980;59:289–295.

Perlman JM, Risser R, Broyles RS. Bilateral cystic leukomalacia in the premature infant: Associated risk factors. Pediatrics 1996;97: 822–827.

Petrie RH, Yeh SY, Maurata Y, et al. Effect of drugs on fetal heart rate variability. Am J Obstet Gynecol 1978;130:294–299.

Phelan JP. Antepartum fetal assessment: Newer techniques. Semin Perinatal 1988;12:57–65.

Phelan JP. The postdate pregnancy: An overview. In: Phelan JP, ed. Postdatism. Clin Obstet Gynecol 1989;32(2):221–227.

Phelan JP. Labor admission test. In: Devoe L, ed. Clinics in Perinatology. Philadelphia, PA: W.B. Saunders Co., 1994;21(4):879–885.

Phelan JP, Ahn MO. Perinatal observations in forty-eight neurologically impaired term infants. Am J Obstet Gynecol 1994;171:424–431.

Phelan JP, Ahn MO. Fetal heart rate observations in 300 term brain-damaged infants. J Matern Fetal Invest 1998;8:1–5.

Phelan JP, Kim JO. Fetal heart rate observations in the brain-damaged infant. Semin Perinatol 2000;24:221–229.

Phelan JP, Lewis PE. Fetal heart rate decelerations during a nonstress test. Obstet Gynecol 1981;57:228–232.

Phelan JP, Smith CV. Antepartum fetal assessment: the contraction stress test. In: Hill A, Volpe JJ, eds. Fetal neurology. New York: Raven, 1989;75–90.

Phelan JP, Smith CV, Broussard P, Small M. Amniotic fluid volume assessment using the four quadrant technique at 36–42 weeks' gestation. J Reprod Med 1987a;32:540–543.

Phelan JP, Ahn MO, Smith CV, Rutherford SE, Anderson E. Amniotic fluid index measurements during pregnancy. J Reprod Med 1987b;32:601–604.

Phelan JP, Ahn MO, Korst L, Martin G. Nucleated red blood cells: A marker for fetal asphyxia? Am J Obstet Gynecol 1995;173: 1380–1384.

Phelan JP, Korst LM, Ahn MO, Martin GI. Neonatal nucleated red blood cell and lymphocyte counts in fetal brain injury. Obstet Gynecol 1998a;91:485–489.

Phelan JP, Ahn MO, Korst L, Martin GI, Wang YM. Intrapartum fetal asphyxial brain injury with absent multiorgan system dysfunction. J Maternal-Fetal Medicine 1998b;7:19–22.

Phelan JP, Kirkendall C, Martin G, Romo M, Korst L. Neonatal neuroimaging and intrapartum FHR patterns in fetal brain injury. Am J Obstet Gynecol 2001;185(6):S94.

Polko LE, McMahon MJ. Burns in pregnancy. Obstet Gynecol Surv 1998;53:50–56.

Porter TF, Clark SL, Dildy GA, et al. Isolated disseminated intravascular coagulation and amniotic fluid embolism. Am J Obstet Gynecol 1996;174:486.

Pritchard JA, Cunningham FG, Pritchard SA. The Parkland Memorial Hospital protocol for treatment of eclampsia: evaluation of 245 cases. Am J Obstet Gynecol 1984;148:951–963.

Reece E, Chervenak F, Romero R, Hobbins J. Magnesium sulfate in the management of acute intrapartum fetal distress. Am J Obstet Gynecol 1984;148:104–106.

Reisman RE. Responding to acute anaphylaxis. Contemp Obstet Gynecol 1989;33:45–57.

Rhodes RW, Ogburn PL. Treatment of severe diabetic ketoacidosis in the early third trimester in a patient with fetal distress. J Reprod Med 1984;29:621–625.

Rigg D, McDonough J. Use of sodium nitroprusside in deliverate hypotension during pregnancy. Br J Anaesth 1981;53:959.

Robertson PA, Sniderman SH, Laros RK, et al. Neonatal morbidity according to gestational age and birth weight from five tertiary care centers in the United States. 1983 through 1986. Am J Obstet Gynecol 1992;166:1629–1645.

Roe vs Wade, 410 U.S. 113, 93 S. Ct. 705 (1973).

Roland EH, Poskitt K, Rodriguez E, Lupton BA, Hill A. Perinatal hypoxic–ischemic thalamic injury: clinical features and neuroimaging. Ann Neurol 1998;44:161–166.

Rosen M, Dickinson MG. The incidence of cerebral palsy. Am J Obstet Gynecol 1992;167:417–423.

Rutherford SE, Phelan JP, Smith CV, Jacobs N. The four quadrant assessment of amniotic fluid volume: An adjunct to antepartum fetal heart rate testing. Obstet Gynecol 1987;70:353–356.

Saling E. Technik der endoskopischen microbluentnahme am feten. Geburtshilfe Frauenheikd 1964;24:464–467.

Saling E, Schneider D. Biochemical supervision of the fetus during labor. J Obstet Gynaecol Br Cwlth 1967;74:799–803.

Sampson MB, Peterson LP. Post-traumatic coma during pregnancy. Obstet Gynecol 1979;53:25–35.

Shaw K, Clark SL. Reliability of intrapartum fetal heart rate monitoring in the postterm fetus with meconium passage. Obstet Gynecol 1988;72:886–889.

Sheehan PQ, Rowland TW, Shah BL, et al. Maternal diabetic control and hypertrophic cardiomyopathy in infants of diabetic mothers. Clin Pediatr 1986;25:226–230.

Shenker L, Post RC, Seiler JS. Routine electronic monitoring of fetal heart rate and uterine activity during labor. Obstet Gynecol 1980;46:185–189.

Skupski DW, Rosenberg CR, Eglinton GS. Intrapartum fetal stimulation tests: A meta-analysis. Obstet Gynecol 2002;99:129–134.

Slomka C, Phelan JP. Pregnancy outcome in the gravida with a Nonreactive nonstress test and positive contraction stress test. Am J Obstet Gynecol 1981;139:11–15.

Smith CV. Vibroacoustic stimulation for risk assessment. Clin Perinatol 1994;21:797–808.

Smith CV, Rufleth P, Phelan JP, et al. Longterm enteral hyperalimentation in the pregnant woman with insulin dependent diabetes. Am J Obstet Gynecol 1981;141:180–183.

Smith J, Wells L, Dodd K. The continuing fall in incidence of hypoxic-ischemic encephalopathy in term infants. Br J Obstet Gynecol 2000;107:461–466.

Stannard L, Bellis A. Maternal anaphylactic reaction to a general anesthetic at emergency cesarean section for fetal bradycardia. Br J Obstet Gynecol 2001;108:539–540.

Strange K, Halldin M. Hypothermia in pregnancy. Anesthesiology 1983;58:460–465.

Theard FC, Penny LL, Otterson WN. Sinusoidal fetal heart rate: ominous or benign? J Reprod Med 1984;29:265–268.

Van Arsdel PP. Drug allergy update. Med Clin North Am 1981;65: 1089–1092.

Visser GHA, deVries LS, Groeneudaul F. How bad is a low pH at birth? Prenat Neonat Med 2001;6:265–266.

Vives A, Carmona F, Zabala E, Fernandez C, Cararach V, Iglesia X. Maternal brain death during pregnancy. Int J Gynecol Obstet 1996;52:67–69.

Weber CE. Postmortem cesarean section: review of the literature and case reports. Am J Obstet Gynecol 1971;110:158–165.

Witter FR, Niebyl JR. Drug intoxication and anaphylactic shock in the obstetric patient. In: Berkowitz RL, ed. Critical care of the obstetric patient. New York: Churchill Livingstone, 1983;527–543.

Yoon BH, Kim CJ, Jun JK. Amniotic fluid interleukin 6: A sensitive test for antenatal diagnosis of acute inflammatory lesions of preterm placenta and prediction of perinatal morbidity. Am J Obstet Gynecol 1995;172:960–970.

43 Fetal effects of drugs commonly used in critical care

Jerome Yankowitz

Consideration given to use of medications in the obstetric critical care setting is somewhat different from other situations. Thoughts about teratogenicity, usually the over-riding concern, are minimized. By definition, the life of the mother, and therefore fetus as well, are in jeopardy. When multiple medications are under consideration fetal effects can be factored in, but usually the main concern is to restore stability to the maternal condition. Analysis of fetal effects of any specific medication is difficult due to the relative rarity of pregnancy complicated by critical illness and the fact that the pregnant woman and her fetus are generally exposed to many medications.

To best evaluate the medications used during critical care, information about the specific etiologies behind the treatment indication and specific drug classes are helpful. Embolism, hypertensive disease, hemorrhage, or infection accounted for over half the cases of 2,475 maternal deaths in the United States from 1974 to 1978 (Dildy & Cotton, 1992). A recent evaluation at an urban hospital (Ho et al., 2002) shows a slightly different distribution, but hypertensive disease, infection, hemorrhage, and underlying medical diseases still account for a high proportion of maternal deaths. The various etiologies tend to converge into final pathways involving hypotension, hypoperfusion, thromboembolism, and ventricular dysfunction (including arrhythmias).

Volume expanders

Initial treatment given to critically ill patients often includes administration of volume replacement. Albumin and other colloid solutions may augment large volume infusion of saline or lactated Ringer's solutions. A search of the major teratogen databases including Teris, Reprotox, Reprotext, and Shepard's shows no data pointing to a teratogenic effect of intravenous administration of saline solutions, lactated Ringer's, albumin, dextran, or hetastarch.

Inotropic agents

Volume expansion alone may often be insufficient to maintain blood pressure in critically ill patients. Inotropic agents that function to increase cardiac output by increasing myocardial contractility, heart rate, peripheral vasodilation, or a combination of these factors, would then be used. This group includes dopamine, dobutamine, isoproterenol, and digoxin.

Dopamine (Intropin) is a naturally occurring catecholamine and a precursor of norepinephrine. No studies regarding teratogenicity are available in the literature. This medication has been successfully used to treat acute renal failure secondary to preeclampsia during pregnancy (Nasu et al., 1996) and in the postpartum period (Mantel & Makin, 1997). Dopamine will generally cause vasodilation of renal and mesenteric vasculature at doses between 2 and 5 μg/kg/min via β_2 and dopaminergic receptors. At doses between 5 and 10 μg/kg/min it will result in increased myocardial contractility and cardiac output via β_1 receptors. At doses beyond 20 μg/kg/min it will cause vasoconstriction via alpha-adrenergic receptors.

Dobutamine (Dobutrex, Inotrex) is a beta-adrenergic sympathomimetic agent that can improve cardiac function. Dobutamine has not been studied in human pregnancy although there are occasional case reports describing its use. More recently there are descriptions of use postpartum both as treatment for cardiomyopathy and as part of evaluation of patients with peripartum cardiomyopathy (Lampert et al., 1997; Chan & Ngan Kee, 1999; Hibbard et al., 1999).

Isoproterenol (isoprenaline, Isuprel) is also a beta-adrenergic sympathomimetic agent. Among 31 women treated with isoproterenol during the first 4 months of pregnancy in the collaborative Perinatal Project (Heinonen et al., 1977) there was no increase in malformations.

Amrinone and milrinone (Primacor) are positive inotropic agents administered intravenously to treat heart failure. There have been no epidemiological studies of congenital anomalies among infants born to women treated with either agent during pregnancy.

Digoxin, one of the cardiac glycosides, is used to treat heart failure and cardiac arrhythmias. Among the infants of 142 women who were treated with digoxin in the first trimester, the frequency of congenital anomalies was no greater than expected (Aselton et al., 1985). The rate of anomalies was also not increased among the 52 women treated with cardiac glycosides in the first trimester or the 129 women treated any time in pregnancy in the Collaborative Perinatal Project (Heinonen et al., 1977).

Antihypertensive agents

Acute antihypertensive therapy is usually given to patients with a diastolic blood pressure over 110 mmHg. The drugs commonly used for treatment of severe hypertension in pregnancy include hydralazine, labetalol, sodium nitroprusside, nitroglycerin, calcium-channel blockers (including nicardipine and nifedipine), and beta-blockers (including atenolol). The Joint National Committee on Prevention, Detection, Evaluation, and Treatment of High Blood Pressure classifies hypertension by degree of blood pressure elevation. Stage 3 includes a systolic BP ≥ 180 mmHg or a diastolic BP ≥ 110 mmHg. This is also classified as severe hypertension or accelerated hypertension and corresponds to the BP criteria for severe preeclampsia (Varon & Marik, 2000).

Hydralazine (Apresoline) has a long history of safety and efficacy in the obstetric setting. It is an arteriolar vasodilator but can also cause sympathetic discharge resulting in tachycardia and increased cardiac output. For many obstetricians it is the preferred parenteral antihypertensive for severe hypertension. The frequency of congenital anomalies was not significantly increased among the children of 136 women treated with hydralazine during pregnancy in the Collaborative Perinatal Project (Heinonen et al., 1977). However, only eight of these women were treated in the first trimester. Fetal distress may be more common among hypertensive pregnant women treated with hydralazine near term (Spinnato et al., 1986; Kirshon et al., 1991). This is probably due to systemic vasodilation and either hypotension or decreased placental perfusion. Thus, pregnant women, particularly those who have intravascular volume depletion, should be monitored closely and intravenous hydration should be considered. If late decelerations occur they often will respond to fluid loading and other conservative measures (Mabie, 1999). Thrombocytopenia, a rare side effect of hydralazine in adults, has been reported in neonates born to women treated with this agent in the third trimester (Widerlov et al., 1980). Hydralazine has been compared to other commonly used antihypertension agents. Some studies have shown this drug to be as efficacious as nifedipine (Derham & Robinson, 1990; Martins-Costa et al., 1992), while other studies have shown it to be less efficacious than nifedipine (Seabe et al., 1989; Fernakel et al., 1991). Similarly in comparison to labetalol, two trials found hydralazine to be the better agent (Ashe et al., 1987; Mabie et al., 1987) and two found labetalol to be preferable (Garden et al., 1982; Michael, 1986).

Labetalol (Normodyne, Trandate) is another commonly used agent for severe hypertension treatment. It is a nonselective beta-blocker and postsynaptic alpha-l-blocker. It can slow heart rate and decreases systemic vascular resistance. There are little published data pertaining to labetalol use and congenital malformations. In one randomized double-blind trial of 152 women with hypertension there were no malformations in either the treatment group or the placebo group (Pickles et al., 1989) although these were second and third trimester exposures. Labetalol has been compared to methyldopa in the treatment of pregnancy-induced hypertension and found to be better tolerated and give more efficient control of BP (El-Qarmalawi et al., 1995). When compared to oral nifedipine in hypertensive emergencies, the same group of authors found that both drugs were effective but nifedipine controlled hypertension more rapidly with a significant increase in urinary output (Vermillion et al., 1999) and nifedipine increased cardiac index whereas labetalol may not (Scardo et al., 1999). The authors did acknowledge that one earlier study raised concerns about an increased rate of myocardial infarction in hypertensive patients treated with short-acting calcium-channel blockers (Psaty et al., 1995). At the time it was felt that this study dealt with elderly patients and had methodological and selection bias problems. However, there is a recently reported case of a pregnant patient treated for preterm labor who had an MI associated with receiving nifedipine (Oei et al., 1999). These studies would support labetalol over the calcium-channel blockers. Several recent studies and reviews do not confirm an increased risk of MI in patients treated with calcium-channel blockers so the final word is not established about this issue.

The calcium-channel blockers include nicardipine for parenteral use and nifedipine for oral or sublingual therapy. Nicardipine (Cardene) is a vasodilator that acts on the vascular smooth muscle by blocking calcium entry into the cells. In a study of 40 hypertensive women treated with oral nicardipine and 20 preeclamptic women treated with intravenous nicardipine there were no adverse outcomes (Carbonne et al., 1993). The same investigators compared nicardipine to metoprolol and felt that nicardipine offered advantages in terms of blood pressure control and Doppler blood flow measurements (Jannet et al., 1994). Nifedipine (Procardia), another calcium-channel blocker, does not appear to cause an increase in the rate of malformations among exposed fetuses (Magee et al., 1996). Caution must be exercised when combining nifedipine with magnesium sulfate since the latter would be administered to preeclamptic patients. There have been reports of the combination causing neuromuscular blockade (Snyder & Cardwell, 1989; Ben-Ami et al., 1994) and severe hypotension (Waisman et al., 1988). As alluded to earlier there is also a concern about cardiac toxicity of the calcium-channel blockers, which may be potentiated by combining with magnesium sulfate (Davis et al., 1997).

Atenolol (Tenormin) is a cardioselective beta-blocker. No reports of birth defects have been associated with this drug, but extensive first trimester experience is not available. In fact a large analysis of published trials involving beta-blocker therapy showed little or no information on teratogenicity for the multiple agents reported including atenolol, labetalol, metoprolol, oxprenolol, pindolol, and propranolol (Magee et al., 2001). With maternal treatment before delivery, neonatal beta-blockade, characterized by bradycardia and hypotension, has been reported (Woods & Morrell, 1982; Rubin et al., 1983, 1984). Treatment with beta-blocking agents has been associated with growth restriction; however, it is not clear whether this is due to the underlying disease or reduction in maternal arterial pressure. Also many of the studies showing an association with growth restriction and other problems were in patients who received the agents for long-term treatment of chronic hypertension rather than use in acute critical care situations. Atenolol was associated with lower birth weight and a trend toward more preterm delivery compared to other antihypertensive drugs as monotherapy or to no therapy, but these effects were more pronounced when the drug was given earlier in pregnancy and for long durations (Lydakis et al., 1999). In an observational retrospective study, it was felt that treatment of hypertension, mostly with atenolol, reduced the risk of severe hypertension and preterm labor. These authors felt that the therapy had to be adjusted in order to avoid an excessive fall in cardiac output or an increase in vascular resistance, as these were associated with reduced fetal growth and not the atenolol per se (Easterling et al., 2001). The same group showed that atenolol prevented preeclampsia in a double-blinded randomized placebo-controlled trial, but did result in infants with birth weights of 440 g less than the placebo group for reasons that were not clear (Lip et al., 1997; Easterling et al., 1999). It is hypothesized that some of the effect is specific to atenolol and due to increasing peripheral vascular resistance in the central fetal circulation. These authors (Lip et al., 1997) further conjectured that pindolol, which results in more maternal vasodilation and improved placental blood flow might be a better choice of beta-blocker. Others have found that atenolol alters fetal hemodynamics to a greater extent than pindolol, potentially making the latter a better choice (Rasanen & Jouppila, 1995). Overall the choice of beta-blocker in a critical care situation (late onset severe hypertension) is probably of less consequence than in long-term treatment of mild to moderate hypertension throughout gestation. In the case of long-term treatment some would say that it is not clear that the risks of beta-receptor blockers justify the benefits and use of other agents may be advisable (Magee et al., 2000; Magee & Duley, 2002).

Sodium nitroprusside (Nipride) is an arteriolar and venular vasodilator. It is a potent antihypertensive agent. This drug is rarely needed to control hypertension in obstetric patients and therefore experience is limited. Given its action to reduce peripheral resistance and reduce left ventricular preload, it leads to reduction in pulmonary congestion. This makes sodium nitroprusside a particularly good agent for the patient with severe hypertension in the setting of acute congestive heart failure and pulmonary edema. There have been theoretic concerns about fetal accumulation of cyanide but this has not been definitively proven. In one case where fetal thiocyanate level was obtained at delivery it was equal to the maternal level of 0.1 μg/ml (Stempel et al., 1982). Given the overall concerns about toxicity this agent should be reserved when other intravenous antihypertensive agents are not available or effective (Varon & Marik, 2000).

Diazoxide (Hyperstat, Proglycem) relaxes smooth muscle and produces vasodilation. There are no epidemiologic studies evaluating teratogenicity and most of the concern about its use centers on the profound hypotension that it may cause. Severe maternal hypotension would reduce uterine blood flow and cause fetal distress or death.

Enalapril (Vasotec) and captopril are in the angiotensin-converting enzyme (ACE) inhibitor family. They can be administered orally or parenterally to treat hypertension. This family of drugs does not appear to be teratogenic when given in the first trimester (Burrows & Burrows, 1998). On the other hand, oligohydramnios, fetal growth retardation and neonatal renal failure, hypotension, pulmonary hypoplasia, and other abnormalities have been described following maternal treatment in the second or third trimester (Lavoratti et al., 1997; Ratnapalan & Koren, 2002). It has been recommended that ACE inhibitors not be used during pregnancy (Barr, 1994). Virtually all adverse outcomes reported to the FDA occurred with second and third trimester exposure (Tabacova et al., 2000).

Cardiac arrhythmias

Several agents are available for treatment of cardiac arrhythmias during pregnancy. Treatment of tachyarrhythmias during pregnancy and lactation can involve a variety of agents including quinidine, procainamide, lidocaine, flecainide, propranolol, amiodarone, verapamil, and digoxin. These latter agents do not reduce placental blood flow, while adenosine can (Tan & Lie, 2001).

Amiodarone (Cordarone) is an antianginal and antiarrhythmic that appears to work by blocking sodium channels in the heart. It is structurally similar to thyroxine and contains 39% iodine by weight. Rarely hyperthyroidism and a 9–17% risk of neonatal hypothyroidism have been associated with its use (Bartalena et al., 2001; Tan & Lie, 2001). Given to two women, one in early gestation and the other after the eighth month, transient neonatal hypothyroidism with no long-term developmental consequences has been described (Grosso et al., 1998). This agent has most frequently been used to treat fetal arrhythmia. Few first trimester exposures have been reported and while there is not a clear increase in malformations, concerns about neurologic development have been raised. When used in the second and third trimester, ultrasound evaluations for thyroid size are suggested. Neonatal thyroid function should be closely evaluated and thyroid hormone replacement provided as needed. In a review of the 64 reported pregnancies in which amiodarone was given to the mother there was no clear increase in malformation, rarely neonatal hyperthyroidism, rarely (3%) neonatal goiter, and most commonly (17%) neonatal hypothyroidism (Bartalena et al., 2001). The reviewed cases did not show a clear impact on IQ but there may be an association with mild neurodevelopmental alteration (Bartalena et al., 2001). Neurodevelopment following in utero amiodarone exposure has recently been reviewed (Magee et al., 1999) and confirms problems in nonverbal learning and other mild deficits in the children studied. Amiodarone can also affect the maternal thyroid function (Martino et al., 2001).

Propranolol (Inderal) is a nonselective beta-adrenergic blocking agent that can be used to treat hypertension, tachydysrhythmia, and hyperthyroidism. No association was found for use in the first trimester in a case–control study of 726 infants with neural tube defects, 578 with cleft lip or palate, 191 with hypospadias, and 4,470 with other congenital anomalies (Czeizel, 1989). Among Michigan Medicaid recipients there was no greater frequency of major congenital anomalies among 274 infants of women given prescriptions for propranolol during the first trimester (F. Rosa, personal communication 1993). Newborns should be observed for up to 48 hours for bradycardia, hypoglycemia and other signs and symptoms of beta-blockade.

Quinidine (Duraquin, Quinaglute, Quinalan, Cardioquin, Quinidex) is another antiarrhythmic drug. It has not been associated with adverse pregnancy outcomes although there have not been epidemiologic studies of congenital anomalies in infants born to women who used quinidine during pregnancy. This agent has been used to treat fetal arrhythmias, in particular tachyarrhythmias, without fetal problems attributable to the drug (Spinnato et al., 1984; Guntheroth et al., 1985).

Procainamide (Pronestyl) is a local anesthetic used as a cardiac antiarrhythmic. It has been used to treat both maternal and fetal arrhythmias without reported teratogenic or other significant untoward fetal or neonatal effects. Reported use of procainamide is generally in case reports for fetal tachyarrhythmias (Hallack et al., 1991; Simpson et al., 1995).

Lidocaine (lignocaine, Xylocaine) is a local anesthetic; it is administered intravenously to treat cardiac arrhythmias—usually ventricular arrhythmias. In the collaborative Perinatal Project (Heinonen et al., 1977) there was no increase in malformations among the children of 293 women who had been treated with lidocaine as a local anesthetic in the early part of pregnancy. No epidemiologic studies of lidocaine given intravenously for cardiac arrhythmias and relation to teratogenic effects have been published.

Flecainide (Tambocor) is an antiarrhythmic agent probably most commonly used in pregnancy to treat fetal arrhythmias. There have been only three case reports of use throughout pregnancy, without demonstrated teratogenic effects (Wagner et al., 1990; Ahmed et al., 1996; Villanovea et al., 1998).

Verapamil (Calan, Isoptin, Verelan) is a calcium-channel blocking agent. There was no association with congenital anomalies in the Hungarian Case–Control Surveillance of Congenital Abnormalities (Czeizel & Rockenauer, 1997), or among women who reported first trimester verapamil use to teratogen information services (Magee et al., 1996). No adverse drug effects were noted among the infants of 137 hypertensive women treated with verapamil in late pregnancy in two trials (Orlandi et al., 1986; Marlettini et al., 1990).

Adenosine is adenine riboside (Adenocard) that has been used to treat certain supraventricular tachycardias. Adenosine acts via the adenosine A1 receptor, predominantly at the SA node, AV node and atrial myocytes. By increasing the outward potassium current the cells are hyperpolarized increasing the threshold for triggering a subsequent action potential (Wilbur & Marchlinski, 1997). Paroxysmal SVT is the most commonly seen sustained arrhythmia in pregnant women. Given its short duration of action, adenosine may have advantages over verapamil or digoxin (Wilbur & Marchlinski, 1997). Adenosine has been used in case reports to treat both maternal and fetal tachycardias. There have been reports of fetal bradycardia following intravenous administration of adenosine to the mother. The mother had paroxysmal supraventricular tachycardia and the fetal bradycardia developed despite her maintaining normal blood pressure (Dunn & Brost, 2000). Adenosine has been directly administered to the fetus to treat fetal tachyarrhythmia (Kohl et al., 1995). Despite recent data that suggest that adenosine is an important modulator of mammalian development (Rivkees et al., 2001), significant negative impact on the fetus and newborn have not been observed.

Sotalol (beta-Cardone, Betapace) is a beta-blocking agent. It has rapid placental transfer which has made it an agent selected to treat fetal arrhythmia (Sonesson et al., 1998; Oudijk et al., 2000). No epidemiologic studies have been published.

Thromboembolic disease

Thromboembolism occurs in 0.5–3.0 per 1,000 pregnancies (Yankowitz, 2001). Usual treatment considerations revolve around use of unfractionated heparin, low molecular weight heparin, and coumarin derivatives. Rarely must there be consideration to use streptokinase and other such agents.

Streptokinase (Streptase, Awelysin, Kinalysin, Kabikinase) is a plasminogen activator used as a fibrinolytic enzyme. It is administered intravenously or intra-arterially to dissolve blood clots in conditions such as pulmonary thromboembolism, deep vein thrombosis, and coronary artery thrombosis. In a review of the 166 pregnant women treated with streptokinase there was no increase in congenital anomalies but only four were known to have been treated in the first trimester (Turrentine et al., 1995).

Urokinase (Abbokinase, Breokinase, Win-kinase) is an enzyme that converts plasminogen to plasmin. It is administered intramuscularly for treatment of pulmonary embolism or coronary artery thrombosis. No epidemiologic studies of congenital abnormalities related to urokinase administration have been performed. There are several reports of urokinase use in pregnancy. One publication deals with first-trimester exposure (La Valleur et al., 1996) and the neonate had no abnormalities. Another case describes use in a woman with extensive cerebral venous thrombosis at 8 weeks, but the outcome of the pregnancy is not given (Chow et al., 2000).

Tissue plasminogen activator (Alteplase) is administered following acute myocardial infarction or as a thrombolytic for pulmonary embolus. No adverse neonatal effects were seen in most cases reporting its use. However, caution about severe maternal and fetal/neonatal hemorrhage is warranted. There are several cases of significant uterine hemorrhage occurring after its use, in the non-English literature. There is also one case of an extensive intracranial hemorrhage and neonatal death in an infant the day after the mother was treated for pulmonary embolism (Baudo et al., 1990). Recently, a massive pulmonary embolism was treated at 12 weeks with tissue plasminogen activator; reportedly a normal neonate was born. These authors reviewed the literature on treatment options including thrombolytic agents and embolectomy during pregnancy (Ahearn et al., 2002). They noted 164 women treated with streptokinase, three with urokinase, and five with recombinant tissue plasminogen activator.

The clinician is much more likely to encounter anticoagulants such as unfractionated heparin, low molecular weight heparin (LMWH), or coumarin derivatives than the thrombolytic agents. Unfractionated heparin is a glycosaminoglycan with a molecular weight of 20,000–40,000. It is a highly charged molecule, characteristics preventing it from crossing the placenta. Heparin binds to antithrombin (AT) increasing AT's ability to inactivate the coagulation factors Iia (thrombin), Xa, and IXa. Although associated with few complications, it can cause heparin-induced thrombocytopenia in as many as 3% of patients at 2 weeks, heparin-induced osteoporosis with long-term use, and bleeding complications in 5–10%. A review of 1,325 pregnancies found that reported high rates of adverse fetal/neonatal outcomes associated with heparin use during pregnancy were largely owed to comorbid conditions of the mother and not the heparin itself (Ginsberg et al., 1989).

Low molecular weight heparin is produced by controlled enzymatic or chemical depolymerization that yields chains with a mean molecular weight of 5,000. It does not cross the placenta and is thought to produce a more predictable anticoagulant response. The American College of Obstetricians and Gynecologists (ACOG, 1998) stated that experience with LMWH use during pregnancy supports the conclusions that patients with history of thromboembolic events or thrombophilic disorders can be treated as effectively with LMWH as with traditional heparin. Overall, LMWH has appeared safe in the management of more than 480 pregnancies (Sanson et al., 1999). Recently, concern has been raised about LMWH use to protect against thrombus formation in pregnant patients with artificial heart valves. Caution should certainly be exercised in this group; depending on the type and location of the valve prosthesis, coumarin derivatives may be necessary.

Warfarin sodium (coumadin) is administered orally and works by depressing vitamin K-dependent clotting factors (II, VII, IX, and X). It has a low molecular weight and readily crosses the placenta, potentially resulting in teratogenic effects (Ramin et al., 1997). In a review of 1,325 pregnancies, a 16.9% incidence of adverse outcomes was reported with use of warfarin. The risk of detrimental fetal effects is dependent on the trimester of exposure and possibly the dose (Vitale et al., 1999). In the first trimester, there is a clearly described teratogenic syndrome. Later in pregnancy detrimental fetal effects can be due to fetal anticoagulation and bleeding.

Endocrine emergencies

Among emergencies of the endocrine system, hyperthyroidism due to autoimmune Graves' disease is the leading cause of thyrotoxicosis in pregnant women. About two of every 1,000 pregnancies have been reported to be complicated by hyperthyroidism (Masiukiewicz & Burrow, 1999). Hyperthyroidism has been associated with low-birth-weight infants, severe preeclampsia, and preterm delivery. The main pharmacologic treatments include the thionamides propylthiouracil (PTU) and methimazole (MMI).

PTU has been the mainstay of treatment in the United States. It can cause fetal and neonatal hypothyroidism and rarely goiter. The rate of malformations is not higher among infants of women treated with PTU (Burrow, 1985; Wing et al., 1994).

Methimazole (Tapazole, Carbimazole), like PTU, is given orally to treat hyperthyroidism. Multiple children with aplasia cutis congenita have been reported following in utero exposure to methimazole (Vogt et al., 1995; Martin-Denavit et al., 2000). On the other hand, the risk of a scalp defect appears to be small as several large series found no cases of aplasia cutis (Wing et al., 1994).

Pheochromocytoma in pregnancy is a rare event (Hamilton et al., 1997). The main pharmacologic intervention for this disorder, phentolamine, is an alpha-adrenoreceptor blocking agent given parenterally to control hypertension. No epidemiologic studies are available in relation to this medication. Whether this agent is specifically required or other antihypertensives can and should be used in this particular clinical situation is open to debate (Hamilton et al., 1997).

Miscellaneous agents

The critically ill pregnant patient may require administration of other pharmacologic agents. Often the severely ill patient is fluid overloaded and diuretic therapy is necessary. Furosemide (Lasix, Novosemide) is a loop diuretic. It has not been associated with fetal malformations but should only be used for significant fluid overload, congestive heart failure, or chronic renal disease. It is not generally used to treat hypertension during pregnancy. Care should be given that the patient has adequate intravascular volume to avoid hypotension and reduced uterine perfusion. Other diuretics are available, with little information related to use in pregnancy.

Nitroglycerin is a smooth muscle relaxant used to treat cardiac failure and, over the last decade, preterm labor. This agent also has been used to treat severe hypertension. No epidemiologic studies of congenital anomalies have been performed. Severe pulmonary edema was reported in a woman given nitroglycerine for tocolysis following fetal surgery (DiFederico et al., 1996). The same group of authors found that the pulmonary edema associated with fetal surgery and nitroglycerin tocolysis has among the most severe, protracted course of cases of pulmonary edema at their institution (DiFederico et al., 1998). Although one pilot study showed nitroglycerin to be a promising tocolytic (Smith et al., 1999), its performance was inferior to magnesium sulfate in another trial (El-Sayed et al., 1999). Other than a more marked decrease in maternal blood pressure, there were no other particularly negative maternal or fetal consequences of nitroglycerin administration.

Finally, the critically ill gravida may require sedation, pain medication, anesthesia, and any of a wide variety of other pharmacologic interventions. There are many safe and effective choices to achieve such goals. If there is sparce information available about an agent that must be used to preserve the mother's life, careful fetal monitoring should be considered, if neonatal survival is a possibility. This monitoring should be done in the context of discussion among the team caring for the woman as to whether it would be feasible to undertake delivery if fetal compromise is noted.

Conclusion

A wide variety of conditions can lead to the need for critical care of the pregnant woman. Some of these medications can have teratogenic effects. Other agents can acutely cause fetal compromise secondary to alterations in maternal blood pressure, uterine perfusion, or direct fetal affects. Care of such patients is clearly a team approach and should involve the intensivists, perinatologists, and other personnel as warranted.

References

Ahearn GS, Hadjiliadis D, Govert JA, Tapson VF. Massive pulmonary embolism during pregnancy successfully treated with recombinant tissue plasminogen activator. Arch Intern Med 2002;162:1221–1237.

Ahmed K, Issawi I, Peddireddy R. Use of flecainide for refractory atrial tachycardia of pregnancy. Am J Crit Care 1996;5:306–308.

American College of Obstetricians and Gynecologists. Anticoagulation with low-molecular-weight heparin during pregnancy. ACOG Committee Opinion No. 211, November 1998.

Aselton P, Jick H, Milunsky A, et al. First-trimester drug use and congenital disorders. Obstet Gynecol 1985;65:451–455.

Ashe RG, Moodley J, Richards AM, Philpott RH. Comparison of labetalol and dihydralazine in hypertensive emergencies of pregnancy. S Afr Med J 1987;71:154–356.

Barr Jr M. Teratogen update: angiotensin-converting enzyme inhibitors. Teratology 1994;50:399–409.

Bartalena L, Bogazzi F, Braverman LE, Martino E. Effects of amiodarone administration during pregnancy on neonatal thyroid function and subsequent neurodevelopment. J Endocrinol Invest 2001;24:116–130.

Baudo F, Caimi TM, Redaelli R, et al. Emergency treatment with recombinant tissue plasminogen activator of pulmonary embolism in a pregnant woman with antithrombin III deficiency. Am J Obstet Gynecol 1990;163:1274–1275.

Ben-Ami M, Giladi Y, Shalev E. The combination of magnesium sulphate and nifedipine: a cause of neuromuscular blockade. Br J Obstet Gynaecol 1994;101:262–263.

Burrow GN. The management of thyrotoxicosis in pregnancy. N Engl J Med 1985;313:562–565.

Burrows RF, Burrows EA. Assessing the teratogenic potential of angiotensin-converting enzyme inhibitors in pregnancy. Aust NZ J Obstet Gynecol 1998;38:3:306–311.

Carbonne B, Jannet D, Touboul C, Khelifati Y, Milliez J. Nicardipine treatment of hypertension during pregnancy. Obstet Gynecol 1993;81:908–914.

Chan F, Ngan Kee WD. Idiopathic dilated cardiomyopathy presenting in pregnancy. Can J Anaesth 1999;46:1146–1149.

Chow K, Gobin P, Saver J, Kidwell C, Dong P, Vinuela F. Endovascular treatment of dural sinus thrombosis with rheolytic thrombectomy and intra-arterial thrombolysis. Stroke 2000;31:1420–1425.

Czeizel A. Teratogenicity of ergotamine. J Med Genet 1989;26:69–70.

Czeizel AE, Rockenauer M. Population-based case-control study of teratogenic potential of corticosteroids. Teratology 1997;56:335–340.

Davis WB, Wells SR, Kuller JA, Thorp JM Jr. Analysis of the risks associated with calcium channel blockade: implications for the obstetrician-gynecologist. Obstet Gynecol Surv 1997;52:198–201.

Derham RJ, Robinson J. Severe preeclampsia: is vasodilatation therapy with hydralazine dangerous for the preterm fetus? Am J Perinatol 1990;7:239–244.

DiFederico EM, Harrison M, Matthay MA. Pulmonary edema in a woman following fetal surgery. Chest 1996;109:1114–1117.

DiFederico EM, Burlingame JM, Kilpatrick SJ, Harrison M, Matthay MA. Pulmonary edema in obstetric patients is rapidly resolved except in the presence of infection or of nitroglycerine tocolysis after open fetal surgery. Am J Obstet Gynecol 1998;179:925–933.

Dildy GA, Cotton DB. Trauma, shock, and critical care obstetrics. In: Reece EA, Hobbins JC, Mahoney MJ, Petrie RH, eds. Medicine of the Fetus and Mother. Philadelphia: PB Lippincott Company, 1992.

Dunn JS, Brost BC. Fetal bradycardia after IV adenosine for maternal PSVT. Am J Emerg Med 2000;18:234–235.

Easterling TR, Brateng D, Schmucker B, Brown Z, Millard SP. Prevention of preeclampsia: A randomized trial of atenolol in hyperdynamic patients before onset of hypertension. Obstet Gynecol 1999;93:725–733.

Easterling TR, Carr DB, Brateng D, Diederichs C, Schmucker B. Treatment of hypertension in pregnancy: effect of atenolol on maternal disease, preterm delivery, and fetal growth. Obstet Gynecol 2001;98:427–433.

El-Qarmalawi AM, Morsy AH, Al-Fadly A, Obeid A, Hashem M. Labetalol vs. methyldopa in the treatment of pregnancy-induced hypertension. Int J Gynecol Obstet 1995;49:125–130.

El-Sayed YY, Riley ET, Holbrook RH, Cohen SE, Chitkara U, Druzin ML. Randomized comparison of intravenous nitroglycerin and magnesium sulfate for treatment of preterm labor. Obstet Gynecol 1999;93:79–83.

Fenakel K, Fenakel B, Appelman Z, et al. Nifedipine in the treatment of severe pre-eclampsia. Obstet Gynecol 1991;77:331–337.

Garden A, Davey DA, Dommisse J. Intravenous labetalol and intravenous dihydralazine in severe hypertension in pregnancy. Clin Exp Hypertens 1982;1:371–383.

Ginsberg JS, Hirsh J, Turner DC, et al. Risks to the fetus of anticoagulant therapy during pregnancy. Thromb Haemost 1989;61:197–203.

Grosso S, Berardi R, Cioni M, Morgese G. Transient neonatal hypothyroidism after gestational exposure to amiodarone: A follow-up of two cases. J Endocrinol Invest 1998;21:699–702.

Guntheroth WG, Cyr DR, Mack LA, et al. Hydrops from reciprocating atrioventricular tachycardia in a 27-week fetus requiring quinidine for conversion. Obstet Gynecol 1985;66(Suppl):29S–33S.

Hamilton A, Sirrs S, Schmidt N, Onrot J. Anaesthesia for phaeochromocytoma in pregnancy. Can J Anaesth 1997;44:654–657.

Hallack M, Neerhof MG, Perry R, et al. Fetal supraventricular tachycardia and hydrops fetalis: Combined intensive, direct, and transplacental therapy. Obstet Gynecol 1991;78:523–525.

Heinonen OP, Slone D, Shapiro S. Birth defects and drugs in pregnancy. John Wright-PSG: Littleton, Mass., 1977.

Hibbard JU, Lindheimer M, Lang RM. A modified definition for peripartum cardiomyopathy and prognosis based on echocardiography. Obstet Gynecol 1999;94:311–316.

Ho EM, Brown JA, Graves W, Lindsay MK. Maternal death at an inner-city hospital, 1949–2000. Am J Obstet Gynecol 2002;187:1213–1216.

Jannet D, Carbonne B, Sebban E, Milliez J, Nicardipine versus metoprolol in the treatment of hypertension during pregnancy: a randomized comparative trial. Obstet Gynecol 1994;84:354–359.

Kirshon B, Wasserstrum N, Cotton DB. Should continuous hydralazine infusions be utilized in severer pregnancy-induced hypertension? Am J Perinatol 1991;8:206–208.

Kohl T, Tercanli S, Kececioglue D, Holzgreve W. Direct fetal administration of adenosine for the termination of incessant supraventricular tachycardia. Obstet Gynecol 1995;85:873–874.

Lampert MB, Weinert L, Hibbard J, Korcarz C, Lindheimer M, Lang RM. Contractile reserve in patients with peripartum cardiomyopathy and recovered left ventricular function. Am J Obstet Gynecol 1997;176:189–195.

La Valleur J, Molina E, Williams PP, Rolnick SJ. Use of urokinase in pregnancy. Two success stories. Postgrad Med 1996;99:269–273.

Lavoratti G, Seracini D, Fiorini P, et al. Neonatal anuria by ACE inhibitors during pregnancy. Nephron 1997;76:235–236.

Lip GYH, Beevers M, Churchill D, Shaffer LM, Beevers DG. Effect of atenolol on birth weight. Am J Cardiol 1997;79:1436–1438.

Lydąkis C, Lip GYH, Beevers M, Beevers DG. Atenolol and fetal growth in pregnancies complicates by hypertension. Am J Hypertension 1999;12:541–547.

Mabie WC. Management of acute severe hypertension and encephalopathy. Clin Obstet Gynecol 1999;42:519–531.

Mabie WC, Gonzalez AR, Sibai BM, Amon EA. A comparative trial of labetalol and hydralazine in the acute management of severe hypertension complicating pregnancy. Obstet Gynecol 1987;70:328–333.

Magee LA, Schick B, Donnenfeld AE, et al. The safety of calcium channel blockers in human pregnancy: A prospective, multicenter cohort study. Am J Obstet Gynecol 1996;174:823–828.

Magee LA, Nulman I, Rover JF, Koren G. Neurodevelopment after in utero amiodarone exposure. Neurotoxicol Teratol 1999;21:261–265.

Magee LA, Elran E, Bull SB, Logan A, Koren G. Risks and benefits of β-receptor blockers for pregnancy hypertension: overview of the randomized trials. Eur J Obstet Gynecol 2000;88:15–26.

Magee LA, Bull SB, Koren G, Logan A. The generalizability of trial data; a comparison of β-blocker trial participants with a prospective cohort of women taking β-blockers in pregnancy. Eur J Obstet Gynecol Reprod Biol 2001;94:205–210.

Magee LA, Duley L. Oral beta-blockers for mild to moderate hypertension during pregnancy. Cochrane Database Sys Rev 2002;Issue 4:1–36.

Mantel GD, Makin JD. Low dose dopamine in postpartum preeclamptic women with oliguria: a double-blind, placebo controlled, randomised trial. Br J Obstet Gynaecol 1997;104:1180–1183.

Marlettini MG, Crippa S, Morselli-Labate AM, et al. Randomized comparison of calcium antagonists and beta-blockers in the treatment of pregnancy-induced hypertension. Curr Ther Res 1990;48:684–692.

Martin-Denavit T, Edery P, Plauchu H, et al. Ectodermal abnormalities associated with methimazole intrauterine exposure. Am J Med Genet 2000;94:338–340.

Martino E, Bartalena L, Bogazzi F, Braverman LE. The effects of amiodarone on the thyroid. Endocrine Rev 2001;22:240–254.

Martins-Costa S, Ramos JG, Barros E, et al. Randomized controlled trial of hydralazine versus nifedipine in pre-eclamptic women with acute hypertension. Clin Ex Hypertens 1992;11:25–44.

Masiukiewicz US, Burrow GN. Hyperthyroidism in pregnancy: Diagnosis and treatment. Thyroid 1999;9:647–652.

Michael GA. Intravenous labetalol and intravenous diazoxide in severe hypertension complicating pregnancy. Aust N Z J Obstet Gynaecol 1986;26:26–29.

Nasu K, Yoshimatsu J, Anai T, Miyakawa I. Low-dose dopamine in treating acute renal failure caused by preeclampsia. Gynecol Obstet Invest 1996;42:140–141.

Oei SG, Oei SK, Brolmann HA. Myocardial infarction during nifedipine therapy for preterm labor. [Letter] New Engl J Med 1999;340:154.

Orlandi C, Marlettini MG, Cassani A, et al. Treatment of hypertension during pregnancy with the calcium antagonist verapamil. Curr Ther Res 1986;39:884–893.

Oudijk MA, Michon MM, Kleinman CS, et al. Sotalo in the treatment of fetal dysrhythmias. Circulation 2000;101:2721–2726.

Pickles CJ, Symonds EM, Broughton PF. The fetal outcome in a randomized double-blind controlled trial of labetalol versus placebo in pregnancy-induced hypertension. Br J Obstet Gynecol 1989;98:38–43.

Psaty B, Keckbert S, Koepsell T, et al. The risk of MI associated with antihypertensive drug therapies. JAMA 1995;247:620–625.

Ramin SM, Ramin KD, Gilstrap LC. Anticoagulants and thrombolytics during pregnancy. Sem Perinatol 1997;21:149–153.

Rasanen J, Jouppila P. Uterine and fetal hemodynamics and fetal cardiac function after atenolol and pindolol infusion. A randomized study. Eur J Obstet Gynecol 1995;62:195–201.

Ratnapalan S, Koren G. Taking ACE inhibitors during pregnancy: Is it safe? Can Fam Phys 2002;48:1047–1049.

Rivkees SA, Zhao Z, Porter G, Turner C. Influences of adenosine on the fetus and newborn. Molec Genet Metab 2001;74:160–171.

Rubin PC, Butters L, Clark DM, et al. Placebo-controlled trial of atenolol in treatment of pregnancy-associated hypertension. Lancet 1983;1:431–434.

Rubin PC, Butters L, Clark D, et al. Obstetric aspects of the use in pregnancy-associated hypertension of the beta-adrenoceptor antagonist atenolol. Am J Obset Gynecol 1984;150:389–392.

Sanson BJ, Lensing AW, Prins MH, et al. Safety of low-molecular-weight heparin in pregnancy: a systematic review. Thromb Haemost 1999;81:668–672.

Scardo JA, Vermillion ST, Newman RB, Chauhan SP, Hogg BB. A randomized, double-blind, hemodynamic evaluation of nifedipine and labetalol in preeclamptic hypertensive emergencies. Am J Obstet Gynecol 1999;181:862–868.

Seabe SJ, Moodley J, Becker P. Nifedipine in acute hypertensive emergencies in pregnancy. S Afr Med J 1989;76:248–250.

Simpson LL, Marx GR, D'Alton ME. Management of supraventricular tachycardia in the fetus. Curr Opin Obstet Gynecol 1995;7:409–413.

Smith GN, Walker MC, McGrath MJ. Randomised, double-blind, placebo controlled pilot study assessing nitroglycerin as a tocolytic. Br J Obstet Gynaecol 1999;106:736–739.

Snyder SW, Cardwell MS. Neuromuscular blockade with magnesium sulfate and nifedipine. Am J Obstet Gynecol 1989;161:35–36.

Sonesson S-E, Fouron J-C, Wesslen-Eriksson E, et al. Foetal supraventricular tachycardia treated with sotalol. Acta Paediatr 1998;87:587–587.

Spinnato JA, Shaver DC, Flinn GS, et al. Fetal supraventricular tachycardia: in utero therapy with digoxin and quinidine. Obstet Gynecol 1984;64:730–735.

Spinnato JA, Sibai BM, Anderson GD. Fetal distress after hydralazine therapy for severe pregnancy-induced hypertension. South Med J 1986;79:559–562.

Stempel JE, O'Grady JP, Morton MJ, Johnson KA. Use of sodium nitroprusside in complications of gestational hypertension. Obstet Gynecol 1982;60:533–538.

Tabacova SA, Vega A, McCloskey C, Kimmel CA. Enalapril: exposure during pregnancy: Adverse developmental outcomes reported to FDA. Teratology 2000;61:520.

Tan HL, Lie KI. Treatment of tachyarrhythmias during pregnancy and lactation. Eur Heart J 2001;22:458–464.

Turrentine MA, Braems G, Ramirez MM. Use of thrombolytics for the treatment of thromboembolic disease during pregnancy. Obstet Gynecol Surv 1995;50:534–541.

Varon J, Marik PE. The diagnosis and management of hypertensive crises. Chest 2000;118:214–227.

Vermillion ST, Scardo JA, Newman RB, Chauhan SP. A randomized, double-blind trial of oral nifedipine and intravenous labetalol in hypertensive emergenices of pregnancy. Am J Obstet Gynecol 1999;181:858–861.

Villanovea C, Muriago M, Nava FG. Arrhythmogenic right ventricular dysplasia: pregnancy under flecainide treatment. Ital Cardiol 1998;28:691–693.

Vitale N, De Feo M, De Santo LS, et al. Dose-dependent fetal complications of warfarin in pregnant women with mechanical heart valves. J Am Coll Cardiol 1999;33:1637–1641.

Vogt T, Stolz W, Landthaler M. Aplasia cutis congenita after exposure to methimazole: a causal relationship? Br J Dermatol 1995; 133:994–996.

Wagner X, Jouglard J, Moulin M, et al. Coadminstration of flecainide acetate and sotalol during pregnancy: lack of teratogenic effects, passage across the placenta, and excretion in human breast milk. Am Heart J 1990;119:700–702.

Waisman GD, Mayorga LM, Camera MI, Vignolo CA, Martinotti A. Magnesium plus nifedipine: potentiation of hypotensive effect in preeclampsia? Am J Obstet Gynecol 1988;159:308–309.

Widerlov E, Karlman I, Storsater J. Hydralazine-induced neonatal thrombocytopenia. N Engl J Med 1980;303:1235.

Wilbur SL, Marchlinski FE. Adenosine as an antiarrhythmic agent. Am J Cardiol 1997;79:30–37.

Wing DA, Millar LK, Koonings PP, Montoro MN, Mestman JH. A comparison of propylthiouracil versus methimazole in the treatment of hyperthyroidism in pregnancy. Am J Obstet Gynecol 1994;170:90–95.

Woods DL, Morrell DF. Atenolol: side effects in a newborn infant. Br Med J 1982;285:691–692.

Yankowitz J. Chapter 24. Anticoagulation in pregnancy. In: Yankowitz J, Niebyl JR, eds. Drug therapy in pregnancy. Philadelphia: Lippincott Williams & Wilkins, 2001

44 Anesthesia for the critically ill parturient with cardiac disease and pregnancy-induced hypertension

Rakesh B. Vadhera

Cardiac diseases and severe preeclampsia are conditions likely to present as life-threatening medical or obstetric emergencies requiring intensive management and aggressive hemodynamic, cardiovascular, and respiratory support. If left untreated, these conditions are likely to lead to a less than optimal maternal and/or fetal outcome. Anesthetic and analgesic techniques in these patients are largely determined by the nature of the presenting illness. Choice of anesthetic technique largely depends upon the patient's airway, intravascular volume and blood pressure (BP), changes in hemodynamics expected from the technique and the dependence upon sympathetic drive, coagulation and bleeding status, and requirements for respiratory support.

Maternal survival always takes priority, and sometimes what is good for the mother can be detrimental for the neonate. Occasionally, general anesthetic techniques must be used, which can lead to neonatal respiratory depression and the requirement for ventilatory support. Fetal well-being is an issue in the antepartum period; therefore, every effort should be made to maintain normal maternal BP and cardiac output (CO), and satisfactory uteroplacental blood flow. Every anesthesia technique is associated with known hazards, so the risks of each technique must be balanced against the possible benefits in the context of the presenting illness.

Cardiac diseases

Maternal cardiac disease complicates 0.5–2% of all pregnancies and remains the leading nonobstetric cause of maternal mortality (Sullivan & Ramanathan, 1985). The 1991–1993 triennial report on Confidential Enquiry into Maternal Deaths in the United Kingdom reported a significant increase in the maternal mortality related to cardiac diseases (Department of Heath, 1996). The relative incidence of congenital cardiac diseases has increased, mainly because of improved diagnostic and surgical techniques, whereas that of rheumatic and other acquired cardiac diseases has decreased (Mangano, 1986). The demands of pregnancy and especially labor can exacerbate heart disease to the point of critical illness, and some of these conditions are associated with very high mortality rates.

General considerations

Providing care for the parturient with cardiac disease is probably the most challenging task for an obstetric anesthesiologist. The anesthesiologist, cardiologist, and obstetrician must work as a team, and the anesthesiologist must be involved as early as possible in order to ensure maternal and fetal safety and maternal comfort at the time of delivery. Inadequate cooperation between specialists involved in patient care was one of the primary reasons for substandard care pointed out in the Confidential Enquiry into Maternal Deaths in the United Kingdom (Department of Health, 1996).

Changes in the heart rate (HR) and rhythm, preload and afterload, and myocardial contractility related to adaptations of pregnancy, stress of labor and delivery, and obstetric and anesthesia intervention (including the effect of drugs) all affect a particular cardiac disease in a specific way. Taking these variables into account, it is frequently possible to anticipate the hemodynamic effect. Left-to-right cardiac shunts (i.e. atrial and ventricular septal defects and patent ductus arteriosus), mitral and aortic regurgitation, and asymptomatic mitral stenosis (MS) are usually well tolerated during pregnancy and contribute between 1% and 10% of the associated maternal mortality (see Table 19.2, p. 253). However, symptomatic MS, MS with atrial fibrillation (AF), severe aortic stenosis (AS), right-to-left shunt, pulmonary hypertension, myocardial infarction (MI), uncorrected tetralogy of Fallot, and peripartum cardiomyopathy become worse as pregnancy progresses, and contribute to significant (17–55%) maternal mortality (Palacios & Joyce, 1988). Based on the hemodynamic changes of each cardiac disease and the implications of drugs and anesthetic techniques, guidelines for the selection of the anesthetic technique to be used are suggested in Table 44.1 (Carvalho, 2000).

Table 44.1 Expected ideal hemodynamic features for the anesthetic techniques used and suggested anesthetic technique in the management of various cardiac diseases in pregnant patients

Disease	Heart rate	Preload	Afterload	Contractility	Technique
Mitral stenosis	M–SD	M–SD	M–SD	M	Regional
Mitral insufficiency	M–SI	M–SD	M–SD	M–SI	Regional
Aortic stenosis	M	M–SI	M–SI	M	General
Aortic insufficiency	M–SI	M–SD	M–SD	M–SI	Regional
Pulmonic stenosis	M	M–SI	M–SI	M	General
Pulmonary hypertension	M	M–SI	M–SI	M	General
Dilated cardiomyopathy	M	M–SD	M–SD	SI	Regional?
Hypertrophic cardiomyopathy	M–SD	M–SI	M	M–SD	General
Left-to-right shunt	M	M–SI	M–SI	M	General
Right-to-left shunt	M	M–SI	M–SI	M	General
Ischemic heart disease	M–SD	M–SD	M–SD	M–SD	Regional?

M, maintain; SD, slight decrease; SI, slight increase.
(Modified by permission from Carvalho J. Cardiovascular disease in the pregnant patient. In: Birnbach DJ, et al. Textbook of Obstetric Anesthesia. New York: Churchill Livingston, 2000:553–564.)

Monitoring during labor and delivery

Asymptomatic New York Heart Association (NYHA) class I and II patients, without any evidence of progressive or worsening cardiac disease and congestive heart failure, usually do not require invasive monitoring (Ostheimer & Alper, 1975; Clark et al., 1985). These patients do require a minimum of five-lead continuous electrocardiogram (EKG) monitoring with ability to monitor two leads (II and V_5) simultaneously in order to detect any ischemia and arrhythmias, a noninvasive BP measurement, and continuous peripheral oxygen saturation monitoring ($S_{P}O_2$). Strict intake and output records of fluids are imperative. Additional invasive monitoring—arterial, central venous (CVP), and pulmonary artery pressures (PAP), with or without continuous mixed venous oxygen saturation—is justified in symptomatic NYHA class III and IV patients and parturients with significant pulmonary hypertension (primary or secondary), right-to-left shunt, severe aortic and mitral valve stenosis, dissecting aortic aneurysm, acute MI, congestive heart failure, pulmonary edema, left ventricular dysfunction, cardiomyopathy, sepsis, and pulmonary embolism (Clark et al., 1985). The risks and benefits must be weighed in each patient whenever invasive monitoring is considered. An arterial line is indicated in all symptomatic patients with moderate to severe valve lesions, congenital heart disease, pump failure, and ischemic coronary disease. A pulmonary artery catheter is useful in more severe cases, such as in patients with an ejection fraction less than 0.4 (40%), a left ventricular end-diastolic pressure greater than 18 mmHg, or a cardiac index less than 2.0 (Johnson & Saltzman, 1996).

Cardiovascular effects of fluids, drugs, and anesthetic techniques

Although the efficacy of preload has been questioned recently, it is still customary to give a large crystalloid fluid bolus (10–20 mL/kg) before initiation of regional anesthesia (Rout et al., 1993). This preload needs to be given rapidly and in large amounts for it to have any prophylactic value against hypotension (Ueyama et al., 1999). Sudden increase in preload is detrimental for parturients with severe MS, peripartum cardiomyopathy, or MI, whereas this increase in preload may have beneficial effects in patients with aortic and mitral regurgitation. Because a fixed, preconceived fluid bolus can be detrimental to a parturient with cardiac disease, it is wise to titrate the fluid requirement guided by the changes in CVP or PAP and match it to slow extension of regional block and vasodilation achieved during regional anesthesia.

Nearly all the drugs used during the peripartum period interfere with cardiovascular function in some way, therefore knowledge of the actions and interactions of each drug and their beneficial or detrimental effect on each cardiac disease is of paramount importance. Drugs that increase or decrease uterine tone, those with chronotropic or inotropic effects, and vasodilators and vasopressors need to be used with extreme caution. Epinephrine, given either as a test dose or added to local anesthetics (LA), causes β-receptor stimulation, which in turn causes an increase in HR and CO and a decrease in the systemic vascular resistance (SVR). Ephedrine, an α- and β-receptor agonist, causes peripheral vasoconstriction with an increase in HR. Phenylephrine, a pure α-receptor agonist, cause intense vasoconstriction and reflex bradycardia.

Drugs, used to either stimulate or relax the uterus, need to be used with caution. Terbutaline, a β_2-receptor agonist, causes hypotension and an increase in HR. Oxytocin (in large doses)

produces vasodilation and hypotension, while methylergonovine or 15-methyl prostaglandin F_2-α may increase pulmonary vascular resistance (PVR) and SVR.

Epidural anesthesia with LAs may be the technique of choice for patients with mitral regurgitation and aortic regurgitation who would benefit from peripheral vasodilation and afterload reduction, but such drugs may be tolerated poorly by patients with a low and fixed CO that is dependent upon maintenance of peripheral resistance (i.e. severe MS, severe AS, and primary pulmonary hypertension). However, sudden changes in SVR, HR, and BP can be avoided by either a careful and slow extension of epidural block with a low concentration of LAs and opiates or the use of intrathecal opiates during the first stage of labor. An additional crystalloid fluid bolus, given prior to the initiation of epidural analgesia, should be used carefully and slowly titrated to the degree of vasodilation and the degree of reduction in BP. Regional anesthesia for a cesarean section is inherently safer for the mother than is general anesthesia, and regional anesthetic techniques are associated with 17 times lower case-related mortality than general anesthesia (Hawkins et al., 1997). Epidural anesthesia is considered to be safer than spinal anesthesia in cardiac patients. Sudden sympathectomy and reduction in SVR with spinal anesthesia could be detrimental. Reduction in SVR with epidural anesthesia is easier to treat with crystalloids and vasopressors. Caution is required when discontinuing epidural LA infusion after delivery, as an increase in peripheral resistance combined with a sudden increase in preload, because of auto transfusion and a lack of aortocaval compression, increase the risk of pulmonary edema.

Intravenous opiates in moderate doses can produce analgesia and relief of anxiety and fear, but they also may produce peripheral vasodilation, hypotension, and respiratory depression. Meperidine produces tachycardia and should be avoided in patients with severe MS or idiopathic hypertrophic subaortic stenosis. Morphine may produce bradycardia. The use of narcotic analgesic agents is not contraindicated in the cardiac patient; however, these considerations must be kept in mind when contemplating their use. Intravenous fentanyl or remifentanil, given either as a continuous infusion or as patient-controlled analgesia, offers cardiovascular stability. Intravenous subanesthetic doses of ketamine (0.25 mg/kg) are useful at the time of delivery, but associated increases in HR and BP can be detrimental to patients with MS and myocardial infarction.

Inhalational analgesia, provided with either nitrous oxide in oxygen or the judicious use of subanesthetic concentrations of various inhalational anesthetic agents, during late labor and delivery produces acceptable pain relief in 40–80% of patients without causing significant hemodynamic changes. High CO, high minute ventilation, and the presence of intracardiac shunts all affect the uptake of anesthetics, which can result in unpredictable anesthetic depth and thus an increased risk of overdose and maternal aspiration.

Maternal cardiovascular stability is the main consideration when planning general anesthesia. For cesarean section, indications for general anesthesia include a parturient with primary or secondary pulmonary hypertension, right-to-left shunt, severe pulmonary and aortic stenosis, hypertrophic cardiomyopathy, coagulation abnormalities, and perhaps left-to-right shunt. A high-dose opiate technique with high inspired oxygen concentration is preferable in parturients with cardiac disease. Although high-dose alfentanil or fentanyl with etomidate and succinylcholine usually obtunds the pressure response to intubation and provides hemodynamic stability, it also causes neonatal respiratory depression. An increase in HR because of the stress related to intubation, light anesthesia, ketamine induction, or use of drugs like terbutaline, atropine, meperidine, phenothiazines, ephedrine, and methergine may be poorly tolerated in patients with MS, MI, and subaortic stenosis. A decrease in SVR with thiopentone and isoflurane is detrimental to patients with severe stenotic lesions and right-to-left or left-to-right shunts. Halothane, a myocardial depressant, should be avoided in cardiomyopathy patients, but may be of benefit in parturients with subaortic stenosis. Vecuronium remains an appropriate nondepolarizing muscle relaxant in most cardiac patients. Hypoxia, hypercapnia, and acidosis increase the PVR, and should be avoided at all costs in patients with right-to-left shunt and pulmonary hypertension.

It is important to consider the prevention of bacterial endocarditis in parturients with congenital and acquired cardiac disease. In a pregnant patient with valvular heart disease, a prosthetic heart valve, any shunt or congenital heart disease, any kind of cardiomyopathy, or mitral valve prolapse and insufficiency, antibiotics should be administered prior to any invasive procedures, including anesthesia and monitoring. In most cases of cardiomyopathy with severely decreased cardiac output consideration should be given to anticoagulation because of the risk of embolism, particularly into the cerebral circulation.

Left-to-right shunt

A small atrial septal defect, ventricular septal defect, or patent ductus arteriosus is usually tolerated well during pregnancy. These three lesions account for approximately 75% of congenital heart disease, but contribute to less than 10% of the observed maternal mortality. A modest degree of left-to-right shunt produced by a small defect in the absence of pulmonary hypertension requires little additional treatment. Small defects are associated with a slight increase in pulmonary blood flow, a slight decrease in PVR, and a normal PAP. Larger defects, on the other hand, lead to marked increases in the pulmonary blood flow and resistance. Eventually, pulmonary hypertension develops. An increase in PAP that approximates systemic pressure can cause bi-directional flow or reversal of flow through the shunt. This is obviously an extremely dangerous situation that may precipitate sudden and devastating hypoxia and acidosis. Goals and management of the larger shunts include the following:

General considerations

Avoid sudden changes (increases or decreases) in the SVR. Pain, stress, dehydration, endogenous catecholamines, aortocaval compression, vasopressors, or any other factor that causes increased SVR worsens the left-to-right shunt and may result in pulmonary hypertension and right ventricular failure. On the other hand, a sudden drop in SVR, BP, and oxygen saturation, and an increase in the PVR might lead to reversal of flow through the shunt in the presence of pulmonary hypertension. A left-to-right shunt is also aggravated by increases in HR and CO. Always use an air entrapment filter with intravenous infusion and with arterial lines. In addition, it is preferable to use saline rather than air to identify the epidural space. Intravenous injection of even a small amount of air can result in a paradoxical embolus. These precautions are also important when dealing with a right-to-left shunt.

Regional anesthesia techniques

A careful and slow extension of the epidural block with low concentrations of LAs and opiates (0.0625–0.125% bupivacaine with 2.5 μg/mL fentanyl) or the use of intrathecal opiates (15–25 μg fentanyl or 5–10 μg sufentanil with 150–500 μg morphine) avoids sudden changes in SVR and is considered safe for labor analgesia in patients with left-to-right shunt. Perineal anesthesia during the second stage of labor or the need for cesarean section requires extension of the epidural block with higher concentrations of LAs, which can cause a decrease in SVR and BP. Decreases in SVR and BP, which are more extensive during spinal anesthesia, should be treated immediately with fluids and phenylephrine. Remember that aggressive use and overuse of phenylephrine might worsen the left-to-right shunt. A pudendal nerve block may be required for comfort during the second stage of labor and for vaginal or assisted vaginal deliveries.

General anesthesia

If general anesthesia is required, avoid increases in SVR, HR, and exacerbation of PVR by hypoxia, acidosis, and hypercarbia. Induction of anesthesia with ketamine, light anesthesia, and treatment of hypotension with phenylephrine should be avoided. Peripheral hypoxia may be a sign of reversal of the shunt. A marked increase in SVR may require vasodilator therapy.

Right-to-left shunts

A right-to-left shunt can either be present at birth as in tetralogy of Fallot (i.e. infundibular pulmonary artery stenosis, right ventricular hypertrophy, overriding of the aorta, and a ventricular septal defect) or develop later in life as Eisenmenger's syndrome (i.e. chronic fixed elevation of PAP close to systemic artery pressure, right ventricular hypertrophy and dysfunction leading to a bidirectional or reversal of flow through a left-to-right shunt). Women with tetralogy of Fallot usually do not reach child-bearing age and become pregnant without corrective surgery. Pregnancy in women with Eisenmenger's syndrome carries a very high risk (23–40%) of mortality, which becomes worse as the pregnancy progresses (Gleicher et al., 1979; ACOG, 1993; Avila et al., 1995). Mortality associated with pregnancy in the Eisenmenger's syndrome patient peaks at delivery and during the first postpartum week. Increase in blood volume and CO and changes in SVR during pregnancy are poorly tolerated. Maternal and fetal progress depends on the severity of pulmonary hypertension. Early recognition, admission, bed rest, oxygen, and drug therapy to reduce PVR improve maternal as well as fetal outcome.

Goals and management of the parturients with right-to-left shunt are extremely challenging and include the following.

General considerations

Although shunt is no longer present in patients with surgical correction, pulmonary stenosis might be present, and a detailed evaluation of the right ventricular outflow is suggested in these patients (echocardiogram and or right heart catheterization if necessary). Pulmonary stenosis in these patients seems to be minor and regional analgesia techniques are usually safe (Carvahlo et al., 1993). Anesthetic management is similar to that used in pulmonary hypertension. In patients with Eisenmenger's syndrome, any increase in the pulmonary artery resistance (because of pain, hypoxia, hypercarbia, and acidosis), increase in PAP (associated with increase in blood volume, preload, or resistance), or decrease in the SVR further worsens the shunt. A drug-induced decrease in the PVR is usually ineffective in this fixed chronic obstruction, but inhaled nitric oxide has shown some promise and improved outcome (Goodwin et al., 1999; Lust et al., 1999; Rosenthal & Nelson-Piercy, 2000).

Monitoring should include EKG, S_pO_2, and arterial and CVP measurements. Continuous S_pO_2 monitoring is extremely useful and is an ideal indicator of changes in shunt fraction (Garber et al., 1988). A difference of S_pO_2 between the right hand and lower extremity is a good guide of shunt fraction in the Eisenmenger's syndrome patient with patent ductus arteriosus (Pollack et al., 1990). An arterial line more precisely allows continuous BP monitoring, acid–base status measurement, and is useful in guiding therapy for reduced SVR and hypotension. The roles of continuous CVP and PAP monitoring are controversial (Devitt et al., 1982; Robinson, 1983). A CVP monitoring device is helpful in following and maintaining preload. Care must be taken to avoid air emboli.

Potential complications deriving from the use of central venous and pulmonary artery catheterization are high risk of arrhythmias, thrombi, paradoxical emboli, pulmonary artery rupture, and PDA occlusion. Patients may benefit only in the presence of aortopulmonary shunt (Foster & Jones, 1984). Pulmonary artery wedge pressure may not reflect left ventricular filling pressures in patients with a ventricular septal defect or a large atrial septal defect, and a CVP may be more useful, especially as the right ventricle is at greater risk of dysfunction (Pollack et al., 1990).

Regional anesthesia

Although the role of regional anesthesia is somewhat controversial, epidural anesthesia for cesarean section and intrathecal opiates for labor analgesia have been successfully used in patients with Eisenmenger's syndrome (Spinnato et al., 1981; Pollack et al., 1990; Ghai et al., 2002). Sympathectomy and a reduction in SVR with LA increase the shunt fraction and must be avoided or treated aggressively. However, an epidural block—slowly and carefully titrated to BP and S_pO_2 changes—and judicious use of volume preload and continuous phenylephrine infusion or small doses of mephenteramine to maintain SVR have been successfully used for cesarean section (Spinnato et al., 1981; Ghai et al., 2002). A dose of 1.5 mg of morphine given intrathecally with careful monitoring for respiratory depression has been successfully used (Pollack et al., 1990). Pudendal nerve block may be required during the second stage of labor and delivery. Concurrent therapy with heparin or prostacyclin precludes using a regional technique.

General anesthesia

A cesarean delivery may serve to avoid the stress of labor and continued insult from the worsening cardiovascular demands of gestation. If general anesthesia is required, a slowly induced high-dose narcotic technique with ketamine or etomidate is recommended. Drugs that either cause myocardial depression (pentothal) or decrease the SVR (isoflurane and oxytocin) should be avoided. Ketamine induction with phenylephrine or norepinephrine infusion maintains the SVR and shunt fraction. The effect of positive pressure ventilation on venous return, ventilation/perfusion mismatching, PAP, and shunt fraction are particularly worrisome. Methylergonovine might be a preferable treatment to increase uterine tone postpartum.

Primary pulmonary hypertension

Peripartum mortality in primary pulmonary hypertension may exceed 60% and is highest following operative delivery (Nelson et al., 1983; Fuster et al., 1984). Hemodynamic features include a mean PAP >25 mmHg in the absence of an intracardiac shunt, right ventricular hypertrophy, heart failure, and a low CO. Patients with pulmonary hypertension often have a reactive pulmonary vasculature, and pulmonary vasodilation can be achieved with prostacycline (10 ng/kg/hr), isoproterenol (0.4 mg/hr), diltiazem (20 mg/hr), adenosine, and inhaled nitric oxide (Nootens & Rich, 1993; Lam et al., 2001; Monnery et al., 2001; Naeije & Vachiery, 2001; Stewart et al., 2001). A pulmonary artery catheter not only helps with definitive assessment of the right ventricle—it also helps guide the treatment. A cardiac index <4.0 L/min/m^2, right atrial pressure >10 mmHg, and PVR >1,000 dyn/sec/cm^{-5} are poor prognostic signs. Goals and basic rules for anesthetic management of a parturient with primary pulmonary hypertension include the following:

General considerations

The most important objectives are to minimize the increase in PVR and avoid any major hemodynamic changes. In addition, seek to prevent pain, hypoxemia (oxygen supplementation throughout labor and the immediate postpartum period), acidosis, and hypercarbia. In addition, one should avoid aortocaval compression, hypovolemia (replace excessive blood loss), and any reduction in venous return, as it reduces right ventricular output, which leads to hypoxia and hence a further increase in PVR. Maintain adequate SVR and myocardial contractility. Intensive monitoring with systemic and pulmonary artery catheters and continuous oxygen saturation is essential. It might be technically more difficult to float a pulmonary artery catheter in the presence of tricuspid regurgitation. Anticipate severe bradycardia and treat it aggressively with atropine, isoproterenol, or transvenous pacing.

Anesthetic techniques

Although regional analgesia/anesthesia has historically been avoided, various regional anesthetic techniques for labor analgesia, such as intrathecal opiates alone or combined with pudendal nerve block (Abboud et al., 1983; Hays et al., 1985; Hawkins et al., 1997), segmental epidural with pudendal nerve block (Sorensen et al., 1982), continuous epidural with either double catheter technique or infusion of low concentration LAs with opiates (Robinson & Leicht, 1988; Slomka et al., 1988), or combined spinal epidural with a combination of intrathecal opiates followed by epidural infusion of low concentration LAs with opiates (Department of Health, 1996), have been described. Although a high, dense block for cesarean section may be hazardous, it has been successfully used (Roessler & Lambert, 1986). General anesthesia probably poses less risk and provides much more stable hemodynamic conditions in these patients.

Mitral stenosis

Mostly acquired from and associated with rheumatic heart fever, MS is the most common valvular lesion seen during pregnancy. A reduction in mitral valve surface area (from 4–6 cm^2 to 1 cm^2) and symptomatic (NYHA class III and IV) patients are risk factors for increased mortality and morbidity. Most of the cardiovascular changes associated with pregnancy, such as increase in HR, blood volume, and CO, and drop in SVR, are detrimental to the parturient with MS. Pregnancy is likely to precipitate acute decompensation in patients with severe MS. Major complications of MS during pregnancy include pulmonary congestion, AF, paroxysmal atrial tachycardia, pulmonary embolism, and pulmonary edema. Maternal mortality during pregnancy in asymptomatic patients is 1% and increases to 15% in patients with NYHA class III and IV and AF. Goals and basic rules for anesthetic management of MS include the following (Clark et al., 1985; Hemmings et al., 1987; Ziskind et al., 1990; Mangano, 1993).

General considerations

Maintain a normal HR and normal sinus rhythm. A rapid ventricular rate decreases the time for diastolic filling through a fixed, obstructed mitral valve, increases the left atrial pressure, and decreases CO. Avoid maternal tachycardia and aggressively treat AF and any acute dysrhythmias, if present. Beta-blockers can be used to control HR. In the presence of AF and a ventricular rate of more than 110 beats/min (bpm), one should consider cardioversion (beginning with 25 watts-seconds) and digoxin (0.5 mg IV followed by 0.25 mg every 2 hr) or propranolol (0.2 mg in repeated doses) until the HR is below 100 bpm. Esmolol crosses the placenta and causes persistent β-blockade with fetal hypoxia and it should be avoided unless essential. Other beta-blockers are preferred (Ducey & Knape, 1992). Try to maintain the afterload and SVR. A sudden decrease in SVR causes a reflex increase in HR and further reduces CO. Myocardial contractility is usually not a problem in patients with MS. Avoid a sudden increase or decrease in preload. Pain, hypoxemia, hypercarbia, and acidosis increase the PVR and exacerbate right ventricular failure. Pushing during the second stage of labor (Valsalva's maneuver) increases the SVR and is helpful.

Analgesia for labor and delivery

Epidural analgesia is considered safe and has been successfully used in patients with severe MS (Clark et al., 1985; Hemmings et al., 1987). Consider and provide an early labor epidural to reduce pain and stress and to suppress pain-related tachycardia and endogenous epinephrine release. Sympathectomy, on one hand, is detrimental, as it reduces the SVR, but on the other hand it is beneficial, as it protects against increases in preload during uterine contractions. Give supplemental oxygen before initiating regional block. Extreme care is needed when considering the amount of preload. Avoid sudden changes in preload by carefully titrating small boluses of crystalloid solutions to gradually effect onset and extension of regional block. In symptomatic patients, a CVP monitor may help to assess the central volume status and allow careful titration between vasodilation and the need for additional fluid boluses. Strongly consider a pulmonary artery catheter in NYHA class III and IV patients and in patients with associated pulmonary hypertension. Avoid the use of epinephrine as a test dose or with LAs. Always extend the epidural block very slowly, preferably with low concentration LAs and opiates. Epidural analgesia, preferably with 0.0625% bupivacaine with 2.5 μg/mL fentanyl, provides adequate analgesia for the first stage of labor and offers the flexibility of providing perineal block for the second stage of labor with 0.125–0.25% bupivacaine.

Adequate analgesia, with minimal changes in HR and SVR, for the first stage of labor can be provided with intrathecal opiates. There is no ideal intrathecal opiate in use at present. Doses of 15–25 μg fentanyl or 5–10 μg sufentanil given intrathecally act immediately but are limited by their short action (2–3 hr); on the other hand, a 150–500 μg dose of morphine is longer acting (approximately 8 hr) but requires an hour to achieve analgesia. A combination of 15–25 μg fentanyl and 150–500 μg morphine provides adequate analgesia for the first stage of labor in most parturients but does not provide any analgesia for the second stage. An alternative approach is to use a combined spinal epidural technique, which offers the advantage of intrathecal administration of opiates for the first stage of labor and offers the flexibility of epidural analgesia with a dilute solution of LA (with or without opiate) for both the late first stage and second stage of labor. Prior presence of a dural hole and administration of intrathecal opiates might reduce the requirement of LAs needed later. If the hypotension does occur, avoid the ephedrine-related increase in HR and treat it with small (50 μg) incremental doses of phenylephrine.

In the parturient unsuitable for regional analgesia, labor analgesia can be provided with a parenteral opiate given either as intermittent boluses or continuous infusion, or as a patient-controlled analgesia infusion. Opiates with rapid onset and a short duration of action, such as fentanyl or remifentanil, are recommended. Meperidine, which may cause tachycardia, and morphine, which may cause venodilation, should thus be avoided. The neonatologist should be informed of the possibility of neonatal depression.

Anesthesia for cesarean section

The need for prehydration with large amounts of crystalloids and the inability to titrate this fluid preload to sudden vasodilation associated with sympathectomy are the reasons spinal anesthesia is contraindicated in patients with MS. Invasive hemodynamic monitoring to adjust the preload, judiciously and carefully titrated crystalloid infusion, slow induction and extension of the epidural block, and treating hypotension with small increments of phenylephrine ensure hemodynamic stability during higher epidural blocks for cesarean section, which are usually well tolerated. If general anesthesia is required, avoid stress response to intubation with β-blockers, opiates, or both. An opiate with etomidate and esmolol is a good maternal choice for induction. It is unclear whether perioperative use of β-blockers like esmolol has any detrimental effect on the fetus since the exposure is usually limited (Larson et al., 1990; Losasso et al., 1991; Ducey & Knape, 1992). The neonatalogist should always be made aware of the use of esmolol. Drugs that increase HR, like ketamine, atropine, pancuronium, and meperidine, should be avoided. Maintain anesthesia with halothane or enflurane in oxygen and avoid light anesthesia (tachycardia), nitrous oxide (increases PAP), and isoflurane (decreases SVR). Morphine is a better choice than meperidine for postoperative pain control. Venodilation associated with morphine reduces the detrimental effects of postpartum autotransfusion.

Postpartum care

Autotransfusion and the lack of aortocaval compression after delivery suddenly expands the blood volume, increases the preload, and can precipitate acute pulmonary edema. Continuous epidural anesthesia and associated sympathectomy in the postpartum period reduce the incidence of pulmonary edema. Diuretics (e.g. furosemide 20–40 mg) given immediately after the delivery reduce the preload without causing much reduction in the afterload. Drugs used for increasing the uterine tone after delivery can have detrimental effects; oxytocin produces vasodilation and methylergonovine or 15-methyl prostaglandin F_2-alpha may increase the PVR. The effect of misoprostol is currently unclear. Increased blood loss associated with a cesarean section is beneficial for these patients. Patients should be kept under close observation (high care or ICU area) for at least 24 hours, and thereafter they should be closely monitored for at least another 48 hours.

Mitral and aortic insufficiency

Most of the cardiovascular adaptations of pregnancy, especially the increase in the blood volume and decrease in the SVR, are beneficial; therefore, mitral and aortic insufficiency are usually well tolerated during pregnancy and contribute to less than 1% of the maternal mortality. In the presence of mitral regurgitation, the resistance to left ventricular emptying is reduced, thus producing a greater outflow to the noncompliant left atrium; this means that any anesthetic technique that encourages forward flow is beneficial. Cardiac output is maintained by an increase in the left ventricular contractility. A slower HR or an increase in SVR in patients with aortic regurgitation worsens the aortic regurgitant fraction and increases the left ventriclar end-diastolic volume. An increase in SVR reduces the forward flow from the left ventricle and increases the flow to the left atrium in patients with mitral regurgitation. Any deterioration in left ventricular contractility or high SVR leads to a dilated left ventricle and a low CO. Long-standing chronic aortic and mitral regurgitation can both lead to an enlarged left atrium, increased pulmonary pressure, and right heart failure. Goals and basic rules for anesthetic management in parturients with mitral regurgitation and aortic regurgitation are very similar and include the following.

General considerations

Prevent pain, stress, dehydration, aortocaval compression, and drug-induced increases in HR and SVR. Avoid drug-induced myocardial depression, as CO is dependent upon ventricular contractility. Avoid a sudden decrease in HR, maintain normal sinus rhythm, and treat any arrhythmias aggressively. Maintain preload and monitor the size of the V wave (if monitoring pulmonary capillary wedge pressure [PCWP]), as it reflects regurgitant flow.

Regional anesthesia

Regional anesthesia is the preferred technique for vaginal deliveries and cesarean section. Sympathectomy helps reduce the SVR and analgesia reduces pain and stress-related increases in the SVR. Intravenous fluids given prior to the block help maintain the preload and prevent hypotension. Hypotension can be treated with additional fluids and ephedrine. Myocardial contractility is maintained, as LAs cause the least myocardial depression.

General anesthesia

During general anesthesia, limit the pressure response to intubation, avoid drug (thiopentone and halothane) induced myocardial depression, avoid bradycardia, and maintain preload. An opiate technique is preferred after delivery of the fetus. Isoflurane or vasodilator infusion may be a useful adjunct. In severe cases, the use of an inotrope may be necessary.

Aortic stenosis

Relatively uncommon during pregnancy, AS can present as valvular, subvalvular, or supravalvular stenosis and is associated with high (17%) maternal mortality (Arias & Pineda, 1978). Valvular stenosis is mostly rheumatic, while subvalvular and supravalvular lesions are congenital in origin, with a bicuspid aortic valve being perhaps the most common congenital anomaly of the heart (ACOG, 1993). AS, mostly asymptomatic in the childbearing age group, becomes hemodynamically significant when the valve area is reduced to one-third of its normal size and becomes severe when the valvular gradient is more than 50 mmHg (ACOG, 1993). The classical triad of symptoms (angina, shortness of breath, and syncope) signifies severe disease and, if uncorrected, a life expectancy of less than 5 years (Lao et al., 1993). The presence of a stenotic valve leads to left ventricular hypertrophy, which may proceed to ventricular dilation. Goals and basic rules for anesthetic management in parturient with severe AS include the following.

General considerations

It is of paramount importance to maintain a normal HR, as either a sudden increase or decrease in HR is detrimental. Arrhythmias are not tolerated well by patients with AS, and aggressive and prompt treatment of any arrhythmia is essential. Decreases in afterload and HR with an inability to increase the stroke volume through a fixed stenosis, excessive increase in HR with a decrease in diastolic filling time, and increases in myocardial oxygen consumption are all tolerated poorly by patients with AS. A drop in CO cannot be compensated with an increase in stroke volume (fixed) and becomes worse if compensated with an increase in HR. Maintain intravascular volume, venous return, and left ventricular filling pressure in patients with AS. Noninvasive monitoring is usually sufficient in mild cases, while monitoring of arterial and central venous (and preferable pulmonary artery) pressures is strongly recommended in severe cases. Monitoring PAP carries the risk of precipitating an arrhythmia.

Analgesia for labor and delivery

The most appropriate anesthetic technique for treating a patient with severe AS is somewhat controversial (Whitfield & Holdcroft, 1998). Although continuous epidural or spinal anesthesia has been safely used, historically, anesthesiologists have avoided the use of regional anesthesia in parturients with severe AS (Easterling et al., 1988; Brian et al., 1993; Colclough et al., 1995). Hypovolemia is a greater threat in these patients than pulmonary edema; thus, adequate prehydration before regional anesthesia can be assured by maintaining the CVP or PCWP at high to normal levels. The presence of aortic regurgitation with AS is beneficial for patients undergoing sympathectomy. A continuous infusion technique—similar to one described for parturients with severe MS—with low-concentration LAs with an opiate, or combined spinal/epidural analgesia with the use of intrathecal opiates are safe techniques. Consider using intravenous opiates in patients where regional analgesia is contraindicated. Analgesia and comfort during second stage and vaginal delivery may be achieved with local infiltration or pudendal nerve block.

Anesthesia for cesarean section

In mild cases of AS, an epidural block that is slowly extended can be used, whereas general anesthesia is probably the safest anesthetic technique to use when managing a patient with severe AS. Although a case of mild AS was successfully managed with a continuous spinal microcatheter, the pros and cons of regional versus general anesthesia for cesarean delivery were highlighted in two recent articles (Brighouse, 1998; Whitfield & Holdcroft, 1998). Carefully administered, both techniques have their advantages. Early preoperative recognition of symptoms and aggressive management and cooperation between teams are essential for improved outcome. Treatment of hypotension, initially with a fluid bolus, and, if needed, later with phenylephrine, is preferable to ephedrine. Avoid sudden vasodilation with terbutaline and a bolus dose of oxytocin. Myocardial depression induced by using pentothal and β-blockers (used to limit the tachycardic response to intubation) can be detrimental.

Peripartum cardiomyopathy

Peripartum cardiomyopathy, mostly presenting as dilating cardiomyopathy of unknown etiology, is a rare and devastating from of heart failure that causes significant morbidity and mortality. The disease primarily affects ventricular contractility with a reduction in ejection fraction, an increase in end-diastolic volume, elevated filling pressures, a decrease in CO, and biventricular hypokinesia. Cardiomegaly is the hallmark of the disease. The disease process, if chronic in nature and caused by Chagas' disease, can cause thromboembolism and intracardiac conduction disturbances (Moraes, 1994). Goals and basic principles for anesthetic management are listed below (George et al., 1997).

General considerations

The most important aspect when caring for these patients is to maintain myocardial contractility and avoid drug-induced myocardial depression. An increase in myocardial con-tractility is beneficial and might require inotropic support in severely compromised patients. A sudden increase in either preload or afterload is harmful, as it may precipitate left ventricular failure. Infusion of a fixed preconceived large crystalloid volume before epidural can be detrimental and lead to pulmonary edema; hence, restricting the preload and volume of infused fluids is advised. Autotransfusion and increased venous return during contractions and after delivery are detrimental. Diuretics may have a role in the immediate postpartum period. Avoid bradycardia, as an increase in diastolic filling time raises the left ventricular end-diastolic volumes and compromises ejection fraction. An arterial line and a CVP monitor must be considered for patients with severe AS.

Regional anesthesia

Carefully titrated continuous epidural or spinal analgesia with low dose and diluted-concentration LAs reduces afterload and venous return with minimal effect on myocardial contractility, thus improving CO. Regional anesthesia has been successfully used for cesarean section as well. The addition of epinephrine to LA solutions might have a beneficial effect by increasing contractility and HR and reducing SVR. Titration of LA and fluid/vasoactive treatment of hypotension, which restricts the rise in preload and helps prevent pulmonary edema, should be based on wedge pressure (George et al., 1997). Parturients with very low ejection fraction might benefit from preinduction dobutamine infusion to increase the contractility and nitroglycerine infusion to reduce the SVR. Continuation of an epidural with low concentration LAs during the immediate postpartum period safeguards against autotransfusion and pulmonary edema while simultaneously providing good analgesia.

General anesthesia

General anesthesia may result in profound myocardial depression and cardiac arrest (McIndoe et al., 1995). Myocardial depression caused by thiopental, volatile agents, and ketamine; bradycardia caused by laryngoscopy, succinylcholine, and halothane; and increased afterload caused by ketamine and light anesthesia are all detrimental. Induction with high-dose fentanyl and etomidate is preferred. Morphine, rather than meperidine, is a good choice for postoperative pain control. Venodilation associated with morphine reduces the detrimental effects of postpartum autotransfusion and increases in the preload.

Obstructive cardiomyopathy

Obstructive cardiomyopathy (also known as idiopathic hypertrophic subaortic stenosis), which is associated with hypertrophic changes in the left ventricle, causes a reduction in ventricular outflow and is symptomatically and hemodynamically very similar to AS. Hypertrophic and obstructive changes around the ventricular inflow may also interfere with the mitral valve function, causing MS or mitral regurgitation. The obstruction is a dynamic one and is caused by increased contractility, hypertrophy, and, ultimately, low compliance of the left ventricle. Increases in CO, left ventricular muscle mass, and HR associated with pregnancy have detrimental effects and may lead to pulmonary edema or a life-threatening arrhythmia. Decreases in preload and afterload are tolerated poorly. A reduction in the contractility and HR improves the obstruction and can be clinically achieved using β-blockers.

General considerations

Pain and stress associated with an increase in HR and aggressive and long trials of labor should be avoided. Drugs to be used with extreme caution include terbutaline, digoxin, epinephrine, ephedrine, diuretics, and methergine.

Anesthesia for labor and delivery

During labor and delivery these patients should be managed in a similar fashion to those presenting with pulmonary or AS. Vasodilation during regional anesthesia is poorly tolerated. Treat hypotension with small doses of phenylephedrine. The volume status of these patients must be followed carefully. The Valsalva maneuver during the second stage of labor should be avoided.

Anesthesia for cesarean section

Cesarean section under regional anesthesia requires extreme caution but is not contraindicated (Boccio et al., 1986; Autore et al., 1999; Recasens et al., 2000). However, single-shot spinal anesthesia and rapid extension of an epidural block should be avoided (Loubser et al., 1984; Baraka et al., 1987). Slowly titrated continuous epidural or spinal block with aggressive BP support combined with fluid therapy guided by hemodynamic monitoring and the use of phenylephrine provides a stable cardiovascular state (Deiml et al., 2000). It is prudent to monitor these patients for 24 hours (the period of maximum increase in the CO) after delivery and provide adequate postoperative analgesia.

During general anesthesia, avoid any pentothal-related reduction in SVR or ketamine-associated increase in HR and contractility. Ketamine and its sympathomimetic side effects are detrimental. Although there have been some concerns about the safety of β-blockers, a rapidly titratable, short-acting β-blocker like esmolol must be considered for controlling HR and contractility during the peripartum period. Low concentrations of halothane with opiates are a good choice, as they cause a reduction in contractility and HR. Avoid isoflurane, as it reduces the SVR.

Myocardial infarction

Although MI is rare during pregnancy, with an incidence of 1 in 10,000 deliveries, mortality rates as high as 30–40% have been reported (Hankins et al., 1985). Infarction is more common in the third trimester and in women over the age of 35. MI during the peripartum and postpartum periods and in younger patients carries a worse prognosis, and care in tertiary facility is essential for reducing mortality. It is obviously difficult to delay the obstetric and anesthetic intervention for 3 months after MI to reduce the incidence of reinfarction and other complications (Rao et al., 1983; Shah et al., 1990); however, if possible, every effort should be made to postpone the delivery for 2 weeks after the acute event. Vaginal delivery seems to be associated with a lower incidence of complications (Hankins et al., 1985). Basic rules and goals specific to the anesthetic management include the following.

General considerations

Continuous monitoring of EKG (specifically the V_5 lead), S_po_2, and noninvasive BP are the basic minimal essentials, while resources for invasive monitoring and support of cardiac functions, including echocardiography, systemic and pulmonary artery catheterization, nitroglycerine and inotrope infusions, should be immediately available. An intra-arterial catheter helps maintain HR and BP near baseline. Patients who have had an infarction within the last 3 months, and in whom there is poor ventricular function, and evidence of valvular dysfunction may require a pulmonary artery catheter to monitor cardiac function. Nitroglycerine infusion (0.5 mg/kg/min) may help provide coronary artery vasodilation and reduce the preload, afterload, and left ventricular workload. Direct-current conversion of arrhythmias with energy levels between 25 and 100 watts-seconds seems to be effective and safe for the fetus.

Anesthesia

The main goal of any anesthetic technique is to avoid tachycardia, maintain normal sinus rhythm, and avoid any sudden increase in CO and left ventricular workload. Continuous epidural anesthesia is an excellent choice for labor and vaginal delivery (Aglio & Johnson, 1990; Soderlin et al., 1994; Busto et al., 1995). Vaginal delivery with good regional analgesia eliminates the stress- and pain-induced tachycardia, reduces maternal catecholamine levels, provides hemodynamic stability, reduces afterload and left ventricular workload, prevents hyperventilation, and maintains coronary blood flow (Rowe, 1974), reduces blood loss, and allows early ambulation. The additive effects of sympathectomy and nitroglycerine can lower the diastolic BP and jeopardize the subendocardial blood flow. If hypotension does occur, it should be treated with phenylephrine. Ephedrine causes an increase in HR and myocardial oxygen consumption, which is detrimental to parturients with MI. Continuous epidural anesthesia and associated sympathectomy in the postpartum period reduce the incidence of pulmonary edema and offset the problems caused by a sudden increase in CO and left ventricular work index.

Pregnancy-induced hypertension

Hypertension complicates about 7–10% of pregnancies (5–10% of which represent severe cases), accounts for 15–19% of all maternal mortality in the United States and the United Kingdom, and is the most common reason for admission of a parturient to ICU (ACOG, 1993; Berg et al., 1996; Department of Health, 1996; Umo-Etuk et al., 1996). The four subtypes of hypertension during pregnancy espoused by the National High Blood Pressure Education Program on High Blood Pressure in Pregnancy (2000) are gestational hypertension, chronic hypertension, preeclampsia, and chronic hypertension with superimposed preeclampsia. Although the precise etiology of preeclampsia is unknown, its widespread effects on various organs must be considered when choosing the optimal anesthetic regimen for each patient.

Preoperative evaluation

As preeclampsia is a multisystem disorder, both the extent and severity of the disease must be assessed during a complete preoperative evaluation, which must include a complete history, a physical examination, a history of previous anesthetics, a list of drugs currently taken (including the ones required for the treatment of hypertension and seizure prophylaxis), and a review of laboratory values. Important considerations to be taken into account before deciding on the anesthetic technique to be used for labor analgesia or cesarean section are intravascular volume status, BP control, drug interactions, electrolyte disturbances, and coagulation abnormality. One must also rule out any cardiac, renal, hepatic, and neurological involvement. Signs and symptoms of severe preeclampsia include BP above 160/110 mmHg, more than 5 g proteinuria, oliguria, cerebral and visual disturbances, epigastric pain, pulmonary edema, and hemolysis, elevated liver enzymes, and low platelet (HELLP) syndrome.

An increasing hematocrit or a hematocrit above 36 may be suggestive of hemoconecentration. In 10% of patients with severe preeclampsia, a microangiopathic hemolytic anemia associated with thrombocytopenia and increased liver enzymes (HELLP) may develop (Vardi & Fields, 1974). It is important to know about the coagulation status in these patients in order to determine the risk of bleeding at the time of delivery and the suitability of the patient for regional anesthesia. Coagulation abnormalities frequently occur in parturients with severe preeclampsia or eclampsia (Pritchard et al., 1976; Schwartz & Brenner, 1983).

Hepatic and renal dysfunction can occur and lead to inadequate production of enzymes and coagulation factors, a decrease in renal blood flow and glomerular filtration (with a rise in blood urea nitrogen and serum creatinine), and a decrease in creatinine clearance. Such dysfunction can also affect pharmacokinetics and drug clearance. Oliguria is common in severe preeclampsia and represents intravascular volume depletion, reduced CO, and renal artery spasm. Drugs like magnesium sulfate, which are excreted through the kidneys, require dose adjustment in patients with a creatinine level above 1.0 mg/dL.

Coagulation and anesthetic implications

Thrombocytopenia (platelet count <100,000/mm^3)—the most common coagulopathy seen in preeclamptic patients—occurs in about 20% of severe cases and may be the presenting symptom in some patients (Pritchard et al., 1976; Schwartz Brenner, 1983; Kelton et al., 1985; Burrows et al., 1987). Platelet count can change rapidly, especially with the worsening of preeclampsia, and should be measured within 4–6 hours of expected anesthetic intervention (Rout, 2001). Because the disease affects platelet function, it is advisable to assess the platelets in patients with a platelet count <100,000/mm^3, as the platelet function is directly related to the severity of the disease (Burrows et al., 1987; Ramanathan et al., 1989). A sudden decrease in platelet count is riskier than a chronic reduction, as seen in idiopathic thrombocytopenic purpura.

Bleeding time, and more recently, thromboelastogram and platelet function analyzers (PFA-100) have been used to define the platelet function. Although prolonged bleeding time has been reported in preeclamptic patients with normal platelet counts, the bleeding time is probably unreliable; as a result, its role and usefulness have been questioned (Kelton et all., 1985; O'Kelly et al., 1992; Rodgers & Levin, 1990).

Most obstetric anesthesiologists would perform a regional technique in preeclamptic patients, when the platelet count is at least 100,000/mm^3. However, more and more anesthesiologists are performing regional techniques when the platelet count is between 80,000/mm^3 and 100,000/mm^3, especially when the benefits seem to outweigh the risks. For patients with a sudden drop in platelet count or a count below 80,000/mm^3, the anesthesiologist must balance the benefit of epidural anesthesia against a remote risk of epidural hematoma.

With an incidence of 1 in 190,000 procedures, epidural hematoma seems to be an extremely rare event (Sullivan & Ramanathan, 1985), even in patients who received epidural anesthesia in the presence of unrecognized thrombocytopenia (Clark et al., 1985; Rasmus et al., 1989; ACOG, 1993). Despite the concerns about abnormal platelet function, there are only a few definitive reports of epidural hematoma in preeclamptic patients after epidural anesthesia (Sullivan & Ramanathan, 1985; Lao et al., 1993).

Although maximum amplitude from a thromboelastogram (Haemoscope Corporation, Skokie, IL) tracing and a closure time from a PFA-100 (Dade Behring, Newark, DE) analyzer have been shown to correlate with a low platelet count, it remains to be seen whether these values can accurately predict the risk of epidural hematoma in clinical settings of parturients with preeclampsia, especially when the platelet count is between 60,000/mm^3 and 100,000/mm^3. Studies looking at maximum amplitude and closure time seem to suggest that platelet function starts to deteriorate below a platelet count of 60,000/mm^3 (Orlikowski et al., 1996; Marietta et al., 2001; Vincelot et al., 2001). Orlikowski and colleagues (Orlikowski et al., 1996) found that the maximum amplitude remained normal until the platelet count decreased to less than 54,000/mm^3 (95% confidence interval 40–75,000/mm^3). Based on their study, they suggested that a platelet count of 75,000/mm^3 should be associated with adequate hemostasis. Initial studies that have primarily focused on expected closure time (Vincelot et al., 2001) have so far shown that closure time may be more sensitive than the maximum amplitude for patients with preeclampsia and thrombocytopenia (Davies et al., 2001a,b). Although to date there are no large randomized trials using preeclamptic patients underway to assure safety of regional anesthesia in patients with low platelet count, most of the studies discussed above indicate that, in the near future, it might become an acceptable and safe practice to look at platelet function and conduct a regional technique at platelet counts as low as 60,000/mm^3.

Disseminated intravascular coagulation is rare in preeclamptic patients and is usually associated with fetal demise, sepsis, or placental abruption. If there are no signs of hemorrhage, placental abruption, or consumptive coagulopathy, routine prothrombin time and activated partial thromboplastin time measurements are of limited value, even in the presence of thrombocytopenia (Prieto et al., 1995). A thromboelastogram might not be able to predict abnormal coagulation (i.e. prothrombin time, activated partial thromboplastin time, and bleeding time) in either normal or preeclamptic parturients (Wong et al., 1995).

Hemodynamic implications

Hemodynamic changes in preeclamptic patients vary and are unpredictable (Benedetti et al., 1980; Hodgkinson et al., 1980; Newsome et al., 1986; Cotton et al., 1988; Bolte et al., 2000, 2001). Historically, a parturient with severe preeclampsia, before any therapeutic intervention, has been considered to be a patient with low intravascular volume, low left and right ventricular filling pressures, low PCWP, high SVR, and a normal to hyperdynamic left ventricular function despite the increase in left ventricular workload (Rafferty & Berkowitz, 1980; Kuzniar et al., 1983; Hays et al., 1985). The changes in SVR in the parturient with severe PIH are variable and have an inverse relationship with CO. Changes in PCWP vary from normal to high and are not as low as historically believed. Furthermore, CVP and PCWP often do not correlate (Cotton et al., 1985a). In patients treated with fluids and/or vasodilators, these findings can be different. Before treatment there seems to be some correlation between the two pressures, which after volume expansion becomes poor (Bolte et al., 2000).

Fluids

Evaluation of a patient's fluid balance must include a strict hourly intake/output chart that includes hourly urine output. Maternal urine output is probably the best way, in the absence of invasive monitoring, to assess the intravascular volume status. It is difficult to predict the preeclamptic patient's response to fluid preload. Rising serum creatinine and oliguria suggest renal function deterioration. This deterioration can be a result of either: (i) high SVR and low PCWP, requiring additional fluids; or (ii) high SVR, normal or elevated PCWP, and elevated CO, requiring fluid restriction and a vasodilator; or (iii) high SVR and PCWP and low CO, requiring an afterload reduction (Clark et al., 1986). Fluid resuscitation after a single fluid bolus challenge, with no improvement in urine output, should be guided by CVP monitoring or pulmonary artery catheterization in parturients with severe PIH and oliguria (Clark et al., 1986).

Pulmonary edema, a significant cause of maternal morbidity and mortality, occurs approximately in 3% of patients with severe preeclampsia (Sibai et al., 1987) and 70% of these cases occur in the postpartum period. The origin of pulmonary edema may be either cardiogenic or non-cardiogenic (Mabie et al., 1988). Severe preeclamptic patients with cardiogenic edema might require CO and/or echocardiography studies to differentiate between a systolic or diastolic dysfunction. Non-cardiogenic pulmonary edema often occurs as a result of a large-volume crystalloid or colloid infusion, low colloid oncotic pressure (Benedetti & Carlson, 1979), increased hydrostatic pressure, and increased pulmonary capillary permeability. Older multiparous parturients with sepsis and chronic hypertension are more prone to develop pulmonary edema. Volume infusion prior to regional anesthesia is unlikely to contribute to pulmonary edema (Sibai et al., 1987). Initial treatment includes fluid restriction, supplemental oxygen, and administration of diuretics. Vasodilation and a reduction in afterload associated with regional anesthesia are beneficial for these patients. Further management may include pulmonary artery catheterization to determine the cause of pulmonary edema and guide the therapy; vasodilators (nitroglycerine) to reduce preload and afterload; inotropes to increase contractility in patients with pump failure; and ventilation support for patients with respiratory failure and refractory pulmonary edema. There is little evidence to suggest that infusion of colloid solutions in severe preeclampsia is any better than crystalloid solutions (Anthony et al., 1996).

Drugs

The therapeutic objective for treating severe hypertension and using antihypertensive drugs in preeclampsia is to prevent maternal morbidity associated with encephalopathy, cerebrovascular accidents, congestive heart failure, and other end-organ damage without compromising cerebral perfusion or jeopardizing uteroplacental blood flow and the fetus. The goal is not the normalization of BP, but rather the reduction of BP to a range that is not at risk for loss of cerebral autoregulation. The threshold for treatment of BP is a diastolic BP of 110 mmHg or a mean arterial BP (MAP) of 125 mmHg. The aim of therapy is to maintain a diastolic BP of 90–105 mmHg and a MAP of 105–125 mmHg (Sibai, 1996). Since most of these patients have a high SVR, the main principle of treatment is to reduce the systemic resistance by using a peripheral vasodilator (i.e. a direct-acting smooth muscle relaxant, an α-adrenoreceptor antagonist, or a calcium-channel blocker). Adequate volume expansion prior to vasodilation may be required to safeguard against a sudden severe drop in BP and a reduction in perfusion (especially to placenta and kidneys), which thus risks oliguric renal failure and fetal compromise.

Hydralazine and labetalol are first-line drugs used in the management of peripartum hypertensive disorders. Although most patients respond well to intermittent boluses of these drugs, a small number require other drugs for the management of refractory hypertension. Hydralazine, a direct acting vasodilator, is given intravenously in small (2.5–5 mg) increments until the diastolic BP is controlled below 110 mmHg. The onset of action is approximately 20 minutes. Hydralazine primarily decreases precapillary arteriolar resistance, but an associated increase in maternal CO and tachycardia interferes with its antihypertensive effects (Cotton et al., 1985b). Though it is widely used and considered very safe, there have been several reports which indicate that hydralazine may decrease uterine blood flow in a significant number of women (Lunell et al., 1983; Lipshitz et al., 1987) and cause fetal distress (Vink & Moodley, 1982) and neonatal thrombocytopenia (Lindheimer & Katz, 1985). The slow onset, delayed peak effect, and compensatory tachycardia make hydralazine a less-than-ideal drug.

Labetalol causes non-selective β-blockade and a selective postsynaptic α-1 blockade with a β/α ratio of 7:1. It has a more rapid onset than hydralazine and lacks the side effects of tachycardia, nausea, headache, excessive hypotension, and decreased uterine blood flow associated with hydralazine (Mabie et al., 1987). Although labetalol crosses the placenta, fetal side effects rarely occur. Caution must be used when administering β-blockers to patients with bronchoconstrictive disorders and compromised myocardial function. It is difficult to achieve a fine control of BP with either hydralazine or labetalol. Esmolol, a pure β-receptor antagonist, crosses the placenta and causes fetal hypoxia and bradycardia effects; as a result, esmolol never gained popularity among anesthesiologists for use in pregnant patients (Ducey & Knape, 1992). Even labetalol has been implicated to cause adverse fetal effects (Klarr et al., 1994). Labetalol in a dose of 1 mg/kg can be used to blunt the stress response of tracheal intubation.

Nitroglycerin and sodium nitroprusside have been used successfully in parturients, but both can cause a precipitous fall in BP in severe preeclamptic patients with reduced blood volume. Their use in severe preeclampsia requires blood volume expansion and more invasive monitoring, including CVP measurement (Naulty et al., 1981; Longmire et al., 1991). Both drugs have a rapid onset of action and are easily titratable because of their very short half-lives. Their use is restricted to patients with intractable hypertension that is not controlled by first-line drugs and for obtunding the hypertensive response to intubation.

Sodium nitroprusside, a potent arterial and venous dilator (Ellis et al., 1982), should be reserved for extreme emergencies secondary to concerns of thiocynate toxicity in neonates and mothers after prolonged use and increases in intracranial pressures. At the same time, sodium nitroprusside infusion for a short period of time seems to be safe. Nitroglycerine, a venodilator, is easier to use than sodium nitroprusside, since it can be used as 50–100 μg boluses, especially during general anesthesia. Associated uterine atony is a limiting factor and restricts the use of nitroglycerin in such patients. The recommended initial infusion dose for both drugs is 0.5–5 μg/kg/min, which is then titrated slowly to response.

Calcium-channel blockers, particularly nifedipine, are gaining importance as safe and effective antihypertensives for use in pregnancy. Nifedipine has been used both for the treatment of chronic hypertension during pregnancy as well as for acute reduction in BP in severe preeclamptic patients at term. Nifedipine, a potent vasodilator, selectively decreases peripheral resistance without reducing CO and affecting HR. Neither fetal effects nor the changes in uteroplacental flow have been reported after either short-term or long-term therapy (Lindow et al., 1988; Hanretty et al., 1989). Nifedipine, if used close to delivery, also relaxes the uterus and increases the chances of postpartum hemorrhage. A major cause of concern is that concurrent use of nifedipine with magnesium sulfate may potentiate the antihypertensive effect and neuromuscular block (Bennett & Edwards, 1997). Nimodipine, a selective cerebral vasodilator calcium-channel blocker, initially thought to be an effective prophylactic agent (Belfort et al., 1993) has been recently shown to be less effective than $MgSO_4$ in seizure prevention. It is now recommended that this agent should be avoided as a primary prophylaxis agent in preeclampsia but it may still have a role in eclampsia therapy especially where severe cerebral vasospasm has been diagnosed. Very limited experience with nicardipine has shown it to be an effective antihypertensive agent in severe preeclampsia and in pregnant women with autonomic hyperreflexia (Carbonne et al., 1993; Kobayashi et al., 1995). So far, nicardipine has not been shown to have any deleterious effects on neonatal outcome or Apgar scores (Carbonne et al., 1993; Jannet et al., 1994, 1997).

Monitoring

Patients with severe preeclampsia might require more invasive monitoring than routine arterial saturation and BP measurement, which is usually dictated by the severity of the hypertension, the expected intervention with vasodilators (like nitroglycerine and sodium nitroprusside), the reduction in intravascular volume status, and the presence of oliguria and pulmonary edema (Cotton et al., 1985; Wasserstrum & Cotton, 1986; Clark & Cotton, 1988). Systemic artery catheterization might be required in patients with a BP above 160/110, with potent vasodilators like nitroglycerine and sodium nitroprusside being used during induction of regional anesthesia in patients with suspected intravascular volume depletion, during induction of general anesthesia (where big swings in BP are expected), in morbidly obese patients, in patients with pulmonary edema, or for repeated blood sampling for repeated labs and arterial blood gas tensions. Selected patients may benefit from the placement of a pulmonary artery catheter to guide hemodynamic and fluid management during labor and/or surgery (Clark & Cotton, 1988). Severe preeclampsia in itself is not an indication for pulmonary artery catheterization. Placement of a pulmonary catheter is indicated in patients with: (i) refractory hypertension and pulmonary edema where conventional therapy has failed; (ii) persistent oliguria/anuria unresponsive to a fluid challenge; and (iii) hemodynamic instability requiring regional anesthesia (Wasserstrum & Cotton, 1986; Clark & Cotton, 1988). In most cases of preeclampsia, decreased urine output or failure to respond to antihypertensive therapy are no longer regarded as indications for insertion of a PA catheter. In such instances a "single-shot" echocardiogram can be useful in defining the cardiac output, ejection fraction, and central venous pressure (Belfort et al., 1994, 1997). These data can then be used in determining the need for further fluid or whether a PA catheter is necessary.

Analgesia for labor and delivery

For labor and vaginal delivery or cesarean section, most obstetric anesthesiologists consider epidural analgesia (with the appropriate monitoring) to be the best and safest choice for patients with severe preeclampsia. Epidural analgesia not only provides the best pain relief, it also attenuates the hypertensive response to pain, reduces endogenous catecholamine levels, improves intervillous blood flow, results in stable CO (Jouppila et al., 1982; Newsome et al., 1986; Ramanathan et al., 1991), and offers the flexibility of augmenting the block for cesarean section later on, if needed (Abboud et al., 1982). An early epidural placement can avoid inducing general anesthesia, if urgent cesarean section is required. Several areas of concern—difficulty in assessing intravascular volume, amount of prehydration, and risk of pulmonary edema with prehydration—must be addressed when considering epidural analgesia. Epidural analgesia does not increase the incidence of maternal hypotension and provokes little changes in pulmonary artery occlusion pressure, CVP, and cardiac index in women hydrated to a pulmonary artery occlusion pressure of 8–12 mmHg (Moore et al., 1985; Newsome et al., 1986). Sibai and colleagues (Sibai et al., 1987) were unable to show any relationship between crystalloid preload given prior to epidural and pulmonary edema. Prudent use of fluids guided by urine output, excessive recent weight gain, positive fluid balance during the previous 24 hours, and invasive monitoring are factors which reduce the risk of precipitous hypotension when using regional anesthesia in preeclamptic patients. A typical crystalloid bolus of 10 mL/kg is acceptable in most patients. Using 0.125% bupivacaine with 2 μg/mL of fentanyl, a fractionated bolus of 10 mL followed by a 10 mL/hr infusion provides excellent analgesia with minimum motor block. Low concentrations of ropivacaine or levobupivacaine may be used instead. However, these drugs are expensive, and their superiority over bupivacaine is yet to be established. Hypotension can be treated, if necessary, with an additional 200–300 mL fluid bolus and 2.5–5 mg of intravenous ephedrine.

The combined spinal epidural technique has been safely used to provide analgesia for labor and delivery in preeclamptic patients (Ramanathan et al., 2001). An initial intrathecal dose of either fentanyl 25 μg or sufentanil 10 μg can be used alone or in combination with a small (1.25–2.5 mg) dose of bupivacaine or morphine (0.25 mg). After initial analgesia, continued analgesia can be achieved with the epidural infusions, as discussed earlier.

Choice of anesthesia for cesarean section

The choice between epidural, spinal, or general anesthesia depends upon the patient's airway assessment, urgency of situation, severity of the disease and hypertension, suspected severe intravascular volume depletion, renal and hepatic involvement, and coagulation status. The anesthesiologist should, however, always be prepared for an emergency cesarean section for worsening maternal or fetal well-being.

Regional anesthesia

Epidural anesthesia for cesarean section is inherently considered safe for both mother and fetus because it: (i) offers cardiovascular stability over general anesthesia (Hodgkinson et al., 1980; Moore et al., 1985) and neuroendocrine stability with less stress for the mother (Ramanathan et al., 1991); (ii) lacks neonatal depression and results in better Apgar scores (Ramanathan et al., 1991; Moodley et al., 2001); and (iii) is associated with less morbidity and mortality when compared to general anesthesia (Hawkins et al., 1997). Spinal anesthesia, on the other hand, has traditionally been contraindicated in severe preeclamptic patients because of the fears that spinal anesthesia produces abrupt and profound hypotension secondary to rapid and complete sympathectomy in patients with restricted intravascular volume and that this could have a detrimental effect on the already compromised fetus. Despite these concerns, recent studies have shown spinal anesthesia to be a safe option (Hood & Curry, 1999). Hood and Curry (1999) demonstrated no difference in hemodynamics after spinal or epidural anesthesia for cesarean section in patients with severe preeclampsia. Proponents of spinal anesthesia believe that in severe preeclamptic patients, spinal anesthesia might still be a better option than a hurried general anesthesia, since it avoids the inherent risks of general anesthesia and intubation, allows for timely cesarean delivery (in 10–15 min) in cases of fetal distress, gives better operating conditions than epidural anesthesia, and does not appear to affect BP variability any worse than general anesthesia (Rout et al., 1998).

Combined spinal epidural anesthesia offers the advantage of a quick onset of action, the use of the minimum spinal dose expected to achieve an anesthetic block, and the flexibility to extend the block if needed. Recently, doses of 7.5 mg and 11.25 mg bupivacaine, used for combined spinal epidural anesthesia, have been found to provide anesthesia without any severe hypotension or other detrimental effects (Wallace et al., 1995; Ramanathan et al., 2001).

General anesthesia

Patient refusal for regional anesthesia, the urgency of the situation, and impaired coagulopathy might necessitate general anesthesia. Three major issues must be considered to ensure maternal and fetal safety: (i) the effect of preeclampsia on airway and laryngeal edema and the possibility of a difficult intubation, which is more common in preeclamptic patients; (ii) maintenance of hemodynamic stability during airway management; and (iii) drug interactions, especially between muscle relaxants and magnesium. Hence, it is prudent to control BP prior to induction of general anesthesia as dramatic and dangerous hypertension can complicate tracheal intubation and cause pulmonary edema or cerebral hemorrhage (Fox et al., 1977). Pressure response to intubation can also cause significant reduction in uterine blood flow, increase myocardial oxygen consumption, and cause cardiac arrhythmias (Jouppila et al., 1979). Several drugs, such as hydralazine (5–10 mg bolus), labetalol (20 mg bolus up to 1 mg/kg), nitroglycerin (50–100 μg bolus), lidocaine (50–100 mg bolus), or short-acting opiates like fentanyl (2 μg/kg) or remifentanil (0.1–0.5 μg/kg/min) have been used to control the hypertensive response to intubation by titrating these drugs to reduce MAP by 20% before intubation. Consider awake fiberoptic intubation in parturients with a difficult airway, especially if there is any contraindication to the use of regional anesthesia. During a comparison of three different techniques in severe preeclamptic patients—epidural, combined spinal epidural, and general anesthesia—Wallace and colleagues (Wallace et al., 1995) found no serious maternal or fetal complications. Each technique has its role and benefits, provided a careful approach is taken.

Conclusion

Early preoperative assessment, good communication among various subspecialties, and a team approach are all important to assure maternal as well as fetal safety. Every effort must be made to avoid any rushed deliveries and emergency cesarean sections without proper patient evaluation and preparation. A carefully conducted early epidural analgesia for labor seems to be safe for most critically ill parturients (except in those patients where a reduction in SVR can be detrimental), and most of the time this epidural can also be safely augmented for cesarean section. Every anesthetic technique offers some advantage, and, more so than the choice of anesthetic, maternal safety depends upon understanding the hemodynamic changes associated with the disease process and its effect on pregnancy, the effect of pregnancy on the disease process, and the effect of a particular anesthetic intervention on the hemodynamic changes.

References

Abboud T, Artal R, Sarkis F, Henriksen EH, Kammula RK. Sympathoadrenal activity, maternal, fetal, and neonatal responses after epidural anesthesia in the preeclamptic patient. Am J Obstet Gynecol 1982;144:915–918.

Abboud TK, Raya J, Noueihed R, Daniel J. Intrathecal morphine for relief of labor pain in a parturient with severe pulmonary hypertension. Anesthesiology 1983;59:477–479.

Aglio LS, Johnson MD. Anaesthetic management of myocardial infarction in a parturient. Br J Anaesth 1990;65:258–261.

American College of Obstetrics and Gynecology. Cardiac disease in pregnancy. ACOG technical bulletin number 168—June 1992. Int J Gynaecol Obstet 1993;41:298–306.

Anthony J, Mantel G, Johanson R, Dommisse J. The haemodynamic and respiratory effects of intravenous nimodipine used in the treatment of eclampsia. Br J Obstet Gynaecol 1996;103:518–522.

Arias F, Pineda J. Aortic stenosis and pregnancy. J Reprod Med 1978;20:229–232.

Autore C, Brauneis S, Apponi F, et al. Epidural anesthesia for cesarean section in patients with hypertrophic cardiomyopathy: a report of three cases. Anesthesiology 1999;90:1205–1207.

Avila WS, Grinberg M, Snitcowsky R, et al. Maternal and fetal outcome in pregnant women with Eisenmenger's syndrome. Eur Heart J 1995;16:460–464.

Baraka A, Jabbour S, Itani I. Severe bradycardia following epidural anesthesia in a patient with idiopathic hypertrophic subaortic stenosis. Anesth Analg 1987;66:1337–1338.

Belfort MA, Carpenter RJ, Jr., Kirshon B, Saade GR, Moise KJ, Jr. The use of nimodipine in a patient with eclampsia: color flow Doppler demonstration of retinal artery relaxation. Am J Obstet Gynecol 1993;169:204–206.

Belfort MA, Rokey R, Saade GR, Moise KJ. Rapid echocardiographic assessment of left and right heart hemodynamics in critically ill obstetric patients. Am J Obstet Gynecol 1994;171(4):884–892.

Belfort MA, Mares A, Saade G, Wen TS, Rokey R. Two-dimensional echocardiography and Doppler ultrasound in managing obstetric patients. Obstet Gynecol 1997;90(3):326–330.

Benedetti TJ, Carlson RW. Studies of colloid osmotic pressure in pregnancy-induced hypertension. Am J Obstet Gynecol 1979;135: 308–311.

Benedetti TJ, Cotton DB, Read JC, Miller FC. Hemodynamic observations in severe pre-eclampsia with a flow-directed pulmonary artery catheter. Am J Obstet Gynecol 1980;136:465–470.

Bennett P, Edwards D. Use of magnesium sulphate in obstetrics. Lancet 1997;350:1491.

Berg CJ, Atrash HK, Koonin LM, Tucker M. Pregnancy-related mortality in the United States, 1987–1990. Obstet Gynecol 1996;88: 161–167.

Boccio RV, Chung JH, Harrison DM. Anesthetic management of cesarean section in a patient with idiopathic hypertrophic subaortic stenosis. Anesthesiology 1986;65:663–665.

Bolte AC, Dekker GA, van Eyck J, van Schijndel RS, van Geijn HP. Lack of agreement between central venous pressure and pulmonary capillary wedge pressure in preeclampsia. Hypertens Pregnancy 2000;19:261–271.

Bolte AC, van Geijn HP, Dekker GA. Management and monitoring of severe preeclampsia. Eur J Obstet Gynecol Reprod Biol 2001;96: 8–20.

Brian JE, Jr., Seifen AB, Clark RB, Robertson DM, Quirk JG. Aortic stenosis, cesarean delivery, and epidural anesthesia. J Clin Anesth 1993;5:154–157.

Brighouse D. Anaesthesia for caesarean section in patients with aortic stenosis: the case for regional anaesthesia. Anaesthesia 1998;53:107–109.

Burrows RF, Hunter DJ, Andrew M, Kelton JG. A prospective study investigating the mechanism of thrombocytopenia in preeclampsia. Obstet Gynecol 1987;70:334–338.

Busto N, Ramos G, Fernandez MJ, Bayon J, del Amo P. Anesthetic management of labor in a pregnant woman with myocardial infarction. Rev Esp Anestesiol Reanim 1995;42:142–144.

Carbonne B, Jannet D, Touboul C, Khelifati Y, Milliez J. Nicardipine treatment of hypertension during pregnancy. Obstet Gynecol 1993;81:908–914.

Carvalho J. Cardiovascular disease in the pregnant patient. In: Birnbach DJ, Gatt SP, Datta S, eds. Textbook of Obstetric Anesthesia. New York: Churchill Livingstone 2000:553–564.

Carvahlo JCA, Mathias RS, Siaulys MM, et al. Anesthesia for cesarean section in patients with surgically corrected Tetralogy of Fallot. Braz J Anesthesiol Int Issue 1993;4:32–34.

Clark SL, Cotton DB. Clinical indications for pulmonary artery catheterization in the patient with severe preeclampsia. Am J Obstet Gynecol 1988;158:453–458.

Clark SL, Phelan JP, Greenspoon J, Aldahl D, Horenstein J. Labor and delivery in the presence of mitral stenosis: central hemodynamic observations. Am J Obstet Gynecol 1985;152:984–988.

Clark SL, Greenspoon JS, Aldahl D, Phelan JP. Severe preeclampsia with persistent oliguria: management of hemodynamic subsets. Am J Obstet Gynecol 1986;154:490–494.

Colclough GW, Ackerman WE, III, Walmsley PM, Hessel EA. Epidural anesthesia for a parturient with critical aortic stenosis. J Clin Anesth 1995;7:264–265.

Cotton DB, Gonik B, Dorman K, Harrist R. Cardiovascular alterations in severe pregnancy-induced hypertension: relationship of central venous pressure to pulmonary capillary wedge pressure. Am J Obstet Gynecol 1985a;151:762–764.

Cotton DB, Gonik B, Dorman KF. Cardiovascular alterations in severe pregnancy-induced hypertension seen with an intravenously given hydralazine bolus. Surg Gynecol Obstet 1985b;161: 240–244.

Cotton DB, Lee W, Huhta JC, Dorman KF. Hemodynamic profile of severe pregnancy-induced hypertension. Am J Obstet Gynecol 1988;158:523–529.

Davies J, Fernando R, Hallworth S. Platelet function in preeclampsia: platelet function analyzer (PFA-100) vs. (TEG). Anesthesiology 2001a;94:A1.

Davies J, Fernando R, Hallworth S. Thrombocytopenia in pregnancy: platelet function analyzer (PFA-100) vs. thromboelastograph (TEG). Anesthesiology 2001b;94:A23.

Deiml R, Hess W, Bahlmann E. Primary cesarean section. Use of phenylephrine during anesthesia in a patient with hypertrophic obstructive cardiomyopathy. Anaesthesist 2000;49:527–531.

Department of Health. Report on confidential enquiry into maternal deaths in the United Kingdom 1991–1993. London: HMSO, 1996.

Devitt JH, Noble WH, Byrick RJ. A Swan–Ganz catheter related complication in a patient with Eisenmenger's syndrome. Anesthesiology 1982;57:335–337.

Ducey JP, Knape KG. Maternal esmolol administration resulting in fetal distress and cesarean section in a term pregnancy. Anesthesiology 1992;77:829–832.

Easterling TR, Chadwick HS, Otto CM, Benedetti TJ. Aortic stenosis in pregnancy. Obstet Gynecol 1988;72:113–118.

Ellis SC, Wheeler AS, James FM, III, et al. Fetal and maternal effects of sodium nitroprusside used to counteract hypertension in gravid ewes. Am J Obstet Gynecol 1982;143:766–770.

Foster JM, Jones RM. The anaesthetic management of the Eisenmenger syndrome. Ann R Coll Surg Engl 1984;66:353–355.

Fox EJ, Sklar GS, Hill CH, Villanueva R, King BD. Complications related to the pressor response to endotracheal intubation. Anesthesiology 1977;47:524–525.

Fuster V, Steele PM, Edwards WD, Gersh BJ, McGoon MD, Frye RL. Primary pulmonary hypertension: natural history and the importance of thrombosis. Circulation 1984;70:580–587.

Garber SZ, Choi HJ, Tremper KK. Use of a pulse oximeter in the anesthetic management of a pregnant patient with Eisenmenger's syndrome. Anesthesiol Rev 1988;15:59.

George LM, Gatt SP, Lowe S. Peripartum cardiomyopathy: four case histories and a commentary on anaesthetic management. Anaesth Intensive Care 1997;25:292–296.

Ghai B, Mohan V, Malhotra N. Epidural anesthesia for cesarean section in a patient with Eisenmenger's syndrome. Int J Obstet Anesthesia 2002;11:44–47.

Gleicher N, Midwall J, Hochberger D, Jaffin H. Eisenmenger's syndrome and pregnancy. Obstet Gynecol Surv 1979;34:721–741.

Goodwin TM, Gherman RB, Hameed A, Elkayam U. Favorable response of Eisenmenger syndrome to inhaled nitric oxide during pregnancy. Am J Obstet Gynecol 1999;180:64–67.

Hankins GD, Wendel GD, Jr., Leveno KJ, Stoneham J. Myocardial infarction during pregnancy: a review. Obstet Gynecol 1985;65:139–146.

Hanretty KP, Whittle MJ, Howie CA, Rubin PC. Effect of nifedipine on Doppler flow velocity waveforms in severe pre-eclampsia. BMJ 1989;299:1205–1206.

Hawkins JL, Koonin LM, Palmer SK, Gibbs CP. Anesthesia-related deaths during obstetric delivery in the United States, 1979–1990. Anesthesiology 1997;86:277–284.

Hays PM, Cruikshank DP, Dunn LJ. Plasma volume determination in normal and preeclamptic pregnancies. Am J Obstet Gynecol 1985;151:958–966.

Hemmings GT, Whalley DG, O'Connor PJ, Benjamin A, Dunn C. Invasive monitoring and anaesthetic management of a parturient with mitral stenosis. Can J Anaesth 1987;34:182–185.

Hodgkinson R, Husain FJ, Hayashi RH. Systemic and pulmonary blood pressure during caesarean section in parturients with gestational hypertension. Can Anaesth Soc J 1980;27:389–394.

Hood DD, Curry R. Spinal versus epidural anesthesia for cesarean section in severely preeclamptic patients: a retrospective survey. Anesthesiology 1999;90:1276–1282.

Jannet D, Carbonne B, Sebban E, Milliez J. Nicardipine versus metoprolol in the treatment of hypertension during pregnancy: a randomized comparative trial. Obstet Gynecol 1994;84:354–359.

Jannet D, Abankwa A, Guyard B, et al. Nicardipine versus salbutamol in the treatment of premature labor. A prospective randomized study. Eur J Obstet Gynecol Reprod Biol 1997;73:11–16.

Johnson MD, Saltzman DH. Cardiac disease. In: Datta S, ed. Anesthetic and Obstetric Management of High Risk Pregnancy. St. Louis: Mosby, 1996:200–245.

Jouppila P, Kuikka J, Jouppila R, Hollmen A. Effect of induction of general anesthesia for cesarean section on intervillous blood flow. Acta Obstet Gynecol Scand 1979;58:249–253.

Jouppila P, Jouppila R, Hollmen A, Koivula A. Lumbar epidural analgesia to improve intervillous blood flow during labor in severe preeclampsia. Obstet Gynecol 1982;59:158–161.

Kelton JG, Hunter DJ, Neame PB. A platelet function defect in preeclampsia. Obstet Gynecol 1985;65:107–109.

Klarr JM, Bhatt-Mehta V, Donn SM. Neonatal adrenergic blockade following single dose maternal labetalol administration. Am J Perinatol 1994;11:91–93.

Kobayashi A, Mizobe T, Tojo H, Hashimoto S. Autonomic hyperreflexia during labour. Can J Anaesth 1995;42:1134–1136.

Kuzniar J, Piela A, Skret A. Left ventricular function in preeclamptic patients: an echocardiographic study. Am J Obstet Gynecol 1983;146:400–405.

Lam GK, Stafford RE, Thorp J, Moise KJ, Jr., Cairns BA. Inhaled nitric oxide for primary pulmonary hypertension in pregnancy. Obstet Gynecol 2001;98:895–898.

Lao TT, Sermer M, MaGee L, Farine D, Colman JM. Congenital aortic stenosis and pregnancy—a reappraisal. Am J Obstet Gynecol 1993;169:540–545.

Larson CP, Jr., Shuer LM, Cohen SE. Maternally administered esmolol decreases fetal as well as maternal heart rate. J Clin Anesth 1990;2:427–429.

Lindheimer MD, Katz AI. Current concepts: Hypertension in pregnancy. N Engl J Med 1985;313:675–680.

Lindow SW, Davies N, Davey DA, Smith JA. The effect of sublingual nifedipine on utero-placental blood flow in hypertensive pregnancy. Br J Obstet Gynaecol 1988;95:1276–1281.

Lipshitz J, Ahokas RA, Reynolds SL. The effect of hydralazine on placental perfusion in the spontaneously hypertensive rat. Am J Obstet Gynecol 1987;156:356–359.

Longmire S, Leduc L, Jones MM, et al. The hemodynamic effects of intubation during nitroglycerin infusion in severe preeclampsia. Am J Obstet Gynecol 1991;164:551–556.

Losasso TJ, Muzzi DA, Cucchiara RF. Response of fetal heart rate to maternal administration of esmolol. Anesthesiology 1991;74:782–784.

Loubser P, Suh K, Cohen S. Adverse effects of spinal anesthesia in a patient with idiopathic hypertrophic subaortic stenosis. Anesthesiology 1984;60:228–230.

Lunell NO, Lewander R, Nylund L, Sarby B, Thornstrom S. Acute effect of dihydralazine on uteroplacental blood flow in hypertension during pregnancy. Gynecol Obstet Invest 1983;16:274–282.

Lust KM, Boots RJ, Dooris M, Wilson J. Management of labor in Eisenmenger syndrome with inhaled nitric oxide. Am J Obstet Gynecol 1999;181:419–423.

Mabie WC, Gonzalez AR, Sibai BM, Amon E. A comparative trial of labetalol and hydralazine in the acute management of severe hypertension complicating pregnancy. Obstet Gynecol 1987;70: 328–333.

Mabie WC, Ratts TE, Ramanathan KB, Sibai BM. Circulatory congestion in obese hypertensive women: a subset of pulmonary edema in pregnancy. Obstet Gynecol 1988;72:553–558.

McIndoe AK, Hammond EJ, Babington PC. Peripartum cardiomyopathy presenting as a cardiac arrest at induction of anaesthesia for emergency caesarean section. Br J Anaesth 1995;75:97–101.

Mangano DT. Anesthesia for the cardiac patient. In: Shnider SM, Levinson G, eds. Anesthesia for Obstetrics. Baltimore: Williams & Wilkins, 1986:345–381.

Mangano DT. Anesthesia for the pregnant cardiac patients. In: Shnider SM, Levinson G, eds. Anesthesia for Obstetrics. Baltimore: Williams & Wilkins 1993:485–523.

Marietta M, Castelli I, Piccinini F, et al. The PFA-100 system for the assessment of platelet function in normotensive and hypertensive pregnancies. Clin Lab Haematol 2001;23:131–134.

Monnery L, Nanson J, Charlton G. Primary pulmonary hypertension in pregnancy; a role for novel vasodilators. Br J Anaesth 2001; 87:295–298.

Moodley J, Jjuuko G, Rout C. Epidural compared with general anaesthesia for caesarean delivery in conscious women with eclampsia. Br J Obstet Gynaecol 2001;108:378–382.

Moore TR, Key TC, Reisner LS, Resnik R. Evaluation of the use of continuous lumbar epidural anesthesia for hypertensive pregnant women in labor. Am J Obstet Gynecol 1985;152:404–412.

Moraes TABPP. Pregnancy in patients with Chagas' disease. Rev Soc Cardiol Estado São Paulo 1994;6:547–551.

Naeije R, Vachiery JL. Medical therapy of pulmonary hypertension. Conventional therapies. Clin Chest Med 2001;22:517–527.

National High Blood Pressure Education Program Working Group on High Blood Pressure in Pregnancy. Report. Am J Obstet Gynecol 2000;183:S1–22.

Naulty J, Cefalo RC, Lewis PE. Fetal toxicity of nitroprusside in the pregnant ewe. Am J Obstet Gynecol 1981;139:708–711.

Nelson DM, Main E, Crafford W, Ahumada GG. Peripartum heart failure due to primary pulmonary hypertension. Obstet Gynecol 1983;62:58s–63s.

Newsome LR, Bramwell RS, Curling PE. Severe preeclampsia: hemodynamic effects of lumbar epidural anesthesia. Anesth Analg 1986;65:31–36.

Nootens M, Rich S. Successful management of labor and delivery in primary pulmonary hypertension. Am J Cardiol 1993;71:1124–1125.

O'Kelly SW, Lawes EG, Luntley JB. Bleeding time: is it a useful clinical tool? Br J Anaesth 1992;68:313–315.

Orlikowski CE, Rocke DA, Murray WB, et al. Thrombelastography changes in pre-eclampsia and eclampsia. Br J Anaesth 1996;77: 157–161.

Ostheimer GW, Alper MH. Intrapartum anesthetic management of the pregnant patient with heart disease. Clin Obstet Gynecol 1975;18:81–97.

Palacios QT, Joyce TH. Cardiac disease. In: James FM, Wheeler AS, Dewan DM, eds. Obstetric Anesthesia: The Complicated Patient. Philadelphia: FA Davis 1988:159–180.

Pollack KL, Chestnut DH, Wenstrom KD. Anesthetic management of a parturient with Eisenmenger's syndrome. Anesth Analg 1990;70: 212–215.

Prieto JA, Mastrobattista JM, Blanco JD. Coagulation studies in patients with marked thrombocytopenia due to severe preeclampsia. Am J Perinatol 1995;12:220–222.

Pritchard JA, Cunningham FG, Mason RA. Coagulation changes in eclampsia: their frequency and pathogenesis. Am J Obstet Gynecol 1976;124:855–864.

Rafferty TD, Berkowitz RL. Hemodynamics in patients with severe toxemia during labor and delivery. Am J Obstet Gynecol 1980;138: 263–270.

Ramanathan J, Sibai BM, Vu T, Chauhan D. Correlation between bleeding times and platelet counts in women with preeclampsia undergoing cesarean section. Anesthesiology 1989;71:188–191.

Ramanathan J, Coleman P, Sibai B. Anesthetic modification of hemodynamic and neuroendocrine stress responses to cesarean delivery in women with severe preeclampsia. Anesth Analg 1991;73:772–779.

Ramanathan J, Vaddadi AK, Arheart KL. Combined spinal and epidural anesthesia with low doses of intrathecal bupivacaine in women with severe preeclampsia: a preliminary report. Reg Anesth Pain Med 2001;26:46–51.

Rao TL, Jacobs KH, El Etr AA. Reinfarction following anesthesia in patients with myocardial infarction. Anesthesiology 1983;59:499–505.

Rasmus KT, Rottman RL, Kotelko DM, et al. Unrecognized thrombocytopenia and regional anesthesia in parturients: a retrospective review. Obstet Gynecol 1989;73:943–946.

Recasens UJ, Boàda PS, Solsona DE, et al. [Elective cesarean section with epidural anesthesia in a pregnant woman with obstructive hypertrophic myocardiopathy]. Rev Esp Anestesiol Reanim 2000;47: 320–322.

Robinson DE, Leicht CH. Epidural analgesia with low-dose bupivacaine and fentanyl for labor and delivery in a parturient with severe pulmonary hypertension. Anesthesiology 1988;68:285–288.

Robinson S. Pulmonary artery catheters in Eisenmenger's syndrome: many risks, few benefits. Anesthesiology 1983;58:588–590.

Rodgers RP, Levin J. A critical reappraisal of the bleeding time. Semin Thromb Hemost 1990;16:1–20.

Roessler P, Lambert TF. Anaesthesia for caesarean section in the presence of primary pulmonary hypertension. Anaesth Intensive Care 1986;14:317–320.

Rosenthal E, Nelson-Piercy C. Value of inhaled nitric oxide in Eisenmenger syndrome during pregnancy. Am J Obstet Gynecol 2000;183:781–782.

Rout CC. Anaesthesia and analgesia for the critically ill parturient. Best Pract Res Clin Obstet Gynaecol 2001;15:507–522.

Rout CC, Rocke DA, Levin J, Gouws E, Reddy D. A reevaluation of the role of crystalloid preload in the prevention of hypotension associated with spinal anesthesia for elective cesarean section. Anesthesiology 1993;79:262–269.

Rout CC, Ward S, Rocke DA. Haemodynamic variability at emergent cesarean section in hypertensive patients—spinal versus general anesthesia. Anesthesiology 1998;88(Suppl):A50.

Rowe GG. Responses of the coronary circulation to physiologic changes and pharmacologic agents. Anesthesiology 1974;41:182–196.

Schwartz ML, Brenner WE. Pregnancy-induced hypertension presenting with life-threatening thrombocytopenia. Am J Obstet Gynecol 1983;146:756–759.

Shah KB, Kleinman BS, Sami H, Patel J, Rao TL. Reevaluation of perioperative myocardial infarction in patients with prior myocardial infarction undergoing noncardiac operations. Anesth Analg 1990;71:231–235.

Sibai BM. Treatment of hypertension in pregnant women. N Engl J Med 1996;335:257–265.

Sibai BM, Mabie BC, Harvey CJ, Gonzalez AR. Pulmonary edema in severe preeclampsia-eclampsia: analysis of thirty-seven consecutive cases. Am J Obstet Gynecol 1987;156:1174–1179.

Slomka F, Salmeron S, Zetlaoui P, et al. Primary pulmonary hypertension and pregnancy: anesthetic management for delivery. Anesthesiology 1988;69:959–961.

Soderlin MK, Purhonen S, Haring P, et al. Myocardial infarction in a parturient. A case report with emphasis on medication and management. Anaesthesia 1994;49:870–872.

Sorensen MB, Korshin JD, Fernandes A, Secher O. The use of epidural analgesia for delivery in a patient with pulmonary hypertension. Acta Anaesthesiol Scand 1982;26:180–182.

Spinnato JA, Kraynack BJ, Cooper MW. Eisenmenger's syndrome in pregnancy: epidural anesthesia for elective cesarean section. N Engl J Med 1981;304:1215–1217.

Stewart R, Tuazon D, Olson G, Duarte AG. Pregnancy and primary pulmonary hypertension: successful outcome with epoprostenol therapy. Chest 2001;119:973–975.

Sullivan JM, Ramanathan KB. Management of medical problems in pregnancy—severe cardiac disease. N Engl J Med 1985;313:304–309.

Ueyama H, He YL, Tanigami H, Mashimo T, Yoshiya I. Effects of crystalloid and colloid preload on blood volume in the parturient undergoing spinal anesthesia for elective Cesarean section. Anesthesiology 1999;91:1571–1576.

Umo-Etuk J, Lumley J, Holdcraft A. Critically ill parturient women and admission to intensive care: a 5-year review. Int J Obstet Anesthesia 1996;5:84.

Vardi J, Fields GA. Microangiopathic hemolytic anemia in severe preeclampsia. A review of the literature and pathophysiology. Am J Obstet Gynecol 1974;119:617–622.

Vincelot A, Nathan N, Collet D, et al. Platelet function during pregnancy: an evaluation using the PFA-100 analyser. Br J Anaesth 2001;87:890–893.

Vink GJ, Moodley J. The effect of low-dose dihydrallazine on the fetus in the emergency treatment of hypertension in pregnancy. S Afr Med J 1982;62:475–477.

Wallace DH, Leveno KJ, Cunningham FG, Giesecke AH, Shearer VE, Sidawi JE. Randomized comparison of general and regional anesthesia for cesarean delivery in pregnancies complicated by severe preeclampsia. Obstet Gynecol 1995;86:193–199.

Wasserstrum N, Cotton DB. Hemodynamic monitoring in severe pregnancy-induced hypertension. Clin Perinatol 1986;13:781–799.

Whitfield A, Holdcroft A. Anaesthesia for caesarean section in patients with aortic stenosis: the case for general anaesthesia. Anaesthesia 1998;53:109–112.

Wong CA, Liu S, Glassenberg R. Comparison of thrombelastography with common coagulation tests in preeclamptic and healthy parturients. Reg Anesth 1995;20:521–527.

Ziskind Z, Etchin A, Frenkel Y, et al. Epidural anesthesia with the Trendelenburg position for cesarean section with or without a cardiac surgical procedure in patients with severe mitral stenosis: a hemodynamic study. J Cardiothorac Anesth 1990;4:354–359.

45 The organ transplant obstetric patient

James R. Scott

Successful pregnancies have been reported in women with virtually all types of organ and tissue allografts now used clinically. However, all transplant patients have significant underlying medical disorders that can adversely affect the outcome. Problems may occur unpredictably, and each group of organ recipients has its own array of specific issues. Pregnancy in transplant patients also represents a natural experiment in immunologic aspects of gestation. The implanted conceptus is itself a graft of living tissue, and it is still not clear how the developing semi-allogeneic placenta and fetus survive the normal immunocompetent maternal environment. Pregnancy in allograft recipients takes place in a relative state of generalized immune deficiency because of the immunosuppressive agents these women must take. This combination of factors presents unique management challenges to the physician.

Organ and tissue transplantation have evolved from a clinical experiment into a contemporary treatment which restores many patients to near-normal life styles. The first reported post-transplant pregnancy was in a woman who had received a kidney from her identical twin sister in 1985 (Murray et al., 1963). Since then, the number of young women with allografts has dramatically increased and thousands have become pregnant (Fig. 45.1). There are no randomized trials that have investigated pregnancy management options for transplant patients, but a great deal has been learned through experience. The largest experience is with patients receiving living donor or cadaver kidney transplants, but many recipients of liver, heart, lung, and pancreas allografts and bone marrow transplants have also become pregnant. Potential problems in these women include adverse effects of immunosuppressive drugs, medical and obstetric complications, and the psychological stress of being both transplant recipient and an expectant mother. Although the prognosis for a live birth is usually good, it is clear that these are high-risk pregnancies that require expert obstetric care.

Pre-pregnancy evaluation

Preconception counseling is desirable for all transplant patients, but it is often difficult to decide how to advise these couples (Scott, 1992; Norton & Scott, 1993; Alston et al., 2001). Any woman contemplating pregnancy after transplantation should be in good health with no evidence of graft rejection (Table 45.1). Medical problems such as diabetes mellitus, recurrent infections, and serious side effects from the immunosuppressive drugs make pregnancy inadvisable. The ideal time for pregnancy is between 2 and 5 years after transplantation when allograft function has stabilized and immunosuppressive medication has been reduced to moderate doses. An assessment of the patient's family support as well as a tactful but honest discussion of the potential pregnancy problems is important. Those of us who have followed many of these patients are aware that the literature may be overly optimistic about pregnancy and long-term prognosis. It is not always appreciated that long-term organ allograft survival rates are not 100%, and many transplant recipients will not live to raise their children to adulthood. About 10% of mothers receiving allografts die within 7 years of pregnancy and 50% within 15 years (Davidson, 1995).

Prenatal care

Kidney transplantation is the prototype, but antepartum care is similar with essentially all other organ allografts. Early diagnosis of pregnancy is important, and a first trimester ultrasound examination is valuable to establish an accurate estimated date of confinement. Antenatal management should be meticulous and includes serial assessment of maternal allograft function, detection of graft rejection episodes, and prompt diagnosis and treatment of infections, anemia, hypertension, and preeclampsia (Table 45.2). Close fetal surveillance is also necessary, and the known risk for fetal growth restriction is monitored by serial ultrasound examinations (Table 45.3).

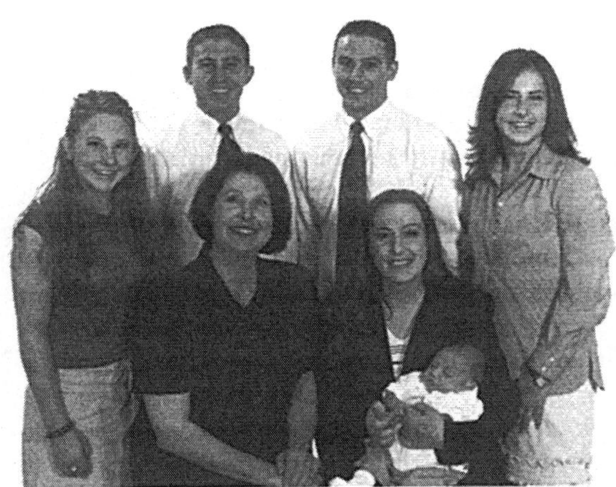

Fig. 45.1 Two generations following renal transplantation. The patient is pictured with her five children and recently born granddaughter.

Table 45.1 Estimated number of pregnancies in transplant patients worldwide, 1958–2001

Kidney	>10,000
Liver	800
Heart	200
Pancreas	200
Lung	40
Bone marrow	200

Table 45.2 Important prognostic factors for optimum pregnancy outcome in transplant patients

Two years since transplant
Good general health and prognosis
Satisfactory graft function with no evidence of rejection
Stable immunosuppressive regimen
No or minimal hypertension and proteinuria
Serum creatinine <2 mg/dL
Family support

The incidence of intraepithelial and invasive cancer of the genital tract in patients taking immunosuppressive drugs is increased, and regular Papanicolaou tests and screening for malignancies are vital components of clinical care. Urinary tract infections are particularly common in kidney transplant patients with up to a twofold increase in the incidence of pyelonephritis. Asymptomatic bacteruria should be treated for 2 weeks with follow-up urine cultures, and suppressive doses of antibiotics may be needed for the rest of the pregnancy. Other bacterial and fungal infections associated with immunosuppression include endometritis, wound infections, skin abscesses, and pneumonia often with unusual organisms such as *Aspergillus*, *Pneumocystis*, *Mycobacterium tuberculosis*, and *Listeria*.

Table 45.3 Classification of fetal risk for immunosuppressive drugs used in transplantation

	Pregnancy category*
Corticosteroids (prednisone)	B
Azathioprine (Imuran)	D
Cyclosporine (Sandimmune, Neoral, SangCya)	C
Tacrolimus (Prograf)	C
Sirolimus, rapamycin (Rapamune)	C
Mycophenolate mofetil (CellCept)	C
Antithymocyte globulin (ATGAM, ATG, Thymoglobulin)	C
Muromonab-CD3 (Orthoclone OKT3)	C
Basilizimab (Simulect)	B
Daclizumab (Zenapax)	C

* A, controlled studies, no risk; B, no evidence of risk in humans; C, risks cannot be ruled out; D, positive evidence of risk; X, contraindicated.

Some patients have become Rh-sensitized from the allograft, and commonly acquired viral infections such as cytomegalovirus (CMV), herpes simplex virus (HSV), human papillovirus (HPV), human immunodeficiency virus (HIV) and hepatitis B (HBV) and C (HCV) pose a risk for both the mother and her fetus. The transplanted graft is a source of CMV, and patients typically receive prophylaxis against CMV for 1–3 months postoperatively when the risk for infection is highest. The greatest risk of congenital infection in the fetus is with primary CMV infection during pregnancy, but recurrent CMV infection in immunosuppressed women has also been reported to cause congenital CMV in the infant (ACOG, 2000). HBV and HCV are usually acquired through dialysis and blood transfusions prior to transplantation. Hepatitis B immune globulin (HBIG) and HBV vaccine should be given to the newborn and are 90% effective in preventing chronic hepatitis. Aciclovir as prophylaxis or treatment of HSV can be used safely during pregnancy.

The management of antepartum obstetric complications is similar to nontransplant patients. However, the risk of infection warrants a more aggressive approach and avoidance of invasive procedures when possible.

Immunosuppression during pregnancy

Many obstetricians are not familiar with immunosuppressive drugs, but it is crucial that they become aware of the impact on pregnancy and potential side effects when caring for these women. Most maintenance immunosuppressive regimens in transplant patients include combinations of daily corticosteroids, azathioprine, cyclosporine, or more recently tacrolimus (FK 506). However, new agents continually become available, multiple drug regimens are common, and both the dose and timing of drug administration require close monitoring during pregnancy. The potential fetal risks for each drug categorized by the US Food and Drug Administration are shown on Table 45.4.

Prednisone is the usual corticosteroid used in transplant patients, and intravenous glucocorticoids are used to treat acute rejection reactions. These anti-inflammatory medications inhibit both humoral and cell-mediated immune responses. Maternal adverse effects include glucose intolerance, hirsutism, acne, weight gain, cushinoid appearance, striae formation, osteonecrosis, osteoporosis, fluid retention, hypertension, severe infections, impaired wound healing, and mood changes. Since prednisone is largely metabolized by placental 11-hydroxygenase to the relatively inactive 11-keto form, the fetus is exposed to only 10% of the maternal dose of the active drug (Levitz et al., 1978). Most patients are maintained on moderate doses of prednisone (10–30 mg/day) that are relatively safe with few fetal effects. However, it is uncertain whether the increased incidence of premature rupture of membranes, preterm birth, preeclampsia, and fetal growth restriction are due exclusively to the underlying condition or whether prednisone might contribute to these complications (Scott, 1977; Cowchock, 1992). There is also growing concern that prolonged exposure to other glucocorticoids, such as dexamethasone and betamethasone used to accelerate fetal lung maturation, may lead to decreased fetal and neonatal somatic and brain growth, adrenal suppression, neonatal sepsis, chronic lung disease, psychomotor delay, and behavioral problems (Abbasi et al., 2000; Esplin et al., 2000; NIH, 2000).

Azathioprine (and its more toxic metabolite 6-mercaptopurine) is a purine analogue whose principal action is to decrease delayed hypersensitivity and cellular cytotoxicity. The primary maternal hazards of azathioprine administration are an increased risk of infection and neoplasia. Maternal liver toxicity and bone marrow depression with anemia, leukopenia, and thrombocytopenia have occurred but usually resolve with a decrease in dose. Between 64% and 90% of azathioprine crosses the placenta in human pregnancies, but the majority is the inactive form thiouric acid (Saarikoski & Seppala, 1973). Classification of azathioprine as category D is based largely on two early series which reported an incidence of congenital anomalies of 9% and 6.4% (Penn et al., 1980; Registration Committee, 1980). No specific pattern has emerged, and further experience has shown that azathioprine is not associated with more congenital malformations than seen in the normal population (Rizzoni et al., 1992; Armenti et al., 2000). Other fetal effects that have occasionally occurred include fatal neonatal anemia, thrombocytopenia, leukopenia, and acquired chromosome breaks. One approach suggested to minimize neonatal effects is to adjust doses to keep the maternal leukocyte count within normal limits for pregnancy (Davison et al., 1985).

Cyclosporine is a fungal metabolite whose major inhibitory effect is on T-cell-mediated responses by preventing formation of interleukin-2 (IL-2). Cyclosporine has improved survival in transplant recipients and is now a standard component of most immunosuppressant regimens. Bone marrow depression is infrequent, but the drug has a propensity for nephrotoxicity and hypertension. Other side effects include hirsutism, tremor, gingival hyperplasia, viral infections, hepatotoxicity, and an increased risk for neoplasia such as lymphomas. Cyclosporine levels drop during pregnancy, but graft function has remained stable in most patients despite decreases in trough levels (Bumgardner & Matas, 1992). Cyclosporine readily crosses the placenta, but there is no evidence of teratogenicity of cyclosporine in the human.

Tacrolimus (FK-506) is a macrolide obtained from streptomyces. The incidence of post-transplant diabetes mellitus with tacrolimus is 11–20%; the median time to onset is 68 days, but it is reversible in up to 50% of patients after 2 years (Pirsch et al., 1997; Miller et al., 2000). Nephrotoxicity and hyperkalemia develop in at least one-third of patients, and neurotoxicities such as headache, tremor, changes in motor function, mental status or sensory function have also been described. Cord blood concentrations are approximately 50% of maternal levels (Winkler et al., 1993), but there is no proven association with congenital malformations to date.

It is apparent that all immunosuppressive drugs cross the placental barrier and diffuse into the fetus during the development of its own immune system. Yet there is no con-

Table 45.4 Representative pregnancy outcome in organ allograft recipients from recent literature (Bumgardner & Matas, 1992; Barrou et al., 1998; Branch et al., 1998; Armenti et al., 1999, 2000; Salooja et al., 2001)

	Graft rejection (%)	Graft loss* (%)	Preeclampsia (%)	Live-born (%)	Mean GA (wkees)	Mean BW (g)	Newborn complications (%)	Neonatal deaths (%)
Kidney (*n* = 630)	12	8	24	79	36	2,504	19	2
Liver (*n* = 66)	11	6	14	85	37	2,755	23	1
Heart (*n* = 47)	24	26	20	74	37	2,543	20	0
Pancreas (*n* = 44)	4	11	25	95	35	2,100	24	0
Lung (*n* = 6)	33	17	NA	50	33	2,202	67	0
Bone marrow (*n* = 99)	—	—	14	79	39	3,130	6	NA

vincing evidence that prednisone, azathoprine, cyclosporine, or tacrolimus produce congenital abnormalities in the human fetus, and they remain the drugs of choice during pregnancy. Other than fetal growth restriction and preterm birth, the majority of offspring born to immunosuppressed mothers have had relatively uncomplicated courses. Respiratory distress syndrome (RDS), increased susceptibility to infection, hypoglycemia, hypocalcemia, adrenal insufficiency, thymic atrophy, bone marrow hypoplasia, transient leukopenia, reduced levels of IgM and IgG, and transiently elevated serum creatinine levels have all been reported, but these conditions are also commonly present in premature infants not exposed to these drugs. Most neonates have also progressed normally through infancy and childhood (Lau & Scott, 1985), but as they reach adulthood there are concerns about the possibility of delayed adverse effects (Scott, 2002). Fetal exposure to immunosuppressive agents could be associated with later development of fertility problems, autoimmune disease, and neoplasia (Classen & Shevach, 1991; Willis et al., 2000; Scott et al., 2002). With newer agents, it may be even more difficult to accurately identify a cause and effect. It is hoped that lower dosages now possible with drug combinations resulting in less exposure to each specific drug will decrease the potential for teratogenesis. However, potentiating effects among drugs as well as unknown interactions in multiple-drug regimens could also result in as yet unrecognized adverse fetal effects. Thus, it is important that all offspring exposed to these agents have long-term follow-up.

Renal transplantation

Approximately 1 in 20 women of childbearing age with a functioning renal allograft becomes pregnant (Alston et al., 2001), and it is estimated that more than 10,000 pregnancies have now occurred. Many women have now had more than one pregnancy, and some have successfully delivered twins and triplets. One patient has had five live births and one spontaneous abortion with no deleterious effect on the kidney evident 25 years after transplantation (Scott et al., 1986) (Fig. 45.1).

If preconception graft function is adequate as evidenced by a plasma creatinine <1.5 mg/dL, the pregnancy can be expected to progress normally until near term. Although the transplanted kidney usually functions satisfactorily during gestation, most patients do not have an increased glomerular filtration rate (GFR) seen in normal pregnant women. GFR instead characteristically decreases during the third trimester, although this has been reversible after delivery except in a few cases. Proteinuria also occurs in 40% of renal transplant in the third trimester, but this characteristically resolves postpartum. If there are no signs of preeclampsia, this proteinuria requires no specific treatment.

Pregnancy is almost always more complicated in patients with elevated creatinine levels and those with chronic rejection episodes. Deterioration in renal function, rejection, and even maternal death have occurred. There is no evidence that pregnancy has a deleterious effect on the transplanted kidney. Rejection of the renal graft with irreversible impairment of renal function during pregnancy or postpartum occurs in 10–20% of women, a risk similar to nonpregnant patients (First et al., 1995). The clinical hallmarks of rejection include fever, oliguria, deteriorating renal function, enlargement of the kidney, and tenderness to palpation. The diagnosis can be difficult because the findings overlap with other disorders such as pyelonephritis, recurrent glomerulopathy, preeclampsia, and nephrotoxicity from immunosuppressant drugs. It is crucial to establish the diagnosis of rejection before initiating additional anti-rejection therapy, and the clinical situation of failing renal function demands prompt hospitalization. Imaging studies such as ultrasound are useful to detect changes in the renal parenchyma and an indistinct corticomedullary boundary indicative of rejection. If the diagnosis is still unclear, renal biopsy is sometimes necessary.

Chronic hypertension and preeclampsia are the most prominent complications in these pregnancies and contribute to the increase in preterm births, fetal growth restriction, and occasional fetal death (Table 45.2). Hypertension is present in at least half of these pregnancies and almost one-third develop preeclampsia. In women with a renal transplant, blood pressure greater than 140/90 mmHg should usually be managed pharmacologically. Most commonly used antihypertensive agents can be continued during pregnancy with little risk to the fetus, but angiotensin-converting enzyme (ACE) inhibitors should be not be used because of adverse effects on the fetus such as oligohydramnios, pulmonary hypoplasia, and neonatal anuria. Calcium-channel blockers are the preferred agents, and they appear to be beneficial in countering the vasoconstrictive effect of cyclosporine. Preeclampsia should be anticipated, and the management is the same as with nontransplant patients.

Patients with systemic diseases require even closer surveillance, but successful pregnancies have occurred in recipients who received their renal allografts for diabetes, type I oxalosis, previous urinary diversion, Fabry's disease, systemic lupus erythematosus, cystinosis, sickle cell disease, Wegener's, and Goodpasture's syndrome (Bumgardner & Matas, 1992). Although renal transplantation allows diabetic women to become pregnant, immunosuppression adds to the complexity of management because of the risk of infection and potentially poor diabetic control. Maternal complications in diabetic transplant patients have included weight-bearing foot fractures, diabetic neuropathy, and vascular complications leading to maternal and fetal death. Neonatal hypocalcemia and hypoglycemia have also been reported in the offspring of these mothers (Bumgardner & Matas, 1992).

Other organ transplantation

Pancreas

Whole or segmental pancreas transplantation is now a treatment option for certain patients with insulin-dependent diabetes mellitus. One-year graft survival rate is approximately 80% with a 5-year graft survival rate of 60%. The 10-year probability of insulin independence is about 90% if the patient has a functioning graft at 5 years (Sutherland & Gruessner, 1995). Findings of pancreatic rejection are pain at the graft site, elevated serum amylase, hyperglycemia, and histologic evidence. Most cases of pancreas transplantation are performed in patients who already have or will receive a kidney allograft at the same time they receive the pancreas. Since many issues are the same, antepartum and intrapartum management are similar to kidney transplant patients. However, the diabetogenic effects of pregnancy, corticosteroids, cyclosporine, and other immunosuppressive drugs can all lead to or aggravate hyperglycemia, macrosomia, and other sequellae in pancreas transplant patients. Euglycemia should be achieved preconception, and glucose tolerance testing (GTT) is warranted prior to 20 weeks, particularly in patients who receive a segmental graft. If hyperglycemia is present, diet and insulin therapy should be instituted at that time. If the GTT screen is normal, it should be repeated at 24–28 weeks as with any pregnant patient. In reality, most pancreas transplant patients have maintained euglycemia throughout pregnancy and labor (Barron et al., 1998). Nevertheless, complications characteristic of diabetes have occurred in these patients including osteoporosis, fractures, diabetic neuropathy, chronic vascular insufficiency, maternal death, stillbirth, neonatal hypocalcemia, and hypoglycemia (Bumgardner & Matas, 1992).

Liver

Improvements in immunosuppressant drug therapy and surgical techniques have resulted in longer life expectancy and many pregnancies in women with liver allografts. Currently, 11% of all patients receiving liver transplants are women of reproductive age, and an additional 15% are younger patients who will survive to and beyond the childbearing age (Casele & Laifer, 1998). Clinical signs suggesting liver rejection are fever, right upper quadrant pain, leukocytosis, elevated serum bilirubin, and aminotransferase levels. Because these tests are nonspecific, suspected graft rejection needs biopsy confirmation. Most rejection episodes can be managed by adjusting the drug regimen. Maternal complications have included elevated liver function tests, rejection, recurrent hepatitis, decreased renal function, urinary tract infection, adrenal insufficiency, and endometritis (Casele & Laifer, 1998; Armenti et al., 1999, 2000). There is also an increased rate of fetal growth restriction, preeclampsia, premature rupture of membranes, preterm birth, cesarean delivery, and neonatal infections (Table 45.4). These complications are in part dependent an maternal health before pregnancy and their management is similar to those in renal transplant patients.

Heart

The first successful pregnancy in a cardiac transplant patient was reported in 1988 (Lowenstein et al., 1988). Since then more than 5,000 women in North America have undergone heart transplants at a current rate of more than 500 per year. The transplanted denervated heart must adapt to the physiologic changes of pregnancy. Arrhythmias may be present, and the denervated heart may not respond to some vasopressors in a predictable way. Only direct acting vasoactive drugs will have an effect, and the transplanted heart may be more sensitive to β-adrenergic agonists due to an increase in β-receptors (Camann et al., 1989). One-third of patents have tricuspid regurgitation 1-year post transplant, and it may worsen with the increased blood volume associated with pregnancy. Almost one-third of cardiac transplant patients have atherosclerotic coronary vessel stenosis by 3 years after the transplant and up to 50% have atherosclerosis at 5 years (Uretshky et al., 1987). Chest pain from myocardial ischemia will not be present since there is no afferent innervation, and paroxysmal dyspnea may be the only presenting symptom. Many signs and symptoms observed in normal pregnancies, including fatigue, dyspnea, and peripheral edema, may be confusing in heart transplant recipients. Many women have had heart transplants for peripartum cardiomyopathy which has not recurred with subsequent pregnancies (Scott et al., 1996). Maternal graft rejection episodes occur in 20–30% of pregnancies, but most are not clinically evident and are diagnosed by routine surveillance biopsies. These biopsies are obtained from the right ventricle guided by either fluoroscopy or echocardiography (Kim et al., 1996). Rejection episodes are usually successful managed by increasing the immunosuppression regimen. The increased incidence of hypertension, preeclampsia, prematurity, and low birth weights are similar to that of other transplant patients (Wagoner et al., 1993; Branch et al., 1998; Armenti et al., 2000) (Table 45.4). It is prudent to involve an anesthesiologist during late second trimester to formulate a well-organized plan for labor and delivery. An important intrapartum consideration is the denervated heart's increased sensitivity to hypovolemia and catecholamines.

Lung

In North America, there are approximately 30 female heart–lung transplant procedures annually. The most frequent indications are congenital heart disease with Eisenmenger's syndrome, primary pulmonary hypertension, and less commonly cystic fibrosis and emphysema. One-year survival rate for heart–lung recipients is 63%, and this decreases to approximately 40% at 5 years (Branch et al., 1998). There are few cases of pregnancy following heart–lung transplantation in the literature (Parry et al., 1997; Trouche et al., 1998; Armenti et al., 2000; Rigg et al., 2000). In addition to the management issues related to heart transplant patients, there are specific issues to be considered in the heart–lung transplant recipient. Diagnosing chronic rejection of the lung allograft may be challenging, but one of the first symptoms can be a mild cough with subsequent deterioration in pulmonary function. Very little is known about the changes that occur in the gravid heart–lung recipient. As a result of the transplant, there is a loss of pulmonary innervation, bronchial arterial supply and pulmonary lymphatics. This denervation leads to compromise of the cough reflex and difficulty protecting the airway. Decreased lung compliance may result in a persistent alveolar–arterial oxygen gradient. Pulmonary edema is a definite possibility in these patients, and excess intravenous hydration should be avoided. Two patients have died postpartum from complications of obliterative bronchiolitis (Rigg et al., 2000).

Bone marrow

The use of stem cell transplantation for women of childbearing age with leukemia and other malignant and nonmalignant hematologic disorders has increased steadily for the past 20 years. Pretransplant conditioning protocols include alkylating agents and irradiation which can cause germ cell injury, ovarian failure, and infertility, but many normal children have been born to women after bone marrow transplantation. Miscarriage, preeclampsia, fetal growth restriction, and preterm birth are the most frequent complications, but most have had relatively uncomplicated pregnancies and deliveries (Sanders et al., 1996; Salooja et al., 2001) (Table 45.2).

Labor and delivery

The timing of delivery is often dictated by events such as premature labor, premature ruptured membranes, or severe preeclampsia. The extraperitoneal location of the transplanted kidney in the iliac fossa usually does not interfere with vaginal delivery. Obstructed labor from soft-tissue dystocia due to the graft or pelvic osteodystrophy are very rare. If the fetal head is not engaged in the pelvis during labor, dystocia can be assessed by ultrasound and computed tomography (CT) scan pelvimetry. There are no particular contraindications to induction, labor, or vaginal delivery in organ graft recipients. Because of an increased susceptibility to infection, vaginal examinations should be kept to a minimum and artificial rupture of membranes and internal monitoring performed only when specifically indicated. Cultures and antibiotics are warranted with the earliest sign of infection.

Delivery by cesarean is based on accepted obstetric indications. Operative deliveries in these patients are managed with prophylactic antibiotics and additional glucocorticoids, and require strict asepsis, careful attention to hemostasis, and good surgical technique. A lower midline vertical incision provides the greatest exposure and avoids the region of the transplanted kidney. A low transverse uterine incision is almost always possible, but the obstetrician should be aware of the anatomic alterations associated with the transplanted kidney to avoid inadvertent damage to the blood supply or urinary drainage. These mothers are usually advised against breastfeeding since the immunosuppressive drugs are detected in breast milk (Norton & Scott, 1993). However, the dosage delivered to the infant is generally small. If a woman decides to breastfeed, she should understand that there is limited information available to make this decision.

Obstetric emergencies

Acute emergencies may arise in transplant patients during pregnancy with severe consequences that require aggressive management and intensive care. These patients are best managed in a tertiary setting where the transplant surgeon, obstetrician, nephrologist, and other subspecialists and intensivists can work together. Most difficult is severe and chronic rejection or allograft vasculopathy with loss of graft function which threatens the life of the mother and fetus. In some cases, patients have deliberately stopped their immunosuppression drugs resulting in acute rejection episodes and even death (Sims, 1991; Scott et al., 1993). Renal allograft patients with deteriorating function may have to be placed back on dialysis therapy for the remainder of the pregnancy, and other organ recipients need a variety of supportive measures including retransplantation. Sepsis and overwhelming infections are also a constant threat to these women, and patients have died of meningitis, pneumonia, gastroenteritis, hepatitis C and B, and AIDS (Bumgardner & Matas, 1992; Scott et al., 1993). With the high incidence of hypertension and preeclampsia, it is not surprising that HELLP syndrome, stroke, and eclampsia have occurred (Bumgardner & Matas, 1992; Norton & Scott, 1993). Other causes of morbidity that have required emergent surgery include rupture of renal vessel anastomosis, mechanical obstruction of the ureter, antepartum bleeding, uterine rupture, small bowel injury at cesarean delivery, severe postparutm hemorrhage, abdominal wound dehiscence, and pelvic abscess (Bumgardner & Matas, 1992; Norton & Scott, 1993).

References

Abbasi S, Hirsch D, Davis J, et al. Effect of single versus multiple courses of antenatal corticosteroids on maternal and neonatal outcome. Am J Obstet Gynecol 2000;182:1243–1249.

Alston PK, Kuller JA, McMahon MJ. Pregnancy in transplant recipients. Obstet Gynecol Survey 2001;56:289–295.

American College of Obstetrics and Gynecology. Perinatal viral and parasitic infections. ACOG Practice Bulletin 2000;20:1–5.

Armenti VT, Wilson GA, Radomski JS, et al. Report from the National Transplantation Pregnancy Registry (NTPR): Outcomes of pregnancy after transplantation. In: Cecka JM, Terasaki PI, eds. Clinical Transplants 1999. UCLA Immunogenetics Center, Los Angeles, CA pp. 111–119.

Armenti VT, Moritz MJ, Radomski JS, et al. Pregnancy and transplantation. Graft 2000;3:59–63.

Barrou BM, Gruessner AC, Sutherland DER, Gruessner RWG. Pregnancy after pancreas transplantation in the cyclosporine era: report from the International Pancreas Transplant Registry. Transplantation 1998;65:524–527.

Branch KR, Wagoner LE, McGrory CH, et al. Risks of subsequent pregnancies on mother and newborn in female heart transplant recipients. J Heart Lung Transplant 1998;17:698–702.

Bumgardner GL, Matas AJ. Transplantation and pregnancy. Transplant Rev 1992;6:139–162.

Camann WR, Goldman GA, Johnson MD, Moore J, Greene M. Cesarean delivery in a patient with a transplanted heart. Anesthesiology 1989;71:618–620.

Casele HL, Laifer SA. Pregnancy after liver transplantation. Sem Perinatol 1998;22:149–155.

Classen BJ, Shevach EM. Evidence that cyclosporine treatment during pregnancy predisposes offspring to develop autoantibodies. Transplantation 1991;51:1052–1057.

Cowchock FS, Reece EA, Bababan D, Branch DW, Plouffe L. Repeated fetal losses associated with antiphospholipid antibodies: A collaborative randomized trial comparing prednisone to low-dose heparin treatment. Am J Obstet Gynecol 1992;166:1318–1327.

Davidson JM. Towards long-graft survival in renal transplantation: Pregnancy Nephrol Dial Transplant 1995;10:85–89.

Davison JM, Dellagrammatikas H, Parkin JM. Maternal azathioprine therapy and depressed haemopoiesis in the babies of renal allograft patients. Br J Obstet Gynaecol 1985;92:233–239.

Esplin M, Fausett M, Smith S. Multiple courses of antenatal steroids are associated with a delay in long-term pyschomotor development in children with birth weights <1,500 grams. Am J Obstet Gynecol 2000;182:S24.

First MR, Combs CA, Weiskittel P, Miodovnik M. Lack of effect of pregnancy on renal allograft survival or function. Transplantation 1995;59:472–476.

Kim KM, Sukhani R, Slogoff S, Tomich PG. Central hemodynamic changes associated with pregnancy in a long-term cardiac transplant recipient. Am J Obstet Gynecol 1996;174:1651–1653.

Lau RJ, Scott JR. Pregnancy following renal transplantation. Clin Obstet Gynecol 1985;28:339–350.

Levitz M, Jansen V, Dancis J. The transfer and metabolism of corticosteroids in the perfused human placenta. Am J Obstet Gynecol 1978;132:363–366.

Lowenstein BR, Vain NW, Perrone SV, et al. Successful pregnancy and vaginal delivery after heart transplantation. Am J Obstet Gynecol 1988;158:589–590.

Miller J, Mendez R, Pirsch JD, Jensik SC. Safety and efficacy of tacrolius in combination with mycophenolate mofetil (MMF) in cadaveric renal transplant recipients. FK506/MMF dose ranging kidney transplant study group. Transplantation 2000;69:875–880.

Murray JE, Reid DE, Harrison JH. Successful pregnancies after human transplantation. N Engl J Med 1963;269:341–348.

National Institutes of Health. Antenatal corticosteroids revisited: repeat courses. NIH Consensus Statement 2000;17:1–18.

Norton PA, Scott JR. Gynecologic and obstetric problems in renal allograft recipients. In: Buchsbaum H, Schmidt J, eds. Gynecologic and Obstetric Urology, 3rd edn. Philadelphia, PA: WB Saunders Co., 1993;657–674.

Parry D, Hextall A, Banner N, Robinson V, Yacoub M. Pregnancy following lung transplantation. Transplant Proc 1997;29:629.

Penn I, Makowski EL, Harris P. Parenthood following renal transplantation. Kidney Int 1980;18:221–233.

Pirsch JD, Miller J, Deierhoi MH, Vincenti D, Filo RS. A comparison of tacrolimus (FK506) and cyclosporine for immunosuppression after cadaveric renal transplantation. FK506 kidney transplant study group. Transplantation 1997;63:977–983.

Registration Committee of the European Dialysis and Transplant Association. Successful pregnancies in women treated by dialysis and kidney transplantation. Br J Obstet Gynecol 1980;87: 839–845.

Rigg CD, Bythell VE, Bryson MR, Halshaw J, Davidson JM. Caesarean section in patients with heart-lung transplants: a report of three cases and review. Int J Obstet Anesth 2000;9:125–132.

Rizzoni G, Ehrich JHH, Broyer M. Successful pregnancies in women on renal replacement therapy: Report from the EDTA Registry. Nephrol Dial Transplant 1992;7:279–287.

Saarikoski S, Seppala M. Immunosuppression during pregnancy: Transmission of azathioprine and its metabolites from mother to fetus. Am J Obstet Gynecol 1973;115:1100–1106.

Salooja N, Szydlo RM, Socie G, et al. Pregnancy outcomes after peripheral blood or bone marrow transplantation: a retrospective survey. Lancet 2001;358:271–276.

Sanders JE, Hawley J, Levy W, et al. Pregnancies following high-dose cyclophosphamide with or without high-dose busulfan or total-body irradiation and bone marrow transplantation. Blood 1996;87:3045–3052.

Scott JR, Branch DW, Holman J. Autoimmune and pregnancy complications in the daughter of a kidney transplant patient. Transplantation 2002;73:815–816.

Scott JR, Branch DW, Kochenour NK, Larkin RM. The effect of repeated pregnancies on renal allograft function. Transplantation 1986; 42:694–695.

Scott JR. Fetal growth restriction associated with maternal administration of immunosuppressive drugs. Am J Obstet Gynecol 1977;128: 668–676.

Scott JR. Risks to the children born to mothers with autoimmune diseases. Lupus 2002;11:655–660.

Scott JR. Pregnancy in transplant recipients. In: Coulam CB, Faulk WP, McIntyre JA, eds. Immunology and Obstetrics. New York: WW Norton Co. 1992;640–644.

Scott JR, Wagoner LE, Olsen SL, Taylor DO, Renlund DG. Pregnancy in heart transplant recipients. Management and outcome. Obstet Gynecol 1993;82:324–327.

Sims CJ. Organ transplantation and immunosuppressive drugs. Clin Obstet Gynecol 1991;34:100–111.

Sutherland DER, Gruessner A. Long-term function (>5 years) of pancreas grafts form the International Pancreas Transplant Registry database. Transplant Proc 1995;27:2977.

Trouche V, Ville Y, Fernandez H. Pregnancy after heart or heart-lung transplantation: a series of 10 pregnancies. Br J Obstet Gynaecol 1998;105:454–458.

Uretshky BF, Murali S, Reddy PS. Development of coronary disease in cardiact transplant patients receiving immunosuppressive therapy with cyclosporine and prednisone. Circulation 1987;76:827–834.

Wagoner LE, Taylor DO, Olsen SL, et al. Immunosuppressive therapy, management, and outcome of heart transplant recipients during pregnancy. J Heart Lung Transplant 1993;12:993–999.

Willis FR, Findlay CA, Gorrie MJ, et al. Children of renal transplant recipient mothers. J Pediatr Child Health 2000;36:230–235.

Winkler ME, Niesert S, Ringe B, Pichlmayr R. Successful pregnancy in a patient after liver transplantation maintained on FK 506. Transplantation 1993;56:1589–1590.

46 Ethics in the obstetric critical care setting

Fidelma B. Rigby

Ethical issues remain a relevant topic in the obstetric setting. This is especially true when one considers that obstetrics often deal with the care of two or more individuals at any one moment. In essence, ethics is "the determination of what ought to be done, all things considered" (Brown & Elkins, 1992). This definition, a form of ethics in action, requires differentiating "what could be done" from "what ought to be done" and calls for special thought regarding nonprofessional factors (Brown & Elkins, 1992). Chervenak and McCullough (1999) describe medical ethics as the "disciplined study of morality in medicine regarding obligations of physicians and institutions to patients and the obligations of patients." They note that medical ethics calls for examining concrete and clinically applicable accounts of how physicians ought to conduct themselves with patients. Tools for answering ethical dilemmas derive from ethical principles that assist practitioners in interpreting and implementing their general moral obligations to protect and promote the interest of the patient (Chervenak & McCullough, 1999).

This chapter first introduces four ethical principles that form the framework for ethical decision-making, i.e. autonomy, nonmaleficence, beneficence, and justice. Boxes 46.1 and 46.2 provide a glossary of ethical terms and review of important legal cases. The doctrine of informed consent and the relative status of the fetus are then examined in relation to the mother. Applications to the critical care setting are then made. Issues involving competency, critically ill patients, and maternal–fetal conflict are addressed. Specific concerns regarding Jehovah's Witness cases are reviewed, and finally letters of condolence are discussed. With the aid of this chapter the reader should have an understanding of how to apply ethical principles to the care of the critically ill obstetric patient.

Ethical principles

Four principles frame the values of the underlying common morality in the community formed by the patient–physician relationship. These principles should guide the approach to the patient in medical ethics (Beauchamp & Childress, 2001). Until the 1960s, the Hippocratic tradition served as the basis for medical ethics discussion in the United States (Brown & Elkins, 1992). Physicians were expected to be beneficent, thereby promoting patient well-being. Beneficence obligates the physician to act in a manner that produces the greater good for the patient. The coinciding ethical principle of nonmaleficence obligated the physician to do no harm (Brown & Elkins, 1992; Beauchamp & Childress, 2001). The technological advances and cultural change that accompanied the 1960s expanded the framework to include respect for autonomy. This principle emphasizes the decision-making capacity of the competent person (Beauchamp & Childress, 2001). The prior assumption that the physician is the main decision-maker came to be shunned as paternalism. The emphasis shifted from the physician making decisions "in the patient's best interests" to the patient's right to self-determination. Patient autonomy rose to the foremost of the ethical principles and tended to overpower other ethical considerations (Brown & Elkins, 1992). More recently, limitations on a patient's absolute autonomy have been raised in light of affirmation of the physician's autonomy, consideration for the physician's character, and efforts to protect physicians from compromising their own principles. These varied emphases merged into a model of shared decision making.

Informed consent

The legal right to informed consent is well summarized in Justice Benjamin Cardozo's ruling in the 1914 case of Schloendorff vs Society of New York Hospital: "Every being of adult years and sound mind has a right to determine what shall be done with his body, and a surgeon who performs an operation without his patient's consent commits an assault for which he is liable in damages" (Schloendorff vs Society of New York Hospitals (1914)). The original concept of informed consent centered on the legal doctrine regarding battery: the harmful or offensive touching of another person (Lo, 2000). This concept of battery for unauthorized surgery applies even if the surgery is appropriately and skillfully done (Lo, 2000). This

Box 46.1 Glossary of ethical and legal terminology

Battery Harmful or offensive touching of another person: physicians may commit battery if they operate without patient's consent.
Beneficence The physician's obligation to act in the patient's best interest.
Competence Capacity to understand and appreciate the nature and consequences of one's actions.
Dependent moral status A moral status which is dependent on someone else's actions.
Ethical principles Guidelines for ethical behavior (i.e. beneficence, autonomy, nonmaleficence)
Independent moral status Having a moral status in and of one's self.
Negligence Breach of duty to the patient from which the patient suffers harm.
Nonmaleficence The physician's obligation to do no harm.
Paternalism Overriding the patient's wishes to act in a way the physician feels would most benefit the patient.
Respect for autonomy Respect for the patient's wishes and right to self-determination.
Substituted judgment When a surrogate decision makes attempts to determine what a patient would have decided.

(Adapted from Chervenak & McCullough, 1994; Anna & Densberger, 1984, Pinkerton, 1996.)

point was underscored in the classic case of Mohr vs Williams in which the consent was obtained for surgery on the patient's right ear (Mohr vs Williams, 1905). However, increased disease was noted in the patient's left ear at the time of surgery. Although appropriate surgery was done on the more severely affected left ear, the courts ruled that the patient had not consented to the surgery and held the physician liable (Mohr vs Williams, as presented in Beauchamp & Childress, 2001).

The breach of informed consent in today's legal setting is more commonly interpreted as a form of negligence (Lo, 2000). Negligence involves a breach of duty to the patient from which the patient suffers harm. In the case of informed consent, negligence occurs when the physician has not disclosed a risk of the surgery and this risk occurs, causing harm to the patient. The patient could then claim that she would not have consented to the surgery if the risk had been disclosed.

Exceptions to this concept of informed consent do occur. In an emergency setting, where the patient is incapable of providing informed consent and there is not time to find a proxy decision maker, doctors may provide lifesaving procedures (as long as they do not go against any known beliefs of the patient) (Lo, 2000). In the case of minors, parental consent is usually needed except when state laws provide for emancipation of minors. Pregnancy is generally one of the conditions that allows minors to consent to procedures on their own behalf. The essence and interpretation of these laws can vary from state to state. For instance, until 2001 at Louisiana Health Sciences Center (LSUHSC) in New Orleans, the interpretation of minor emancipation in pregnancy was such that pregnant minors could consent for procedures directly related to the pregnancy and for the procedures done on their newborn. They could consent for an epidural for cesarean section but needed parental consent for a labor epidural because the latter was considered an elective procedure by the anesthesiology team.

Other exceptions to informed consent occur. One of these rare exceptions may include a waiver of informed consent. In this case, a patient with a serious illness specifically requests that the physician make decisions regarding treatment options the patient does not feel capable of making (such as surgery vs radiation treatment). As Lo points out, self-determination is undermined when reluctant patients are forced to engage in decision-making against their wishes. Shared decision-making is a goal but not an absolute requirement in this particular setting. Physicians should be aware that such patients can change their minds and choose to actively participate in a later phase of their therapy (Lo, 2000).

The American College of Obstetrics and Gynecology was among the first specialty societies to establish an ethics committee (Brown & Elkins, 1992). The concept of informed consent evolved in the 1970s when the central concern for the medical well-being of the patient evolved to include increasing concern for the autonomy of the patient in making medical decisions (ACOG, 1992). In the 1980s, the concept of shared decision-making evolved (ACOG, 1992). The issue of informed consent was addressed by ACOG in its 1992 ACOG Ethics Committee Opinion regarding the "Ethical Dimensions of Informed Consent." In this bulletin, two main aspects of informed consent are addressed: free consent and comprehension. Free consent is defined as an act that is intentional and voluntary by which the individual is authorized to act in certain ways. For medicine free consent means the patient freely authorizes a medical intervention (ACOG, 1992). "Consent" implies that no coercion is present. "Free" implies that the person is choosing among alternatives.

The bulletin also emphasizes the element of comprehension, i.e. an awareness and understanding of the information regarding one's care and the possibilities that surround it (ACOG, 1992). The ideal of informed consent works best in a relationship of mutual respect and is best seen as a process, as opposed to a task of getting the patient to sign the consent form. In the critical care setting, decisions are often made under periods of stress with limited time. Special effort must

Box 46.2 Summaries of important medical–legal cases

Case	Summary
Informed Consent	
Mohr vs Williams (1904)	Physician was held accountable for operating on opposite ear without consent.
Schloendorff vs Society of New York Hospital (1914)	Judge Cardozo's classic case where patient was not properly informed. re: nature of surgery.
In the Matter of Karen Quinlan (1976)	Court permitted withdrawal of respirator in first "right to die" case, introduced "substituted judgment" stand and spurred evolution of ethics committees.
Lane vs Candura (1987)	Case affirmed competency of woman who declined amputation of her gangrenous leg.
Superintendent of Belchertown v. Bouvia (1983)	Court granted right of patient with cerebral palsy to refuse nutrition.
Cruzan vs Missouri Department of Health (1990)	Courts permitted parents to withdraw feeding tube from patient with persistent vegetative state: spurred development of living wills.
Maternal–Fetal Conflict	
Smith vs Brennan (1960)	Court permitted neonate to sue for damages inflicted during gestation.
Jefferson vs Griffer Spalding Hospital Authority (1981)	Court ordered cesarean section for patient with complete previa at term.
Re: Madyin (1986)	Court ordered cesarean after 60 hours of ruptured membranes.
Re: A.C. (1990)	Patient with terminal cancer underwent court ordered cesarean with subsequent demise of mother and neonate. Appeals Court overturned decision.
Baby Doe vs Mother Doe (1999)	Court declined to order cesarean section for placental insufficiency, citing re: A.C. as precedent Supreme Court Case.
Supreme Court Cases	
Roe vs Wade (1973)	Landmark decision permitting abortion in first trimester with regulation in second and third trimesters.
Colauttiv vs Franklin (1979)	Supreme Court invalidated statute that required postviability termination using least destructive techniques.
Webster vs Reproductive Health Services (1989)	Court permitted ultrasounds of fetus 12 weeks undergoing termination.
Planned Parenthood vs Casey (1992)	Court permitted restrictions on abortions after viability.
Jehovah's Witness	
Raleigh-Fitkin (1964)	Court gave permission for forced transfusion of pregnant woman but she left hospital before transfusion.
Georgetown Hospital Case (1964)	Court ordered transfusion to prevent abandonment of young child.
Application of Jamaica Hospital (1985)	Court ordered transfusion at 18 weeks' gestation in pregnant women with esophageal varices.

be made to allow the patient (or the designated surrogate) to help in the decision process as much as possible.

Competency

Informed consent presupposes the patient's competency. Competency questions lead to ethical dilemmas when the patient refuses life-sustaining interventions. In Lane vs. Candura, a 77-year-old widow with diabetes refused amputation of a gangrenous lower leg (Lane vs Candura, 1978). She was considered competent when she consented to the earlier amputations of her toe and then a portion of her foot. When she initially vacillated and then firmly and repeatedly declined the further amputation, her competency was called into question. Although the lower court ruled against her, the appeals court ruled in her favor, stating, "Mrs. Candura's decision may be regarded by most as unfortunate but . . . it is not the uninformed decision of a person incapable of appreciating the nature and consequence of her act." (Lane vs Candura in Annas, 1984). Thus the mere fact that she was declining a life-saving operation did not in itself make her incompetent.

Ethical guidelines must allow for decision making to proceed when the patient is judged to be incompetent. The Karen Quinlan case in 1976 was pivotal in the evolution of the substituted judgement standard in these cases. Karen Quinlan was a 22-year-old woman in a persistent vegetative state. She was initially intubated and placed on a respirator using consent to treatment implied by the emergency doctrine (Sanbar, 2001). As the vegetative state continued without hope of recovery, her father petitioned to be named her legal guardian so that he could ask that she be taken off the respirator. The court ruling discussed the right to privacy, which includes a right to decline treatment. The court decided the father could exercise this right on his daughter's behalf. The question that needed to be addressed was, "What would the patient decide if the patient were able to decide?" (In the Matter of Karen Quinlan, 1976). Decision-makers for the patient were expected to "render their best judgment" (Lo, 2000). This expectation became known as the "substituted judgment standard" (Lo, 2000). The complications surrounding this case spurred the development of ethics committees (Lo, 2000). This case in particular made clear the limitations of medicine in predicting the outcome of critically ill patients, as Karen Quinlan lived for years after being removed from the respirator (Lo, 2000).

Further evolutions in the ethical and legal response to critically ill patients occurred in the Cruzan, Brophy, and Bouvia cases. Cruzan was a young woman in a persistent vegetative state following a 1983 motor vehicle accident. In 1986, her parents asked that her gastrostomy feeding tube be discontinued because she had previously stated that she "didn't want to live" as a "vegetable" (Cruzan vs Missouri Dept. of Health, 1990 as presented in Lo, 2000). In 1990, the Supreme Court affirmed the Missouri court ruling that states may require life-sustaining interventions in cases where there is no clear convincing evidence that the incompetent patient would refuse such. Many states allow the family to make decisions on the patient's behalf but the Supreme Court ruled that states could intervene on the patient's behalf to continue life-sustaining measures if there were no clear indications of the patient's preferences (Lo, 2000). Ironically, the court was repetitioned after more evidence of Cruzan's wishes was discovered. In this phase of the proceedings, the State of Missouri withdrew from the proceedings and Cruzan's attending physician no longer challenged the removal of the feeding tube. The Court then ruled that the tube could be removed (Cruzan vs Missouri Dept of Health adapted from Lo, 2000). This case was a landmark case involving the refusal of treatment and spurred the development of living wills and advance directive statures.

The Brophy case in 1986 also confirmed the right for patients' families to allow the removal of feeding tubes in patients in persistent vegetative states (Brophy vs New England Sinai Hospital, 1986). Brophy was a firefighter who fell into a persistent vegetative state following a ruptured aneurysm in 1983. In 1985 his wife petitioned the court to remove his feeding tube and in 1986 a four to three decision by the Supreme Judicial Court of Massachusetts affirmed that the tube could be removed (Brophy vs New England Sinai Hospital, 1986 adapted from Beauchamp, 2001).

The Bouvia case presented the judicial system with the issue of removing a feeding tube from a competent patient who was not terminally ill (Bouvia vs Superior Court, 1986). Elizabeth Bouvia was a 26-year-old woman with cerebral palsy. Her disease left her with only limited use of her right hand such that she could operate an electric wheelchair but could only eat when fed by another person. In 1983 the courts originally upheld the hospital's right to feed her due to the onerous effect her refusal to eat would have had on the staff and other patients (Annas & Densberger, 1984). She went to court again 2 years later and lost again. However, this decision was overturned by the appeals court which held "a person of adult years and in sound mind has the right, in the exercise of control over his own body, to determine whether or not to submit to lawful medical treatment . . . It follows that such a patient has the right to refuse any medical treatment, even that which may save or prolong her life" (Bouvia vs Superior Court, 1986). Thus the Bouvia case permitted withdrawal of nutrition from a competent patient with a nonterminal illness.

We will address how these cases and ethical principles should influence our approach to critically ill obstetric patients in the sections below after addressing the status of the fetus.

Status of the fetus

One of the special aspects of obstetric medic ethics is that there are two patients involved: the mother and fetus. The status of the fetus can significantly influence the approach to ethical issues surrounding the pregnancy. The debate regarding the moral/legal/political status of the fetus as a person has been going on since antiquity (Brown & Elkins, 1992). Many authors have addressed this issue during the last two decades (Leiberman, 1979; Fost et al., 1980; Fletcher, 1981; Chervenak et al., 1984; Gillon, 1988; Abrams, 1989; Chervenak & McCullough, 1989, 1997; Mahoney, 1989; Newton, 1989; Strong & Garland, 1989; Beller & Zlatnik, 1992; Mattingly, 1992; Botkin, 1995). Three main views can be distinguished in much of today's debate regarding fetal status: the fetus never has normal status, has independent moral status, or has dependent moral status.

One view is that the fetus never has moral status. Annas argues that there is no justification for considering forced treatment of pregnant women because the fetus has no independent moral status and maternal autonomy concerns should therefore prevail in any situation (Annas, 1982, 1987).

Problems with this view have become more evident as knowledge of fetal status and beneficial prenatal fetal interventions have become more common. The expanding ability to treat the fetus has encouraged viewing the issue of the fetus as a patient. The idea of a graded moral status for the fetus has been introduced as a way to relieve this dilemma. Brown and Elkins credit Fletcher with introducing the concept of the fetus as a patient (Fletcher, 1981; Brown & Elkins, 1992). In this 1981 editorial in JAMA, he identified several important ethical dilemmas in the emerging field of fetal therapy. Central to his analysis was the pressure to consider the fetus as a separate entity in that specific interventions were becoming possible on its behalf. Since that time many authors have addressed this issue of fetal status (Fost et al., 1980; The Fetus as Patient, 1981; Chervenak et al., 1984; Gillon, 1988; Abrams, 1989; Chervenak & McCullough, 1989, 1997; Mahoney, 1989; Newton, 1989; Strong & Garland, 1989; Beller & Zlaknik, 1992; Mattingly, 1992; Botkin, 1995).

McCullough and Chervenak have developed a framework to discuss the issue of fetal status by presenting the concepts of independent and dependent moral status of the fetus (McCullough & Chervenak, 1994). They argue that the fetus is a being who can be reliably linked to later "achieving" independent moral status as its development progresses. Knowing when to confer "independent moral status" is the problematic issue. They hold that the fetus does not have subjective interests per se due to the immaturity of its central nervous system. Therefore, there can be no autonomy-based obligations to the fetus (McCullough & Chervenak, 1994). They conclude that there are, therefore, no fetal rights in the sense that the fetus itself can "generate" these rights.

This conclusion leads McCullough and Chervenak to propose a dependent moral status for the viable fetus in that viability is the first important step the fetus achieves in progressing towards an independent moral status (McCullough & Chervenak, 1994). The age at which the fetus achieves independent moral status could vary in different countries but in the US it is approximately 24–25 weeks. Viability means that the fetus can begin to have "interests" that deserve to be protected/promoted by obstetric interventions (McCullough & Chervenak, 1994). The potential protection of the fetus, however, can only occur when the pregnant woman presents the fetus to the health-care team when she seeks prenatal care. To McCullough and Chervenak's viewpoint, the dependent moral status of the fetus obligates the pregnant woman to take reasonable risks to protect the fetus. She is not obligated to take unreasonable risks (McCullough & Chervenak, 1994).

According to this view of fetal moral status, the previable fetus has no claim on the pregnant woman or her physician to remain in utero because the fetus requires the use of the pregnant woman's body to achieve viability. The fetus needs the pregnant woman to make an autonomous decision in order for the "patient" status to be conferred during the previable period (McCullough & Chervenak, 1994). The pregnant woman has no ethical obligation to present her previable fetus to her physician. If and only if she presents her fetus to the physician for treatment, is the physician then obligated to protect and promote fetal interests. Thus the previable fetus in this view has only dependent moral status (McCullough & Chervenak, 1994). If the mother is undecided regarding her views toward the fetus, McCullough and Chervenak recommend using Pascal's wager (if you are unsure regarding the existence of God then it would make more sense to act as if God exists) and proceeding in ways that promote full fetal benefit (until the mother withholds the status from her fetus). This view of the fetus as having dependent moral status provides a useful framework to look at the issues, which confront the physician during dilemmas in critical care obstetric settings.

Practical applications of ethical principles to high-risk obstetrics

Maternal–fetal conflict

Advocates of strong maternal autonomy

One's approach to the issue of maternal–fetal conflict is largely defined by how one approaches the status of the fetus. Strong maternal autonomy advocates such as Annas argue that it is an assumption in Anglo-American law that every competent adult is at liberty to consent or to refuse any proposed medical treatment. This legal right to refuse treatment is viewed by Annas as part of the common law right to self-determination and associated with the constitutional right to privacy (Annas & Densberger, 1984). He notes that forcing compliance with medical advice would give the fetus status as a patient which is not correct as the fetus can only be treated (without the mother's consent) by drastically curtailing the mother's liberties (Annas, 1987). He warns against using an "outcome" approach to judge competency in cases of maternal–fetal conflict wherein the mother's competency comes into question only when her wishes go against the beliefs of her doctors (Annas & Densberger, 1984). Annas outlines questions he considers helpful in assessing patient competency.

Can the patient describe:
1 her current medical problem;
2 the therapy suggested for the problem;
3 the risks associated with the recommended therapy;
4 the risks associated with foregoing this therapy;
5 the other available therapies and their risks/benefits?

(Adapted from Annas & Densberger, 1984.)

Annas notes that if the patient is not decisive and treatment is immediately needed to save her life or prevent severe damage, then reasonable treatment can be done as this promotes society's general interest in health. However, if a question persists and nonemergent treatment is indicated, then evaluation of the patient for competency is called for. If the patient is determined incompetent, then a proxy decision-maker must be identified. When psychiatric assistance is needed, it is important to note that psychiatry determines whether the patient is competent to make treatment decisions. The psychiatric evaluation should not play a direct role in determining which treatment to use, but should only be used to determine whether the patient is competent to decide among the different treatment options (Annas & Densberger, 1984). Annas argues that the unusual case of a pregnant woman's refusal to consent to an intervention that would benefit her fetus should always be honored. He notes that this may seem callous to the rights of fetuses, but this is the price society should be prepared to pay in order to protect the rights of all competent adults (Annas, 1982).

Other authors also argue for full maternal autonomy for resolving ethical conflicts that arise during pregnancy. Mahowald bases her arguments on four issues: the right to informed consent, the right of bodily integrity, the questionable personhood of the fetus, and the maternal risks in undergoing forced treatments such as cesarean section. Mahowald agrees with Annas that forcing women to undergo any treatment for the sake of the fetus marks women as "unequal citizens" equivalent to "fetal containers" (Mahowald, 1989). Rhoden also advocates strong maternal autonomy, noting that there is a "quantum leap in logic" between the oft-cited Roe vs Wade decision where prohibitions on abortions were allowed when the fetus reached viability. Rhoden notes that there is a marked difference between prohibiting destruction and requiring surgical preservation (Rhoden, 1987).

Harris supports strong maternal autonomy and proposes that fetal needs exist only as a projection by a third party (i.e. the physician). This projection can become problematic. It has been estimated that up to one-third of court-ordered interventions use wrong medical judgment (Harris, 2000).

Advocates of fetal rights

In contrast to those who believe the fetus never has moral status, there are advocates of fetal rights. Strong is supportive of fetal rights in maternal–fetal conflict cases. He proposes intervention with treatments that pose insignificant or no health risks to the mother or treatments that would promote her interests in life/health. He advocates interventions that protect fetal life or prevent serious harm to the fetus. He surpasses some other authors in finding supportive compelling reasons to override maternal autonomy. These other reasons include preventing abandonment of dependent children, preserving the ethical integrity of physicians, and promoting the well-being of the community. As an example he sanctions the transfusion of blood in a Jehovah's Witness at term if the pregnant woman has multiple dependent children and there are no other people to assume care of the children (Strong & Carson, 1987; Strong, 1991).

Review of prominent court cases

Background: Roe vs Wade

The groundwork for maternal and fetal rights cases was in many ways laid by the Supreme Court's 1973 decision in Roe v. Wade (Roe vs Wade, 1973). Roe vs Wade changes the status assigned to the fetus as the fetus progresses through the three trimesters. In the first trimester, a woman's right to privacy is emphasized. The first-trimester fetus is noted to lack personhood (as defined by the 14th Amendment) and no societal obligations to the fetus are granted. This landmark decision establishes that during the first trimester, no states can interfere with the right of the pregnant woman to have an abortion. In the second trimester, increasing regulation of pregnancy termination is permitted to safeguard the mother's health. In the third trimester, stricter restrictions by the states are permitted to protect the rights of the viable fetus. Ironically it is this protective language regarding the third-trimester fetus that has been increasingly used by fetal advocates to justify interventions for the fetus at this stage (Rhoden, 1987). The Supreme Court has revisited this issue in several cases since Roe vs Wade.

Cases affirming maternal autonomy

Several cases have settled in favor of maternal autonomy. One of the more celebrated of these cases is the Angela Carder case in 1990 (re: AC, 1990). Angela Carder had developed bone cancer at age 13 but was felt to be in remission when she married at the age of 27 and subsequently became pregnant. When she reached 25 weeks' gestational age, Angela was discovered to have metastases to her lungs and was admitted to the hospital for further work-up. At 26 weeks' gestational age, Angela's condition began to deteriorate and she decided that she would undergo chemotherapy with the goal of reaching 28 weeks before delivery might be indicated. However, her condition degenerated rapidly and one day later the question of whether the fetus should be delivered earlier was raised (re: AC as noted in Mohaupt & Sharma, 1998). Her feelings about the pregnancy were noted to be equivocal and the hospital sought a declaratory judgment regarding a caesarean delivery for the fetus. A hearing was convened at the bedside but Angela was not coherent at the time and the judge ruled in favor of proceeding with the cesarean section. A short time later Angela and her attending obstetrician had communications that strongly suggested she did not want the surgery performed (re: AC as noted in Brown, 2001).

A session was reconvened at the bedside. The attending obstetrician and Angela's family were opposed to the cesarean section. The counsel for the District of Columbia suggested that Angela's current refusal did not change the situation because the court would not have been called in the first place had she consented for the surgery. The judge agreed and reaffirmed his order that the cesarean section be performed. Less than 1 hour later, a three-judge panel heard arguments for a stay of the procedure. Angela's lawyer argued that the surgery would likely end his client's life and that it should not be done without her consent. The lawyer for the fetus argued that fetal concerns should outweigh maternal concerns because the mother was clearly going to die soon, but the fetus had a chance for life. It was argued that the fetus had a better chance of survival than the mother. The three-judge panel denied the request for a stay but reserved the right to file an opinion at a later date. The fetus was delivered via cesarean section and lived just a few hours. Angela died 2 days later without awakening from the surgery. The D.C. Court of Appeals reviewed the case (although the outcome was long decided) and vacated the lower court's decision, arguing that substituted judgment by one of the family members should have been used if Angela's competency was in question. They ruled against the court-ordered cesarean section (re: AC as noted in Brown, 2001).

A more recent case has also favored maternal autonomy: Baby Doe vs Mother Doe (re: Baby Doe, 1994). This case involved a woman at 36 weeks of gestation who was thought to have placental insufficiency so severe that the fetus would die in utero or be severely damaged unless it was delivered via cesarean section immediately. The mother expressed her faith in God's healing powers and declined the cesarean section. The attending physician and hospital took the case to the Cook County State Attorney who brought it to court. The Court of Appeal's decision strongly reaffirmed the right of a competent pregnant woman to decline invasive medical treatments. They could find no other case in which any person has an obligation to undergo invasive surgery for the sake of another. The Carder case was cited as a precedent (re: Baby Doe as presented in Pinkerton & Finnerty, 1996).

The Supreme Court has revisited the maternal versus fetal rights issue several times. In 1979, in Colautti vs Franklin, the Court ruled in favor of maternal rights and invalidated a state statute that had protected the fetus by requiring that post-viability abortions be done in a manner least destructive to the fetus (Colautti vs Franklin, 1979). The statute had required that a more destructive abortion technique was permitted only if it were indispensable to the life of the mother. The Supreme Court ruled that this language was too restrictive (Colautti vs Franklin as reported in Rhoden, 1987).

Cases affirming fetal rights

Several court cases have granted the fetus or neonate certain rights relative to that of the mother. One of the frequently cited cases is Jefferson vs Griffen (Jefferson vs Griffen, 1981). This case involved a woman diagnosed with a complete placenta previa at term. The hospital asked the court for permission to perform a cesarean section and give blood if necessary should the patient present to the hospital. The trial court gave permission for all medical procedures deemed necessary to preserve the life of the unborn child, but the order was only valid if the mother sought admission to Griffen Hospital. The Georgia Department of Human Resources then petitioned the Juvenile court for temporary custody of the child. The petition was granted with a ruling that the Georgia Department of Human Resources could give permission for the cesarean section. The Supreme Court of Georgia then ordered Jefferson to undergo a cesarean section due to the state's compelling interest in preserving life after viability. Most accounts of this case note that the patient left the hospital but subsequently delivered successfully via a vaginal delivery (Pinkerton & Finnerty, 1996; Mohaupt & Sharma, 1998).

The Smith vs Brennan case involved a neonate, but applied to injuries sustained during the gestational period (Smith vs Brennan, 1960). This case recognized the right of a child after birth to sue for damages for injuries wrongfully inflicted by a third party prior to birth (Nelson & Milliken, 1988). Some have interpreted this case as a basis for the fetus' legal right to develop without injury. The pertinent section said, "justice requires that the principle be recognized that a child has a legal right to begin life with a sound mind and body." (Smith vs Brennan as noted in Nelson & Milliken, 1988). Nelson disagrees with this view, noting that the case refers to a child *after* birth who has a right to sue for damages but who had no such rights as a fetus. The wording of the case does explicitly state that this decision applied to an injured, live-born child. The decision makes explicit that it was "immaterial whether before birth the child is considered a person in being" that could have definite legal rights (Smith vs Brennan, 1960 as referenced in Nelson, 1988).

In the Maydun case, a 19-year-old primagravida at term was transferred to Georgetown University Hospital from an outlying hospital following 48 hours of labor with ruptured membranes and failure to progress (re: Maydun, 1986). She insisted upon a vaginal delivery. She was observed until the duration of ruptured membranes reached 60 hours, at which time a cesarean section was again recommended. The patient and her husband declined the procedure, noting that they understood the infection risk to the fetus and that as a Muslim woman she had the right to determine if a risk to her fetus warranted the risk to her own health from the cesarean section. The hospital then requested from the courts a sanction to allow delivery by cesarean section. The court ruled that, while a competent adult does have the right to refuse treatment on religious grounds, the state has a compelling interest to ensure the health of the viable fetus. The court ruled that parents do not have the right to make a martyr of the unborn child and ordered the hospital to take medically necessary steps, including a cesarean if needed (in re: Maydun as presented in Pinkerton & Finnerty, 1996).

The Supreme Court has also had several post-Roe-vs-Wade rulings that have supported fetal rights. In 1989, the Court decided in Webster vs Reproductive Health Services that a Missouri statute was constitutional (Webster vs Reproductive Health Services, 1989). This law required ultrasound, prior to termination, for gestations of at least 20 weeks. The statute was deemed constitutional because the Roe vs Wade decision affirmed the state's interest in protecting potential human life after a certain gestational age. To justify this interpretation, the Court had to modify the first-, second-, and third-trimester framework of Roe vs Wade in order to permit testing as early as 20 weeks (Mohaupt & Sharma, 1998). In 1992 the Court again took up the abortion issue in Planned Parenthood v. Casey (Planned Parenthood of Southeastern Pennsylvania vs Casey 1992 as reported in Lo, 2000). In this case, the court affirmed that states may ban abortions after viability has been reached as long as there are exceptions to protect the life and health of the mother and there are not excessive restrictions placed prior to viability. For example, if the state has parental notification laws, then judicial reviews for juveniles must be made available (Planned Parenthood vs Casey as reported in Lo, 2000). Thus the Supreme Court has both affirmed maternal autonomy, particularly in clearly previable fetuses, and has granted restrictions on the practice of abortion, especially as the fetus nears viability.

Special considerations following case reviews

There are drawbacks to placing an emphasis too strongly on either maternal or fetal rights. This section discusses problems with maternal autonomy and fetal rights viewpoints. A case is then presented in which a seemingly bad outcome (forcibly restraining a woman for cesarean section) ended with a good outcome for both mother and fetus.

Problems with emphasizing maternal autonomy viewpoint

One of the strongest arguments for giving priority to maternal autonomy is the seemingly discriminatory nature of the application of court-ordered interventions for minority women. However, a closer review of the situation highlights concerns about this viewpoint.

Many strong maternal autonomy advocates refer to Kolder's study of the practice of court-ordered interventions (Kolder et al., 1987). This study of court-ordered cesarean sections noted that 81% of the cases studied involved African American, Hispanic, or Asian women. Of this study population 44% were not married and 24% did not speak English as their first language (Kolder et al., 1987). Harris suggests that the consideration of forced treatment of pregnant women can be regarded as racism masked as fetal protection (Harris, 2000). Kolder's study is to be commended as it is the most complete review of the demographics of women in the situation of court-ordered interventions. However, a closer look at the study population also reveals the difficulty in adequately addressing this issue. As Nelson makes clear, Kolder's study only questioned maternal–fetal medicine fellowship heads (preferably in University settings) or (in their absence) residency directors (Nelson & Milliken, 1988). Although there was an 83% response rate, significant selection bias can be introduced by studying the population in this manner. For instance, there were five states (Alaska, Idaho, Montana, North Dakota, and Wyoming) that were not represented. The patient population of the hospitals studied (preferably university centers or at least those with residency programs) would also have a disproportionate number of minority or non-English speaking patients. It would be helpful to know if the proportion of patients for whom court-ordered interventions were contemplated differed in general from the patient population in these medical centers. The study is a good first step in quantifying a difficult demographic situation, but the use of its demographics to condemn the practice of seeking court interventions does not take into account the biases that may have been introduced by the types of programs surveyed for this study.

One must also be cautious regarding the "reported" outcomes of the maternal autonomy cases. The Jefferson case is often cited as ending with the safe vaginal delivery of the child. What is not usually presented in this scenario is that the patient voluntarily returned to her original hospital where another ultrasound was obtained several days later. This ultrasound showed the previa was no longer present, and she labored under the care of the original hospital, which had earlier sought a cesarean delivery (Berg, 1981).

When courts decline to intervene, the outcome can sometimes be poor. Elkins reports another case in 1975 where a 27-year-old primagravida was seen by Planned Parenthood and requested pregnancy termination (Elkins et al., 1989). She was noted to be 30–34 weeks with blood pressures of 180/110 and was transferred to a tertiary care center. A decision was made the following morning to induce labor. Internal monitoring found no variability with late decelerations. The scalp pH was noted to be 7.09. The patient was advised that her baby needed to be delivered abdominally, but she declined, stating that she did not want the baby. The hospital attorney was unsuccessful in getting any of the three judges he contacted to hear the case. Oxytocin was begun and the fetal heart tracing continued to worsen with severe late decelerations and longer periods of bradycardia. A sister of the patient was summoned to the hospital but was unable to convince the patient to undergo a cesarean section. A second scalp pH was noted to be 6.71. Labor continued and finally a stillborn female infant weighing 2,140 g was delivered (Elkins et al., 1989).

Problems with advocating fetal rights

In contrast, there have been cases where court orders have effected the opposite of their intention. Strong (1991) cites the case of Barbara Jefferies, a 33-year-old Michigan woman with a placenta previa who declined cesarean delivery on religious grounds. The court ordered the police to escort the patient to the hospital but the patient had fled to another state.

Forcible restraint with good outcome

There are also cases where severe fetal harm may be avoided with timely court interventions. Elkins reports a case involving a 24-year-old primagravida who presented at 34 weeks with thick meconium (Elkins et al., 1989). She had recently left another hospital against medical advice because a cesarean section had been recommended. She presented with severe hypertension (160/110 mmHg) and 3+ proteinuria. The fetal heart tracing showed no variability with recurrent late decelerations and episodic severe bradycardia. The patient repeatedly declined all recommendations for cesarean delivery. She was noted to have a flat affect and did not wish to discuss her decision. Her mother noted that her daughter had been in a similar state for several weeks during which she would not communicate with her either. Serial fetal scalp blood sampling was performed which noted progressive acidemia (pH drop from 7.1 to 6.96). After 4 hours, a juvenile court judge was contacted on behalf of the fetus and a court order obtained to proceed with cesarean section. The patient needed to be restrained while general anesthesia was given. A four-pound male infant was delivered with Apgars of 2, 5, and 7 at 1, 5, and 10 minutes. The postoperative course was uneventful, and the infant did well after an initial period of seizures. After the surgery the patient said she now understood why the surgery was necessary. At 1 year follow-up the patient and her child appeared to be doing well (Elkins et al., 1989).

As the cases above have illustrated, there can be problems with either a strict maternal autonomy or fetal rights viewpoint. Maternal advocates may rely on minority bias and ultimately good outcomes for mother and fetus to help justify their position, but with a closer examination, these factors may be misleading. The maternal advocate's approach can also result in the unnecessary death of a fetus that is viable. On the other hand, a strict adherence to fetal rights can result in unintended consequences such as maternal flight to avoid a court order. The next section critiques viewpoints that address both issues.

Compromise views regarding maternal–fetal conflict

Fortunately, the vast majority of maternal–fetal interactions in the context of a viable fetus do not result in maternal–fetal conflict. However, the potential for scenarios such as those mentioned above does exist, especially in the high-risk setting, and the obstetrician must be prepared to deal with complex ethical situations. Three more balanced responses to maternal–fetal conflict situations should be considered: the ACOG, the American Academy of Pediatrics (AAP), and Chervenak and McCullough. These views are examined in regard to risks to pregnant women, risks to the fetus without the procedure, effect of the procedure on the fetus, and special considerations. The different viewpoints are summarized in Table 46.1.

The APP revised its statement on maternal–fetal conflict in 1999. The new statement requires that the proposed treatment

Table 46.1 Considerations for treatment of fetus without maternal consent

Reference	Risk to pregnant woman	Risk to fetus without procedure	Effects of procedure on fetus	Special considerations
ACOG, 1999 Committee Opinion	High probability that treatment helps or has very little risk for pregnant woman	High probability of serious harm to fetus	High probability that treatment will significantly decrease fetal harm	Always consult ethics committee before considering legal approach
AAP, 1999 Statement	Negligible risk to health/well-being of pregnant woman	Serious harm	Effective treatment that prevents irrevocable and substantial fetal harm	No less invasive way to help the fetus
Chervenak & McCullough, 1985	Mortality risk and risk of disease/injury/disability to pregnant woman reliably low or manageable	High probability of saving life or preventing serious and irreversible disease/injury/disability for viable fetus	Treatment reliably has low mortality and low or manageable risk of serious disease/injury/disability to fetus	Do not force pregnant woman but use court order to help persuade
Strong, 1991	Insignificant or no health risk *or* would promote her health	Serious fetal harm/death	Prevent serious fetal harm	Promote well-being of community. Prevent abandonment of dependent children. Preserve ethical integrity of physician

of the mother against her will should be of negligible risk to the health and well-being of the pregnant woman. The treatment should prevent irrevocable and substantial fetal harm and be effective therapy (AAP, 1999).

The ACOG revised its statement on maternal–fetal conflict in 1999 as well. The revision, by referring to "patient choice" rather than "maternal–fetal conflict" deemphasizes the idea of conflict between mother and fetus. The Committee Opinion asserts that there needs to be high probability the treatment will help or cause minimal harm to the mother. It also requires that there be a high probability of serious harm to the fetus and a high probability that treatment will significantly decrease fetal harm. The statement strongly recommends that an ethics committee be consulted before appealing to a court case (ACOG, 1999).

Chervenak and McCullough are two authors who deal extensively with maternal–fetal conflict. They present a thorough approach to maternal–fetal conflict that complements the guidelines proposed by ACOG and AAP. Chervenak and McCullough require that: (i) the mortality risk and the risk of disease, injury, or disability to the pregnant woman be reliably low or manageable in order to consider coercing the intervention; and (ii) there be a high probability that the procedure will be life saving or will prevent serious or irreversible damage to a viable fetus. They expect that the treatment will also reliably have a low mortality or have a manageable risk of serious injury to the fetus (Chervenak et al., 1994).

Chervenak and McCullough address the issue of the possible use of court orders in the case of a woman with a well-documented complete placenta previa at term who is demanding to be delivered via the vaginal route. They address the argument that court-ordered cesarean sections can never be ethically justified. They state that no physician should be justified in accepting a patient's refusal of cesarean section in the case of a complete previa at term because of the unreliability of the patient's clinical judgement. They note that physicians are justified in resisting a patient's exercise of her positive right if the fulfilling of her positive right would contradict the physician's best clinical judgment and negate all beneficence-based interests of the woman and her fetus. A woman does not have a right to make her physician practice medicine that is against the physician's best clinical judgment. They argue that a court-ordered cesarean in this instance does not treat a woman as a "mere instrument" to benefit her fetus, one of Rhoden's claims (Rhoden, 1987), because in this case the cesarean benefits the woman as well. There is no violation of her autonomy without justification because a pregnant woman who has taken a pregnancy to term has an ethical obligation to accept reasonable risks on behalf of her fetus. An exercise of someone's positive and negative rights can be limited when the exercise of those rights brings certain serious harm to others. They argue that the woman's fear of surgery cannot be used to justify her claim because her claim is an irrational fear and irrational beliefs disable the exercise of autonomy. Even objections on religious grounds can be overcome in that courts have ordered the treatment of pediatric patients over the religious objections of their parents.

Chervenak and McCullough then turn to arguments to justify court intervention in the case of complete previa at term. They note that the use of a state's power to enforce a pregnant woman's beneficence-based obligations to her fetus at term is justified when the net risk to her is nonexistent. Maternal autonomy rights are not absolute in this case and can be constrained by the probability of severe, preventable harm to third parties. Judge Belson stated this obligation succinctly in his commentary in the Angela Carder case:

> A woman who carries a child to viability is in fact a member of a unique category of persons. Her circumstances differ fundamentally from those of other potential patients for medical procedures that will aid another person, for example, a potential donor of bone marrow for transplant. This is so because she has undertaken to bear another human being, and has carried an unborn child to viability. Another unique feature of the situation we address arises from the singular nature of the dependence of the unborn child upon the mother . . . The expectant mother has placed herself in a special category of person who is bringing another person into existence, and upon whom that other person's life is totally dependent. Also, uniquely, the viable unborn child is literally captive within the mother's body. No other potential beneficiary of a surgical procedure on another person is in that position.
>
> (In re: AC as reported in McCullough & Chervenak, 1994)

As Chervenak and McCullough state, the primary moral relationship of a pregnant woman and her viable fetus is one of obligation as opposed to unrestrained freedom. The analogous relationship is that of a parent to a child rather than a potential organ donor and recipient. Legal issues can also be framed in terms of the legal obligations of parents to their children in terms of child neglect and abuse cases. They conclude that, in cases similar to that of a placenta previa at term, there are cases when ethical and legal court sanctions can be sought for cesarean delivery. Whether physical force can be used to perform the surgery is not clearly defined. They oppose the use of force in this situation if there is no time to obtain a court order, but do not address the issue if the court order is obtained. They also stop short of condoning court orders for cesarean delivery in cases where there is no clear benefit for the mother (i.e. fetal distress cases). Their criteria for intervention include that the mortality risk to the pregnant woman be very low and the risk of injury or handicap be low or manageable. They acknowledge that any attempt to go beyond these criteria faces a "considerable, perhaps daunting, burden of proof" (McCullough & Chervenak, 1994).

Suggestions for managing maternal–fetal conflict

The above sections have dealt with court cases and theories regarding how to deal with maternal–fetal conflicts. In their 1996 article, Pinkerton and Finnerty present a logical outline for preparing for and dealing with issues of maternal–fetal conflict by using a proactive team approach that attempts to deal with these issues across departmental lines (Pinkerton & Finnerty, 1996). This has become the model at the University of Virginia Health Sciences Center. They developed a subcommittee of the hospital ethics committee consisting of representatives of the departments of obstetrics and gynecology, pediatrics, anesthesiology, family medicine, ethics committee, and hospital counsel. All subcommittee members reviewed relevant literature on maternal–fetal conflict and guidelines were then developed. The guidelines were discussed in the individual departments and finally discussed with the full ethics committee. Many diverse opinions were noted and many revisions occurred over the course of 1 year. The guidelines evolved from being a staunch advocate of full maternal autonomy to including references to some instances where court-mandated interventions could be considered. Separate guidelines were developed for incompetent women. The final consensus was that the courts should be used very rarely and maternal autonomy should prevail in almost all instances (Pinkerton & Finnerty, 1996). The purpose of the guidelines was to provide a framework to foster communication between the patient and the health-care team members. Unresolved conflicts could then be mediated by the ethics consultation service. If the conflict remained unresolved then the ethics committee and departmental representatives were available for assistance. Only after these avenues had failed was turning to the courts considered (Pinkerton & Finnerty, 1996).

Although the process of developing these guidelines was long and difficult, the end result was a greater appreciation for the nuances of cases and the judicial decisions surrounding them. This increased awareness should decrease the likelihood of resorting to the courts for assistance. Should a court order a direct intervention, the policy stated that physical force should not be used in its implementation. The court order should rather be used to help persuade the patient to agree to the intervention (Pinkerton & Finnerty, 1996).

A common theme among many authors is the responsibility of ethics committees to help mediate in difficult situations. To do so in a viable manner for high-risk obstetric cases, the ethics committee needs to have members available on an emergency basis. At Louisiana State University Health Sciences Center (LSUHSC) in New Orleans, one member carries a beeper so that response can be immediate if necessary. Also important in this process is an awareness and appreciation for the role of the ethics committee. The more the ethics committee is involved in service to the hospital community (i.e. by sponsoring workshops and lectures), the more people will feel comfortable approaching the committee. It is also important to let patients and their family members know that the committee is available and to allow, if possible, their direct access to its services as well (Brown, 2001).

Issues regarding brain death

Background

Cesarean sections were first used to deliver the living fetus from dead mothers (Dillon et al., 1982; Loewy, 1987). In Greek mythology, Asklepios (the famous Greek physician and Apollo's son) was said to be delivered from his dead mother in this manner (Loewy, 1987). In the fourth century BC Susruta's Samhita recommended cesarean delivery when the woman's life was in great danger or she had died. Pliny the Elder was said to have been delivered by postmortem cesarean in 23 AD. The Babylonian Talmud recommended opening the abdomen immediately to deliver the child of a mother who died in childbirth. Postmortem cesarean section was practiced in Hellenistic times by Roman authorities and in 17th century Venice (Loewy, 1987). In approximately 700 BC Numa Popilus forbade burial of a pregnant woman before the child was removed. This edict, which may have been used to rescue a live child or allow separate burial of the child, became part of the Roman's King's Law (Lex Regia) which in turn became the Emperor's Law or Lex Caesare, which may be the origin of the term *cesarean*. It is unlikely that Julius Cesar was delivered in this manner because there are references to his mother being alive 40 years later. In 1280 the Council of Cologne required postmortem cesareans to allow for baptism and proper burial of children from mothers who had died (Dillon et al., 1982; Loewy, 1987). Not until approximately 1500 were cesareans performed successfully to save a mother and child. Jacob Nufer, a Swiss sow gelder, accomplished such a delivery (Loewy, 1987).

Only in the past century have cesarean sections been used regularly to save both mother and child (Dillon et al., 1982). Ironically, improvements in the care of critically ill obstetric patients have brought us full circle, making it now possible to contemplate postmortem sections in which the mother has been brain dead for prolonged periods of time. With intensive care, it is possible to prolong fetal maturation in a mother who would otherwise have been declared dead and taken off life support. Rapid evacuation of the uterus (especially after 5 minutes of a full code with no significant response from the mother) is still recommended in mothers with a fetus of significant size impeding blood flow during a code situation.

This section deals with cases of fatally ill women who can be stabilized with life support techniques. In some of these cases, care of the mother with monitoring of the fetus allows for fetal growth. The means for providing a rapid abdominal delivery at the bedside is reviewed.

There is a significant moral distinction between a rapid postmortem cesarean section and maintaining viability solely for the sake of the fetus. Some would have concerns about using brain-dead mothers as incubators, merely as a means to justify an end. However, the moral value of brain-dead pregnant women can also be viewed as secondary moral status (Loewy, 1987). The brain-dead mother's worth is secondary in that she has symbolic worth and value for others but cannot have actual or potential harm or benefit directly herself (Loewy, 1987). On the other hand, the fetus has real and symbolic value. Its real moral value is based on its potential for being harmed or benefited. The symbolic value can be derived from its role as a symbol of renewal or continuity of life. The concept of "flesh of her flesh" underscores the continuity of her life and could justify the prolonged use of brain-dead mothers to continue fetal life (Loewy, 1987). The embryo can be viewed as having inherent interests, with the discussion focusing on where those interests lie relative to those of the mother. With a brain-dead mother, her interests still exist, but in a secondary status (Loewy, 1987). With technological advances, there comes an increasing probability of success defined as a viable infant who is not severely damaged. However, such cases must still be considered experimental, therefore the risks and benefits cannot be clearly outlined. Informed consent from the patient's surrogate decision-maker is critical in deciding courses of action (Loewy, 1987). The job of the high-risk pregnancy team is to coordinate the response and give this decision-maker the information required to proceed.

Case studies regarding brain damaged pregnant women

Decision to withdraw support

In 1982 Dillon and colleagues presented two cases. The first case involved a 30-year-old patient at 18 weeks who developed severe herpes simplex virus (HSV) encephalitis. An EEG on the seventh hospital day showed suppression of left-sided slow-wave activity. On the tenth hospital day, the patient had stable vital signs but was totally unresponsive and had no reaction to caloric stimulation. Ultrasound confirmed an active fetus. After much debate between her physicians and consultant, a discussion between her physician and family concluded that she should be removed from life support. In this case the decision was made to withdraw treatment (Dillon et al., 1982).

Decision to continue support (short interval)

The second case Dillon presented involved a 24-year-old unmarried primigravida at 23 weeks who was admitted to a local hospital in status epilepticus. She had had a seizure disorder since 5 years of age and took anti-epileptic medication throughout the pregnancy. She was diagnosed with meningoencephalitis and treated with IV antibiotics and steroids. Her condition initially improved but then worsened. On the 15th hospital day, she was readmitted into the intensive care unit and again given IV steroids and subsequently required intubation. By the 17th hospital day, her pupils were fixed and dilated. Reflexes were absent. The fetal heart tracing continued to be normal and an ultrasound showed an appropriately grown 25-week fetus. She was transferred to the maternity division where her vital signs were stable. Evoked brainstem potentials found no activity and the diagnosis of brain death was made on the 19th day. The decision was made to maintain life support until the patient became hemodynamically unstable or fetal distress developed. On day 23, significant fluctuations in blood pressure started to develop and by day 24 her blood pressure dropped to 60/30 mmHg despite fluids and pressors. The fetal heart rate tracing deteriorated. A bedside cesarean section was performed with delivery of a 930 g female infant with 8 and 8 Apgars. The infant was discharged from the nursery at 3 months of age weighing 2,000 g (Dillon et al., 1982).

Thus the mother was admitted to the hospital severely ill at 23 weeks, declared brain dead at 25 weeks and an extra 6 days of intrauterine life was accomplished through relatively intensive support measures. Given the above experience, and a review of the literature, Dillon noted that at less than 24 weeks no continued life support be offered. Between 24 and 27 weeks he suggested that intensive support be considered and recommended delivery for all fetuses greater than 28 weeks.

It is important in such cases that one be prepared for emergency cesarean delivery. Obstetric personnel should review with the ICU staff the immediate steps that would be needed in such a case. A rapid response by the obstetric and pediatric teams should also be assured. Table 46.2 summarizes the suggested equipment.

Decision to support (prolonged interval)

In 1988 Field et al. reported a case in JAMA regarding a 27-year-old primigravida maintained from 22 to 31 weeks in a brain-dead state with subsequent delivery of a 1,440 g fetus, noted to be normal at an 18-month follow-up. The mother had rapid progression over 2 days to brain death via the Harvard criteria. The father of the child wished to maintain full support until viability. Full ventilatory support was used and regulated by frequent use of arterial blood gases. Maximum effort was directed toward treating hypotension, temperature

Table 46.2 Suggested equipment for emergency cesarean in ICU setting

Maternal equipment	Infant equipment
Surgical drapes	Warmer
Cesarean section instrument tray	Blankets
Suction	Infant identification kit (i.e. ID Bands, footprint sheet)
Bovie with grounding pad (optional)	Blood tubes for cord blood
Gloves/gowns/masks	Cord blood gas kit
Sutures	Suction/laryngoscope/endotracheal tube
Laps	Neonatal resuscitation medications
Cord clamps/bulb suction	

fluctuations, diabetes insipidus, hypothyroidism, and cortisol deficiencies. Nasogastic feedings were unsuccessful and TPN was started to maintain 9,500 kJ/day. Fetal heart tones were monitored every shift and serial ultrasounds were obtained. Steroids were given weekly after 26 weeks. Antepartum fetal surveillance was initiated. On day 58 given the lack of fetal growth and recurrent septicemia, the decision was made for delivery. A 1,440 g fetus was delivered with Apgars of 8 and 8 at 1 and 5 minutes. Maternal ventilatory support was discontinued and cardiac activity soon ceased. The neonate was discharged home after a 3-week stay (Field et al., 1988).

Decision to maintain support in vegetative state with complicated family dynamics

Webb presented the case of a 24-year-old primipara, who at 12 weeks of gestation in 1995 declared her desire to have an elective termination (Webb & Huddleston, 1996). At 14 weeks of gestation, she took an overdose of her mother's insulin. The father of the child was unknown. After several days of care there was no significant recovery of brain function. Some family members inquired about the feasibility of an abortion in this setting. They were interested in pursuing this course even if it would not improve the clinical outcome of the patient. The ethics committee was consulted, prompting the patient's mother to have further discussions with other family members. The patient's mother decided not to terminate the pregnancy because she then felt that, had the patient not been depressed, she would not have desired termination. At 16 weeks cerebral imaging showed "toxic injury" and the EEG was "severely abnormal" (Webb & Huddleston, 1996). She was diagnosed to be in a chronic vegetative state with little chance of recovery. It was decided to withdraw all treatment (except nutrition) and give her DNR status. At 23 weeks, pneumonia was diagnosed and ultrasound showed a normal size fetus. The ethics committee was reconsulted and met with the obstetric and medical teams and with family members. It was determined that care could be given that would help the fetus as long as there was a chance of a normal outcome. Antibiotics and other medications could be provided. Fetal monitoring was to start at 28 weeks. At 31 weeks late decelerations and vaginal bleeding were noted. An abruption was diagnosed and cesarean section was performed with delivery of a 2,240 g fetus with Apgars of 4 and 7. The mother died on postoperative day three. The baby developed bronchopulmonary dysplasia and was discharged from the hospital at 2 months of age. At 5 months the child was noted to be "otherwise apparently well" (Webb & Huddleston, 1996).

Conflict between a pregnant woman's parents and the father of the baby

Fost, in a 1994 Hasting Center Report article, commented on a scenario in which a 20-year-old unmarried female was found to be brain dead following head trauma in a motor vehicle accident. She was 15 weeks pregnant at the time. The father of the baby wished to continue life support but her parents were opposed. There was no evidence of advance directives or other indications of what the patient would have wanted. In this scenario, Fost recommends maintaining the woman on life support for a few days if the concerned parties are in disagreement. While the parents are the legal next of kin (since the patient is unmarried), the father's wishes should be taken into account. Fost recommends discussion with the parents and the father regarding the feasibility of maintaining the patient until viability. He advocates careful evaluation of the fetus to insure no anomalies are present. If no consensus can be reached, he recommends involvement of the ethics committee to help resolve the issue. He hopes that, with appropriate counseling and mediation, no one will feel compelled to attempt to take the issue to court (Fost, 1996).

Guidelines for management in the severely brain damaged pregnant woman

For any pregnant patient with severe neurological involvement, an attempt to support the fetus while aggressively pursuing maternal diagnosis and prognosis should be done. As noted earlier, the exception to this management is acute anoxia due to maternal cardiac arrest that is unresponsive to immediate resuscitative efforts. In these cases, rapid delivery of the fetus can significantly improve maternal survival (Webb & Huddleston, 1996).

The etiology and extent of the injury as well as its prognosis are necessary before making decisions regarding fetal status (Webb & Huddleston, 1996). This assessment may take time, as the improvement (or lack thereof) over time may be crucial in determining the extent of injury as well as the prognosis. A team approach is critical in managing these complex medical and ethical cases. It is important for the obstetric team to discuss and agree on plans and options with the consultants before talking with the family. Frequent discussions are needed to keep the family updated. It is also important to keep the nurses and residents updated on changes in the patient's status (Webb & Huddleston, 1996).

When the patient is deemed incapable of consent, a neurologist should be consulted to assess mental status and to determine the patient's state of chronic brain damage (coma, stupor, or chronic vegetative state) (Table 46.3). A commonly used diagnosis of brain death is often the one adopted in 1981 by the President's Commission for the Study of Ethical Problems in Medicine and Biomedical and Behavioral Research (1981). These criteria called for the irreversible cessation of circulatory or respiratory function or the irreversible cessation of all functioning of the brain (including the brain stem). Table 46.4 describes some of the tests used for this determination. Studies that can be useful for documentation of clinical findings include EEG, brainstem evoked potentials, and cerebral blood flow studies (Halevy & Brody, 1993).

When a patient is deemed incompetent, identify who

Table 46.3 States of brain damage

Stupor	Coma	Chronic vegetative state	Brain death
Patient can be aroused *only* by vigorous or continuous stimulation	Patient cannot be aroused by any stimulus	Intermediate state Can be initial presentation or can evolve Patient has brain stem function without cerebral function (has sleep–wake cycles, opens eyes to verbal stimuli, normal respiratory control but no apparent understanding or discrete localizing motor responses)	Irreversible cessation of circulatory/respiratory function, *or* Irreversible cessation of *all* functions of brain, including brain stem (President's Commission for the Study of Ethical Problems in Medicine and Biomedical and Behavioral Research, 1981)

(From Webb, G, Huddleston, J. Management of the pregnant woman who sustains severe brain damage. *Clin Perinatol* 1996;23:453–464.)

Table 46.4 Brain death criteria and tests

Need to exclude reversible causes of coma (i.e. drug toxicity, hypothermia)
Allow time for brain to recover function
Cerebral criteria: no clinical response to stimuli
Brain stem criteria:
No response to cranial nerve testing. Absence of reflexes: papillary/corneal/oculocephalic/oculovestibular/oropharyngeal
Apnea test for respiratory function
Studies to help document lack of brain function:
EEG
Brain stem evoked potential study

(From Halevy A, Brody B. Brain death: reconciling definitions, criteria and test. Ann Intern Med 1993;119:519–525.)

speaks for the patient. If there is no advance directive, the person who is the next of kin should provide guidance for what decisions the patient would have made. The medical team needs to be updated by legal counsel regarding the right-to-die and living will statutes applicable in their state (Webb & Huddleston, 1996). Many such statutes have pregnancy clauses that change their interpretation during pregnancy (Burch, 1995). There may also be hospital bylaws addressing these situations. Requesting input from an ethics committee can also be helpful (Webb & Huddleston, 1996).

Assessment of fetal status is also important. Establishment of estimated gestational age by ultrasound and electronic fetal heart rate monitoring should be performed as soon as feasible. Fetal brain function in the older fetus can be indirectly assessed by beat-to-beat variability, accelerations, or biophysical profile. Serial sonography may reveal more regarding developmental brain injury. Intrauterine growth restriction (IUGR) can be a sign of early first or second trimester injury. Microcephaly can be due to anoxia and decreased cortical growth can cause enlarged cerebral ventricles. Periventricular leukoencephalopathy can sometimes be seen and MRI can be used to assess the fetal brain (Webb & Huddleston, 1996).

The effort spent in keeping the pregnant woman alive for fetal growth must also be assessed in terms of fetal status. If there is no evidence of fetal harm, then directive counseling for fetal benefit may be appropriate. If evidence of significant fetal injury develops (such as microcephaly or IUGR), then aggressive versus nonaggressive interventions may be recommended (Webb & Huddleston, 1996).

The mother's autonomy, beneficence, and nonmaleficence should be balanced. In the brain-dead patient, maternal autonomy concerns remain important (as expressed through maternal proxy) but can be seen as secondary moral claims compared to those of the fetus. One would not wish to violate the tenet of nonmaleficence by prolonging maternal death but should also consider beneficence based claims for the fetus. In the case of first-trimester fetuses or mid-to-late second-trimester fetuses with hard to control maternal conditions, the issue of nonmaleficence toward the fetus must be considered. If there is little chance of the fetus reaching viability in a relatively intact state, then the claim of nonmaleficence for the fetus may favor withdrawing maternal life support so as to avoid simply postponing fetal death (Webb & Huddleston, 1996). As the cases above illustrate, it can be relatively easy to manage a fetus in a patient in a chronic vegetative state but much more challenging when more extensive brain damage has occurred. Counseling for the patient's proxy must then take into account the fetal status just after the injury. Subsequent evaluations of the fetus must be conducted. The gestational timing of the injury is important. Informed consent for the patient's proxy is key to any endeavors involving prolonged maternal support as this must still be considered an experimental procedure in many regards (Webb & Huddleston, 1996). As technology progresses and cases accumulate, they may become less experimental.

In summary, the first ethical tasks in these cases are to clarify maternal diagnosis and to assess the prognosis for both the mother and the chances for relatively intact survival for the fetus. An appropriate proxy decision-maker must be identified and provided with appropriate information to guide informed consent. Extensive efforts must be made to educate this person and to empathize with the family (Webb & Huddleston, 1996). Consultation with the ethics committee and legal guidance as to the applicability of living will statutes in pregnancy can also be helpful.

Management to the Jehovah's Witness

Patient

This last section will address treatment of the Jehovah's Witness pregnant patient. The history of this religious faith and the origins of its tenets regarding blood transfusions are reviewed. Important legal cases regarding Jehovah's Witnesses are introduced. Finally, general guidelines for the management of these patients are given.

Background

To properly address the ethical issues which accompany the care of Jehovah's Witness patients, the background of their religion and its tenets regarding blood product transfusion should be understood. Jehovah's Witnesses are a fundamentalist Christian sect founded in Philadelphia in 1884 that emphasizes a literal reading of the Bible (Jonsen, 1986; Sacks & Koppes, 1994). There are currently about 2 million worldwide members with half of these in the United States (Elkins, 1994). This religious faith concentrates on prophecies regarding the end of this world and the coming reign of Jehovah. Converts tend to come from the working class and have limited educational background (Jonsen, 1986). They are characteristically deeply devout with a great commitment to the tenets of their faith. One of these tenets causing controversy is the refusal to acknowledge the authority of any earthly establishment. Therefore, controversies have arisen in the past regarding not pledging allegiance to the flag or taking oaths of loyalty. They are also conscientious objectors to military service (Jonsen, 1986).

Prior to 5 July, 1945 there were no explicit prohibitions regarding blood product transfusion. It was on this date that an article in *The Watchtower*, the official journal for Jehovah's Witnesses, forbade the taking of blood into the body. The penalty for doing so would be loss of eternal life in God's Kingdom (Sacks & Koppes, 1994). The basis for this proclamation was the reviewed interpretations of several Biblical passages (Genesis 9: 3–4, Leviticus 17: 13–14, Acts 15: 19–21). The Christian writing Acts of the Apostles restated the Hebrew scripture's prohibition against eating blood or flesh with blood in it (Macklin, 1988): "And whatsoever man there be among you, that eateth any manner of blood: I will even set my face against that would that eateth blood and will cut him off from amongst his people." (Leviticus 17: 10–14.) The first leaders of the newly founded Christian faith meeting in Jerusalem appealed to this prohibition when they instructed non-Jewish converts to observe Jewish law insofar as it required abstinence "from things polluted by idols, from fornication and from what is strangled and from blood" (Acts 15: 19–21 as noted in Jonsen, 1986). The article in *The Watchtower* forbids the taking of blood into the body by any route: "the issue for Jehovah's Witnesses involves the most fundamental principle on which they as Christians base their lives. Their relationship with their creator and God is at stake" (Jonsen, 1986). The Jehovah's Witness who violates this tenet not only jeopardizes his or her eternal future but more immediately risks being "disfellowshipped", excommunication and shunning by family and friends. This risk may be influenced by how vigorously the member resists the transfusion (Sacks & Koppes, 1994). It is clear that this tenet of faith is definite, absolute, and important to practitioners of this religion (Jonsen, 1986).

However, several points remain unclear. Why was this tenet expanded to include the routes of intake that were not oral? Why was the proclamation done at this particular time? Who was in charge of the decision for this proclamation? Was it a governing board or an individual? Is it just blood that is forbidden or are certain blood components and organ transplants also forbidden? (Jonsen, 1986; Sacks & Koppes, 1994). Can this sin be forgiven? Are they still guilty if they are unconscious and/or it is given against their will? (Macklin, 1988). These issues are not addressed in the tract that Jehovah's Witnesses give to their physicians. Some have even addressed these questions to Church authorities and been given different answers (Macklin, 1988).

What constitutes a forbidden product is not entirely clear. Whole blood, packed red blood cells, plasma, and platelets seemed to be banned but the transfusion of albumin, immune serum globulin and antihemophilic preparations, and organ transplants appear to be left to the conscience of the individual member (Sacks & Koppes, 1994). Even within these guidelines, there appears to be individual variations. For instance, a confidential questionnaire of one Witness congregation noted that some would accept plasma and one person would accept autotransfusion (Sacks & Koppes, 1994).

Despite their reluctance to accept blood component therapy, Jehovah's Witnesses actively seek medical care and have been in the forefront of developing artificial blood components and other pharmacological methods of helping the body increase its blood count (i.e. erythropoietin). There are alternatives that many Witnesses will accept which can lessen the risk of surgeries where a large blood loss is expected. For example, open heart surgery has been successfully performed on Witnesses who underwent extracorporeal dilution of their blood. This technique can be acceptable as long as the blood is always in physical continuity with their circulatory systems. It involves removing a portion of their blood and diluting it with an intravenous solution, then returning it back to their circulatory system. The blood lost at surgery will be more dilute and, volume for volume, the patient will be able to tolerate larger losses of volume during the surgery (Sacks & Koppes, 1994).

Legal cases regarding treatment of Jehovah's Witnesses

The issue of court-ordered transfusions in cases of pregnant Jehovah's Witnesses has been addressed. In Raleigh Fitkin-Paul Morgan Hospital vs Anderson, a woman at 32 weeks' gestation was thought to be at high risk for hemorrhage prior to birth and a transfusion was recommended (Raleigh Fitkin-Paul Morgan Hospital vs Anderson, 1964). She declined on religious grounds because she was a Jehovah's Witness. The issue went to court and the initial trial court upheld her refusal. The hospital then appealed to the New Jersey Supreme Court. By this time, the woman had left the hospital against medical advice. However, the New Jersey Supreme Court determined that the unborn child was "entitled to the law's protection" and that blood could be given "if necessary to save her life or the life of her child, as the physician in charge at the time may determine" (Elias & Annas, 1987; Raleigh Fitkin-Paul Morgan Hospital vs Anderson as described in Elkins, 1994). This case determined that the First Amendment embodied two freedoms: the freedom to believe and the freedom to act on those beliefs. The court held that only the first of these two concepts is absolute. The second concept in this case is limited by the child's right to live (Elkins, 1994). This case has been criticized for the shortness of the opinion and the fact that the judgment was not enacted as the patient left the hospital (Elias & Annas, 1987).

In re: Jamaica Hospital in 1985, the New York Supreme Court addressed the issue of a Jehovah's Witness who was 18 weeks pregnant and bleeding extensively from esophageal varices (re: Jamaica Hospital, 1985). The mother refused blood. She was noted to be the single mother of 10 children with her only relative being a sister who was unavailable at the time. The court allowed the transfusion to protect the fetus (Strong, 1991). It decided that a person does have the right to refuse medical treatment but that the state is permitted (under Roe vs Wade) to interfere with reproductive choices when it has a compelling interest. The court acknowledged that, in the case of a nonviable fetus, the interest is not compelling but rather "significant." This interest was felt to outweigh the patient's right to refuse a blood transfusion and she was ordered to receive blood (re: Jamaica Hospital, 1985 as presented in Mohaupt & Sharma, 1998).

In the Georgetown Hospital case, the court also ordered a transfusion for a nonpregnant woman who was the sole provider for a 7-month-old child. This decision aimed to prevent child abuse and abandonment (Application of the President and Directors of Georgetown College Hospital, as presented in Elkins, 1994). There have been inconsistent decisions involving patients without dependents or those who are not the sole providers for their children (Elkins, 1994). There have been frequent rulings in favor of intervention for transfusions for the children of Jehovah's Witness against their parents' wishes (Elkins, 1994). The courts have ruled that parents cannot make martyrs of their children (Cain, 1994). It is now commonplace for court orders for transfusion to be given in the case of children.

There have also been case of successful lawsuits against physicians who have knowingly transfused Witness patients in emergency settings. In a Canadian case, a 57-year-old woman was brought unconscious to the emergency room with multiple injuries from a motor vehicle accident. In searching her belongings, a nurse located a note in her wallet that stated she was a Jehovah's Witness and never wished to receive blood products. It was signed but not dated or witnessed. The treating physician decided to proceed with the blood transfusion despite this note. The patient recovered and sued, alleging battery. The court noted that the transfusion was necessary to save the patient's life but the physician knowingly did so against her wishes. The court could not absolve the physician from respecting the patient's wishes on the basis that the wishes were unreasonable. The patient was awarded $20,000 (Malette vs Shulman as presented in Sanbar, 2001). Not many successful lawsuits of this nature have been reported. This may be due to pretrial settlements or to feelings on the part of the Witness that the injuries inflicted cannot be compensated by monetary awards (Sacks & Koppes, 1994).

Guidelines for approaching Jehovah's Witness patients

One of the more important aspects in dealing with adult or emancipated Witness patients is for the physician to be honest regarding whether he or she can respect their wishes regarding transfusion of blood products. If it would be impossible for the physician to allow the patient to die without a transfusion then he or she needs to be honest at the first patient encounter and if possible find an alternative physician to assume care. It is important to determine the exact wishes of the Witness patient regarding which blood products are acceptable. There are local and individual variations in Witness' interpretation of the prohibition and it is important to ascertain what products would be acceptable in individual cases. Maximizing acceptable alternatives to blood product therapy, such as erthypoietin treatments and hemodilution of blood prior to major surgeries, should be emphasized. Remember that Jehovah's Witnesses are in general very active and compliant in seeking alternatives to replacement therapy. This conversation should occur as early as possible in the care of the patient. In the critical care setting, this may not always be possible to do in early gestation. The conversation should occur in private and the presence of family or church members may unduly influence the patient in a potential life or death situation where the decision should belong to the patient. There are also Jehovah Witness patients who will allow transfusion if they do not sign a consent form putting their wishes in writing. This obviously would put the physician in a very awkward position later if the patient were transfused and then stated that a previous conversation with the physician never occurred. Whether to transfuse in this situation would be up to the individual physician. Other Witness patients may accept transfusions and consent in writing but not wish any family or church members to know they have done so. All conversations of this nature should be clearly documented in the patient chart so that anyone who assumes care of the patient is aware of the patient's wishes.

The physician should acquire support of other members of the health-care team. The anesthesiology team needs to be aware of the patient's wishes and be willing to honor them.

Other issues can develop after this initial conversation. It is important to affirm that the patient's wishes remain the same when faced with imminent loss of life during a critical bleeding episode. If the patient's wishes have previously been clearly documented, efforts to confirm these wishes should not come across as attempts to change the patient's mind, but rather as offers to reassess the beliefs when facing a life-threatening hemorrhage. It is important to keep in mind that most of the Witness population are dealing with much more than a life or death situation. They feel the use of blood products can prevent them from reaching eternal salvation. There is also the very real concern regarding being isolated from their community.

A more difficult situation occurs when there is no time for conversation during a life-threatening hemorrhage (i.e. the patient is unconscious). This is especially difficult when dealing with a Witness who is unknown to the medical team and is only identified by a card in the wallet. In these cases, patient autonomy should probably prevail and the patient's wishes against transfusion be honored. As noted above, doctors have been successfully sued in these cases, but the amounts awarded have been relatively small, probably indicative of the court's recognition that the physicians were trying to save the lives of the involved patients. Prior documentation regarding alternatives such as autotransfusion devices may be helpful in these situations. Considerations such as leaving the patient intubated significantly longer after surgery can also be effective in minimizing the workload on the patient's metabolism (personal communication, Gary Dildy III, November 2001).

Jehovah's Witness patients who are minors represent another special category. In general, the courts have been quick to allow transfusions of minors against parental wishes. However, most states consider pregnancy to place minors in an emancipated category, which would give them the same decision making capacities as adults. Even in nonemancipated minor cases, there has been a trend to allow more autonomy as the patient approaches the age of emancipation and is clearly able to articulate her beliefs (Cain, 1994).

Some physicians and courts have placed the pregnant Jehovah's Witness in a special category, especially when the fetus is viable. The presence of the fetus is used to justify transfusions in these settings, with the feeling that the transfusion is not as much an assault as a cesarean delivery on the patient's autonomy. By comparison, a transfusion is a more minor procedure. This author finds such reasoning troubling. To the Witness, the blood transfusion is much more of an assault than is cesarean delivery. In the case of a viable fetus with a hemorrhaging mother, delivery of the baby would seem to be a more ethical alternative than a blood transfusion.

Thus, care of the Jehovah's Witness in the critical care setting entails many ethical issues. It is important to respect the patient's autonomy and to exercise beneficence by understanding the alternative treatments the patient may allow consideration. If one has trouble caring for the patient within these limitations, it is imperative to inform the patient and assist in obtaining alternative care.

Letter of condolence

It is fitting to conclude a chapter on ethics in high-risk obstetrics with a reminder that a physician's duty to his patient does not end with the death of the patient. There remains one final responsibility, to assist the family members who are left behind. The idea of writing a letter of condolence was recently presented by Bedell, Cadenhead, and Graboys in the New England Journal of Medicine (Bedell et al., 2001). This responsibility was an accepted part of a physician's practice in 19th century America. Bedell et al. illustrate with this letter from Dr James Jackson to Mrs Louisa Higgonson in 1892 (Bedell et al., 2001):

> My Dear Friend,
>
> I need not tell you how much I have sympathized with you. I think I realize in some measure how much you will miss Dear Aunt Nancy for a long time—for the rest of your life. I know that she has been a part of you . . . mind as well as body was duly exercised, and she always had stock from which she poured out stores for the delight of her friends,—stores of wit and wisdom, affording pleasure with profit to all around her.
>
> How constantly will the events of life recall her to our minds—realizing what she said or did under interesting and important circumstances—or perhaps suggesting imperfectly what she would have said under new and unexpected occurrences.
>
> For you my dear friend I implore God's blessing.
>
> Your old friend,
>
> J. Jackson

A letter of condolence can be a great help to the family during their grieving process. This is particularly true when the death is unexpected or comes after complications that occurred during hospitalization (Bedell et al., 2001). The loss of a fetus, and even more so of a mother, could fall into this category. This letter can be of great assistance to the family in dealing with the anger that naturally accompanies such a loss (Bedell et al., 2001). This letter can be much more comforting than expressions of sympathy given in person or via telephone in that it can be referenced over and over. The absence of a visible sign of sympathy can be quite distressing to the family. Bedell mentions a family member who felt strongly about this: "After my mom died, the doctor never even wrote me. He ran and hid" (Bedell et al., 2001). Bedell, Cadenhead, and Graboys encourage all physicians, house staff, and fellows who have had personal contact with their deceased patients to write condolence letters.

Suggestions for writing condolence letters

Phrases to avoid

Expressions that de-emphasize the loss or suffering: "it was meant to be"; "I know how you must feel"; "it is better that she died".

Avoid revisiting the medical details of the death (also helps to avoid legal liability issues).

Suggestions for inclusion

Begin with a direct expression of sorrow for the loss, such as "I would like to send you our condolences on the death of your wife."

Include a personal memory of the patient and/or a reference to her family or work. References to the patient's achievements, devotion to family, character, or strength during the hospitalization are also helpful.

Mention the strength the patient received from the family's love.

Tell the family that it was a privilege to participate in the care of their loved one.

Let the family know your thoughts are with them in their hour of need (Bedell et al., 2001).

The above suggestions are meant simply as guidelines for helping start a letter of condolence. The letter may be a few short sentences or a more detailed description of the physician–patient relationship. The physician should write the type of letter with which he or she is most comfortable. As Bedell, Cadenhead, and Graboys point out, "the letter of condolence is a professional responsibility of the past that is worth reviving" (Bedell et al., 2001). Such a letter provides a sense of comfort to the patient's family and affects positively the family's interactions with physicians in the future. On the other hand, a failure to communicate our sadness at the loss can be seen as a lack of interest or concern.

Conclusion

This book has detailed how to technologically deal with many of the high-risk situations that confront us in the care of our critically ill obstetric patients. This chapter helps the physician take a step back from the technology and look at the patient and her family as individuals who need to be dealt with at more levels than just the technological ones. Doing so is not always an easy process, especially when balancing the physician's ethical responsibility of beneficence with the patient's right to autonomy. Identifying possible ethical conflicts early in the decision process and clarifying these issues through communication can often help resolve them. Ethics committees can be helpful when communication between the physician, the patient, and her family is at an impasse. Rarely, if ever, should the courts be called upon to help in this decision process. The old French proverb to "Cure sometimes, help often and comfort always" is especially applicable to the ethical dilemmas that face the high-risk obstetrician. When the best medical technologies do not result in the best outcome, it is also important to remember that a thoughtful letter of condolence can further the healing process.

Acknowledgments

The author wishes to thank Doug Brown, PhD, Thomas Nolan, MD, Cliona Robb, Esq., Ginger Vehaskari, PhD, and Ms Betty Rowe for their invaluable assistance in preparation of the manuscript.

References

Abrams F. Polarity within beneficence: additional thoughts on nonaggressive obstetric management. JAMA 1989;261:3454–3455.

AC as noted in Doug Brown, Maternal Fetal Topic II, Clinical Ethics for Practitioners Symposium, "Hard Choices at the Beginning of Life, November 16, 2001, Nashville, TN.

American Academy of Pediatrics Committee on Bioethics. Fetal therapy—ethical considerations. Pediatrics 1999;103:1061–1063.

American College of Obstetricians and Gynecologist, Committee on Ethics Opinion 108. Ethical Dimensions of Informed Consent. Washington, DC: ACOG, 1992: No. 108.

American College of Obstetricians and Gynecologists, Committee on Ethics Opinion 214. Patient Choice and the Maternal-Fetal Relationship. Washington, DC: ACOG, 1999: No. 214.

Annas G. Forced cesareans: the most unkindest cut of all. Hastings Cent Rep 1982;16–17, 45.

Annas GJ, Densberger JE. Competence to refuse medical treatment: autonomy vs. paternalism. Toledo Law Review 1984;15:561–592.

Annas, G. Protecting the Liberty of Pregnant Patients. N Engl J Med 1987;316:1213–1214.

Application of the President and Directors of Georgetown College Hospital, F2d 1000 (1964).

Baby Doe v. Mother Doe, 632 NF2d 326 (III App 1 Dist 1994).

Beauchamp T, Childress J. Principles of Biomedical Ethics, 5th edn. New York: Oxford University Press, 2001:57–164.

Bedell SE, Cadenhead K, Graboys TB. The doctor's letter of condolence. N Engl J Med 2001;344(15):1162–1164.

Beller F, Zlatnik G. The beginning of human life: medical observations and ethical reflections. Clin Obstet Gynecol 1992;35:720–727.

Berg RN. Georgia Supreme Court orders Caesarean Section—mother nature reverses on appeal. J Med Asso Ga 1981;70:451–543.

Botkin J. Fetal Privacy and Confidentiality. Hastings Cent Rep 1995;32–39.

Bouvia v. Superior Court, 179 Cal. App. 3d 1127, 225 Cal Rpt. 297 (Ct. App. 1986).

Brophy v. New England Sinai Hospital, Inc. 497 N.E. 2d 626 (Mass. 1986).

Brown D. Maternal Fetal Topic II, Re: AC Clinical Ethics for Practitioners Symposium, Hard Choices at the Beginning of Life, November 16, 2001, Nashville, TN.

Brown D, Elkins T. Ethical issues in obstetrics cases involving prematurity. Clin Perinatol 1992;19:469–481.

Burch TJ. Incubator or Individual: The legal and policy deficiencies of Pregnancy Clauses in Living Wills and Advance Health care Directive Statutes. Maryland Law Rev 1995;54:528–570.

Cain J. Exploring Medical–Legal Issues in Obstetric and Gynecology. Refusal of Blood Transfusion, 1994;62–64.

Calautti v. Franklin 439 U.S. 379 (1979).

Chervenak FA, McCullough FB. Perinatal ethics: a practical method of analysis of obligations to mother and fetus. Obstet Gynecol 1985;66:442–446.

Chervenak F, McCullough L. Nonaggressive obstetric management: an option for some fetal anomalies during the third trimester. JAMA 1989;261:3439–3440.

Chervenak F, McCullough L. The Limits of Viability. J Prenat Med 1997;25:418–420.

Chervenak F, McCullough L. Ethical and Legal Issues. In: Danforth's Obstetrics and Gynecology, 8th edn. Philadelphia: Lippincott, Williams and Wilkins, 1999:939–953.

Chervenak F, Farley A, Walters L, Hobbins JC, Mahoney MJ. When is termination of pregnancy during the third trimester morally justifiable? N Engl J Med 1984;310:501–504.

Cruzan v. Missouri, Department of Health 497 U.S. 261 110 S. Ct. 2842 (1990).

Dillon W, Lee R, et al. Life support and maternal brain death during pregnancy. JAMA 1982;248:1089–1091.

Elias S, Annas G. Reproductive Genetics and the Law. Chicago Yearbook Medical Publishers, 1987;83–120,143–271.

Elkins T. Exploring Medical-Legal Issues in Obstetrics and Gynecology. Washington DC: Association of Professors of OB/GYN, 1994;35–38.

Elkins T, Andersen H, et al. Court-ordered Cesarean section: an analysis of Ethical concerns in compelling cases. Am J Obstet Gynecol 1989;161:150–154.

Field D, Gates E, et al. Maternal brain death during pregnancy: medical and ethical issues. JAMA 1988;260:816–822.

Fletcher J. The fetus as patient: Ethical issues. JAMA 1981;246–772.

Fost N. Case Study: The Baby in the Body. Hastings Cent Rep 1996;31–32.

Fost N, Chudwin D, Wikler, D. The Limited Moral Significance of "Fetal Viability". Hastings Cent Rep 1980;10–13.

Gillon R. Pregnancy, obstetrics and the moral status of the fetus. J Med Ethics 1988;14:3–4.

Halevy A, Brody B. Brain death: Reconciling definitions, criteria and test. Ann Intern Med 1993;119:519–525.

Harris L. Rethinking maternal–fetal conflict: gender and equality in perinatal ethics. Obstet Gynecol 2000;96:786–791.

In the Matter of Karen Quinlan 70 N.J. 10, 335A, 2d 647, cert. Denied U.S. 922 (1976).

Jefferson v. Griffen Spalding Hospital Authority, Ga., 274 S.F. 2d 457 (1981).

Jonsen A. Blood transfusions and Jehovah's Witnesses: The impact of the patient's unusual beliefs in critical care. Crit Care Clin 1986;2(1):91–99.

Kolder V, Gallagher J, Parson M. Court ordered obstetrical interventions. N Engl J Med 1987;316:1192–1196.

Lane v. Candura 6 Mass. App. Ct 377, 376 N.E. 2d 1232 (1978).

Leiberman J, Mazor M, et al. The fetal right to live. Obstet Gynecol 1979;53:515–517.

Lo B. Resolving Ethical Dilemmas: A Guide for Clinicians, 2nd edn. Philadelphia: Lippincott, Williams and Wilkins, 2000:19–29; 181–188.

Loewy E. The pregnant brain dead and the fetus: must we always try to wrest life from death? Am J Obstet Gynecol 1987;157:1097–1101.

McCullough L, Chervenak F. Ethics in Obstetrics and Gynecology, New York: Oxford University Press, 1994:96–129;241–265.

Macklin R. The Inner Workings of an Ethics Committee: Latest Battle over Jehovah's Witnesses. Hastings Cent Rep 1988;15–20.

Mahoney M. The Fetus as Patient. West J Med 1989;150:459–460.

Mahowald M. Beyond abortion: Refusal of caesarean section. Bioethics 1989;3:106–121.

Malette v. Shulman 630 R. 2d, 243, 720R. 2d, 417 (O.C.A.).

Mattingly, S. The Maternal Fetal Dyad: Exploring the Two-Patient Obstetric Model. Hastings Cent Rep 1992;13–18.

Maydun. 114 Daily Wash I. Rptr 2233 (DC Super Ct 1986).

Mohaupt S, Sharma K. Forensic Implications and Medical-Legal Dilemmas of Maternal Versus Fetal Rights. J Forensic Sci 1998; 43(5)985–992.

Mohr v. Williams, Minn, 261,265;104 N.W. 12, 15 (1905).

Nelson L, Milliken N. Compelled medical treatment of pregnant women: Life, liberty and law in conflict. JAMA 1988;259:1060–1068.

Newton E. The fetus as a patient. Med Clin North Am 1989;73:517–540.

Pinkerton J, Finnerty J. Resolving the Clinical and Ethical Dilemma Involved in Fetal-Maternal Conflicts. Am J Obstet Gynecol 1996;175:289–295.

Planned Parenthood of Southeastern Pennsylvania v Casey 112 U.S. 674 (1992).

President's Commission for the Study of Ethical Problems in Medicine and Biomedical and Behavorial Research. Guidelines for the determination of death. Report of the Medical Consultants on the Diagnosis of Death to the President's Commission. JAMA 1981;246(19).

Raleigh Fitkin-Paul Morgan Hospital v. Anderson 42. NJ421, 201 A2d, 537 cert. Denied 377 US 985 (1964).

Re: AC, District of Columbia, 573 A. 2d 1235 (D.C. App. 1990).

Re: Jamaica Hospital, 491 NYS 2d 898 (1985).

Re: Maydun, 114 Daily Wash L. Rptr 2233 (DC Super Ct 1986).

Rhoden N. Cesareans and Samaritans. Law Med Health Care 1987;15:118–125.

Roe v. Wade: United States Supreme Court: 35 LED 2d 147 (1973).

Sacks DH, Koppes RH. Caring for the female Jehovah's Witness: Balancing medicine, ethics, and the First Amendment. Am J Obstet Gynecol 1994;170(2):452–455.

Sanbar S, Firestone M, Gibofsky A. Legal Medicine, 5th edn. St Louis: Mosby, 2001;292, 341.

Schloendorff v. Society of New York Hospitals. 211 N.Y. 125, at 129, 105 N.E. 92, at 93 (1914).

Smith v. Brennan 157 A 2d 497 (NJ 1960).

Strong C. Ethical conflicts between mothers and fetus in obstetrics. Clin Perinatol 1987;14:313–328.

Strong C. Court ordered treatment in obstetrics: The ethical views and legal framework. Obstet Gynecol 1991;78:861–868.

Strong C, Garland A. The moral status of the near-term fetus. J Med Ethics 1989;15:25–27.

Webb G, Huddleston J. Management of the pregnant woman who sustains severe brain damage. Clin Perinatol 1996;23:453–464.

Webster v. Reproductive Health Services, Daily Appellate Report, July 6, 1989;8724.

Appendix 1
Physiologic tables and formulas

Normal third-trimester physiologic values

Hemodynamics abbreviation	Definition	Normal value/units
BSA	Body surface area	m^2
MAP	Mean systemic arterial pressure	84–96 mmHg
CVP	Central venous pressure	4–10 mmHg
PA	Mean pulmonary artery pressure	10–17 mmHg
PCWP	Mean pulmonary capillary wedge pressure	6–12 mmHg
CO	Cardiac output	5.5–7.5 L/min
SVR	Systemic vascular resistance	1,000–1,400 dynes/sec/cm^{-5}
PVR	Pulmonary vascular resistance	55–100 dynes/sec/cm^{-5}
HR	Heart rate	75–95 bpm (beats/min)
SV	Stroke volume	60–100 mL/beat
LVSWI	Left ventricular stroke work index	40–55 gM/m^2
EF	Ejection fraction	0.67
EDV	End-diastolic volume	70–75 mL/m^2
COP	Colloid oncotic pressure	16–19 mmHg
COP-PCWP	Colloid oncotic pressure–wedge pressure gradient	8–14 mmHg
$P_{A}O_2$	Mean partial pressure of oxygen in the alveolus	104 mmHg
$P_{a}O_2$	Partial pressure of oxygen in arterial blood	106–108 mmHg (first trimester); 101–104 mmHg (third trimester)
$P(A\text{-}a)O_2$	Alveolar–arterial, gradient	25–65 mmHg with $F_{I}O_2 = 1.0$
$P_{A}CO_2$	Partial pressure of carbon dioxide in the alveolus	40 mmHg
$P_{a}CO_2$	Partial pressure of carbon dioxide in arterial blood	35 mmHg
$P_{\bar{v}}O_2$	Partial pressure of oxygen in mixed venous blood	Varies, dependent upon cardiac output, $F_{I}O_2$ and oxygen consumption from approximately 35–40 mmHg
$P_{\bar{v}}CO_2$	Partial pressure of carbon dioxide in mixed venous blood	40–50 mmHg
$S_{a}O_2$	Oxyhemoglobin saturation of arterial blood	98% (room air)
$S_{\bar{v}}O_2$	Oxyhemoglobin saturation of mixed venous blood	75% (room air)
$C_{a}O_2$	Arterial oxygen content	18–22 mL/dL
$C_{\bar{v}}O_2$	Mixed venous oxygen content	14–17 mL/dL
$C_{(a\text{-}v)}O_2$	Arteriovenous oxygen content difference	4–6 mL/100 mL
O_2 extraction ratio		0.25
VO_2	Oxygen consumption	270–320 mL/min
VCO_2	Carbon dioxide production	240–280 mL/min
R	Respiratory quotient	0.8
FRC	Functional residual capacity	2,000 mL
VC	Vital capacity	65–75 mL/kg
Ventilation		11–13 L/min
IF	Inspiratory force	75–100 cmH_2O
EDC	Effective compliance	35–45 mL/cmH_2O
V_D	Dead space	150 mL
V_T	Tidal volume	500 mL
V_D/V_T	Dead space to tidal volume ratio	0.30–0.35
$\dot{Q}_s/Q_t$	Right-to-left shunt (percent of cardiac output flowing past nonventilated alveoli or the equivalent)	3.3%
Flow volume loops (mean)		
$\dot{V}_{50}$	Instantaneous flow at 50% VC	3.5 L/sec
$\dot{V}_{25}$	Instantaneous flow at 25% VC	1.5 L/sec
$\dot{V}_{50R}$	Expiratory/inspiratory flow at 50% VC	1.0
$\dot{V}_{25R}$	Expiratory/inspiratory flow at 25% VC	0.5
$V_{50/25}$	Ratio of exp. flow at 50% VC to exp. flow at 25% VC	2.3

Useful formulas

$$MAP = 2 \cdot (\text{diastolic pressure}) + (\text{systolic pressure})/3$$

$$CI(L/min/m^2) = \frac{\text{Cardiac output [L/min]}}{\text{Body surface area [m}^2\text{]}}$$

$$SVR(dynes/sec/cm^{-5}) = \frac{MAP\,[mmHg] - CVP\,[mmHg] \times 79.9}{\text{Cardiac output [L/min]}}$$

$$PVR\,(dynes/sec/cm^{-5}) = \frac{MPAP\,[mmHg] - PCWP\,[mmHg] \times 79.9}{\text{Cardiac output [L/min]}}$$

$$SV\,(mL/beat) = \frac{\text{Cardiac output}}{\text{Heart rate}}$$

$$SVI\,(mL/min/m^2) = \frac{\text{Stroke volume}}{\text{Body surface area}}$$

$$RVSWI\,(gM/m^2) = SVI \times MPAP\,[mmHg] \times 0.0136$$

$$LVSWI\,(gM/m^2) = SI \times MAP\,[mmHg] \times 0.0136$$

$$C_{(a\text{-}v)}O_2\,(mL/100\,mL \text{ or vol\%}) = C_aO_2 - C_vO_2$$

$$\dot{V}O_2\,(mL/min/m^2) = CI \times C_{(a\text{-}v)}O_2 \times 10$$

$$RQ = \frac{\dot{V}CO_2}{\dot{V}O_2}$$

$$O_2\,\text{avail}\,(mL/min/m^2) = CI \times C_aO_2 \times 10$$

$$\dot{Q}_s/\dot{Q}_t\,(\%) = \frac{Cco_2 - C_aO_2}{Cco_2 - C_vO_2} \times 100$$

$$\dot{Q}_s/\dot{Q}_t\,(\%) = \frac{0.0031 \times P_{(A-a)}O_2}{[C_{(a-v)}]O_2 + (0.0031 \times P_{(A-a)}O_2)} \times 100$$

$$EDC\,(mL/cmH_2O) = \frac{\text{Tidal volume [mL]}}{\text{Peak airway pressure [cmH}_2\text{O]}}$$

$$V_D/V_T = \frac{P_aCO_2 - P_{\bar{E}}CO_2}{P_aCO_2}$$

$$P_{(A\text{-}a)}O_2\,(mmHg) = P_AO_2 - P_aO_2$$

$$C_aO_2 = [Hgb]\,(1.34)S_aO_2 + (P_aO_2 \times 0.0031)$$

(S_aO_2 = Arterial saturation)

$$C_{\bar{v}}O_2 = [Hgb]\,(1.34)S_{\bar{v}}O_2 + (P_v\bar{O}_2 \times 0.0031)$$

($S_{\bar{v}}O_2$ = Percent saturation of mixed venous blood)

$$\frac{\dot{Q}_s}{\dot{Q}_t} = \frac{C_{c'}O_2 - C_aO_2}{C_{c'}O_2 - C_{\bar{v}}O_2}$$

$$C_{\dot{c}}O_2 = (1.34)\,[Hgb]\,100\%\text{ saturation} + 0.0031\,P_aO_2$$

$$P_AO_2 = (P_B - P_{H_2O})\,F_iO_2 - {}_PCO_2/0.8$$

(P_{H_2O} = Water vapor pressure)

(P_B = Barometric pressure)

Body surface area calculation

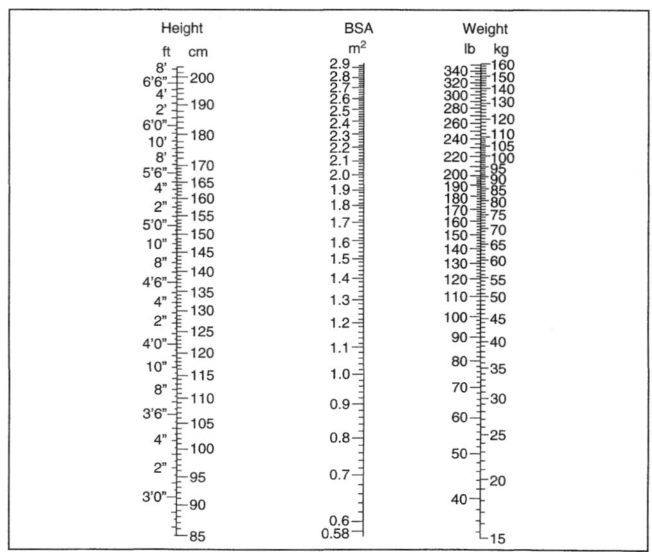

DuBois nomogram for calculating the body surface area of adults. To find body surface of a patient, locate height in inches (or centimeters) on scale 1 and weight in pounds (or kilograms) on scale 3 and place straight edge (ruler) between these two points.

EKG changes in pregnancy*

	1TM	2TM	3TM	D	PP
Heart rate (bpm)	77	79	87	80	66
QT interval(s)	0.378	0.375	0.361	0.362	0.406
QT_C interval(s)	0.424	0.427	0.431	0.414	0.423
PR interval(s)	0.160	0.160	0.155	0.155	0.160
P wave					
Duration (s)	0.092	0.092	0.091	0.091	0.096
Amplitude (mm)	1.9	1.9	2.0	2.0	1.9
Axis (degrees)	40	38	38	41	35
QRS complex					
Duration (s)	0.074	0.074	0.074	0.076	0.077
Amplitude (mm)	11.5	11.5	12.4	12.2	11.2
Axis (degrees)	49	46	40	44	44
T wave					
Duration (s)	0.168	0.171	0.165	0.166	0.176
Amplitude (mm)	3.4	3.5	3.4	3.6	3.5
Axis (degrees)	27	25	22	33	34

1TM, first trimester; 2TM, second trimester; 3TM, third trimester; D, 1–3 days after delivery; PP, 6–8 weeks postpartum.

*Mean EKG measurements during normal pregnancy, delivery, and postpartum in 102 patients

(Reprinted with permission from Carruth JE, Mirvis SB, Brogan DR, et al. The electrocardiogram in normal pregnancy. Am Heart J 1981;6:1075.)

Modified Glasgow Coma Score (GCS)*

Sign	Evaluation	Score
Eye opening	Spontaneous	4
	To speech	3
	To pain	2
	None	1
Best verbal response	Oriented	5
	Confused	4
	Inappropriate	3
	Incomprehensible	2
	None	1
Best motor response	Obeys commands	6
	Localizes pain	5
	Withdrawal to pain	4
	Flexion to pain	3
	Extension to pain	2
	None	1

* GCS < 8 = severe brain injury; GCS < 7 = immediate intubation.
(Modified from Jennett B. Assessment of severity of head injury. J Neurol Neurosurg Psychiatry 1976;39:647–655.)

Serum osmolality calculation

$$\text{Osmolality (mosm/kg)} = 2[\text{Na(mEq/L)}] + \text{K(mEq/L)} + \frac{\text{Urea (mg/dL)}}{2.8} + \frac{\text{Glucose (mg/dL)}}{18}$$

Coagulation factor requirements for hemostasis

Coagulation factor	Requirement (% of normal)
Prothrombin	40
Factor V	10–15
Factor VII	5–10
Factor VIII	10–40
Factor IX	10–40
Factor X	10–15
Factor XI	20–30
Factor XII	0
Prekallikrein	0
High-molecular-weight kininogen	0
Factor XIII	1–5

(Reproduced with permission from Orland MJ, Saltman J, eds. Manual of medical therapeutics, 25th ed. Boston: Little, Brown, 1986:277.)

Plasma coagulation factors in pregnancy

Factor	Name	Change in pregnancy
I	Fibrinogen	4.0–6.5 g/L
II	Prothrombin	100–125%
IV	Ca^{H}	
V	Proaccelerin	100–150%
VII	Proconvertin	150–250%
VIII	Antihemophilic factor A (AHF)	200–500%
IX	Antihemophilic B (Christmas factor)	100–150%
X	Stuart Prower factor	150–250%
XI	Antihemophilic factor C	50–100%
XII	Hageman factor	100–200%
XIII	Fibrin-stabilizing factor	35–75%
	Antithrombin III	75–100%
	Antifactor Xa	75–100%

(Modified from Romero R. The management of acquired hemolytic failure in pregnancy. In: Berkowtiz RL, ed. Critical care of the obstetric patient. New York: Churchill Livingstone, 1983.)

The coagulation cascade

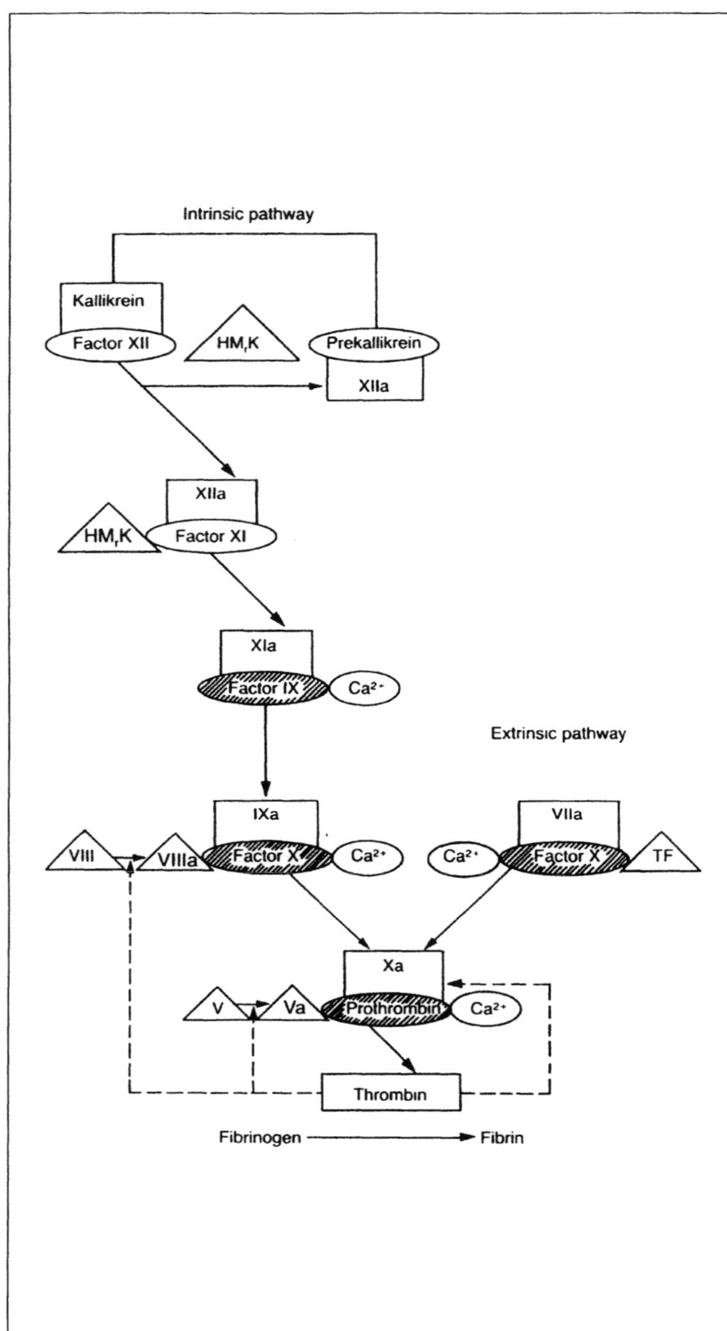

Ovals represent inactive protease precursors. Rectangles represent active proteases. Nonenzymatic protein cofactors are represented by triangles. Hatched ovals represent factors which are felt to be activated on a tissue phospholipid surface. The feedback reactions accelerate the coagulation process. (Reproduced with permission from Orland MJ, Saltman J, eds. Manual of medical therapeutics, 25th ed. Boston: Little, Brown 1986: 272.)

Anemia: differential diagnosis

Anemia type	Peripheral smear
Iron deficiency	Hypochromic microcytic
Anemia of chronic disease	Microcytic/normocytic
Thalassemia	Target cells, anisocytosis, microcytic
B_{12}/folate deficient	Macrocytic, hypersegmented PMNs
Microangiopathic hemolysis anemia	Normocytic schistocytes, helmet cells
Sickling disorders	Normocytic sickled cells

PMN, polymorphonuclear neutrophils.

Pulmonary function in pregnancy

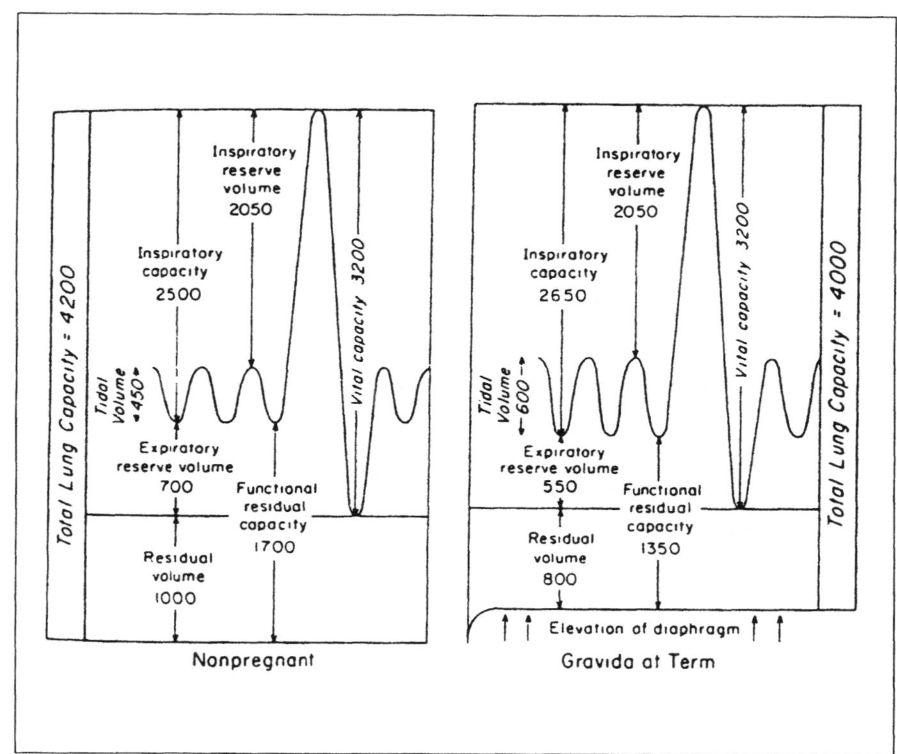

Pulmonary volumes and capacities in the nonpregnant state and in the gravida at term. (Courtesy of Bonica JJ. Principles and practice of obstetric analgesia and anesthesia. Philadelphia: F.A. Davis Company, 1967.)

Oxygenation throughout pregnancy

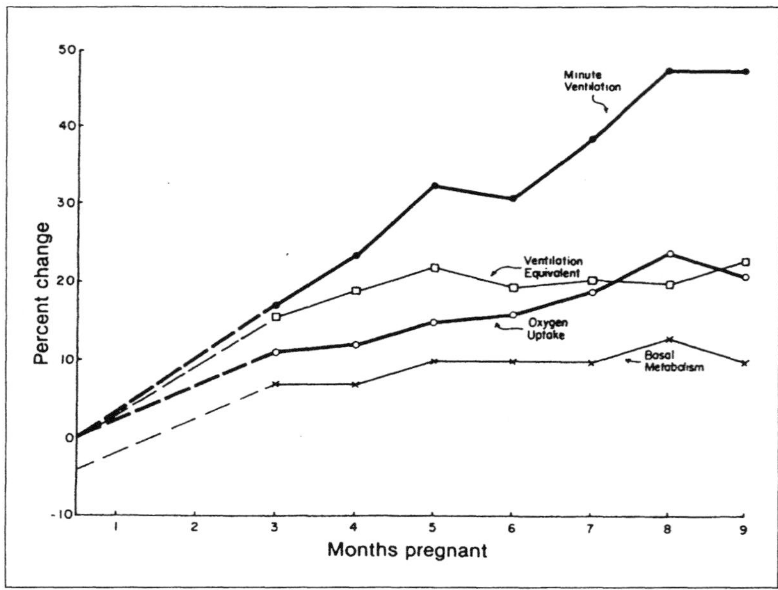

Percentage changes of minute volume, oxygen uptake, basal metabolism, and the ventilation equivalent for oxygen at monthly intervals throughout pregnancy. (Reproduced by permission from Prowse CM, Gaensler EA. Respiratory and acid-base changes during pregnancy. Anesthesiology 1965;26:381.)

Postpartum hematocrit and blood volume changes

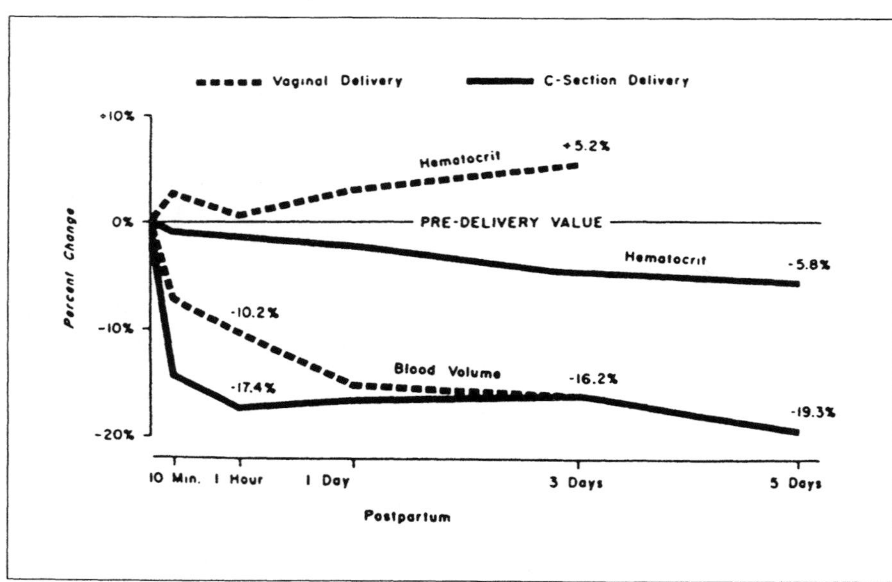

Percentage changes in blood volume and venous hematocrit following vaginal delivery or cesarean section. (Reproduced by permission from Metcalfe J, Ueland K. Heart disease and pregnancy. In: Fowler NO, ed. Cardiac diagnosis and treatment, 3rd edn. Hagerstown, MD: Harper & Row, 1980:1153–1170.)

Body water distribution

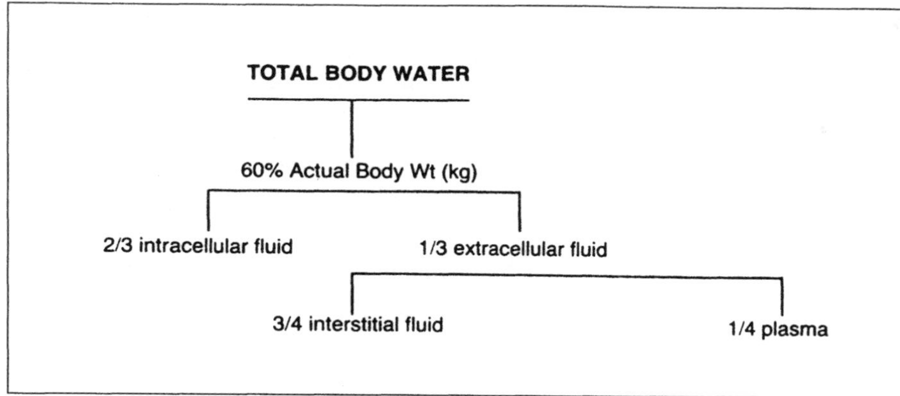

Electrolyte content of body fluids

Sweat or gastrointestinal secretion	Electrolyte concentration (mEq/L)					Replacement amount for each liter lost			
	Na^-	K^-	H^-	Cl^-	HCO_3^-	Isotonic saline (mL)	5% D/W (mL)	KCl* (mEq)	$NaHCO_3$† (mEq)
Sweat	30–50	5		45–55		300	700	5	
Gastric secretions	40–65	10	90‡	100–140		300	700	20§	
Pancreatic fistula	135–155	5		55–75	70–90	250	750	5	90
Biliary fistula	135–155	5		80–110	35–50	750	250	5	45
Ileostomy fluid	120–130	10		50–60	50–70	300	700	10	67.6
Diarrhea fluid	25–50	35–60		20–40	30–45		1,000	35	45

* Caution should be used in administering potassium faster than 10 mEq/hr.
† One ampule of 7.5% $NaHCO_3$ contains 45 mEq HCO_3^-.
‡ Variable (e.g., achlorhydria).
§ Administration of more than the observed gastric loss of potassium is often required because of enhanced urinary potassium excretion in alkalosis.
(Reproduced with permission from Orland MJ, Saltman J, eds. Manual of medical therapeutics, 25th edn. Boston: Little, Brown, 1986:43.)

Appendix 2
Drugs, devices, and fluid therapy

Guidelines for the institution and discontinuation of mechanical ventilation

Parameter	Normal range	Indication for ventilatory assistance	Indication for weaning
Mechanics			
Respiratory rate	12–20	>35	<30
Vital capacity (mL/kg of body weight)	65–75	<15	12–15
FEV_1 (mL/kg of body weight)	50–60	<10	>10
Inspiratory force	75–100	<25	>25
Oxygenation			
P_ao_2 (mmHg)	100–75 (room air)	<70 (on mask O_2)	—
$P_{(A-a)}o_2$ ($F_io_2 = 1.0$)	25-65	450	<400
Ventilation			
P_aco_2 (mmHg)	35–45	>55	—
V_D/V_T	0.25–0.40	>0.60	<0.58

Oxygen delivery systems

Delivery	Common flow (L/min)	Inspired O_2 concentration (%)	Comments
Nasal cannula	1–6	24–44	Inspired O_2 concentration increases by approximately 4% for each 1 L/min flow; exact F_io_2 is uncertain
Face mask	8–10	40–60	Oxygen flow should be higher than 5 L/min to avoid accumulation of exhaled air
Face mask with oxygen reservoir	6–10	60–100	Inspired O_2 concentration increases by 10% for each 1 L/min flow
Venturi mask	—	24, 28, 31, 35, 40, 50	Provides constant controlled F_io_2
Mouth-to-mouth	—	17	—
Mouth-to-mask	10–15	50–80	—

Vitamin requirements in pregnancy (compared with standard intravenous vitamin preparation)

Vitamin	RDA	MVI-12
A	800 μg RE	3,300 USP (retinol)*
D	400 IU (10 μg cholecalciferol)	200 USP units†
E (de-alpha-tocopherol acetate)	10 mg a-TE	10 USP units*
Ascorbic acid	70 mg	100 mg
Thiamine (B_1)	1.5 mg	3.0 mg
Riboflavin (B_2)	1.6 mg	3.6 mg
Pyridoxine (B_6)	2.2 mg	4.0 mg
Niacin	17 mg	40.0 mg
Pantothenic acid	4–7 mg‡	15.0 mg
Biotin	30–100 μg‡	60 μg
Folic acid	400 μg	400 μg
B_{12}	2.2 μg	5 μg
K	0.03–1.5 μg/kg (RDA)	–§

* Equivalent to recommended daily allowance (RDA).
† May require additional supplementation for women with a history of poor intake.
‡ Estimated safe and adequate daily dietary intakes in nonpregnant adults (RDA).
§ Must be added to vitamin regimens.
(Reproduced with permission from Nutrition Support Dietetics, 2nd edn. American Society for Parenteral and Enteral Care, Silver Springs, MD, 1993.)

Mineral and trace element requirements in pregnancy

Mineral	Enteral nutrition	Parenteral nutrition
Calcium	1,200 mg	200–250 mg (9.6–12.5 mEq)
Phosphorus	1,200 mg (38 mm)	30–45 mm
Magnesium	450 mg (37.5 mEq)	10–15 mEq
Zinc	15 mg	2.55–3.0 mg
Copper	1.5–3.0 mg*	0.5–1.5 mg
Manganese	2.0–5.0 mg*	0.15–0.8 mg
Iodine	175 μg	50 μg†
Selenium	65 μg	20–40 μg‡
Iron	10 + 30–60 mg supplemental iron	3–6 mg
Chromium	0.05–0.2 mg*	10–15 μg

* Estimated safe and adequate daily intakes in nonpregnant adults.
† Assuming 80% absorption.
‡ Recommended intravenous dose for stable adults.
(Reproduced with permission from Nutrition Support Dietetics, 2nd edn. American Society for Parenteral and Enteral Nutrition, Silver Springs, MD, 1993.)

Insulin preparations and properties

Type	Action (hours)*		
	Onset	Peak	Duration
Rapid			
Regular (crystalline)	0.3–1	2–4	6–8
Semilente	0.5–1.0	2–6	10–12
Intermediate			
NPH	1–2	6–12	18–24
Lente	1–2	6–12	18–24
Slow			
Ultralente	3–8	18–24	36
Protamine zinc	3–8	14–24	36

* These are approximate figures. There is significant variation from patient to patient and from dose to dose in the same patient.

Topical corticosteroid preparations

Low potency	Medium potency	High potency
Hydrocortisone 0.5%	Triamcinolone acetonide 0.1%	Fluocinonide 0.05%
Hydrocortisone 1%	Betamethasone dipropionate 0.05%	Halcinonide 0.1%
Desonide 0.05%	Betamethasone valerate 0.1%	Desoximetasone 0.25%
	Fluocinolone acetonide 0.025%	
	Flurandrenolide 0.05%	

Glucocorticoids

Steroid action	Available tablet size (mg)	Relative anti-inflammatory effect	Relative mineralocorticoid effect	Duration
Hydrocortisone	5, 10, 20	1.0	1.0	S
Prednisone	1, 2.5, 5, 10, 20, 50	4.0	0.8	I
Prednisolone	5	4.0	0.8	I
Methyl-prednisolone	2, 4, 8, 16, 24, 32	5.0	0.5	I
Dexamethasone	0.25, 0.5, 0.75, 1.5, 4, 6	25.0	0.0	L
Betamethasone	0.6	25.0	0.0	L

S, short; I, intermediate; L, long.

Narcotics: relative potency

Drug	Potency relative to morphine	Oral 1 : 1 parenteral potency
Hydromorphone	6.0	1 : 5
Morphine	1.0	1 : 6
Oxycodone	1.0	1 : 2
Pentazocine (Talwin)	0.25	1 : 3
Meperidine (Demerol)	0.15	1 : 3
Codeine	0.1	2 : 3

Commonly used agents for hemodynamic manipulation*

Drug	Method of preparation	Microdrop concentration† (μg/μgtt)	Begin at low dosage† (μg/kg/min)	Progress to high dosage† (μg/kg/min)	Comments
Dopamine (Inotropin, single strength)	1 amp (200 mg) in 250 mL	13.3	5 (26)‡	20 (105)‡	Renal 0–3 μg/kg/min Mixed renal/beta 3–7 μg/kg/min Renal/beta/alpha >7 μg/kg/min
Dopamine (Inotropin, double strength)	2 amps (400 mg) in 250 mL	26.6	5 (13)‡	20 (52)‡	
Dobutamine (Dobutrex)	1 amp (250 mg) in 250 mL	16.6	5 (21)‡	—	NEJM 1979;300:17.
Epinephrine	2 amps (2 mg) in 250 mL	0.13	0.01 (5)‡	0.20 (100)‡	Beta 0.01–0.03 μg/kg/min Mixed 0.03 μg/kg/min Alpha >0.15 μg/kg/min
Isoproterenol (Isuprel)	1 large amp (1 mg) in 250 mL (*or* 5 small amps in 250 mL)	0.066	0.01 (10)‡	0.30 (300)‡	
Phenylophrine (Neosynephrine)	1 amp (10 mg) in 250 mL	0.66	0.1‡ (11)	0.7 (74)‡	Practically, pure alpha
Norepinephrine (Levophed)	2 amps (8 mg) in 250 mL	0.53	0.05 (7)‡	1 (132)‡	
Phentolamine (Regitine)	1.5 amps (7.5 mg) in 250 mL	0.5	0.5 (70)‡	20 (2,800)‡	
Nitroprusside (Nipride)	1 bottle (50 mg) in 250 mL	3.3	0.4 (8)‡	5 (106)‡	Toxic 8 μg/kg/min, or acute toxicity 1.5 mg/kg over 3-hour period
Nitroglycerin	50 mg in 250 mL via millipore filter	3.3	0.4 (8)‡	1.5; may go up to 5 in awake patients (106)‡	No known metabolic toxicity as yet

* Some guidelines are approximate and modulated by clinical response and indications.
† Microdrop (μgtt) is provided by an infusion apparatus giving 60 drops per mL.
‡ Microdrops per minute for a 70-kg patient.

Commonly used agents for chronic hypertension during pregnancy

Agent	Starting daily dose (mg)*	Dosing interval (hr)*	Maximum daily dose (mg)*
Methyldopa	500–1,000	6–12	3,000
Hydralazine	40	6	400
Atenolol	50	24	100
Propranolol	160	12	640
Labetalol	200	12	2,400
Nifedipine†	30–60	24	120

* Doses are shown as *daily doses* and must be divided.
† Short-acting nifedipine is not FDA approved for treatment of hypertension.

Commonly used agents for severe acute hypertension during pregnancy

Agent	Dosing	Maximum dose
Hydralazine	5–10 mg IV every 20 min	20–30 mg
Labetalol	20 + 40 + 80 + 80 mg IV every 10 min	220 mg
Nifedipine*	10 mg PO and repeat in 30 min	20 mg
Nitroprusside	0.25 μg/kg/min IV, increase 0.25 μg/kg/min every 5 min	5 μg/kg/min

* Short-acting nifedipine is not FDA approved for treatment of hypertension.

Blood component therapy

Product	Volume (mL)	Content	Shelf life
Whole blood	450	All blood components	35 days No granulocytes or platelets after 24 hours Decreased but functionally adequate levels of factors V and VIII for 1–2 weeks
Packed red blood cells	250	Red cells only	35 days
Fresh frozen plasma	200–250	All stable and labile clotting factors	1 year
Cryoprecipitate	50	Factors V, VIII: C, VIII: Von Willibrand, XIII, fibronectin fibrinogen	1 year
Platelets	50 (per pack)	Platelets	5 days

Electrolyte equivalencies

$NaCl$	58 mg/mEq
$NaHCO_3$	84 mg/mEq
KCl	75 mg/mEq
$KHCO_3$	100 mg/mEq
$MgSO_4 \cdot 7\,H_2O$	123 mg/mEq
$CaCO_3$	50 mg/mEq
$CaCl_2 \cdot 2\,H_2O$	73 mg/mEq
Ca gluconate$_2 \cdot 1\,H_2O$	224 mg/mEq

Intravenous fluids

	Osmolality (mosm/kg)	Glucose concentration (g/L)	Na (mEq/L)	Cl (mEq/L)
5% dextrose/water	252	50	—	—
10% dextrose/water	505	100	—	—
50% dextrose/water	2,520	500	—	—
0.45% NaCl	154	—	77	77
0.9% NaCl	308	—	154	154
Lactated Ringer's solution*	272	—	130	109

* Also contains K (4 mEq/L), Ca (3 mEq/L), and lactate (28 mEq/L).

Solution for total parenteral nutrition (TPN) in pregnancy

Pharmacy orders

Aminosyn 2, 8.5%	454.0 mL
Dextrose, 50%	516.0 mL
Lypholyte II	20.0 mL
Sodium phosphate (4.0 mEq/mL)	4.0 mL
MVI	5.5 mL
Trace elements*	0.7 mL
Make 2 bottles, send 500 mL of lipid emulsion 10%	

* Add 800 μg folic acid and 6 mg iron to one bottle daily.

Nursing orders

1 Run TPN bottles at 80 mL per hour

2 Run lipid 10% emulsion at 125 mL per hour until 500 mL of lipid have been infused

3 Routine monitoring (weight, intake and output (I&O), and urinary glucose every 6 hours)

Each bottle of TPN (total volume 1,000 mL) supplies the following:

Aminosyn 2, 8.5%	454 cm^3 (38.6 g protein)
Dextrose, 50%	516 cm^3 (end concentration 25.8%)
	1.03 cal/mL TPN
Sodium	51.0 mEq
Potassium	20.0 mEq
Calcium	4.5 mEq
Magnesium	5.0 mEq
Zinc	3.5 mg
Copper	0.7 mg
Manganese	0.4 mg
Chromium	7.0 μg
Chloride	35.0 mEq
Acetate	29.5 mEq
Phosphate	24.0 mEq
MVI-12	5.5 cm^3
Folic acid	800 mg
Iron	6 mg

Sample TPN solution in pregnancy for 63-kg woman, height 168 cm, age 23 years.

Calories

Using the Harris–Benedict equation, these factors calculate a basal energy expenditure (BEE) of 1,461 kcal/day. Since calorie and protein requirements parenterally are the same as for a pregnant woman being fed orally or enterally, we used the factor of 1.5 × BEE to calculate caloric need.

Patient's BEE (1,461) × 1.5 – 2,192 + additional kcal for 2nd + 3rd trimester (300 kcal/day) – 2,500 kcal/day

Protein

The current recommended dietary allowance (RDA) for protein has been reduced to an additional 10 g/day.

Feeding 1 g/kg/day would provide 63 g of protein for this patient on her ideal weight. An additional 10 g were added to her TPN for a total of 73 g or 1.2 g/kg/day.

Fats

The requirement for essential fatty acids (EFA) is slightly increased in pregnancy to 4.5% of total calories. It is important to use a fat emulsion that contains both linoleic and linolenic acids. Liposyn is the brand of fat emulsion used in this TPN order and it is composed of 60% essential fatty acids.

Electrolytes and trace elements

Most standard packs provide adequate amounts except for folate and iron. The iron can be safely infused intravenously, dependent upon rate and dosage.

Index

Page numbers in *italic* refer to figures, numbers in **bold** refer to tables

Printed in the United States of America/BNB